Pathology
OF THE Skin

Pathology
OF THE Skin

Editors

Evan R. Farmer, MD
Associate Professor of Dermatology and Pathology
Director, Dermatopathology and Oral Pathology Laboratory
Johns Hopkins University School of Medicine
Baltimore, Maryland

Antoinette F. Hood, MD
Associate Professor of Dermatology and Pathology
Division of Dermatopathology and Oral Pathology
Johns Hopkins University School of Medicine
Baltimore, Maryland

APPLETON & LANGE
Norwalk, Connecticut/San Mateo, California

0-8385-7715-6

Notice: Our knowledge in clinical sciences is constantly changing. As new
information becomes available, changes in treatment and in the use of drugs
become necessary. The author(s) and the publisher of this volume have taken
care to make certain that the doses of drugs and schedules of treatment are
correct and compatible with the standards generally accepted at the time of
publication. The reader is advised to consult carefully the instruction
and information material included in the package insert of each drug or
therapeutic agent before administration. This advice is especially
important when using new or infrequently used drugs.

90 91 92 93 94 / 10 9 8 7 6 5 4 3 2 1

Prentice Hall International (UK) Limited, *London*
Prentice Hall of Australia Pty. Limited, *Sydney*
Prentice Hall Canada, Inc., *Toronto*
Prentice Hall Hispanoamericana, S.A., *Mexico*
Prentice Hall of India Private Limited, *New Delhi*
Prentice Hall of Japan, Inc., *Tokyo*
Simon & Schuster Asia Pte. Ltd., *Singapore*
Editora Prentice Hall do Brasil Ltda., *Rio de Janeiro*
Prentice Hall, *Englewood Cliffs, New Jersey*

Library of Congress Cataloging-in-Publication Data
Pathology of the skin/[edited by] Evan R. Farmer, Antoinette F. Hood.
    p. cm.
    ISBN 0-8385-7715-6
    1. Skin—Diseases. 2. Skin—Histopathology. I. Farmer, Evan R.
II. Hood, Antoinette F.
    [DNLM: 1. Skin Diseases—pathology. WR 105 P297]
RL95.P35 1990
616.5'07—dc20
DNLM/DLC
for Library of Congress   89–18568
                                                            CIP

Production Editor: Christopher J. Bacich
Cover Designer: Janice Barsevich
Acquisitions Editor: William R. Schmitt
Designer: Steve Byrum

PRINTED IN THE UNITED STATES OF AMERICA

Dedication

This book is dedicated to the memory of our friend and colleague
L. Stefan Levin, DDS, MSD
1939–1989

CONTRIBUTORS

Edward Abell, MD
Associate Professor of Dermatology and Pathology
Department of Dermatology
University of Pittsburgh
Pittsburgh, Pennsylvania

Karl H. Anders, MD
Assistant Clinical Professor of Pathology and Laboratory
  Medicine
University of California, Los Angeles School of Medicine
Los Angeles, California

Wilma F. Bergfeld, MD
Head, Section of Dermatopathology
Department of Pathology

Head, Section of Clinical Dermatologic Research
Department of Dermatology
Cleveland Clinic
Cleveland, Ohio

Jag Bhawan, MD
Professor of Dermatology and Pathology
Department of Dermatology
Boston University School of Medicine
Boston, Massachusetts

Martin M. Black, MD
Consultant Dermatologist
Department of Dermatology
St. Thomas Hospital
London, United Kingdom

Robert A. Briggaman, MD
Professor and Chairman
Department of Dermatology
University of North Carolina School of Medicine
Chapel Hill, North Carolina

Walter H.C. Burgdorf, MD
Professor and Chairman
Department of Dermatology
University of New Mexico at Albuquerque
Albuquerque, New Mexico

Marc D. Chalet, MD
Associate Professor of Medicine (Dermatology)
Director of Dermatopathology
University of California, Los Angeles School of Medicine
Los Angeles, California

Thomas M. Chesney, MD
Director of Training
Department of Pathology
Baptist Memorial Hospital
Memphis, Tennessee

Wallace H. Clark, Jr., MD
Professor of Dermatology and Pathology
University of Pennsylvania School of Medicine
Philadelphia, Pennsylvania

Philip H. Cooper, MD
Professor of Dermatology and Pathology
University of Virginia Health Sciences Center
Charlottesville, Virginia

David E. Elder, MD, ChB
Professor of Pathology and Laboratory Medicine
Division of Surgical Pathology
University of Pennsylvania School of Medicine
Philadelphia, Pennsylvania

Evan R. Farmer, MD
Associate Professor of Dermatology and Pathology
Director, Dermatopathology and Oral Pathology Laboratory
Johns Hopkins University School of Medicine
Baltimore, Maryland

James P. Fields, MD
Associate Professor of Medicine and Pathology
Division of Dermatology
Vanderbilt University Medical Center
Nashville, Tennessee

Marian C. Finan, MD
Atlanta Dermatopathology and Pathology Associates
Atlanta, Georgia

Patricia M. Fishman, MD
Department of Pathology and Medicine (Dermatology)
New York Hospital—Cornell University Medical Center
New York, New York

James E. Fitzpatrick, MD
Department of Dermatology
Fitzsimmons Army Medical Center
Aurora, Colorado

Kenneth J. Friedman, MD
Assistant Professor of Dermatology
Division of Dermatopathology and Oral Pathology
Johns Hopkins University School of Medicine
Baltimore, Maryland

Loren E. Golitz, MD
Professor of Dermatology and Pathology
University of Colorado Health Sciences Center

Director of Dermatopathology
Chief of Dermatology
Denver General Hospital
Denver, Colorado

DuPont Guerry, IV
Professor of Medicine
University of Pennsylvania School of Medicine
Philadelphia, Pennsylvania

Ruth Hanno, MD
Assistant Professor of Medicine/Dermatology
University of South Florida College of Medicine
Tampa, Florida

Ken Hashimoto, MD
Professor and Chairman
Department of Dermatology
Wayne State University
Detroit, Michigan

John T. Headington, MD
Professor of Pathology and Dermatology
Department of Pathology
University of Michigan Medical School
Ann Arbor, Michigan

R. Jeffrey Herten, MD
Assistant Clinical Professor of Dermatology and
  Dermatopathology
University of California, Irvine
Irvine, California

Antoinette F. Hood, MD
Associate Professor of Dermatology and Pathology
Division of Dermatopathology and Oral Pathology
Johns Hopkins University School of Medicine
Baltimore, Maryland

Thomas D. Horn, MD
Assistant Professor of Dermatology
Division of Dermatopathology and Oral Pathology
Johns Hopkins University School of Medicine
Baltimore, Maryland

Sharon R. Hymes, MD
Clinical Assistant Professor
Department of Dermatology
University of Texas Medical School at Houston
Houston, Texas

Michael J. Imber, MD
Instructor in Pathology
Dermatopathology Unit
Department of Pathology
Massachusetts General Hospital
Boston, Massachusetts

Myles S. Jerdan, MD
North Georgia Dermatopathology Laboratory
Marietta, Georgia

Waine C. Johnson, MD
Clinical Professor of Dermatology
University of Pennsylvania School of Medicine
Philadelphia, Pennsylvania

Grace F. Kao, MD
Senior Pathologist of Dermatopathology
Department of Dermatopathology
Armed Forces Institute of Pathology
Washington, DC

Abdul-Ghani Kibbi, MD
Assistant Professor of Dermatology
American University of Beirut Medical Center
New York, New York

Amal Kurban, MD
Professor of Dermatology
Boston University School of Medicine
Boston, Massachusetts

T.H. Kwan, MD
Assistant Professor of Pathology
Harvard Medical School

Associate Pathologist
Beth Israel Hospital
Boston, Massachusetts

W. Clark Lambert, MD, PhD
Associate Professor of Pathology and Medicine
New Jersey Medical School
Newark, New Jersey

Gilles Landman, MD
Assistant Professor
Faculdade de Medicina do ABC
Santo Andre, Sao Paulo, Brazil

L. Stefan Levin, DDS, MSD*
Assistant Professor
Joint Appointment in Dermatology
Associate Professor
Division of Dentistry and Oral and Maxillofacial Surgery
Johns Hopkins University School of Medicine
Baltimore, Maryland

---

* Deceased

Lee G. Luna, MD
Vice President
American Histolabs, Inc. Cold Center
Gaithersburg, Maryland

John C. Maize, MD
Professor of Dermatology
Medical University of South Carolina
Charleston, South Carolina

N. Scott McNutt, MD
Professor of Pathology and Medicine (Dermatology)
New York Hospital—Cornell University Medical Center
New York, New York

John S. Metcalf, MD
Associate Professor of Dermatology and Pathology
Departments of Dermatology and Pathology
Medical University of South Carolina
Charleston, South Carolina

Wayne M. Meyers, MD, PhD
Chief, Mycobacteriology
Armed Forces Institute of Pathology
Washington, DC

Beno Michel, MD
Clinical Professor of Dermatology
Assistant Clinical Professor of Pathology
Head of Cutaneous Pathology and Immunofluorescence
   Laboratory
Case Western Reserve School of Medicine
Cleveland, Ohio

Martin C. Mihm, Jr., MD
Professor of Pathology
Harvard Medical School

Chief of Dermatopathology
Department of Pathology
Massachusetts General Hospital
Boston, Massachusetts

Jess H. Mottaz
University of Minnesota Medical School
Minneapolis, Minnesota

George F. Murphy, MD
Professor of Dermatology and Pathology
Department of Dermatology
University of Pennsylvania School of Medicine
Philadelphia, Pennsylvania

Thomas G. Olsen, MD
Associate Professor of Dermatology
Wright State University School of Medicine
Dayton, Ohio

Susan C. Parker, MRCP
Dowling Skin Unit
United Medical and Dental Schools of Guy's and
   St. Thomas' Hospitals
St. Thomas Hospital
London, United Kingdom

James W. Patterson, MD
Associate Professor of Pathology and Dermatology
Medical College of Virginia
Richmond, Virginia

Neal S. Penneys, MD, PhD
Professor of Dermatology and Pathology
Department of Dermatology and Cutaneous
   Surgery
University of Miami School of Medicine
Miami, Florida

Margot S. Peters, MD
Assistant Professor
Senior Associate Consultant
Department of Dermatology
Mayo Medical School
Rochester, Minnesota

Somsak Poomeechaiwong, MD
Department of Pathology
Chulalongkorn Faculty of Medicine
Chantaburi, Thailand

Philip G. Prioleau, MD
Clinical Associate Professor of Medicine
Assistant Professor of Pathology
Cornell University Medical College
New York, New York

Justin Roscoe, MD
Instructor in Dermatology
Johns Hopkins University School of Medicine
Baltimore, MD

Daniel J. Santa Cruz, MD
Director of Cutaneous Pathology
Department of Dermatopathology
St. John's Mercy Medical Center

Associate Professor of Pathology
Washington University Medical School
St. Louis, Missouri

Karen A. Sherwood
Assistant Professor
Division of Dermatology
University of Southern California School
   of Medicine
Los Angeles, California

Kurt S. Stenn, MD
Professor of Dermatology and Pathology
Department of Pathology
Yale University School of Medicine
New Haven, Connecticut

Jerome B. Taxy, MD
Associate Pathologist
Lutheran General Hospital
Park Ridge, Illinois

Robert M. Taylor, MD
Assistant Professor of Pathology and
    Dermatology
Johns Hopkins University School of Medicine

Staff Pathologist
The Francis Scott Key Medical Center
Baltimore, Maryland

Mathew C. Varghese, MD
Assistant Professor of Medicine
Cornell University Medical College
New York, New York

Thomas R. Wade, MD
Assistant Professor of Dermatology and
    Pathology
Emory University School of Medicine
Atlanta, Georgia

Clifton R. White, MD
Associate Professor of Dermatology and Pathology
University of Oregon Health Sciences Center
Portland, Oregon

Mark R. Wick, MD
Professor of Pathology
Division of Surgical Pathology
Washington University School of Medicine
St. Louis, Missouri

Alvin S. Zelickson, MD
Clinical Professor of Dermatology
University of Minnesota Medical School
Minneapolis, Minnesota

CONTENTS

PREFACE

During our academic lifetimes we have had the opportunity to watch the exciting evolution of dermatopathology as a defined subspecialty—carved from the clinical halls of dermatology and the microscope benches of pathology. We watched the growth of a marriage between two disparate entities, and like most marriages, there was strain as the entities gradually fused to form a couple. No other subspecialty of pathology is as dependent on the clinician for an accurate definition of disease, because no other organ can be scrutinized hour by hour for observable change, and no other organ can be biopsied sequentially for microscopic evidence of change. Ready accessibility of the skin to photographic documentation and biopsy has lent new meaning to the concept of clinical–pathological correlation. The necessity for a fundamental understanding of the clinical aspects of dermatologic disease as well as the basic principles of pathology led to the establishment of subspecialty boards in dermatopathology, and examinations that emphasized combined training—in the clinic and at the microscope.

Early textbooks in dermatopathology reflected the genius of a few superior intellects able to combine their knowledge in the two fields and write about those experiences in a manner that was understandable to the uninitiated. These textbooks have earned their places on library shelves. Walter F. Lever with his *Histopathology of the Skin,* now in its seventh edition, perhaps best exemplifies a brilliant student of the gross and microscopic aspects of skin disease. Hamilton Montgomery's two volume text, *Dermatopathology,* gave new meaning to the concept of detailed description. The Armed Forces Institute of Pathology greats Helwig, Graham, and Johnson created a masterful text, *Dermal Pathology,* with particularly notable chapters on epidermal neoplasia and fungal infections. Sadly the last two books are no longer being published and are increasingly difficult to find. More recently the charismatic presence of A. Bernard Ackerman has forced each of us to reassess the standards of excellence in textbooks, having produced one of the most beautifully illustrated and at the same time uniquely organized book in dermatopathology, *Histologic Diagnosis of Inflammatory Skin Diseases.*

The specialty continues to evolve. New diseases are recognized and described, old diseases are redefined with the use of histochemistry and immunohistochemistry. Academic dermatopathologists have focused their research on limited areas or specific diseases, thereby creating miniexperts within the field. It becomes more and more difficult for one dermatopathologist to be all things to all people at all times. This book arose from our perceived need for a text that utilized the expertise of our colleagues and friends in dermatopathology integrating their knowledge into one tome. This book was therefore conceived as a thorough, authoritative, and scholarly survey of dermatopathology that would present information in a practical format useful to dermatopathologists, pathologists, and dermatologists in practice and in training.

To accomplish this we selected authors who represent an international array of experts in dermatopathology. Each author is an experienced writer and investigator who has written landmark articles, monographs, or review articles in a particular area of interest. A total of 64 authors contributed to the book. They are a heterogeneous lot, representing all the acknowledged schools of dermatopathology, with broad and diverse backgrounds and training. It is a tribute to the field of dermatopathology that there are so many well trained, investigative, academically oriented dermatopathologists with selective expertise. Their expertise made a multiauthored text possible and a multiauthored book necessary for accurate dissemination of knowledge.

As editors we provided guidelines for these authors in an attempt to produce balanced and parallel chapters. As expected, some authors were easier to guide than others. Each provided us with superb compilations of personal experience in a particular field, high quality photomicrographs illustrating the written material and up-to-date references. Most importantly, each provided us with an approach to a specific histologic problem, a means to sort through a difficult problem and derive a solution, i.e., a diagnosis. If this book achieves its goal and is successful it will be because of the efforts put forth by the individual authors. To each author we extend our heartfelt thanks, and with our thanks, the sincere hope that each person is pleased with the completed team effort.

The organization of this book attempts to blend the traditional disease-oriented approach of pathology with the more modern pattern-recognition approach. The book is divided into ten sections. Section I provides important background material for the beginning student of dermatopathology, and we recommend that this section be read in its entirety by individuals relatively new to the field. Material covered in this section includes normal histology of the skin, histochemistry, immunopathology, and electron microscopy. Special reference is also made to specimen preparation and to common artifacts that occur when preparing tissue for microscopic examination. Sections II through IV deal with inflammatory disorders, Section V with non-inflammatory disorders, and Section VI with pigmentary disorders. A large section is devoted to neoplasia, and smaller sections deal with cysts, disorders of the mucous membranes, and disorders of the appendages.

While full credit for this book goes to the authors, there are many others whose contributions must be mentioned. We are indebted to our early mentors in dermatology who encouraged us to strive for excellence: George W. Hambrick, Jr., Thomas B. Fitzpatrick, and Irwin M. Freedberg. We each were inspired by great thinkers and teachers in the field of dermatopathology: Elson B. Helwig, Martin C. Mihm, Jr., and Wallace H. Clark, Jr. Thomas T. Provost has provided both of us with an environment conducive to the production of scholarly work, and has given us his unfailing support throughout the endeavor. Bonnie Weissfeld contributed her magnificent organizational skills; she and Mumtaz Kammerer graciously took us through multiple revisions of our own chapters. Pete Lund was personally responsible for many photomicrographs in the book. Susan Edmunds was extremely helpful with the editing of several of the chapters in the earlier sections. Our executive editor, William Schmitt, always was near when we needed him, and that was quite often in the early stages of the book. He was especially helpful when we were learning how to be editors, and the text was subtitled "Will this marriage survive co-editorship?" And last, but never least, we thank our children Sheri, Susan, Eliza, Evan, and Molly for being the wonderful people they are and for allowing us to do what we enjoy so much.

Evan R. Farmer, MD
Antoinette F. Hood, MD
March, 1990

SECTION I
General Considerations

CHAPTER 1
The Normal Histology of the Skin

Kurt S. Stenn and Jag Bhawan

Any unit of biologic organization is defined by the interface structure separating it from the environment. At the organismal level, it is the integument, or skin, that establishes the unit. For the organism, the integument stands as a protective front, as well as a means of sending signals to and receiving signals from the environment. To serve these ends, skin has evolved into a deceptively simple structure that becomes more complex and interesting as we study it. It consists of three layers: an impermeable multilayered epithelium, the *epidermis,* a tough, durable but porous layer, the *dermis,* and a soft, lipid-rich, deep layer, the *subcutis.* To complement the function of this basic structure, epidermal redundancies, the cutaneous adnexa, have evolved. In general, although the skin manifests bilateral symmetry, the heterogeneity of skin from site to site is striking and can be described at histologic, cytologic, or biochemical levels, for example, the varied epidermal, dermal, and subcutaneous histologies of the scalp, palms, and abdomen (Fig. 1–1), the varied mitotic potential of epidermal basal cells, and the differing metabolic activities of the subcutaneous fat in the forearm and abdominal girth. Such heterogeneity is one of the central themes of skin biology. Heterogeneity of this structure appears to be critical to its function and to the unique topologic expression of its diseases.

The purpose of this chapter is to present a short review and update of the histology and biology of skin relevant to the student of dematopathology. We recognize at the outset that such a chapter cannot be complete, but we hope that it will offer a perspective and direction for further study. More detailed general references to skin histology, biology and biochemistry are available.[1–4]

EMBRYOLOGY OF SKIN

The ontogeny or morphogenesis of human skin displays features reminiscent of cutaneous phylogeny[5–7c] (Table 1–1). Like simple, water-dwelling invertebrates, the skin of the embryo also is simple. Initially, its outer surface consists of a single epithelial layer. With time, the epidermis becomes double-layered, then 3–4 layers thick and, by 6 months, multilayered and cornified. The embryonic dermis is an ill-defined, cell-rich, and glycosaminoglycan-rich stroma spanning from the epidermis to muscle fascia without regional morphologic distinction. At birth, it is a collagen-rich structure with embedded mesenchymal cells, adnexa, and distinct papillary and reticular dermal zones.

Like other organs, skin formation is conceived as occurring within two periods: a period of organogenesis (months 1 and 2), the *embryonic period,* and a period of growth and differentiation (month 3 to term), the *fetal period.* In general, the growth and maturation of epidermis and its derivatives precede that of the dermis, and maturation occurs in a cephalad-to-caudad and dorsal-to-ventral direction.

The embryo has a simple integument during the first 2 months of life when the anlagen of most organs form. During this stage, the single-layered epidermis becomes double-layered, acquiring a deep basal and a superficial periderm layer. The cells of both strata have the capacity to divide. The periderm, a transient and unique cell layer that covers the epidermis until it is stratified and cornified is, in early morphogenesis, made of flat epithelial cells with abundant glycogen-filled cytoplasm and intercellular desmosomes. Its surface is covered with microvilli that project into the amniotic cavity and later broaden to become blebs. These projections serve to expand the epidermal surface and thus its contact with amniotic fluid. Because analogous villous and vesicular structures are seen in other active secretory epithelia and because of isotopic water transport studies,[8] it is believed that periderm serves to conduct substances across the epidermis.[9] At the end of the sixth fetal month, the periderm flattens to a thin layer, microvilli decrease in number, and the surface blebs disappear. Concomitantly, an osmotic gradient (due to urea nitrogen and creatinine) develops between the amniotic fluid and the fetal–maternal plasma, and the amniotic fluid takes on the ionic character of dilute urine. These events suggest a role for periderm in equilibrating amniotic and maternal fluids

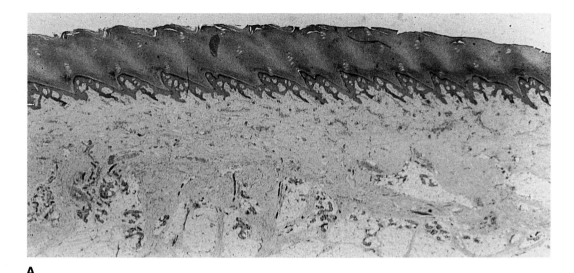

A

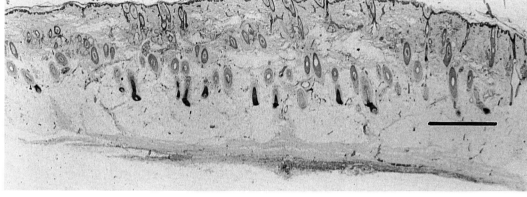

B

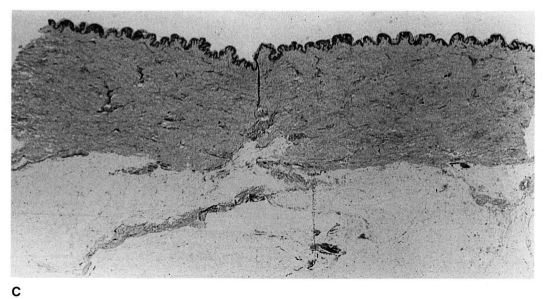

C

Figure 1–1. Regional variation of skin. **A.** Plantar skin. **B.** Scalp skin. **C.** Abdominal skin.

TABLE 1–1. EMBRYOGENESIS OF HUMAN SKIN

Structure	Embryonic Period		Fetal Period				
	\ Month of Gestation						
	1	2	3	4	5	6	7
Epidermis							
Str. basale	→———————————————————————————————→						
Periderm	→——————————————————————————→						
Str. intermedium (stratification of epidermis)		→————————————————————————→					
Str. granulosum					→——————————→		
Str. corneum (acral skin)				→————————————————→			
Str. corneum (truncal skin—inter-follicular epidermal keratinization)						→————→	
Desmosomes	→———————————————————————————————→						
Tight junctions	→——————————————————————————→						
Hemidesmosomes				→————————————————→			
Pemphigus–pemphigoid antigen				→————————————————→			
A, B, H blood group antigens				→————————————————→			
Immigrant cells							
Melanocytes with premelanosomes		→————————————————————————→					
Melanocytes with melanin-synthesizing melanosomes				→————————————————→			
Transfer of melanin to keratinocytes						→————→	
Langerhans cells				→————————————————→			
Merkel cells				→————————————————→			
Epidermal appendages							
Pilosebaceous apparatus							
Hair follicle anlage				→————————————————→			
Hair tract cornified (keratinization of the piliary canal)					→——————————→		
Hair shaft on surface				→————————————————→			
Sebaceous anlage and first secretion				→————————————————→			
Sebaceous duct cornified					→——————————→		
Apocrine gland function				→————————————————→			
Eccrine gland function						→——→	
Cornification of eccrine duct (intraepidermal)						→————→	
Dermis							
Papillary and reticular regions defined				→————————————————→			
Dermal papillae formed				→————————————————→			
Dermal–subcutis boundary defined			→————————————————————→			
Panniculus adiposus formed				→————————————————→			
Collagen present			→————————————————————→			
Elastin microfibrils			→————————————————————→			
Elastin matrix				→————————————————→			
Nail							
Nail fold and matrix established			→————————————————————→			
Keratinization of nail dorsal ridge			→————————————————————→			
Nail plate forms				→————————————————→			

Adapted from Holbrook and Wolf.[6]

in the young fetus. Moreover, a major barrier to epidermal fluid transport appears in the skin of the 6-month-old fetus concomitantly as the periderm sloughs and the epidermis cornifies.

During the third fetal month, an intermediate cell layer forms in the epidermis between the periderm and the basal layers. Keratins unique to each of these layers are now detectable: keratins k5 and k14 in the basal layer, keratins k1 and k10 in the intermediate cells, and keratins k8 and k19 in the periderm.[10] The intermediate cells are better differentiated than the basal cells. They have more desmo-

somes, and their keratin filaments are organized into bundles.

During the final 3 months of gestation, the full complement of adult epidermal layers is present, the periderm is shed, and the epidermal adnexa become functional. The dermal–epidermal interface shows early rete ridge and dermal papilla formations, which become better defined in childhood. With adolescence, the adnexa grow, mature hair develops regionally, and apocrine and sebaceous glands begin secreting. The embryonic dermis consists of mesenchymal cells widely separated by stroma rich in glycosami-

TABLE 1–2. HISTOLOGIC FEATURES OF AGING HUMAN SKIN

Epidermis	Dermis	Appendages
Flattened dermal–epidermal junction	Atrophy (loss of dermal volume)	Depigmented hairs
Variable thickness	Fewer fibroblasts	Loss of hair
Occasional nuclear atypia	Fewer mast cells	Conversion of terminal to vellus hairs
Fewer melanocytes	Fewer blood vessels	Abnormal nailplates
Fewer Langerhans cells	Shortened capillary loops	Fewer glands
	Abnormal nerve endings	

From Gilchrist.[11]

noglycans and fine collagen fibrils. This stroma gives the fetal dermis its high water content (90% wt/vol). As the mesenchymal cells start to produce mature collagen, the dermal hyaluronic acid concentration falls, and the content of dermal sulfated glycosaminoglycans rises. Elastic microfibrils are seen in the fetus, but elastin itself is not synthesized at this time. It is remarkable that a mature complement of elastin is not seen in the dermis until about 6 months after birth. At about 6 months also, the subcutis becomes defined.

With aging and senescence, the development of skin, in a sense, reverses itself[11] (Table 1–2). The epidermis and dermis thin, melanocytes decrease in density, and the dermal–epidermal junction smooths out with reduction of the rete ridges and the dermal papillae. Moreover, the vascular networks within the dermis and about the adnexa attenuate. The organized cutaneous sensory end organs atrophy, dermal collagen becomes more heavily crosslinked, and elastin

fibers become thicker. In old age, hair follicles and the sebaceous, apocrine, and eccrine glands atrophy. Eventually, the adnexa may disappear. With time, the skin loses much of its protective, sensory, and communicative properties.

EPIDERMIS

More than any other cutaneous structure the epidermis graphically demonstrates the biologic principle of structural equilibrium: preservation of form but not substance. The epidermis is a stratified squamous epithelium that, while maintaining its shape and thickness, grows relatively rapidly, cleanses its surface by shedding itself, and serves as a resistant surface cover and permeability barrier. It grows from the basal layer, structures itself in the spinous layer, establishes the permeability barrier in the granular layer, and sheds itself in the outer cornified layer (Fig. 1–2).

Because it is a very difficult tissue to study kinetically,[12] we do not know with certainty how the epidermis grows. We do recognize that in order to maintain a structure of constant thickness, the epidermis coordinates its desquamation and growth. Although most epidermal growth occurs in the basal layer, about 30% of the growing cells are found suprabasally.[13] Not all the cells in the lower epidermis or the basal layer, however, are mitotically active. It is not surprising, then, that the basal epidermal cells are not homogeneous. Although a large percentage of these cells actively proliferate, there is a significant number (up to 60%) that divide very slowly. In this regard, epidermal cells of the basal layer have a unique morphology[14] (Fig. 1–3). At the base of the rete, the basal cells have a smooth inferior surface and are pigmented, cuboidal, and small. They prolif-

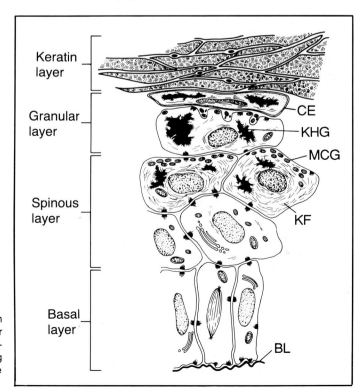

Figure 1–2. Sketch of the epidermis showing its four strata: keratin layer (Keratin layer), granular layer (Granular layer), spinous layer (Spinous layer), basal layer (Basal layer)—and its pattern of differentiation: basal lamina (BL), keratin filament (KF), membrane coating granule (MCG), Keratohyaline granule (KHG), cornified envelope (CE) (Adapted from Montagna and Parakkal.)

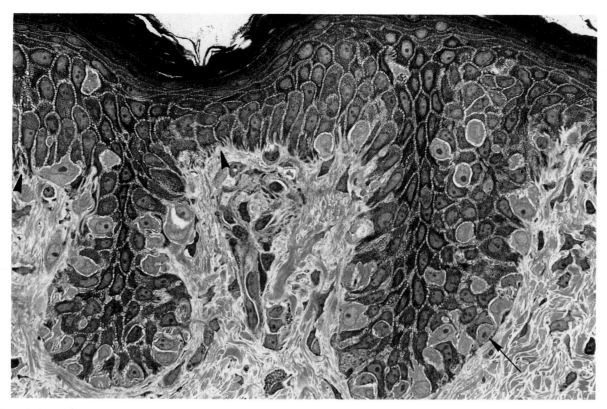

Figure 1–3. Photomicrograph of superficial lentiginous skin. This 1 μm thick section clearly shows the serrated basal cells (arrowheads) above the dermal papillae and the nonserrated basal cells at the base of the rete. Note the presence of lightly staining melanocytes (arrow) (toluidine blue, ×1000).

erate slowly while the cells above them incorporate label more rapidly. The basal cells above the dermal papillae, in contrast, have serrated inferior surfaces and are poorly pigmented, columnar, and rather large. They proliferate slowly. It is the cells of the rete that are generating. In general, the cells of the deep rete appear to represent the stem cells and transient amplifying cells of the epidermis, whereas the cells above the dermal papillae are mostly postmitotic and serve a sustentacular role by means of their inferior serrated margin. Because basal cells are heterogeneous in their growth potential and because we have been unable to measure their growth rate directly, we do not know the precise intermitotic time of normal human basal cells. For understanding dermatopathology, the location of the dividing cell population in the basal layer is significant. If that population of cells were randomly distributed in the basal layer, one would expect to find a uniformly thickened epidermis in the hyperproliferative states. Instead, one finds a prominent rete pattern (as in psoriasis), an observation that adds credence to the concept of a nonrandom distribution of dividing basal cells. Currently, considerable experimental work is being done defining the molecules that stimulate and slow[15] epidermal growth.

In general, one daughter cell of every cell division leaves the basal layer to differentiate. The mechanism for this emigration is not entirely clear. Although a passive mechanism such as growth pressure would appear most

likely, some evidence has been presented to suggest that active cell motility could play a role.[16] Once a cell leaves the basal layer, it takes about 14 days to reach the stratum corneum and another 14 days to transit the stratum corneum and desquamate.[17]

After leaving the basal layer, the keratinocyte becomes postmitotic and begins to differentiate. As the keratinocyte matures and moves upward, it acquires an increasingly smaller nuclear/cytoplasmic ratio and changes shape from cuboidal to tetrakeidecahedral (14-sided polygon) to flattened hexagonal plates, the squames.[18] These morphologic changes give rise to the characteristic strata of the epidermis: stratum basale, stratum spinosum, stratum granulosum, and stratum corneum.

On differentiating, the keratinocyte acquires a rigid cytostructure and a system by which it firmly attaches to neighboring cells in all three dimensions. To this end, the cell employs two important structural systems: the keratin filament–filaggrin–desmosome complex and the cornified envelope. In this discussion, the term "keratin" is used specifically to refer to the well-characterized proteins making up the keratin filaments. The term "keratinization" and "cornification," however, are used here as they are used in dermatologic parlance to refer to the process or state of complete differentiation of the keratinocyte. In this sense, the words "keratinization" and "cornification" refer more generally to the development of both structural systems:

the keratin filament–filaggrin–desmosome complex and the cornified envelope.

Three filament cytoskeletal networks are found in all eukaryotic cells, including the keratinocyte: microfilaments (7 nm), microtubules (25 nm), and intermediate filaments (10–15 nm). Keratin, which makes up one member of the related class of intermediate filament proteins[19] (in addition to vimentin, desmin, glial fibrillary acidic protein, lamins, and neurofilament proteins), manifests a seven amino acid residue repeat that bestows on the polypeptide the ability to form coiled-coil α-helical dimers. At least 20 distinct keratin proteins are recognized (about 10 of which are found in epidermis) ranging in molecular weight from 40 to 68 kD[20] (Fig. 1–4). The keratins arise as a multigene family of polypeptides that are expressed in different sets during different routes of differentiation. For a given epithelial tissue, the specific keratins fingerprint that tissue with regard to form and state of differentiation.[21] For the epidermis, keratins of increasing molecular weight are synthesized as cells differentiate and migrate from the basal layer (e.g., keratins k5 and k14 are synthesized by basal cells, and keratins k1 and k10 are synthesized by suprabasal cells). All human keratins can be divided into an acidic (type I) and a basic (type II) subfamily. In filament formation, one member of the acidic subfamily and one member of the basic subfamily pair. In pairing, it is the general rule that the basic (type II) keratin member is larger than the acidic (type I) member by 8kD.[21]

As the epidermal cell matures, its cytoplasm becomes packed with keratin filaments. The filaments extend from one side of the cell to the other, nesting the nucleus and forming a structural framework for the cytoplasm. At either end, the filaments appear to insert into desmosomes.

Desmosomes are discrete 0.3–0.5 μm diameter regions of the epithelial cell plasma membrane that are structurally specialized, on their cytoplasmic face, to form membrane anchorage sites for keratin filaments and, on their intercellular face, to mediate strong cell–cell cohesion. Such a structural combination makes the desmosome–keratin system particularly well suited to impart tensile strength and mechanical resistance to the epidermis. Desmosomes, then, consist of two regions: a cytoplasmic and an intercyto-

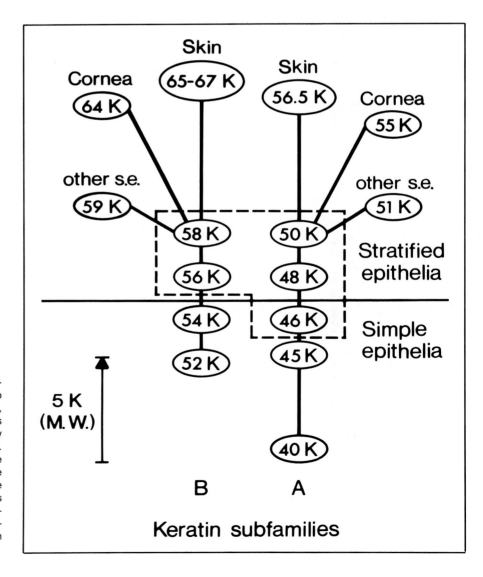

Figure 1–4. Diagram of the two keratin families. The keratins are organized into two groups: the B, or basic, family and the A, or acidic, family. In the diagram, the keratins are sketched within their respective family in the order of increasing molecular weight. Those keratins found in simple epithelia are listed below the horizontal line, and those found in stratified squamous epithelia are above the line. The dashed box encloses those keratins found in all stratified squamous epithelia. The numbers refer to molecular weight of the keratin (K) expressed in kilodaltons. (*From Cooper et al.*[21])

plasmic zone. On the cytoplasmic surface of each interacting plasma membrane, there is a dense plaque associated with inserting keratin filaments. Between the plasma membranes of the contacting cells in apparent continuity with the attachment plaque, poorly characterized filaments extend across the intercellular space. Eight major polypeptides have been isolated from desmosomes.[22] By means of monoclonal antibodies, these proteins have been localized within the desmosome to the two regions: those protein constituents found intracellularly, the desmoplakins, and those found extracellularly, the desmogleins. In contrast to the desmoplakins, the desmogleins are heavily glycosylated, an observation accounting for the glycosylation of the intercellular (desmogleal) area. That antibodies to desmoglein I occur in pemphigus foliaceus and appear to induce acantholysis illustrates the importance of these molecules to epidermal integrity.[23] Because the desmosome is a well-recognized marker for epithelium and epithelium-derived tumors, antibodies to desmosomal proteins are used currently as an additional marker for the light microscopic study of tumors.[24]

As keratinocytes move outward, they accumulate nonmembrane-bounded, basophilic, so-called keratohyaline granules, which characterize the stratum granulosum[24a] (Fig. 1–5). The keratohyaline granules are composed of a high-molecular weight (600 kD), histidine-rich, phosphorylated, electron-dense precursor form of the protein filaggrin.[25] Conversion of the precursor, profilaggrin, to filaggrin is thought to occur enzymatically during the transition of a granular cell to a cornified cell. That filaggrin, a 50 kD protein, functions as a keratin matrix protein in vivo is suggested by in vitro studies in which added filaggrin causes keratin filaments to aggregate and form organized bundles.[26] Profilaggrin, in contrast, does not have this aggregating property. Filaggrin, however, may not have a permanent structural role in the stratum corneum, since shortly after its formation, it is broken down (in the stratum corneum) to a concentrated pool of free amino acids, which are further metabolized to urocanic acid (from histidine) and pyrrolidone carboxylic acid.[27] Since the former may act as an ultraviolet light blocker and the latter as a hygroscopic compound providing hydration to the stratum corneum at low environmental humidities, it is possible that filaggrin serves the epidermis in addition to its filament-aggregating role. Filaggrin metabolism entails many steps: synthesis of a large histidine-rich precursor protein, phos-

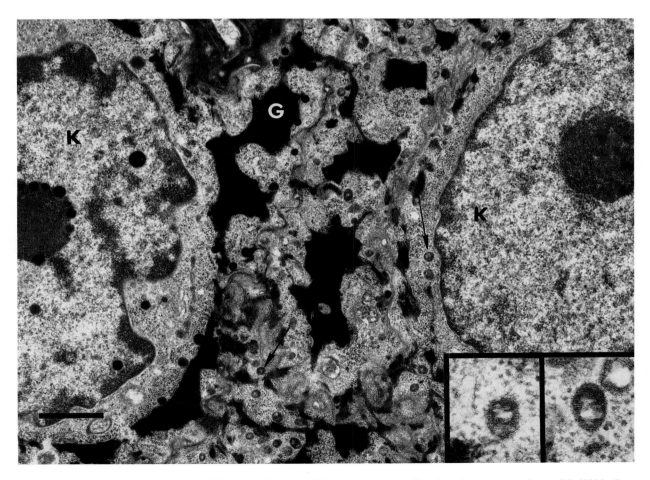

Figure 1–5. Electron micrograph of epidermis at the level of the granular layer. Two keratinocytes are shown (K). Within the keratinocyte cytoplasm are keratohyaline granules (G) and membrane coating granules (Odland bodies) (arrows and inset) (bar = 1μm for photography and a bar equivalent of 4.1 μm for the inset.

phorylation of the precursor, formation of keratohyaline granules, dephosphorylation and limited proteolysis of the precursor to yield the active, keratin filament-aggregating protein, filaggrin, and, finally, complete proteolysis with some modification to yield sun-shielding and water-binding chemical derivatives. The interplay of this complex system and the diseases of keratinization are currently under study. Once formed, keratin bundles are further stabilized by disulfide crosslinks and by mooring insertions into desmosomes and the cornified envelope.

As a keratinocyte moves into the granular layer, its membrane region thickens in all areas from 8–15 nm due to the formation of the cornified envelope along the cytoplasmic side. Like keratin, this structure gives stability and chemical resistance to the epidermis, but unlike keratin, it is resistant to disulfide-breaking reagents. The stability of the cornified envelope to reducing and denaturing reagents is due to the extensive ε-(γ-glutamyl)lysyl isopeptide crosslinks among its constituent peptides.[28] Two distinct proteins have been identified within the cornified envelope: involucrin, a 92 kD protein isolated from cultured epidermal cells,[29] and keratolinin, a 36 kD protein isolated from epidermis.[30] Both these proteins serve as substrates for a keratinocyte-specific, calcium-sensitive transglutaminase. Although this transglutaminase is localized to the granular layer, the envelope proteins are first found in the cells of the stratum spinosum. The extremely insoluble, chemically resistant, and relatively impermeable cornified envelope, then, is made of protein monomers synthesized in the lower epidermis and crosslinked by a calcium-dependent transglutaminase localized in the granular layer.

If an isolated epidermal preparation is exposed to an aqueous dye either from the outer cornified surface or the inner basal layer surface, the dye will penetrate the epidermis only as far as the granular layer. At this level, there is a barrier to hydrophilic materials. In fact, a dramatic ultrastructural change occurs in the interkeratinocyte region at about the level of the granular layer: the lamellar bodies (membrane-coating granules, Odland bodies, keratinosomes, cementosomes) are secreted into the intercellular space (Fig. 1–5). The lamellar body, a 0.2–0.3 μm diameter ovoid organelle that is synthesized primarily within the spinous cells, moves to the apex and periphery of the granular cells, fuses with the plasma membrane, and secretes its contents into the intercellular space. Since the granule is rich in glycolipids and sterols, the intercellular space becomes lipid rich and hydrophobic, a change that correlates with the development of a hydrophobic barrier at this level. Because the cells of the upper stratum granulosum and stratum corneum are protein rich (being packed with structural protein) and the plasma membranes and intercellular space are lipid rich, the upper epidermis is conceived as having the metaphorical structure of brick and mortar, protein bricks and lipid mortar.[31]

As the cells of the stratum corneum mature and differentiate further, their lipid content changes qualitatively. In the basal layer, the constituent lipids resemble those of other epithelia, being mostly phospholipids. Higher up in the lower stratum corneum, phospholipids now make up a minor component, and the predominant lipids are neutral lipids, glucosylceramides, and cholesterol sulfate. In the outermost layers of the stratum corneum, the lipids are once again modified: the more polar glucosylceramides are converted to ceramides, and cholesterol sulfate is converted to cholesterol. Because in disease states where cholesterol sulfate accumulates in the epidermis the cornified layer does not desquamate normally (as in recessive X-linked ichthyosis, were there is a steroid sulfatase deficiency), it is assumed that as cholesterol sulfate is hydrolyzed to cholesterol and glucosylceramide is hydrolyzed to ceramide, keratinocyte attachments break down and the cells desquamate.[32] Although the actual mechanism is unknown, we recognize that the processes of epidermal disintegration (desquamation) are not passive. They appear to require as active a biochemical mechanism as keratinization itself.

The predominant epidermal cell is the keratinocyte, which, through very creative mechanisms, plays the central role in epidermal structure. The keratinocyte is, however, not the only epidermal cell. Other epidermal resident cells—melanocytes, Merkel cells, Langerhans cells—that contribute significantly to epidermal function are discussed in the following sections.

DERMAL–EPIDERMAL JUNCTION

All epithelia interface the stroma upon which they rest by a specialized region called the basement membrane zone (BMZ) or, in the case of the epidermis, the dermal–epidermal junction.[33] This interface region has at least three important functions: to give support to the basal cells of the epidermis, to moor the epidermis to the underlying dermis, and to serve as a zonal barrier to cells and molecules that are localized in one or the other compartment.

By light microscopy, the BMZ, best appreciated after staining for glycoproteins, appears as a thin, well-defined sheet just below the epidermis. By electron microscopy, however, the BMZ is more complex. It encompasses the lower portion of the basal cell, several distinct underlying layers, and a system of communicating filaments that stretch from the basal cell into the upper dermis (Fig. 1–6).

Basal cells attach to the BMZ at least in part by point junctions with the morphology of half desmosomes, hemidesmosomes. Like the desmosome, the hemidesmosome consists of a dense plaque and an associated bundle of keratin filaments. Unlike a desmosome, however, the hemidesmosome lacks a mirror image of itself at the junction. Even though they have some similarities, these two point junctions actually differ in specific function, morphology, and biochemistry. Recent work indicates, for example, that bullous pemphigoid antigen is present intracellularly in the area of the dense plaque of the hemidesmosome.[34] In contrast, this antigen is not found in desmosomes.

Subjacent to basal cells is an electron-clear layer of approximately 20–40 nm width, the lamina lucida, which parallels the inferior basal cell surface. Below this is a granular, somewhat more electron-dense layer of about 30–60 nm width, the lamina densa (or basal lamina). The lamina densa is thickest below hemidesmosomes, whereas the lamina lucida is thicker between hemidesmosomes. (It is notable that the glycoprotein-rich BMZ seen by light microscopy actually is a zone beneath the lamina densa.) Fine, as yet uncharacterized, filaments, called anchoring filaments, course from the hemidesmosome through the lamina lucida

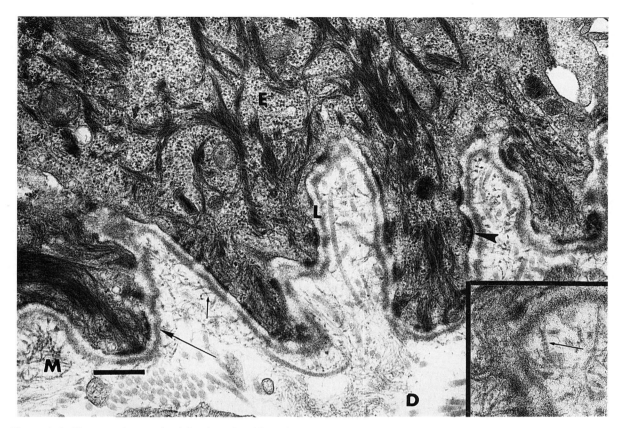

Figure 1–6. Electron micrograph of the dermal–epidermal junction. The epidermis, rich in keratin filaments, interacts with the dermis (D) across the lamina lucida (L), and lamina densa (arrow). In the area of a hemidesmosome (arrowhead), there are fine anchoring filaments coursing across the lamina lucida and a thickening of the lamina densa. Anchoring fibrils (small arrow) and dermal microfibrillar bundles (M) extend from the lamina densa to the underlying dermis (bar = 0.5 μm). **Inset.** The banded pattern on the anchoring fibrils (arrow) (bar equivalent = 0.85μm).

to the lamina densa. Anchoring fibrils appear to attach to the lower aspect of the lamina densa and extend perpendicularly into the upper papillary dermis. Anchoring fibrils are made of type VII collagen.[35] Anchoring fibrils vary in density from region to region; they are denser in leg and thigh skin than in arm skin. In regions of the BMZ overlying dermal papillae, characteristic microfibrillary bundles, as yet chemically ill-defined, filamentous structures, extend from the lamina densa into the dermis.

Although their structural and physiologic functions are less certain, many specific and unique molecular species have been identified in the BMZ (Table 1–3) that currently are used by means of immunologic techniques to categorize cutaneous diseases. The lamina lucida, for example, contains the large, cruciate, glycoprotein, laminin. The lamina densa contains, among other constitutents, basement membrane collagen (type IV) and heparan sulfate proteoglycan. Perhaps related to its supportive role in the lamina densa, type IV collagen has a netlike tertiary structure. In analogy to the renal glomerulus, heparan sulfate of the cutaneous BMZ also may serve as a sieve regulating the molecular traffic in this area.

The BMZ, then, is an interface between the dermis and epidermis. It acts as a mooring structure and a barrier to the escape of cells and large molecules from the dermis and to the movement of epidermal cells into the dermis.

It also appears to serve as a zone through which pass epidermal and dermal cytokines, molecules that influence the growth and differentiation of tissues at variable distances.[36]

Although dramatic examples of dermal–epidermal interactions are found in the skin, the specific mechanisms involved (physical or chemical) are not yet obvious. For example, at an ultrastructural level, hemidesmosomes appear to form preferentially at sites of dermal anchoring fibrils, suggesting an inductive role for anchoring fibrils in hemidesmosome formation.[37] In a series of classic experiments, Billingham and Silvers[38] found that the dermis influences the character of the overlying epidermis, so that when plantar dermis was transplanted under truncal epidermis, that epidermis acquired characteristics of the sole.

Histopathologically, examples of dermal–epidermal interactions are well known, e.g., the prominent epidermal hyperplasia associated with tuberculosis verrucosa cutis, granular cell tumor, or dermatofibroma.

PIGMENTATION

Central to the protection of skin from electromagnetic radiation is pigmentation.[39] Although predominantly the result of the presence of melanins in the epithelial cells of epidermis and hair, skin coloration also is caused by carotenoids

TABLE 1–3. IDENTIFIED MOLECULAR ELEMENTS OF THE BASEMENT ZONE

Microscopic Structure	Molecular Element	Properties	Synthesizing Cell
Hemidesmosome tonofilament	Keratin	Nonglycosylated proteins of 40–68 kD	Basal cell
Attachment plaque	Pemphigoid antigen	Glycoprotein with 220–240 kD subunits; unique to stratified squamous epithelium[104]	Basal cell
Lamina lucida	Laminin	Glycoprotein with 3A-chains (220 kD) and 1B-chains (440 kD), which binds collagen and heparan sulfate	Basal cell
	Cicatricial pemphigoid antigen	Found in stratified squamous epithelium and some mucosa	Basal cell
Lamina densa	Type IV collagen	540 kD protein forming a chicken wire structure	Basal cell
	KF-1	A noncollagenous 72 kD antigen in the lamina densa of stratified squamous epithelium but not in the BMZ of dermal blood vessels or appendages	?
	LH7-2	Antigen in the lamina densa of stratified squamous epithelium (not vascular BMZ)	?
	Nidogen[105]	Ubiquitous lamina densa component; noncollagenous; self-aggregating protein of 150 kD	?
	Heparan sulfate proteoglycan	400–600 kD; 70% protein and 30% heparan sulfate	?
Anchoring fibrils	Type VII collagen	Forms segment long spacing banded fibril defined by monoclonal antibodies	?
	AF-1 AF-2	?	?

Adapted from Fine.[33]

in the epidermis, oxyhemoglobin in dermal capillaries, and deoxyhemoglobin in dermal venules. Nevertheless, it is generally accepted that melanin pigmentation plays the most important protective role in geographic regions with high solar radiation and that lightly melanized individuals are more likely to develop skin malignancies than their heavily pigmented neighbors.

Melanins are high molecular weight, chemically inert, polymerized oxidation products of tyrosine. In humans, the cutaneous melanins are categorized as eumelanins and pheomelanins. Eumelanins range in color from brown to black, have a high molecular weight, contain less than 6% sulfur, and are insoluble. Pheomelanins are reddish brown macromolecular pigments distinguished from eumelanins by their solubility in dilute alkali and high sulfur content (greater than 8%). Both forms arise as a result of the action of the aerobic copper-containing oxidase, tyrosinase, on tyrosine and dihydroxyphenylalanine. Oxidation of the latter leads to the formation of dopaquinone, which subsequently cyclizes and polymerizes to form eumelanin. Although the chemical details of these complex molecules are beginning to be defined, the molecular structure of the melanins is still unknown.[40] The melanins absorb strongly throughout the ultraviolet and visible range of electromagnetic radiation. They filter light by converting radiative energy into heat. Ironically, irradiated melanin also can generate deleterious chemical species, such as superoxide, which can oxidize melanin and kill the cell housing that melanin.[41]

Melanins are synthesized and packaged within neural crest-derived dendritic cells, melanocytes. Migrating from the neural crest, undifferentiated melanocyte precursors first appear in human skin during the eighth week of fetal life.[6] Those melanocytes that rest on the basal lamina of the epidermis, mucosa, and hair follicles are secretory and distribute their pigment to a family of epithelial cells (Fig. 1–7). Those that are found in the dermis and noncutaneous regions, such as the eye, inner ear, and vestibular system, are continent and do not discharge their melanin into surrounding cells.

For any individual within a given animal species, the number of melanocytes per unit area of skin is constant. Thus, it has been found that the density of cutaneous melanocytes in the heavily pigmented human races equals that of the lightly pigmented races.[42] Actual color differences are produced by the amount of melanin synthesized by the melanocyte, how it is packaged, and how it is transferred.

Melanin is packaged and transferred from the melanocyte in melanosomes. The melanosome appears to be a

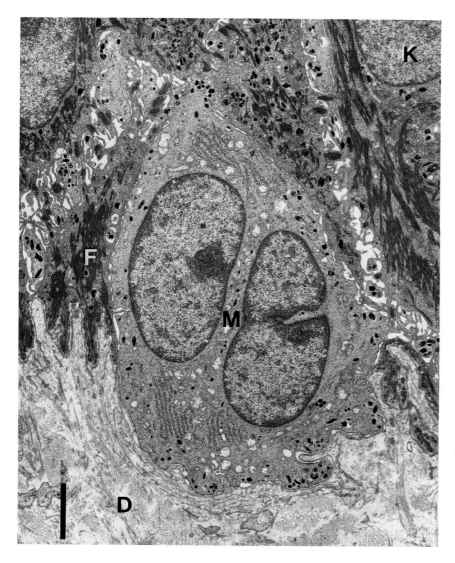

Figure 1–7. Electron micrograph of melanocyte at the epidermal–dermal junction. This melanocyte (M) is surrounded by mature keratinocytes (K) containing keratin filaments (F). Notice here the basement membrane zone, the dark cytoplasmic melanosomes, and the dendrites of the melanocyte between the keratinocytes (bar = 2 μm).

Golgi-derived laminated 0.7 μm × 0.3 μm vesicle. A convincing demonstration of how the melanosome is assembled is not yet available. One attractive hypothesis is that tyrosinase is synthesized on the endoplasmic reticulum and later incorporated into a Golgi-derived vesicle, the melanosome. In the beginning, the inner lamellae of the immature melanosomes do not contain tyrosinase. Later, melanization of the immature melanosome begins only after a second structure, a coated-vesicle containing tyrosinase, releases its contents into the melanosome.[43] The extent of melanosome pigmentation is described by four stages of melanosome development: in stage 1, the melanosome is a spherical, membrane-delineated vesicle: in stage 2, the organelle is oval and shows numerous filaments with a distinctive periodicity; in stage 3, the internal structure becomes obscured by melanin deposits; in stage 4, the organelle becomes melanin-packed and thus completely opaque without discernible internal structure (Fig. 1–8).

By means of its abundant dendritic projections, the basal layer melanocyte distributes melanosomes, and thus pigment, to a family of keratinocytes (Fig. 1–9). In humans, one melanocyte appears to be associated with 36 keratinocytes, and this association is referred to as the epidermal melanin unit.[44] The epidermal melanin unit is thought to serve as the basic system for the organization and control of melanin pigmentation in humans and animals. The number of such units varies between different regions of human skin, but the ratio of melanocyte/keratinocyte is invariant. Most of the dendritic projections contact basally situated keratinocytes. However, a few stretch up to the stratum spinosum. In lightly pigmented Caucasoids, the melanosomes within melanocytes are mostly immature; i.e., very few stage III or IV melanosomes are present. In more heavily pigmented Caucasoids, stage I, II, and III melanosomes are found about the nucleus, but stage IV melanosomes are found in the dendrites. In heavily pigmented Negroids, stage IV melanosomes are found about the nucleus as well as in the dendrites. The passage of melanosomes from the melanocyte dendrite to the keratinocyte requires active phagocytosis of the dendritic tip by the keratinocyte (Fig. 1–9). Melanosome transfer, therefore, involves a cytophagic process and a melanosome dispersal step. By a highly effi-

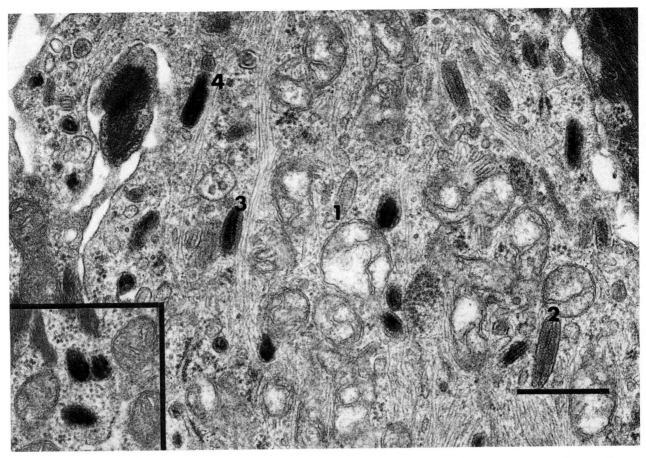

Figure 1–8. Electron micrograph of melanocytic cytoplasm showing multiple melanosomes in various stages of maturation. The stages are labeled 1 through 4; the most immature and least melanized is stage 1 (bar = 0.5 μm). **Inset.** Several fully melanized melanosomes and surrounding mitochondria (bar equivalent = 0.45).

cient, though poorly understood mechanism melanin is distributed to the generative population of basal cells in a supranuclear position—an optimal location for absorbing incoming radiation and protecting the mitotically active nucleus. In Caucasoids and Mongoloids, the keratinocyte takes up melanosomes within aggregated groups surrounded by membrane. By contrast, in Negroids, not only are the melanosomes larger but also they are taken up one at a time and are singly situated in the cytoplasm. Once redistributed in keratinocytes, melanosome aggregates are slowly degraded by cytoplasmic enzymes. By the time the keratinocyte reaches the horny layer, all its melanosomes are dispersed singly or fragmented.

Many factors contribute to the normal modulation of melanin pigmentation. Skin color intensity is determined by the total number of melanosomes present in the cells of the epidermis, the rate of melanogenesis, and the rate of transport of melanosomes into epidermal cells. The tanning that occurs after ultraviolet radiation is due to an increased number of both melanocytes and melanosomes. Hormones influence cutaneous pigmentation; for example, ACTH, testosterone, and estrogen stimulate melanization.

With aging, there is a dilution of skin pigmentation because of a decreased number of melanocytes. It is widely recognized that multiple genes influence coloration in mice,[45] and undoubtedly a similar complexity exists in humans.

DERMIS

Dermal Stroma

Cutaneous strength is due to the dermis, without which skin would be a water-impermeable, though soft, friable, and tenuous cover. The range in dermal thickness from region to region accounts for its variable leatherlike character. It is a deceptively simple-appearing layer of the skin consisting of a complex organization of connective tissue with subregions, vessels, nerves, and resident cells. The dermis consists of two compartments. That one interfacing a basement membrane (e.g., epidermal, adnexal, vascular) and consisting of fine fibers is referred to as the "papillary dermis" (below the epidermis) or the "adventitial dermis" (about the adnexa and vessels). The one making up the

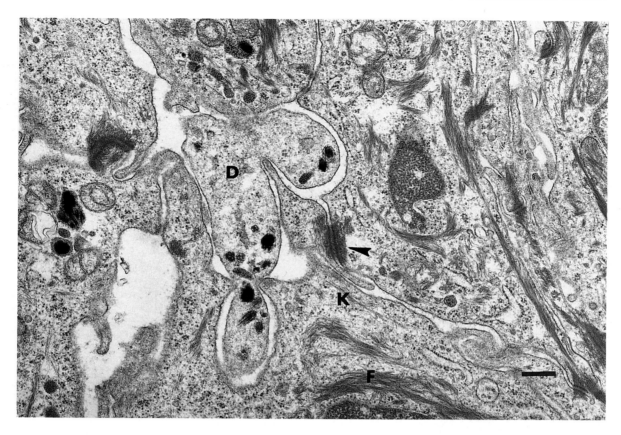

Figure 1–9. Electron micrograph of a melanocytic dendrite (D) in the process of being phagocytosed by at least one surrounding keratinocyte (K). Notice the included keratin filaments (F) and the desmosomes (arrowhead) (bar = 0.5 μm).

structural bulk of the dermis lying deep to the papillary dermis and consisting of coarse fibers is referred to as the "reticular dermis." By microscopy, the fibers of both compartments appear to course randomly in three dimensions, although functionally they provide very specific vectorial properties, as demonstrated by the greater ease of stretching the skin in one direction over another. Histologically, the dermis appears to be a rigid, tightly packed structure. This appearance is misleading, however, since it behaves functionally like a gel. Indeed, invading cells or worms can move through dermis by motility alone without digesting connective tissue structures.[46]

Although it is morphologically simple and apparently quiescent, we are beginning to recognize that the dermis also is much more complex and metabolically active than it would appear. Dermal structure is provided by a group of interacting interstitial and basement membrane collagens, a complex of amorphous and microfibrillary elastin structures, and glycosaminoglycans (GAGs). The predominant interstitial collagens of the dermis, type I and type III, are present in about the same ratio in the papillary and reticular dermis (80–98:2–20%, type I:type III[47]). In general, type III collagen fibrils are smaller in diameter than type I, and they organize into smaller bundles. That collagen fibrillogenesis is influenced by environmental factors (such as surrounding GAGs) and posttranslational modification (such

as glycosylation) may explain the morphologic (fine fibers versus coarse fibers) differences of these compartments in view of their molecular similarity. Intermixed among these major collagens are other minor species (e.g., procollagen types I and III, α1-trimer collagen). Why there are different collagen types and how they interact are questions not yet answered, although such interactions must be stable and numerous.

By electron microscopy, one can see between the collagen bundles a prominent population of fine microfibers, some of which are associated with the densely packed, amorphous elastin protein. The microfibrils in the papillary dermis, referred to as "oxytalan" bundles, run perpendicular to the epidermis and join, at the lower papillary dermis, elaunin fibers.[48] The latter fibers form a horizontal plexus about the level of the papillary–reticular dermal interface and are associated with variable amounts of elastin matrix. In the deep reticular dermis, elastin consists predominantly of amorphous matrix and relatively few microfibrils. A protein component of the microfibril has been identified and named fibrillin.[49] In contrast to axially oriented collagen bundles, which are nonextensible, elastin fibers, made of a crosslinked, randomly positioned molecule, can be stretched to twice their length and have a characteristic snap on recoil.[50]

The elastic properties of skin seen clinically are a func-

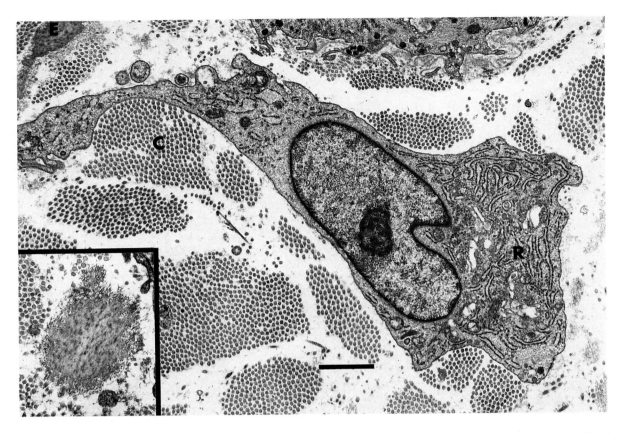

Figure 1–10. Electron micrograph of synthetically active dermal fibroblast as evidenced by its abundant rough endoplasmic reticulum (R). In the dermis are collagen bundles (C) and elastin (E) (bar = 2 μm). **Inset.** Elastin matrix and the associated microfibrils (bar equivalent = 3.6 μm).

tion not only of the elastic fiber system but also of the gel properties of the dermis. It is the proteoglycans and GAGs that give turgor to dermis through the high water-binding capacity of these polymers.[51] In embryonic dermis, the predominant GAG is hyaluronic acid (this GAG also accumulates in many disease states, such as myxedema and focal mucinosis), but as the dermis accumulates fibrous matrix, proteoglycans appear: heparin sulfate, heparin, chrondroitin-4-sulfate, and chondroitin-6-sulfate. The proteoglycans interact with collagen and other matrix molecules, and they influence collagen fibrillogenesis and dermal cellular interactions.

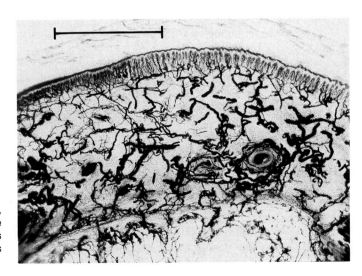

Figure 1–11. Blood vessel supply to the skin. For this preparation, skin was perfused with dye and then prepared for histology. Notice the coarse vessels of the reticular dermis compared to the fine vessels of the papillary dermis. The outer epidermis is not apparent in this preparation (bar = 2 mm). (*Courtesy of R. Winkelmann.*)

The dermis normally contains a population of resident cells that supports the slow normal turnover of the dermis and serves as a primary defense mechanism. Within dermal stroma are mesenchymal cells traditionally referred to as fibroblasts (Fig. 1–10). These cells synthesize all the collagen types, elastin, GAGs, proteoglycans, and collagenase. Although one fibroblast may synthesize two types of collagen simultaneously,[52] fibroblasts of the dermis are not uniform. Those of the papillary and reticular dermis differ in their growth[53] and synthetic properties.[54] Although traditionally labeled fibroblasts, most of the apparent mesenchymal cells of the dermal stroma are in fact highly dendritic and share properties of the mononuclear phagocytic system.[55] Not only do these cells serve a role in dermal homeostasis, but they also play a role in the immune response. About the dermal vessels and adnexa are a few resident helper T cells, macrophages, Langerhans cells, and mast cells. These cells, normally in small number, also may be present in the interadnexal stroma.

Blood Vessels

Vessels of the dermis serve the function of heat regulation and nutrition. Because the very rich vascular plexuses of the skin can potentially deliver a blood volume far in excess of its nutritional needs, the primary function of cutaneous blood flow is thermoregulatory. Arising from branches of musculocutaneous arteries, there are two major horizontal dermal plexuses, a deep one at the level of the dermal–subcutis junction and a superficial one at the papillary and reticular dermis junction[56,57] (Fig. 1–11). Direct vertical vascular channels that link these two plexuses give off side branches that provide blood to the adnexa. The venules within the deep plexus contain valves, in contrast to the venules of the superficial plexus.[58] Capillary loops branch off of the arterial vessels of the superficial plexus and project into the dermal papilla. The capillary loops have arterial characteristics within the confines of the dermal papilla but acquire venous properties as they leave the papilla and join the venous channels of the superficial plexus. (In contrast, in psoriasis the capillary within the dermal papilla has venous characteristics.[56]

Ultrastructurally, the arterial capillaries have homogeneous-appearing basement membranes, whereas the venous capillaries have multilayered basement membranes. This differential character to the wall of venous and arterial capillaries would appear to be important, since it is the venous limb of the capillary that is most sensitive to histamine and thus the site of inflammatory cell and exudate release. Dermal vessel blood flow is controlled by arteriovenous anastomoses that are normal vascular channels connecting the arterial and venous sides of the circulation within the superficial and deep plexuses. Arteriovenous anastomoses are composed of a modified arterial segment, venous segment, and, in some areas, intermediate segment. The simplest anastomosis shows only muscular thickening of the vessel segments. In the fully developed anastomosis, found characteristically in acral skin, the intermediate portion is tortuous and shows a fully developed glomus body. About 60% of cutaneous blood volume passes through these

shunts.[59] The shunt portion of the vessel has no elastic tissue and contains a very rich, mainly cholinergic nerve supply. Blood flow is regulated at these points by a direct tissue response to the stimulus (e.g., cold), by sympathetic innervation, and by circulating pressor agents.

Lymphatics

Cutaneous lymphatics[60] serve to provide a conduit for clearing protein and fluid, as well as cells (such as macrophages), from the tissue. Moreover, the afferent immune response depends on lymphatic patency to carry lymphocytes, Langerhans cells, and antigens to the effector organs.

Under normal conditions, lymphatics of skin are not obvious by light microscopy, since they are invariably collapsed. Even when distended, they may be difficult to distinguish from blood vessels. Lymphatics in the uppermost dermis are endothelium-lined, thin-walled, and blindly ending capillaries. They are distinguished from the blood vessels of the superficial plexus by their thin walls, prominent endothelial cell nuclei, and elastin-free valves (in contrast, veins of the superficial plexus do not contain valves; moreover where dermal veins contain valves, i.e., in the deep plexus, they also contain elastin).

Ultrastructurally, the upper dermal lymphatic, made almost entirely of endothelial cells, has an incomplete basement membrane that separates the endothelium from the surrounding connective tissue. The anchoring filaments of the lymphatic wall (to be distinguished from the anchoring fibrils of the lamina densa), which appear to be identical to the microfilaments associated with elastin, connect the lymphatic wall with the surrounding dermal stroma. Although there is no elastin within the lymphatic wall, the upper lymphatics are surrounded by a rim or cuff of elastic fibers. Smooth muscles are found in the larger lymphatics of the deep dermis. As the dermal stroma accumulates fluid, the anchoring filaments pull the lymphatics open and effect drainage. Cells, proteins, and fluids are cleared by their passive movement through the connective tissue into the lymphatic channels. Directional flow is established in the opened channels by the system of valves, which assures one-way flow back into the blood circulation.

Nerve Supply

Innervation of the skin is largely through myelinated branches of the musculocutaneous nerves that arise segmentally from spinal or cranial nerve trunks.[61] These nerves branch in the dermis to form a deep and superficial plexus. Epineurial connective tissue surrounds small branches. Perineurial and endoneurial sheaths surround fiber bundles, and Schwann cells surround individual fibers. The extent to which nerves retain their sheaths depends on their terminal distribution.

Nerves of the skin have both somatic sensory and sympathetic autonomic fibers that distribute together. The sympathetic nerves branch to innervate the sweat glands, smooth muscle of vessel walls, and the arrector pili muscle. The sensory fibers, which may have specialized or free

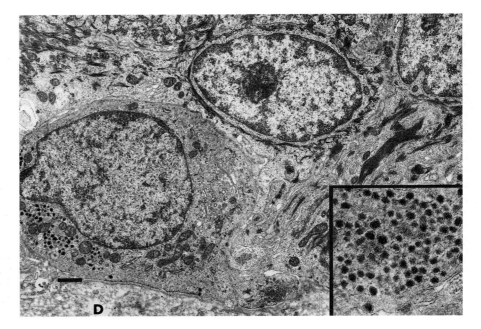

Figure 1–12. Electron micrograph of Merkel cell in basal layer of epidermis. Separated from the dermis (D) by the elements of the basement membrane is the Merkel cell. Notice the eccentric placement of the neurosecretory granules in the lower left of the cytoplasm (bar = 1 μm). The neurosecretory granules are shown at a higher power in the **inset** (bar equivalent = 2.4 μm).

endings, are variably distributed, resulting in the regional difference in sensory acuity. Although sensory nerves generally supply the skin segmentally, autonomic nerves do not follow the dermatomes precisely because the postganglionic fibers destined for the skin arise in several different spinal nerve synapses.

The cutaneous sensory receptors can be divided into two groups: those with free nerve endings (penicillate, papillary, hair follicle-associated, and Merkel cell-associated) and those with encapsulated endings (Meissner's, Pacinian, Ruffini). Because they are so widespread, free terminals are the most important of the cutaneous receptors. Free receptors are found in the dermis at all levels, but they are particularly numerous in the papillary dermis just beneath the epidermis. In fact, more than 60% of dermal papillae contain free receptors.[62] Each neurite supplies a discrete area of skin in a punctate pattern. Pencillate fibers are the major component of the subepidermal neural network in hairy skin. They are unmyelinated and serve in the perception of touch, temperature, pain, and itch, but they provide a rather diffuse sensory discrimination because of their overlapping innervation. Free nerve endings in nonhairy acral skin (palms and soles) provide more precise localization and project individually into the dermal papillae without overlapping distribution. Papillary endings occur at the orifice of follicles. They branch from nerves that innervate the follicle at a deeper level. They appear to be receptors of cold sensation. Hair follicle-associated free nerve receptors arise from myelinated axons in the deep dermal plexus. They branch into longitudinal and circular fibers that encircle the hair follicle about the level of the sebaceous gland and apparently respond to the bending and movement of hairs.

Free nerve endings are associated also with Merkel cells, a unique cell located in the basal epidermis[63] (Fig. 1–12). This cell sits on the basement membrane and forms desmosomal contacts with keratinocytes. It is identified by its association with intraepidermal free nerve endings and its cytoplasmic neurosecretory granules, which collect at the cell pole adherent to the nerve. Although Merkel cells have some neural properties (they contain neuron-specific enolase), they are epithelial in their desmosomal formations and cytoplasmic keratin filaments.[64] As a nerve radical approaches a Merkel cell, it loses its sheath and inserts into the cell. Because as it approaches the epidermis a nerve divides into multiple branches, one nerve may contact up to 50 Merkel cells. This resulting complex receptor, referred to as a *Haarscheibe* (Pinkus corpuscle, hederiform ending), is irregularly present in human skin on hairy, glabrous, and acral areas forming adjacent to eccrine ducts or hair follicles (e.g., neck, dorsal forearm) but showing considerable variation in location and number from individual to individual.

The three corpuscular receptors have a capsule and an inner core with both neural and nonneural elements. The capsule is a continuation of the perineurium, and the core includes preterminal and terminal portions of the nerve fiber surrounded by laminated coats of Schwann cells. These receptors are classified by the character of their inner core. The Ruffini corpuscle lacks a lamellated inner core. It occurs in the subcutaneous tissue of acral skin, but its occurrence is rare. It is a spindle-shaped structure lying parallel to the long axis of the limb, having a capsule of 4–5 layers of perineurium and an inner core of nerve terminals and connective tissue surrounded by a capsular space filled with fluid. Meissner's corpuscle, which has an asymmetrical lamellated core, is located within the uppermost dermal papilla and oriented perpendicular to the surface. One to six individual unmyelinated axons enter the base of the capsule, lose their myelin covering, ramify, and terminate in bulbous endings surrounded by lamellae. Mucocutaneous end organs are similar to Meissner's corpuscles, but these are located between hairy skin and mucous membranes, e.g., lips, glans penis, clitoris, and perianal skin. Pacinian corpuscle, an oval to round nerve ending located in many parts of the body but with the greatest number on acral (digit) skin, is distinguished by its symmetrical, lamellated inner core. This terminal is surrounded by 30–80 concentric lamellae separated from each other by spaces containing proteinaceous fluid, collagen, blood vessels, and some free cells. Typically, one axon extends from a digital nerve to the corpuscle without branching. They are usually found in the deep dermis or subcutis associated with blood vessels. Pacinian corpuscles serve as rapidly adapting mechanoreceptors responding to vibrational stimuli.

SUBCUTIS

Below the densely packed connective tissue of the dermis is the loosely packed adipose tissue of the subcutis, which extends to the level of the fascial planes.[65] The adipose cells are mesenchymally derived and organized into lobules separated by their loose fibrous connective tissue septae. Within these septae course nerves, vessels, and lymphatics that serve the skin. The subcutis contains the largest volume of fat tissue in the body. It serves as a cushion to physical trauma, an insulation to temperature fluctuation, and an energy reservoir. There is a slow turnover of the constituent adipose tissue in this compartment because of cell growth and death.

The nature of the subcutis varies from site to site (Fig. 1–1). For example, it is characteristically thick in abdominal skin and thin in eyelid skin; it contains fibrous dermal projections in arm skin and embedded hair follicles in the scalp. It varies with sex: women have a thicker subcutis in pubic and thigh skins, whereas men have a thicker subcutis in the epigastric, posterior neck, and upper arm skins. Underlying this morphologic heterogeneity is the demonstration that fat cells from different sites of the same individual show differences in metabolic activity.[66]

CUTANEOUS APPENDAGES

Pilosebaceous Apparatus

Hair

The epidermal appendages arose phylogenetically as redundancies of stratified squamous epidermis. The homologous redundancy appeared as a flat scale in fish and reptiles and a flat or cylindrical protrusion in birds and mammals. Hair, unique to mammals, is a solid cylindrical fiber made of tightly packed, coherent, and cornified epithelial cells.[67] It is formed at the base of an epidermal invagination, the follicle (L., *folliculus* a small bag). The follicle arises as an epithelial bud from the primitive epidermis and grows down as a solid finger into the dermis. As it grows down, it forms an angle with the surface epidermis in such a way that the shaft points caudad and lies parallel to the cephalad–caudad axis. Along the caudad edge of the follicle at about the middermis, the follicular epithelium forms a bulge to which a mesenchymal product, the muscle of the hair follicle (arrector pili), attaches. Immediately above this muscle, a sebaceous gland forms and above that, in specific areas, an apocrine gland. When it is fully formed, the hair follicle consists of three regions: the inferior follicle, or the root, extending from the bulb-shaped deepest end to the insertion of the muscle, the isthmus, or midfollicle, extending from the muscle to the sebaceous duct, and the infundibulum, or upper follicle, extending from the sebaceous duct to the epidermal surface.

Like the life of a cell that undergoes growth and resting periods, hair growth and thus the structure of the hair follicle show distinct growing (anagen), regressing (catagen), and resting (telogen) phases (Fig. 1–13). Since it is the portion of the hair follicle forming the shaft, the inferior follicle shows the most dramatic changes during the growth cycle. In contrast, that portion of the follicle above the muscle is relatively permanent and apparently unaffected by the changes occurring below it. What physiologic factors stimulate the spontaneous cycle remain obscure. We do recognize, however, some influencing factors; for example, systemic insults, such as nutritional deficiency, severe stress (trauma, surgery, infection), and hormonal alteration (e.g., thyroid disease, pregnancy), may induce the follicle to stop growing and enter telogen. Although trauma to an individual follicle (e.g., traction) may stimulate the cycle (i.e., from telogen to anagen), cutting the shaft has no influence.[68] It is well established that hair follicle formation in the embryo and hair shaft formation in the adult are strongly influenced by the mesenchymal component of the lower hair follicle, the dermal papilla. Removing the dermal papilla from an adult follicle abrogates the ability of that follicle to form a shaft. Conversely, isolated dermal papillae have the property of inducing hair follicle formation when appropriately placed under follicular epithelium.[69,70] Moreover, dermal papilla cells grown in culture will induce hair shaft formation when inserted into the base of a follicle from which the papilla had been removed.[71]

The follicle is made of tapering concentric cylinders of cells (Fig. 1–14). Some of these cylindrical layers form a sleeve for the hair shaft, and others form the shaft itself.[71a] The external root sheath (ERS), present as the outermost portion of the follicle, is thickest at the top, where it shows epidermal characteristics, and thinnest at the follicle base, where the sheath epithelium is glycogen-rich. The deep portion of the ERS has been named the trichilemma (Gr., *lemma*, a husk) because it is the outermost epithelial layer of the lower follicle.

The cells of the central lower follicle (bulb) form the hair shaft, which consists of a narrow central medulla, a thick cortex, and a cuticle made of a single layer of overlapping cells. As cortical cells leave the basal layer, they take up melanin from resident melanocytes and thus give color to the shaft. Initially, the cells are cuboidal, but as they are pushed (by growth pressure) upward, they differentiate to become elongated, compacted, and cornified. The tightly coherent cells fill with vertically aligned keratin filaments, which pack in the absence of prominent cytoplasmic gran-

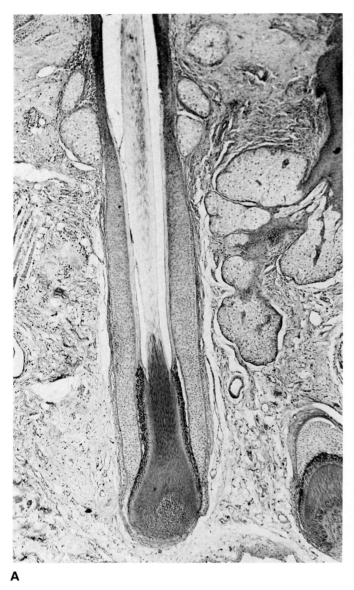

A

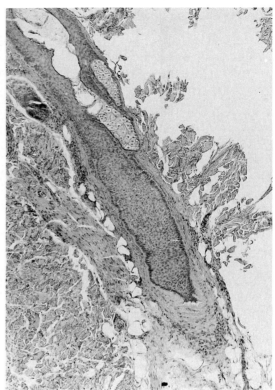

B

Figure 1–13. Composite micrograph of anagen (**A**), catagen (**B**), and early telogen (**C**) hair follicles.

C

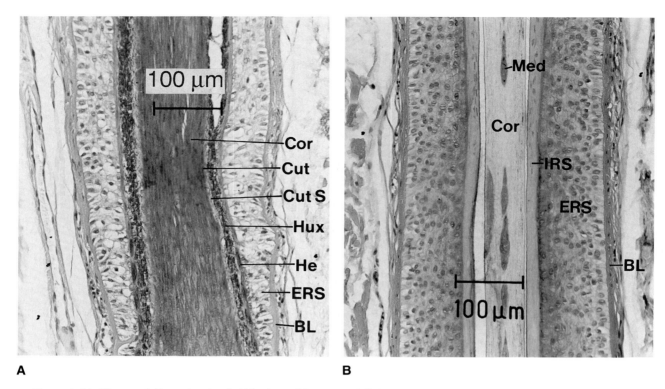

Figure 1–14. Micrograph illustrating detailed histology of the anagen follicle just above the bulb (**A**) and just below the sebaceous duct (**B**). Labeled are the cortex (Cor) and medulla (Med) of the shaft, the cuticle of the shaft (Cut), and the cuticle of the internal root sheath (Cut S), the internal root sheath (IRS) and its layers, Huxley's layer (Hux) and Henle's layer (He), the external root sheath (ERS), and the basal lamina (BL).

ules. The process of cornification appears to be similar to that in the epidermis, but it involves a different set of proteins (low sulfur keratins, high sulfur proteins, and high glycine/tyrosine proteins[72]) it occurs in the absence of a granular layer, and it does not terminate in the desquamation of the cornified cells. Finally, the hair shaft is bounded by a single, but overlapping, cylindrical layer of cells, the cuticle of the hair shaft.

Separating the ERS from the shaft is the internal root sheath (IRS). The IRS has three cylindrical cell layers, namely (extending from inside to outside), the cuticle of the internal sheath, Huxley's layer, and Henle's layer. Henle's cells are the first to cornify in the hair follicle and apparently provide a mold for the formative shaft. This layer also may provide the sliding plane along which the shaft moves. Huxley's layer is usually two cells in thickness, but this may vary. These cells keratinize in the presence of prominent intracytoplasmic granules, the trichohyaline granules. Huxley's layer also serves to mold the hair shaft and appears to be responsible for any cross-sectional asymmetry of the shaft.[73]

The hair shaft is moored to the sheath predominantly by the interlocking cuticular cells of the shaft and internal sheath. The cuticular layer of both structures is made of a single sheet of overlapping, keratinized cells. However, the cuticle cells of the shaft point downward, and those of the sheath point upward. The nature of cuticle cell placement thus gives to the shaft and the IRS surface a directionality and a mechanism for a durable and rigid interaction.

The anagen, or growth, phase of the hair cycle varies from site to site. For scalp hair it is relatively long (2–6 years), but at other sites where the shaft is shorter, the growth phase also is shorter.[74] At the end of the growth phase, the lower hair follicle cells degenerate through a process of single-cell cornification, apoptosis,[75] and the whole lower follicle regresses to the level of the follicle muscle. This regressing process, the catagen phase, lasts 4–6 weeks in the scalp. At the end of catagen, the shaft is firmly moored to the lower, now club-shaped, follicle, the epithelial cells are not growing, and the epithelium of the lower follicle shows features of the upper ERS. This is the quiescent phase of the cycle, telogen (in the scalp, telogen lasts 3–4 months). At the proper, as yet undefined, signal, the resting germ cells of the telogen follicle start dividing, move down into the dermis once again as a solid core, and form a tapered hair shaft that eventually reaches the surface and pushes the old resting club hair out. This growing, or anagen, phase of the cycle is recognized to have six subphases.[76]

The number of follicles in the skin appears to be fixed, with no new follicle formation occurring after birth. The initial hair produced by the fetus is very fine, nonmedullated, lightly pigmented, and variable in length (lanugo hair). Adult hair shafts very in length, thickness, and pig-

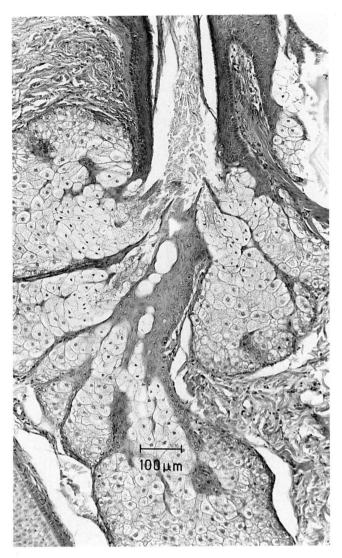

Figure 1–15. Micrograph of sebaceous gland. Notice the single basal layer of this multilobulated structure and the holocrine secretion of the sebaceous cells at the entrance to the duct.

mentation. Large hair follicles (terminal follicles) produce long, thick, medullated, pigmented, so-called terminal shafts, and small follicles (vellus follicles), which are thin and short, produce short, thin, nonpigmented, nonmedullated, so-called vellus shafts. The type of shaft formed often is influenced by the ambient androgen concentration.[77] Some follicles are highly androgen sensitive (e.g., facial and body), some follicles grow with puberty (e.g., axillary and pubic), some follicles regress with androgens (specifically, scalp hair in the susceptible individual), and some follicles are independent of androgens (e.g., eyebrow or eyelid hair). Although the size of mature follicle differs, the density of hair follicles essentially is equal between the sexes of equivalent genetic background, e.g., a brother and sister.

Sebaceous Gland

As the hair shaft moves along the pilary canal, it passes the sebaceous duct and is coated by the lipid-rich secretions of this gland.

The sebaceous gland arises as an outgrowth from the original pilosebaceous peg (13–15 weeks gestation). Except for acral skin, sebaceous glands are found in all areas. On the head and neck, they are large and form multiacinar structures; on the lateral trunk, they are small and form uniacinar structures. The secretory epithelium grows from the periphery of the lobule where basaloid cells divide, moves toward the duct, and differentiates by accumulating foamy cytoplasmic lipid vacuoles and losing cytoplasmic organelles (Fig. 1–15). Within the sebaceous duct and pilary canal, the lipid-laden cells rupture, and the sebaceous product is released as a clear oily product, sebum. Sebum contains glycerides and free fatty acids (57.5%), wax esters (26%), squalene (12%), and a small amount of cholesterol and cholesterol esters.[78]

Because it is a holocrine product, sebum production, which is continuous, depends entirely on the growth of the sebaceous acinar basal cells. The period from cell division to cell rupture is about 14 days.[79] Evidence for neural control of sebaceous secretion has not been found, although temperature may increase sebum flow. In both men and women, gonadal androgen secretion stimulates sebaceous gland growth and, thus, its secretion.[77]

Apocrine Gland

Although the apocrine gland[80,81] is commonly thought to be restricted to very specific regions, i.e., the axilla, mammary line, inguinal region, umbilicus, eyelid, and ear, it is, in fact, irregularly found wherever hair is present. So, except for acral skin of the hand and foot, where pilosebaceous structures are not found, apocrine glands may be found in any cutaneous region.

These glands develop between 15 and 20 weeks of intrauterine life as the most superior bud on the primitive pilosebaceous germ. From the level of the infundibulum, the bud grows down into the deep mesenchyme. In the majority of follicles, where the mature gland is not found, the rudimentary germ atrophies after birth. The gland becomes fully developed in adolescence.

The secretory portion of the apocrine gland is made of one cell type, which rests in part on the basal lamina and in part on a myoepithelial cell (Fig. 1–16). The apocrine secretory cell contains two types of granules: an electron-dense large granule of probable Golgi origin and a smaller, round electron-lucent granule of apparent mitochondrial origin. It is generally agreed that the secretory granules are not discharged from the cell as granules, since they break up in the luminal cytoplasm and concentrate in the apical cap. Apocrine secretion is stimulated by local or systemic adrenergic agents. Although human apocrine glands have an associated nerve supply, the neural role in apocrine secretion is unclear. Apocrine secretion, in contrast to eccrine secretion, is not continuous (the secretions are stored), is characterized by long refractory periods after stimulation and release, and is not coordinated. Therefore, one might find in a microscopic field contiguous contracted and dilated

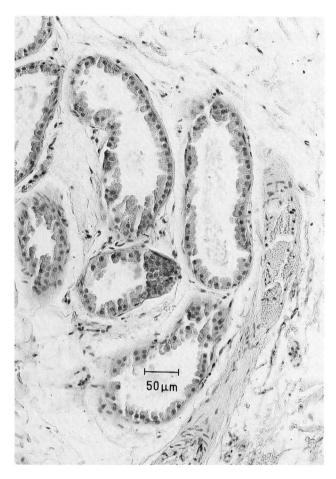

Figure 1–16. Micrograph of apocrine gland.

secretory portions of apocrine glands. Although cleavage of the apocrine cap, so-called apocrine secretion, is characteristic, these glands also demonstrate merocrine and holocrine secretory processes.

In contrast to the double layers of the eccrine duct, the apocrine duct is often made of three cell layer: a luminal, a middle (variably present), and a basal layer. The luminal cells have surface microvilli, and the luminal cytoplasm contains bundles of keratin filaments, giving a hyaline appearance to the inner duct by light microscopy. Myoepithelial cells are not found in the apocrine duct.

Little is known with confidence about the contents of apocrine secretion.[81] The secretion is described as viscid and milky pale, but the color has been observed as clear white, gray, reddish, yellowish, and black. It is protein rich and lipid poor. Apocrine secretions are thought to be odorless on release and acquire their characteristic smell with bacterial degradation. Without critical experimental evidence, except that they are released with adrenergic stress, these secretions have been considered to be phermones.[82] In fact, a physiologic role for this gland in humans is not yet apparent.

Eccrine Gland

Developing as a downgrowth of the primitive embryonic epidermis, the eccrine gland in the adult consists of the following parts: secretory segment, coiled duct, straight duct, intraepidermal coil, and eccrine pore[83,84] (Fig. 1–17).

The secretory coil is surrounded by a basal lamina that enwraps one discontinuous layer of myoepithelial cells. The gland is made of glycogen-containing, clear serous cells and a lesser number of dark, granule-containing mucous cells. Serous cells extend to the periphery and contact either the basal lamina or myoepithelial cells, whereas mucous cells are more commonly found along the luminal border and have smaller basal laminal contacts. With respect to the basal lamina, serous cells have a pyramidal shape and mucous cells an inverted pyramid shape. Both cells have secretory functions. The main function of the serous cell is to produce the precursor of sweat. The lateral border of this cell is richly plicated. Between the resulting villous

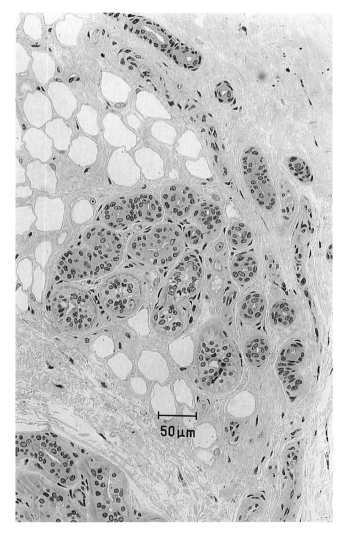

Figure 1–17. Micrograph of eccrine gland, secretory and ductal portions.

projections, an intercellular channel is formed that opens to the basal interface. Although there are desmosomes between mucous cells and serous cells, there are virtually no desmosomes in this channel region so that the resulting structure actually is an open route through which interstitial fluid can travel from the basal surface to the lumen. At the luminal end, however, the channel is closed by tight junctions.

General principles of eccrine sweat secretion have been established. When cholinergic nerves are stimulated by heat or emotion, acetylocholine is secreted. This mediator penetrates the basal lamina and enters the intercellular channels. As acetylcholine depolarizes the infolded serous cell membranes, sodium ions flow into the cell, and interstitial fluids follow. At its luminal end, tight junctions enable the intercellular channel to maintain its own osmotic pressure gradient against serous cells and the gland lumen. As the sodium ion osmotic gradient draws fluid into the serous cell and saturates it, the sodium pump across the luminal membranes become functional, sodium ion is transported into the lumen, and serous cell secretory fluid follows the sodium gradient. This secreted material is isotonic to serum with regard to sodium ion content. The secretory product of the mucous cells is a cell granule that arises in the Golgi region, passes though the cytoplasm, and then goes into the extracellular space. Although these cells contain glycoproteins and mucopolysaccharides, their exact contribution to sweat is not yet established.

The coiled duct distal to the transitional portion is made of two cell layers: the luminal cells, which bear microvilli and have a broad luminal band of tonofilaments, and the basal cells. It is here, in the coiled duct, that most of the reabsorption of precursor isotonic sweat occurs. In this segment, sodium ion is taken up from the precursor sweat in excess of water so that the final sweat becomes hypotonic.

The straight duct also consists of two cylindrical layers of cells connected by desmosomes. The luminal cytoplasm of the inner cell contains densely packed keratin filaments. Finally, the acrosyringium enters the epidermis within a rete ridge. At its lowest portion, the acrosyringium is composed of a single inner layer of luminal cells, which contain keratohyaline granules, surrounded by epidermal cells. Within the upper epidermis, the acrosyringial cells keratinize. Throughout the epidermis, the eccrine ductal cells remain distinct from the epidermal cells.

Nail

Serving as a protective cover and support for the tip of the digit, the nail apparatus arises as a derivative of the primitive epidermis[85] (Fig. 1–18). Beginning during the late second fetal month, rectangular grooves form along the lateral and proximal margins of the distal digit tip by the invagination of the primitive epidermis. Although portions of the nail apparatus begin to keratinize as early as the third month (hair follicle keratinization does not begin before the fourth month), mature nail plate does not appear before the fourth month, and its formation is not complete before the fifth month.

The matrix, an epithelial invagination along the proximal margin of the nail apparatus, is solely responsible for the formation of the nail plate.[86] As the germinative part of the nail, the matrix is made of a stratified squamous epithelium of basal cells that sit on connective tissue just above the periosteum of the distal digit. The basal cells possess desmosomes, hemidesmosomes, and multiple interdigitations. With nail plate differentiation, the cells leave

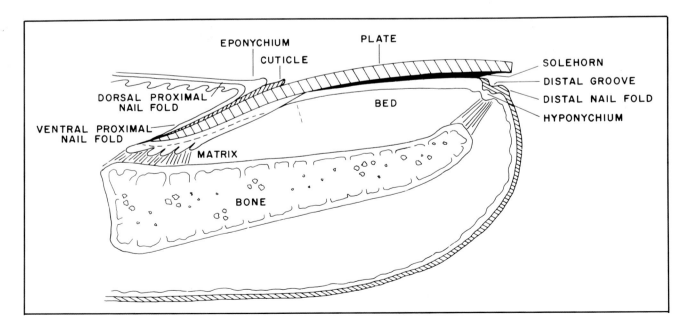

Figure 1–18. Diagrammatic representation of a sagittal section of nail. (*Courtesy of Dr. Aldo Gonzalez-Serva.*)

the basal region and push outward, they fill and pack with keratin filaments in the absence of keratohyalin, they make and discharge membrane-coating granules, they form cornified envelopes, and they lose their cytoplasmic organelles. Like the hair cortex, the nail plate, then, is composed of tightly coherent epithelial cells that are filled with keratin filaments lying parallel to the nail surface and oriented perpendicular to the direction of growth. The filaments are packed in a cytoplasmic matrix of high sulfur-containing proteins. The nail plate moves distally entirely by growth pressure arising from the matrix. The nail bed epithelium plays a passive role in this movement.[87]

In the fetus, the nail plate, a translucent, fully keratinized sheet, contains three layers that are less apparent in the adult: a thin, dorsal layer derived from the dorsal matrix found at the deep ventral portion of the proximal nail fold, a thick, intermediate portion derived from the central part of the matrix, and a thin, ventral portion derived from the ventral matrix. The layers of the nail plate in the adult can be distinguished chemically by the differential disulfide and sulfhydryl content[88] and ultrastructurally by the character of the cellular interdigitations.[89] Since it is the ventral matrix that appears as the lunula, it is not surprising that the shape of the distal nail parallels the distal lunula.

The nail plate is embedded by upfoldings of the surrounding skin, which form the lateral and proximal nail folds. The keratin layer of the proximal fold adheres to the surface of the nail plate as the cuticle. The nail plate adheres to and moves over the nail bed, which consists of a thin (2–3 cells) epidermis that lacks a granular layer. The bed epidermis has an undulating rete pattern that runs parallel to the direction of the nail plate growth and gives to the plate its characteristic subtle ribbing. Capillaries feeding the nail bed course along the rete parallel to the direction of growth. Moreover, glomus bodies, which serve to shunt blood away from the periphery, lie parallel to the capillaries. In the nail bed, dermis connective tissue bundles radiate from the periosteum of the digit to the epidermis. Although nail bed skin manifests no true subcutis or pilosebaceous structures, the dermis here, as elsewhere, contains elastic fibers, a small amount of fat, blood vessels, lymphatics, and unencapsulated and encapsulated nerve endings.

The hyponychium extends from the nail bed to the distal groove. It keratinizes like the epidermis with a granular layer and desquamating surface cells.

THE SKIN AS AN IMMUNOLOGIC ORGAN

Since it is the outermost surface, it is reasonable to suppose that the skin would provide for the host, besides its static protective structure, an active system of defense. Such a function is provided by a component of the immune system that is initiated and developed in the skin. For many years, immunologists recognized the skin as a privileged site in terms of experimental antibody production. They knew that placing antigens in the skin was a very effective way of generating antibodies. The concept of the skin as an immunologic organ, however, is new.[90] Currently, this aspect of skin biology is developing at such a pace that any comprehensive statement is, paradoxically, limited.

It is becoming clear that the immunologic elements of the skin involve more than the cells we traditionally consider to be part of the lymphoid system. Besides dermal lymphocytes and mast cells, we now recognize that mononuclear phagocytes, dendritic cells, Langerhans cells, and keratinocytes are part of this interacting system.

In general, to muster a primary immunologic defense, six key steps must be effected[91]: (1) the antigen must be encountered, (2) it must be recognized as foreign, (3) immune cells must be activated, (4) accessory immune cells (e.g., phagocytes) and molecules (e.g., complement) must be deployed, (5) the response must discriminate between self and nonself, and (6) the response must be regulated to balance the reaction to the particular antigenic load imposed. Although the skin and its draining lymph nodes have the elements to complete the steps of an immune response, in this discussion, only the afferent limb of that response, involving Langerhans cells and keratinocytes, is considered. Reviews of this field are available.[92,93]

In 1869, using a gold chloride stain, Paul Langerhans identified a second dendritic cell of the epidermis that was situated above the basal layer (in contrast to the melanocyte, another dendritic cell, which is found at the level of or below the basal layer) and appeared to him to serve a neural function. About a century later, Birbeck pointed out that by electron microscopy this cell has unique characteristics: (1) it has an irregular surface membrane lacking desmosomes, (2) it has clear cytoplasm by light microscopy lacking keratin filaments, melanosomes, and premelanosomes, (3) it has an irregularly folded nucleus, and (4) it bears a unique and characteristic inclusion, the Birbeck granule (Fig. 1–19). This granule, which has become the sine qua non of Langerhans cells, is rod-shaped at one end and bleb-shaped at the other, giving it a tennis racket morphology overall. Although the function of this granule is as yet unclear, studies suggest that it arises as a product of cell membrane endocytosis[94,95] and that it may be involved in the processing of antigens by Langerhans cells.[96]

Approximately 3–4% of all epidermal cells are Langerhans cells. Besides the epidermis, they are found in the epithelium of skin appendages, oral mucosa, esophagus, and uterine cervical mucosa. They are found in lower density in the dermis, thymus, and lymph nodes.

Soluble antigen recognition by T lymphocytes requires an initial uptake and processing of that antigen by macrophagelike cells. Like other cells of the phagocytic–monocytic cell lineage, the Langerhans cell (or its precursor) arises in the bone marrow[97,97a] and functions as an antigen presenting cell. The Langerhans cell is perfectly suited for this function. As a dendritic-shaped cell contacting a family of keratinocytes in the midepidermis, it is ideally situated to survey the skin surface for foreign antigens. The Langerhans cell bears on it membranes receptors for the Ia region of type II major histocompatibility antigens, a marker important to accessory cell–T lymphocyte interaction. Like the mononuclear phagocytes, Langerhans cells also express receptors for the Fc portion of the IgG molecule and the C3 component of complement. Under the proper stimulus, it secretes inter-

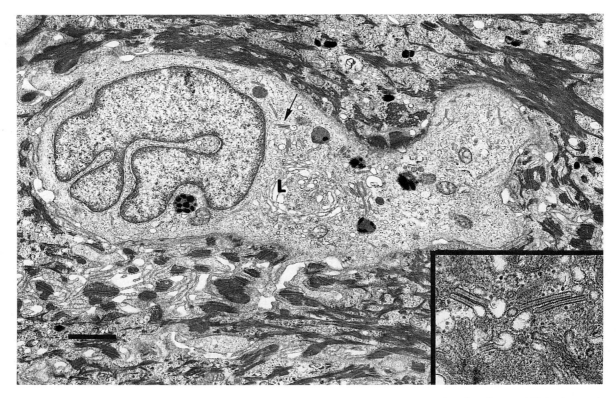

Figure 1–19. Electron micrograph of Langerhans cell within the epidermis. Notice the convoluted nucleus and Birbeck granules (arrow) within the Langerhans cell (bar = 1 μm). The surrounding keratinocytes show many desmosomes and keratin bundles. **Inset.** Detailed structure of the Birbeck granule (bar equivalent = 3.2 μm).

leukin 1 (IL-1) a molecule that stimulates the immune response of T lymphocytes.[98] The Langerhans cell also carries antigens identified by monoclonal antibodies generated to lymphocytes. For example, it expresses the antigen for monoclonal antibody T4, an antigen common to helper T lymphocytes and monocytes, and the antigen for monoclonal antibody T6, an antigen found on immature but not mature thymocytes. The function of the latter antigens is not known, but they may facilitate the ability of the Langerhans cell to initiate the immune response to certain foreign substances.

In a seminal study, Sauder et al.[98] discovered that epidermal cells in the absence of Langerhans cells produce a cytokine, ETAF, that stimulates the growth of T lymphocytes. This unexpected discovery presented for the first time the idea that the keratinocyte itself can modulate the immune response and that the keratinocyte is capable of producing cytokines, soluble mediators of cell activity. Subsequent studies have shown that keratinocytes produce IL-1 and that a molecule identical to monocyte IL-1 is at least one component of the ETAF preparation of Sauder.[99,100] Since this initial discovery, the keratinocyte has been found to produce other immunoactive cytokines: a thymopoietin-like molecule[101] and a granulocyte macrophage colony-stimulating factor.[36] The cytokine function of the keratinocyte has been reviewed.[102] That the keratinocyte contains receptors for immunoregulatory molecules[103] underscores its central role in cutaneous immune activities.

REFERENCES

1. Bereiter-Hahn J, Maltoltsy AG, Richards KS. *Biology of the Integument. II. Vertebrates.* Berlin: Springer Verlag; 1986.
2. Goldsmith LA, ed. *Biochemistry and Physiology of the Skin. I, II.* New York: Oxford University Press; 1983.
3. Jarrett A, ed. *The Physiology and Pathophysiology of the Skin. 1–9.* New York: Academic Press; 1976–1986.
4. Montagna W, Parakkal F. *The Structure and Function of Skin.* New York: Academic Press; 1974.
5. Holbrook KA. Structure and development of the skin. In *Pathophysiology of Dermatologic Diseases.* Soter NA, Baden HP, eds. New York: McGraw-Hill; 1984: 3–43.
6. Holbrook KA, Wolff K. The structure and development of skin. In: Fitzpatrick TB, Eisen AZ, Wolff K, Freedberg IM, Austen KF, *Dermatology in General Medicine.* New York: McGraw-Hill; 1987: 93–131.
7. Krey AK, Moshell AN, Dayton DH, Sawyer RH, Holbrook KA. Morphogenesis and malformations of the skin. NICHD/NIADDK Research Workshop *J Invest Dermatol.* 1987; 88:464–473.
7a. Bereiter-Hahn J, Maltoltsy AG, Richards KS. *Biology of the Integument. I Invertebrates.* Berlin: Springer-Verlag, 1984.
7b. Montagna W. Cutaneous comparative biology. *Arch Dermatol.* 1971; 104:577–591.
7c. Spearman RIC. *The Integument: A Textbook of Skin Biology.* Cambridge: Cambridge University Press; 1973.
8. Parmley TH, Seeds AE. Fetal skin permeability to isotopic water (THO) in early pregnancy. *Am J Obstet Gynecol.* 1970; 108:128–131.

9. Riddle CV. Intramembranous response to cAMP in fetal skin. *Cell Tissue Res.* 1985; 241:687–689.

10. Dale BA, Holbrook KA, Kimball JR, Hoff M, Sun T-T. Expression of epidermal keratins and filaggrin during human fetal skin development. *J Cell Biol.* 1985; 101:1257–1269.

11. Gilchrest BA. *Skin and the Aging Process.* Boca Raton, Fla: CRC Press; 1984: 17–35.

12. Wright N, Alison M. *The Biology of Epithelial Cell Populations. I.* Oxford: Clarendon Press; 1984: 283–345.

13. Penneys NS, Fulton JE, Weinstein GD, Frost P. Location of proliferating cells in human epidermis. *Arch Dermatol.* 1970; 101:323–327.

14. Lavker RM, Sun T-T. Heterogeneity in epidermal basal keratinocytes: Morphological and functional correlations. *Science.* 1982; 215:1239–1241.

15. Reichelt KL, Elgjo K, Edminson PD. Isolation and structure of an epidermal mitosis inhibiting pentapeptide. *Biochem Biophys Res Commun.* 1987; 146:1493–1501.

16. Etoh H, Taguchi YH, Tabachnick J. Movement of beta irradiated epidermal basal cells to the spinous-granular layers in the absence of cell division. *J Invest Dermatol.* 1975; 54:431–435.

17. Rothberg S, Crounse RG, Lee JL. Glycine C-14 incorporation into the proteins of normal stratum corneum and the abnormal stratum corneum of psoriasis. *J Invest Dermatol.* 1961; 37:497–504.

18. Menton D. A minimum-surface mechanism to account for the organization of cells into columns in the mammalian epidermis. *Am J Anat.* 1976; 145:1–22.

19. Steinert PM, Steven AC, Roop DR. The molecular biology of intermediate filaments. *Cell.* 1985; 42:411–419.

20. Moll R, Franke WW, Schiller DL, Geiger B, and Krepler R. The catalog of human cytokeratins: Patterns of expression in normal epithelia, tumors and cultured cells. *Cell.* 1982; 31:11–24.

21. Cooper D, Schermer A, Sun T-T. Classification of human epithelia and their neoplasms using monoclonal antibodies to keratins: Strategies, applications, and limitations. *Lab Invest.* 1985; 52:243–256.

22. Guidice GJ, Cohen SM, Patel NH, Steinberg MS. Immunological comparison of desmosomal components from several bovine tissues. *J Cell Biochem.* 1984; 26:35–45.

23. Stanley JR, Klaus-Kouton V, Sampaio SAP. Antigen specificity of fogo selvagem autoantibodies is similar to North American pemphigus foliaceus and distinct from pemphigus vulgaris autoantibodies. *J Invest Dermatol.* 1986; 87:197–201.

24. Moll R, Cowin P, Kapprell H-P, Franke WW. Desmosomal proteins: New markers for identification and classification of tumors. *Lab Invest.* 1986; 54:4–25.

24a. Jessen H. Two types of keratohyaline granules. *J Ultrastr Res.* 1970; 33:95–115.

25. Dale BA. Filaggrin, the matrix protein of keratin. *Am J Dermatopath.* 1985; 7:65–68.

26. Dale BA, Holbrook KA, Steinert PM. Assembly of stratum corneum basic protein and keratin filaments in macrofibrils. *Nature.* 1978; 276:729–731.

27. Scott IR, Harding CR, Barrett JG. Histidine-rich protein of the keratohyaline granules: Source of the free amino acids, urocanic acid and pyrrolidone carboxylic acid in the stratum corneum. *Biochim Biophys Acta.* 1982; 719:110–117.

28. Peterson LL, Wuepper KD. Epidermal and hair follicle transglutaminases and crosslinking in skin. *Mol Cell Biochem.* 1984; 58:99–111.

29. Rice RH, Green H. The cornified envelope of terminally differentiated human epidermal keratinocytes consists of crosslinked protein. *Cell.* 1977; 11:417–422.

30. Zettergren JG, Peterson LL, Wuepper KD. Keratolinin: The soluble substrate of epidermal transglutaminase from human and bovine tissue. *Proc Natl Acad Sci USA.* 1984; 81:238–242.

31. Elias PM. Epidermal lipids, barrier function, and desquamation. *J Invest Dermatol.* 1983; 80:44s–49s.

32. Williams ML. The ichthyoses—Pathogenesis and prenatal diagnosis: A review of recent advances. *Pediatr Dermatol* 1983; 1:1–24.

33. Fine J-D. The skin basement membrane zone. *Adv Dermatol.* 1987; 2:283–303.

34. Westgate GE, Weaver AC, Couchman JR. Bullous pemphigoid antigen localization suggests an intracellular association with hemidesmosomes. *J Invest Dermatol.* 1985; 84:218–224.

35. Sakai LY, Keene DR, Morris NP, Burgeson RE. Type VII collagen is a major structural component of anchoring fibrils. *J Cell Biol.* 1986; 103:1577–1586.

36. Kupper TS, Birchall N, McGuire JS, Lee F. Induction of granulocyte macrophage colony stimulating factor gene expression by interleukin 1 in human keratinocytes. *Clin Res.* 1987; 35:581.

37. Gipson IK, Grill SM, Spurr SJ, Brennan SJ. Hemidesmosome formation in vitro. *J Cell Biol.* 1983; 97:849–857.

38. Billingham RE, Silvers WK. Studies on the conservation of epidermal specificities of skin and certain mucosas in adult mammals. *J Exp Med.* 1967; 125:429–446.

39. Quevedo WC, Fitzpatrick TB, Szabo G, Jimbow K. Biology of melanocytes. In Fitzpatrick TB, Eisen AZ, Wolff K, Freedberg IM, Austen KF, eds. *Dermatology in General Medicine.* New York: McGraw-Hill; 1987:224–251.

40. Proto G. Recent advances in the chemistry of melanogenesis in mammals. *J Invest Dermatol.* 1980; 75:122–127.

41. Riley PA. Melanin and melanocytes. In: Jarrett A, ed. *The Physiology and Patholophysiology of the Skin.* London: Academic Press; 1974; 3:1107–1108.

42. Szabo G. The number of melanocytes in human epidermis. *Br Med J.* 1954; 1:1016–1017.

43. Turner WA, Taylor JD, Tchen TT. Melanosome formation in the goldfish: The role of multivesicular bodies. *J Ultastruct Res.* 1975; 51:16–31.

44. Fitzpatrick TB, Breathnach AS. Das Epidermale Melanin Einheit System. *Dermatol. Wechenschr.* 1963; 147:481.

45. Silvers WK. *The Coat Colors of Mice.* Basel: Springer Verlag; 1979.

46. Jarrett A. The physical nature of the dermis in living skin. In: Jarrett A, ed. *The Physiology and Pathophysiology of the Skin.* London: Academic Press; 1974:873–893.

47. Weber L, Kirsch E, Muller P, Krieg T. Collagen type, distribution, and macromolecular organization of connective tissue in different layers of human skin. *J Invest Dermatol.* 1984; 82:156–160.

48. Cotta-Pereira G, Rodrigo FG, Bittencourt-Sampaio S. Oxytalan, elaunin, and elastic fibers in the human skin. *J Invest Dermatol.* 1976; 66:143–148.

49. Sakai LY, Keene DR, Engwall E. Fibrillin, a new 350 kD glycoprotein, is a component of extracellular microfibrils. *J Cell Biol.* 1986; 103:2499–2509.

50. Partridge SM. Isolation and characterization of elastin. In: Balazs EA, ed. *Chemistry and Molecular Biology of the Intercellular Matrix.* New York: Academic Press; 1970:593.

51. Silbert JE. Structure and metabolism of proteoglycans and glycosaminoglycans. *J Invest Dermatol.* 1982; 79:31s–37s.

52. Gay S, Martin GR, Muller PK, Timpl R, Kuhn K. Simultaneous synthesis of types I and III collagen by fibroblasts in culture. *Proc Natl Acad Sci USA.* 1976; 73:4037–4040.

53. Harper RA, Grove G. Human skin fibroblasts derived from papillary and reticular dermis: Differences in growth potential in vitro. *Science.* 1979; 204:526–527.

54. Buckingham RB, Prince RK, Rodnan GP, Taylor F. Increased collagen accumulation in dermal fibroblast cultures from patients with progressive systemic sclerosis (scleroderma). *J Lab Clin Med.* 1978; 92:5–21.

55. Headington JT. The dermal dendrocyte. *Adv Dermatol.* 1986; 1:159–171.

56. Braverman IM, Yen A. Ultrastructure of the human dermal microcirculation II. The capillary loops of the dermal papillae. *J Invest Dermatol.* 1977; 68:44–52.

57. Yen A, Braverman IM. Ultrastructure of the human dermal microcirculation: The horizontal plexus of the papillary dermis. *J Invest Dermatol.* 1976; 66:131–142.

58. Braverman IM, Keh-Yen A. Ultrastructure of the human dermal microcirculation. IV. Valve containing collecting veins at the dermal–subcutaneous junction. *J Invest Dermatol.* 1983; 81:438–442.

59. Brakkee AJ, Vendrik AJ. Arteriovenous shunts in peripheral vascular systems. *Pflugers Arch.* 1970; 314:170.

60. Ryan TJ, Mortimer PS, Jones RL. Lymphatics of the skin. Neglected but important. *Int J Dermatol.* 1986; 25:411–419.

61. Sinclair D. *Mechanisms of Cutaneous Sensation.* Oxford: Oxford University Press; 1981.

62. Cauna N. Fine morphological characteristics and microtopology of the free nerve endings of the human digital skin. *Anat Rec.* 1980; 198:643–656.

63. Gould VE, Moll R, Moll I, Lee I, Franke W. Neuroendocrine (Merkel) cells of the skin: Hyperplasias, dysplasias, and neoplasms. *Lab Invest.* 1985; 52:334–352.

64. Saurat JH, Didierjean L, Skalli O, Siegenthaler G, Gabbiani G. The intermediate filament proteins of rabbit normal epidermal Merkel cells are cytokeratin. *J Invest Dermatol.* 1984; 83:431–435.

65. Spearman RIC. Structure and function of subcutaneous tissue. In: Jarrett A, ed. *The Physiology and Pathophysiology of the Skin.* New York: Academic Press; 1982; 7:2251–2281.

66. Hirsch J, Goldrick B. Metabolism of human adipose tissue in vitro. In: *Handbook of Physiology. Section 5 Adipose Tissue.* 1965:455–470.

67. Rook A, Dawber R. *Diseases of the Hair and Scalp.* Oxford: Blackwell Scientific; 1982:1–48.

68. Ghadially FN. Effect of trauma on growth of hair. *Nature.* 1958; 181:993.

69. Oliver RF. The experimental induction of whisker growth in the hooded rat by implantation of dermal papillae. *J Embryol Exp Morphol.* 1967; 18:43–51.

70. Pisansarakit P, Moore GPM. Induction of hair follicles in mouse skin by rat vibrissa dermal papillae. *J Embryol Exp Morphol.* 1986; 94:113–119.

71. Horne KA, Jahoda CAB, Oliver RF. Whisker growth induced by implantation of cultured vibrissae dermal papilla cells in the adult rat. *J Embryol Exp Morphol.* 1986; 97:111–124.

71a. Epstein WL, Maibach HI. Cell proliferation and movement in human hair bulbs. *Adv Biol Skin.* 1969; 9:83–97.

72. Fraser RBD, MacRae TP, Rogers GE. *Keratins—Their Composition, Structure, and Biosynthesis.* Springfield, Ill: Charles C. Thomas; 1972.

73. Priestley GC, Rudall KM. Modifications in the Huxley layer associated with changes in fiber diameter and output. In: Lyne AG, Short BF, eds. *Biology of the Skin and Hair Growth.* New York: American Elsevier; 1965:165–170.

74. Saitoh M, Uzuka M, Sakamoto M. Human hair cycle. *J Invest Dermatol.* 1970; 54:65–81.

75. Weedon D, Strutton G. Apoptosis as the mechanism of the involution of hair follicles in catagen transformation. *Acta Derm Venereol (Stockh).* 1981; 61:335–369.

76. Chase HB. Growth of the hair. *Physiol Rev.* 1954; 34:113–126.

77. Ebling FJG. Hair follicles and associated glands as androgen targets. *Clin Endocrine Metab.* 1986; 15:319–339.

78. Downing DT, et al. Variability in the chemical composition of human surface lipids. *J Invest Dermatol.* 1970; 53:322–327.

79. Downing DT, Strauss JS. On the mechanism of sebaceous secretion. *Arch Dermatol Res.* 1982; 272:343–349.

80. Craigmyle MBL. *The Apocrine Glands and the Breast.* Chichester, England: John Wiley & Sons; 1984.

81. Hurley HJ, Shelley WB. *The Human Apocrine Sweat Gland in Health and Disease.* Springfield, Ill: Charles C. Thomas; 1960.

82. Morris D. *The Naked Ape.* New York: Dell Publishing Co; 1967:64–65.

83. Hashimoto K. The eccrine gland. In: Jarrett A, ed. *The Physiology and Pathophysiology of the Skin.* New York: Academic Press; 1978; 5:1543–1573.

84. Sato K. The physiology and pharmacology of the eccrine sweat gland. In: Goldsmith ZA, ed. *Biochemistry and Physiology of the Skin.* Oxford: Oxford University Press; 1983:596–641.

85. Dawber RPR, Baran R. Structure, embryology, comparative anatomy and physiology of the nail. In: Baran R, Dawber RPR, eds. *Diseases of the Nails and Their Management.* Blackwell Scientific; 1984:1–23.

86. Zaias N, Alvarez J. The formation of the primate nail plate: An autoradiographic study in squirrel monkey. *J Invest Dermatol.* 1968; 51:120.

87. Zaias N. The movement of the nail bed. *J Invest Dermatol.* 1967; 48:402–403.

88. Jarrett A, Spearman RIC. The histochemistry of the human nail. *Arch Dermatol.* 1966; 94:652–657.

89. Parent D, Achten G, Stouffs-Vanhoof F. Ultrastructure of the normal human nail. *Am J Dermatopathol.* 1985; 7:529–535.

90. Katz SI. The skin as an immunologic organ. *J Am Acad Dermatol.* 1985; 13:530–536.

91. Nossal GJV. The basic components of the immune system. *N Engl J Med.* 1987; 316:1320–1325.

92. Choi KL, Sauder DN. The role of Langerhans cells and keratinocytes in epidermal immunity. *J Leukocyte Biol.* 1986; 39:343–358.

93. Stingl G, Wolff K. Langerhans cells and their relation to other dendritic cells and mononuclear phagocytes. In: Fitzpatrick TB, Eisen AZ, Wolff K, Freedberg IM, Austen KF, eds. *Dermatology in General Medicine.* New York: McGraw-Hill; 1987:410–426.

94. Takahashi S, Hashimoto K. Derivation of Langerhans' cell granules from cytomembranes. *J Invest Dermatol.* 1985; 84:469–471.

95. Takigawa M, Iwatsuki K, Yamada M, Okamoto H, Imamura S. The Langerhans' cell granule is an adsorptive endocytic organelle. *J Invest Dermatol.* 1985; 85:12–15.

96. Hanau D, Fabre M, Schmidt DA, et al. Human epidermal Langerhans cells internalize by receptor-mediated endocytosis T6 (CD1 "NA1/34") surface antigen. Birbeck granules are involved in the intracellular traffic of the T6 antigen. *J Invest Dermatol.* 1987; 89:172–177.

97. Katz SI, Tamake K, Sachs DH. Epidermal Langerhans cells are derived from cells originating in bone marrow. *Nature.* 1979; 282:324–326.

97a. Basset F, Soler P, Hance AJ. The Langerhans' cell in human pathology. *Ann NY Acad Sci.* 1986; 465:324–339.

98. Sauder DN, Dinarella CA, Morhenn VB. Langerhans cell production of interleukin 1. *J Invest Dermatol.* 1984; 82:605–607.

99. Bell TB, Harley CB, Stetsko D, Sauder DN. Expression of mRNA homologous to interleukin 1 in human epidermal cells. *J Invest Dermatol.* 1987; 88:375–379.

100. Kupper TS, Ballard D, Chua AO, et al. Human keratinocytes contain mRNA indistinguishable from monocyte interleukin 1 alpha and beta mRNA: Keratinocyte epidermal cell-derived

thymocyte activating factor is identical to interleukin 1. *J Exp Med.* 1986; 164:2095–2100.

101. Chu AC, Patternson JAK, Goldstein G, Berger CL, Takezaki S, Edelson RL. Thymopoietin-like substance in human skin. *J Invest Dermatol* 1983; 81:194–197.

102. Kupper TS. Interleukin-1 and other human keratinocyte cytokines: Molecular and functional characterization. *Adv Dermatol.* 1988; 3:293–306.

103. Nickoloff BJ. Binding of I-125 gamma-interferon to cultured human keratinocytes. *J Invest Dermatol.* 1987; 89:132–135.

104. Stanley JR, Hawley-Nelson P, Yuspa S, et al. Characterization of bullous pemphigoid antigen: A unique basement membrane protein of stratified squamous epithelia. *Cell.* 1981; 24:897–903.

105. Caughman SW, Kreig T, Timpl R, Hintner H, Katz SI. Nidogen and heparan sulfate proteoglycan: Detection of newly isolated basement membrane components in normal and epidermolysis bullosa skin. *J Invest Dermatol.* 1987; 89:547–550.

CHAPTER 2
Specimen Preparation

Lee G. Luna

This chapter provides what the author considers the best available methods for performing the basic processes in histopathologic technique as they apply to dermatopathology. Production of high-quality microscopic tissue sections depends, of course, on good fixation, processing, microtomy, and staining.

Because many factors can affect the end product when taking a raw tissue specimen to finished slide, the skill and careful attention of the personnel involved in each step of the process are critical. One can have the best equipment, facilities, and working conditions, but unless the technical staff is intently involved in every facet of their daily work, preparations will suffer greatly. This is especially true when dealing with tissue specimens of skin, which because of the complexity of the skin, require the use of different techniques from those employed with most other organs. Although not all techniques available for the study of skin are given here, the procedures presented should be sufficient to produce excellent slides of most skin specimens.

GROSS SECTIONING OF TISSUE SPECIMENS

Obviously, good slides begin with good grossing procedures. Although the choice of instruments and techniques is left to the individual, there are several points that should be kept in mind during this aspect of tissue processing.

The gross sectioning of skin specimens is best performed with knives that have a Teflon-coated facet or similar type coating. Grossing specimens with this type of knife reduces resistance somewhat as the knife travels through the keratin and layers of collagen in the skin, resulting in reduced tissue compression. Specimens destined for fixation in formalin-type fixative and paraffin embedding should be no thicker than 4 mm. Thinner specimens and shorter fixation exposure periods may be required with nonformalin fixatives (see remarks in the discussion of each fixative). The use of processing–embedding cassettes to contain the specimen during processing will help insure safe indentification, processing, embedding, cutting, and filing. Likewise, careful attention should be given to any requirement that might preclude placing the tissue in formalin fixative and embedding in paraffin.

Gross sectioning of skin should be performed in a manner that includes all aspects of the specimen, that is, pathologic aspects as well as all normal tissues from the stratum corneum to the fat cells near the hypodermis. Protruding hair should be trimmed off as close to the skin surface as possible to reduce damage to the cutting edge of the microtome knife or disposable blade being used for sectioning.

Finally, skin specimens should not be allowed to dry before fixation. For this reason, tissues should be placed in the fixative of choice immediately on removal from the host. If this is not possible, the specimen may be placed temporarily between gauze pads that have been saturated with normal saline solution. Exposure should be limited, however, and the specimen should be transferred to the chosen fixative as quickly as possible.

FIXATION

Skin consists of three dissimilar layers, the epidermis, dermis, and subcutaneous layer, each of which presents equally different problems to the histotechnologist and histotechnician. One of the principal problems is selection of a fixative that penetrates quickly and preserves well all the different tissues and cellular elements from the stratum corneum to the adipose tissue of the subcutaneous layer. The fixatives described will fulfil the fixation needs of the dermatopathologist. The formulas given are for making the smallest amount of solution possible.

Phosphate-buffered Formalin

Formaldehyde, concentrated 37–40%	10.0	mL
Distilled water	90.0	mL
Sodium phosphate, monobasic	0.4	g
Sodium phosphate, dibasic, anhydrous	0.65	g

This is the most useful fixative in histotechnology. The buffering of the solution prevents the formation of formic acid, which causes formalin crystal to form. Formalin crystals, when present in tissue, can pose staining problems with silver reactions, since these crystals reduce silver nitrate readily, a reduction that can simulate reduced pathologic pigments. Hematoxylin and eosin staining is good after this fixative is used but not as good as when unbuffered formalin has been used. Most special stains, including most immunochemical stains, can be performed after use of this fixative. Tissue may remain in this formalin solution for years, with only minor alteration in tissue constituents and staining reactions. Tissue shrinkage is minimal.

Formalin Sodium Acetate Solution

Formaldehyde, concentrated 37–40%	10.0 mL
Sodium acetate	2.0 g
Distilled water	90.0 mL

This fixative is the best substitute for 10% phosphate-buffered formalin. It penetrates tissue as well as does buffered formalin, and formalin pigment is not produced. However, the pH of the solution becomes more acid soon after tissue is placed in it.

10% Formalin Solution

Formaldehyde, concentrated 37–40%	10.0 mL
Distilled water	90.0 mL

It is not surprising that this unbuffered formalin fixative continues to be used in many laboratories. Staining with hematoxylin and eosin is generally better than that with buffered formalin fixatives, probably because of the acid pH of the solution. This same factor results in the tissue being fixed somewhat harder, which aids in microtomy. It has the disadvantages that the acidity of the solution causes dissolving of calcium and iron from specimens that may contain these products, and formalin pigment will be produced throughout the section (Fig. 2–1). The formation of methylene glycol (the actual fixing agent of formaldehyde) takes several days in unbuffered solutions. Therefore, unbuffered fixative solutions should be made at least 3 days before the date they are expected to be needed.

Sodium Acetate–Mercuric Chloride–Formalin (B-5)

Distilled water	90.0 mL
Mercuric chloride	6.0 g
Sodium acetate (anhydrous)	1.25 g
Formaldehyde, concentrated 37–40%	10.0 mL

(Concentrated formaldehyde is added to the solution just before use.)

Fixation with mercuric chloride–formalin mixtures appears to be adequate in 4 to 8 hours, but even rodent livers are not overhardened in 6 to 7 days. Tissues should be transferred directly to and stored in 70% or 80% alcohol. This fixative has been found to be excellent for many purposes, including skin specimens. As indicated, fixation is fairly rapid.

Bouin's Solution

Picric acid, saturated aqueous solution	75.0 mL
Formaldehyde, concentrated 37–40%	25.0 mL
Glacial acetic acid	5.0 mL

Fix blocks from 4 to 8 hours depending on the size. It is important to wash in several changes of 50% alcohol for 2 to 4 hours, agitating constantly, to ensure proper

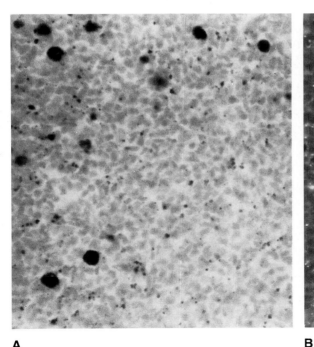

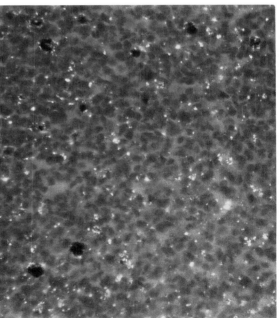

A   **B**

Figure 2–1. Formalin pigment granules deposited in tissue. **A.** Light microscopic appearance of granules. **B.** Polaroscopy-positive granules (H&E, ×400).

removal of the picric acid. Store in 70% alcohol. (*Note:* The removal of picric acid from tissues is essential in order to ensure proper staining of the tissue sections. It has been shown that tissues undergo deleterious effects, as evidenced in the staining, when the picric acid has not been properly removed and remains in the tissue throughout the entire processing cycle.) This fixative has been used successfully for skin specimens, but overfixation of specimens in always a possibility. In this case, poor staining of nuclear substances may result.

> **Zenker's Solution**
> Distilled water   100.0 mL
> Mercuric chloride   5.0 g
> Potassium dichromate   2.5 g
> Sodium sulfate   1.0 g
> Add 5 ml of glacial acetic acid to 95 ml
>   of Zenker's solution before use.

This mixture has been used since 1894, when Zenker suggested the addition of mercuric chloride to Muller's fluid to improve the fixation of nuclei. Small pieces (4 mm in thickness) usually are fixed completely in 6 to 8 hours. Tissues preserved by this method stain well with many staining techniques. Wash in running water for 2 hours.

As with Bouin's fixation, care should be exercised not to fix skin specimens for extended periods of time, since subsequent staining may be a problem.

There are numerous other fixatives that are useful in specific circumstances in dermatopathology. They are not included here but can be found in most books on histopathologic technique. It is important that the reader be aware that immunochemical staining and other special stains may require specific fixatives. For this information, see the chapters dealing with those subjects.

REMOVAL OF PIGMENTS AND PRECIPITATES

This information on removal of pigments and precipitates is limited to melanin, Zenker's crystals, and formalin pigment. For more detailed information, the reader is referred to the books listed in the Bibliography, especially *Histological Procedures and Special Stains: A Practical Guide.*

Melanin Pigment Removal

Melanin is a pigment of the skin, hair, eyes, substantia nigra of the brain, and various tumors. Its removal from cells often is beneficial, since it allows good visibility of the cell constituents.

1. Deparaffinize slides in two changes of xylene 2 minutes each, two changes of absolute alcohol 2 minutes each, and two changes of 95% alcohol 2 minutes each.
2. Rinse in distilled water.
3. Place slides in 0.25% potassium permanganate for 30 minutes.
4. Wash well in running tap water.

5. Place slide in 5% aqueous oxalic acid for 2 minutes.
6. Wash well in tap water and rinse in distilled water before staining by preferred methods.

Formalin Pigment Removal

Formalin pigment (precipitate) is a brown to black crystal produced by the interaction of formic acid (present in unbuffered formalin) and hemoglobin (Fig. 2–1). The removal of this pigment is important to prevent false silver reactions that may be confused with normal or pathologic pigments.

1. Deparaffinize slides in two changes of xylene 2 minutes each, two changes of absolute alcohol 2 minutes each, and two changes of 95% alcohol 2 minutes each.
2. Rinse in distilled water.
3. Place in the following solution for 30 minutes
   Alcohol, 95% 50.0 mL
   Ammonium hydroxide, 28% 15.0 mL
4. Wash slides in running tap water for 5 minutes before staining by preferred method.

Mercuric Chloride Precipitate

Fixatives containing mercuric chloride deposit a crystalline precipitate (Fig. 2–2) within tissue that should be removed. As in the case with formalin pigment, this precipitate will

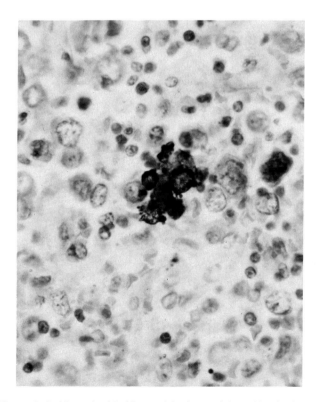

Figure 2–2. Mercuric chloride precipitation and deposition in tissue associated with Zenker's fixative (H&E, ×400).

react with silver methods, which, in turn, may cause staining problems.

1. Deparaffinize slides in two changes of xylene 2 minutes each, two changes of absolute alcohol 2 minutes each, and two changes of 95% alcohol 2 minutes each.
2. Place in Gram's or Lugol's iodine solution for 15 minutes.

           Gram's Iodine Solution

Iodine	1.0 g
Potassium iodide	2.0 g
Distilled water	300.0 mL

3. Rinse in tap water.
4. Place in 5% aqueous sodium thiosulfate for 3 minutes.
5. Wash in tap water for 5 minutes before staining by preferred method.

TISSUE PROCESSING

This facet of histologic technique is as important as good fixation. Indeed, nothing affects the quality of the final section than poor processing; an improperly processed section simply will not cut well. Here, too, one must consider the diversified tissue of the skin, each of which will be impregnated with paraffin differently.

Well-processed tissue depends on the proper removal of extractable water from the tissue with a good dehydrating agent, such as isopropyl or ethyl alcohol. The alcohol, in turn, must be removed from the specimen by a clearing agent. In most instances, the clearing agent is xylene. Since xylene is a paraffin solvent, it also prepares the specimen for accepting paraffin, which is used for impregnating tissue structures. The impregnation of tissue structures results in the formation of a paraffin matrix that allows the microtome blade to cut the section with little distortion.

The processing schedule used must be based to some extent, on the size of the skin specimen. Most small (1 to 2 mm) biopsies can be processed in 4 hours, 3 to 4 mm sections can be processed in 8 hours, and specimens measuring 4 mm or thicker should be processed on a 12-hour schedule. The agents used for processing are not discussed here, since there are a number of good dehydrating, clearing, and impregnating media available, and often the choice is based on personal preference. The agents used in the processing schedules in this chapter are my preferences.

Likewise, the type of processing equipment used must be left to each individual laboratory. For various reasons, however, the closed tissue processing systems are preferred, since these systems provide one or all of the following aids to tissue processing: moderate heat, vacuum, pressure, and time controls. This does not mean that the standard, time-proven tissue processors are not adequate. In fact, they are extremely well suited for processing skin specimens, with the proper schedule.

The orientation of tissue specimens during embedding is of utmost importance in dermatopathology. Every effort must be made to orient all skin specimens properly during the embedding process. Proper embedding will ensure that the cut section will include the lesion, epidermis, dermis, and subcutaneous fat cells if present. Figure 2–3 provides some suggestion of proper embedding to ensure the least amount of cutting artifacts. The black solid line represents the epidermis of skin specimens.

4½-Hour Processing Schedule
(For use only with closed tissue processing systems and specimens that are 1 to 2 mm thick)

Formalin, phosphate buffered, 10%	25 minutes*
Formalin, phosphate buffered, 10%	25 minutes
Isopropyl alcohol, 80%	15 minutes
Isopropyl alcohol, 95%	15 minutes
Isopropyl alcohol, 95%	20 minutes
Isopropyl alcohol, 100%	15 minutes
Isopropyl alcohol, 100%	20 minutes
Xylene	30 minutes
Xylene	30 minutes
Paraffin	35 minutes
Paraffin	40 minutes

Embed in paraffin of choice

* It is assumed that specimens have been exposed to formalin fixation for several hours before this step.

8-Hour Processing Schedule
(To be used with specimens 3 to 4 mm thick)

Formalin, phosphate buffered, 10%	60 minutes*
Formalin, phosphate buffered, 10%	60 minutes
Isopropyl alcohol, 80%	30 minutes
Isopropyl alcohol, 95%	30 minutes
Isopropyl alcohol, 95%	30 minutes
Isopropyl alcohol, 100%	30 minutes
Isopropyl alcohol, 100%	60 minutes
Xylene	30 minutes
Xylene	60 minutes
Paraffin	30 minutes
Paraffin	60 minutes

Embed in paraffin of choice

* It is assumed that specimens have been exposed to formalin fixation for several hours before this step.

12-Hour Processing Schedule
(To be used with specimens 4 to 6 mm thick)

Formalin, phosphate buffered, 10%	3 hours*
Alcohol, 80%	1 hour
Alcohol, 95%	1 hour
Alcohol, 95%	1 hour
Alcohol, 100%	1 hour
Alcohol, 100%	1 hour
Xylene	1 hour
Xylene	1 hour
Paraffin	½ hour
Paraffin	1 hour
Paraffin	½ hour

Embed in paraffin of choice

* It is assumed that specimens have been exposed to formalin fixation for several hours before this step.

Tissue Section Slide Detachment

A problem facing many laboratories relates to sections falling off slides during the performance of routine as well

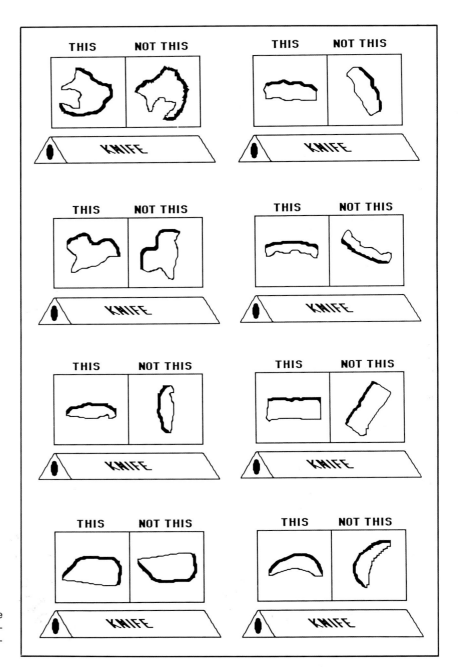

Figure 2–3. This diagram demonstrates the suggested method for embedding skin specimens. The thick, black area represents the epidermis.

as special staining procedures. Some of the more common reasons are discussed.

Inadequate Adhesion

Inadequate section adhesion often results from improper application of adhesives. For example, if one uses granular gelatin by sprinkling it on the surface of the flotation bath, an excessive amount may be removed during the surface cleaning with the paper towel. This is particularly true if the gelatin is not mixed adequately.

Overexpansion

Sections frequently fall off slides because of overexpansion in the flotation bath. This occurs when the waterbath is

excessively hot, and the section expands beyond its normal size and is picked up on a slide in this extended condition. When the section shrinks to its original shape during the drying and staining phases, the adhesive bonds are broken. This allows liquids to enter between the section and the slide, causing the section to break loose and fall off the slide.

Alkaline Solutions

Few people realize that protein (egg albumin) section adhesive bonds are broken when slides are exposed to alkaline solutions (e.g., ammoniacal silver), causing sections to come off slides. The bonds of protein adhesives do not break easily in acid solutions.

Enzyme Action

The use of enzymes, such as diastase and amylase, to digest glycogen in the periodic acid-Schiff technique causes sections to fall off slides. This is also true of enzymes, such as trypsin, used in immunochemical staining.

Section Adhesives

There are many section adhesives for various purposes. Those adhesives that are best suited routinely attaching sections of skin specimens to glass microscopic slides are presented here. These are gelatin and Elmer's Glue adhesives. For more comprehensive information on section adhesives see *Histological Procedures and Special Stains: A Practical Guide.*

Gelatin Adhesive

The amount of gelatin that should be used in making this adhesive depends on the size of the flotation bath in which it is made. In a large bath (approximately 800 mL capacity), use enough gelatin granules to cover completely the surface of a quarter. In a smaller bath (approximately 400 mL capacity), use enough gelatin to cover the surface of a nickel. These amounts are estimates and may need to be adjusted to suit specific circumstances. It is extremely important that all the gelatin granules dissolve in the flotation bath to achieve proper section adhesion. This may be accomplished by performing the following steps in the order presented.

1. Sprinkle the gelatin granules on the bottom of the empty flotation bath.
2. Slowly pour hot (almost boiling) water into the flotation bath. Some of the gelatin granules will remain on the botton surface, and others will float to the top of the water. Let this stand for approximately 10 minutes, then stir well.
3. Clear the surface of the flotation bath of extraneous material by laying a piece of paper on top of the water and gently drawing it across the entire length of the container. It is important to clean the flotation bath daily (and any utensils used in it) to prevent the growth of bacteria.

This gelatin adhesive solution will work well with most skin specimens. However, for sections containing a fair amount of keratin or bone it may be necessary to use the gelatin–formalin procedure that follows.

Gelatin–Formalin Adhesive

1. Pick up sections from the flotation bath containing the gelatin solution on a clean glass slide.
2. Drain the slide of excess water by placing it in a vertical position at room temperature for approximately 1 minute.
3. Place the slide in a Coplin jar containing approximately 5 ml of concentrated (37%) formalin. Make certain the formalin does not come in contact with the tissue section(s). Tightly cover the jar and place it in an oven at 60°C for 45 to 60 minutes.
4. Remove the slide from the Coplin jar and dry it in the conventional way, overnight on a slide warmer or for 30 minutes in a 60°C oven.

Elmer's Glue Adhesive

Elmer's Glue has achieved some popularity as a section adhesive, particularly in those cases destined for enzyme treatment and subsequent immunochemical staining of paraffin-embedded sections. The following procedure gives good results even with specimens containing bone and keratin.

1. Make up a 10% aqueous solution of Elmer's Glue in a Falcon conical tube or similar container.
2. Dip the slide into the tube container and wipe the excess glue from the *back* of the slide. Then dip the slide underneath the section in the flotation bath, and gently tease the section onto the slide.
3. Quickly draw the section up from the flotation bath and drain the slide in a vertical position for a few seconds. Allow it to dry in the conventional manner, on a slide warmer overnight or in a 60°C oven for 30 minutes. After drying, the slide will be white where excess glue remains, but this will not interfere with the staining of the tissue section(s). (*Note:* It is important to remember to keep the tube containing the glue solution in the refrigerator when it is not in use.)

Elmer's Glue Adhesive Solution

An Elmer's Glue solution also can be used in the flotation bath as a routine section adhesive.

Elmer's Glue, general purpose	15.0 mL
Distilled water	100.0 mL

(Add 12 teaspoons to an 800 ml flotation bath and 6 teaspoons to a 400 ml bath.)

Add the suggested amount to the flotation bath and stir well. Sections are placed on the surface of the water in the flotation bath and picked up in the conventional manner. Slides are dried in a 60°C oven for 30 minutes or in a slide warmer overnight.

MICROTOMY: PREPARATION OF SECTIONS

Of all variables that might affect results in microtomy, the skill and knowledge of the technician are paramount. From years of practical experience, he or she must have learned to recognize poorly processed specimens, gained a knowledge of tissue-softening methods, and be able to select and use the correct cutting instrument (microtome) and other necessary tools.

The advent of disposable sectioning blades has, to some extent, eliminated the need for knife sharpeners and conventional microtome blades. In my opinion, a conventional microtome blade is needed only when cutting sections of thick keratin (toenails) or calcified material. All other skin specimens usually can be cut with a disposable blade. Although most disposable blades perform well, one should try several brands in order to select the one that best serves the purpose. I prefer Accu-Edge disposable microtome blades. (Miles, Inc., Diagnostic Division, Elkhart, IN).

Several things should be remembered when sectioning specimens. First, be sure all screws on both the microtome

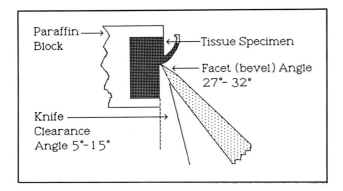

Figure 2–4. This schematic demonstrates the clearance angle necessary for obtaining good compression-free sections.

and blade holder are tightened properly. The paraffin block must be oriented correctly for sectioning. The blade must be used at the proper angle, which generally leaves a clearance of between 5° and 15° (Fig. 2–4). Likewise, the paraffin block must be properly aligned on the microtome to obtain a complete section without excessive use of tissue. Next, rough cutting to expose the entire surface of the specimen must be done carefully. If the rough cutting results in thick sections, holes may be gouged in the specimen (Fig. 2–5). These so-called moth-eaten effect holes in the tissue sections can be readily identified by their characteristic serrated edges.

Water must be reintroduced into the specimen before sectioning to prevent horizontal tissue microvibrations and other cutting artifacts. The introduction of moisture into

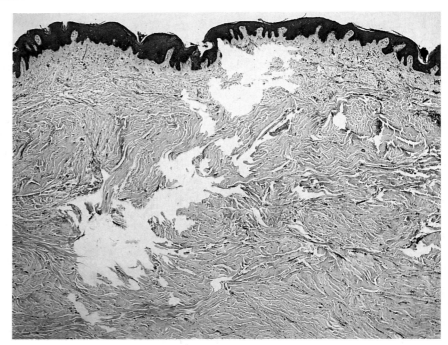

Figure 2–5. Moth-eaten artifact seen in thick sections (H&E, ×35).

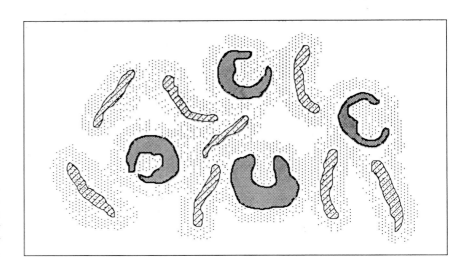

Figure 2–6. A schematic representation of globular protein (horseshoe shape) and albumin protein (bars). The dots on and around the protein represent water molecules. This bound water must be reinforced by the introduction of water with the aid of a piece of water-soaked cotton.

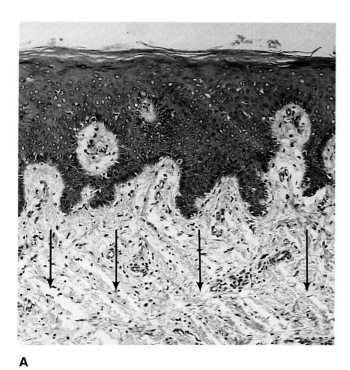

A

Figure 2–7. Examples of knife lines in tissue sections. (**A.** H&E, ×125. **B.** H&E, ×35).

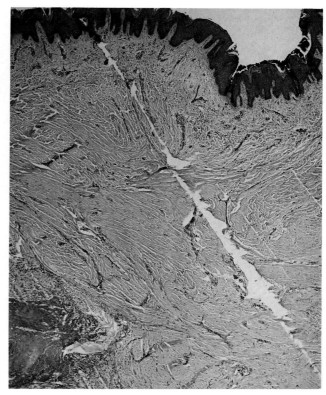

B

tissue protein is very important, since tissue must recapture some of the water removed during dehydration, clearing, and paraffin impregnation (Fig. 2–6). Without this reintroduced water, tissue will not cut well primarily because of its inability to bend and cut clean at the molecular level as the apex of the microtome blade advances. The resultant

effect is that tissue molecules break and shatter as the knife apex advances causing some, if not all, of the artifacts often seen in skin sections (Figs. 2–7, 2–8, 2–9, 2–10, 2–11). The difference between cutting a piece of tissue before the introduction of moisture as opposed to that with moisture can be compared to cutting uncooked vs. cooked spaghetti.

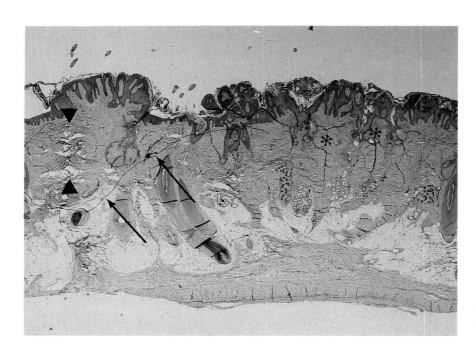

Figure 2–8. Multiple artifacts, including fiber strand (arrows), folds (asterisk), and moth-eaten appearance (arrowheads) (H&E, ×12).

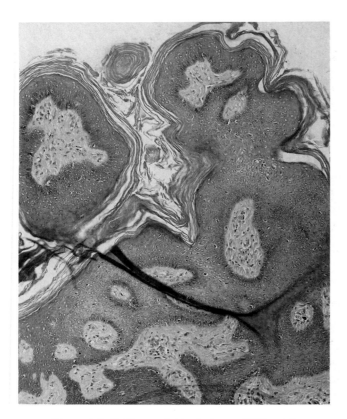

Figure 2–9. Folds or wrinkles in tissue (H&E, ×12).

in the need for moisture if high-quality sections are to be obtained. For example, the stratum corneum will, under normal circumstances, require a great deal of moisture, whereas the sebaceous glands require none. Collagen requires moderate amounts and smooth muscle tissue requires very little. The cells of the stratum germinativum require no moisture, but the cells of the stratum granulosum do.

Application Of Moisture

Moisture may be applied to the rough cut face (surface) of the paraffin block by several means. The easiest and least time-consuming method is to simply dip one's thumb in the flotation water bath and rub it on the surface of the block. This action is repeated only two or three times over a period of 5 to 10 seconds if the specimen was not overly processed. However, thick cornified material will require longer wetting with a water-soaked piece of cotton or soaking with something other than water. Alternatively, 5% aqueous solution of ammonium hydroxide serves the purpose very well. A piece of cotton is soaked in the solution and placed on the face of the block until the proper consistency is achieved. The length of time required will depend on the thickness of the cornified material. Since the moisture on the face of the block helps the blade cut more smoothly, this step should be performed routinely on all skin specimens.

Hematoxylin and Eosin Staining

The routine hematoxylin and eosin (H & E) stain is, in fact, the most important staining procedure in anatomic pathology. Moreover, many of the inconsistencies in quality that are found in H & E staining are directly attributable

On the one hand, the spaghetti breaks and shatters, causing uneven cut ends of the strands, whereas in the second case, a clean, neat cut can be made through the strands. One must keep remembering that skin consists of many dissimilar tissues and this factor plays an important part

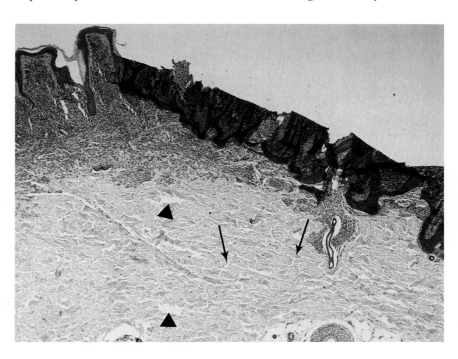

Figure 2–10. Foldover artifact, moth-eaten appearing holes (arrowhead), and parched earth or crackling effect (arrows) (H&E, ×45).

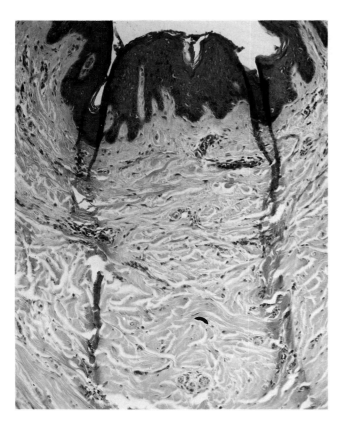

Figure 2–11. Tissue wrinkles and parched earth effect (H&E, ×30).

to the technician performing the stain. Because it is performed routinely, technicians frequently neglect to ensure that all factors that can affect the outcome have been accounted for. The following guidelines should prove helpful in achieving consistent, high-quality H & E staining of skin specimens.

First, in selecting a hematoxylin solution, preference should be given to a progressive hematoxylin solution. Mayer's and Gill's hematoxylin solutions are the most useful, since they are compounded to be specific for nuclear chromatin with very little background staining. This type of stain also eliminates the often incurred problem of over- or understaining of tissue structures.

On the other hand, if one prefers to use a regressive hematoxylin solution (such as Harris' hematoxylin), the technician must be an expert at decolorizing sections properly in order to achieve high-quality cell constituent deferential results. Furthermore, there are situations in which a progressive hematoxylin is not appropriate. Decalcified tissue or specimens that have remained in acid fixative for an extended period will not stain well with progressive hematoxylins. In these instances, a regressive hematoxylin must be used.

In addition to the type of hematoxylin used, careful consideration must be given to the choice of the counterstain as well. The three preferred counterstains for use with skin specimens are alcohol eosin, eosin-phloxine, and picric acid-phloxine-safran.

In general the staining results will be different depending on which counterstain is selected. Alcoholic eosin produces a pinkish to red cytoplasmic stain with very little tinctorial difference of the various tissue components. On the other hand, eosin-phloxine gives good tinctorial differentiation of the various tissue elements. For example, muscle will stain darker red than collagen, and some inclusion bodies also will be more prominent and stain a deep red in most instances. It is for this reason that I prefer this counterstain for skin specimens. Finally, the picric acid-phloxine-safran counterstain results in an even wider spectrum of colors that can be used for differentiation of tissue constituents. Results are nuclei blue, red cells vermilion pink, collagen yellow, muscle red, and other tissue structures varying colors depending on the fixative used.

It is important for the technician to realize that these counterstains can reveal entities that could aid in making a diagnosis. Therefore, one must strive to decolorize these counterstains properly. The most important key is the tissue exposure period in alcohol immediately after the application of the counterstain. Therefore, the times designated in the following staining procedures should be strictly adhered to.

Mayer's Hematoxylin and Eosin-Phloxine Stain

Mayer's Hematoxylin Solution

Hematoxylin	1.0 g
Distilled water	1000.0 mL
Sodium iodate	0.2 g
Ammonium or potassium alum	50.0 g
Citric acid	1.0 g
Chloral hydrate*	50.0 g

* (50 ml of glycerin may be substituted for chloral hydrate with no appreciable difference seen in staining results. This may be desirable, since chloral hydrate is a controlled substance.

Dissolve the alum in water; add and dissolve the hematoxylin in this solution. Add the remaining ingredients and shake well to ensure that all are completely dissolved. The final solution will have a reddish violet color and a winelike smell.

Stock Eosin Solution

Eosin Y, water soluble	1.0 g
Distilled water	100.0 mL

Stock Phloxine Solution

Phloxine B	1.0 g
Distilled water	100.0 mL

Eosin-Phloxine Working Solution

Stock eosin solution	100.0 mL
Stock phloxine solution	10.0 mL
Alcohol, 95%	780.0 mL
Acetic acid	4.0 mL

All stock eosin-phloxine solutions have a shelf life of 1 year if kept tightly sealed. The eosin-phloxine working solution has a shelf life of 6 months, due primarily to the evaporation rate of the alcohol.

Ammonia Water Solution

Ammonium hydroxide	0.25 mL
Distilled water	100.0 mL

Staining Procedure

1. Xylene	2 minutes
2. Xylene	2 minutes
3. Isopropyl alcohol, 100%	1 minute
4. Isopropyl alcohol, 100%	1 minute
5. Isopropyl alcohol, 95%	1 minute
6. Isopropyl alcohol, 95%	1 minute
7. Isopropyl alcohol, 70%	1 minute
8. Rinse slide in water	
9. Drain slide well (to prevent excessive solution carryover)	
10. Mayer's hematoxylin solution	15 minutes
11. Wash in running water	30 seconds
12. Blue in ammonia water	3 dips
13. Wash in tap water	5 minutes
14. Drain slide well (to prevent excessive water carryover)	
15. Eosin-phloxine working solution	1 minute
16. Isopropyl alcohol, 95%	2 minutes
17. Isopropyl alcohol, 95%	3 minutes
18. Isopropyl alcohol, 100%	2 minutes
19. Isopropyl alcohol, 100%	1 minute
20. Xylene	1 minute
21. Xylene	2 minutes
22. Xylene	2 minutes
23. Mount coverglass with resinous medium	

Results: If the procedure has been followed accurately, the tissue's nuclear chromatin will stain blue, with some signs of metachromasia. The cytoplasm will be visible in various shades of pink to red depending on which tissue structure is being demonstrated. It is important to recognize that the H & E staining procedures presented here can be performed much faster than outlined if desired. However, high-quality reproducible results in rapid staining of H & E slides are possible only if the technician takes special care to ensure such results.

Harris' Hematoxylin and Eosin Stain

This also is an excellent staining procedure for skin specimens, particularly those that have been decalcified or have been overexposed to acid fixative solutions. This also applies to tissues that have undergone some autolytic changes.

Harris' Hematoxylin Solution

Hematoxylin crystals	5.0 g
Alcohol, 100%	50.0 mL
Ammonium or potassium alum	100.0 g
Distilled water	1000.0 mL
Mercuric oxide (red)	2.5 g

Dissolve the hematoxylin in the alcohol and the alum in the water with the aid of heat. Remove from heat and mix the two solutions. Bring this solution to a boil as rapidly as possible (limit this heat to less than 3 minutes and stir often). Remove from heat and slowly add the mercuric oxide. Reheat to a simmer until it becomes dark purple; remove from heat and slowly place the container in a basin of cold water until cool. The stain is ready for use as soon as it cools. The addition of 2 to 3 mL of glacial acetic acid for every 100 mL of solution increases the precision of the nuclear stain.

1% Stock Alcoholic Eosin

Eosin Y, water soluble	1.0 g
Distilled water	20.0 mL
Dissolve and add:	
Alcohol, 95%	80.0 mL

Eosin Working Solution

Eosin stock solution	1 part
Alcohol, 80%	3 parts

Just before use, add 0.5 mL of glacial acetic acid to each 100 mL of stain and stir.

Acid Alcohol Solution

Hydrochloric acid	10.0 mL
Alcohol, 80%	90.0 mL

Ammonia Water Solution

Ammonium hydroxide	0.25 mL
Distilled water	100.0 mL

Staining Procedure

1. Xylene	2 minutes
2. Xylene	2 minutes
3. Isopropyl alcohol, 100%	1 minutes
4. Isopropyl alcohol, 100%	1 minute
5. Isopropyl alcohol, 95%	1 minute
6. Isopropyl alcohol, 95%	1 minute
7. Isopropyl alcohol, 70%	1 minute
8. Harris' hematoxylin	3–10 minutes
9. Rinse in tap water	
10. Acid alcohol	Several dips
11. Wash in running tap water	5 minutes
12. Ammonia water	5 dips
13. Wash in tap water	2 minutes
14. Working eosin solution	1 minute
15. Isopropyl alcohol, 95%	2 minutes
16. Isopropyl alcohol, 95%	2 minutes
17. Isopropyl alcohol, 100%	1 minute
18. Isopropyl alcohol, 100%	2 minutes
19. Xylene	2 minutes
20. Xylene	2 minutes
21. Mount coverglass with resinous medium	

Results: Nuclear chromatin will be blue, with some signs of metachromasia; cytoplasm will be pink. The cytoplasmic stain may vary in tinctorial properties depending on how well the counterstain was differentiated.

Mayer's Hematoxylin-Phloxine-Safran Stain

This method is useful for color differentiation of various tissue components and for that reason may be valuable to some laboratories processing skin specimens.

Mayer's Hematoxylin Solution
(See page 39)

Saturated Aqueous Picric Acid
Picric acid	2.0 g
Distilled water	100.0 mL

Phloxine B Solution
Phloxine B	1.5 g
Distilled water	100.0 mL

Alcoholic Safran Solution
Safran du gatinais	2.0 g
Alcohol, 100%	100.0 mL

Add the safran to the alcohol, stopper the bottle well, and place in a 60° C oven to allow extraction of the dye. This process may take several days (in most instances 1 week). The solution container should always be kept in the 60° C oven when not in use.

Staining Procedure
1. Xylene — 2 minutes
2. Xylene — 2 minutes
3. Isopropyl alcohol, 100% — 1 minute
4. Isopropyl alcohol, 100% — 1 minute
5. Isopropyl alcohol, 95% — 1 minute
6. Isopropyl alcohol, 95% — 1 minute
7. Isopropyl alcohol, 70% — 1 minute
8. Rinse slide in water
9. Place in aqueous picric acid — 5 minutes
10. Rinse in tap water until all the yellow color of the picric acid is removed
11. Mayer's hematoxylin — 15 minutes
12. Wash in running tap water — 10 minutes
13. Phloxine B solution — 2 minutes
14. Wash in tap water — 5 minutes
15. Isopropyl alcohol, 100% — 3 changes
16. Alcoholic safran solution — 5 minutes
17. Isopropyl alcohol, 100% — 1 minute
18. Isopropyl alcohol, 100% — 2 minutes
19. Xylene — 2 minutes
20. Xylene — 2 minutes
21. Mount coverglass with resinous medium

Results: Nuclear chromatin will be blue with some signs of metachromasia; red cells vermilion pink; bone yellow; cartilage yellowish green; muscle red; collagen yellow. It should be recognized that various useful colors will be present on different tissue constituents, especially if different fixatives are used.

BIBLIOGRAPHY

The following books are recommended for those wishing to read beyond the scope of the practical information presented here.

Bancroft JD, Cook HC. *Manual of Histological Techniques.* New York: Churchill-Livingstone, 1984

Hayat MA *Fixation for Electron Microscopy.* New York: Academic Press, 1981.

Kiernan JA. *Histological and Histochemical Methods: Theory and Practice.* New York: Pergamon Press, 1981

Luna LG: *Histological Procedures and Special Stains: A Practical Guide.* Gaithersburg, Md: Center for Histotechnology Training, 1988.

CHAPTER 3

Histochemistry and Special Stains

Waine C. Johnson

Histopathology is based primarily on microscopic observations made available by staining of tissue elements, thus giving the form and pattern that we recognize as normal or altered tissues. The hematoxylin and eosin stain is used almost universally as the routine staining method. Tissue affinity with hematoxylin, a natural dye in use since 1863, is partially due to the dye's basic character that gives rise to combination with acidic substances, such as nucleic acids. In this chapter, consideration is given to inorganic substances, simple polysaccharides, mucosaccharides, proteins, lipids, enzymatic studies, and stains for tissue elements and organisms. The indications and use of the techniques in cutaneous pathology are discussed.

INORGANIC SUBSTANCES

Histochemical methods have been described for detecting many inorganic substances, but only those elements that commonly occur in abnormal quantities in skin are discussed in this chapter. Unless otherwise stated, formalin fixation and paraffin sections are satisfactory for use with these procedures.

Iron

The Prussian blue reaction, or Perls' iron stain, is used most commonly for detection of ferric iron. The reaction is based on the combination of ferric ions in tissue with ferrocyanide in acid solution, which results in ferric ferrocyanide as a blue precipitate. The reaction will not demonstrate iron when it exists in the form of hemoglobin, ferritin, or any ferrous forms. Microincineration is necessary to convert all iron-containing compounds to ferric oxide, which then can be demonstrated by the Prussian blue reaction.

Iron as demonstrated by the Prussian blue reaction is present in normal skin in the secretory granules of a limited number of apocrine sweat glands. Extravasation of red blood cells with degradation into hemosiderin is the common cause of abnormal deposits of iron in skin. If a biopsy is being performed to establish a diagnosis of hemochromatosis, a site other than the leg should be chosen, since hemosiderin may be found frequently in the skin of the legs. Localized brown-to-blue-black discolorations of the skin have been reported in patients receiving long-term minocycline hydrochloride therapy. This material stained both with the Prussian blue reaction for iron and with the Fontana-Masson silver technique for melanin, and there was unstained pigment in addition that was thought to be a metabolic derivative of minocycline.[1] Pigmentation in sun-exposed sites in patients taking chlorpromazine was negative for iron but showed the presence of melanin and chlorpromazine.[2]

Calcium

The von Kossa staining method is based on recombination of silver with an anion salt, which may be carbonate, phosphate, oxalate, or others, and the subsequent reduction to metallic silver that is carried out by exposure to light. Those salts remaining in tissue sections after routine processing are almost always calcium salts. Urates and uric acids are the only serious sources of error, and they can be removed by dissolving them in lithium carbonate solutions.[3] The alizarin red S stain gives a specific reaction for the calcium ion, although other metals (barium, cadmium, strontium, and lead) also may form colored products with alizarin. Since other metals are not normally present in significant amounts in skin, this test is relatively specific for calcium. Calcium oxalate gives a negative or a weak reaction with alizarin red, but incineration will convert it to the oxalate, which will give a positive reaction.

Calcium deposits in tissue can be removed before embedding with a 5% solution of ethylenediaminetetraacetic acid. Calcification of skin is seen in a number of abnormal processes, including tumors and chronic inflammation.

Silver

In unstained tissue sections and hematoxylin and eosin-stained sections, silver appears as brown-black granules, which apparently represent a silver–protein complex. Silver may be demonstrated on darkfield examination as a bright white material. Sites of predilection for silver deposits in argyria are the lamina propria and basement membranes of the sweat glands, the stroma surrounding the pilosebaceous apparatus, arrectores pilorum muscles, nerves, elastic fibers, and endothelial cells and walls of blood vessels. The granules can be removed or decolorized by 1% potassium ferrocyanide in a 20% sodium thiosulfate solution.

SIMPLE POLYSACCHARIDES

Glycogen is the only member of this group remaining in animal tissue sections after formalin fixation, routine processing, and paraffin embedding. Glycogen is composed of D-glucosyl units in branched forms through 1,4- and 1,6-glucosidic linkages. The most common and practical method for glycogen detection is the periodic acid-Schiff (PAS) reaction with and without diastase digestion. Theoretically, any substance containing 1,2-glycol groupings or the equivalent amino or alkylamino derivative that does not diffuse away and is present in sufficient concentration should give a positive reaction. Acutal substances shown to be reactive to PAS include glycogens, starches, cellulose, mucosaccharides, glycolipids, unsaturated lipids, and phospholipids. In usage, one section is treated by the PAS reaction and an adjacent section is treated by diastase digestion followed by the PAS reaction. Diastase digestion usually is performed by exposing tissue sections to a 0.5% solution of freshly prepared diastase for 20 minutes. Any reactive sites in the PAS section that are nonreactive in the diastase-PAS section indicate the presence of glycogen.

The PAS reaction for glycogen usually is negative in the normal epidermis, except for small amounts about the orifices of the sweat glands and pilosebaceous follicles.[4] The outer root sheath of the pilosebaceous follicle, especially the middle third, is rich in glycogen, whereas glycogen is absent in the inner root sheath. The cuticle of the cortex above the hair bulb and the medulla cells approximately halfway up the follicle contain glycogen. The peripheral areas of the sebaceous glands contain glycogen, and the amount decreases as the cells accumulate lipid toward the center of the gland. The clear cells of the eccrine sweat gland show a strong positive reaction for glycogen, the dark cells may show small amounts of positive material, and the eccrine ducts contain a moderate amount of glycogen.[5] Glycogen usually is absent, or is present in only minute quantities, in the apocrine sweat gland. Glycogen accumulates within the epidermis in response to various stimuli, including mechanical injury, radiation injury, and numerous pathologic conditions. Accumulation of glycogen may result from a variety of changes in metabolic demands associated with either an increased production or a diminished use. In some instances, the storage of glycogen seems to bear an inverse ratio to the mitotic activity of the tissue.

A large amount of glycogen is seen routinely in certain tumors, such as a keratoacanthoma, and lesser amounts usually are present in squamous cell carcinomas.[6]

MUCOSACCHARIDES

A mucosaccharide, or mucosubstance, is a hexosamine-containing saccharide that may or may not be combined with protein and includes mucins of connective tissue and of epithelial origin. Most mucosaccharides of skin are acid in character and are referred to as glycosaminoglycans (acid mucosaccharides). The glycosaminoglycans include hyaluronic acid, heparin, chondroitin sulfate, dermatan sulfate, and keratin sulfate. Hyaluronic acid is the predominant nonsulfated glycosaminoglycan in skin. Glycoproteins are predominantly protein but also have a carbohydrate component, which may be acidic (usually sialic acid), or a neutral component. Substances present in normal skin that may represent neutral glycoprotein include basement membrane material and the so-called secretory granules of apocrine glands. These latter substances are PAS-reactive and diastase-resistant and give negative reactions with stains for acidic groups. Neutral buffered aqueous formalin is a satisfactory fixative for most glycosaminoglycans and sialomucins in skin.

Colloidal Iron Stain

Colloidal iron technique modifications of the Hale iron stain as described by Reinhart and Abul-Haj and Mowry have been used.[4] The basic principle involved is the exposure of tissue sections to a colloidal iron solution, washing the sections, and demonstrating the bound iron by the Prussian blue method. If the presence of preexisting iron is suspected, a control stain also must be run. A positive reaction probably is based on binding of colloidal iron by acid groups. These acid groups include the carboxyl and sulfate groups of the glycosaminoglycans and sialomucins and the phosphate groups of nucleic acids. A positive result produces a blue color, although this may be changed by a counterstain; for example, use of a yellow counterstain results in a green color. In formalin-fixed and paraffin-embedded tissue sections, a positive reaction usually means the presence of glycosaminoglycans, sialomucin, or nucleic acids. The colloidal iron technique often is used in combination with hyaluronidase and other enzymatic digestions.

Alcian Blue Stain

This stain, as described by Mowry, consisted of a solution of alcian blue in 3% acetic acid in combination with a nuclear fast red counterstain. The use of solutions at various pH values aids in the distinction between sulfated and nonsulfated acid mucosubstances.[7] We have used a phosphate buffer solution with a pH of approximately 2.5 and 0.5 It is necessary to use a buffer solution of the same pH value as the staining solution for the first rinse. The technique for preparing these solutions has been published.[4] At pH 2.5, most glycosaminoglycans and sialomucins give a blue color, and nucleic acids usually produce a less intense blue. At low pH values (0.5), only strongly acid substances, such as sulfated glycosaminoglycans, give a positive reaction; these include chondroitin sulfate, dermatan sulfate, and heparin.

Periodic Acid-Schiff Reaction

The PAS reaction is not affected significantly by variation in pH of the staining solutions, although some difference in color may be seen.[7] The mechanism of the reaction was discussed under Simple Polysaccharides. Hyaluronic acid does not give a positive PAS reaction. Most sialic acid-containing mucosubstances, chondroitin sulfate, and mast cell granules react positively. Substances other than glycogen and mucosubstances may contain 1,2-glycol groups and give a positive reaction. Other reactive substances include glycogens, starches, cellulose, unsaturated lipids, and phospholipids.

Aldehyde-Fuchsin Stain

This method was described by Gomori as a technique for elastic tissue, but it was found that the method also stains certain mucosubstances.[4] The pH of the staining solution appears to affect the aldehyde-fuchsin stain, and staining at pH values below 1 indicates the presence of sulfated acid mucosubstances. Hyaluronic acid does not stain or stains only weakly by the aldehyde-fuchsin stain, many of the sialomucins stain at pH 1.7 (the pH of the stain as described in the original description), and sulfated acid mucosubstances stain at the lower pH values.

Mucicarmine

This technique was established by Mayer in 1896 and modified by Southgate in 1927. It has been recommended for epithelial mucins and for the capsule in cryptococcosis. No detailed studies have been carried out in recent years, and the mechanism of staining has not been explored in detail.

Toluidine Blue for Metachromasia

Toluidine blue stain for metachromasia is a technique often used at pH values of 1.5 and 3.0. At the higher pH value, most acid mucosubstances will show metachromasia, and at the lower pH values, probably only sulfated substances show metachromasia. Because of problems with loss of metachromasia in dehydration with alcohols, it is necessary to examine the sections immediately after rinsing, drying, and mounting the sections in a permanent mounting medium without dehydration in alcohols and xylene. Many dermatopathologists find it easier just to use the alcian blue stain at varying pH values, since the result is essentially the same and the technique is simpler.

Diamine Methods

Spicer has reported the use of a mixture of the meta and para isomers of N,N-dimethyl-*m* or *p*-phenylenediamine for demonstration of various mucosubstances. Periodate oxidation, varying the concentrations of diamine and iron, control of pH, and combining with other methods were used to distinguish between some sulfated and nonsulfated glycosaminoglycans.[4]

Alcian Blue–Alcian Yellow

Carlo suggested staining with alcian blue at pH 0.5, rinsing, and then staining with alcian yellow at a pH of 2.5 to demonstrate sulfated and nonsulfated glycosaminoglycans in the same section.[4] The alcian yellow does not show as intense a color as does the alcian blue stain.

Antihyaluronectin–Hyaluronectin Immune Complexes

This is a relatively new and specific technique based on the high affinity of hyaluronectin for hyaluronic acid, using antihyaluronectin–hyaluronectin immune complexes.[8] This can be used to determine accurately the locations of hyaluronic acid in tissues.

Enzymes Used for Mucosubstances

Diastase
A 0.5% freshly prepared aqueous solution of diastase used for 20 minutes will remove glycogen from tissue sections. Comparing sections digested with diastase and undigested sections, followed by the PAS method, will demonstrate glycogen. Diastase digestion on PAS sections is used routinely when looking for fungi, which are PAS positive and diastase resistant.

Bacterial Hyaluronidase
This enzyme will remove hyaluronic acid from tissue sections.

Bovine Testicular Hyaluronidase
Using this technique for 1 hour at 37°C removes most hyaluronic acid and relatively little chrondroitin sulfate. Hyaluronidase digestion ordinarily is used in conjunction with the colloidal iron technique, but it can be used with any method that demonstrates the presence of acid groups.

Ribonuclease Digestion
This enzyme can be used to remove some ribonucleic acids that may, at times, be confused with acid mucosaccharides stained with the colloidal iron technique or alcian blue.

Application of Methods

Normal Skin

The extracellular interfibrillar ground substance shows reactions that indicate that the main material is hyaluronic acid. [4,9,10] Normal skin shows a variable amount of ground substance in different sites of the body, with the fingers and toes showing a greater concentration than other areas (Table 3–1). The greater concentration is seen in the papillary dermis and about adnexal structures. In general, there is more hyaluronic acid in the dermis of infants and children than in adults. The ground substance of the dermal hair papillae and the connective tissue sheath about the lower part of the follicle shows evidence of a sulfated acid mucosaccharide in addition to hyaluronic acid. [4] Much of the chondroitin sulfate found on analysis of whole skin was associated mainly with the fibrillar elements (collagen and elastin).

Using the previously mentioned techniques, the following findings have been described. Mast cells show reactions indicating a sulfated acid mucosaccharide thought to be heparin within the granules (Table 3–1). There is no histochemical evidence to suggest the presence of hyaluronic acid in human mast cells.

Within the walls of larger blood vessels in the lower dermis and subcutaneous tissue, observed reactions are interpreted as representing a combination of hyaluronic acid and a sulfated mucopolysaccharide, chondroitin sulfate. Between the epidermal cells, histochemical reactions indicate the presence of hyaluronic acid and possibly a sialomucin. The outer root sheath of hair follicles also show reactions indicating the presence of hyaluronic acid. The dermal papillae of anagen hair show evidence of sulfated mucopolysaccharide as well as hyaluronic acid. In the apex of the cells and in the lumens of apocrine sweat glands, there is a nonsulfated, hyaluronidase-resistant material that probably is a sialomucin. Within the cytoplasm of the dark cells of eccrine sweat glands and attached to the cell membranes, there is material showing similar histochemical reactions, probably also a sialomucin. The so-called secretory granules of the apocrine gland show reactions indicating an absence of acid substances. These granules contain a neutral mucosaccharide or glycolipid. Within the cutaneous nerve sheath, there is a relatively large amount of mucin that shows reactions including one indicating hyaluronic acid.

Myxoid Group

The conditions considered under primary myxomatous diseases include generalized myxedema, localized myxedema, papular mucinosis or lichen myxedematosus, myxoid cyst, and focal mucinosis. [11,12] The mucin present in all of these conditions as determined by histochemical methods is hyaluronic acid. The altered epithelial cells in the outer root sheath and sebaceous glands in follicular mucinosis show histochemical evidence of hyaluronic acid similar to that seen in the outer root sheaths of normal hair follicles. [13] Several conditions that can be considered as secondary mucinoses show an increase in hyaluronic acid but also show other significant histologic features. This group includes lupus erythematosus, Degos' disease (malignant papulosis), palisading granulomas, and miscellaneous conditions. The presence of increased hyaluronic acid may be seen in up to 80% of biopsies from patients with acute and discoid lupus erythematosus and serves as an important aid in separating this disease from polymorphic light eruption. [14] Dermatomyositis may show similar histologic features to those seen in acute lupus erythematosus. In general, granu-

TABLE 3–1. HISTOCHEMICAL REACTIONS FOR ACID MUCOPOLYSACCHARIDES OF THE NORMAL SKIN

| Material | Colloidal Iron | | Alcian Blue | | PAS Positive Diatase Resistant | Aldehyde-Fuchsin | | Toluidine Blue | |
	Without Hyaluronidase Digestion	With Hyaluronidase Digestion 1 h at 37° C	pH 2.7–3	pH 0.4–1		pH 1.7	pH ≤ 1	pH 3	pH 1.5
Ground substance	4+*	− to ±	4+	−	−	− to ±	−	4+	−
Mast cells	4+	4+	4+	4+	4+	4+	4+	4+	4+
Blood vessel walls	4+	3+	4+	3+	−	3+	2+	3+	2+
Apex of cell and lumen, apocrine	4+	4+	4+	−	4+	4+	−	4+	−
Secretory granules, apocrine	−†	−†	−	−	4+	−	−	−	−
Cytoplasm of secretory cells, eccrine	4+	4+	4+	−	− to 2+	− to +	−	+ to −	−
Interstices of epidermal cells	3+	− to ±	3+	−	−	−	−	±	−
Dermal papilla of anagen hair	4+	4+	4+	4+	−	4+	4+	4+	4+
Nerves	4+	− to ±	4+	−	−	− to ±	−	+	−

* 4+, strongly positive; 3+, moderately strongly positive; 2+, moderately positive; +, weakly positive; ±, trace reaction; −, negative.
† Except those containing iron.
From Johnson WC, Helwig EB. Histochemistry of the acid mucopolysaccharides of skin in normal and in certain pathologic conditions. Am J Clin Pathol. 1963, 40:123–131.

loma annulare shows a greater amount of hyaluronic acid than does necrobiosis lipoidica.

Neoplasms

The presence or absence of mucin associated with neoplasms often has been helpful in establishing a diagnosis. For instance, the mucin present in adenoid basal cell carcinoma is principally sulfated acid mucosaccharides.[15] The mucin associated with the pseudoglandular spaces of adenoid squamous cell carcinoma shows properties of hyaluronic acid.[16] Metastatic adenocarcinomas from the breast, bronchus, and colon showed reactions we interpreted to represent a sialomucin. Mammary and extramammary Paget's disease shows mucoid cells with reactions consistent with a sialomucin. This is helpful in distinguishing the individual, migrating, atypical pagetoid cells from cells of Bowen's disease and cells of superficial spreading malignant melanoma. The use of immunoperoxidase markers has extended the study of mucins in identifying many neoplasms.

LIPIDS

Lipids are a chemically heterogeneous group of substances with the common characteristic of solubility in organic solvents, i.e., in lipid solvents. A formol-calcium fixation for periods of not greater than 2 or 3 days is the preferred fixative if one knows before taking the biopsy that lipid studies are needed.[4] This may be prepared by using 10 mL of 40% formaldehyde, 1 g of anhydrous calcium chloride, and 90 mL of distilled water. After formol-calcium fixation, most lipid studies must be performed on cryostat (frozen) sections. The most common use of lipid studies in skin is to identify material in the skin as being lipid and to determine if this is a natural lipid or an exogenous lipid. Since all natural lipids contain unsaturated groups, methods for staining these unsaturated groups are very useful. Such methods include the bromine-silver technique, osmic acid, and PAS reaction of Lilly. A combination of general methods for lipids, such as a Sudan dye (oil-red-O), will show the presence of a lipid material. If the lipid is then negative with methods for unsaturated groups, such as the bromine-silver method, this indicates a foreign lipid that has been injected into the skin. The condition described as sclerosing lipogranuloma most commonly involving the genitalia has been proven to be a paraffin oil granuloma. Examples of paraffin oil granuloma have been seen also in patients who thought they were having silicone oil injected into their legs.[17]

AMINO ACIDS AND PROTEINS

The Feulgen reaction consists of mild acid hydrolysis, leaving a reactive aldehyde group that shows up purple by Schiff's reagent. This is an excellent method for demonstrating deoxyribonucleic acid (DNA) and is useful for demonstration of DNA viral inclusions, such as those seen in verruca vulgaris and molluscum contagiosum. This reaction also is used for evaluation of DNA in nuclei of tumors and other cells.

A method for detecting citrulline (carbaminodiacetyl reaction) has been described, and this amino acid is seen in the inner root sheath of human hair.[18] The presence of citrulline in tumors, detected by this method, indicates a pilar origin for the tumor.

ENZYME HISTOCHEMISTRY

Enzyme histochemical studies have been used for demonstration of anatomic structures, normal and abnormal. Examples include excellent visualization of the small blood vessels using alkaline phosphatase and visualization of nerves using cholinesterase. Enzyme histochemistry also has been used for the study of normal and pathologic metabolism, as an aid in diagnosis of enzyme defects, and to relate tumors to possible anatomic structures of origin. Enzyme histochemistry has been replaced recently by the immunoperoxidase methods, which can be done on paraffin-embedded tissue, whereas frozen sections are required for enzyme histochemistry.

Phosphatases

Using the azo-dye method, alkaline phosphatase activity has been demonstrated in endothelial cells of blood vessels, the dermal hair papillae, and intercellular canaliculi of eccrine sweat glands. Some activity has been seen in the cytoplasm and the cytoplasm of apocrine glands.[4] The activity of the intercellular canaliculi appears to be joined with the adjacent capillary plexus, suggesting that the canaliculi transport nutrients to the eccrine gland. The alkaline phosphatase technique has been very useful in studying abnormal capillaries of the skin in psoriasis and in studying blood vessels related to various tumors. It also can be used to distinguish capillaries with positive endothelial cells from lymphangiomas, which are not alkaline phosphatase positive.

Using the azo-dye technique, intense activity in acid phosphatase has been described in the upper stratum spinosum, granular layer, and stratum corneum, about the hair in the upper pilary canal, in the secretory granules of apocrine glands and melanocytes, and in fibrocytes. Moderate activity was seen in sebaceous glands and eccrine sweat glands, and a mild to minimal activity has been seen in other epithelial cells. The activity of acid phosphatase may be changed with disease processes, including increased activity associated with tumors.

Cholinesterase

Cholinesterase has been used in thick sections to study cutaneous nerves. It also has been used to study metabolism of tumors and normal constituents of the skin. Using acetylthiocholine iodide as a substrate, there is activity demonstrated in blue nevus cells and many nevus cells in the dermis in both intradermal and compound nevi. These dermal nevus cells show cytoplasmic processes that appear to be directly connected with nerve fibers. Using this method, nerve fibers have been described as extending into the epidermis.[18]

Tyrosinase (Dopa-oxidase)

The technique for evaluating dopa-oxidase activity has been used extensively in the past to study melanocytes and melanin formation. As with all enzyme histochemistry tests, it has the drawback of having to be performed on frozen sections. Vitiligo can be diagnosed by demonstration of the absence of dopa-oxidase cells.

Dehydrogenases

These enzymes act to transfer electrons from one molecule to another in the living cell and represent the major sources of energy in tissues, as well as synthetic and degradative processes. Five major pathways and an example of each are glycolytic pathway, lactic dehydrogenase; pentose cycle (hexose monophosphate shunt), glucose-6-phosphate dehydrogenase; Krebs cycle, succinic dehydrogenase; glutamate cycle, glutamic dehydrogenase; oxidation of fatty acids, β-hydroxybutyrate dehydrogenase. Most methods are based on reduction of tetrazolium salts and appropriate controls.

Glucose-6-Phosphate Dehydrogenase

With this enzyme, normal skin shows (1) an intense reaction in the sebaceous glands, (2) a moderate reaction in Huxley's layer and cuticle of the inner root sheath in the lower third of the follicle and inner layers of the outer root sheath in the upper part of the follicle, the hair matrix, the granular layer, and upper stratum spinosum of the epidermis, the apex of apocrine sweat gland cells, and (3) minimal to mild activity of fibrocytes, endothelial cells, and eccrine sweat glands.[4] Prematurely keratinizing cells, such as those seen in Bowen's disease, give an intense reaction. Melanocytes, basal epidermal cells, eccrine duct cells, and tumors arising from these cells are nonreactive, which is in sharp contrast to the intense activity of these structures and tumors derived from them with succinic dehydrogenase.

Succinic Dehydrogenase

In normal skin, the activity of succinic dehydrogenase is intense in the basal cell layer and lower stratum spinosum, outer root sheaths of upper follicles, eccrine sweat glands and ducts, apocrine sweat glands, matrix of hair follicles, dermal hair papillae, and fibrocytes. It is moderately intense in melanocytes and sebaceous glands, and it is moderate in arrectores pilorum muscles and endothelial cells of small blood vessels.[4] Basal cell carcinomas, tumors arising from eccrine structures, such as eccrine porosyringoma, and tumors of melanocytic origin, such as nevi and melanoma, show intense activity.

Aminopeptidases

A simultaneous coupling azo-dye method is commonly used, for example, a mixture of L-leucyl-β-naphthylamine and D,l-alanyl-β-naphthylamide and fast red violet LB salt, similar to the technique described by Burstone.[4] Normal human skin shows an intense reaction with aminopeptidase in the dermal hair papillae, the secretory granule of the apocrine sweat glands, and eccrine sweat glands. A moderate to strong reaction is seen in fibrocytes, walls of blood vessels, the outer root sheath of the follicles, and the basal cell layer. The connective tissue near these sites also shows moderate activity, and the possibility of diffusion giving rise to the epithelial localization described must be considered. Moderate activity occurs in the arrectores pilorum muscles and at the periphery of the sebaceous glands. The central areas of the sebaceous glands, the subcutaneous fat, stratum corneum, and hair, do not react. The stroma of certain tumors, such as basal cell carcinoma, shows intense activity. Histiocytic infiltrations, such as those occurring in juvenile xanthogranuloma, show intense activity in the cytoplasm.

OTHER SPECIAL STAINS

Elastic Tissue Stains

Elastic fibers may be demonstrated more or less specifically by use of either crystal violet, orcein in acid alcohol, resorcin-fuchsin, or aldehyde-fuchsin. Hart's elastic stain is based on resorcin-fuchsin, and the elastic tissue stains black. Weigert's elastic stain also is based on resorcin-fuchsin but uses iron hematoxylin and van Gieson's counterstain.[19]

Reticulum Stain

Snook's reticulum stain is based on reduction of silver nitrate to gray or black silver. Wilder's stain also is based on silver solution but has some differences in technique. These methods stain reticulin fibers.

Amyloid Stains

No staining technique is specific for amyloid, but PAS with diastase digestion and crystal violet are probably the most useful in paraffin sections. A greater amount of amyloid can be demonstrated in fresh, unfixed cryostat sections than on paraffin sections using the same staining technique.[20] Behnnold's Congo red stains amyloid pink to red and will give a red to green dichroism on polarization. Crystal violet stain shows amyloid as a purplish violet. Sirius red stains amyloid pink to red. With thioflavin T stain, amyloid gives a yellowish appearance under a fluorescent microscope. Recent studies confirm the presence of sulfated proteoglycans in amyloid.[21]

Fontana-Masson Silver Method

This is used for identification of melanin pigment, but other reducing groups will cause reduction or precipitation of silver nitrate as black metallic silver. Argentaffin granules and formalin pigment also give a positive result.

Stains for Acid-Fast Organisms

The Ziehl-Neelsen acid-fast stain uses carbolfuchsin solution, acid alcohol, sulfuric acid, and methylene blue, and acid-fast bacilli appear red. Fite's acid-fast stain is preferred by some for lepra bacilli and is similar to the Ziehl-Neelsen stain, except sections are soaked in xylene-peanut oil before staining.

Stains for Gram-Positive and Gram-Negative Organisms

Specific names attached to various modifications of this technique include Brown and Brenn, Brown-Hopps, Mac-Callum-Goodpasture, and Taylor's method. The Brown and Brenn method includes crystal violet solution, sodium bicarbonate, Gram's iodine, ether-acetone, basic fuchsin, and picric acid-acetone solution. Gram-positive organisms appear blue, and gram-negative organisms appear red.

Warthin-Starry Stain

The solutions include silver nitrate and hydroquinone, and the method is used primarily for spirochetes and Donovan bodies. Organisms stain black as with other techniques. Adequate controls must be used and details followed carefully, since the method is difficult and the pH of solutions is very important.

Grocott-Gomori Methenamine-Silver Nitrate Method

With this method, fungi and certain bacteria stain black, mucin stains gray, and the inner parts of mycelia and hyphae may appear rose.

Giemsa Stain

Bacteria appear blue, and rickettsia appear purple. Mast cell granules also are stained.

REFERENCES

1. McGrae JD, Zelickson AS. Skin pigmentation secondary to minocycline therapy. *Arch Dermatol.* 1980;116:1262–1265.
2. Johnson WC. Histochemistry of the skin. In:Spicer S, ed. *Histochemistry in Pathologic Diagnosis.* New York: Marcel Dekker Inc, 1987:665–694.
3. McGee-Russell SM. Histochemical methods for calcium. *J Histochem Cytochem.* 1958;6:22–42.
4. Johnson WC. Histochemistry of skin. In: Helwig EB, ed. *The Skin.* Baltimore: Williams & Wilkins Co; 1971: chap 7. International Academy of Pathology Monograph No 10.
5. Johnson, WC. Histochemisty of the cutaneous adnexa and selected adnexal neoplasms. *J Cutan Pathol.* 1984;11:352–356.
6. Johnson WC, Graham JH. Keratoacanthoma: A histochemical study. *Am J Pathol.* 1966;48:6A–7A.
7. Johnson WC, Johnson FB, Helwig EB. Effects of varying the pH on reactions for acid mucopolysaccharide. *J Histochem Cytochem.* 1962;10:684.
8. Girard N, Delpech A, Delpech B. Characterization of hyaluronic acid on tissue sections with hyaluronectin. *J Histochem Cytochem.* 1986;34:539–541.
9. Johnson WC. Histochemistry of cutaneous ground substance. *Meth Achiev Exp Pathol.* 1966;1:33–51.
10. Johnson WC, Helwig EB. Histochemistry of the cutaneous interfibrillar ground substance. *J Invest Dermatol.* 1964;42:81–85.
11. Johnson WC, Graham JH, Helwig EB. Cutaneous myxoid cyst: A clinicopathological and histochemical study. *JAMA.* 1965;191:15.
12. Johnson WC, Helwig EB. Cutaneous focal mucinosis. *Arch Dermatol.* 1966;93:13.
13. Johnson WC, Higdon RS, Helwig EB. Alopecia mucinosa. *Arch Dermatol.* 1959;79:395–406.
14. Panet-Raymond G, Johnson WC. Lupus erythematosus and polymorphous light eruption: Differentiation by histochemical procedures. *Arch Dermatol.* 1973;108:785–787.
15. Johnson WC, Helwig EB. Histochemistry of primary and metastatic mucus-secreting tumors. *Ann NY Acad Sci.* 1963;106:794–803.
16. Johnson WC, Helwig EB. Adenoid squamous cell carcinoma (adenoacanthoma): A clinicopathologic study of 155 patients. *Cancer.* 1966;19:1639.
17. Johnson WC. Foreign body and lipid granulomas. In: Graham JH, Johnson WC, Helwig EB, eds. *Dermal Pathology.* Hagerstown, MD: Harper & Row, 1972:433–449
18. Johnson WC. Histochemistry of the skin. In: Graham JH, Johnson WC, Helwig EB, eds. *Dermal Pathology.* Hagerstown, MD: Harper & Row, 1972:75–117.
19. Luna LG. *Manual of Histologic Staining Methods of the Armed Forces Institute of Pathology.* 3rd ed. New York: McGraw-Hill; 1968.
20. Potter BS, Johnson WC. Primary localized amyloidosis cutis: Tumefactive type. *Arch Dermatol.* 1971;103:448–451.
21. Snow AD, Willmer J, Kisilevsky R. A close ultrastructural relationship between sulfated proteoglycans and AA amyloid fibrils. *Lab Invest.* 1987;57:687–698.

CHAPTER 4
Immunopathology

Neal S. Penneys

Arriving at a diagnosis in pathology rests on the recognition of morphologic changes in a tissue specimen. Pathologists recognize that there are limitations to the extent that diagnoses can be made on information present in routinely processed sections, and these limitations have led to the development of a variety of special stains that facilitate recognition and diagnosis. In immunohistology, very specific special stains are used to determine the presence or absence of individual antigens in tissue.

IMMUNOFLUORESCENT TECHNIQUES

The field of practical immunohistology began with the report of Coons et al. describing the binding of fluorescein isothiocyanate-labeled antibody to specific antigen.[1] Immunohistology using fluorescein-labeled antibodies has advanced to a great degree the diagnosis and management of a variety of dermatologic conditions. There are two general classes of immunofluorescent examinations, direct immunofluorescence and indirect immunofluorescence. In the first technique, skin biopsies are examined directly for the presence of the antigen. The specimen usually is placed in a transport medium, such as Michel's solution. In the laboratory, frozen sections are taken from the tissue specimen and are exposed to fluorescein isothiocyanate-labeled antibody of the desired specificity (e.g., anti-IgG, anti-IgA). After a period of incubation, the slides are washed and mounted for examination with a fluorescent microscope. In indirect immunofluorescence, serum is submitted to the laboratory for demonstration of specific antibodies. For primary dermatologic diseases, the serum is tested on a suitable substrate, such as monkey esophagus, for the presence of antibodies to a variety of antigens, including those associated with pemphigus and pemphigoid. The technical aspects of performing these procedures can be obtained from the excellent text of Beutner et al.[2]

IMMUNOENZYME TECHNIQUES

The success of immunofluorescent techniques has emphasized the need for immunohistochemical reagents that can be used without the drawbacks of fluorescein-labeled reagents, i.e., the need for specialized microscopy, the dark background needed to visualize the excitation of fluorescein, technical needs such as frozen or specially collected tissues, poor morphologic result, and the lack of permanence of sections. A number of immunoenzyme techniques, therefore, have been developed. These methods are predicated on the linking of an enzyme, such as horseradish peroxidase, glucose oxidase, or alkaline phosphatase, to specific antibody. Binding is visualized by adding the appropriate substrate for the enzyme and a chromogen.[3] Once the basic idea of enzyme-antibody linkage was defined, a number of modifications involving second- and third-stage reagents, such as the indirect method, peroxidase-antiperoxidase method, and avidin-biotin method, were developed to increase the applicability and sensitivity of the method, to conserve primary antibody, and to decrease the background associated with these reactions. Advantages of these methods include the ability to counterstain with a variety of agents, to study materials in paraffin blocks (if the antigen under study is preserved after formalin fixation and paraffin embedding), to identify more than one antigen by multiple-labeling studies, to use standard microscopy, and to obtain good morphologic results in stained sections. Methodology in this field is dynamic and continually advancing. Source materials on methodology can be obtained from two excellent current texts[4,5] as well as primary sources.[6]

There is beauty in the simplicity of the concept that underlies immunohistology, that is, the amplication and visualization of the binding of an antibody to an antigen, and in the directness and specificity of these techniques. However, there are limitations to the day-to-day application of these methods using routinely fixed and embedded tissues. Many antigens that would be of diagnostic value are not stable with formalin fixation. Furthermore, many antigens that are retained may decay after prolonged periods in fixative, a variable that may not be under the control of the laboratory because of delays in arrival of the specimen and other reasons. Consequently, sections should have internal positive controls, particularly specimens of poorly differentiated neoplasms that may or may not be expressing an antigen. Fortunately, the most commonly used markers for the analysis of skin tumors identify structures that are present routinely in the same section. A second variable is the expertise of the technician who prepares the sections and the investigator who interprets them. Appropriate internal and external controls must be included in each assay. Biologic reagents should be used at maximally dilute concentrations to minimize background. Experience is helpful in the interpretation of both positive and negative findings. Each antibody will have a unique binding pattern in the skin, with areas of both specific and nonspecific adherence. For example, many primary antibodies nonspecifically adhere to keratinous material. Nonspecific and specific patterns may be present in the same sections; for example, antibody to bovine papillomavirus common antigen nonspecifically binds to the cytoplasm of keratinocytes but has a specific pattern in infected cells overlying the nucleus. Occasionally, loss of tissue antigen occurs during routine fixation. Before assuming that a tumor cell is not expressing an antigen, normal structures that express the antigen in the same tissue section should be examined to see if the antigen has been retained.

The introduction and development of immunohistochemical methods have led to a significant advance in the ability to recognize, classify, and understand the pathogenesis of a variety of disparate skin processes, ranging from the identification of poorly differentiated tumors to the clarification of autoimmune diseases. Antigens that are stable with formalin fixation, such as keratin epitopes,[7-9] S100 protein,[10-12] carcinoembryonic antigen (CEA),[13-15] epithelial

membrane antigen (EMA),[16] salivary mucin,[17] kappa and lambda chains,[18] leukocyte common antigen,[19] von Willebrand's-related antigen,[20] myelin basic protein,[21] and a variety of markers that identify the site of origin of a metastatic tumor (prostate-specific antigen,[22] and thyroglobulin),[23] can be used on a daily basis for the evaluation of routine specimens (Table 4-1). The majority of tissue markers, however, are lost during the fixation process, and fresh tissue specimens must be collected for frozen sections. Evaluation of lymphoreticular neoplasms and the composition of inflammatory infiltrates usually requires frozen sections for the analysis of applicable epitopes. There is an endless series of research applications in dermatology for these techniques. Many of the applications described here are also discussed elsewhere in this text.

APPLICATIONS

Histogenesis of Skin Lesions

The demonstration of a unique antigen within a neoplasm can be an elegant means of inferring the parent cell type toward which the tumor cell is differentiating, accepting the proviso that tissues not histogenetically related may, on occasion, share common antigens. Furthermore, the absence of an antigen does not exclude potential relationships between a tumor cell and a parent cell type. Absence of a marker may be secondary to poor differentiation, loss of antigen during fixation, and technical factors.

Epidermal, Adnexal, and Melanocytic Neoplasms

The most common applications are to identify poorly differentiated neoplasms in the skin. Poorly differentiated neoplasms may arise from all cellular components in the skin. In reality, however, effective identification of the majority of neoplasms that occur in the skin can be obtained with relatively few primary antibodies that identify stable anti-

TABLE 4-1. COMMONLY USED ANTIGENS IN DIAGNOSTIC DERMATOPATHOLOGY

Antibody	Clonality	Normal Structures	Tumor
Prekeratin	P*	Epidermis and adnexae	Squamous cell carcinoma
PKK-1	M	Sweat gland epithelium	Paget's cells
S100 protein	P	Melanocytes, Langerhans cells, Schwann cells	Melanoma, histiocytosis X
Carcinoembryonic antigen	P	Sweat gland epithelium	Paget's cells, sweat gland neoplasms, metastatic lesions
Neuron-specific enolase	P	Nerve, muscle	Merkel cell tumors
Epithelial membrane antigen	P	Sebaceous cells	Paget's cells, sweat gland and sebaceous neoplasms
Synaptophysin	P	—	Merkel cell tumors
Epithelial mucin	M	Eccrine duct	Sweat gland tumors
Type IV collagen	P	Basement membrane	Kaposi's sarcoma (early)
Factor VIII-related antigen	P	Blood vessels	Vascular tumors

* P, polyclonal; M, monoclonal.

gens in epidermal and adnexal keratinocytes, melanocytes, and fibrohistiocytes.

As specific antigenic markers become available, the algorithm for the analysis of poorly differentiated tumors will change and expand. At the present time, a polyclonal antibody to prekeratin may be sufficient to identify a poorly differentiated squamous cell carcinoma arising from epidermal or adnexal keratinocytes. However, antibodies for keratin epitopes unique for adnexal structures and tumors derived from adnexal structures eventually will be available and allow more precise categorization of squamous cell carcinomas related to adnexal structures. Antigens in a neoplasm that suggest sweat gland differentiation are CEA (decorates both eccrine and apocrine glands), EMA (decorates primarily apocrine gland), and a monoclonal antibody that identifies an epitope in eccrine duct and acrosyringium.[17]

S100 protein, an acidic protein originally purified from ox brain, currently is the most sensitive marker in the skin for identification of melanocytes, Schwann cells, Langerhans cells, certain cells in the eccrine coil, and tumors derived from these cells in routinely processed tissue. The use of this marker is important in identifying amelanotic malignant melanoma, assessing tumor depth when the deep margins of the tumor are obscured by infiltrate, seeing melanocytes in infiltrates, identifying desmoplastic melanocytes, and identifying small foci of microinvasion, particularly in lentigo maligna melanoma.[24] Limitations of this marker include its inability to separate nevus cells from atypical melanocytes in melanomas that are associated with a benign intradermal nevus and its relative lack of specificity. It is hoped that there will soon be reliable monoclonal antibodies to markers retained in fixed tissue that are specific for melanoma cells and that differentiate nevus cells from atypical melanocytes in malignant melanomas.

An area where immunohistology is quite useful is in the differentiation of Paget's or extramammary Paget's disease from melanoma in situ and squamous cell carcinoma in situ, all of which may be characterized by the presence of atypical, pale-staining cells in the epidermis. Paget's cells contain CEA,[15] PKK-1 (a keratin not routinely expressed in epidermis), and EMA, whereas pagetoid keratinocytes and melanocytes generally do not (Fig. 4–1). Melanocytes contain S100 protein, whereas the other two cell types do not. These stains are much more reliable than are histochemical stains for mucin and acid mucopolysaccharide.

Merkel cell or trabecular cell carcinoma is an uncommon, poorly differentiated neuroendocrine neoplasm primary to the skin, lacking in a distinctive clinical appearance, and often arising in the head and neck area. The neoplasm has a significant risk of metastasis. Histologic differential diagnosis is inaccurate, and it is difficult to exclude a metastatic small cell carcinoma from other body sites. Neuron-specific enolase, prekeratin, and a variety of other markers, including vasoactive intestinal polypeptide (VIP), somatostatin, met-enkephalin, neurofilaments, EMA, and others, have been advocated as useful in the analysis of this tumor.[25–29] The results of these studies are confusing and do not address the issue of primary site of the neoplasm. Synaptophysin, a newly available marker, may be of use in identifying these neoplasms.[30] Many of these markers

are episodically expressed in this neoplasm, and electron microscopy is still the method used for absolute confirmation.

Atypical Spindle Cell Lesions

The majority of atypical spindle cell lesions in the skin are either desmoplastic malignant melanomas or poorly differentiated squamous cell carcinomas. These lesions are usually identifiable by their content of S100 protein and keratin, respectively. Less commonly seen are dermatofibrosarcoma protruberans, fibrosarcoma, malignant schwannoma, leiomyosarcoma, and malignant fibrous histiocytoma (atypical fibroxanthoma). Reliably expressed markers for fibrohistiocytic cells are not available, although antibodies against lysozyme, alpha$_1$-antitrypsin, factor XIIIa, and antichymotrypsin have been used with variable success. In our laboratory, a neoplasm differentiating toward a fibrohistiocytic cell (atypical fibroxanthoma) might have the following immunohistochemical profile: prekeratin negative, S100 protein negative, CEA/EMA negative, lysozyme, antichymotrypsin, and alpha$_1$-antitrypsin and factor XIIIa variably positive.

Neoplasms Metastatic to the Skin

The field of immunohistology offers the exciting prospect of identifying metastatic lesions by their content of a specific marker antigen. Several markers already exist. Metastatic thyroid carcinoma, prostate carcinoma, and carcinoid tumor to the skin have been confirmed by their contents of thyroglobulin, prostate-specific antigen, and serotonin, respectively. Metastatic amelanotic melanoma can be considered if the tumor cells contain S100 protein.

Analysis of Lymphoreticular Neoplasms

Most markers available for the categorization of lymphoreticular neoplasms are lost during routine fixation.[31–34] Antibodies to kappa and lambda chains, leukocyte common antigen (a cell membrane protein present on all leukocytes), and S100 protein can be used in formalin-fixed tissue to determine monoclonality in a plasmacellular infiltrate, to determine if an infiltrate is composed of leukocytes, or to determine if an infiltrate is composed of Langerhans cells, as in histiocytosis X. Other markers must be examined in frozen sections. Since T cell lymphomas are the most common lymphoreticular neoplasm to involve the skin, immunohistology usually is applied to these lesions to see if the neoplasm is composed of T helper or T suppressor phenotype. A number of recent publications have documented the application of these techniques in the evaluation of cutaneous lymphomas other than mycosis fungoides.[34]

RESEARCH

Immunohistologic techniques represent a research tool of incredible magnitude. These techniques permit the analysis of the components of cellular infiltrates and their changes

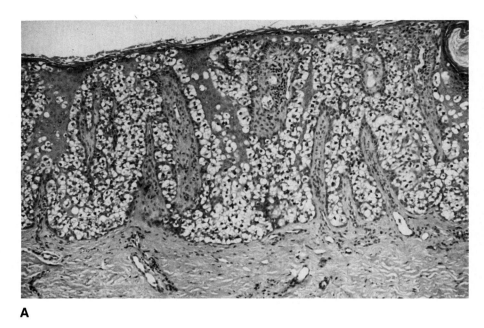

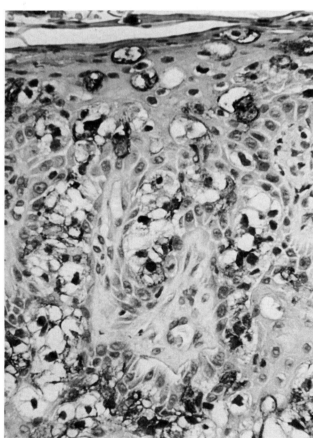

Figure 4–1.A. Extramammary Paget's disease (H&E, ×40). **B.** Extramammary Paget's disease stained by the avidin-biotin method for epithelial membrane antigen (H&E, ×200).

with time.[35] Langerhans cells can be identified and quantitated in paraffin-embedded tissues.[36] Viral antigens, such as those expressed by cytomegalovirus, herpes virus, and papillomavirus, can be detected in tissue specimens.[37,38] Each new antibody reagent represents an opportunity to ask new questions about the dynamic expression of antigens in tissue specimens. There are no limits to the use of these methods, and their applications will be with us for many years to come.

Tests in the future will permit the examination of the gene, rather than the gene product, in tissue sections. These studies will be performed by in situ detection of DNA sequences using DNA probes with attached markers to visualize their binding.[39] Biotinylated probes are now available for a number of DNA sequences. These probes are stable and can be a very sensitive means for the detection of unique gene sequences (such as viral sequences) in the genome of the cell. The success of these methods rests on denaturation of the nuclear contents and successful amplification of the bound DNA probe. Routine chromophores, such as diaminobenzidine, can then be used with counterstains to visualize the tissue.

REFERENCES

1. Coons AH, Creech HJ, Jones RN. Immunological properties of an antibody containing a fluorescent group. *Proc Soc Exp Biol Med.* 1941;47:200–202.

2. Beutner EH, Chorzelski TP, Kumar V. *Immunopathology of the Skin.* 3rd ed. New York: John Wiley and Sons; 1987.

3. Trojanowski J, Obrocka M, Lee V. A comparison of eight different chromogen protocols for the demonstration of immunoreactant neurofilaments or glial filaments in rat cerebellum using the peroxidase-antiperoxidase method and monoclonal antibodies. *J Histochem Cytochem.* 1983;31:1217–1223.

4. Sternberger LA: *Immunocytochemistry.* 2nd ed. New York: John Wiley and Sons; 1979.

5. Taylor CR. *Immunomicroscopy: A Diagnostic Tool for the Surgical Pathologist.* Philadelphia: WB Saunders; 1986.

6. Hsu SM, Raine L, Fanger H. A comparative study of the peroxidase-antiperoxidase method and an avidin-biotin complex method for studying polypeptide hormones with radioimmunoassay antibodies. *Am J Clin Pathol.* 1981;75:734–738.

7. Penneys NS, Nadji M, Ziegels-Weissman J, et al. Prekeratin in spindle cell tumors of the skin. *Arch Dermatol.* 1983;119:476–479.

8. Schlegel R, Banks-Schlegel S, Pinkus G. Immunohistochemical localization of keratin in normal human tissues. *Lab Invest.* 1980;42:91–96.

9. Warhol MJ, Pinkus G, Banks-Schlegel S. Localization of keratin proteins in the human epidermis by a postembedding immunoperoxidase technique. *J Histochem Cytochem.* 1983;31:517–526.

10. Nakajima T, Kameya T, Watanabe S, et al. An immunoperoxidase study of S100 protein distribution in normal and neoplastic tissues. *Am J Surg Pathol.* 1982;6:715–726.

11. Nakajima T, Watanabe S, Sato Y, et al. Immunohistochemical demonstration of S100 protein in malignant melanoma and pigmented nevus, and its diagnostic application. *Cancer.* 1982;50:912–918.

12. Kahn H, Baumal R, Marks A. The value of immunohistologic studies using antibodies to S100 protein in dermatopathology. *Int J Dermatol.* 1984;23:38–44.

13. Penneys N, Nadji M. Carcinoembryonic antigen in benign sweat gland tumors. *Arch Dermatol.* 1982;118:225–227.

14. Penneys NS, Nadji M, Ziegels-Weissman J, Katabchi M, Morales A. Carcinoembryonic antigen in sweat gland carcinomas. *Cancer.* 1982;50:1608–1611.

15. Nadji M, Morales A, Girtanner RE, et al. Paget's disease of the skin: A unifying concept of histogenesis. *Cancer.* 1982;50:2203–2206.

16. Heyderman E, Graham RM, Chapman DV, et al. Epithelial markers in primary skin cancer: An immunoperoxidase study of the distribution of epithelial membrane antigen (EMA) and carcinoembryonic antigen (CEA) in 65 primary skin carcinomas. *Histopathology.* 1984;8:423–434.

17. Penneys NS, Matsuo S. A monoclonal antibody which identifies an epitope in eccrine ducts. *J Cutan Pathol.* 1986;13:458.

18. Barr RJ, Sun NC, King DF. Immunoperoxidase staining of cytoplasmic immunoglobulins. *J Am Acad Dermatol.* 1980;3:58–62.

19. Warnke RA, Gatter KC, Falini B. The diagnosis of human lymphoma using monoclonal antileukocyte antibodies. *N Engl J Med.* 1984;309:1275–1281.

20. Nadji M, Morales AR, Ziegels-Weissman J, et al. Kaposi's sarcoma: Immunohistochemical evidence for an endothelial origin. *Arch Pathol Lab Med.* 1981;105:274–275.

21. Penneys NS, Adachi K, Ziegels-Weissman J, et al. Granular cell tumors of the skin contain myelin basic protein. *Arch Pathol Lab Med.* 1983;107:302–303.

22. Nadji M, Tabei SZ, Castro A, et al. Prostatic origin of tumors. An immunoperoxidase study. *Am J Clin Pathol.* 1980;73:735–737.

23. Rico J, Penneys NS. Metastatic follicular carcinoma of the thyroid to the skin: A case confirmed by immunohistochemistry. *J Cutan Pathol.* 1985;12:103–105.

24. Penneys NS. Microinvasive lentigo maligna melanoma. *J Cutan Pathol.* 1986;13:459.

25. Battifora H, Silva EG. The use of antikeratin antibodies in the immunohistochemical distinction between neuroendocrine (Merkel cell) carcinoma of the skin, lymphoma, and oat cell carcinoma. *Cancer.* 1986;58:1040–1046.

26. Gu J, Polak JM, Tapia FJ, et al. Neuron-specific enolase in the Merkel cells of mammalian skin. *Am J Pathol.* 1981;104:63–68.

27. Drukoningen M, De Wolf-Peeters C, Van Limbergen E, Desmet V. Merkel cell tumor of the skin: An immunohistochemical study. *Hum Pathol.* 1986;17:301–307.

28. Merot Y, Margolis RJ, Dahl D, et al. Coexpression of neurofilament and keratin proteins in cutaneous neuroendocrine carcinoma cells. *J Invest Dermatol.* 1986;86:74–77.

29. Hartschuh W, Weihe E, Yanaihara N, et al. Immunohistochemical localization of vasoactive intestinal polypeptide (VIP) in Merkel cells of various mammals: Evidence for a neuromodulator function of the Merkel cell. *J Invest Dermatol.* 1983;81:361–364.

30. Miettinen M. Synaptophysin and neurofilament proteins as markers for neuroendocrine tumors. *Arch Pathol Lab Med.* 1987;111:813–818.

31. Wirt DP, Grogan TM, Jolley CS, et al. The immunoarchitecture of cutaneous pseudolymphoma. *Hum Pathol.* 1985;16:492–510.

32. McMillan ME, Peters S, Jackson I, et al. Immunoperoxidase examination of cutaneous infiltrates of mycosis fungoides and large-plaque parapsoriasis with OKT10. *J Am Acad Dermatol.* 1984;10:457–461.

33. Bhan AK, Harris NL. The immunohistology of normal and neoplastic lymphoid tissues. In: Murphy GF, Mihm MC, Jr, eds. *Lymphoproliferative Disorders of the Skin.* Boston: Butterworths; 1986:31–72.

34. Ralfkiaer E, Saati T, Bosq J, Delsol G, Gatter K, Mason D. Immunocytochemical characterisation of cutaneous lymphomas other than mycosis fungoides. *J Clin Pathol.* 1986;39:553–563.

35. Gawkrodger DJ, McVittie E, Hunter JAA. Immunophenotyping of the eczymatous flare-up reaction in a nickel-sensitive subject. *Dermatologica*. 1987;175:171–177.

36. Penneys NS, Kott-Blumenkranz R, Buck BE, Nadji M, Gould E, Ibe M. S100 protein-containing dendritic cells in fetal and newborn epidermis and thymus. *Pediatr Dermatol*. 1986;3:226–229.

37. Civantos J, Penneys N, Ziegels-Weissman J. Kaposi's sarcoma: Immunoperoxidase staining for cytomegalovirus. *AIDS Res*. 1984;1:121–125.

38. Penneys NS, Mogollon RJ, Nadji M, Gould E. Papillomavirus common antigens. *Arch Dermatol*. 1984;119:859–861.

39. Grody WW, Cheng L, Lewin K. In situ viral DNA hybridization in surgical pathology. *Hum Pathol*. 1987;18:535–543.

CHAPTER 5
Methodology for Use of Electron Microscopy in Dermatopathology

Alvin S. Zelickson and Jess H. Mottaz

HISTORY

The first electron microscope was developed in the early 1930s by Max Knoll and Ernst Ruska in Berlin, Germany. It was a very crude two-stage instrument that at first was hardly an improvement over the best light microscope of the time.[1] With this instrument, the first electron micrograph was obtained. The highest magnification obtainable was 17×, considerably less than that attainable with a good light microscope. Hillier, in 1946, presented a paper demonstrating 1 nm resolution with the electron microscope.[2] In 1947, Hillier and Ramberg introduced the first compensated objective lens for the electron microscope.[3] This is considered one of the most significant contributions toward obtaining resolving powers close to the theoretical limit of 0.28 nm. The electron microscope has been and continues to be a very important research tool, but in addition, it is invaluable as a diagnostic tool in all fields of surgical pathology.[4]

TISSUE PREPARATION

The methods used in obtaining tissue samples for electron microscopy differ from those used in light microscopy. Improper handling technique is the single major reason for tissue damage resulting in material that cannot be optimally evaluated at the electron microscopic level. To obtain the ultimate in ultrastructural evaluation and interpretation of a specimen, familiarity with and strict adherence to the accepted techniques used in electron microscopy are imperative. Damage and alteration of fine structure apparent at the electron microscopic level of examination begin immediately on removing the tissue from the body. Therefore, extreme care must be taken to get the biopsy specimen into the fixative as soon as possible with the least amount of mechanical damage.[5] To avoid any undo damage to the tissue, it is recommended that a very sharp cutting instrument be used and that forceps not be used to handle the tissue. After the knife or punch biopsy instrument has penetrated through the epidermis and dermis into the subcutis, the tissue should be lifted gently, and the base of the specimen should be cut with a curved fine point scissors. With the tissue still on the tips of the scissors, it should be placed into the fixative, and the scissors should then be moved until the tissue is free in the fixative.

Minute cytologic alterations of the fine structure not discernible with the light microscope become a very important factor in meaningful electron microscopy. The initial fixation of the tissue takes place in a 2.5% buffered solution of electron microscope grade glutaraldehyde chilled to 4° C. After 2 hours of fixing in the glutaraldehyde, the tissue is cut with a de-oiled razor blade into slices 1 mm thick. To keep tissue from drying during the cutting, place the specimen in a few drops of fixative placed on a square of dental wax. If desired at this point, a portion of the sample can be cut off and processed in paraffin for light microscopy. If the tissue is not going to be processed beyond this point for a while, it can be held for some time in the buffer (only) solution. Because of their caustic nature, great care should be exercised to avoid personal contact with any of the fixatives.

Because the gluteraldehyde, although an adequate fixative, does not give much contrast or density to the tissue and does not reveal membranes well, the tissue must be further fixed and stained with a 1% solution of osmium tetroxide.[6] This is done not only to increase contrast and density but also to aid in further staining of the membranes (Fig. 5–1). Osmium is an extremely toxic substance and must be handled in a properly vented hood area. The length of time the tissue remains in the osmium tetroxide can vary from 1 to 3 hours. The osmium is buffered to the same pH with the same buffer solution as was used for the glutaraldehyde.[7] At this point, the tissue is washed several times with the buffer solution, after which it can be held an indefinite period of time in the buffer solution before the embedding process is continued.

The next steps involve the actual embedding process and, once started, must be carried to completion.[8,9] This generally is done by passing the tissue through a series

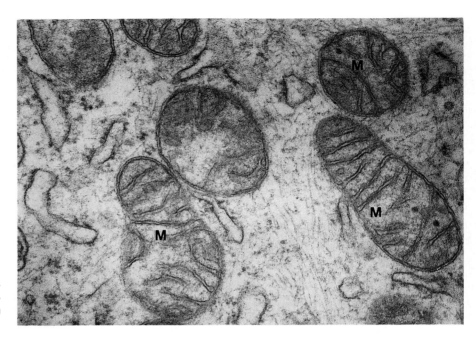

Figure 5–1. High magnification of mitochondria (M) from tissue first fixed with glutaraldehyde and further fixed and stained with osmium tetroxide.

of graded alcohols, 50%, 70%, 95%, and 100%, over a period of 1 hour.[10] At no time during this stage should the tissue be allowed to dry out. This is followed by four 15-minute changes of 100% alcohol. Equal amounts of 100% alcohol and resin embedding mixture are added to the last change. This is mixed well and allowed to stand for 15 minutes, with occasional mixing. Another quantity of embedding mixture is added, and the mixture is shaken and allowed to stand for one-half hour. All of the liquid is drained from the tissue, fresh resin is added, the mixture is allowed to stand for one-half hour. The tissue is now fully infiltrated with resin and is ready to be embedded in polyethylene capsules, such as Beem capsules. These capsules are used as containment vessels when polymerizing the resin, and they are later removed. Before the tissue and the resin are placed in the capsules, small paper rings with identification numbers are placed in the capsules. The capsules are filled three-quarters full with the embedding mixture, and the tissue samples are placed in the capsules so that the cross-section of the tissue lies flat on the bottom of the capsule. The material is then polymerized in an oven at 60° C for about 8 hours, depending on the embedding material used.

Thick Sections

To ready the tissue for viewing in the electron microscope, it is advisable to prepare thick sections (1 to 1.5 μm). Taking thick sections is a fast method to determine if the tissue is properly oriented and appropriately trimmed and permits a preliminary evaluation of tissue preservation. Sections from the plastic block usually are taken with a glass knife using the same ultratome sectioning instrument used for thin sectioning. The sections are floated on water in a trough that has been prepared on the glass knife. The sections are removed from the water surface with a small wire loop,

placed on a glass slide, loosely covered with a coverslip, and examined with a phase microscope. Placing a drop of xylene under the coverslip aids in viewing the specimen by providing additional contrast and by enhancing detail. Thick sections can be stained with toluidine blue, paragon stain, and methylene blue, among others. If at this point the embedded tissue is properly oriented, properly preserved, and exhibits an area of interest, ultrathin sections can be cut for viewing with the electron microscope.

Ultrathin Sections

Ultrathin sections (60 to 70 nm) usually are cut with the aid of a diamond knife mounted in an ultratome, although well-prepared glass knives also are used. As the sections are cut, they are floated on a trough of water and are picked up on a fine mesh copper grid. Occasionally and for certain special conditions, grids made of other metals are used. If extra support is needed, the grids can be coated with a very thin coating of Formvar. Formvar, a thin transparent plastic material, should then be coated with an extremely thin layer of evaporated carbon with a thickness of no more than 2 nm. This film will add mechanical strength and stability under the electron beam, something that is lacking in Formvar film.

STAINING

Generally, tissue embedded in any one of the several resins, Epon, Spurr, or Araldite, does not yield sections with sufficient contrast to be seen well in the electron microscope, so a poststaining or section staining process usually is needed. A common section stain used to enhance contrast is a lead citrate or uranyl acetate stain.[11,12] A staining dish can be made by placing a square of dental wax on the bottom of a Petri dish. A warm glass rod is used to make several depressions in the wax. Into these depressions, a small drop of the prepared staining solution is placed. A grid, tissue side down, is then carefully placed on a drop of stain, the staining dish is covered and the grid is allowed to remain on the stain for a specified time depending on the stain being used. After the time has lapsed, one grid at a time is removed and gently washed under a stream of distilled water to remove all excess stain. Grids are placed on a piece of filter paper and are covered to dry. Special care should be used to avoid letting the specimen become dry during or after the staining process until the last washing step has been completed.

Staining can be done at several different times during tissue preparation. During fixation, staining is accomplished with osmium, potassium permanganate, uranyl acetate, or ruthenium tetroxide. Staining during washing can be done with iron chloride for nucleic acids or phosphotungstic acid for certain membranes and for elastin. Phosphotungstic acid, uranyl acetate, uranyl nitrate, and potassium permanganate are among those stains that can be used during the dehydration steps. The number of stains and different compounds used in electron microscopy are extensive, and an excellent reference on this subject is Hayat's book.[13]

After the stained grids are dried completely, they can be placed in the specimen holder of the electron microscope and viewed on the fluorescent screen of the scope. Photographs of areas of special interest are taken on film or photographic plates.

Cytochemical Staining

Cytochemical staining has been used for conventional light microscopy, and with the advent of the electron microscope, techniques were adapted for use with this instrument. Cyto-chemical techniques may be used for enzyme localization. To make the technique applicable to electron microscopy, a procedure had to be devised to form electron-dense deposits at the enzyme sites. Specific techniques apply for each specific application, and an investigator is advised to consult the original literature before undertaking an electron microscopic cytochemical project. Information of general interest on this subject is contained in articles by Holt and Hicks[14] and by Sabatini et al.[15]

Dopa Reaction Stain

The dopa reaction stain introduced by Bloch[16] and later modified by Laidlow and Blackberg[17] has been widely used in studies involving melanin synthesis. Dopa stain has been used in ultrastructural studies to follow melanin synthesis through the melanocyte in normal tissue[18] and in diseased tissue.[19] The dopa staining procedure requires that the tissue be fixed for 2 to 3 hours, followed by overnight incubation in a freshly prepared dopa medium, and then fixed in osmium and embedded (Fig. 5–2).

AUTORADIOGRAPHY

Autoradiography is a cytochemical means of tagging a specific chemical in vivo that was first used in light microscopy. The techniques used in electron microscopy follow those used in light microscopy. Radioactive isotopes are applied either by injection into animals or, in a few instances, by means of in vitro incubation of tissue pieces. Because of the high resolution of autoradiographic techniques in electron microscopy, it is possible to localize the incorporation of radioactivity in cell organelles. Although autoradiographic resolution does not approach maximum resolutions

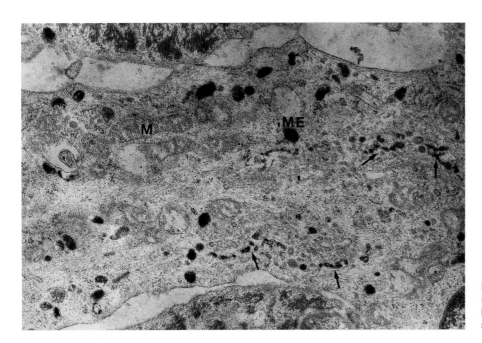

Figure 5–2. Melanocyte treated with dopa reaction stain. Reaction product (arrows) can be seen in the Golgi region. ME, melanosomes; M, mitochondria.

obtainable with the electron microscope, it is possible to achieve resolutions in the neighborhood of 0.01 nm. A time sequence study of a labeled melanin precursor made it possible to visualize the progression of the melanin through the cell until its incorporation into the final end product, a melanin granule[20] (Fig. 5–3). For general autoradiography, the tissue is fixed and embedded as outlined for regular transmission electron microscopy. Thin sections are taken and mounted on grids especially coated with Formvar. The use of titanium grids has been recommended because they are not affected by the photographic solutions. After the sections have been placed on the coated grids, they are coated with a photographic emulsion.

Several methods are used to coat the sections with the emulsion, but the method of Hay and Revel[21] has proved to be most successful and is described here. Glass microscope slides are dipped in a 1% collodion solution and allowed to dry. A small strip of double-stick cellophane tape is placed on the lower half of the slide. On top of this tape is placed a strip of black plastic electrical tape with the adhesive side up. Holes slightly smaller than the diameter of the grid are punched in the electrical tape before attaching it to the cellophane tape. Grids with sections are placed on the electrical tape over the holes. The slides are then dipped in photographic emulsion prepared by adding

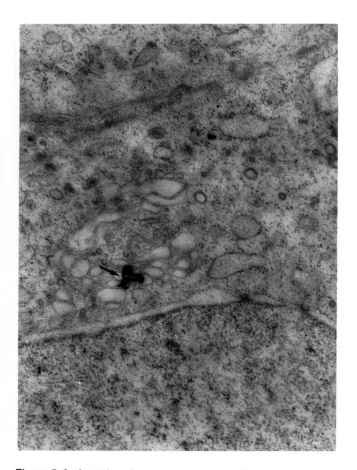

Figure 5–3. A section of melanoma injected with tritiated dopa. An exposed silver grain (arrow) can be seen in the Golgi area.

solid emulsion to distilled water held at a constant temperature of 45°C. When the emulsion is thoroughly melted in the water, the container is covered and inverted several times to mix. Test slides are then dipped, dried, and developed to test for background. On achieving satisfactory test results in the background test slides, slides bearing grids with radioactive, thin section are dipped into the same emulsion. The dipped slides are hanged in a light-tight container and are allowed to dry. After all slides and grids are dry, they are transferred to a covered black slide box sealed with black plastic electrical tape. Each box should contain a small amount of Drierite in a container with dust. The boxes are placed in the refrigerator for an exposure period of usually 2 to 3 weeks. The exposure time depends on many variables, and only an experimental series of test slides can establish the time exactly.[22] The slides are removed after the determined exposure time and developed photographically. During development, a long spaghettilike strand of silver grows from each irradiated silver bromide crystal, which is seen in the electron microscope. The contrast is improved for viewing by removing the gelatin[23] and staining the grids. Staining is sometimes done before applying the emulsion. After removing the gelatin and staining, the sections are coated with a very thin layer of evaporated carbon. At all times during this process, the manufacturer's instructions on use, handling, and processing of the emulsion should be followed carefully.

IMMUNOELECTRON MICROSCOPY

One of the many applications of immunoelectron microscopy is to demonstrate the specific localization of ferritin-labeled antibodies on the surface of Langerhans cells. This technique has been performed to aid in the establishment of the Langerhans cell lineage. In preparing the tissue, care must be taken to strike a compromise between preserving the cellular structure and preventing the loss and secondary location of antigens. A fixative that yields the greatest preservation of the fine structure causes a reduction in immunoreactivity. A fixative to consider is a low concentration glutaraldehyde. Methods of preparation vary as much as the many applications. An indepth search of the literature would be in order before embarking on an immunoelectron microscopy study.

ELECTRON MICROSCOPY OF PARAFFIN-EMBEDDED TISSUE

Occasionally, tissue is embedded in paraffin, and it is later determined that electron microscopy is needed. If it is not possible or convenient to obtain fresh tissue, the paraffin-embedded tissue can be reembedded in plastic. The quality of the tissue is somewhat diminished, but usually meaningful information can be obtained. A small portion of the paraffin-embedded tissue is cut from the paraffin block. The piece removed is placed in xylene to remove all paraffin. The tissue is then rehydrated by placing it in decreasing concentrations of alcohol. The tissue is postfixed in osmium, and the embedding procedure is continued as outlined previously. It is also possible, but much more difficult, to reprocess paraffin-embedded hematoxylin and eosin sections. When working with sections, the same procedure is used as with the larger pieces, except the sections remain on the slide and are embedded in the resin while they are on the slide. After the resin has hardened, the section is separated from the glass slide and mounted on a hardened resin blank to be mounted and sectioned in an ultramicrotome.

REFERENCES

1. Knoll M, Ruska E. Beitrag zur Geometrischen Elektronenptik I and II. *Annalen Der Physik* 1932; 12 (5th Series): 607–640, 641–661.

2. Hillier J. Further improvements in the resolving power of the electron microscope. *J App Physics*. 1946;17:307–309.

3. Hillier J, Ramberg EG. The magnetic electron microscope objective. Contour phenomena and the attainment of high resolving power. *J App Physics*. 1947;18:48.

4. Zelickson AS, ed. *Clinical Use of Electron Microscopy in Dermatology*. 4th ed. Minneapolis: Bolger; 1985.

5. Johannessen JV, ed. *Electron Microscopy in Human Medicine, 1. Instrumentation and Techniques*. New York: McGraw-Hill; 1978.

6. Sabatini DD, Bensch K, Barrnett RJ. Double fixation procedure of glutaraldehyde and osmium tetroxide. *J Cell Biol*. 1963;11: 19–31.

7. Kuthy E. Csapo Z. Peculiar artifacts after fixation with glutaraldehyde and osmium tetroxide. *J Microsc*. 1977;107:177.

8. Luft JH. Epon 812 embedding mixture. *J Biophys Biochem Cytol* 1961;9:409.

9. Spurr AR. Spurr low viscosity embedding medium. *J Ultrastruct Res*. 1969;26:31.

10. Glauert A. Fixation and embedding of biological specimens. In: Desmond HK, ed. *Techniques for Electron Microscopy*. Philadelphia: FA Davis; 1965.

11. Reynolds ES. Lead Citrate at high pH. *J Cell Biol*. 1963;17:208.

12. Venable JH, Coggeshall R. Simplified lead citrate stain. *J Cell Biol*. 1965;25:407.

13. Hayat MA. *Positive Staining for Electron Microscopy*. New York: Van Nostrand Reinhold; 1975.

14. Holt SJ, Hicks RM. Studies on formalin fixation for electron microscopy and cytochemical staining purposes. *J Biophys Biochem Cytol*. 1961;11:31.

15. Sabitini DD, Bensch K, Barrnett RJ. Cytochemistry and electron microscopy, the preservation of cellular ultrastructure and enzymatic activity by aldehyde fixation. *J Cell Biol*. 1963;17:19.

16. Bloch B. Das pigment. In Jadassohn J, ed. *Handbuch der Haut und Geschlechtskraukheiten, I*. Berlin: Springer; 1927:434.

17. Laidlow GF, Blackberg SN. Melanoma studies II. A simple technique for dopa reaction. *Am J Pathol*. 1932;8:491.

18. Mishima Y. Electron microscopy of melanin synthesis in intradermal nevus cells. *J Invest Dermatol*. 1962;39:369.

19. Hunter JAA, Mottaz JH, Zelickson AS. Melanogensis: Ultrastructural histochemical observations on ultraviolet-irradiated human melanocytes. *J Invest Dermatol*. 1970;54:213.

20. Zelickson AS, Hirsch HM, Hartman JF. Melanogenesis: An autoradiographic study at the ultrastructural level. *J Invest Dermatol*. 1964;43:327.

21. Hay ED, Revel JP. Autoradiographic studies of the origin of the basement lamella in *Ambystoma*. *Dev Biol*. 1963;7:152.

22. Glaubert AM. Section staining, cytology, autoradiography and immunochemistry for biological specimens. In: Kay DH, ed. *Techniques for Electron Microscopy*. Philadelphia: FA Davis; 1965.

23. Meek GA, Moses MJ. Localization of tritiated thymidine in HeLa cells by electron autoradiography. *J R Soc* 1963;81:187.

SECTION II
Non-Infectious Predominantly Superficial Inflammatory Diseases

CHAPTER 6
Spongiotic Dermatitis

Edward Abell

Spongiotic dermatitis represents a primary inflammatory process that involves the epidermis and its adventitial dermis. This pathological reaction, which is synonymous with eczematous dermatitis, predominantly involves the surface epidermis and papillary connective tissues. It may also occasionally occur in the infundibular portion of follicular structures, especially in atopic dermatitis, but only in quite rare situations does the process involve deeper parts of the follicle and its adjacent adventitial dermis. The changes observed by microscopy are created by permeation of the tissues by inflammatory cells and fluid (plasma transudate) and its distortion and damage by this process. The histopathology is altered subsequently by the tissue response to this inflammatory injury, whether this represents healing or adaptation or a combination of the two. The histopathologic appearance will vary, therefore, depending not only on the severity of the injurious stimulus but also with the time at which the biopsy sample has been obtained in the evolving lesion. This variability in pathology is most easily appreciated perhaps by consideration of contact allergic dermatitis. Although poison ivy dermatitis commonly provokes a dramatic vesicobullous reaction of short duration, allergic dermatitis to topically applied preparations such as lanolin is likely to produce a quite subtle eczematous response, which may persist unsuspected for years.

It can readily be appreciated that spongiotic dermatitis, in almost all situations, is characterized by epidermal changes in association with a cellular infiltrate involving the perivascular tissue of the superficial plexus vessels (venules). It represents, essentially, an "epidermatitis." As the common cellular component of all of these reactions contains lymphocytes and histiocytes, the dermal infiltrate is of little or no diagnostic help to a pathologist and only when other inflammatory cells appear (e.g., eosinophils) can the infiltrate help to discriminate among the various dermatitic disorders. The diagnostically useful determinants in this group of disorders will therefore usually be found in the epidermis, if present at all.

It is still useful to deal with spongiotic dermatitis in a generic sense under the categories of acute, subacute, and chronic before attempting to define what characteristic features are associated with the individual clinical disorders. This arrangement permits a general description of the way in which the dermatitic disorders evolve and is also helpful when considering a differential diagnosis. For additional histopathologic considerations of general and specific aspects of dermatitis the reader should review other tests,[1–3] to which this author has been greatly indebted on many occasions.

ACUTE DERMATITIC REACTIONS

An acute dermatitic reaction may be thought of as arising without warning on an unsuspecting epidermis, more or less abruptly. It distorts a previously normal epidermis, but the pathological picture will not usually include changes that could be considered adaptive or reactive.

The inflammation is detected microscopically by the appearance of excessive tissue fluid within the epidermis, at first between the cell walls and then within the cells themselves. It is this tissue fluid overload that distorts the normal cellular architecture to produce a spongelike appearance (spongosis), which characterizes this phase of the reaction. Fluid accumulation in the intercellular spaces creates an appearance of white zones between the cells. Microscopically, these zones can be seen to be crossed by numerous fine and uniformly spaced dark lines (intercellular bridges or prickles), which represent the stretch desmosomal attachments and look like flexible railroad tracks (Fig. 6–1). It is this appearance that suggested the term *prickle cell* for the maturing cells of the malpighian layer. Fluid accumulation within the cells is visualized by cytoplasmic swelling and the appearance of a clear space close to the nucleus (Fig. 6–2). With further accumulation of fluid within the epidermis, the integrity of the cell membranes becomes compromised and disruption occurs. Allowed to progress, this process leads to the development of small cavities (vesicles) (Fig. 6–3), and in unusual circumstances or in certain anatomic sites (e.g., palms and soles), true blisters or bullae may develop (see Figs. 6–17 and 6–18). These vesicles or bullae may contain cells and fluid exudate, though some

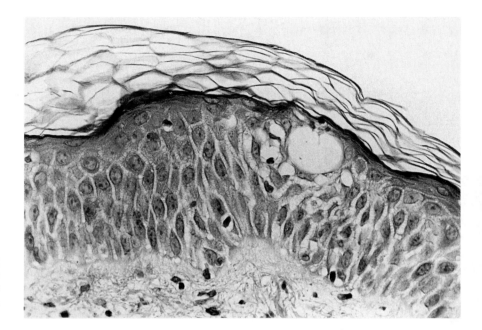

Figure 6–1. Acute dermatitis (vesicular id reaction). Very early lesion with intense intercellular edema and bridges, minimal exocytosis, and normal stratum corneum (H&E, ×160).

of this may not be retained in the tissue sections after processing.

At first, epidermal edema is the most prominent finding, but it is always accompanied by mononuclear cells. Their number can vary markedly, even in examples of the same type of dermatitis. The reaction at this early stage will exist beneath a normal-appearing stratum corneum, but the result of sufficient spongiotic dermatitic reaction is always to alter the keratinization process to some degree, depending on the severity of that reaction. The distortion of stratum corneum is the visual representation of the injury created by the inflammation on the normal maturation of the keratinocytes.

If the acute dermatitic reaction develops only to this stage and then resolves, a situation that might for instance

occur in a single episode of contact allergic dermatitis due to poison ivy, then the pathologic changes of the repair and resolution phase will ensue. Substantial vesicles or blisters often discharge their fluid content onto the surface, where it may dry and form a crust. If discharge to the surface does not occur, then the inspissated proteinaceous fluid is incorporated into an altered stratum corneum and will form a scale crust. With significant injury, there will usually be loss of the granular layer at the injured site and formation of a parakeratotic (nucleated) stratum corneum (Fig. 6–4). Where only minor or minimum dermatitic damage has occurred, the spongiotic edema may be reabsorbed without dramatic alteration of the keratinization process.

The migration of mononuclear inflammatory cells into

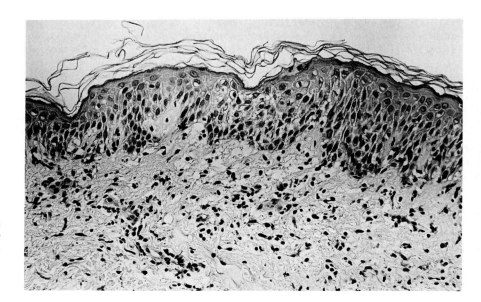

Figure 6–2. Acute dermatitis (positive patch test). Very early lesion showing intercellular edema but also clear spaces adjacent to nuclei representing the development of intracellular edema in center of epidermis (H&E, ×80).

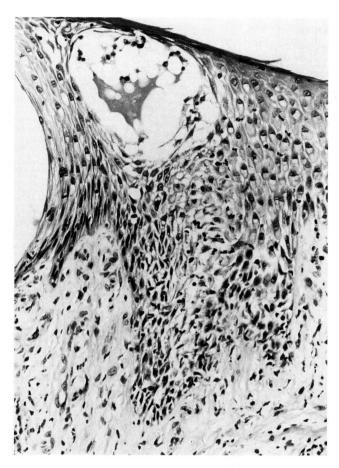

Figure 6–3. Acute dermatitis (allergic contact dermatitis) with vesicle developing above an area of intense intercellular and intracellular edema. Note mononuclear cell exocytosis (H&E, ×160).

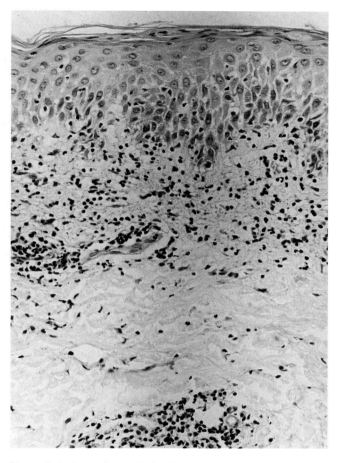

Figure 6–4. Acute dermatitis (positive patch test). Mild early lesion beginning to develop parakeratosis. Note diffuse exocytosis of mononuclear cells with intercellular edema and superficial dermal infiltrate (H&E, ×80).

the epidermis (exocytosis) tends to follow and reflects the severity of the spongiotic edema. If there is apparent thickening (acanthosis) of the epidermis in the acute phase reaction, it is created by the accumulation of inflammatory fluid and cellular swelling and not due to cellular proliferation. This occurs in later stages when resolution or healing has begun. Epidermal cells injured by a dermatitic process accumulate glycogen in their cytoplasm, as can be demonstrated by the periodic acid-Schiff (PAS) stain (Fig. 6–5) and confirmed by diastase digestion.

The dermal changes are largely confined to a diffuse papillary edema, dilation of capillary vessels, and a predominantly perivascular accumulation of lymphocytes and histiocytes following the pattern of the superficial plexus vessels (see Fig. 6–4).

SUBACUTE DERMATITIC REACTIONS

A subacute dermatitic reaction represents a spongiotic dermatitic inflammatory process that has persisted and evolved

during a period of time. It does not arise after a single application of an allergen to a sensitized skin, but would certainly evolve if allergen were reapplied several times. Its development necessitates some adaptation by the epidermis, specifically, an increase in the epidermal cell population derived through mitotic division to create true hyperplasia—acanthosis by increase in cell numbers. Acute dermatitic changes are present together with this acanthotic reaction, indicating a continuation of the active injurious process. The persistence of this process and of injury to keratinocyte maturation leads to replacement of the normal, basketweave pattern of stratum corneum by a parakeratotic scale (Figs. 6–6 and 6–7).

The active dermatitic process, represented by focal edema and mononuclear cell exocytosis, is usually seen scattered throughout the involved epidermis, and the foci are frequently seen at different stages of development (see Figs. 6–6 and 6–7). The stratum corneum is always abnormal, parakeratosis being the almost consistent result of this inflammatory injury. As the spongiotic reaction is focal, so is the parakeratosis, often appearing in small symmetric

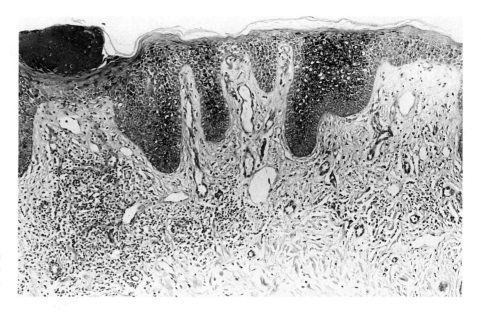

Figure 6–5. Subacute dermatitis ("stasis dermatitis"). Note irregular glycogen deposition in areas of epidermal spongiosis (PAS, ×40).

mounds at the surface. The stratum corneum between the areas of parakeratotic scale, in the early phases of subacute dermatitis, may retain its basket-weave appearance, but as the reaction persists, this is almost always replaced by compact orthokeratotic scale. Minimal persistent dermatitis may generate little or no parakeratosis, but the stratum corneum does not return to normal, instead remaining as a compact scale. This is perhaps most well illustrated in the eczematous dermatitis seen in mild atopic dermatitis, in which the pathologic change may simulate a mildly inflamed ichthyosis. Mild spongiotic epidermal injury therefore may produce only a compact hyperkeratosis. Granular layer changes may be quite variable also. Adjacent to and

above the site of severe spongiotic change, the granular layer may be absent or markedly diminished. In mild to minimum dermatitis, the granular layer may be focally reduced but in other areas show some prominence or thickening. Only in situations of severe uniform inflammatory injury, as seen in severe phototoxic dermatitis, will whole zones of the granular layer be absent.

The overall architectural change in the epidermis also tends to reflect the nature, persistence, and severity of the spongiotic reaction. The acanthosis may be mild and involve an epidermis that shows a normal overall arrangement of the rete ridge pattern, or in persistent severe disease it may mimic psoriasis by pronounced elongation of the rete

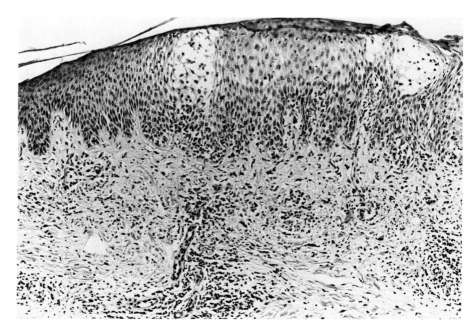

Figure 6–6. Subacute dermatitis (nummular dermatitis). Early lesion with small vesicles and diffuse spongiotic change of epidermis, acanthosis (increase of cells and edema), diffuse exocytosis, and loose but compact scale (H&E, ×80).

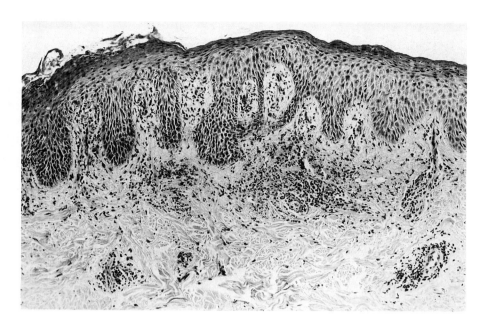

Figure 6–7. Subacute dermatitis (nummular dermatitis). Psoriasiform epidermal hyperplasia with diffuse edema, exocytosis, and confluent parakeratotic scale and a superficial perivascular dermal infiltrate (H&E, ×40).

structures (see Fig. 6–7). This latter pattern is most often seen in established nummular or discoid dermatitis.

The subacute spongiotic dermatitic process, whether of endogenous or exogenous origin, appears to affect the epidermis in a markedly uneven pattern. Uniform injury can be induced by phototoxic reactions and less frequently by contact with severe irritants or caustics. However, these are unusual situations for the pathologist and are most often so clinically obvious that biopsy is not performed and few specimens are therefore available for review.

Although the epidermis undergoes this substantial inflammatory injury, the papillary dermal changes are inconsequentially different from those seen in the acute process. Somewhat less edema may be apparent in the papillary zone. Except in certain special situations, which will be described in subsequent sections under the diagnostic headings, the dermal infiltrate remains more or less the same.

CHRONIC DERMATITIC PROCESSES

A chronic dermatitic process arises where a dermatitic process has persisted for long periods of time. It represents a clinical and pathologic picture of combined persistent injury together with the adaptive response of the epidermis and dermis, which is usually easily interpreted from the pathologic manifestations. As with dermatitis as a whole, variability is to be anticipated so that chronic spongiotic dermatitis may be minimum, mild, or severe. The clinical conditions that are represented by this process include lichenified dermatitis, lichen simplex chronicus, and neurodermatitis.

Acanthosis is always present, and so also is some degree of alteration of the stratum corneum, be it compact orthokeratosis or parakeratosis. The granular layer is prominent and often markedly thickened. Spongiosis is still variable, is usually mild in the chronic stage, and development of vesicles or bullae would be quite exceptional. Conversely, the inflammatory process may be so minimum as to be almost imperceptible and remain only as minimal intercellular edema. Intercellular edema then becomes the only visible manifestation of disease activity (Fig. 6–8). This situation is most easily exemplified by the mild lichenified dermatitis seen in atopic dermatitis (see Fig. 6–14).

In lichen simplex chronicus or neurodermatitis, the spongiotic process can be more obvious, with foci of mild spongiosis and rarely tiny areas of microvesication.

As with all types of dermatitis, pruritus is present and histologic signs of excoriation are to be expected in biopsy specimens. In the chronic form of dermatitis, these signs should be anticipated; indeed, it is the persistence of the external injury of rubbing, friction, and excoriation that appears to lead to much of the persistent epidermal hyperplasia. The external trauma is probably in large measure also responsible for the alteration in the papillary dermal connective tissue seen in these disorders. This pathology is appreciated as thickened collagen fiber oriented vertically in the papillary dermis. The papillary and reticular dermis, therefore, may appear to blend together. An increased number of fibroblasts may be apparent. These changes reach their full expression and development in nodular prurigo (Fig. 6–9).

The dermal infiltrate may be sparse or quite dense. When it is sparse, histiocytes are frequently prominent. When the skin is heavily excoriated, the infiltrate often appears to be focal and dense and may occasionally demonstrate a few plasma cells. Melanin pigment released from the injured epidermis is often found in dermal melanophages.

CONTACT DERMATITIS, ALLERGIC AND IRRITANT

Clinical Features

Except for those occasions when the clinical features are subtle, dermatitis of exogenous origin is recognized by its

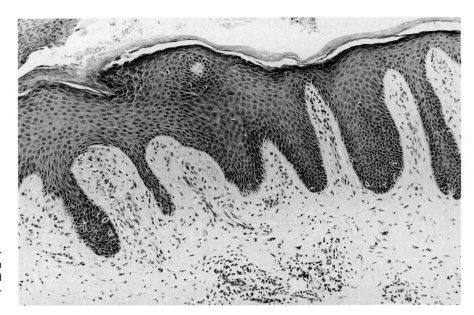

Figure 6–8. Chronic dermatitis (lichen simplex chronicus). Prominent acanthosis with minimal intercellular edema, a thickened granular layer, and parakeratotic and compact orthokeratotic scale (H&E, ×80).

clinical pattern of presentation. The distribution can be related to the epidermal application or direct contact with some substance or material. When dermatitis of this type is suspected, investigation requires a detailed clinical history and confirmation by skin patch testing. Appropriate testing must be performed with insight into the chemicals involved. It is important to know whether they are likely to produce irritation, allergy or both, so that open or closed patch testing can be performed with appropriate concentrations of test chemicals. As the clinical expression of contact dermatitis is protean, the reader is referred to specialty texts.[4–6] Briefly, some appreciation of the clinical diversity can be given. Acute vesicular or bullous reactions are commonly evoked by potent allergens (e.g., poison ivy reactions). Less potent allergens may provoke plaques of

erythema with scale or scale crust, as in nickel allergy associated with jewelry. Minimum erythema and scaling can be produced by low-grade allergic dermatitis to components of medications (e.g., lanolin). These latter reactions may often complicate an underlying primary dermatitis of another type. The histopathologic changes reflect this widely diverse clinical picture.

Irritant contact dermatitis tends to produce milder but persistent dermatitic reactions, which are therefore most often biopsied in the subacute or chronic dermatitic phase. No absolute differentiation of irritant and allergic contact dermatitis can be made, but certain pathologic features occasionally allow consideration of one over the other reaction.

The pathophysiologic mechanisms of acute contact dermatitis are among the most well understood of all of the

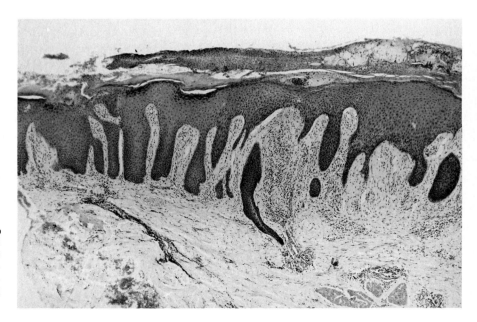

Figure 6–9. Chronic dermatitis (prurigo nodularis). Prominent but irregular epidermal acanthosis, scale crust incorporated into confluent parakeratotic scale, and dense dermal collagen in papillary zone with proliferation of fibroblasts. A diffuse upper dermal infiltrate is present (H&E, ×16).

dermatitic processes and have been considered as the classic type IV immunologic response in the skin. In the induction of the allergic contact reaction, Langerhans' cells are of primary importance. Silberberg first visually documented the apposition of lymphocytes with epidermal Langerhans' cells in 1973[7] and proposed their involvement in the induction of cutaneous allergy of this type.[8] Subsequent work has confirmed the role of Langerhans' cells in antigen recognition in the skin.[9,10] Sensitization of lymphocytes may occur locally in the skin or possibly in the lymph nodes.[11] Rechallenge by allergen is a sensitized host generates a lymphoid reaction within the epidermis with release of lymphokines, and these chemical mediators appear to be involved in the generation of the inflammatory response.[12] Epidermal cells are also able to generate cytokines,[13,14] which may contribute to generation of the inflammatory cell response.

Histologic Features

If a biopsy specimen of a positive patch test reaction is obtained in its early stages of evolution, the pathologic picture is that of a developing acute spongiotic reaction (see Figs. 6–2 and 6–4), with prominent edema, microvesication, and exocytosis of mononuclear cells. This reaction may also produce a copious mononuclear cell infiltrate within the epidermis, therefore mimicking mycosis fungoides. This condition has been called the spongiotic simulant of mycosis fungoides (Fig. 6–10).[15]

In early but established lesions of severe allergic contact dermatitis, the histopathology is that of acute spongiotic or vesicular dermatitis (Figs. 6–3 and 6–11).[16] An occasional neutrophil may be seen in the vesicle of severe reactions, even in the absence of dermatophyte fungi. Eosinophils may be present in substantial numbers in the dermis and may accompany the edema fluid into the epidermis. In addition, basophils accumulate and degranulate in the dermis in the early phase.[17,18]

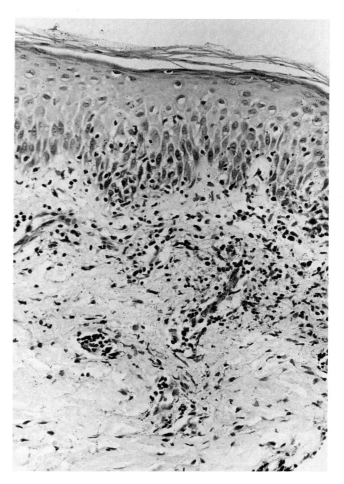

Figure 6–10. Acute dermatitis (positive patch test, 24 hours). Note aggregation of mononuclear cells in the lower third of the epidermis, simulating early patch stage mycosis fungoides (H&E, ×160).

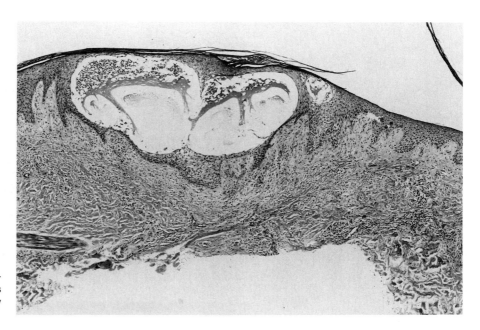

Figure 6–11. Acute dermatitis (allergic contact dermatitis, poison ivy). Large vesicles have developed, with many inflammatory cells in vesicle fluid (H&E, ×16).

Contact allergic dermatitis therefore is one of the several causes of eosinophilic spongiosis. This latter condition is most well developed in the vesicular stage of incontinentia pigmenti. The same type of reaction, but in a less severe and more diffuse form, can be associated with the prodromal infiltrated plaque stage of several bullous dermotoses,[19] particularly pemphigus, but less often bullous pemphigoid and herpes gestationis and also in the epidermis overlying an arthropod bite reaction. It is therefore not of itself a diagnostically specific finding. Epidermal infiltration by eosinophils in an appropriate spongiotic dermatitic setting may suggest that a contact allergic dermatitis is present rather than an irritant one.

Less specifically but much more frequently, contact allergic dermatitis biopsy specimens show a pathologic configuration of subacute spongiotic dermatitis, often attended by mild to moderate epidermal hyperplasia (Fig. 6–12). In older lesions, the pathologic changes are essentially similar to and often not separable from those of nummular or discoid dermatitis. When the condition persists, a chronic stage may be reached; a mildly inflamed lichen simplex chronicus pattern of reaction is then found. Eosinophils may be seen in all phases of the allergic dermatitic reaction.

In severe forms of contact irritant dermatitis, spongiotic inflammatory changes tend to be more prominent in the upper half of the malpighian layer and keratinocytes may become significantly ballooned. Individual necrotic keratinocytes may be seen, and confluent areas of epidermal cell degeneration can occasionally be found superficially in severe cases. The dermal infiltrate may contain sparse neutrophils, and these may also be prominent among the exocytotic cells, especially when the epidermis is severely damaged. These reaction patterns can be difficult or impossible to separate from phototoxic contact dermatitis (see Fig. 6–22), but the latter, when fully developed, will usually demonstrate a deep perivascular mononuclear infiltrate. Similarly, photoallergic reactions are indistinguishable from

contact allergic dermatitis, except when a deep perivascular infiltrate is present.

ATOPIC DERMATITIS

Clinical Features
The clinical expression of atopic dermatitis varies at different ages. Beginning in the first few months of life, the eruption tends to involve the head, neck, and upper trunk. Subsequently, in childhood the dermatitis favors the flexures, especially the antecubital and popliteal, which frequently become significantly lichenified. In adults, more widespread involvement of the skin may occur, but flexure patterns are often maintained. Secondary bacterial infection and folliculitis are common. Many cases, particularly the milder forms, resolve spontaneously at or after puberty. In the adult form, severe cases exceptionally evolve into erythroderma.

Histologic Features
The pathologic pattern varies very considerably.[20,21] Biopsy specimens usually reveal a dermatitis in subacute or chronic phase, but severity can be quite variable. No single pathologic description could possibly cover all the variations without repeating the entire story of spongiotic dermatitis. Epidermal hyperplasia is pronounced in the severe chronic cases, and bacterial colonization of scale crust is frequently seen in exacerbations associated with secondary sepsis. In the mild, persistent low-grade atopic states often associated with a disproportionate pruritus, the pathologic picture may be quite unimpressive. Mild acanthosis, hyperkeratosis with slight spongiosis, small foci of parakeratosis, and little cellular exocytosis constitute a common finding and represent features of modestly inflamed lichenification. Specific involvement of the follicular infundibular epithelium is present in some cases (Fig. 6–13),[22] and a diffuse dermal, usually

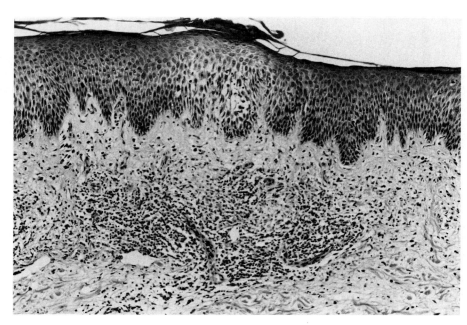

Figure 6–12. Subacute dermatitis (allergic contact dermatitis). Note similarity to lesion of Figure 6–6 (H&E, ×40).

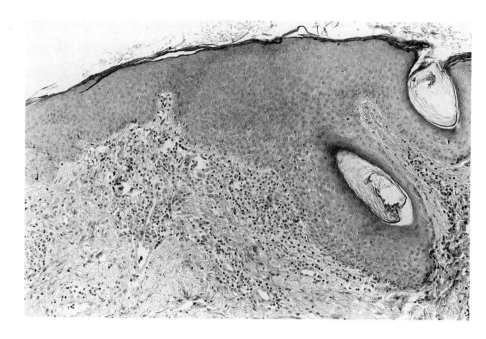

Figure 6–13. Subacute dermatitis (atopic dermatitis). Note mild edema and exocytosis of infundibulum and slightly acanthotic surface epidermis with compact scale (H&E, ×80).

sparse eosinophil infiltrate is also common; neither feature, however, is constant enough to be considered diagnostic. In chronic cases, the picture is that of lichen simplex chronicus with prominent dermal fibrosis occurring secondary to the persistent rubbing and friction (Fig. 6–14). Signs of excoriation should be anticipated in this condition, either as shallow erosions or focal ulcerations. Ichthyosis vulgaris, usually of relatively mild degree, can be present with atopic dermatitis, and follicular retention of keratin can produce pathological changes of keratosis pilaris. Immunologic phenotyping of the dermal lymphocytes in atopic dermatitis shows them to be predominantly T helper/inducer cells.[23]

NUMMULAR (DISCOID) DERMATITIS

Clinical Features

Nummular dermatitis presents round or oval coin-sized patches of intensely itchy dermatitis, usually on the arms and legs. Vesicles may be obvious at the onset of the rash, accompanied by considerable crusting. The condition often tends to affect elderly men and young adult women. No precise cause is known.

Histologic Features

Biopsy specimens taken in the very early stages reveal an

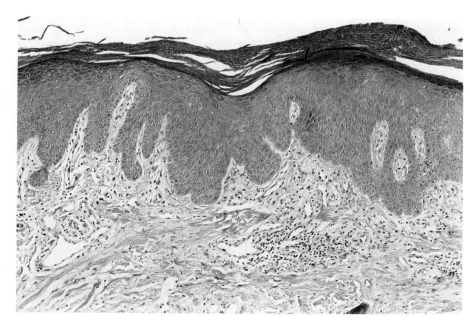

Figure 6–14. Chronic dermatitis (atopic dermatitis). Pathologic changes are those of early lichen simplex chronicus (see Fig. 6–8) (H&E, ×80).

acute spongiotic or vesicular dermatitis, but this is not often seen because patients usually seek advice after the initial phase is over. Biopsy specimens are therefore taken most frequently in the established plaque phase and characteristically show a subacute dermatitis, very often with marked epidermal hyperplasia frequently of psoriasiform proportions (Fig. 6–15). Indeed, psoriasis may be a major differential diagnostic consideration. The elongation of the rete ridges may be less uniform than in an established plaque psoriasis, and there is usually some retention of the granular layer. Indeed, hypergranulosis may be present focally. Because regeneration of the granular layer in psoriasis often occurs quite rapidly after topical therapy with corticosteroids, and because many psoriasis cases may develop secondary irritant dermatitis, some biopsy specimens defy separation. The papillary dermal infiltrate in this condition is not specifically remarkable, but thick collagen fibers may be formed in the chronic or later stages of the condition. In its subacute stage, it is indistinguishable from the subacute forms of contact dermatitis.

SEBORRHEIC DERMATITIS

Clinical Features
Seborrheic dermatitis also presents in different patterns at different ages. In infancy, the eruption is a diffuse, oozing, scaly erythema characteristically involving the head and neck, from which it may become more widespread, tending to be exaggerated in the flexures. In adulthood, men are predominately afflicted. The condition often affects the scalp, the folds of the face and ears, the sternal chest, midback, and major flexures of the trunk. The name *seborrheic* arose because of the condition's predilection to affect the major areas of sebaceous gland activity and also because of the greasy yellow appearance of the retained scales. There is considerable debate about the role of sebaceous glands in this condition. The yellow color of the scale material, however, is derived from plasma exudate and not from

sebaceous material. Secondary infection or colonization by bacteria or yeast organisms is very common.

Histologic Features
The histopathology can reflect all these clinical changes. In milder form, the biopsy results may be entirely nonspecific—usually a mild subacute dermatitis. Certain features, especially in the more florid cases, help the pathologist to consider this condition, particularly the tendency for the spongiotic reaction to involve follicular orifices. Psoriasiform epidermal hyperplasia may evolve but is accompanied by spongiosis. If retained in processing, scale crust may be prominent, and exocytosis of mononuclear cells, occasionally with some neutrophils, may occur into this thick, horny layer. Parakeratosis is often prominent. Substantial neutrophil exocytosis into the stratum corneum may occur in florid cases and tends to aggregate in and immediately adjacent to the follicular orifice. This appearance can be quite specific for seborrheic dermatitis.[24]

The concept of intermittent squirting of the fluid and cellular material through the tips of the dermal papillae has been proposed by Pinkus and Mehregan to explain this prominent exudative process, and they have suggested that the pathophysiological mechanism is not dissimilar to that seen in psoriasis.[25]

Perioral dermatitis is a papular erythematous eruption of face. It may simulate seborrheic dermatitis pathologically because biopsy specimens from patients with this condition often show a subacute spongiotic dermatitis of the infundibular portion of the follicle as well as of the surface epidermis.[26] Biopsy material is usually received in the differential diagnostic context of rosacea versus lupus erythematosus.

EXFOLIATIVE DERMATITIS (ERYTHRODERMA)

Clinical Features
Whole-body dermatitis may arise in many different ways,

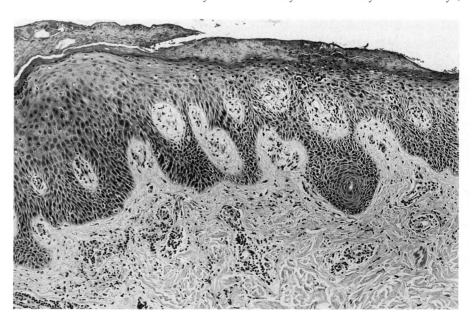

Figure 6–15. Subacute dermatitis (nummular dermatitis). Psoriasiform epidermal hyperplasia with diffuse spongiotic edema, irregular loss of the granular layer, and scale crust (H&E, ×80).

and the precise pathophysiological mechanism in any single case is obscure even when the underlying associated factors are well known. The most common causes include drug reactions, (including lichenoid drug reactions), the generalization of previously established dermostosis such as psoriasis, dermatitis, and pityriasis rubra pilaris, together with a large idiopathic group. Much less frequently, this condition can arise in association with an underlying lymphoma but especially in mycosis fungoides and the Sézary syndrome. *Exfoliative dermatitis* is the clinical term used when the erythematous skin is obviously shedding scale; *erythroderma* is the term used when scale shedding is less obvious. The condition is associated with high epidermal cell mitotic rate and is, therefore, to a greater or a lesser extent an epidermal hyperplasia.

Histologic Features

The pathological picture may reflect the underlying cause, especially when this is psoriasis or pityriasis rubra pilaris. However, this conclusion cannot be depended on because the lesions may become quite markedly spongiotic and therefore appear dermatitic.[27]

Otherwise, biopsy specimens are characterized by variable degrees of epidermal hyperplasia and by the development of thick orthokeratotic and parakeratotic scale and a mild to moderate but uniformly diffuse epidermal edema. Papillary dermal edema is often very prominent also. In drug-induced erythroderma, eosinophils may be present in the infiltrate, which may also show a tendency to involve the deeper vessels. Particular attention should be paid to the dermal mononuclear cell infiltrate and any exocytosis of the epidermis in cases referred with this diagnosis because of the association with lymphomas of the cutaneous T-cell type.[27,28] The finding of sufficient numbers of large lymphoid cells in either situation, especially when these cells demonstrate large crenated nuclei, should raise suspicion of mycosis fungoides. The tendency for these cells to aggregate in the lower half of the malpighian zone (Pautrier's abscess) is also a cardinal sign of development of this type of cutaneous lymphoma. Even when cutaneous T-cell lymphoma is established, the skin pathology may not demonstrate characteristic findings (Fig. 6–16). Exfoliative dermatitis can evolve into a persistent low-grade state, in which the biopsy specimens show a picture of lichen simplex chronicus, though edema is usually more obvious throughout all the tissues.

DYSHIDROTIC DERMATITIS (POMPHOLYX)

Clinical Features

Dyshidrotic dermatitis, a condition of unknown cause, presents with itchy vesicles and blisters on the palms and soles. Any relationship with sweat glands is entirely fortuitous, and the name represents a misnomer. The reaction occurs occasionally in atopics and occasionally as a manifestation of an id reaction (see below) or in association with demonstrable dermatophyte fungus in the overlying stratum corneum. In the chronic form, the vesicles appear in crops on a background of scaling, fissured erythema.

Histologic Features

This condition, at onset, is always an acute vesicular reaction that, because of the thick epidermis and stratum corneum, frequently evolves into substantial blistering (Fig. 6–17). A true subacute phase pathologically is often found, but even when the disease progresses without remission for months and years, the vesicular or bullous phase is usually present in the biopsy specimen. Rarely dermatophyte organisms can be found in the overlying stratum corneum, and it is always prudent to look for them. As the vesicles develop, intense spongiotic changes usually occur at the side and beneath the accumulating intraepidermal fluid (Fig. 6–18). This marginal spongiosis ultimately appears to become obliterated, perhaps by the pressure of the vesicular fluid. Exocytosis into the vesicle is normally only mild to moderate and mononuclear in type, but neutrophils occa-

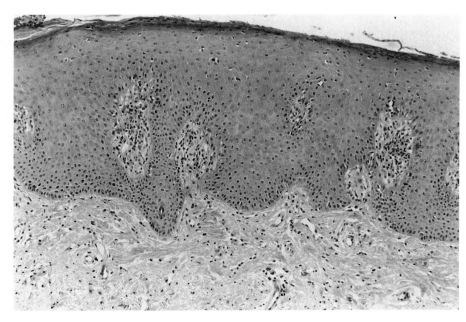

Figure 6–16. Erythoderma (Sézary syndrome). Note acanthosis with mild diffuse edema but sparse dermal infiltrate and minimal exocytosis. This biopsy specimen gives no hint of the primary diagnosis, but when uniform change of this type is present erythroderma should be considered (H&E, ×80).

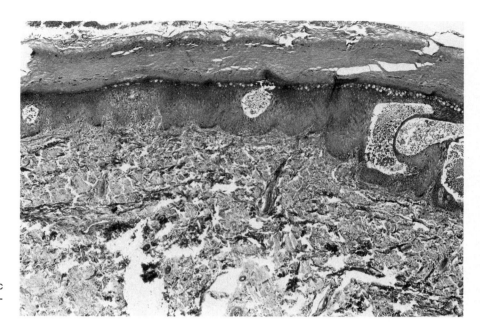

Figure 6–17. Acute dermatitis (dyshidrotic dermatitis). Numerous large vesicles are developing in acral epidermis (H&E, ×16).

sionally are present even when dermatophyte fungi cannot be demonstrated. Biopsy specimens are sometimes seen to have vesicles or small bullae of apparent dyshidrotic type, which accumulate large numbers of neutrophils and become vesicopustules. This condition can very closely mimic pustular psoriasis, and the pattern of pathologic change has been labeled pustulosis palmaris et plantaris.[29] The relationship of this condition to either dyshidrotic dermatitis and genuine pustular psoriasis is not clear.[30]

In persistent cases, the stratum corneum becomes severely disorganized by irregular areas of parakeratosis and exudate. The dermal inflammatory reaction is not specifically helpful in this condition, though eosinophils can occasionally be present in the dermal infiltrates. In very rare incidences, this reaction can be a manifestation of contact allergic dermatitis.

AUTOSENSITIZATION OR ID REACTION

Clinical Features

Autosensitization or id reaction is a poorly understood condition. It appears to represent an acute spongiotic reaction that is associated with an active but distant focus of inflammatory dermatitis. Id reactions have been linked to extensive dermatophyte infection of the feet and also with primary sites of inflamed, often secondarily infected, eczematous dermatitis, particularly those involving the leg or foot. Inflamed and impetigenized dermatitis associated with stasis or venous dermatitis is a typical example of a primary focus. Id reactions most often involve the fingers, palms, backs of hands, and volar aspects of the forearms, but other sites can be afflicted. The condition is itchy, erythematous, and may have detectable vesicles. When fungi or bacterial infection can be demonstrated at the primary site, these are never present at the site of the id or secondary reaction. Other forms of id reaction associated with dermatophyte infection have been observed and described clini-

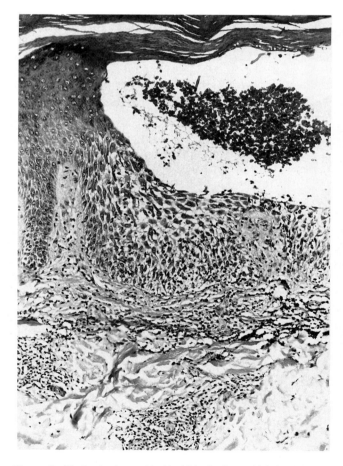

Figure 6–18. Acute dermatitis (dyshidrotic dermatitis). Vesicle lies over intense spongiotic change in acral epidermis. Note similarity to Figure 6–3 (H&E, ×160).

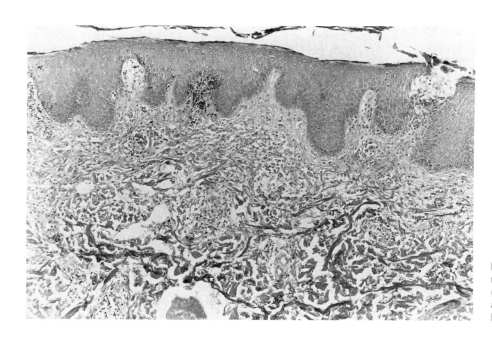

Figure 6–19. Subacute dermatitis (pityriasis rosea). A small vesicle is present at edge (right) of active lesion; parakeratotic scale and focal capillary hemorrhage are toward lesion center (middle) (H&E, ×40).

cally as erythemas, urticarial reactions, and every erythema nodosum. The pathologic changes of these reactions are not discussed here.

Pathologic changes in a developing id reaction are those of a mild, entirely nonspecific acute spongiotic or vesicular dermatitis (see Fig. 6–1). This is the only id reaction that can be recognized microscopically.

PITYRIASIS ROSEA

Clinical Features

The cause of pityriasis rosea is unknown, but the eruption is one of the most easily recognized and is one of the more common dermatoses. The lesion begins as a single scaly red patch (herald patch). A widespread truncal eruption follows about 10 to 14 days later and is often described as having an inverted fir tree pattern. Individual lesions are oval, pink or dull red, and macular; they produce branlike scales. The condition can clinically mimic secondary luetic disease. The so-called inverse pityriasis rosea follows a peripheral distribution on the limbs. Spontaneous resolution is the rule, usually within 6 to 8 weeks.

Histologic Features

Biopsy specimens from established patches of pityriasis rosea show mild to moderately severe subacute spongiotic dermatitis. Focal areas of microvesication are typical, and mounds of parakeratotic scale usually develop at the surface in the immediately adjacent epidermis (Fig. 6–19).[31,32] The dermal infiltrate may be mild or moderate in degree, but striking extravasation of red blood cells may be present around papillary capillaries (Fig. 6–20).[33,34] Despite the fact that purpura is not clinically apparent, this erythrocyte extravasation may even extend into the overlying epidermis. Eosinophils are exceptional, as also are multinucleate epidermal cells.[33] In the milder forms, the spongiotic changes can be quite mild or minimal; in this situation, the condition

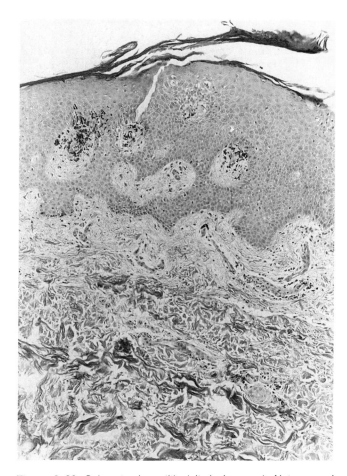

Figure 6–20. Subacute dermatitis (pityriasis rosea). Note mound of parakeratotic scale and mild spongiotic edema, with focal extravasation of red blood cells extending into the epidermis (H&E, ×80).

can be difficult to differentiate from the superficial forms of gyrate erythema. Because almost all cases of secondary luetic disease have a deep perivascular component and obvious plasma cells, adequate biopsies of pityriasis rosea rarely cause a diagnostic dilemma.

INCONTINENTIA PIGMENTI

Clinical Features

Incontinentia pigmenti almost exclusively affects girls, the trait being thought to be lethal in males. The initial phase of the X-linked genodermatosis presents with small blisters at birth or shortly thereafter and is quite brief, rarely lasting more than a few months. Only in this stage is the histopathology that of an acute vesicular spongiotic dermatitis. The vesicles are scattered over the trunk and limbs and may be arranged linearly. The disorder then evolves through a verrucous to a pigmentary stage, the latter being more persistent. Resolution within a couple of decades is usual.

Histologic Features

In this early phase, the characteristic histopathology is that of a vesicle or small blister developing in the middle of the malpighian layer and associated with intense eosinophil exocytosis that fills the vesicle cavity (Fig. 6–21).[35] In the later, vesicular period, anticipating the development of the verrucous phase, single or small clusters of dyskeratotic cells may appear in the epidermis between the vesicles.[36,37] The dermis also demonstrates eosinophils with mononuclear cells. Mihm and colleagues have described basophils in the dermal reaction also and indicate that these, together with eosinophils and mast cells, are in a stage of partial degranulation.[38] Peripheral blood leukocytosis and eosinophilia may be present.

PHOTODERMATITIS, PHOTOALLERGIC, AND PAPULOVESICULAR LIGHT ERUPTIONS

Clinical Features

As an essential component, light energy is required to generate these reactions. These clinical entities are therefore most often, but not exclusively, confined to the exposed areas of the face, neck, chest, and hands. Phototoxic reactions to topically applied compounds (e.g., perfumes) containing psoralen compounds may have a distribution that is unusual at first sight but can usually be elucidated by a detailed history. Information concerning drug ingestion is most important, as this factor can be easily overlooked. Phototoxic and photoallergic reactions are often difficult to separate clinically and, unfortunately, often impossible pathologically also. Toxic reactions are most often indurated erythemas at first, but then considerable scale crust is produced. Photoallergic reactions are characteristically more vesicular or papulovesicular at the onset. Overlaping clinical situations are frequent.

Histologic Features

Photoallergic contact dermatitis and allergic contact dermatitis are not separable histopathologically.[39] Similarly, phototoxic contact dermatitis and irritant contact dermatitis are similar. When very severe, phototoxic dermatitis may cause an acute spongiotic reaction of the upper half of the malpighian layer, with extensive disorganization and necrosis of the epidermal cells (Fig. 6–22). However, both types of photoreactions may show a dermal mononuclear infiltrate that involves the deep dermal vessels also. Photoallergic drug reactions show a moderate or severe subacute spongiotic dermatitis that also is not distinguishable from photocontact allergic dermatitis.

Papulovesicular light eruption represents a group of

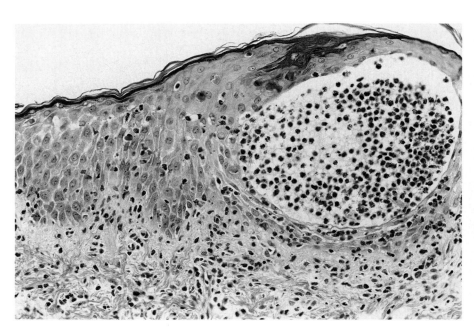

Figure 6–21. Vesicular lesion of incontinentia pigmenti. Note numerous eosinophils and mononuclear cells filling intraepidermal vesicle (H&E, ×160).

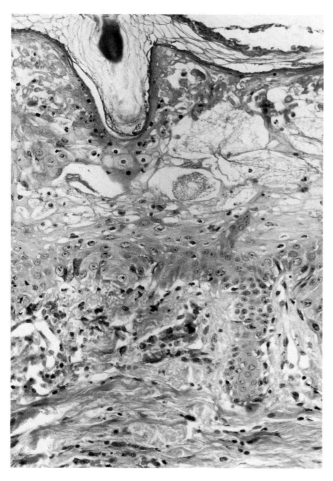

Figure 6–22. Acute dermatitis (severe phototoxic dermatitis). Note extensive degeneration and necrosis of upper two thirds of epidermis, together with intense vesicular and spongiotic alteration, (H&E, ×160).

disorders that are currently poorly understood. In most adult forms, the reaction is purely a dermal inflammation with little or no epidermal involvement. This entity is discussed elsewhere. A few cases, especially those in children, do have a true spongiotic dermatitic component, and vesicles or small blisters are usual. Many cases of this type resolve at puberty or become less severe or more papular in type. A specific form called hydroa estivale leads to scarring and may represent, in part at least, undiagnosed cases of erythropoietic protoporphyria.[40] Spongiotic dermatitic reactions occur in this type of condition, and intraepidermal vesicles and bullae can arise.

MISCELLANEOUS ENTITIES

Biopsy specimens taken from patients with so-called venous stasis (venous hypertension) dermatitis often show a mild to moderate spongiotic dermatitis in addition to an increase in thick-walled capillary vessels in the papillary dermis (see Fig. 6–5). (Contact dermatitis should not be lightly dis-

counted in this situation, as the condition is underdiagnosed and frequently coexists with stasis change.) The cause of stasis dermatitis is not understood, but it is a common clinical problem that is infrequently submitted for biopsy. When biopsy is necessary, a thin elipse often heals without difficulty whereas punch biopsy can be very slow to heal. Biopsy specimens frequently show heavy hemosiderin pigment in dermal macrophages, and fibrosis in established lesions is usual and often extends deeply into the reticular zone.

Acute and subacute spongiotic dermatitis is quite commonly associated with arthropod bites and is found over scabietic papules. Both reactions usually show significant numbers of eosinophils but have infiltrates that almost invariably extend perivasicularly into the deep dermis. Where shave biopsy specimens are taken from such lesions, however, the histologic changes can very closely resemble contact allergic dermatitis. When eosinophils are not present in substantial numbers, other forms of subacute dermatitis can be mimicked.

Dermatophyte infections may produce a spongiotic or vesicular dermatitic reaction, not only in acral sites but also elsewhere. Neutrophils usually accompany this process, but otherwise the reaction can resemble other forms of subacute dermatitis. Neutrophil exocytosis extending into the stratum corneum should always stimulate a search for fungi or yeast organisms.

REFERENCES

1. Civatte A. *Atlas D'Histopathologie Cutanee*. Paris, France: Masson, 1957:5–41.
2. Mehregan AH. *Pinkus' Guide to Dermatohistopathology*. East Norwalk, Conn: Appleton & Lange; 1986:99–110.
3. Lever WF, Schaumberg-Lever G. *Histopathology of the Skin*. Philadelphia, Pa. JB Lippincott; 1983:93–101.
4. Cronin E. *Contact Dermatitis*. Edinburgh, Scotland: Churchill Livingstone, 1980.
5. Fisher AA. *Contact Dermatitis*, 3d ed. Philadelphia, Pa: Lea & Febiger, 1986.
6. Maibach HI, Gellin GA. *Occupational and Industrial Dermatology*. Chicago, Ill: Year Book Medical Publishers; 1982.
7. Silberberg I. Apposition of mononuclear cells to Langerhans cells in contact allergic reactions. *Acta Derm Venerol*. 1973; 53:1–12.
8. Silberberg I, Baer RL, Rosenthal SA. The roll of Langerhans cells in allergic contact hypersensitivity: a review of findings in man and guinea pigs. *J Invest Dermatol*. 1976; 66:210–217.
9. Toews GB, Bergstresser PR, Streilein JW. Langerhans cell density determined whether contact hypersensitivity or unresponsiveness follows skin painting with DNFB. *J Immunol*. 1980; 124:455–461.
10. Streilein JW, Bergstresser PR. Two antigen presentation pathways, only one of which requires Langerhans cells, lead to the induction of contact hypersensitivity, abstracted. *J Invest Dermatol*. 1983; 80:302.
11. Friedlander MH, Baer H. The roll of the regional lymph node in sensitization and tolerance to simple chemicals. *J Immunol*. 1972; 109:1122–1130.
12. Pick E, Turk JL. Interactions between "sensitized lymphocytes" and antigen in vitro. IV: studies of the mechanism of release of skin reactive and macrophage migration inhibitory factors. *Immunology*. 1972; 22:39–49.

13. Luger TA, Stadler BM, Katz SI, et al. Epidermal cell derived thymocyte-activating factor. *J Immunol.* 1981; 127:1493–1498.

14. Sauder DN, Carter C, Katz SI, et al. Epidermal cell production of thymocyte-activating factor (ETAF). *J Invest Dermatol.* 1982; 79:34–39.

15. Ackerman BA, Breza TS, Capland L. Spongiotic simulants of mycosis fungoides. *Arch Dermatol.* 1974; 109:218–220.

16. Dvorak HF, Mihn MC, Dvorak AM. Morphology of delayed type hypersensitivity in man. *J Invest Dermatol.* 1976; 67:391–401.

17. Dvorak HF, Mihm MC. Basophilic leukocytes in allergic contact dermatitis. *J Exp Med.* 1972; 135:235–254.

18. Dvorak AM, Mihm MC, Dvorak HF. Degranulation of basophilic leukocytes in allergic contact dermatitis reactions in man. *J Immunol.* 1976; 116:687–695.

19. Knight AG, Black MM, Delaney JJ. Eosinophilic spongiosis: clinical, histologic and immunofluorescent correlation. *Clin Exp Dermatol.* 1976; 1:141–153.

20. Sedlis E, Prose P. Infantile eczema with special reference to the pathologic lesion. *Pediatrics.* 1959; 23:802–811.

21. Mihm MC, Soter NA, Dvorak HF, et al. The structure of normal skin and the morphology of atopic eczema. *J Invest Dermatol.* 1976; 67:305–312.

22. Ofuji S, Uehara M. Follicular eruptions of atopic dermatitis. *Arch Dermatol.* 1973; 107:54–55.

23. Lueng DYM, Bhan AK, Schneeberger EE, et al. Characterization of the mononuclear cell infiltrate in atopic dermatitis using monoclonal antibodies. *J Allergy Clin Immunol.* 1983; 71:47–56.

24. Ackerman AB. *Histologic Diagnosis of Inflammatory Skin Disease.* Philadelphia, Pa: Lea & Febiger, 1978; 278.

25. Pinkus H, Mehregan AH. The primary histologic lesion of seborrheic dermatitis and psoriasis. *J Invest Dermatol.* 1966; 46:109–116.

26. Marks R, Black MM. Perioral dermatitis: a histopathologic study of 26 cases. *Br J Dermatol.* 1971; 84:242–247.

27. Nicolis GD, Helwig EB. Exfoliative dermatitis. *Arch Dermatol.* 1973; 108:788–797.

28. Winkelmann RK, Perry HO, Muller SA, et al. The pre-Sezary erythroderma syndrome. *Mayo Clin Proc.* 1974; 49:588–589.

29. Uehara M, Ofugi S. The morphogenesis of pustulosis palmaris et plantaris. *Arch Dermatol.* 1974; 109:518–520.

30. Clayton R, Goodwin P, Fry L. DNA synthesis and mitosis in uninvolved epidermis in persistent palmo-plantar pustulosis. *Br J Dermatol.* 1976; 94:603–606.

31. Panizzon R, Bloch PH. Histopathology of pityriasis rosea Gilbert: Qualitative and quantitative light-microscopic study of 62 biopsies of 40 patients. *Dermatologica.* 1982; 165:551–558.

32. Bunch LW, Tilley JC. Pityriasis rosea: a histologic and serologic study. *Arch Dermatol.* 1961; 84:79–86.

33. Ackerman AB. *Histologic Diagnosis of Inflammatory Skin Disease.* Philadelphia, Pa: Lea & Febiger; 1978:233–235.

34. Verbov J. Purpuric pityriasis rosea. *Dermatologica.* 1980; 160;141–144.

35. Epstein S, Vedder JS, Pinkus H. Bullous variety of incontinentia pigmenti (Block-Sulzberger). *Arch Dermatol Syphilol.* 1952; 65:557–567.

36. Caputo R, Gianotti F, Innocenti M. Ultrastructural findings in incontinentia pigmenti. *Int J Dermatol.* 1975; 14:46–55.

37. Schaumberg-Lever G, Lever WF. Electron microscopy of incontinentia pigmenti. *J Invest Dermatol.* 1973; 61:151–158.

38. Mihm MC, Murphy GF, Kwan TH, et al. Characterization of the nature of the inflammatory infiltrate of the vesicular stage of incontinentia pigmenti. In Fitzpatrick TB, Kukita A, Morikawa F, et al, eds. *Biology and Diseases of Dermal Pigmentation.* Tokyo, Japan: University of Tokyo Press; 1981:163–174.

39. Ackerman AB. *Histologic Diagnosis of Inflammatory Skin Disease.* Philadelphia, Pa: Lea & Febiger; 1978:226–227.

40. Bickers DR, Demar LK, DeLeo V, et al. Hydroa vacciniforme. *Arch Dermatol.* 1978; 114:1193–1196.

CHAPTER 7
Psoriasiform Dermatitis

Thomas R. Wade and Marian C. Finan

In the various inflammatory skin diseases, the epidermis may react in several distinct patterns, one of which is psoriasiform epidermal hyperplasia. By definition, the term *psoriasiform* means "like or in the shape of psoriasis."[1] Histologically, psoriasiform epidermal hyperplasia refers to an even elongation of the epidermal rete ridges in conjunction with thinning and elongation of the dermal papillae.

Psoriasiform dermatoses include those diseases that histologically demonstrate this rather characteristic pattern of epidermal hyperplasia. These diseases can be classified as follows: (1) diseases that show psoriasiform epidermal hyperplasia as a characteristic histologic feature, (2) diseases in which psoriasiform epidermal hyperplasia is a frequent histologic feature, and (3) diseases having psoriasiform epidermal hyperplasia as an occasional histologic feature (Table 7–1). The various diseases classified into these groups, although demonstrating certain common histologic features, may be totally unrelated and of various causes.

DISEASES THAT SHOW PSORIASIFORM EPIDERMAL HYPERPLASIA AS A CHARACTERISTIC HISTOLOGIC FEATURE

PSORIASIS

Clinical Features
Psoriasis is a common skin disorder, initially recognized more than two centuries ago by Willan and Hebra.[2] In its most typical form, the disease is characterized by rounded, well-circumscribed, erythematous patches and/or plaques of various sizes. The patches/plaques are covered by abundant whitish scales. The lesions have a predilection for the extensor surfaces of the extremities, knees, elbows, scalp, sacral area, and nails. Eruption often is symmetrical. The number of lesions may vary from a single spot to hundreds of lesions. In severe cases, the disease may encompass the entire skin surface and present as an exfoliative erythroderma.[3] Guttate psoriatic lesions are of similar clinical appearance to the more well-formed plaque-type lesions of psoriasis, but are of smaller size and often less coloration.

In addition to the typical patch/plaque type of psoriasis (psoriasis vulgaris), there are other variants of psoriasis in which pustules are an integral part of the clinical picture. These include the localized forms of pustular psoriasis (three types recognized) and generalized pustular (Zumbusch's) psoriasis.[4]

Histologic Features
The histologic findings in psoriasis vary with the type and age of the lesion from which the biopsy specimen is obtained.[5] The histology of an active, typical psoriatic plaque (Fig. 7–1) shows classic findings.[6,7] The epidermis shows typical psoriasiform hyperplasia characterized by regular elongation of the rete ridges with thickening of their lower portion. The suprapapillary plate is thinned, and the granular zone is thinned to absent. Neutrophils are present, often scattered throughout the epidermis (spongiform pustules). Overlying hyperkeratosis with focal parakeratosis is noted, and collections of neutrophils are present within the stratum corneum. The dermal papillae show thinning, elongation, and edema. The vessels within the papillae are tortuous and dilated. Within the dermis is a superficial perivascular inflammatory cell infiltrate of lymphocytes, histiocytes, and scattered neutrophils.

Older, long-standing plaques of psoriasis show histologic features that are similar to those noted earlier. However, the neutrophilic component seen within the epidermis, dermis, and stratum corneum is less pronounced. In addition, the stratum corneum often shows confluent parakeratosis.

Early guttate lesions of psoriasis have a distinctly different histologic picture from those previously described.[8] The characteristic finding of psoriasiform epidermal hyperplasia is absent, and the degree of epidermal hyperplasia is minimal. In addition, the granular zone is largely preserved. A characteristic finding is neutrophils within the epidermis (spongiform pustules), beneath the stratum corneum (sub-

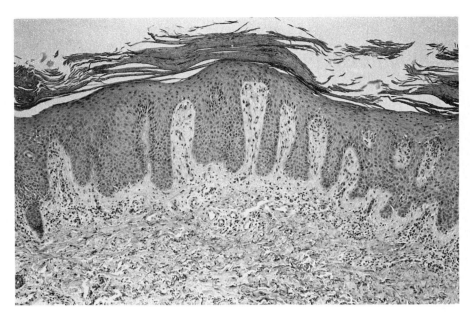

Figure 7–1. Psoriasis. **A.** This fully developed plaque shows characteristic features of hyperkeratosis with parakeratosis and focal collections of neutrophils, psoriasiform epidermal hyperplasia, a diminished to absent granular layer, dilated vessels within the papillary dermis, and a superficial inflammatory cell infiltrate (H&E, ×90).

corneal pustules), and within the stratum corneum associated with moundlike areas of parakeratosis (Fig. 7–2).[5] The papillary dermis shows mild, focal edema with dilated, tortuous vessels and a sparse superficial infiltrate of lymphocytes, histiocytes, and neutrophils. Extravasated erythrocytes are also present within the papillary dermis.

The histologic manifestations of erythrodermic psoriasis often include features that allow a definitive diagnosis of psoriasis. In many instances, however, the changes of typical psoriasis are not found and an absolute diagnosis of the underlying disease process cannot be made.[3]

Both the generalized and localized types of pustular

TABLE 7–1. PSORIASIFORM DERMATOSES

Diseases that show psoriasiform epidermal hyperplasia as a characteristic histologic feature:
    Psoriasis
    Reiter's syndrome
    Lichen simplex chronicus
    Prurigo nodularis
    Pityriasis rubra pilaris
    Inflammatory linear verrucous epidermal nevus
    Lamellar ichthyosis
    Pellagra
    Acrodermatitis enteropathica
    Necrolytic migratory erythema
Diseases that show psoriasiform epidermal hyperplasia as a frequent histologic feature:
    Contact dermatitis
    Nummular dermatitis
    Seborrheic dermatitis
    Secondary syphilis
    Mycosis fungoides
    Pityriasis rosea, herald patch
Diseases that show psoriasiform epidermal hyperplasia as an occasional histologic feature:
    Dermatophytosis and candidiasis, scaling lesions
    Scabies, Norwegian type

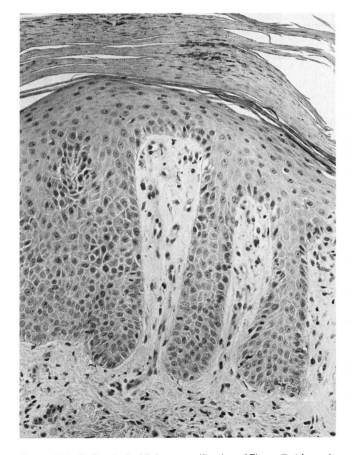

Figure 7–1. B. Psoriasis. Higher magnification of Figure 7–1A, again showing the hyperkeratosis, parakeratosis and neutrophils, psoriasiform hyperplasia, and typical changes within the papillary dermis (H&E, ×225).

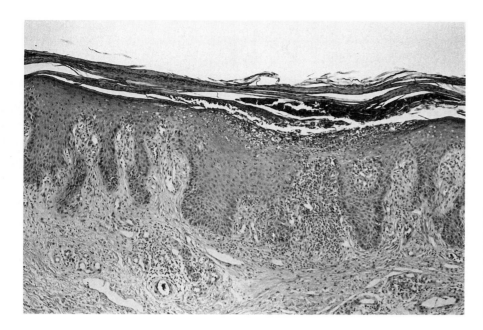

Figure 7–2. Psoriasis, guttate lesion. **A.** This lesion shows evidence of psoriasiform hyperplasia, with the presence of neutrophils both within the epidermis and beneath the stratum corneum (spongiform and subcorneal pustules) and within the stratum corneum. Again, the dermis shows dilated vessels within the papillae and a superficial inflammatory cell infiltrate (H&E, ×90).

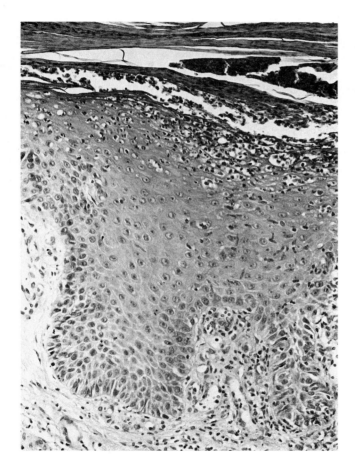

Figure 7–2. B. Psoriasis, guttate lesion. A higher magnification of Figure 7–2A showing the location of the neutrophils within both the epidermis and stratum corneum (H&E, ×225).

psoriasis share certain histologic features and may be histologically indistinguishable from each other.[9] Each is characterized by the presence of spongiform pustules within the epidermis. These pustules vary in size from small micropustules to large macropustules. The epidermis often shows psoriasiform hyperplasia. Overlying the epidermis is hyperkeratosis with parakeratosis and collections of neutrophils. The superficial dermis shows an infiltrate of lymphocytes, histiocytes, and neutrophils.

Differential Diagnosis

The active, well-developed plaque of psoriasis should present little difficulty in histologic diagnosis. Long-standing lesions of psoriasis may, however, be indistinguishable from other disease processes that show psoriasiform epidermal hyperplasia and often cannot be reliably differentiated from them (e.g., chronic contact dermatitis, chronic nummular dermatitis, chronic seborrheic dermatitis). Certain lesions of cutaneous dermatophytosis and candidiasis may also show prominent psoriasiform hyperplasia, with the presence of neutrophils within both the epidermis and stratum corneum. The presence of hyphal elements within the cornified layer is a key diagnostic finding.

The differential diagnosis of the pustular variants of psoriasis include various diseases in which collections of neutrophils are found within the epidermis. Diseases that may show this feature include subcorneal pustular dermatosis (Sneddon-Wilkinson disease), impetigo, and keratoderma blennorrhagicum (Reiter's disease).

Last, certain lesions of secondary syphilis may show psoriasiform epidermal hyperplasia as well as numerous collections of neutrophils within both the epidermis and stratum corneum (especially rupial syphilis). Unlike psoriasis, this disease often is manifested by a superficial and

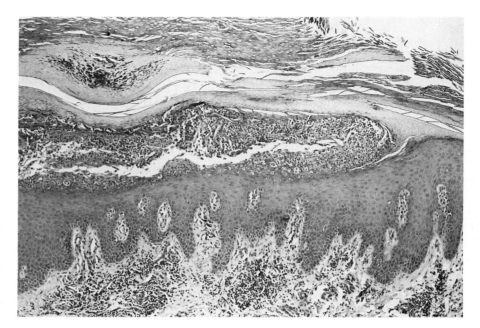

Figure 7–3. Pustular dermatitis. **A.** This lesion shows features of a pustular dermatitis with neutrophils present within the epidermis, subcorneal area, and intracorneal area. In addition, the epidermis shows psoriasiform hyperplasia. A moderately dense inflammatory cell infiltrate is seen within the dermis (H&E, ×90).

deep perivascular and lichenoid inflammatory infiltrate of lymphocytes, histiocytes, and plasma cells.

REITER'S SYNDROME

Clinical Features

Reiter's syndrome has classically been defined as a triad consisting of arthritis, urethritis, and conjunctivitis. However, the presence of mucocutaneous lesions in more than two thirds of patients has led some authors to regard this syndrome as a tetrad of symptoms.[10] More than 90% of cases occur in males, with onset most frequently during the third to fourth decades. Any one of the triad signs may occur first, accompanied by fever, malaise, and/or weight loss. Other organ systems that may be involved include the gastrointestinal, cardiovascular, and musculoskeletal systems. Epidemiologic evidence supports an infectious cause.[11] A genetic predisposition is also suggested.[12] Close clinical and histologic similarities between psoriasis and Reiter's syndrome have suggested that these diseases may be part of a pathologic continuum.[10]

Cutaneous, oral, and penile lesions may be found. The most characteristic mucocutaneous lesions, referred to as keratoderma blennorrhagica, consist of hyperkeratotic, scaling papules and plaques, often with a vesicular or pustular component on an erythematous base and involving the acral regions symmetrically, including the nail beds. Penile lesions, known as balanitis circinata, usually appear as red to hyperpigmented patches with central clearing. Oral lesions, characteristically transient and painless and involving buccal, palatal, and lingual mucosa, appear as nonspecific erosions or erythematous patches. Lesions on the lingual mucosa simulate geographic tongue. Psoriasiform lesions may also occur on the general body surface.

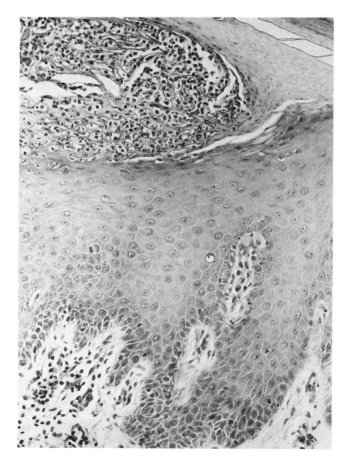

Figure 7–3. B. Higher magnification shows that most of the neutrophils have a subcorneal location. These changes can be seen in any of the variants of pustular psoriasis (H&E, ×225).

Histologic Features

Early lesions of Reiter's syndrome may show many or all of the histologic features typical of psoriasis vulgaris or pustular psoriasis, including psoriasiform epidermal hyperplasia, hyperkeratosis with extensive parakeratosis, and the presence of neutrophils within both the stratum corneum and the epidermis (spongiform pustules). The spongiform pustule, often occurring as a macropustule as in pustular psoriasis, may be quite massive and is considered to be the most characteristic histological feature of Reiter's syndrome (Fig. 7–3). Massive hyperkeratosis with very thick parakeratosis in which are embedded numerous neutrophils may also be seen, particularly in late lesions of Reiter's. The suprapapillary plate may appear thickened rather than thinned as in typical psoriasis, because of marked edema of the papillary dermis.[13] In very acute cases, vesiculation and spongiosis may occur as a result of this extensive edema.[13,14] A moderate, predominantly perivascular infiltrate may be seen in the superficial dermis, often containing significant numbers of neutrophils.

Differential Diagnosis

Lesions of Reiter's syndrome may be histologically indistinguishable from those of psoriasis vulgaris or the various forms of pustular psoriasis, including acrodermatitis continua and impetigo herpetiformis. In these instances, reliance on clinical data becomes obligatory. Features that when present may aid in the diagnosis of Reiter's include (1) massive hyperkeratosis, most typically found in late lesions; (2) thickening of the suprapapillary plate caused by extensive dermal edema; (3) a more pronounced and acute inflammatory reaction in the superficial dermis; and (4) the presence of spongiosis, with or without serous crust formation. It should be recalled, however, that the rupioid variety of psoriasis may show the same massive hyperkeratosis, with a large number of neutrophils within the horny layer, as is seen in later lesions of Reiter's.

LICHEN SIMPLEX CHRONICUS/ PRURIGO NODULARIS

Clinical Features

Lichen simplex chronicus is a reaction pattern of the skin occurring in response to chronic rubbing and/or scratching. Clinically, the lesions appear as circumscribed, lichenified papules and plaques, located most frequently on the nape of the neck and extremities, although they may occur elsewhere. Lesions are sometimes scaly and hyperpigmented, and secondary excoriation is common, as pruritus is a constant feature.

Prurigo nodularis is usually regarded as an exaggerated form of lichen simplex chronicus in which nodule formation occurs in response to chronic rubbing and scratching of discrete foci. Clinically, the lesions are single or multiple firm, dome-shaped, hyperkeratotic nodules, situated chiefly on the extremities. Erosion or ulceration is variably present.

Histologic Features

The histopathology of both lichen simplex chronicus and prurigo nodularis reflects the effects of chronic rubbing and scratching. Characteristic findings in lichen simplex chronicus include (1) psoriasiform epidermal hyperplasia, which may be either regular or irregular; (2) prominent hypergranulosis; (3) hyperkeratosis, primarily orthokeratosis, with small foci of parakeratosis; (4) dermal fibrosis, manifested as thickened collagen bundles oriented in vertical streaks in the papillary dermis[15]; and (5) a mild to moderate superficial perivascular dermal infiltrate, consisting primarily of lymphocytes and histiocytes, with occasional stellate and multinucleated fibroblasts, plasma cells, melanophages, and eosinophils (Fig. 7–4).

Spongiosis is occasionally present. More prominent parakeratosis, erosion, and ulceration are seen in cases in which scratching is pronounced. The papillary dermis may be massively thickened, up to 20 times its usual size.[15] Ectasia of vessels of the papillary dermis, with slight thickening of their walls, is frequently observed. A high percentage of mast cells in the inflammatory infiltrate has been described in some cases.[16] Silver impregnation techniques have demonstrated Schwann cell proliferation.

The changes noted in lichen simplex chronicus tend to be more pronounced in prurigo nodularis (Fig. 7–5). Epidermal hyperplasia may appear pseudoepitheliomatous and may involve hair follicles and acrosyringia. Doyle and colleagues[17] emphasized the presence of mast cells within the epidermis and dermis. Proliferations of dermal Schwann cells, with both hypertrophy and hyperplasia of dermal nerve fibers and occasional neuroma-schwannoma formation, have been repeatedly emphasized in prurigo nodularis.[18] It remains unclear whether these neural changes are a primary finding, causing the pruritus characteristic of prurigo nodularis, or are secondary to the chronic trauma of scratching.

Differential Diagnosis

Psoriasis is frequently included in the differential diagnosis of lichen simplex chronicus, as both share a similar pattern of epidermal hyperplasia. In psoriasis, however, one characteristically sees significant parakeratosis, hypogranulosis, neutrophils within the stratum corneum, thinning of suprapapillary plates, and tortuosity of capillaries of the papillary dermis—findings not characteristic of lichen simplex chronicus. The elongated rete ridges in lichen simplex chronicus tend to terminate in points rather than clubs, as in psoriasis.[19] In addition, the coarse, fibrotic collagen found in lichen simplex chronicus is absent in psoriasis.

The histology of lichen simplex chronicus may be superimposed on many pruritic dermatoses, such as contact dermatitis and nummular dermatitis, making differentiation of these diseases difficult. Hypertrophic lichen planus may be indistinguishable from lichen simplex chronicus, when the lichenoid infiltrate and degeneration of the basal layer found in the active stage of lichen planus are no longer present. Their focal presence, however, may suggest the diagnosis.

Prurigo nodularis shares with keratoacanthomas of the multiple type the presence of pronounced epidermal hyperplasia. However, the presence of marked dermal fibrosis in the former, among other features, should prove helpful in differentiating the two conditions.

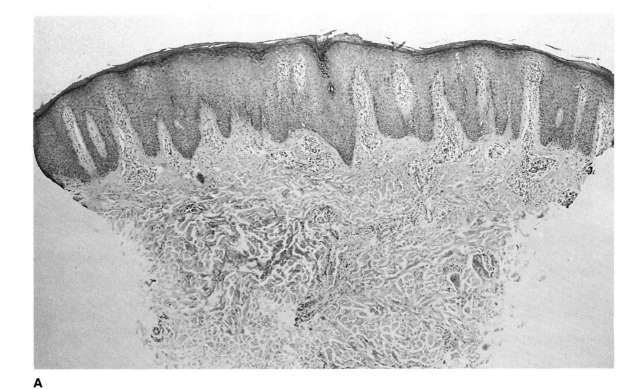

Figure 7–4. Lichen simplex chronicus. **A.** Low-power view showing compact hyperkeratosis, psoriasiform hyperplasia with focal prominence of the granular layer, and a superficial lymphohistiocytic infiltrate (H&E, ×45). **B.** Higher magnification showing to better advantage the thickened papillary dermis (H&E, ×90).

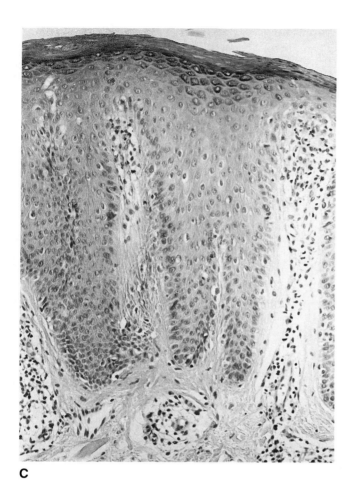

C

Figure 7–4. C. (*Continued*) Still higher magnification of Fig. 7–4A showing the collagen oriented in vertical streaks parallel to the elongated epidermal rete pegs, vessel ectasia and numerous fibroblasts. (H&E, ×225).

PITYRIASIS RUBRA PILARIS

Clinical Features

Pityriasis rubra pilaris (PRP) is an uncommon, chronic cutaneous disorder characterized by (1) prominent follicular plugging with follicular and perifollicular papules, (2) disseminated scaling plaques of erythroderma, and (3) extensive keratoderma of the palms and soles. Although the acuminate (tapered or pointed) follicular papule, with its central horny plug, is often regarded as the clinical hallmark of the disease, it is an inconstant sign and may be found in other disease processes. It is found most frequently on the dorsal hands, especially over the phalanges, but may be found elsewhere. Through coalescence of papules, orange-red plaques evolve on the trunk and extensor extremities, characteristically trapping within them islands of normal skin. Pruritus is uncommon.

The disease has traditionally been classified into two types—a hereditary (juvenile) form and an acquired form, with the latter generally occurring in adults.[20] More recently, Griffiths has subdivided this disease into five groups after analysis of clinical features and prognoses, with the classic adult type being most common, followed by a distinctive circumscribed type affecting children.[21] In general, PRP may persist from a few months to a lifetime, with spontaneous remissions occurring most frequently in the classic adult type.

Histologic Features

Characteristic findings in fully developed lesions of PRP include the following: (1) alternating orthokeratosis and parakeratosis in both vertical and horizontal directions,[22] (2) prominent conical keratotic plugs in follicular infundibula with frequent parafollicular parakeratosis, (3) psoriasiform epidermal hyperplasia, which may be regular or irregular, and (4) a mild to moderate perivascular lymphohistiocytic infiltrate in the superficial dermis. The hyperkeratosis in PRP most commonly appears in lamellar array but at times has a basket-weave appearance, particularly in early cases. The granular layer tends to be thickened in the vast majority of cases, with a tendency to its focal loss at the shoulders of the follicles in cases in which parakeratosis is prominent.[23] Occasional keratinization of the acrosyringium may be observed.[24] Spongiosis tends to be focal and slight, when present. The capillaries of the superficial dermis may be dilated but are not tortuous, as is seen in psoriasis. Occasional neutrophils and eosinophils may be seen in the superficial dermis,[23] along with lymphocytes and histiocytes (Fig. 7–6).

The presence or absence of these findings depends, in part, on the age of the lesion from which the biopsy specimen is obtained, as well as its site. Follicular plugging, in which remnants of a hair shaft may be seen, is deemed to be the most important diagnostic feature. However, unless the biopsy is obtained from a site where hair follicles

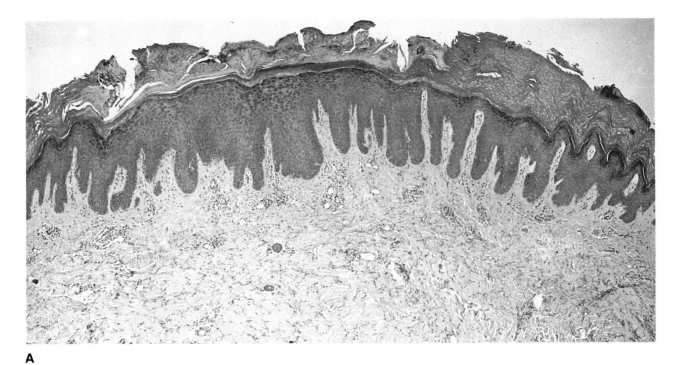

A

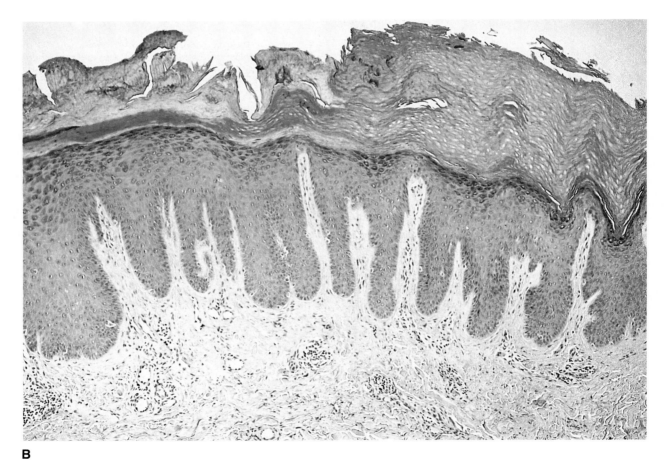

B

Figure 7–5. Prurigo nodularis. **A.** The histologic features are similar to those seen in lichen simplex chronicus, only more accentuated (H&E, ×45). **B.** Marked hyperkeratosis with focal parakeratosis, hypergranulosis, irregular psoriasiform hyperplasia, and prominent thickening of the papillary dermis, again with vertically streaked collagen (H&E, ×90).

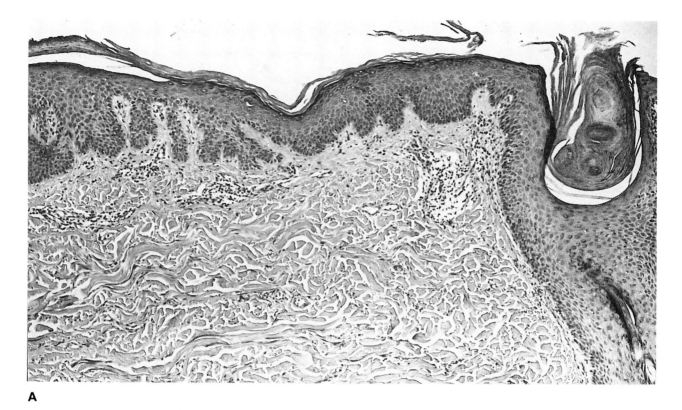

A

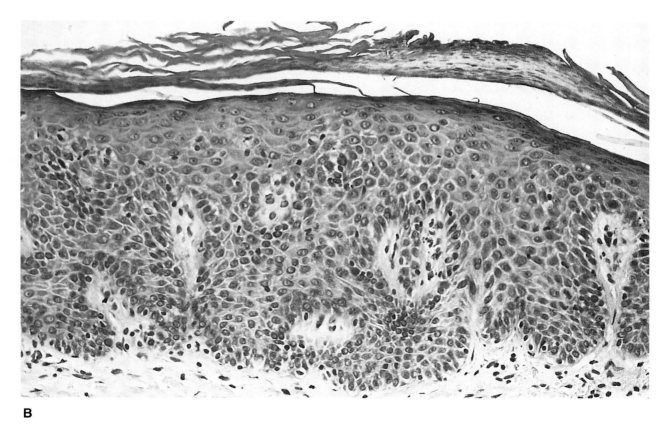

B

Figure 7–6. Pityriasis rubra pilaris. **A.** This lesion shows hyperkeratosis with a follicular plug. The epidermis shows mild psoriasiform hyperplasia, and a superficial perivascular lymphohistiocytic infiltrate is present. (H&E, ×90). **B.** Higher magnification of Figure 7–6A showing areas of alternating orthokeratosis and parakeratosis in the thickened stratum corneum (H&E, ×225).

are numerous and unless characteristic acuminate follicular papules are observed, this finding may be absent.

Soeprono recently studied 55 cases of PRP histologically and noted characteristic findings in stages that he called early, fully developed, and late.[25] He observed that a helpful feature in differentiating PRP from psoriasis at various stages has been the difference in epidermal proliferative patterns. In this detailed study, the histological features found most helpful in the diagnosis of PRP throughout most of the course of the disease included (1) alternating orthokeratosis and parakeratosis in vertical and horizontal directions, (2) focal or confluent hypergranulosis, (3) thickened suprapapillary plates, (4) broad rete ridges, (5) narrow dermal papillae, and (6) a sparse superficial perivascular infiltrate, composed primarily of lymphocytes. In early and late lesions, orthokeratosis in lamellar array tended to predominate over parakeratosis, while in fully developed lesions the parakeratosis tended to be more prominent. Suprabasal mitotic figures were observed more often in fully developed lesions. In fully developed erythrodermic lesions, the stratum corneum tended to be thinned or absent, with accompanying hypogranulosis and the occasional presence of plasma cells.[25]

Differential Diagnosis

Psoriasis vulgaris shares many common histologic features with PRP. These include the presence of orthokeratosis, parakeratosis, psoriasiform epidermal hyperplasia, suprabasalar mitotic figures, variable foci of spongiosis, dilated capillaries in the papillary dermis, and a superficial perivascular inflammatory infiltrate. However, psoriasis may be differentiated, in most instances, on the basis of a number of additional features, including (1) the presence of neutrophils within the stratum corneum, characteristically absent in PRP; (2) thin, elongated rete ridges with thin suprapapillary plates and broad dermal papillae, in contrast to the broader, shorter rete ridges with thick suprapapillary plates and narrow dermal papillae of PRP; (3) hypogranulosis, in contrast to the hypergranulosis most characteristic of PRP; and (4) tortuosity of the capillaries in the papillary dermis, a finding absent in PRP.[8] Although suprabasal mitotic figures may be found in both entities, they are more frequent and prominent in lesions of psoriasis.[25]

Phrynoderma and keratosis pilaris, like PRP, show hyperkeratosis with follicular plugging. Phrynoderma, however, lacks the epidermal hyperplasia, parakeratosis, and superficial dermal inflammatory infiltrate seen in PRP.[26] Keratosis pilaris similarly lacks these features.

INFLAMMATORY LINEAR VERRUCOUS EPIDERMAL NEVUS

Clinical Features

Inflammatory linear verrucous epidermal nevus (ILVEN) was initially described by Altman and Mehregan in 1971[27] as a clinicopathologic entity distinct from other forms of epidermal nevus. Clinically, ILVEN appears as a persistent, pruritic linear eruption consisting of multiple erythematous scaling papules, often coalescing into linear plaques that may appear verrucoid, psoriasiform, lichenified, or excori-

ated. Other characteristic clinical features include an early age at onset, a female predominance, and frequent involvement of the lower extremity.[28] As with other epidermal nevi, occasional associations with congenital malformations of the skeletal and/or other organ systems have been described.[29,30]

Histologic Features

The characteristic histologic features of ILVEN include (1) psoriasiform epidermal hyperplasia; (2) well-defined foci of parakeratosis overlying areas of hypogranulosis, alternating with foci of orthokeratosis overlying areas of hypergranulosis; (3) a mild to moderate lymphohistiocytic infiltrate within the superficial dermis, with a primarily perivascular distribution; and (4) ectasia of the superficial dermal vessels (Fig. 7–7).

Although not all of these features may be present in a particular biopsy specimen, the pattern of keratinization is believed by some authors to be distinctive and specific for ILVEN.[31] The demarcation between the two types of keratinization tends to be very sharp at both the level of the granular layer and the stratum corneum. When the two types of keratinization alternate at short intervals and are readily apparent in the biopsy specimen, the diagnosis may be easily defined. However, when they alternate at broad spatial intervals, the diagnosis may be difficult or impossible to make on histological findings alone.

Differential Diagnosis

A number of entities considered in the clinical differential diagnosis of ILVEN (e.g., linear lichen planus, linear Darier's disease, and lichen striatus) can be readily ruled out on histopathologic grounds. Linear psoriasis is probably most often confused with ILVEN, because parakeratosis, loss of the granular layer, and regular psoriasiform epidermal hyperplasia can be observed in both diseases. The alternating keratinization pattern of ILVEN may prove helpful. However, it may be difficult or impossible to rule out psoriasis in cases in which the keratinization alternates at broad intervals within a single biopsy specimen showing, for example, only the pattern of agranulosis with parakeratosis. In such cases, multiple biopsies may be necessary. Unfortunately, a distinction may not be possible, rendering the need for assessment of clinical features such as the presence or absence of typical psoriasiform lesions elsewhere.

In biopsy specimens showing hypergranulosis with orthokeratosis as the sole pattern of keratinization, a resemblance to lichen simplex chronicus is suggested. When areas of agranulosis with accompanying parakeratosis are very narrow, a resemblance to the cornoid lamella seen in various types of porokeratosis may be noted. In both of these instances, accessory histological features must be carefully studied, and again multiple biopsies may prove helpful.

LAMELLAR ICHTHYOSIS

Clinical Features

Lamellar ichthyosis is a congenital disease present either at birth or apparent shortly thereafter. The disease is characterized by broad, grayish-brown scales associated with er-

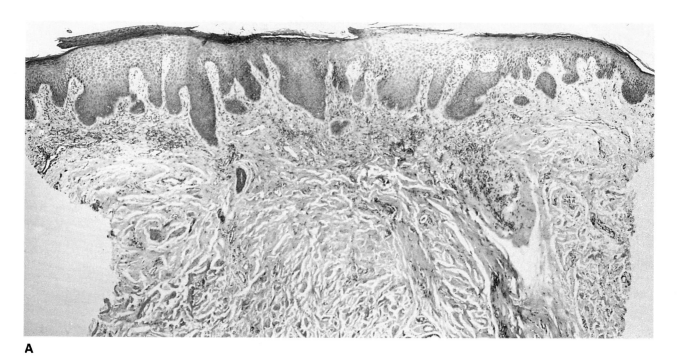

A

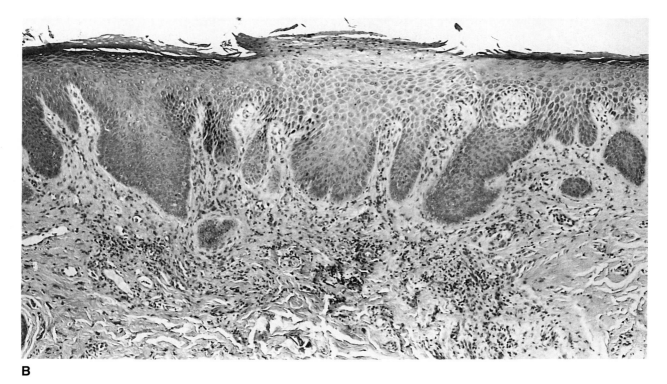

B

Figure 7–7. Inflammatory linear verrucous epidermal nevus. **A.** Low power view showing psoriasiform epidermal hyperplasia. The thickened stratum corneum shows characteristic areas of parakeratosis overlying areas of hypogranulosis, alternating with foci of orthokeratosis and relative hypergranulosis (H&E, ×45). **B.** Closer view of Figure 7–7A to show the well-demarcated zone of parakeratosis/hypogranulosis juxtaposed to the adjacent orthokeratotic stratum corneum. Note also the superficial dermal infiltrate and telangiectases (H&E, ×90).

ythema. In mild cases, only the antecubital and popliteal areas and the neck may be involved. Hyperkeratosis of the palms and soles is often present.

Histologic Features

The epidermis shows psoriasiform hyperplasia with a normal or thickened granular layer.[32] The stratum corneum shows moderate hyperkeratosis with a pattern of compact, laminated orthokeratosis. Within the dermis, a sparse superficial perivascular lymphohistiocytic infiltrate is present. In addition, the superficial dermal vessels are dilated.

Differential Diagnosis

The findings within the stratum corneum are a key feature in the diagnosis of lamellar ichthyosis and help to differentiate it from other psoriasiform processes. Differentiation from other forms of ichthyosis is possible because of the presence of psoriasiform epidermal hyperplasia (not seen in ichthyosis vulgaris or X-linked ichthyosis) in conjunction with the presence of a normal or thickened granular layer (thinned or absent in ichthyosis vulgaris).[33]

PELLAGRA

Clinical Features

Certain deficiency diseases may also show features of psoriasiform hyperplasia as part of their histological picture. In pellagra, a vitamin deficiency, the cutaneous eruption occurs on the face, neck, wrists, and dorsum of the hands and is influenced by the action of light. The lesions are well demarcated and present as areas of erythema, occasionally with vesicles. In older lesions, the skin becomes thickened, hyperpigmented, and scaly.

Histologic Features

The histologic features of early lesions usually show only a mild, superficial perivascular inflammatory infiltrate of lymphocytes and histiocytes around dilated vessels. The latter are seen especially in the papillary dermis. If vesiculation occurs, the split is usually located at the dermoepidermal junction.[34]

Older lesions show mild psoriasiform epidermal hyperplasia with pallor of the keratinocytes, especially within the upper portions of the epidermis. The stratum corneum is thickened, and confluent parakeratosis is present.[35] Again, within the dermis, there is dilatation of the superficial blood vessels and a sparse superficial perivascular infiltrate of lymphocytes and histiocytes (Fig. 7–8).

ACRODERMATITIS ENTEROPATHICA

Clinical Features

Acrodermatitis enteropathica, caused by zinc deficiency, is characterized by alopecia, gastrointestinal symptoms, and cutaneous lesions that involve the extremities and periorificial areas. The disease usually begins in infancy. The primary skin lesions are vesiculobullous, usually with pustule formation. With time, the lesions may become psoriasiform.[36]

Histologic Features

The psoriasiform lesions of acrodermatitis enteropathica show psoriasiform epidermal hyperplasia. Within the epidermis, scattered dyskeratotic cells are often present. The overlying stratum corneum shows hyperkeratosis with parakeratosis. A sparse superficial perivascular lymphohistiocytic infiltrate is present within the dermis.

NECROLYTIC MIGRATORY ERYTHEMA

Clinical Features

Necrolytic migratory erythema is the dermatosis associated with glucagonoma syndrome, a distinctive syndrome in which weight loss, anemia, diabetes mellitus, and mucocutaneous lesions occur secondary to glucagon-secreting tumors of the pancreatic islets,[37] resulting in amino acid deficiency. The cutaneous lesions most commonly present as erosions with surface crusts and are present in the groin, perineum, buttocks, distal extremities, and periorificial portions of the face. These lesions begin as small erythematous patches in which blisters form, with subsequent rupture and erosion. The lesions often appear as psoriasiform, scaly plaques.[38]

Histologic Features

A biopsy of early lesions shows characteristic changes of pyknotic and dyskeratotic keratinocytes within the upper portions of the epidermis.[38] These abrupt changes can result in both clefting and vesicle formation within the epidermis. Other areas may show intracellular edema of the superficial keratinocytes.[39] Neutrophils are often present within the involved portion of the epidermis. In addition to these changes, the epidermis may show evidence of psoriasiform hyperplasia.[38] There is a sparse, superficial infiltrate of lymphocytes and histiocytes around the vessels in the papillar dermis (Fig. 7–9).

Differential Diagnosis

Histologically, these three deficiency diseases show similar changes, and they require careful differentiation from each other. Thorough examination should, however, facilitate this process. In acrodermatitis enteropathica, there is an absence of intraepidermal edema and spongiosis. Lesions of pellagra typically show confluent parakeratosis. Neutrophils are often present within the epidermis (sometimes as spongiform pustules) in lesions of necrolytic migratory erythema.

DISEASES IN WHICH PSORIASIFORM EPIDERMAL HYPERPLASIA IS A FREQUENT HISTOLOGIC FEATURE

Certain dermatoses, when subacute to chronic and long-standing, manifest features of psoriasiform epidermal hyperplasia. Three such diseases are contact dermatitis, nummular dermatitis, and seborrheic dermatitis. In their acute phases, these disease processes show epidermal spongiosis as the primary pathologic finding. As such, they are considered to be spongiotic dermatoses and are discussed in detail

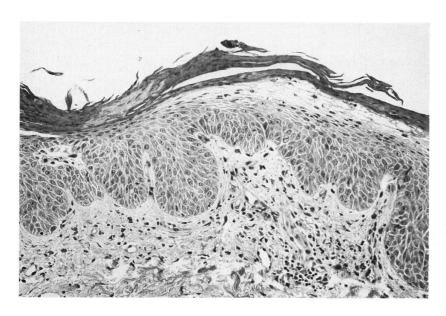

Figure 7–8. Pellagra. This lesion is characterized by hyperkeratosis with confluent parakeratosis, mild psoriasiform epidermal hyperplasia with pallor of the keratinocytes in the superficial epidermis, and a sparse superficial lymphohistiocytic infiltrate and dilated superficial vessels (H&E, ×225).

elsewhere (Chapter 6). If these diseases persist for prolonged periods of time, however, the degree of epidermal spongiosis decreases and the epidermis becomes progressively more hyperplastic, having a psoriasiform pattern.

CONTACT DERMATITIS, NUMMULAR DERMATITIS, SEBORRHEIC DERMATITIS

Clinical Features

Lesions of both subacute and chronic contact dermatitis are characterized by erythematous patches and plaques with overlying scale. Lesions of long-standing nummular dermatitis also have a patch or plaque-like appearance and are usually sharply demarcated, with overlying scale or scale crust. Pruritus is usually severe in both disease processes, and as a consequence of chronic scratching and rubbing, the lesions usually show lichenification. Lesions of seborrheic dermatitis usually present as brownish-red areas that are often sharply demarcated, with overlying yellowish or reddish-yellow scaling. In the subacute to chronic stages, the lesions become more indurated (psoriasiform). Pruritus is also a feature of this disease, and lesions may become lichenified. An exfoliative erythroderma has been noted

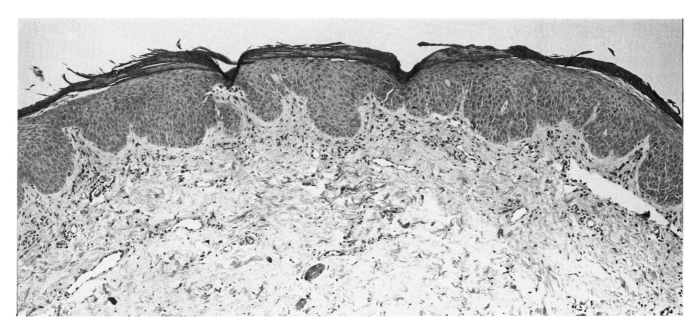

Figure 7–9. Necrolytic migratory erythema. There is mild psoriasiform epidermal hyperplasia with focal intracellular edema of the superficial keratinocytes, as well as hyperkeratosis with parakeratosis. The dermis shows a sparse superficial infiltrate of lymphocytes and histiocytes (H&E, ×90).

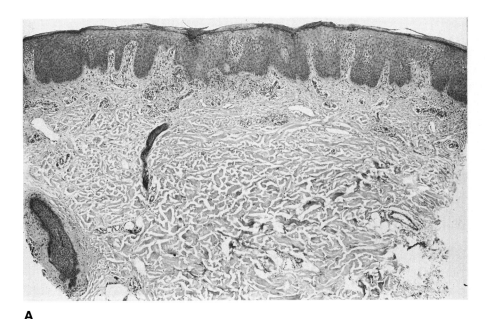

A

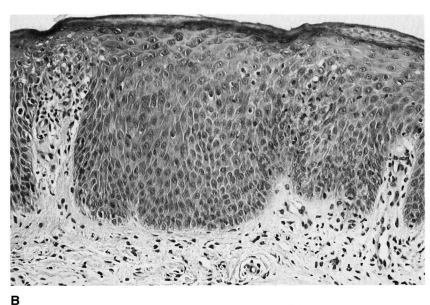

Figure 7–10. Nummular dermatitis, subacute. **A.** The key histologic feature is psoriasiform epidermal hyperplasia with spongiosis. Usually there is associated hyperkeratosis with focal scale-crusts. Similar changes are seen in lesions of subacute contact dermatitis (H&E, ×45). **B.** Higher magnification showing the areas of focal spongiosis and surface scale crust (H&E, ×225).

B

in severe cases of both contact dermatitis and seborrheic dermatitis.

Histologic Features

The histologic features of contact dermatitis and nummular dermatitis are similar in both the subacute and chronic forms of the disease.[40] In the subacute stage (Fig. 7–10), psoriasiform epidermal hyperplasia is accompanied by focal spongiosis. The stratum corneum reveals focal parakeratosis with areas of serous exudate in which inflammatory cells are present (scale-crust). Within the dermis is found a superficial, perivascular inflammatory infiltrate of lymphocytes, histiocytes, and varying numbers of eosinophils. Edema of the papillary dermis is also present.

Chronic contact dermatitis and chronic nummular dermatitis again show features of psoriasiform epidermal hyperplasia (Fig. 7–11). Focal parakeratosis is present. A superficial perivascular infiltrate of lymphocytes and histiocytes is noted within the dermis. The collagen within the papillary dermis is often thickened and oriented in vertical streaks. These latter changes are similar to those seen in lesions of lichen simplex chronicus.

Subacute seborrheic dermatitis shows mild psoriasiform epidermal hyperplasia with focal spongiosis. The stratum corneum shows focal parakeratosis and collections of neutrophils, the latter often associated with scale-crust present adjacent to follicular ostia. The follicles often are plugged with parakeratotic material. The dermis shows a mild, superficial perivascular inflammatory cell infiltrate of lymphocytes and histiocytes. In chronic seborrheic dermatitis, the

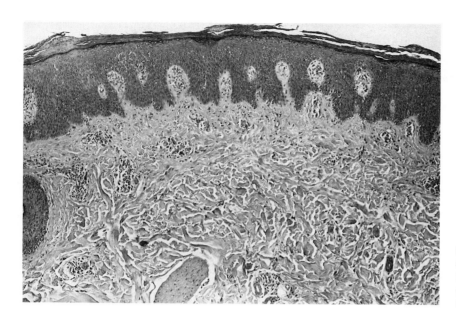

Figure 7–11. Contact dermatitis, chronic. This lesion shows hyperkeratosis with focal parakeratosis, psoriasiform epidermal hyperplasia (without spongiosis), and a superficial perivascular lymphohistiocytic infiltrate (H&E, ×90).

histologic features are similar but the epidermis shows more prominent psoriasiform hyperplasia and spongiosis is absent (Fig. 7–12).

Differential Diagnosis
Each of these three diseases in the chronic form may present difficulty in differential diagnosis, both among each other and with other disease processes that have psoriasiform epidermal hyperplasia as a prominent histologic feature. In the subacute stage, the finding of epidermal spongiosis is a helpful clue for differentiation, at least with respect to psoriasis. The histologic features of contact dermatitis and nummular dermatitis in both the subacute and chronic forms are essentially identical, thus reliable histologic differentiation is not possible.

SECONDARY SYPHILIS

Clinical Features
The cutaneous lesions of secondary syphilis are many and varied. One of its clinical patterns presents as lesions that resemble those of psoriasis, with scaly erythematous plaques. These lesions may be generalized in location.

Histologic Features
The most common histologic pattern of secondary syphilis is a superficial and deep perivascular infiltrate that may obscure the dermoepidermal interface area in conjunction with overlying epidermal hyperplasia (Fig. 7–13).[41] The epidermis may show irregular hyperplasia but quite often has a psoriasiform pattern. Neutrophils are often present, some-

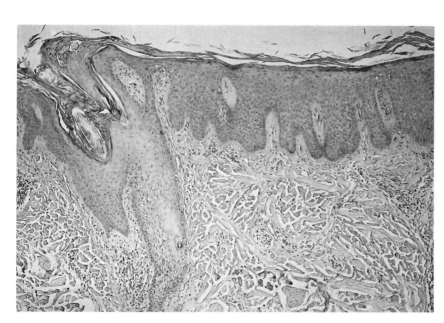

Figure 7–12. Seborrheic dermatitis, chronic. This lesion shows psoriasiform epidermal hyperplasia with overlying hyperkeratosis and focal parakeratosis. Note the follicular plug with parakeratotic material (H&E, ×90).

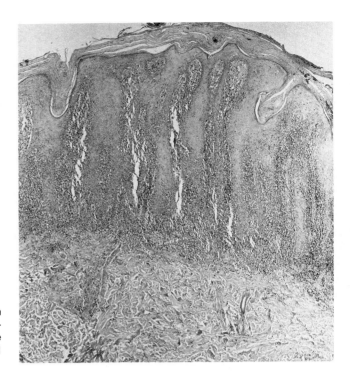

Figure 7–13. Secondary syphilis. Hyperkeratosis is present with both parakeratosis and focal scale-crust. The epidermis shows irregular psoriasiform hyperplasia, and a dense lichenoid inflammatory cell infiltrate obscures the interface area. In addition, inflammation is seen around the dermal vessels (H&E, ×90).

times as small microabscesses. Overlying hyperkeratosis is present, often attended by focal scale-crust formation. The dermis shows a superficial and deep perivascular inflammatory cell infiltrate of lymphocytes, histiocytes, and plasma cells. The plasma cell component, in some cases, may be quite prominent. In addition, inflammation obscures the dermoepidermal junction in a lichenoid pattern. Many of the dermal blood vessels have plump endothelial cells.

Differential Diagnosis
Psoriasiform lesions of secondary syphilis may be differentiated from psoriasis by the pattern, intensity, and composition of the dermal inflammatory cell infiltrate. Differentiation from lesions of mycosis fungoides may be made by the absence of atypical mononuclear cells that are present within the dermal infiltrate in mycosis fungoides and the vascular changes present in secondary syphilis.[42]

MYCOSIS FUNGOIDES

Clinical Features
Mycosis fungoides is typically divided into three stages: an erythematous or patch stage, a plaque stage, and a tumor stage.[43] In the plaque stage, the lesions may resemble psoriasis. These lesions are erythematous, scaling, and usually well demarcated from surrounding normal skin. An element of central clearing is often present.

Histologic Features
Biopsies of plaque lesions show a perivascular infiltrate of mononuclear cells, both superficial and deep within the dermis. In addition, the infiltrate is also present within

the papillary dermis, having a lichenoid pattern. The epidermis frequently shows a pattern of psoriasiform epidermal hyperplasia (Fig. 7–14). Lymphoid cells are usually present within the epidermis, either singly or in collections. Some of these mononuclear cells are almost always atypical and have convoluted nuclei. Similar atypical cells are also present within the dermis.[44] Overlying the epidermis is hyperkeratosis, usually with focal parakeratosis and scale-crust.

In long-standing plaques, the papillary dermal collagen is often thickened (similar to changes seen in lesions of lichen simplex chronicus). The dermal infiltrate may be mixed with scattered eosinophils and plasma cells, in addition to lymphocytes, histiocytes, and atypical lymphoid cells.

Differential Diagnosis
Lesions of plaque-stage mycosis fungoides and psoriasiform secondary syphilis may show some histologic similarity. In mycosis fungoides, the infiltrate shows atypical cells and the vascular changes seen in secondary syphilis are not found.

PITYRIASIS ROSEA, HERALD PATCH

Clinical Features
The herald patch of pityriasis rosea is usually larger than the succeeding lesions. Like the other lesions, it is characterized as an oval, erythematous, or salmon-colored macular or papular lesion with surface scale.

Histologic Features
The herald patch of pityriasis rosea usually shows psoriasiform epidermal hyperplasia with overlying focal parakeratosis (Fig. 7–15). Mild focal spongiosis may be present. Within

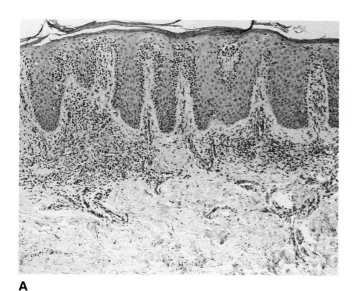

A

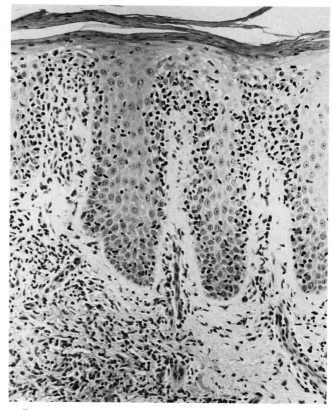

B

Figure 7–14. Mycosis fungoides. **A.** This plaque lesion shows psoriasiform hyperplasia of the epidermis, associated with a lichenoid infiltrate of mononuclear cells (H&E, ×90). **B.** A higher magnification showing psoriasiform epidermal hyperplasia with mononuclear cells, both singly and in small collections, within the epidermis (H&E, ×225).

the dermis is a superficial and deep perivascular inflammatory cell infiltrate of lymphocytes and histiocytes.[45] These changes differ from the histology of the typical eruptive lesions that develop later.

Differential Diagnosis
Differentiation between the herald patch of pityriasis rosea and other mild spongiotic, psoriasiform eruptions such as contact dermatitis or nummular dermatitis may be difficult. The presence of an inflammatory infiltrate that is usually deep as well as superficial is a helpful clue.

DISEASES SHOWING PSORIASIFORM EPIDERMAL HYPERPLASIA AS AN OCCASIONAL HISTOLOGIC FEATURE

DERMATOPHYTOSIS AND CANDIDIASIS: SCALING LESIONS

Clinical Features
The main clinical features of these two diseases are discussed elsewhere. Both diseases may present as scaly plaques.

Histologic Features
In the plaquelike lesions of both dermatophytosis and candidiasis, the histologic features are similar if not indistinguishable. Both may show psoriasiform epidermal hyperplasia,

ranging from slight to marked. Overlying the epidermis, there is usually compact hyperkeratosis with focal areas of parakeratosis. Neutrophils are present within the stratum corneum and may also be found within the epidermis. Within the dermis is seen a superficial perivascular infiltrate of lymphocytes and histiocytes (Fig. 7–16A).

The key diagnostic feature of both dermatophytosis and candidiasis is the presence of hyphal elements within the orthokeratotic portion of the stratum corneum. These can often be demonstrated with hematoxylin and eosin stained sections; however, special stains such as periodic acid-Schiff and silver methenamine facilitate their demonstration (Fig. 7–16B).

Differential Diagnosis
The differential diagnosis is described in the section on psoriasis.

SCABIES

Clinical Features
Most cases of scabies present with few, if any, visible clinical lesions. The characteristic lesion is a burrow, occurring mainly on the palms, sides of the fingers, the web spaces, the flexor surfaces of the wrists, the external genitalia of men, and the nipples of women. In certain susceptible persons, a more severe, widespread eruption referred to as Norwegian scabies may develop.[46] This latter form of scabies

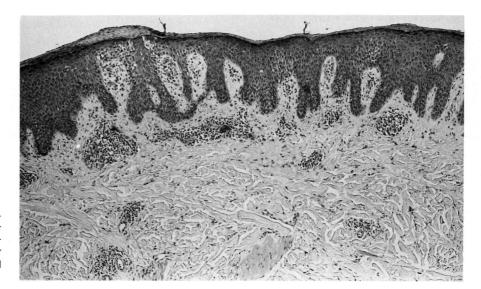

Figure 7–15. Pityriasis rosea, herald patch. This lesion shows psoriasiform epidermal hyperplasia, slight spongiosis, and focal parakeratosis. Within the dermis is a perivascular lymphohistiocytic infiltrate, usually superficial and deep (H&E, ×90).

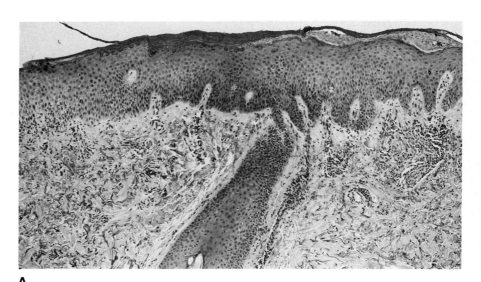

A

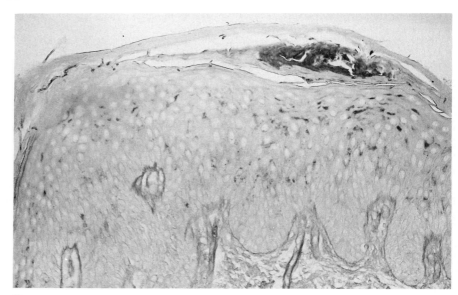

Figure 7–16. Cutaneous dermatophytosis. **A.** The epidermis shows psoriasiform hyperplasia with overlying hyperkeratosis, parakeratosis, and focal neutrophils. Focal mild spongiosis is also present within the epidermis (H&E, ×90). **B.** Higher magnification showing hyphal elements within the stratum corneum (PAS, ×225).

B

may present as an erythroderma with numerous scaling and crusted areas.

Histologic Features

Norwegian scabies shows evidence of psoriasiform epidermal hyperplasia. At times, neutrophils are present within the epidermis, often in small collections. Marked hyperkeratosis is accompanied by prominent parakeratosis and foci of scale-crusts. In addition, numerous mites are present within the cornified layer.[47] Within the dermis there is a superficial and deep inflammatory cell infiltrate of lymphocytes, histiocytes, and eosinophils.

Differential Diagnosis

The histologic diagnosis of Norwegian scabies should present little difficulty because of the numerous mites present within the cornified layer. These are readily identified on routine staining with hematoxylin and eosin.

REFERENCES

1. Leider M, Rosenblum M. *A Dictionary of Dermatological Words, Terms, and Phrases*. 3rd ed. West Haven, Conn: Dome; 1976:349.
2. Farber EM. Historical commentary. In: Farber EM, Cox AJ, Nall L, et al, eds. *Psoriasis*. Proceedings of the Third International Symposium (Stanford University, 1981). New York, NY: Grune & Stratton; 1982.
3. Abrahams I, McCarthy JT, Sanders SL. 101 cases of exfoliative dermatitis. *Arch Dermatol*. 1963; 87:96–101.
4. Baker H, Ryan TJ. Generalized pustular psoriasis. *Br J Dermatol*. 1968; 80:771–793.
5. Ackerman AB, Ragaz A. *The Lives of Lesions. Chronology in Dermatopathology*. New York, NY: Masson; 1984:181–191.
6. Soltani K, Van Scott EJ. Patterns and sequence of tissue changes in incipient and evolving lesions of psoriasis. *Arch Dermatol*. 1972; 106:484–490.
7. Ackerman AB. *Histologic Diagnosis of Inflammatory Skin Diseases*. Philadelphia, Pa: Lea & Febiger; 1978:250–256.
8. Cox AJ, Watson W. Histologic variations in lesions of psoriasis. *Arch Dermatol*. 1972; 106:503–506.
9. Lever WF, Schaumburg-Lever G. *Histopathology of the Skin*. 6th ed. Philadelphia, Pa: JB Lippincott; 1983:145–146.
10. Perry HO, Mayne JG. Psoriasis and Reiter's syndrome. *Arch Dermatol*. 1965; 92:129–136.
11. Keat A. Reiter's syndrome and reactive arthritis in perspective. *N Engl J Med*. 1983; 309:1606–1615.
12. Morris R, Metzger AL, Bluestone R, et al. HLA-W27 a clue to the diagnosis and pathogenesis of Reiter's syndrome. *N Engl J Med*. 1974; 290:554–556.
13. Pinkus H, Mehregan AH. *A Guide to Dermatohistopathology*. 3rd ed. Englewood Cliffs, NJ: Prentice Hall; 1981:105–107.
14. Montgomery H. *Dermatopathology*. New York, NY: Harper & Row; 1967:326–332.
15. Ackerman AB. *Histologic Diagnosis of Inflammatory Skin Diseases*. Philadelphia, Pa: Lea & Febiger; 1978:256–257.
16. Mikhail GR, Miller-Milinska A. Mast cell population in human skin. *J Invest Dermatol*. 1964; 43:249–254.
17. Doyle JA, Connolly SM, Hunziker N, et al. Prurigo nodularis: a reappraisal of the clinical and histologic features. *J Cutan Pathol*. 1979; 6:392–403.
18. Pinkus H, Mehregan AH. *A Guide to Dermatohistopathology*. 3rd ed. Englewood Cliffs, NJ: Prentice Hall; 1981:95–96.
19. Montgomery H. *Dermatopathology*. New York, NY: Harper & Row; 1967:190.
20. Davidson CL, Winkelmann RK, Kierland RR. Pityriasis rubra pilaris: a followup study of 57 patients. *Arch Dermatol*. 1969; 100:175–178.
21. Griffiths WAD. Pityriasis rubra pilaris. *Clin Exp Dermatol*. 1980; 5:105–112.
22. Ackerman AB. *Histologic Diagnosis of Inflammatory Skin Diseases*. Philadelphia, Pa: Lea & Febiger; 1978:263–266.
23. Niemi KM, Kousa M, Storgards K, et al. Pityriasis rubra pilaris. *Dermatologica*. 1976; 152:109–118.
24. Barr RJ, Young EM Jr. Psoriasiform and related papulosquamous disorders. *J Cutan Pathol*. 1985; 12:412–425.
25. Soeprono FF. Histologic criteria for the diagnosis of pityriasis rubra pilaris. *Am J Dermatopathol*. 1986; 8:277–283.
26. Lever WF, Schaumberg-Lever G. *Histopathology of the Skin*. 6th ed. Philadelphia, Pa: JB Lippincott; 1983:432.
27. Altman J, Mehregan AH. Inflammatory linear verrucose epidermal nevus. *Arch Dermatol*. 1971; 104:385–389.
28. Hodge SJ, Barr JM, Owen LG. Inflammatory linear verrucose epidermal nevus. *Arch Dermatol*. 1978; 114:436–438.
29. Golitz LE, Weston WL. Inflammatory linear verrucose epidermal nevus. *Arch Dermatol*. 1979; 115:1208–1212.
30. Adrian RM, Baden HP. Analysis of epidermal fibrous protein in inflammatory linear verrucous epidermal nevus. *Arch Dermatol*. 1980; 116:1179–1180.
31. Dupre A, Christol B. Inflammatory linear verrucose epidermal nevus: a pathological study. *Arch Dermatol*. 1977; 113:767–769.
32. Vandersteen PR, Muller SA. Lamellar ichthyosis. *Arch Dermatol*. 1972; 106:694–701.
33. Ackerman AB. *Histologic Diagnosis of Inflammatory Skin Diseases*. Philadelphia, Pa: Lea & Febiger; 1978:270.
34. Moore RA, Spies TD, Cooper ZK. Histopathology of the skin in pellagra. *Arch Dermatol Syphilol*. 1942; 46:106–111.
35. Ackerman AB. *Histologic Diagnosis of Inflammatory Skin Diseases*. Philadelphia, Pa: Lea & Febiger; 1978:269.
36. Wells BT, Winkelmann RK. Acrodermatitis enteropathica: reports of six cases. *Arch Dermatol*. 1961; 84:40–52.
37. Leichter SB. Clinical and metabolic aspects of glucagonoma. *Medicine (Baltimore)*. 1980; 59:100–113.
38. Kahan RS, Perez-Figaredo RA, Neimanis A. Necrolytic migratory erythema. *Arch Dermatol*. 1977; 113:792–797.
39. Sweet RD. A dermatosis specifically associated with a tumor of pancreatic alpha cells. *Br J Dermatol*. 1974; 90:301–308.
40. Ackerman AB. *Histologic Diagnosis of Inflammatory Skin Diseases*. Philadelphia, Pa: Lea & Febiger; 1978:260–262.
41. Jeerapaet P, Ackerman AB. Histologic patterns of secondary syphilis. *Arch Dermatol*. 1973; 107:373–377.
42. Cochran RIE, Thomson J, Fleming KA, et al. Histology simulating reticulosis in secondary syphilis. *Br J Dermatol*. 1976; 95:251–254.
43. Sanchez JL, Ackerman AB. The patch stage of mycosis fungoides. *Am J Dermatophatol*. 1979; 1:5–26.
44. Lever WF, Schaumburg-Lever G. *Histopathology of the Skin*. 6th ed. Philadelphia, Pa: JB Lippincott; 1983:739–741.
45. Ackerman AB. *Histologic Diagnosis of Inflammatory Skin Diseases*. Philadelphia, Pa: Lea & Febiger; 1978:331.
46. Dick GF, Burgdorf WHC, Gentry WC. Norwegian scabies in Bloom's syndrome. *Arch Dermatol*. 1979; 115:212–213.
47. Fernandez N, Torres A, Ackerman AB. Pathologic findings in human scabies. *Arch Dermatol*. 1977; 113:320–324.

CHAPTER 8
Lichenoid Dermatitis

Evan R. Farmer

The term "lichen" includes a group of plants composed of symbiotic combinations of algae and fungi. These plants are flat in shape and tend to be found in groups on the surface of rocks and tree trunks. There is a resemblance of various skin diseases to the morphology of lichens; hence the names lichen planus, lichen amyloidosus, and so on. The prototype of this group of disorders is lichen planus on both clinical and histologic grounds.

A lichenoid dermatitis or lichenoid tissue reaction is one that has the histologic features of (1) vacuolar alteration of the basal cell layer of the epidermis or epithelium and (2) a bandlike distribution of a mononuclear cell infiltrate in the dermis in close proximity to the epidermis or epithelium.[1] Lichenoid dermatitis comprises a group of fairly well defined entities, such as lichen planus and lichenoid drug eruption. Lichenoid tissue reaction is a term used to characterize this pattern of inflammation and may be seen as part of another process, such as an area of lichenoid tissue reaction in seborrheic keratosis. I use the term lichenoid tissue reaction also as a histologic signout when the features both clinically and histologically do not allow a more definitive diagnosis.

The purpose of this chapter is to present an approach to diagnosis of the various disorders included in the classification of lichenoid dermatitis. The features of lichen planus are developed as a prototype, and then the differences exhibited by the other disorders are discussed. Emphasis is placed on the following features.

1. Epidermal changes
2. Intensity of infiltrate
3. Cellular composition of the infiltrate
4. Presence or absence of a deep infiltrate

Not all clinically lichenoid lesions have a lichenoid histologic pattern (lichen simplex chronicus), and not all lesions having a lichenoid histologic pattern have a lichenoid clinical appearance (halo nevus). However, in general, the correlation is good.

The pathogenesis of a lichenoid tissue reaction is unknown, but there is increasing evidence that cell-mediated immunity, particularly involving T lymphocytes, is the mechanism.[2-6] Damage to the keratinocytes in the basal cell layer with formation of vacuolated cells and apoptotic (dyskeratotic) cells is an early event.[7] There may be a role for Langerhans' cells in these immunologic events, since they are increased in lichen planus and decreased in lichenoid chronic graft-versus-host (GVH) disease.[8] The exact role of the Langerhans' cell in lichenoid tissue reactions remains to be clarified. Recent studies suggest that various cytokines may play a significant role.[9] With the ongoing damage at the basal cell layer, there is a decrease in keratinocyte proliferation as documented by cell turnover studies, probably accounting for the hypergranulosis and lack of significant parakeratosis. Once the inflammatory infiltrate is removed either spontaneously or by therapy, there is rapid restitution of the basal cell layer with loss of the vacuolization, reorientation of the basal cells to their normal position, and no continued formation of apoptotic cells. The previously formed apoptotic cells are removed from the epidermis by migration to either the surface or dermis, or they are ingested and degraded by macrophages or adjacent keratinocytes. Melanin is deposited in the dermis during the inflammation, engulfed by macrophages, and slowly degraded. The role of immunoreactants, which are present at the dermal–epidermal junction, is not known.

LICHEN PLANUS

Clinical Features
The primary lesion in lichen planus is a violaceous, polygonal papule, which when multiple tends to coalesce into plaques. There is a characteristic distribution involving the flexural surfaces, especially the wrists and ankles, but the lesions may become generalized. Pruritus is a common and distressing symptom. Mucous membrane involvement, follicular involvement with scarring alopecia, nail dystrophy, atrophic lesions, bullae, and other unusual variants may occur.[10-14] The cause is unknown, although in individual cases, emotional stress has been thought to play a role.

Histologic Features

The epidermis shows acanthosis, hypergranulosis, orthohyperkeratosis, vacuolization of the basal cell layer, apoptosis of basal and suprabasal cells, and exocytosis of lymphocytes into the lower one third. There is usually a dense bandlike infiltrate of lymphocytes filling a normal to widened papillary dermis in direct apposition to the basal cell layer. This infiltrate tends to obscure the dermal–epidermal junction (Fig. 8–1). Apoptotic cells or apoptotic cell fragments also may be found migrating through the epidermis or singly or clustered in the upper dermis. Occasional satellite lymphocytes may be present adjacent to these apoptotic cells. Melanocytes are disrupted in the basal cell layer, with defective melanin transfer to the keratinocytes and with melanin being deposited into the upper dermis both as free particles and within melanophages. Rarely, plasma cells and eosino-

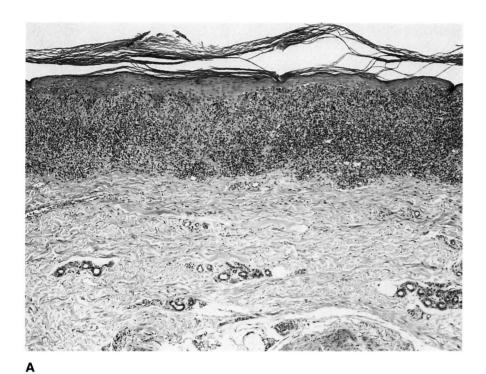

A

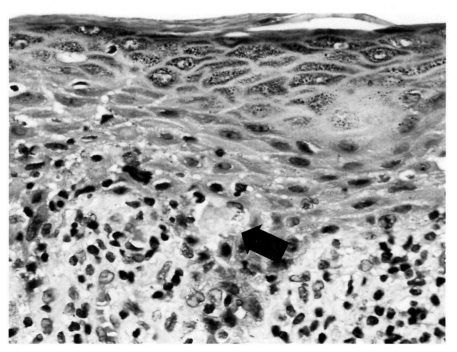

B

Figure 8–1. A. Lichen planus. This specimen shows the typical widened papillary dermis filled with lymphocytes in direct apposition to a mildly thickened hyperkeratotic epidermis and obscuring the dermal–epidermal junction. Note the absence of a perivascular infiltrate (H & E, ×55). **B.** Higher power view showing hypergranulosis, basal cell layer cytoplasmic vacuolization, infiltration of the lower third of the epidermis by lymphocytes, and colloid bodies (arrow) (H & E, ×480).

phils may be present, but they are sufficiently infrequent to allow their presence to be considered as a differential point in favor of an alternative diagnosis. As noted, when the lesion heals (resolution of inflammatory infiltrate), there is rapid reformation of a normal appearing epidermis probably over a 1- to 2-day period. The apoptotic cells stop developing and are cleared over a few days from the epidermis but may remain in the dermis for longer. The melanophages persist for at least several months, accounting for the prolonged postinflammatory hyperpigmentation. No scarring occurs from a noninfected or nonulcerated cutaneous lesion of lichen planus.

Similar features are present in the mucous membranes, except that the normal parakeratotic stratum corneum is replaced by orthokeratosis, and there is a tendency for the epithelium to ulcerate.[15] In my opinion, the evidence that lichen planus is a significant premalignant lesion in the oral mucous membrane is weak.[16]

The same pattern of inflammation is developed in the follicular epithelium and involving the nail, except that the end result is scarring with loss of the follicle or with nail dystrophy. Follicular lichen planus may develop independently without associated epidermal changes (Fig. 8–2). Bullous lesions may develop at the dermal–epidermal junction and generally are rare.

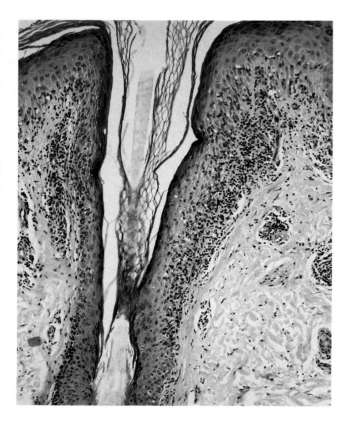

Figure 8–2. Follicular lichen planus. This specimen shows lichenoid involvement of the follicular wall with a bandlike lymphoid infiltrate. The interfollicular epidermis is spared. There is an associated mild perivascular lymphocytic infiltrate (H & E, ×75).

Differential Diagnosis
Lichen planus is one of the few inflammatory skin diseases that may be generally diagnosed based on the histologic features alone. However, an identical pattern may be seen in solitary lichen planus (also known as lichenoid keratosis), in the lichenoid phase of chronic GVH reaction, and occasionally in lichenoid drug reactions. Therefore, clinicopathologic correlation always should be made.

LICHENOID DRUG REACTION

Clinical Features
The primary lesion is a violaceous papule that closely resembles lichen planus or completely mimics it, including there being oral lesions.[17–22] The lesions tend to be widespread, however, without as much predilection for the flexural regions. I have not seen follicular or nail involvement but would not be surprised if it did occur. The lesions usually resolve when the drug is withdrawn, and hyperpigmentation remains, as in lichen planus. An exception to this resolution is the eruptions resulting from the use of some antimalarial agents.

Histologic Features
The features may be identical or quite similar to lichen planus but usually have more than just a rare eosinophil or plasma cell in the bandlike infiltrate. A superficial or a superficial and deep perivascular lymphocytic infiltrate also may be present.

Figure 8–3 is a specimen from a patient receiving gold therapy; however, the implicated drugs do not give individual distinctive features to allow the drug to be identified from the histopathologic reaction pattern.

Differential Diagnosis
In addition to lichen planus, lichenoid drug eruption must be differentiated from secondary syphilis, lichenoid chronic GVH disease, and lupus erythematosus. Endothelial cell swelling usually is more pronounced in syphilis, but lichenoid chronic GVH disease and lupus erythematosus require clinicopathologic correlation.

Lichenoid Phase of Chronic Graft-versus-Host Disease

Clinical Features
The lichenoid phase of chronic GVH disease usually develops around day 100 after an allogeneic bone marrow transplant, but I have seen cases as early as day 45.[23–25] It may or may not be preceded by acute GVH disease.

The primary lesion is a violaceous papule that tends to coalesce into plaques that either are localized or cover wide areas of the body. The dorsum of the hands and feet, the extensor surfaces of the forearms, and the face seem to be involved frequently. Oral and ocular mucosal lesions are present as well as associated sicca signs and symptoms. The lesions resolve with either hyperpigmentation or hypopigmentation.

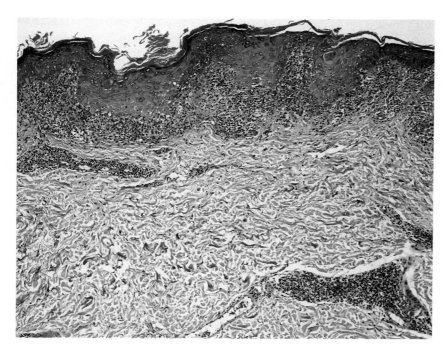

Figure 8–3. Lichenoid drug reaction. The specimen shows a bandlike papillary dermal infiltrate with overlying epidermal changes similar to those of lichen planus. In addition, there is a prominent superficial and deep perivascular lymphocytic infiltrate (H & E, ×75).

Histologic Features

The histologic features are essentially identical to those of lichen planus except that there usually is less of an inflammatory infiltrate (Fig. 8–4).[23–26] The predominant cell in the infiltrate is a lymphocyte comprising a mixture of CD-4- and CD-8-positive T cells. The oral mucous membrane lesions are associated with an underlying lymphocytic and occasional plasma cell infiltrate in the minor salivary glands. This also has been observed in some cases of lichen planus. Follicular involvement may be seen. Therefore, on histologic grounds alone, the lichenoid phase of chronic GVH disease cannot be differentiated from lichen planus and requires clinicopathologic correlation.

SECONDARY SYPHILIS

Clinical Features

Syphilis is caused by infection with the spirochete *Treponema pallidum* and, when untreated, evolves through three stages.

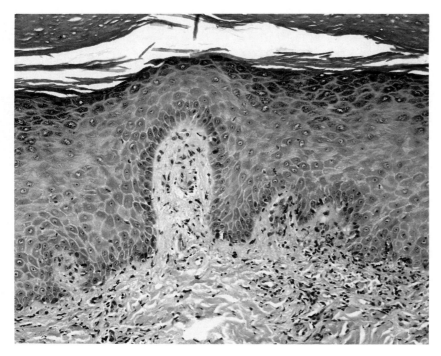

Figure 8–4. Lichenoid phase of chronic graft-versus-host disease. The histologic features are identical to lichen planus except for a much less dense lymphocyte infiltrate (H & E, ×135).

Secondary syphilis usually occurs several weeks after the appearance of primary chancre, and the two stages may overlap. These lesions are violaceous to brown-red papules that are widely disseminated, with a predilection for the palms and soles. Mucous membrane patches, generalized lymphadenopathy, fever, and fatigue variably occur.[27-30]

Histologic Features

The pattern differs from lichen planus by having a tendency to develop parakeratosis and a perivascular infiltrate in addition to the bandlike infiltrate (Fig. 8–5A). I find endothelial cell swelling to be a significant helpful feature suggesting and favoring the diagnosis of syphilis (Fig. 8–5B). Plasma

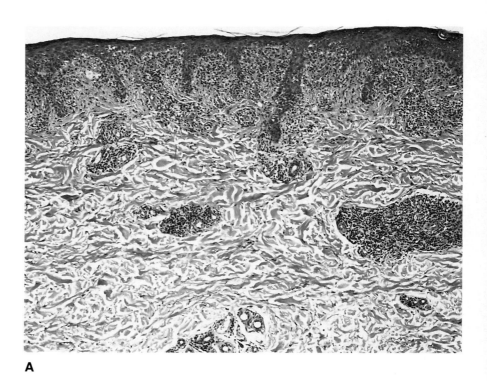

A

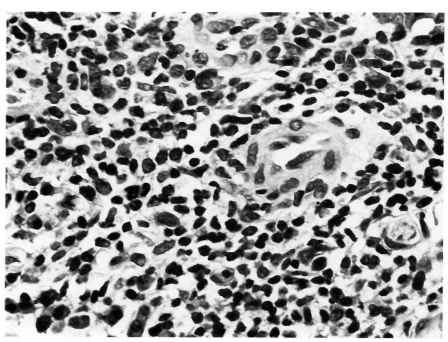

B

Figure 8–5. Secondary syphilis. **A.** This specimen shows a bandlike infiltrate filling the papillary dermis, with associated elongated rete. In addition, there is a prominent perivascular infiltrate (H & E, ×65). **B.** There is a dense perivascular lymphocytic and plasma cell infiltrate with endothelial cell swelling (H & E, ×450).

cells are typically present, but up to 25% of biopsies may not show them. Some cases also may have eosinophils in the infiltrate. Spirochetes are identifiable in the sections by Warthin-Starry or Dieterle staining.

Differential Diagnosis

Syphilis should always be considered in the differential diagnosis of a lichenoid tissue reaction whenever there is a perivascular infiltrate irrespective of whether there are plasma cells. Endothelial cell swelling seems to be the most helpful feature in differential diagnosis, since it tends not to be present in the other lichenoid disorders. To establish the diagnostic clinicopathologic correlation firmly, identification of the spirochete or a positive serologic test for syphilis should be obtained. There recently have been a few cases of serologically negative syphilis in patients with the acquired immunodeficiency syndrome (AIDS), and the spirochetes were demonstrated in biopsy.[31]

LUPUS ERYTHEMATOSUS

Clinical Features

Patients with lupus erythematosus have a wide variety of skin lesions, but some are small violaceous to erythematous papules suggestive of lichen planus. In addition, these patients may develop a lichenoid tissue reaction in discoid lesions or in the lesions usually associated with subacute chronic lupus erythematosus (SCLE) or systemic lupus erythematosus (SLE). Lupus erythematosus is discussed in more detail in Chapters 9 and 14.

Histologic Features

Most cases of lupus erythematosus show the typical features of lupus erythematosus, as discussed in Chapters 9 and 14, but a few show a pattern with a prominant bandlike infiltrate in focal areas (Fig. 8–6A).[32–35] This bandlike infiltrate almost always is accompanied by a perivascular lymphocytic infiltrate, which is helpful in differentiating lupus erythematosus from lichen planus. Lupus erythematosus usually does not have as regular an acanthotic epidermis with a well-developed sawtoothed pattern but tends to have some areas of atrophy interspersed with the acanthosis (Fig. 8–6B). Otherwise the epidermis in lupus erythematosus may be atrophic, acanthotic, or even relatively normal but almost always has some areas of vacuolization of the basal cell layer. I find that the presence of a lymphocytic infiltrate involving the eccrine glands or the presence of plasma cells points to the diagnosis of lupus erythematosus (Fig. 8–6C). Deposits of hyaluronic acid within the reticular dermis is another helpful feature, since this does not tend to occur in the other forms of lichenoid dermatitis discussed in this chapter.

In my opinion, the debate over the existence of an overlapping entity that shares features of lupus erythematosus and lichen planus is not settled.[36,37] I believe that most of these patients are shown to have lupus erythematosus on long-term follow-up.

LICHEN NITIDUS

Clinical Features

Lichen nitidus is a cutaneous disorder of unknown cause characterized by a distinctive primary lesion, a small normopigmented papule usually 1 to 2 mm in diameter. The papules generally are randomly distributed over the body surface, including the genitalia. They usually are asymptomatic. The lesions tend to be numerous, occasionally develop a linear pattern, but do not tend to fuse and form plaques.[38–40]

Histologic Features

The prominent feature is a focal infiltrate involving the papillary dermis confined by two adjacent elongated retia and consisting of lymphocytes and histiocytes (Fig. 8–7). Occasional giant cells are present. The overlying epidermis is thinned, with basal cell vacuolization. apoptotic cells usually are less in number than in lichen planus. If the section is wide enough, two or more areas of the focal infiltrate may be included, but they do not tend to fuse. Variants of lichen nitidus have been described.[41–43]

Differential Diagnosis

The tight focal infiltrate is the main differentiating point between lichen nitidus and lichen planus. These two entities are now regarded as separate but may coexist in a given patient.

LICHENOID KERATOSIS

Clinical Features

A lichenoid keratosis, also termed a lichen planuslike keratosis, is a benign lesion of unknown cause that is frequently misdiagnosed as nevi or basal cell carcinomas because the lesions are solitary violaceous to brown papules usually on the upper extremities or thorax. There is some evidence to suggest that lichenoid keratosis is a stage of a regressing lentigo.[44–49]

Histologic Features

These lesions tend to show the same features as lichen planus except for a tendency to have more parakeratosis and less of a sawtooth configuration to the epidermis (Figs. 8–8, 8–9). Some of the lesions have keratinocyte atypia in association with solar elastosis, and in these cases I use the designation "lichenoid actinic keratosis."

Differential Diagnosis

The diagnosis of lichenoid keratosis is made by a clinicopathologic correlation of the presence of a solitary lesion with the previously noted features. The lack of development of the other typical lesions will exclude lichen planus.

POIKILODERMA

Clinical Features

The term "poikiloderma" refers to patches that have mottled hyperpigmentation and hypopigmentation in a retiform

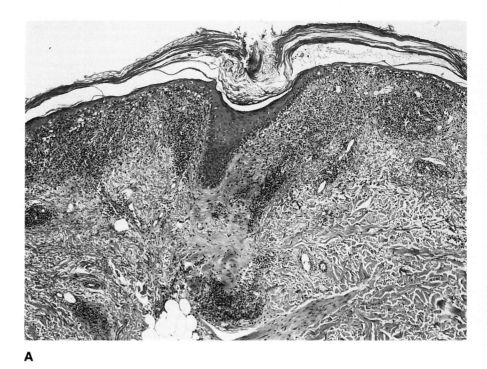

A

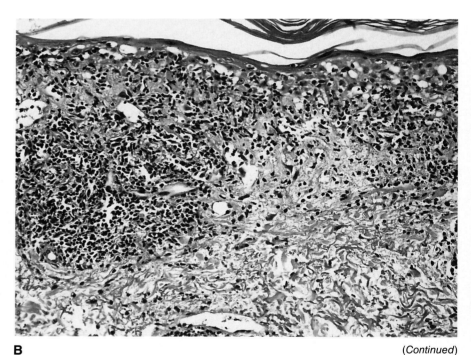

B

Figure 8–6. Lupus erythematosus. **A.** This specimen shows hyperkeratosis, follicular plugging, epidermal atrophy, a bandlike papillary dermal infiltrate, telangiectasia, and a superficial and deep perivascular lymphocytic infiltrate (H & E, ×55). **B.** Higher power view showing the epidermal atrophy, cytoplasmic vacuolization of the basal cell layer, and obscuring of the epidermal–dermal junction by the lymphocytic infiltrate (H & E, ×185).

(Continued)

(netlike) pattern, epidermal atrophy, telangiectasia, and scale. Poikiloderma may be seen as a feature of cutaneous T cell lymphoma (mycosis fungoides type), connective tissue diseases, or as part of genetic syndromes.[50–55]

Histologic Features
The epidermis is atrophic, with orthohyperkeratosis, basilar vacuolization, and apoptotic cell formation. There is a band-like lymphocytic infiltrate in the papillary dermis. In cases associated with cutaneous T cell lymphoma, the lymphocytes show nuclear hyperconvolutions, hyperchromatism, and exocytosis into the epidermis (Fig. 8–10). Otherwise, the features are identical to those in atrophic lichen planus. In cases associated with lupus erythematosus or dermatomyositis, there may be increased hyaluronic acid deposition in the reticular dermis.

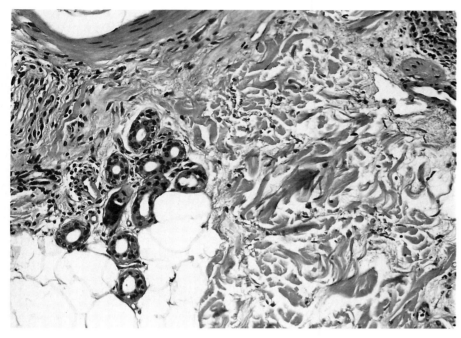

Figure 8–6 C. (*continued*) This area shows a sparse lymphocyte infiltrate among the eccrine glands and splaying of the collagen bundles by hyaluronic acid (H & E, ×185).

C

Differential Diagnosis

Almost all of my recent cases have been associated with cutaneous T cell lymphoma (mycosis fungoides type). The lack of lymphocytic epidermotropism and the presence or absence of increased dermal hyaluronic acid are the helpful differentiating features.

LICHENOID TISSUE REACTION

Clinical Features

A lichenoid tissue reaction may be used as a category of diagnosis when the histologic features or a clinicopathologic correlation does not permit a more definitive diagnosis. Many of these cases represent an inflammatory response in a previously existing epidermal or melanocytic tumor. The diagnosis of a lichenoid tissue reaction usually is not made clinically.[46,56–58]

Histologic Features

Within a preexisting tumor, there is a focus of vacuolization of the basal cell layer, apoptosis, and a bandlike lymphocytic infiltrate, hugging the epidermis (Fig. 8–11). Melanophages may be present in the upper dermis. This reaction is common in many benign tumors and is suggestive of regression or the host's attempt to control the growth. A lichenoid keratosis is probably a later stage of this phenomenon.

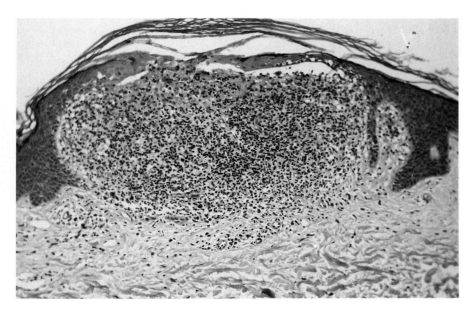

Figure 8–7. Lichen nitidus. This specimen shows the typical, focal lymphoid infiltrate in the papillary dermis limited by elongated, curved retia. The epidermis directly overlying the infiltrate tends to be atrophic (H & E, ×185).

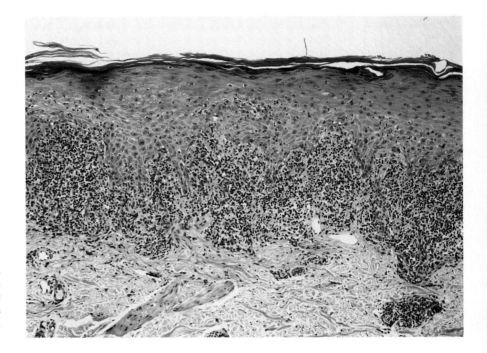

Figure 8–8. Lichenoid keratosis. This specimen shows the typical pattern of lichen planus with the addition of a mild superficial perivascular infiltrate. The diagnosis was made by clinicopathologic correlation (H & E, ×90).

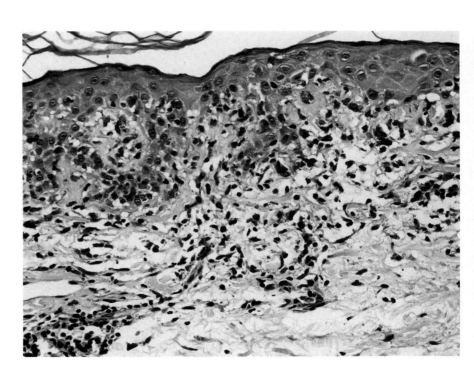

Figure 8–9. Lichenoid keratosis. This lichenoid keratosis developed from a preexisting lentigo. Note the elongated hyperpigmented rete partially obscured by the lymphoid infiltrate (H & E, ×270).

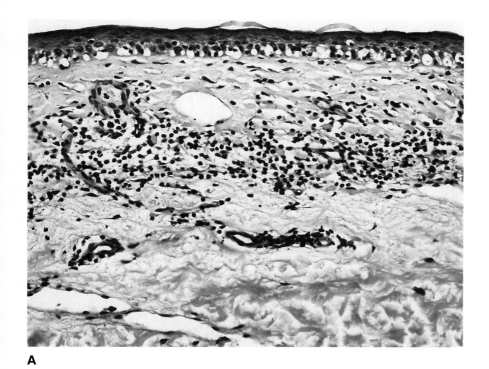

A

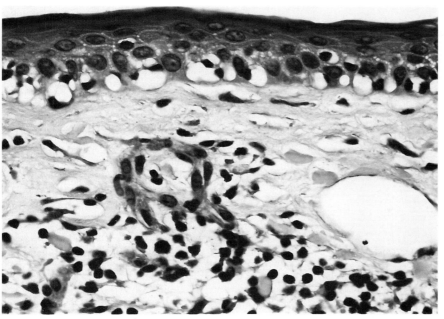

B

Figure 8–10. Poikiloderma. **A.** This specimen is from a case of cutaneous T cell lymphoma (mycosis fungoides type) and shows epidermal atrophy and a bandlike lymphocytic infiltrate with epidermotropism (H & E, ×235). **B.** Higher power view of the epidermis showing the infiltrating lympocytes (H & E, ×450).

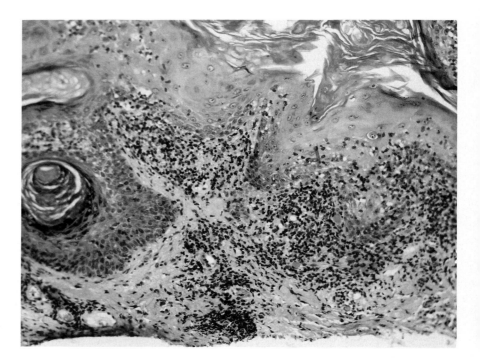

Figure 8–11. Lichenoid tissue reaction. This specimen shows an area of a seborrheic keratosis with a focus of lichenoid tissue reaction. The lymphocytes tend to be confined to the lower half of the epidermis and are arranged in a bandlike pattern in the papillary dermis (H & E, ×135).

REFERENCES

1. Pinkus H. Lichenoid tissue reactions: A speculative review of the clinical spectrum of epidermal basal cell damage with special reference to erythema dyschromicum perstans. *Arch Dermatol.* 1973;107:840–846.

2. Kofoed ML, Wantzin GL. Familial lichen planus: More frequent than previously suggested? *J Am Acad Dermatol.* 1985;13:50–54.

3. Morhenn VB. The etiology of lichen planus: A hypothesis. *Am J Dermatopathol.* 1986;8:154–156.

4. Shiohara T. The lichenoid tissue reaction: An immunological perspective. *Am J Dermatopathol.* 1988;10:252–256.

5. Shiohara T, Moriya N, Tsuchiya K, et al. Lichenoid tissue reaction induced by local transfer of Ia-reactive T-cell clones. *J Invest Dermatol.* 1986;87:33–38.

6. Shiohara T, Moriya N, Tanaka Y, et al. Immunopathologic study of lichenoid skin diseases: Correlation between HLA-DR-positive keratinocytes or Langerhans cells and epidermotropic T cells. *J Am Acad Dermatol.* 1988;18:67–74.

7. Weedon D, Searle J, Kerr JFR: Apoptosis: Its nature and implications for dermatopathology. *Am J Dermatopathol.* 1979;1:133–144.

8. Ragaz A, Ackerman AB. Evolution, maturation, and regression of lesions of lichen planus: New observations and correlations of clinical and histologic findings. *Am J Dermatopathol.* 1981;3:5–25.

9. Shiohara T, Moriya N, Mochizuki T, et al. Lichenoid tissue reaction (LTR) induced by local transfer of Ia-reactive T-cell clones. II. LTR by epidermal invasion of cytotoxic lymphokine-producing autoreactive T cells. *J Invest Dermatol.* 1987;89:8–14.

10. Miyagawa S, Ohi H, Muramatsu R, et al. Lichen planus pemphigoides-like lesions induced by cinnarizine. *Br J Dermatol.* 1985;112:607–613.

11. Prost C, Tesserand F, Laroche L, et al. Lichen planus pemphigoides: An immuno-electron microscopic study. *Br J Dermatol.* 1985;113:31–36.

12. Hanno R, Mathes BM, Krull EA. Longitudinal nail biopsy in evaluation of acquired nail dystrophies. *J Am Acad Dermatol.* 1986;14:803–809.

13. Samman PD. The nails in lichen planus. *Br J Dermatol.* 1961;73:288–292.

14. Dilaimy M. Lichen planus subtropicus. *Arch Dermatol.* 1976;112:1251–1253.

15. Andreasen JO: Oral lichen planus. II. A histologic evaluation of ninety-nine cases. *Oral Surg Oral Med Oral Pathol.* 1968;25:158–166.

16. Silverman S Jr, Gorsky M, Lozada-Nur F. A prospective follow-up study of 570 patients with oral lichen planus: Persistence, remission, and malignant association. *Oral Surg Oral Med Oral Pathol.* 1985;60:30–34.

17. McKenna WB. Lichenoid dermatitis following gold therapy. *Br J Dermatol.* 1957;69:61.

18. Matta ML, Winer LH, Wright ET. Histopathology of drug eruptions. *Arch Dermatol.* 1960;82:56–61.

19. Almeyda J, Levantine A. Lichenoid drug eruptions. *Br J Dermatol.* 1971;85:604–607.

20. Maltz BL, Becker LE. Quinidine-induced lichen planus. *Int J Dermatol.* 1980;19:96–97.

21. Wiesenfeld D, Scully C, MacFadyen EE. Multiple lichenoid drug reactions in a patient with Ferguson-Smith disease. *Oral Surg Oral Med Oral Pathol.* 1982;54:527–529.

22. Reinhardt LA, Wilkin JK, Kirkendall WM. Lichenoid eruption produced by captopril. *Cutis.* 1983;31:98–99.

23. Saurat JH, Gluckman E, Burrel A, et al. The lichen planus-like eruption after bone marrow transplantation. *Br J Dermatol.* 1975;92:675–681.

24. Shulman HM, Sale GE, Lerner KG, et al. Chronic cutaneous graft-versus-host disease in man. *Am J Pathol.* 1978;91:545–570.

25. Farmer ER. Human cutaneous graft-versus-host disease. *J Invest Dermatol* 1985;85 (suppl):124–128.

26. Farmer ER. The histopathology of graft-versus-host disease. *Adv Dermatol.* 1986;1:173–188.

27. McNeely MC, Jorizzo JL, Solomon AR Jr, et al. Cutaneous

secondary syphilis: Preliminary immunohistopathologic support for a role for immune complexes in lesion pathogenesis. *J Am Acad Dermatol.* 1986;14:564–571.

28. Winchell SA, Tschen JA, McGavran MH: Follicular secondary syphilis. *Cutis.* 1985;35:259–261.

29. Alessi E, Innocenti M, Ragusa G. Secondary syphilis. Clinical morphology and histopathology. *Am J Dermatopathol.* 1983; 22:200–203.

30. Jorizzo JL, McNeely MC, Baughn RE, et al. Rabbit model of disseminated syphilis: Immunoblot and immunohistologic evidence for a role of specific immune complexes in lesion pathogenesis. *J Cutan Pathol.* 1988;15:150–160.

31. Hicks CB, Benson PM, Lupton GP, Tramont EC. Seronegative secondary syphilis in a patient with the human immunodeficiency virus (HIV) with Kaposi's sarcoma. *Ann Intern Med.* 1987;107:492–495.

32. Montgomery H. Pathology of lupus erythematosus. *J Invest Dermatol.* 1939;2:343–359.

33. Ellis FA, Bundick WR. Histology of lupus erythematosus. *Arch Dermatol Syph.* 1954;70:311–324.

34. Prunieras M, Montgomery H. Histopathology of cutaneous lesions in systemic lupus erythematosus. *Arch Dermatol.* 1956;74:177–190.

35. Hood AF, Farmer ER. Histopathology of cutaneous lupus erythematosus. *Clin Dermatol.* 1985;3:36–48.

36. Davies MG, Gorkiewicz A, Knight A, et al. Is there a relationship between lupus erythematosus and lichen planus? *Br J Dermatol.* 1977;96:145–154.

37. Plotnick H, Burnham TK. Lichen planus and coexisting lupus erythematosus versus lichen planus-like lupus erythematosus: Clinical, histologic, and immunopathologic considerations. *J Am Acad Dermatol.* 1986;14:931–938.

38. Weiss RM, Cohen AD. Lichen nitidus of the palms and soles. *Arch Dermatol.* 1971;104:538–540.

39. Fox BJ, Odom RB. Papulosquamous diseases: A review. *J Am Acad Dermatol.* 1985;12:597–624.

40. Wall LM, Heenan PJ, Papadimitriou JM. Generalized lichen nitidus: A case report. *Australas J Dermatol.* 1985;26:36–40.

41. Eisen RF, Stenn J, Kahn SM, Bhawan J. Lichen nitidus with plasma cell infiltrate. *Arch Dermatol.* 1985;121:1193–1194.

42. Madhok R, Winkelmann RK. Spinous, follicular lichen nitidus associated with perifollicular granulomas. *J Cutan Pathol.* 1988;15:245–248.

43. Banse-Kupin L, Morales A, Kleinsmith DA. Perforating lichen nitidus. *J Am Acad Dermatol.* 1983;9:452–456.

44. Goldenhersh MA, Barnhill RL, Rosenbaum HM, Stenn KS. Documented evolution of a solar lentigo into a solitary lichen planus-like keratosis. *J Cutan Pathol.* 1986;13:308–311.

45. Frigy AF, Cooper PH. Benign lichen keratosis. *Am J Clin Pathol.* 1985;83:439–443.

46. Berman A, Herszenson S, Winkelmann RK. The involuting lichenoid plaque. *Arch Dermatol.* 1982;118:93–96.

47. Lumpkin LR, Helwig EB. Solitary lichen planus. *Arch Dermatol.* 1966;93:54–55.

48. Barranco VP. Multiple benign lichenoid keratoses simulating photodermatoses: Evolution from senile lentigines and their spontaneous regression. *J Am Acad Dermatol.* 1985;13:201–206.

49. Tan CY, Marks R. Lichenoid solar deratosis—Prevalence and immunologic findings. *J Invest Dermatol.* 1982;79:365–367.

50. Ayedemir EH, Onsun N, Ozan S, Hatemi HH. Rothmund-Thomson syndrome with calcinosis universalis. *Int J Dermatol.* 1988;27:591–592.

51. Lindae ML, Abel EA, Hoppe RT, Wood GS. Poikilodermatous mycosis fungoides and atrophic large-plaque parapsoriasis exhibit similar abnormalities of T-cell antigen expression. *Arch Dermatol.* 1988;124:366–372.

52. Shuttleworth D, Marks R. Epidermal dysplasia and skeletal deformity in congenital poikiloderma (Rothmund-Thomson syndrome). *Br J Dermatol.* 1987;117:377–384.

53. David M, Shanon A, Hazaz B, Sandbank M. Diffuse, progressive hyperpigmentation: An unusual skin manifestation of mycosis fungoides. *J Am Acad Dermatol.* 1987;16:257–260.

54. Colver G, Mortimer P, Dawber R. Premycotic poikiloderma, mycosis fungoides and cutaneous squamous cell carcinoma. Two cases and a discussion of their relevance. *Int J Dermatol.* 1986;25:376–378.

55. Fulk CS. Primary disorders of hyperpigmentation. *J Am Acad Dermatol.* 1984;10:1–16.

56. Weedon D. The lichenoid tissue reaction. *J Cutan Pathol.* 1985;12:279–281.

57. Berman A, Winkelmann RK. Inflammatory seborrheic keratoses with mononuclear cell infiltration. *J Cutan Pathol.* 1978;5:353–360.

58. Winkelmann RK, Harris RB. Lichenoid delayed hypersensitivity reactions in tattoos. *J Cutan Pathol.* 1979;6:59–65.

CHAPTER 9
Interface Dermatitis

Antoinette F. Hood and Evan R. Farmer

The term "interface dermatitis" refers to a characteristic combination of changes occurring in the epidermis and papillary dermis, which includes basilar vacuolization, dyskeratosis, and a variably intense superficial perivascular or interstitial predominantly mononuclear cell infiltrate. These histologic features are shared by a diverse group of diseases (Table 9–1).

Basilar vacuolization, also known as vacuolar alteration of the basal layer and liquefaction degeneration, is characterized by the presence of minute vacuoles below and occasionally above the basement membrane zone. Occasionally, these vacuoles may coalesce to form small clefts or even bullae. There is little known about the pathogenesis of this vacuolization phenomenon.

Dyskeratosis, or apoptosis, refers to eosinophilic hyalinized changes within individual keratinocytes associated with pyknosis, and ultimate loss of the nucleus. Apoptosis is referred to by some investigators as "programmed cell death." This finding is not specific for any dermatologic entity, but it is seen regularly in interface dermatitis and lichenoid tissue reactions. In some diseases, individual dyskeratotic cells are distinctly and intimately associated with one or more lymphocytes. Lymphocytic satellitosis in the past was considered to be pathognomonic of graft-versus-host disease, but it actually may be seen in many diseases with epidermal dyskeratosis. It is somewhat intriguing to contemplate selective specificity of this type of cell injury and to speculate why one specific cell is targeted while another neighboring keratinocyte is not affected.

ERYTHEMA MULTIFORME

Clinical Features
Erythema multiforme is an acute, self-limiting episodic eruption with a broad spectrum of clinical severity. The name is somewhat misleading, for although the appearance of the disease varies from person to person, an individual patient usually displays a relatively monomorphous type of lesion. Erythema multiforme is a relatively common disor-

der and is seen most frequently between the ages of 10 and 30 but it may occur in any age group. Depending on the extent of mucosal involvement, it is divided into two subsets: minor and major.

The lesions begin as discrete, blanchable, erythematous macules and papules that are usually asymptomatic but may be associated with a burning sensation or pruritus. The characteristic pathognomonic target, or iris lesion, consists of a central dark red area (occasionally with a blister) surrounded by an inner pale ring and an outer peripheral erythematous rim. The lesions are most prominent over the distal extremities, particularly the extensor surfaces. Palms and soles are involved frequently. Mucosal involvement, particularly the oral mucosa, is common. If mucosal involvement is extensive and extends to the ocular surfaces, the designation is erythema multiforme major, or Stevens-Johnson syndrome. Erythema multiforme major frequently is associated with bullous cutaneous lesions and systemic toxicity and fever.

New lesions occur in crops, and older lesions may remain stable, enlarge, coalesce, or develop blisters. Individual lesions last 2 to 3 weeks, and an entire episode usually lasts 4 to 6 weeks. Residual postinflammatory hyperpigmentation may persist for months.

The pathogenesis of erythema multiforme is unknown, but it is generally thought to be a hypersensitivity reaction.[1] There are well-documented associations between erythema multiforme and herpes simplex infection, *Mycoplasma* infection, and ingestion of long-acting sulfonamides. Less well documented associations have been reported with other infectious agents, medications, neoplasia, and radiation. In approximately 50% of patients, no precipitating factor can be determined.

Histologic Features
In erythema multiforme, there are microscopic changes in both the epidermis and the dermis.[2] Depending on the clinical expression, one histologic feature occasionally may predominate,[3,4] but in general, there is a mixture of findings. Early lesions, in the macular or papular stage, show only

TABLE 9–1. DISORDERS HISTOLOGICALLY CHARACTERIZED BY AN INTERFACE DERMATITIS

Erythema multiforme
Toxic epidermal necrolysis
Fixed drug eruption
Lupus erythematosus
Dermatomyositis
Drug eruption, morbilliform type
Phototoxic dermatitis
Graft-versus-host disease
Viral exanthem

mild epidermal changes, including slight intercellular edema, rare dyskeratotic cells, and basal vacuolization. In the upper dermis, there is a perivascular lymphohistiocytic infiltrate, and lymphocytes may be seen marginating along the dermal–epidermal junction. Fully formed, mature lesions (Fig. 9–1) show an increased number of dyskeratotic keratinocytes, occasionally occurring in clusters, exocytosis of lymphocytes, and an increase in intercellular edema to produce apparent thickening or acanthosis of the epidermis. Papillary dermal edema may be mild to moderate, and there is a moderately intense superficial perivascular and interstitial mononuclear cell infiltrate associated with some endothelial cell swelling and occasional extravasation of erythrocytes. The general consensus is that eosinophils and neutrophils are not present in any significant numbers in the infiltrate of erythema multiforme.

Bullae are produced by the coalescence of vacuoles to produce a subepidermal cleft.[3] The roof of the bulla often is composed of a necrotic epidermis. In the epidermis lateral to the blister, however, the characteristic dyskeratotic cells are present singly or in clusters. The dermal changes usually are similar to those described previously.

A comparison of biopsies obtained from herpes simplex-associated erythema multiforme and drug-induced erythema multiforme showed more acanthosis, intercellular edema, exocytosis, and dermal inflammation in erythema multiforme precipitated by viral infection. Drug-associated disease showed more dyskeratosis and less dermal inflammation.[5]

Differential Diagnosis

The histologic changes seen in early and mature lesions of erythema multiforme may be similar to those seen in drug eruption, viral exanthems, lupus erythematosus, and some light eruptions. Fixed drug eruptions cannot be differentiated from erythema multiforme. Morbilliform drug eruptions usually (but not always) may be differentiated by the presence of eosinophils. Viral exanthems are not well characterized histologically but, in general, have less dyskeratosis and less dermal inflammation than erythema multiforme. Lupus erythematosus is characterized by a periappendageal and perivascular infiltrate that usually extends deeper into the reticular dermis than the infiltrate associated with erythema multiforme. Light eruptions have only focal, usually mild, dyskeratosis and otherwise usually can be differentiated on a clinical basis.

TOXIC EPIDERMAL NECROLYSIS

Clinical Features

Toxic epidermal necrolysis (TEN) is a potentially life-threatening mucocutaneous reaction characterized by widespread erythema and epithelial detachment. Because it shares many clinical and histologic features with erythema multiforme, it is considered by some authors to be part of the spectrum of that disease, although others believe it is a separate entity.

TEN occurs most commonly in adults, but all age groups may be affected. Multiple etiologic agents have been

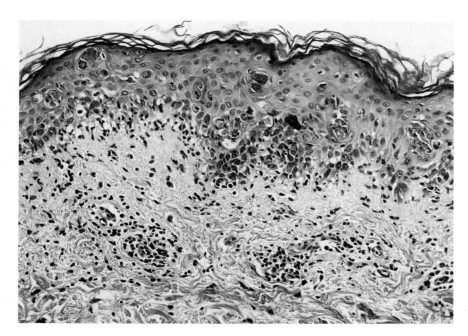

Figure 9–1. Erythema multiforme. A characteristic interface dermatitis with prominent basal vacuolization and a mild superficial mononuclear cell infiltrate. Dyskeratotic cells are scattered singly and in clusters throughout the epidermis (H&E, ×165).

incriminated in the etiology of TEN, but definite associations are rare. Drugs, especially sulfonamides, butazones, and hydantins, have been implicated most frequently.

The clinical manifestations include a diffuse macular and papular erythematous eruption that rapidly becomes confluent and widespread. The patients characteristically describe the lesions as being painful or burning. Vesicles and bullae form and rupture. Mild pressure on erythematous areas may produce detachment of the epidermis (Nikolsky's sign). As a result, there may be large areas of exposed dermis resembling a burn, with the expected risks of infection and fluid and electrolyte problems. Mucosal involvement usually is extensive and severe. Systemic involvement also has been described. Mortality rates range from 25% to 50%.

Histologic Features

Very early lesions show single cell dyskeratosis, basal vacuolization, and a scant superficial perivascular mononuclear cell infiltrate. In the more mature lesion, there is complete separation of the epidermis from the dermis, and the roof of the subepidermal bulla usually is necrotic (Fig. 9–2). Dermal vessels may show endothelial cell swelling, but there is no vasculitis.

Rapid diagnosis is facilitated by frozen tissue examination of either a sheet of exfoliating skin or a biopsy of an intact bulla. Full-thickness epidermal necrosis is characteristic of TEN and differentiates this disorder from the more benign staphylococcal scalded skin syndrome.

Differential Diagnosis

Histologically, it may not always be possible to differentiate TEN from erythema multiforme or widespread fixed drug eruption. Erythema multiforme tends to have a more intense inflammatory infiltrate, and fixed drug eruption tends to have more melanophages in the upper dermis.

FIXED DRUG REACTION

Clinical Features

Fixed drug eruptions are characterized by the appearance of well-demarcated, round to oval erythematous plaques that occasionally vesiculate and may be associated with a burning or painful sensation. The inflammatory phase is followed by hyperpigmentation, often intense and persistent. Readministration of the offending agent results in recurrence of the eruption, usually in the same location. The most commonly involved sites include the genitalia, hands, feet, and face. Many drugs have been implicated as a cause of fixed drug eruption, but the most frequent offenders are tetracycline, phenolphthalein, barbiturates, analgesics, and oral contraceptives. The pathogenesis of the reaction is not well understood.[6]

Histologic Features

The histologic changes seen in a fixed drug eruption are similar to those described for erythema multiforme and include dyskeratosis, basal vacuolization, dermal edema,

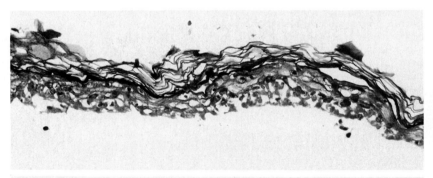

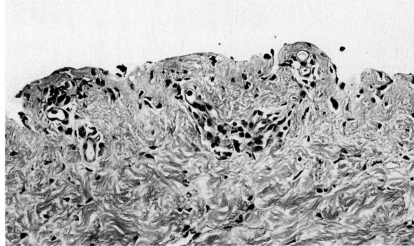

Figure 9–2. Toxic epidermal necrolysis. Composite photomicrograph showing necrotic epidermis completely separated from underlying dermis. Note paucity of dermal infiltrate (H&E, ×210).

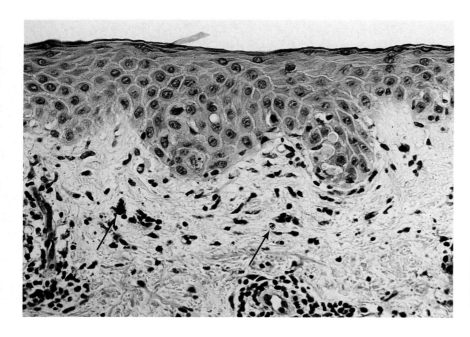

Figure 9–3. Fixed drug eruption. Dyskeratosis, basal vacuolization, papillary dermal edema, superficial perivascular mononuclear cell infiltrate, and pigment incontinence (arrows) (H&E, ×280).

and a perivascular and interstitial lymphohistiocytic infiltrate. Eosinophils may be present. Subepidermal vesicles and bullae with overlying epidermal necrosis may occur. Older and recurrent lesions have melanin deposition in the upper dermis (Fig. 9–3).

The presence of eosinophils or melanin is helpful in differentiating fixed drug eruption from erythema multiforme, light eruptions, and lupus erythematosus.

LUPUS ERYTHEMATOSUS

Clinical Features

Lupus erythematosus is a heterogeneous inflammatory disorder with a broad spectrum of clinical manifestations in the skin. Based on the morphologic features of the cutane-

ous lesions, serologic data, and symptomatology, three subsets of the disease have been defined—chronic cutaneous lupus erythematosus (CCLE), subacute cutaneous lupus erythematosus (SCLE), and acute cutaneous lupus erythematosus (ACLE)—but considerable overlap in features may occur, and these subsets are not absolute (Table 9–2).

Chronic Cutaneous Lupus Erythematosus

Clinical Features

The most common form of CCLE is discoid lupus erythematosus. Discoid lesions are characteristically well demarcated, scaly papules and plaques with prominent dilated follicular openings. Early and active lesions are erythematous; older lesions usually exhibit alterations in pigmentation (hyperpigmentation, hypopigmentation) and atrophy. Discoid le-

TABLE 9–2. MAJOR SUBSETS OF LUPUS ERYTHEMATOSUS

Feature	CCLE	SCLE	ACLE
Clinical forms	Localized Generalized Hypertrophic Lupus profundus	Papulosquamous (psoriasiform) Annular-polycyclic	Facial (malar) erythema Widespread erythema of head, neck, upper trunk, extensor arms, and back of hands Bullous or TEN-like lesions Vasculitic lesions
Clinical features	Usually localized, chronic scarring lesions of head, neck, and upper extremities 5% incidence of associated ACLE	Widespread, nonscarring lesions in photosensitive distribution, usually above waist Severe renal disease uncommon	Transient (hours to days) erythema, and macular or indurated lesions
Serology	5–10% ANA positive	70% ANA positive 40–60% have + Ro and La antibodies	>90% ANA positive
Ig depostion along dermal–epidermal junction	+80% involved skin; may be negative if lesions are <3 months old	+50% lesional skin	+95% lesional skin; +75% nonlesional skin (lupus band test)

sions are typically limited in number and are localized to the head, particularly the ears, scalp, and face. However, a generalized form of the disease occurs with lesions above and below the neck. More than 90% of patients with CCLE have disease that is confined to the skin, and progression of localized discoid CCLE to the systemic LE is rare. Discoid lesions are present in up to 25% of patients with systemic, acute lupus erythematosus. Patients with CCLE rarely have significantly elevated antinuclear antibody (ANA) tests.

Verrucous or hypertrophic lesions are a less common manifestation of CCLE and usually are seen in conjunction with discoid lesions. Verrucous lupus erythematosus, as the name suggests, is characterized by elevated scaly erythematous papules, nodules, or annular plaques that are most frequently located on the extremities. Clinically, these lesions may be confused with keratoacanthoma, prurigo nodularis, lichen planus, and squamous cell carcinoma.

Lupus profundus, or panniculitis, may occur as a form of CCLE, often associated with concomitant discoid lesions, or it may occur in association with systemic LE. The lesions occur as subcutaneous nodules on the head, trunk, forearms, buttocks, and thighs. Ulceration, especially after trauma, is common.

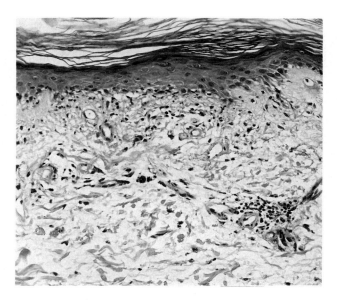

Figure 9–4. Lupus erythematosus. Basal vacuolization, papillary dermal edema, and perivascular mononuclear cell infiltrate (H&E, ×220).

Subacute Cutaneous Lupus Erythematosus

Clinical Features
The lesions associated with SCLE are nonscarring, mildly scaly, erythematous, telangiectatic lesions distributed over the upper trunk, the V-area of the neck, and the extensor surface of the arms. Two morphologic patterns have been described: (1) papulosquamous lesions resembling psoriasis and (2) annular lesions. Approximately 75% of patients with SCLE have positive ANAs, and over 60% have circulating cytoplasmic antibodies to the Ro/SSA antigen. Antibodies to double-stranded DNA, RNP, and Sm are not commonly found.

Acute Cutaneous Lupus Erythematosus

Clinical Features
This form of lupus erythematosus is associated with systemic disease. ACLE lesions are characteristically transient, erythematous, and only mildly scaly. They may occur in the characteristic butterfly malar erythematous eruption or as more diffuse erythematous lesions scattered over the head, upper trunk, and extensor surfaces of the extremities. Discoid lesions, panniculitis, bullous lesions, vascular lesions (palpable purpura, livedo reticularis, urticaria), and alopecia also may be seen in association with ACLE. Patients with ACLE usually have positive ANA and anti-DNA antibody tests, hypocomplementemia, hypergammaglobulinemia, anemia, and leukopenia.

Common Findings

Histologic Features
The histologic changes seen in individual lesions correlate better with the morphology and the age of the lesion than with the specific clinical subset or with serologic findings.[7]

The histologic features common to most lesions of lupus erythematosus include vacuolar alteration of the basal layer, a perivascular mononuclear cell infiltrate, edema of the papillary dermis, and extravasation of erythrocytes (Fig. 9–4).[8–11]

Vacuolar alteration of the basal layer is characterized by the presence of minute vacuoles between and beneath basal cells. This finding, which may be very subtle, becomes more apparent when the basement membrane zone is visually intensified with PAS stain. The vacuoles often are present along the basal layer of the epidermal appendages, especially the hair follicles. Along with the vacuolar alteration is often an alteration in the basal cells themselves. These normally columnar cells lose their vertical orientation, become more polyhedral or cuboidal in configuration, and thus assume a squamotized appearance (Fig. 9–5).

The composition of the perivascular infiltrate is mononuclear cell with a prominence of lymphocytes. Immunohistochemical studies have shown that the numbers of helper and suppressor cells are approximately equal in number.[12] Occasional histiocytic cells and plasma cells may be present.

The infiltrate may be present only in the upper dermis or throughout the papillary and reticular dermis (Fig. 9–6). The intensity of the infiltrate varies from mild to marked. In addition to a perivascular accumulation of cells, lymphocytes may be seen between vessels, occasionally in a bandlike pattern, and around appendages (Fig. 9–7). Extension into the panniculus is not uncommon. Endothelial cell swelling often is seen in association with the perivascular mononuclear cell infiltrate. The presence of endothelial cell swelling, lymphocytes, fibrin deposition, and extravasation of erythrocytes is often referred to as a lymphocytic vasculitis (Fig. 9–8). These histologic changes may accompany macular or papular purpuric lesions or may be seen in otherwise typical lupus erythematosus lesions.

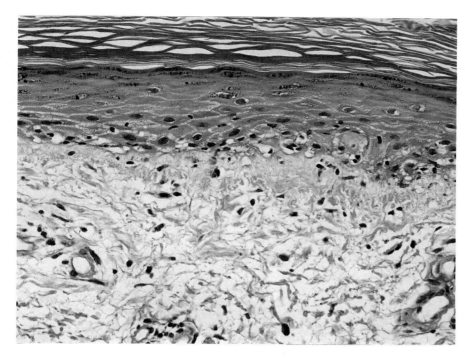

Figure 9–5. Lupus erythematosus. Basal vacuolization, dyskeratosis, squamatization of basal cell layer, vascular ectasia, and papillary dermal edema (H&E, ×300).

Papillary dermal edema is a common histologic feature in all forms of lupus erythematosus, although it may be quite mild in some cases. Dermal edema is manifested simply by separation of the fine collagen fibers and widening of the papillary dermis.

Extravasation of erythrocytes usually is not apparent clinically or noted at the time of skin biopsy. Dermal hemorrhage may be very mild or quite pronounced.

Variable Histologic Changes

Many other histologic findings noted in biopsies of lupus erythematosus lesions correlate with the morphology of the lesion or the duration of the lesion (Figs. 9–9, 9–10, 9–11). Dyskeratosis and vascular ectasia may be present in early and older lesions. Hyperkeratosis typically is present in mature lesions of CCLE and SCLE, often alternating with small focal areas of parakeratotic scale. Epidermal atrophy is typical of older lesions of CCLE but may be seen alternating with acanthosis in SCLE. Similarly, basement membrane zone thickening, follicular dilatation, keratin plugging, pigment incontinence, and sclerosis all are features characteristically seen in mature CCLE lesions. Hyaluronic acid deposition is seen in all forms of lupus erythematosus and may be mild to prominent.

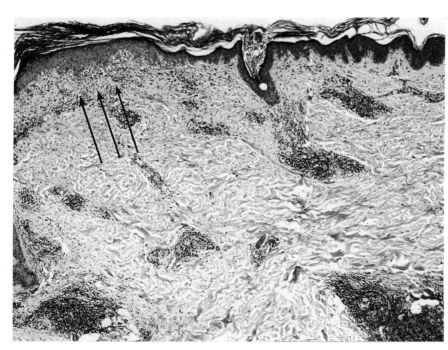

Figure 9–6. Lupus erythematosus. A superficial and deep perivascular infiltrate with focal interface changes (arrows) (H&E, ×50).

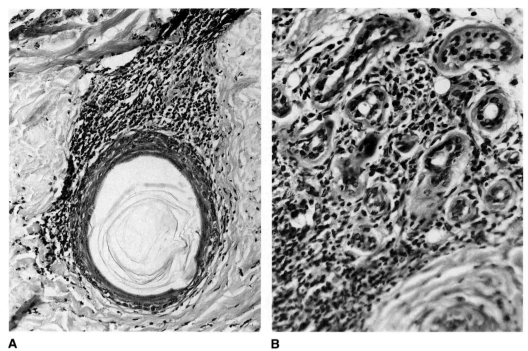

Figure 9–7. Lupus erythematosus. Periadnexal inflammation. **A.** Perifollicular lymphocytic infiltrate (H&E, ×210). **B.** An intense mononuclear cell infiltrate around eccrine ducts in the reticular dermis (H&E, ×320).

A

B

Although the combination of these histologic features often is sufficient to establish the diagnosis of lupus erythematosus, they cannot reliably predict the clinical subset of the disease.

Vesiculobullous Lupus Erythematosus

Two histologic patterns have been described in association with bullous lesions of lupus erythematosus. The most widely accepted pattern is that of a subepidermal bulla

beneath and lateral to which there is a predominantly neutrophilic infiltrate (Figs. 9–12, 9–13).[13,14] The composition and distribution of the infiltrate may make it entirely indistinguishable from that of dermatitis herpetiformis or linear IgA bullous dermatosis. This neutrophil-rich blister is seen in patients with ACLE and systemic disease, and the lesions often arise on apparently normal appearing skin. Direct immunofluorescence of lesional and adjacent nonlesional skin shows a granular deposition of IgM or IgM in the basement membrane zone in all cases and IgA deposition in

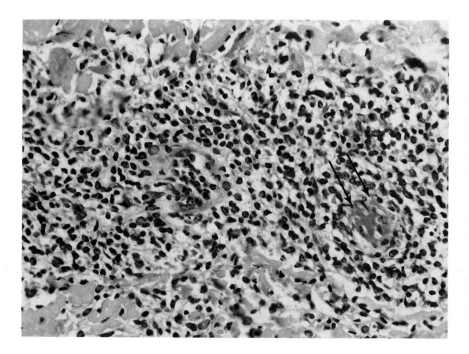

Figure 9–8. Lupus erythematosus. Intense perivascular mononuclear cell infiltrate with endothelial cell swelling and luminal obliteration secondary to fibrin deposition (arrows) (H&E, ×370).

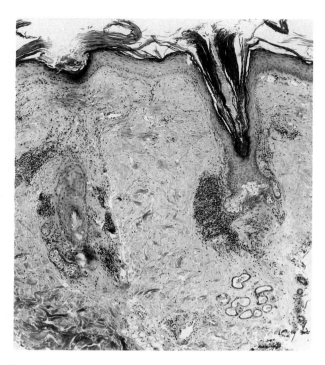

Figure 9–9. Lupus erythematosus. Orthohyperkeratosis, mild epidermal acanthosis, and follicular dilatation with a hyperkeratotic plug (H&E, ×100).

over half the cases.[15] Immunoelectron microscopy has localized the immunoreactants beneath the basal lamina, the same area where immunoglobulins are deposited in other forms of cutaneous lupus erythematosus.[16] This finding supports the concept that the blisters are part of the spectrum of lupus erythematosus rather than being the independent occurrence of LE and another primary blistering disease.

A less common inflammatory response is that of a lymphocytic infiltrate beneath a subepidermal bulla. This pattern usually is seen in association with a long-standing lesion of cutaneous lupus erythematosus.

Verrucous or Hypertrophic Lupus Erythematosus.

Two histologic patterns have been described in association with verrucous lesions of lupus erythematosus. The first pattern resembles a keratoacanthoma, with a central keratin-filled cuplike central depression with surrounding acanthotic epidermis, dyskeratosis, and a patchy, bandlike, perivascular and periappendageal mononuclear cell infiltrate (Fig. 9–14). The second pattern, resembling lichen planus, is characterized by hyperkeratosis, hypergranulosis, irregular acanthosis, and a prominent bandlike dermal mononuclear cell infiltrate. The presence of a deep dermal perivascular and periappendageal infiltrate helps differentiate lesions of verrucous or hypertrophic lupus erythematosus from keratoacanthoma and lichen planus.[17,18]

Lupus Panniculitis.

The subcutaneous fat may be involved as an extension of the dermal infiltrate from an overlying lesion, or it may occur without overlying epidermal and dermal changes.[19] In either situation, the inflammation tends to be more prominent in the lobular portion of the fat and is composed of lymphocytes, histiocytic cells, and occasional plasma cells (Fig. 9–15). Various vascular changes may be present, including endothelial cell hypertrophy, thrombosis, calcification, and concentric peripheral laminated collagen deposition, which produces an onion skin appearance (Fig. 9–16).[20,21] Focal fat necrosis may occur and is associated with fibrin deposition and a neutrophilic infiltrate. Subsequent

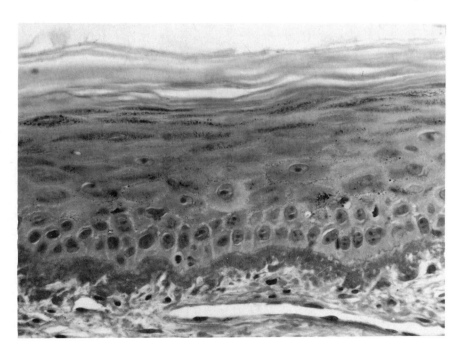

Figure 9–10. Lupus erythematosus. Hyperkeratosis, melanin granules scattered throughout the epidermis, thickened basement membrane zone, and ectatic dermal vessel (PAS, ×450).

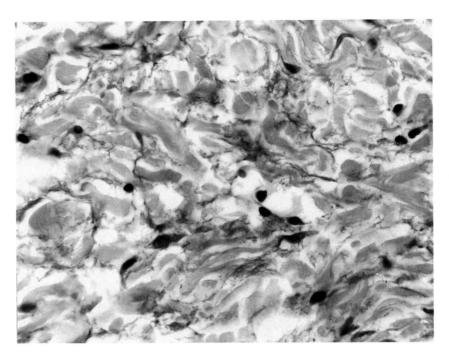

Figure 9–11. Lupus erythematosus. Fibrillar and granular deposition of hyaluronic acid throughout the reticular dermis (H&E, ×370).

hyalinization of fat lobules may produce a diffuse eosinophilic glassy appearance. Focal hyaluronic acid deposition often is visible with routine staining but is markedly enhanced by special stains, such as colloidal iron or alcian blue.[22]

Lymphoid follicles with germinal centers have been described. The combination of a lobular panniculitis with vessel wall changes and lymphoid follicles is strongly suggestive of the diagnosis of lupus panniculitis.[23]

DERMATOMYOSITIS

Clinical Features

Dermatomyositis is a systemic inflammatory disease of connective tissue characterized by acute and chronic inflammation of striated muscle and a characteristic cutaneous eruption. When skin findings are absent, the disease is referred to as "polymyositis." The dermatitis may precede the myositis, or vice versa. Proximal muscle weakness usually is

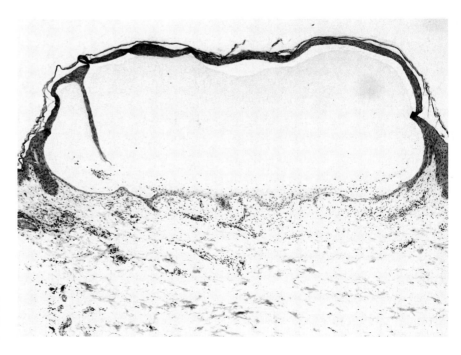

Figure 9–12. Bullous lupus erythematosus. Low-power view showing subepidermal vesicle formation with mild inflammatory infiltrate at base and sides of the blister (H&E, ×95).

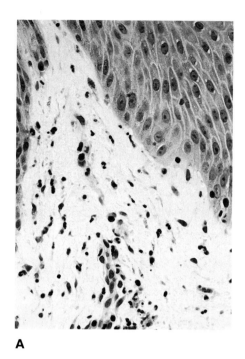

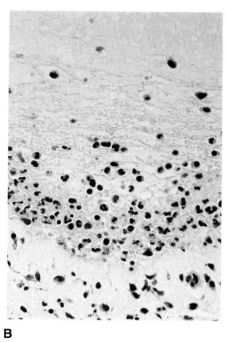

A   B

Figure 9–13. Bullous lupus erythematosus. Neutrophilic infiltrate at lateral edge of blister **(A)** and base of blister **(B)** (H&E, ×320).

prominent early in the course of the disease, and patients typically have difficulty climbing stairs, getting out of bed, and lifting their arms over their heads. Mild muscle tenderness may be present, but frank myalgias occur uncommonly.

A characteristic cutaneous manifestation is a violaceous periorbital macular discoloration that is most prominent on the upper eyelids. This change has been described as a heliotrope erythema. The dermatitis that occurs is an erythematous, scaly, flat or elevated eruption that is usually present on the face, neck, and extensor surfaces of the extremities. The localization of lesions on the knuckles, elbows, and knees is known as Gottron's sign. Areas of poikiloderma (atrophy, telangiectasia, hyperpigmentation,

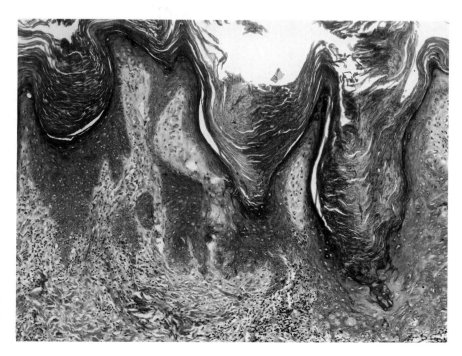

Figure 9–14. Verrucous lupus erythematosus. Hyperkeratosis, papillomatosis, and a patchy perivascular and bandlike mononuclear cell infiltrate (H&E, ×100).

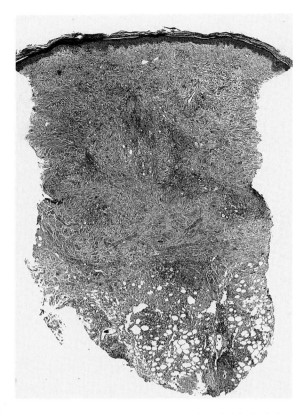

Figure 9–15. Lupus panniculitis. A predominantly lobular inflammation is seen in association with a moderately intense perivascular dermal infiltrate (H&E, ×20).

and hypopigmentation) also may occur in dermatomyositis, as may periungual erythema and telangiectasia. The latter changes are not unique to dermatomyositis, however, and may be seen also in other connective tissue diseases, such as lupus erythematosus and scleroderma.[24]

Patients with dermatomyositis have elevated levels of serum creatine phosphokinase (CPK) and urine creatine. Electromyography is helpful in confirming the occurrence of a myopathy and excluding a neuropathy. However, the definitive diagnostic test remains the muscle biopsy. A variety of changes may be present in the muscle biopsy, including segmental necrosis of muscle fibers, mononuclear cell inflammation between fibers and around venules, loss of striations, and an eosinophilic hyalinization of muscle fibers.

Histologic Features

A biopsy from a typical cutaneous lesion will show variable hyperkeratosis, acanthosis or atrophy, and vacuolar alteration of basal cells. Dermal changes include vascular ectasia, a mild perivascular mononuclear cell infiltrate, and hyaluronic acid deposition (Fig. 9–17).[25,26] These findings are similar to those seen in biopsy specimens of lupus erythematosus, and it is usually impossible to differentiate the two disorders on a histologic basis.

DRUG ERUPTIONS, MORBILLIFORM TYPE

Clinical Features

Adverse reactions to drugs are manifested in the skin by a wide variety of morphologic and histologic patterns. The

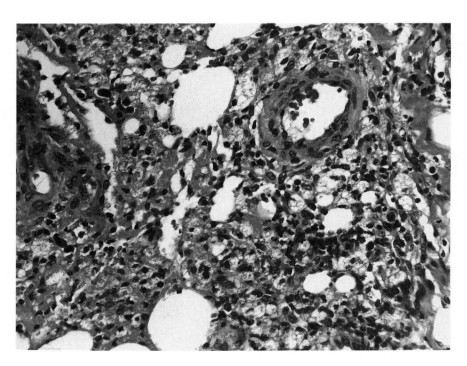

Figure 9–16. Lupus panniculitis. A dense lobular infiltrate of mononuclear cells. Vessel walls are thickened (H&E, ×280).

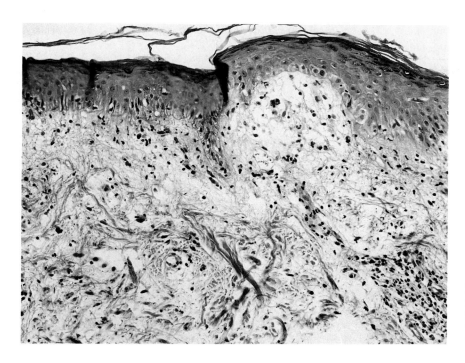

Figure 9–17. Dermatomyositis. Basal vacuolization, squamatization of the basal layer, marked papillary dermal edema, and a mild perivascular and interstitial mononuclear cell infiltrate (H&E, ×165).

most common drug-induced reaction is the morbilliform eruption. Morbilliform drug eruptions are characterized by a blanchable symmetrical macular and papular erythematous eruption that usually is widespread and frequently involves the palms and soles. Individual lesions may coalesce to form large areas of confluent erythema. Occasionally, if the eruption is allowed to progress, an erythroderma may result. The eruption often is pruritic and may be associated with fever. The drugs most frequently associated with a morbilliform pattern of eruption include antibiotics (particularly trimethoprim-sulfamethoxazole, ampicillin, amoxicillin), and allopurinol. Lesions usually appear within the first week of therapy but may be delayed as long as 2 weeks after a medication has been stopped. Although it is usually necessary to stop the offending agent before resolution of the eruption will occur, occasionally the rash clears while the patient is still taking the medication.

Histologic Features
The histologic changes in a morbilliform drug eruption include variable but usually mild dyskeratosis, vacuolar alteration of the basal cell layer, blood vessel ectasia, and a mild to moderately intense perivascular infiltrate composed of lymphocytes and occasional eosinophils. The histologic features are not sufficiently characteristic to determine the causative drug.

Differential Diagnosis
Drug eruptions must be differentiated histologically from pityriasis lichenoides et varioliformis acuta, lupus erythematosus, and dermatomyositis. There is less epidermal damage in drug eruptions compared to the other three diseases and usually there are eosinophils present.

PHOTOTOXIC DERMATITIS

Clinical Features
A phototoxic reaction occurs when a photosensitizing agent interacts with ultraviolet radiation and absorbs energy. This energy is released into tissue and produces damage. The photosensitizing agent may be a systemically administered drug or a topically applied chemical. Clinically, a phototoxic reaction is manifested by a severe, acute burn, with erythema, edema, and occasionally blister formation. This reaction occurs a few hours after exposure to ultraviolet light and is limited to those areas exposed to light. The eruption gradually resolves, with desquamation and hyperpigmentation. Phototoxic reactions are not allergic in nature and, therefore, may occur in any individual receiving the appropriate amount of the drug and the appropriate irradiation. The action spectrum of most phototoxic reactions is in the 320 to 340 nm (UVA) range, but a few agents will react to 290 to 320 nm (UVB) or even visible light.[27,28] Some of the chemicals known to produce phototoxic reactions are demeclocycline, phenothiazines, sulfonamides, amiodarone, and nonsteroidal anti-inflammatory agents.

Histologic Features
The histologic changes observed in a phototoxic reaction include dyskeratosis (occasionally marked), vacuolar alteration of the basal layer, vascular ectasia, and dermal edema (Fig. 9–18). A minimal to mild perivascular inflammatory reaction is present.

Differential Diagnosis
In contrast to hypersensitivity drug eruptions, phototoxic reactions tend to have marked dyskeratosis and a lack of

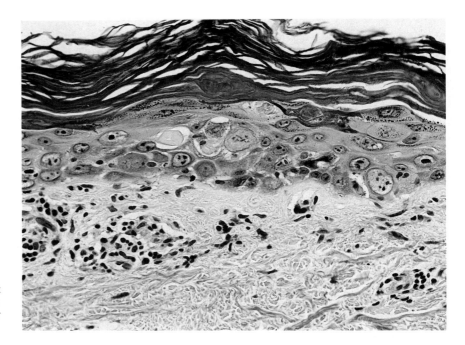

Figure 9–18. Phototoxic eruption. Prominent dyskeratosis, squamotization of the basal layer, and a mild superficial perivascular mononuclear cell infiltrate (H&E, ×280).

eosinophils. At times, it may be difficult or impossible to separate a phototoxic reaction from lupus erythematosus in a lupus erythematosus patient with photosensitivity.

GRAFT-VERSUS-HOST DISEASE

Clinical Features

Immunocompetent cells infused into an immunosuppressed individual are capable of reacting against tissue antigens in the host and producing specific damage to the cells or tissue that is known as graft-versus-host (GVH) disease. GVH disease is seen most frequently following allogeneic bone marrow transplantation but has been described following leukocyte-rich transfusions[29] and solid tumor transplantation containing leukocytes.[30] Recently GVH disease has been described both in animals and in humans who have been infused with their own (syngeneic) cells.[31,32] The current belief is that GVH disease is produced by cytotoxic T lymphocytes.[33]

Acute and chronic forms of the disease have been described that presumably are due to different immunologic mechanisms. Multiple organs may be affected, but the most commonly involved are the skin, gastrointestinal tract, and liver. Morbidity and mortality from GVH disease depend on the severity of the disease and the organs involved. The ability to recognize and aggressively treat GVH disease has significantly improved survival of bone marrow transplant recipients.

Acute cutaneous GVH disease usually occurs 10 to 21 days after marrow transplantation coexistent with marrow recovery. Earliest symptoms include pruritus and a mild discomfort when pressure is exerted on the palms and soles. The initial eruption is a faint blanchable macular erythema present on the upper trunk, neck, hands, and feet. Diffuse erythema of the pinna of the ears and also periungual er-

ythema are characteristic early signs. Coalescence of macules or papules produces confluent areas of involvement. Blisters may occur, especially on the palms and soles. Widespread erythema with blister formation has been described that simulates toxic epidermal necrolysis.

Chronic GVH reaction occurs months to 2 years after marrow transplantation and may or may not be preceded by acute cutaneous GVH disease. Two distinct forms of chronic GVH disease occur in the skin: lichenoid and sclerodermoid.

Lichenoid cutaneous GVH disease is characterized by violaceous papules occurring most commonly on the distal extremities, particularly the palms and soles. The lesions closely resemble those of lichen planus but are somewhat less sharply demarcated and less angulated than are classic lichen planus lesions. These lesions are associated with generalized xerosis and follicular prominence.

Sclerodermoid GVH disease is the later of these two stages and is manifested by localized or diffuse dermal sclerosis. Ulcerations, dyspigmentation, diminished sweating, joint contractures, and alopecia are frequently associated findings. The degree of involvement and severity varies considerably.

Acute GVH Disease

Histologic Features

One to two days preceding a clinically detectable eruption histopathologic abnormalities may be observed in the skin. The earliest alteration consists of focal vacuolar change in the basement membrane zone of the epidermis and hair follicle epithelium. Often in association with the vacuolar change, a scant superficial perivascular mononuclear cell infiltrate will be seen in the papillary and upper reticular dermis. This infiltrate, which is quantitatively variable, is composed predominantly of mononuclear cells. Although

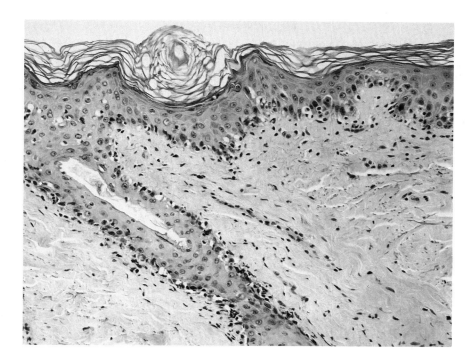

Figure 9–19. Acute graft-versus-host disease. Basal vacuolization involving the epidermis and follicular epithelium. Loss of basal cell polarity gives the basal layer a squamatized appearance (H&E, ×165).

mononuclear cells are primarily distributed around vessels of the superficial venular plexus, exocytosis of individual cells into the epidermis and follicular epithelium commonly occurs. As the reaction progresses, the vacuolar changes become more pronounced (Fig. 9–19), intercellular edema is observed, and there is loss of polarity of epidermal cells in the lower epidermis. Individual dyskeratotic cells appear in the basal cell layer, lower stratum malpighii, and follicular epithelium (Fig. 9–20). Occasionally, mononuclear cells may be seen in close apposition to the dyskeratotic cells, the so-called satellite lymphocytes. Dyskera-

totic cells with adjacent lymphocytes are not specific for GVH disease and may be seen in many other inflammatory interface or lichenoid tissue reactions. In severe acute GVH disease, the vacuoles coalesce to form subepidermal clefts, microvesicles, and even bullae (Fig. 9–21).[34–37] Saurat et al[38] devised a grading system based on the degree of epidermal alteration to quantify the histologic changes in cutaneous GVH disease (Table 9–3). Additional epidermal changes that may be caused by GVH disease, chemotherapy, or irradiation include compact laminated orthohyperkeratosis, epidermal atrophy with flattening of the rete

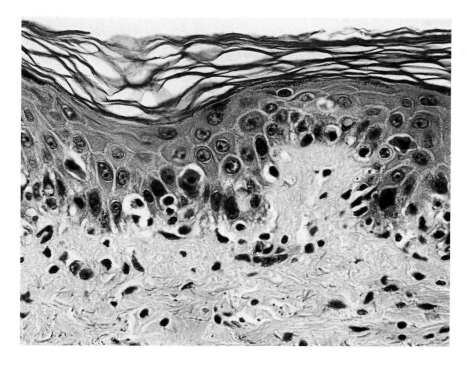

Figure 9–20. Acute graft-versus-host disease. Basal vacuolization and dyskeratosis of individual keratinocytes (H&E, ×440).

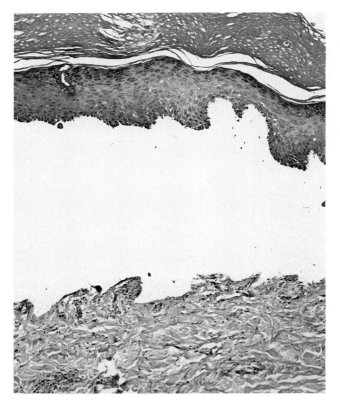

Figure 9–21. Acute graft-versus-host disease. Separation of epidermis and dermis and scant superficial perivascular mononuclear cell infiltrate (H&E, ×85).

ridges, and unevenly distributed melanin granules within keratinocytes.

In association with the perivenular mononuclear cell infiltrate, there is marked endothelial cell swelling and narrowing of the vascular lumina. Dermal hemorrhage is common and may be caused by thrombocytopenia or incompetent vessel walls. Leukocytoclastic vasculitis is not seen as a feature of cutaneous GVH disease. Melanin granules, free and within melanophages, are often present in the papillary dermis.

TABLE 9–3. HISTOPATHOLOGIC GRADING SYSTEM FOR ACUTE CUTANEOUS GRAFT-VERSUS-HOST REACTION

Grade	Histopathologic Features
0	Normal epidermis or epidermal changes of other cutaneous disorders
1	Focal or diffuse vaculolar alteration of the basal cell layer
2	Dyskeratotic squamous cells in epidermis or hair follicle epithelium
3	Subepidermal cleft or microvesicle formation
4	Complete separation of the epidermis from the dermis

Note: To confirm the diagnosis of acute cutaneous graft-versus-host reaction, there should also be an associated mononuclear cell infiltrate involving the epidermis or hair follicle epithelium.

Adapted from Saurat et al.[38]

As acute GVH disease resolves, the basal vacuolar changes diminish, the dyskeratotic cells move upward to be shed with the stratum corneum, the perivascular inflammatory infiltrate decreases, and endothelial cell swelling subsides. Dermal scarring and loss of elastic tissue do not occur unless there has been a superimposed pyoderma, viral infection, or other traumatic event.

Histopathologic changes similar to those in acute cutaneous GVH disease occurring in patients receiving allogeneic bone marrow transplants have been reported also in patients receiving syngeneic bone marrow transplants or autologous (stored marrow reinfused into the same individual) bone marrow transplants.[31,32] These changes, which usually are mild and transient, consist of vacuolar alteration of the basal cell layer, dyskeratosis, and a scant superficial perivenular lymphocytic infiltrate similar to that seen in allogeneic-induced GVH disease.

In summary, to establish the diagnosis of acute GVH disease, we require the following features involving either the epidermis, hair follicle epithelium or oral mucosa: vacuolar alteration of the basal cell layer, dyskeratotic cells, and an associated mononuclear cell infiltrate that involves the superficial vascular plexus and invades the epidermis or epithelium. Vacuolar alteration and occasional dyskeratotic cells in the absence of an associated inflammatory infiltrate may be seen as a consequence of chemotherapy and by themselves are not diagnostic of GVH disease. If the diagnosis is in doubt histologically, we recommend additional biopsies from several sites, obtained over time, to establish or rule out the diagnosis of GVH disease.

Lichenoid Chronic GVH Disease

Histologic Features

Examination of biopsies from well-developed lichenoid lesions show hyperkeratosis (which is generally orthokeratotic), hypergranulosis, moderate irregular acanthosis, and moderate vacuolar changes in the basal cell layer (Fig. 9–22). Individual eosinophilic dyskeratotic keratinocytes with or without nuclei are present in the basal layer and lower stratum malpighii. The follicular epithelium shows changes similar to those observed in the epidermis. In the papillary and upper reticular dermis, there is a mild perivascular and interstitial infiltrate composed of lymphocytes, mononuclear cells, melanophages, and rarely a few plasma cells. Inflammatory cells occasionally are seen in the epidermis but are confined to the basal cell layer or lower stratum malpighii.[34,38]

Lichenoid GVH disease can be histologically distinguished from lichen planus only by its scant, predominantly perivenular infiltrate. The epidermal changes in the two diseases are identical.

Sclerodermoid GVH Reaction

Histologic Features

Biopsy specimens from sclerodermoid lesions exhibit a thickened reticular dermis composed of hypertrophic, densely packed, brightly eosinophilic collagen bundles (Fig.

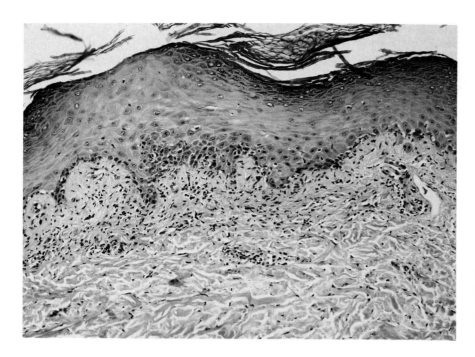

Figure 9–22. Chronic graft-versus-host disease, lichenoid type. Irregular acanthosis, hypergranulosis, basal vacuolization, perivascular and interstitial mononuclear cell infiltrate confined to the papillary and upper reticular dermis (H&E, ×120).

9–23). In many cases, the normal distinction between the papillary and reticular dermis is lost, and the papillary dermis is replaced entirely by thick sclerotic collagen fibers. Hair follicles disappear, and eccrine glands lose their surrounding fat and become entrapped in dense collagen. Arrector pili muscles and eccrine ducts are relatively spared until late in the course of the disease. A variable perivascular and periadnexal mononuclear cell infiltrate is present. This infiltrate is composed of lymphocytes, mononuclear cells, and occasional plasma cells and melanophages. An inflammatory infiltrate is not observed along the dermal–subcutaneous junction, as is seen in morphea. The overlying

epidermis shows hyperkeratosis, keratotic plugging, hypergranulosis, irregular acanthosis or epidermal atrophy, occasional dyskeratotic cells, and diminished melanin in the basal cell layer. Except for the epidermal changes and the lack of infiltrate at the dermal–subcutaneous junction, the histologic changes observed in the sclerodermoid lesions of chronic GVH disease are quite similar to changes present in the lesions of progressive systemic scleroderma and morphea.[34,39] We also have seen a bullous variant of sclerodermoid GVH disease with the cleft being formed in the upper dermis probably secondary to edema.[40]

Electron microscopic examination of the dyskeratotic

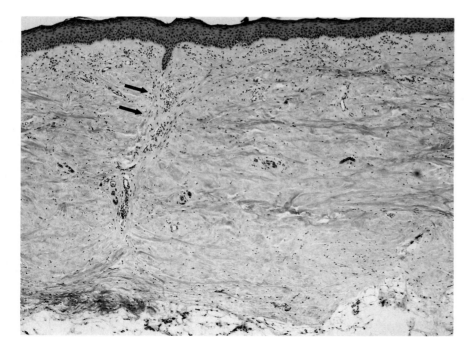

Figure 9–23. Chronic graft-versus-host disease, sclerodermatoid type. Thickened reticular dermis with loss of pilosebaceous unit (arrows). The epidermis appears normal, and there is a scant perivascular lymphocytic infiltrate (H&E, ×45).

cells seen in humans with acute cutaneous GVH disease demonstrated dense aggregation of tonofilaments and cytoplasmic organelles and loss of desmosomes.[41,43] Some of these degenerating or dyskeratotic cells appear to be phagocytized by neighboring keratinocytes,[43] a process also known as apoptosis. Direct contact of lymphocytes with degenerating keratinocytes has been observed by some authors[41] but not by others.[42]

Although deposition of C3 and IgM has been reported in a few patients with acute cutaneous GVH disease, it is not a consistent finding, and it is difficult to attribute an important role to these immunoreactants in the pathogenesis of the disease.[44-46] Examination of skin biopsies from patients with chronic GVH disease reveals more consistent findings. IgM was seen deposited along the dermal–epidermal junction in a globular pattern analogous to that of lichen planus[45] or in a linear fashion.[44,46] Whether the deposition of immunoreactants plays a role in the pathogenesis of the disorder or is merely an epiphenomenon is not known at this time.

REFERENCES

1. Huff JC, Weston WL, Tonnesen MG. Erythema multiforme: A critical review of characteristics, diagnostic criteria, and causes. *J Am Acad Dermatol.* 1983;8:763–775.

2. Ackerman AB, Penneys NS, Clark WH. Erythema multiforme exudativum: Distinctive pathological process. *Br J Dermatol.* 1971;84:554–566.

3. Orfanos CE, Schaumberg-Lever G. Lever WF. Dermal and epidermal types of erythema multiforme: A histologic study of 24 cases. *Arch Dermatol.* 1974;109:682–688.

4. Lever WF: My concept of erythema multiforme. *Am J Dermatopathol.* 1985;7:141–142.

5. Howland WW, Golitz LE, Weston WE, et al. Erythema multiforme: Clinical, histopathologic, and immunologic study. *J Am Acad Dermatol.* 1984;10:438–446.

6. Korkij WK, Soltani K. Fixed drug eruption. A brief review. *Arch Dermatol.* 1984;120:520–524.

7. Jerdan MS, Hood AF, Moore W, et al. Histopathologic comparison of the subsets of lupus erythematosus. *Arch Dermatol.* 1990;126:52.

8. Hood AF. Pathology of cutaneous lupus erythematosus. *Adv Dermatol.* 1988;3:153–170.

9. Prunieras M, Montgomery H. Histopathology of cutaneous lesions in systemic lupus erythematosus. *Arch Dermatol.* 1956;74:177–190.

10. Ellis FA, Bundick WR. Histology of lupus erythematosus. *Arch Dermatol Syph.* 1954;70:311–324.

11. Montgomery H. Pathology of lupus erythematosus. *J Invest Dermatol.* 1939;2:343–359.

12. Synkowski DR, Provost TT. Characterization of the inflammatory infiltrate in lupus erythematosus lesions using monoclonal antibodies. *J Rheumatol.* 1983;10:920–924.

13. Hall RP, Lawley TJ, Smith HR, et al. Bullous eruption of systemic lupus erythematosus. Dramatic response to dapsone therapy. *Ann Intern Med.* 1982;97:165–170.

14. Penneys NS, Wiley HE. Herpetiform blisters in systemic lupus erythematosus. *Arch Dermatol.* 1979;115:1427–1428.

15. Camisa C, Sharma HM. Vesiculobullous systemic lupus erythematosus. Report of two case and review of the literature. *J Am Acad Dermatol.* 1983;9:924–933.

16. Tani M, Shimiza R, Ban M, et al: Systemic lupus erythematosus with vesiculobullous lesions. Immunoelectron microscopic studies. *Arch Dermatol.* 1984;120:1497–1501.

17. Uitto J, Santa Cruz DJ, Eisen AZ, et al. Verrucous lesions in patients with discoid lupus erythematosus. Clinical, histopathological, and immunofluorescence studies. *Br J Dermatol.* 1978;98:507–520.

18. Santa Cruz DJ, Uitto J, Eisen AZ, et al. Verrucous lupus erythematosus: Ultrastructural studies on a distinct variant of chronic discoid lupus erythematosus. *J Am Acad Dermatol.* 1983;9:82–90.

19. Tuffanelli DL. Lupus erythematosus panniculitis (profundus). Clinical and immunologic studies. *Arch Dermatol.* 1971;103:231–242.

20. Sanchez NP, Peters MS, Winkelmann RK. The histopathology of lupus erythematosus panniculitis. *J Am Acad Dermatol.* 1981;5:673–680.

21. Winkelmann RK. Panniculitis and systemic lupus erythematosus. *JAMA.* 1970;21:472–475.

22. Isumi AK, Takiguchi P. Lupus erythematosus panniculitis. *Arch Dermatol.* 1983;119:61–64.

23. Harris RB, Duncan SC, Ecker RI, et al. Lymphoid follicles in subcutaneous inflammatory disease. *Arch Dermatol.* 1979;115:442–443.

24. Callen JP. Dermatomyositis. *Dermatol Clin.* 1983;1:461–473.

25. Janis JF, Winkelmann RK. Histopathology of the skin in dermatomyositis: A histologic study of 55 cases. *Arch Dermatol.* 1968;97:640–650.

26. Hanno R, Callen JP. Histopathology of Gottron's papules. *J Cutan Pathol.* 1985;12:389–394.

27. Epstein JH. Photosensitivity: I. Mechanisms. *Clin Dermatol.* 1986;4:81–87.

28. Epstein JH. Adverse cutaneous reactions to the sun. In: Malkinson FD, Pearson RW, eds. *Year Book of Dermatology.* Chicago: Year Book Medical Publishers; 1971:5–43.

29. Brubaker DB. Transfusion-associated graft-versus-host disease. *Hum Pathol.* 1986;17:1085–1088.

30. Burdick JF, Vogelsang GB, Smith WJ, et al. Severe graft-versus-host disease in a liver transplant recipient. *N Engl J Med.* 1988;318:689–691.

31. Hood AF, Black LP, Vogelsang GB, et al. Acute graft-versus-host disease following autologous and syngeneic bone marrow transplantation. *Arch Dermatol.* 1987;123:745–750.

32. Einsele H, Ehninger G, Schneider EM, et al. High frequency of graft-versus-host-like syndromes following syngeneic bone marrow transplantation. *Transplant.* 1988;45:579–585.

33. Santo GW, Hess AD, Vogelsang GB. Graft-versus-host reactions and disease. *Immunol Rev.* 1985;88:169–192.

34. Farmer ER. The histopathology of graft-versus-host disease. *Adv Dermatol.* 1986;1:173–188.

35. Hymes SR, Farmer ER, Lewis PG, et al. Cutaneous graft-versus-host rection. Prognosis features seen by light microscopy. *JAAD.* 1985;12:468–474.

36. Sale GE, Lerner KG, Berker EA, et al. The skin biopsy in the diagnosis of acute graft-versus-host disease in man. *Am J Pathol.* 1977;89:621–636.

37. Elliott CJ, Sloane JP, Sanderson KV, et al. The histological diagnosis of cutaneous graft versus host disease: Relationship of skin changes to marrow purging and other clinical variables. *Histopathology.* 1987;11:145–155.

38. Saurat JH, Gluckman E, Bussel A, et al. The lichen planuslike eruption after bone marrow transplantation. *Br J Dermatol.* 1975;93:675–681.

39. Shulman HM, Sale GE, Lerner KG, et al. Chronic cutaneous graft-versus-host disease in man. *Am J Pathol.* 1978;92:545–570.

40. Hymes SR, Farmer ER, Burns WH, et al. Bullous scleroderma-like changes in chronic graft-versus-host disease. *Arch Dermatol.* 1985;121:1189–1192.

41. Grogan TM, Odom RB, Brugess JH. Graft-versus-host reaction. *Arch Dermatol.* 1977;118:806–812.

42. Gallucci BB, Shulman HM, Sale GE, et al. The ultrastructure of the human epidermis in chronic graft-versus-host disease. *Am J Pathol.* 1979;95:643–654.

43. De Dobbeleer GD, Ledoux-Corbusier MH, Achten GA. Graft vs host reaction: An ultrastructural study. *Arch Dermatol.* 1975;111:1597–1602.

44. Tsoi MS, Storb R, Jones E, et al. Deposition of IgM and complement at the dermoepidermal junction in acute and chronic cutaneous graft-versus-host disease in man. *J Immunol.* 1978;120:1485–1492.

45. Saurat JH, Bonnetblanc JM, Gluckman E, et al. Skin antibodies in bone marrow transplanted patients. *Clin Exp Dermatol.* 1976;1:377–384.

46. Farmer ER, Provost TT, Tutschka PJ, et al. Cutaneous graft-versus-host reactions: A prospective sequential immunopathologic study in man. *Clin Res.* 1979;27:241A.

CHAPTER 10

Intraepidermal Vesicular, Bullous, and Pustular Dermatoses

Beno Michel and Wilma F. Bergfeld

Intraepidermal vesicular, bullous and pustular dermatoses can result from a variety of mechanisms producing physical and biochemical injury to the epidermal architecture and to individual keratinocytes. The epidermal injury can result from spongiosis or intracellular edema, ballooning degeneration or intercellular edema, acantholysis or loss of intercellular bridges and epidermal necrolysis.

This chapter discusses the acantholytic disorders, such as pemphigus foliaceous, fogo selvagem, pemphigus erythematosus, pemphigus vulgaris, pemphigus vegetans, eosinophilic spongiosis, Darier's disease, Hailey-Hailey disease (familial benign chronic pemphigus), and transient acantholytic dermatosis. Diseases of children, such as acropustulosis of infancy, toxic erythema of newborn, and incontinentia pigmenti, also are discussed (Tables 10–1 and 10–2).

PEMPHIGUS

Clinical Features

The term ''pemphigus'' is now used to describe a group of autoimmune intraepidermal blistering disorders characterized by circulating autoantibodies against antigens present on the surface of keratinocytes, also known as intercellular antibodies (ICS), and by the presence of tissue-fixed immunoglobulins demonstrated by direct immunofluorescence studies on the cell surface of keratinocytes and in the intercellular spaces of the epidermis.

Histologic Features

Histologically, pemphigus is divided into pemphigus foliaceous, fogo selvagem (Brazilian disorder), and pemphigus erythematosus, in which cases acantholysis occurs through the stratum granulosum, and pemphigus vulgaris, in which the intraepidermal split and acantholytic process develop above the basal cell layer. Pemphigus vegetans refers to a verrucous form of pemphigus arising primarily in the intertriginous areas, such as the axillae and the groin.

PEMPHIGUS FOLIACEOUS

Clinical Features

In pemphigus foliaceous there are superficial vesicles and blisters that break readily, leaving either shiny denuded skin or crusted or weeping areas. The lesions spread peripherally (positive Nikolsky sign) and are present primarily in a seborrheic distribution involving the face, chest, and back, although other parts of the body may be affected. In some cases, the lesions can become confluent, causing a generalized erythroderma that mimics an exfoliative dermatitis. A rare form may occur as grouped vesicles and has been reported as pemphigus herpetiformis. An endemic form present in Brazil is known as fogo selvagem and is clinically indistinguishable from pemphigus foliaceous, although at times it is more extensive.

Histologic Features

Using light microscopy, the epidermis shows a split either through the stratum granulosum or between the stratum corneum and the stratum granulosum. At times, individual keratinocytes remain attached to the stratum corneum (Fig. 10–1A). A subcorneal blister may form with acantholytic cells present within the blister cavity (Fig. 10–1B). Early lesions show no inflammatory reaction, and only the split and the acantholytic cells are present. Over a period of time, a secondary inflammatory infiltrate develops, with accumulation of polymorphonuclear leukocytes and occasional eosinophils present within the blister cavity. At this point, the differential diagnosis would include impetigo and subcorneal pustular dermatosis. Older lesions may develop hyperkeratosis, parakeratosis, and slight acanthosis.

Differential Diagnosis

In impetigo, the inflammatory infiltrate is rather intense, and the number of acantholytic cells, if there are any, is small. In pemphigus foliaceous, although the inflammatory

TABLE 10–1. IMMUNOLOGIC ACANTHOLYTIC DISEASES

Disease	H&E Location	DIF[a]	IIF[a]	Locations
Pemphigus foliaceus and fogo selvagem (Brazilian pemphigus)	Split below stratum corneum or through stratum granulosum, acantholysis	ICS	ICS[b]	Face, trunk
Pemphigus erythematosus	Split below stratum corneum or through stratum granulosum, acantholysis	ICS + BM	ICS + ANA	Face, trunk
Pemphigus vulgaris	Suprabasilar split with acantholytic cells	ICS	ICF[c]	Oral musoca, face, trunk, extremities
Pemphigus vegetans (verrucal variant of pemphigus vulgaris)	Suprabasilar split and acantholysis; acanthosis cells; intraepidermal abscesses with eosinophils	ICS	+ICS	Intertriginous areas; axillae and groin

[a] DIF, direct immunofluorescence; IIF, indirect immunofluorescence.
[b] Titer higher on guinea pig esophagus.
[c] Titer higher on monkey esophagus.

TABLE 10–2. NONIMMUNOLOGIC ACANTHOLYTIC DISORDERS

Disease	H&E	Site
Darier's disease	Focal acantholysis, multiple corps ronds and grains	Trunk, palms and soles, oral mucosa
Hailey-Hailey disease (benign mucous membrane pemphigus)	Extensive acantholysis; rare corps ronds and grains	Intertriginous areas, trunk
Transient acantholytic disorder (Grover's disease)	Focal acantholysis; variable number of corps ronds and grains; overlapping features with Hailey-Hailey disease, pemphigus vulgaris, pemphigus foliaceous, and spongiotic dermatitis	Trunk
Acantholytic dyskeratosis, focal and papular (generic term including multiple entities)	Focal acantholysis; rare corps ronds; acantholytic cells	Trunk, mucous membranes

[a] Direct and indirect immunofluorescence negative.

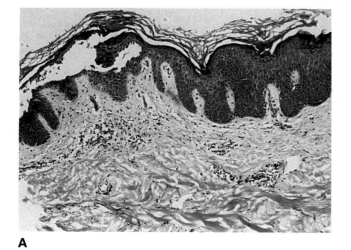

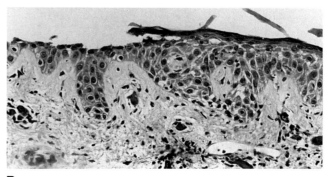

A **B**

Figure 10–1.A. Pemphigus foliaceous, demonstrating a split within the stratum granulosum (H&E, ×20). **B.** Pemphigus foliaceous, demonstrating a superficial epidermal split and intercellular edema associated with a mild chronic mononuclear dermal infiltrate (H&E, ×40).

infiltrate may be intense, the number of acantholytic cells is greater than in impetigo. Bacterial culture would be useful in confirming the diagnosis of impetigo. In the presence of an intense inflammatory infiltrate, a subcorneal pustule may form, and subcorneal pustular dermatosis would become a consideration in the differential diagnosis. Direct and indirect immunofluorescence studies would be helpful in diagnosing pemphigus foliaceous. Direct immunofluorescence tests would be positive for tissue-fixed immunoglobulins (IgG and C3), and with indirect immunofluorescence tests, approximately 70% of the cases would be positive for circulating antiepidermal antibodies in pemphigus foliaceous compared to impetigo and subcorneal pustular dermatoses, which are negative by both direct and indirect immunofluorescence studies. Fogo selvagem would be identical to pemphigus foliaceous by light microscopy and immunofluorescence. The dermis in both pemphigus foliaceous and fogo selvagem would show primarily a perivascular mononuclear cell infiltrate with occasional polymorphonuclear leukocytes and eosinophils.

PEMPHIGUS ERYTHEMATOSUS

Clinical Features
An uncommon variant of pemphigus foliaceous is known as pemphigus erythematosus (Senear-Usher syndrome), in which there are erythematous, scaly, and crusted lesions of the face and chest similar to those in pemphigus foliaceous. In addition, however, a more intense butterfly erythema with follicular plugging resembling lupus erythematosus is present on the face. The disease may coexist with lupus erythematosus or myasthenia gravis with thymoma. Penicillamine-induced pemphigus erythematosus has been reported.

Histologic Features
Light microscopy shows a split through the stratum granulosum, with acantholysis similar to that in pemphigus foliaceous. In addition, however, follicular plugging may be present, and some dyskeratosis of the cells in the granular cell layer has been described. The dermis shows a mixed inflammatory infiltrate.

Differential Diagnosis
This variant can be distinguished from pemphigus foliaceous by direct immunofluorescence studies of perilesional sun-exposed skin. The presence of immunoglobulins at the epidermal–dermal junction (lupus band) in addition to the intercellular fluorescence seen in pemphigus is characteristic of pemphigus erythematosus. Serum studies in pemphigus erythematosus may show both antinuclear and pemphigus antibodies.

IgA PEMPHIGUS FOLIACEOUS

A number of cases recently have been diagnosed clinically and by light microscopy as pemphigus foliaceous, with tissue fixed IgA instead of IgG in the upper epidermis demonstrated by direct immunofluorescence. Two of the seven cases had circulating pemphigus antibodies of the IgA class. Clinically, the lesions appeared as flaccid vesicles of the axilla, trunk, and extremities. These cases appear to belong to the spectrum of pemphigus foliaceous.

PEMPHIGUS VULGARIS

Clinical Features
Pemphigus vulgaris is characterized by the presence of flaccid blisters that develop on normal noninflammatory skin. The lesion breaks readily, leaving a glistening denuded surface. The epidermis detaches peripherally due to trauma (Nikolsky sign). When confluent, lesions can cover large areas of the body and become easily crusted and secondarily infected. Frequently, blisters will start in the oral cavity and be the earliest symptom of the disease. Other mucous membrane, such as the genitalia and the rectal mucosa, may be affected. The conjunctiva is only rarely involved.

Histologic Features
The early lesions of pemphigus vulgaris occur with a suprabasilar split with occasional acantholytic cells (Fig. 10–2A). Later, the epidermis may show some acanthosis and spongiosis. Occasionally, the split may occur two or three layers above the basal cell layer within the stratum malpighii. Acantholytic cells in pemphigus have a characteristic appearance, consisting of single or multiple cells separated from the adjacent keratinocytes. The nucleus is small and hyperchromatic and frequently is surrounded by a halo. The cytoplasm is homogeneous.

The base of the blister may show a tombstone arrangement of basal cells (Fig. 10–2B). The adjacent epidermis occasionally shows spongiosis with an infiltrate of eosinophils and is known as eosinophilic spongiosis. When eosinophilic spongiosis is present without acantholysis, it may represent a precursor to pemphigus or pemphigoid or be the result of an insect bite. As such, it is not pathognomonic for pemphigus but may represent an early marker of pemphigus even before acantholysis develops.

In pemphigus foliaceous as well as pemphigus vulgaris, acantholysis may extend into the outer root sheaths of the hair. The dermis shows a patchy perivascular mononuclear cell infiltrate with occasional polymorphonuclear leukocytes and eosinophils.

Biopsies obtained from lesions of pemphigus vulgaris of the buccal mucosa and also at times from skin lesions may show total loss of the surface epidermis. However, even in these cases, the basal cell layer remains attached to the dermis, and a correct diagnosis is still possible.

Acantholytic cells can be demonstrated rapidly by cytologic examination (Tzanck smear). Cells scraped from the base of a blister, spread on a microscope slide, and stained with Giemsa or Fite stain can help identify the presence of acantholytic cells. However, this technique cannot distinguish between pemphigus foliaceous and pemphigus vulgaris.

The absence of marked acanthosis with elongation of the rete ridges and the absence of a delapidated brickwall

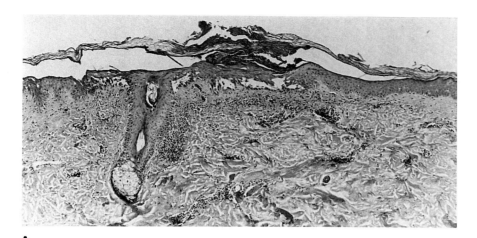

A

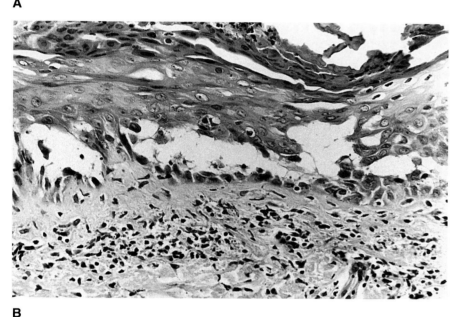

B

Figure 10–2. A. Pemphigus vulgaris, demonstrating a suprabasilar split (H&E, ×20). **B.** Pemphigus vulgaris, demonstrating acantholytic suprabasilar split with acantholysis (H&E, ×40).

appearance helps distinguish pemphigus vulgaris from familial pemphigus (Hailey-Hailey disease). Demonstration of tissue-fixed immunoglobulins in the intercellular space by direct immunofluorescence studies and of circulating antiepithelial antibodies helps confirm the diagnosis of pemphigus in questionable cases.

Immunofluorescence: Diagnostic Procedures
Skin biopsies for direct immunofluorescence tests should be obtained from the normal skin adjacent to a lesion. Lesional biopsies may result in a false negative test. A serologic test is used to distinguish between pemphigus vulgaris and pemphigus foliaceous. It was demonstrated that sera from pemphigus vulgaris cases gave higher titers and stronger immunofluorescent staining reactions on monkey esophagus, whereas sera obtained from pemphigus foliaceous or fogo selvagem patients gave strong reactions on guinea pig sections.

PEMPHIGUS VEGETANS

Clinical Features
Pemphigus vegetans represents a rare verrucous variant of pemphigus vulgaris and is characterized clinically by verrucous plaques of intertriginous areas, such as the side of the neck, the axillae, and the groin.

Histologic Features
Histologically, there is hyperkeratosis, parakeratosis, and marked acanthosis with spongiosis (Fig. 10–3A). Suprabasilar splits with acantholytic cells are noted (Fig. 10–3B). Within the epidermis, there are abscesses filled with polymorphonuclear leukocytes and eosinophils. The dermis shows an intense mixed inflammatory infiltrate. Direct immunofluorescence studies usually are confirmatory and are characterized by the presence of IgG and C3 in the intercellular space.

Pemphigus vegetans has been subclassified into the Neumann type and the Hallopeau type. In the Neumann type, early lesions are similar to those of pemphigus vulgaris and subsequently develop features of pseudoepitheliomatous hyperplasia, with acanthosis and downward proliferation of keratinocytes as well as verrucous changes. Acantholysis that is present in the early stages may disappear. Abscesses filled with eosinophils, however, persist as characteristic features even after the acantholytic cells are no longer present. In the Hallopeau variant of pemphigus vegetans, the lesions start as pustules, with suprabasilar clefts, acantholytic cells, and eosinophils. Eosinophilic spongiosis may be present. The term "pemphigus vegetans" must be restricted to those cases with histologic changes consistent with pemphigus vegetans but in which direct immunofluorescence studies demonstrate the presence of tissue-fixed immunoglobulins in the intercellular space (IgG and C3). Verrucous lesions of intertriginous areas that are negative for immunofluorescence studies are classified under a variety of terms, e.g., blastomycosis-like pyoderma or pyoderma vegetans. The exact nosologic status of the latter entities remains unclear. The patients with Hallopeau type pemphigus vegetans are thought to have a more benign disease, which will respond to lower doses of corticosteroids and enter into prolonged remission. The Neumann type is thought to follow the course of pemphigus vulgaris.

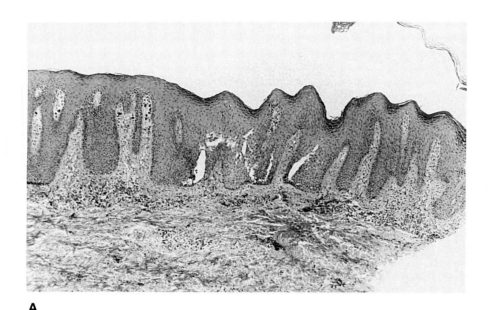

A

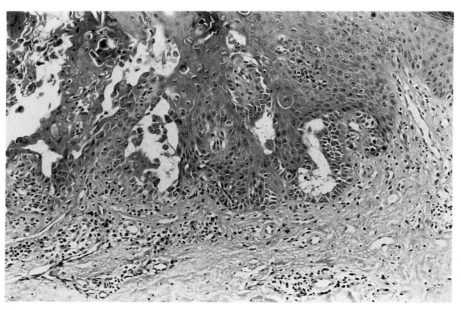

B

Figure 10–3. A. Pemphigus vegetans. Epidermal acanthosis, hyperkeratosis with suprabasilar splits (H&E, ×20). **B.** Pemphigus vegetans. Suprabasilar splits with acantholytic cells and mixed inflammatory cells and epidermal acanthosis (H&E, ×40).

DARIER'S DISEASE: KERATOSIS FOLLICULARIS

Clinical Features

Darier's disease generally is a dominantly inherited disease, although sporadic de novo cases, probably representing mutations, can occur. The lesions are small, frequently follicular papules with keratotic crusts. Confluent lesions may form plaques, some of which become verrucous in nature in the hypertrophic variant of the disease. A rare linear form also has been reported. The lesions usually develop during adult life, although they may start in childhood, and generally affect the so-called seborrheic areas of the face, chest, and back. The arms and legs, including the palms and soles, also can be affected. In rare instances, oral lesions are present.

Histologic Features

Light microscopic findings consist of hyperkeratosis, parakeratosis, follicular plugging, and irregular acanthosis with papillomatosis (Fig. 10–4A). Grains consisting of cells composed of small pyknotic nuclei surrounded by eosinophilic shrunken cytoplasm are present in the stratum corneum (Fig. 10–4B). Corps ronds consisting of large cells containing a small dark nucleus surrounded by a clear halo and basophilic shrunken cytoplasm are present in the stratum granulosum. Multiple splits develop above the basal cell layer, resulting in lacunae or intraepidermal blisters. Within the blister cavity, acantholytic cells are present singly or in groups of cells that have lost their attachment to the adjacent keratinocytes. Villous projections consisting of dermal papillae covered with one layer of keratinocytes may protrude into the blister cavity, resembling those seen in Hailey-

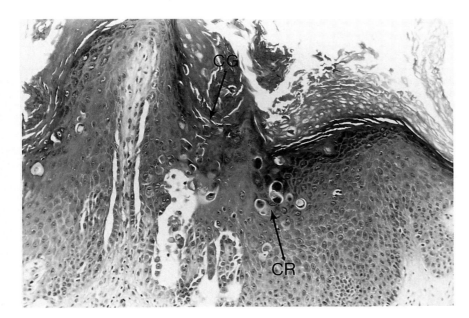

A

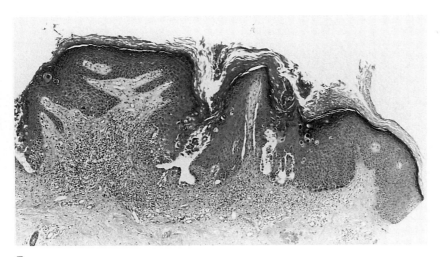

B

Figure 10–4. A. Darier's disease, showing follicular plugging with localized acanthosis, suprabasilar split with acantholytic cells, corps ronds (CR), and grains (CG) (H&E, ×20). **B.** Darier's disease, showing prominent corps ronds and grains, follicular plugging, and a suprabasilar split (H&E, ×40).

Hailey disease. Downward proliferation of anastomosing sheets of keratinocytes may be present.

In the hypertrophic variant, the degree of acanthosis is increased markedly and may resemble pseudoepitheliomatous hyperplasia. Lacunae and acantholytic cells usually are present.

The dermis in Darier's disease generally shows a moderate perivascular mononuclear cell infiltrate. In the hypertrophic variant, however, if secondary infection is present, the dermal infiltrate may be more extensive and contain polymorphonuclear leukocytes as well.

Differential Diagnosis

Pemphigus vulgaris, Hailey-Hailey disease, and transient acantholytic dermatosis must be considered in the differential diagnosis.

Pemphigus vulgaris, which shows suprabasilar acantholysis, does not occur with grains and corps ronds and can be ruled out easily. If any doubt exists on clinical or light microscopic grounds, direct immunofluorescence studies, which are positive in pemphigus and negative in Darier's disease, can be considered.

Hailey-Hailey disease may have great similarities to Darier's disease. However, the lesions in Darier's disease generally are focal in nature and show the presence of normal skin between the foci of Darier's disease, whereas the lesion in Hailey-Hailey disease is confluent. In addition, the number of grains and corps ronds is greater in Darier's disease, which is a useful diagnostic criterion.

Difficulty may arise in distinguishing between transient or persistent acantholytic dermatosis and Darier's disease. At times, the lesions may be histologically indistinguishable, and only clinicopathologic correlation results in accurate diagnosis. Occasionally, transient acantholytic dermatosis in addition to histologic features of Darier's disease also

may show features of Hailey-Hailey disease, pemphigus vulgaris or foliaceous, or an eczematous dermatitis. The presence of mixed histologic findings generally favors a diagnosis of transient acantholytic dermatosis.

Darier-like changes may be found in isolated lesions, e.g., warty dyskeratoma, focal acantholytic dyskeratoma, or within actinic or seborrheic keratosis. These represent incidental findings not indicative of Darier's disease elsewhere.

HAILEY-HAILEY DISEASE: FAMILIAL BENIGN CHRONIC PEMPHIGUS

In April 1939, brothers Howard Hailey and Hugh Hailey of the Department of Dermatology of Emory University School of Medicine in Atlanta reported on the cutaneous findings of two brothers aged 35 and 31. These patients had an unclassified recurrent eruption over a period of 9 and 10 years, respectively.

Clinical Features

Clinically, Hailey-Hailey disease, a dominantly inherited disorder, is characterized by vesicles and bullae that become denuded or crusted. Dry lesions show deep painful fissures. The neck, axillae, inframammary area, and the groin and perineum are commonly affected areas, although the trunk and extremities also can be involved. Unusual clinical variants have been reported as hyperkeratotic, verrucous, neurodermatitic, or papular. The disease is chronic, with periods of remission and exacerbation.

Histologic Features

Light microscopy shows suprabasilar lacunae formation in early lesions, with gradual development of suprabasilar

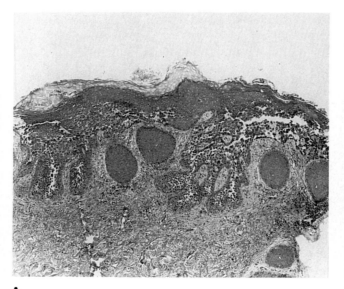

A

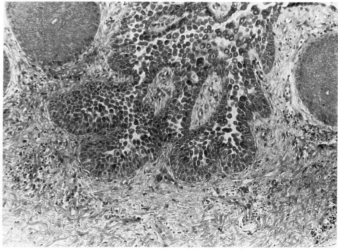

B

Figure 10–5. A. Hailey-Hailey disease, demonstrating acantholysis, intercellular edema, dilapidated brickwall, and a suprabasilar split (H&E, ×20). **B.** Hailey-Hailey disease demonstrating downward proliferation of epidermal strands with prominent intraepidermal edema and acantholysis (H&E, ×40).

vesicles and bullae with acantholysis. There is downward proliferation of epidermal strands. Villi consisting of dermal papillae covered with one or several layers of keratinocytes may protrude into the blister cavity. Extensive intercellular edema results in partial acantholysis, which is referred to as "dilapidated brickwall" appearance and is characteristic of the disease (Fig. 10–5A,B). Occasional grains and corps rond may be found. The dermis shows a mixed perivascular inflammatory infiltrate.

Typical acantholytic cells similar to those in pemphigus vulgaris may be present. Direct and indirect immunofluorescence may be required to distinguish between pemphigus vulgaris, which has positive tissue-fixed and circulating autoantibodies, and Hailey-Hailey disease, which does not.

Transient acantholytic dermatosis may show findings resembling Hailey-Hailey disease and must be considered in the differential diagnosis. The changes, however, are focal in nature, and clinicopathologic correlation usually results in the correct diagnosis. The upper layers of the epidermis may show occasional corps ronds and grains, but these usually are few in numbers and should not create confusion with Darier's disease.

TRANSIENT ACANTHOLYTIC DERMATOSIS (GROVER'S DISEASE)

Clinical Features
In 1970, Grover described transient acantholytic dermatosis (TAD) as a unique clinicopathologic entity. The patients had pruritic, edematous papules and vesicles with excoriations. The lesions were primarily on the trunk, although extremities also could be affected. The palms, soles, and mucous membranes usually are spared. Histologically, the lesions showed epidermal acantholysis. In 1977, Chalet et al. expanded the histologic spectrum to include several patterns, i.e., Darier-like, Hailey-Hailey-like, pemphigus-like, and cases with spongiosis and acantholysis.

Although initially TAD was thought to be more common in men, both sexes are affected. Pruritus can be intense. Sun exposure was incriminated as a precipitating factor in earlier cases, but more recent studies point to the importance of heat and sweat in triggering the eruption.

The lesions may be transient, explaining the original terminology, or they may persist for months or years and have been described under the term "persistent acantholytic dermatosis."

Histologic Features
Typical Lesions. The classic changes consist of slight hyperkeratosis, occasional parakeratosis, and acanthosis with focal spongiosis. Suprabasilar splits with suprabasilar or midepidermal acantholysis are present. Excoriations frequently are noted. The dermis shows a mixed lymphohistiocytic infiltrate with occasional eosinophils.

Darier Type. The histologic changes resemble those described for the typical lesions. In addition, however, grains, corps ronds and elongation of rete ridges similar to those seen in Darier's disease are present (Fig. 10–6).

Hailey-Hailey Type. The lesions show the focal changes described for the classic lesions but in addition show areas of dilapidated brickwall appearance typical of Hailey-Hailey disease.

Pemphigus Type. In addition to the typical changes of subcorneal splits and acantholysis similar to those in pemphigus foliaceous, more extensive suprabasilar acantholysis similar to pemphigus vulgaris may be present. Direct and indirect immunofluorescence studies in these patients always are negative.

Spongiotic Type. In these cases, the degree of spongiosis is more marked, sometimes resulting in intraepidermal vesicles with acantholytic cells.

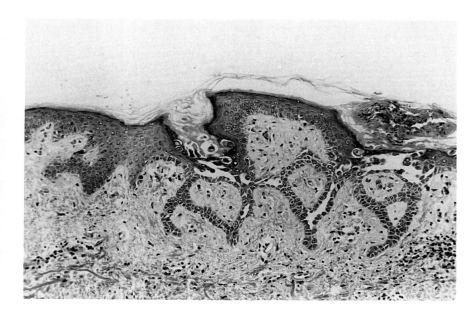

Figure 10–6. Grover's disease (Darier type). Elongation of rete ridges, with suprabasilar split and prominent corps ronds (H&E, ×20).

Two features are typical of transient and persistent acantholytic dermatosis: (1) the circumscribed focal nature of the histologic changes and (2) the coexistence of mixed histologic findings either in the same section or in different sections obtained from the same block. The presence of changes resembling those in Darier's disease, Hailey-Hailey disease, and pemphigus in the same section or the same block usually is indicative of TAD unless proven otherwise by either clinicopathologic correlations or immunofluorescence tests.

Differential Diagnosis

TAD is distinguished from Darier's disease clinicopathologically, since there are only a few scattered, smooth or excoriated lesions in TAD, whereas in Darier's disease, there are multiple crusted lesions. Hailey-Hailey disease affects primarily the flexural areas (neck, axilla, groin), whereas TAD affects mostly the trunk and extremities. Histologically, TAD shows focal changes, whereas Hailey-Hailey disease shows extensive changes. Pemphigus vulgaris is clinically distinct by the presence of mucous membrane lesions and histologically by the presence of more extensive involvement compared to the focal involvement of TAD. Similarly, pemphigus foliaceous shows extensive clinical and histologic changes. In doubtful cases, direct and indirect immunofluorescence tests that are positive in pemphigus and negative in TAD can be used. The spongiotic type can be distinguished from eczematous dermatitis by the presence of acantholytic cells.

FOCAL ACANTHOLYTIC DYSKERATOSIS

Focal acantholytic dyskeratosis was used by Ackerman in 1972 to describe a heterogeneous group of disorders of the skin and mucous membranes with common light microscopic findings.

The histologic changes consisted of suprabasilar clefts, acantholytic and dyskeratotic cells, hyper- and parakeratosis, and proliferation of basal cells. In addition to Darier's and Grover's disease, included in this classification, various solitary lesions also were included in this group. It is a useful classification for the purpose of organizing different disease entities with similar microscopic findings.

INFANTILE ACROPUSTULOSIS

Clinical Features

Infantile acropustulosis (IA) is an uncommon, recurrent, pruritic acral pustular dermatosis of uncertain etiology that affects infants and young children. It is most commonly seen in black, male infants. Clinically, it is notoriously unresponsive to common anti-inflammatory agents, antibiotics, and antipruritic drugs. Sulfapyridine recently has been noted to be helpful. On occasion, infantile acropustulosis is associated with atopic dermatitis. Several reports suggest concomitant or antecedent infantile scabies associated with IA. Differential diagnosis of IA has included viral exanthemas, infantile scabies, toxic erythema of the newborn, transient neonatal pustular melanosis, congenital cutaneous candidiasis, and staphylococcal impetigo.

Clinically, the acral lesions first appear as 1–3 mm inflammatory papules that evolve to vesicopustules. The lesions commonly occur in crops and are extremely pruritic. The clinical course is variable, with intermittent remissions and exacerbations. Relapses are particularly common in the summer. Spontaneous resolution is noted by 2–3 years of age.

Histologic Features

Histologically, the early papule demonstrates spongiosis, focal epidermal necrosis (necrolysis), eosinophilic dyskeratosis, and exocytosis of neutrophils and eosinophils. This is associated with a mild superficial mixed perivascular inflammatory infiltrate. The older lesions are distinctive subcorneal and intraepidermal vesicopustules containing predominantly neutrophils and, occasionally, eosinophils (Fig. 10–7A,B). Rarely, eosinophils are the predominant cells. PAS- and Gram-stained microbial cultures are negative for fungi and bacteria. Direct immunofluorescence is negative.

Differential Diagnosis

Differential diagnosis of vesiculopustular eruptions of infants and children includes several disorders (Table 10–3). Within the immediate neonatal period, the major diagnostic considerations are toxic erythema of the newborn, transient neonatal pustular melanosis, and congenital cutaneous candidiasis. Toxic erythema of the newborn appears shortly after birth in 50% of infants, with erythematous patches studded with vesicopustules containing predominantly eosinophils. These lesions are transient and disappear within 2–5 days.

Transient neonatal pustular melanosis, etiology unknown, appears at birth as a nonpruritic, neutrophilic pustule and primarily involves the chin, neck, lower back, and acral sites, namely, the palms and soles. These pustules disappear within 1–3 days, leaving melanotic macules with a small, fine, scaly collarette that lasts for months.

Congenital candidiasis appears as a generalized maculopapular eruption that evolves to a vesicopustular eruption within a few days. KOH preparations and cultures of the pustules reveal *Candida albicans*.

After the neonatal period, the differential diagnosis of vesicopustular dermatosis of childhood expands and includes infantile scabies, bullous impetigo, and viral exanthemas. From pruritic papules, vesiculopapules, or vesicle pustules of scabies, mites, ova, and scybala can be demonstrated, confirming the diagnosis of scabies. Examination of family members for similar mites is helpful in confirming the diagnosis.

INCONTINENTIA PIGMENTI

Clinical Features

Incontinentia pigmenti (IP) is a rare, inherited, largely sex-limited neurocutaneous syndrome characterized by triphasic cutaneous eruption and dental and central nervous system defects.

The characteristic cutaneous lesions appear in three

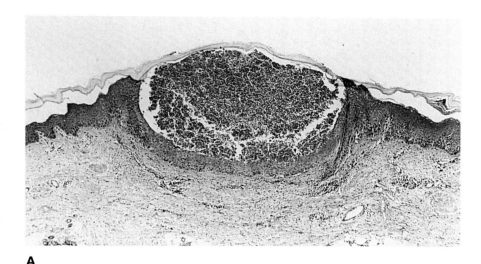

A

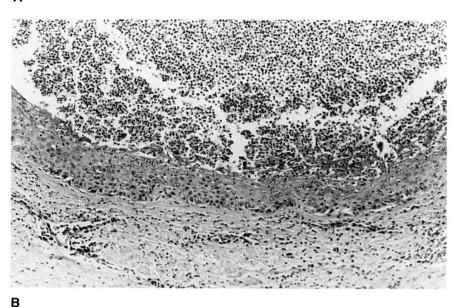

B

Figure 10–7. A. Infantile acropustulosis. An older lesion demonstrating an intraepidermal pustule (H&E, ×20). **B.** Infantile acropustulosis, demonstrating a pustule containing an admixture of acute inflammatory cells (H&E, ×40).

stages: the acute stage (vesicular bullous) and two chronic stages (verrucal and pigmented). A cutaneous eruption is most prominent on the trunk and extremities. Associated disorders include pegged or widely spaced teeth, hypodontia, strabismus, astigmatism, partial alopecia, mental retardation, seizure disorders, and spina bifida.

IP is sex-lined and is lethal to males. IP demonstrates one-half chromosome mutation associated with immunologic defects noted with increased epidermal eosinophilic chemotactic factors and associated peripheral eosinophilia and leukocytosis, defective neutrophilic chemotaxis, and abnormal lymphocyte function.

Histologic Features

In the acute, papulovesicular or urticarial stage, the epidermis is slightly acanthotic and demonstrates eosinophilic spongiosis with minute epidermal microabscesses. Occasionally, eosinophilic dyskeratotic keratinocytes are observed. Frequently, small microabscesses containing eosinophils are seen within the dermal papillae, and, occasionally, eosinophils are seen streaming out of the small papillary dermal vessels into the epidermis (Fig. 10–8A,B). In addition, within the papillary dermis, edema and mixed perivascular infiltrates are observed. In summary, eosinophils and neutrophils can be observed both within the dermis and within the epidermal abscesses. A touch preparation of a vesicle demonstrates increased eosinophils and neutrophils.

In the chronic, verrucous stage, there is mild-to-moderate acanthosis, with frequent clonal collections of eosinophilic dyskeratotic cells, some of which appear in the area of the acrosyringium (Fig. 10–8C). Macrophages have been

TABLE 10–3. DIFFERENTIAL LABORATORY FEATURES OF VESICULOPUSTULAR ERUPTIONS OF INFANCY

Vesiculopustular Eruption	Wright or Giemsa Stain	Gram Stain for Bacteria	Culture	Wet Mount with KOH or Oil	Histology
Infantile acropustulosis	PMN and/or EOS[a]	Negative	Negative	Negative	Eosinophilic dyskeratosis EOS, PMN (EPI/DER)
Toxic erythema of newborn	EOS	Negative	Negative	Negative	Spongiotic necrosis EOS, abscess (EPI)
Transient neonatal pustular melanosis	PMN	Negative	Negative	Negative	PMN abscess (EPI)
Congenital cutaneous candidiasis	PMN	Negative	Candida albicans	Pseudohyphae and spores	PMN abscess (EPI)
Scabies	PMN	Negative	Negative	Mites, ova, or scybala	PMN (EPI/DER) EOS
Staphylococcal impetigo	PMN	Gram-positive cocci	Staphylococcus aureus	Negative	PMN abscess (EPI)
Incontinentia pigmenti	EOS	Negative	Negative	Negative	*Acute stage* EOS spongiosis EOS dyskeratosis

[a] PMN, neutrophilic polymorphonuclear leukocytes; EOS, eosinophils; EPI, epidermis; DER, dermis.
Modified from Hayden and Quackenbush. J Fam Pract. 1984;18:929.

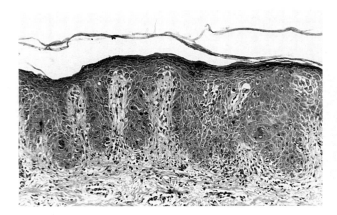

A

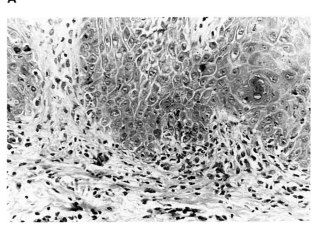

B

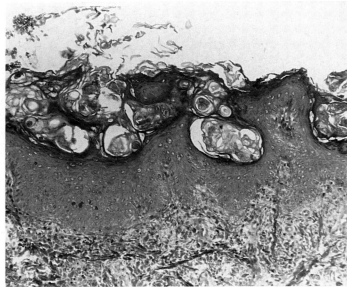

C

Figure 10–8. A. Incontinentia pigmenti. Epidermal acanthosis, elongation of rete ridges, focal dyskeratotic cells, subtle spongiosis, and exocytosis of eosinophils (H&E, ×20). **B.** Incontinentia pigmenti, demonstrating epidermal spongiosis, exocytosis of eosinophils, and dyskeratotic cells (H&E, ×40). **C.** Incontinentia pigmenti, demonstrating the chronic verrucous stage with hyperkeratosis, papillomatoses, and epidermal acanthosis (H&E, ×20).

identified phagocytizing these abnormal keratinocytes. In this chronic stage, a few eosinophils and neutrophils may be observed within the epidermis.

In the last chronic stage, the pigmentary stage, the epidermis may be normal or slightly acanthotic, with a normal distribution of melanocytes or increased basilar melanosis. Within the papillary dermis, melanophages can be observed that most likely represent postinflammatory hyperpigmentation. In a recent study, the pigmentary stage of IP was not observed even though clinically there was abnormal reticulated pigmentation. There was, however, evidence of dermal sclerosis, decreased elastic fibers, and diminished adnexal structures.

Differential Diagnosis

Because of the numerous eosinophils and neutrophils arising in stages 1 and 2 with evidence of degeneration of melanocytes and keratinocytes, the eosinophilic chemotatic factors within the epidermis were hypothesized to be and later demonstrated to be a prerequisite for the accumulation of these cells. Similar eosinophilic chemotactic factors have been observed in other autoimmune diseases, for example, pemphigus vegetans and lichen planus pemphigoides. Similarities between the verrucous stage of IP and autoimmune diseases, e.g., hypertrophic lichen planus, atrophic lichen planus, poikiloderma, and graft-versus-host reactions, have been observed clinically.

REFERENCES

1. Beutner EH, Chorzelski TP, Bean SF. *Immunopathology of the Skin.* 2nd ed. New York: John Wiley & Sons; 1979.
2. Beutner EH, Chorzelski TP, Kumar V. *Immunopathology of the Skin.* 3rd ed. New York: John Wiley & Sons; 1987.
3. Beutner EH, Chorzelski TP, Wilson RM, et al. IgA pemphigus foliaceus. A report of two cases and review of the literature. *J Am Acad Dermatol.* (in press)
4. Furtado TA. Histopathology of pemphigus foliaceous. *Arch Dermatol.* 1959;80:66–71.
5. Knight AG, Black MM, Delaney JJ. Eosinophilic spongiosis: Clinical, histologic and immunofluorescent correlation. *Clin Exp Dermatol.* 1976;1:141–153.
6. Lever WF. *Pemphigus and Pemphigoid.* Springfield, Ill: Charles C Thomas; 1965.
7. Maciejowska E, Jablonska S, Chorzelski T. Is pemphigus herpetiformis an entity? *Int J Dermatol.* 1987;26:571–577.
8. Sabolinski ML, Beutner EH, Krasny S, et al. Substrate specificity of anti-epithelial antibodies of pemphigus vulgaris and pemphigus foliaceous sera in immunofluorescence tests on monkey and guinea pig esophagus sections. *J Invest Dermatol.* 1987;88:545–549.
9. American ML, Ahmed AR. Pemphigus erythematosus, Senear-Usher syndrome. *Int J Dermatol.* 1985;24:16–25.
10. Chorzelski T, Jablonska S, Blaszczyk M. Immunopathological investigation in the Senear-Usher syndrome (coexistence of pemphigus and lupus erythematosus). *Br J Dermatol.* 1968;80:211–217.
11. Thorvaldsen J. Two cases of penicillamine-induced pemphigus erythematosus. *Dermatologica.* 1979;159:167–170.
12. Ahmed AR, Blose DA. Pemphigus vegetans: Neumann type and Hallopeau type. *Int Dermatol.* 1984;23:135–141.
13. Kuo TT, Wang CN. Charcot-Leyden crystals in pemphigus vegetans. *J Cutan Pathol.* 1986;13:242–245.
14. Gottlieb SK, Lutzner MA. Darier's disease. *Arch Dermatol.* 1969;100:50–53.
15. Ishibashi Y, Kajiwara Y, Andoh I, et al. The nature and pathogenesis of dyskeratosis in Hailey-Hailey and Darier's disease. *J Dermatol.* 1984;11:335–353.
16. Weathers DR, Olansky S, Sharpe LO. Darier's disease with mucous membrane involvement. *Arch Dermatol.* 1969;100:50–53.
17. Hailey H, Hailey H. Familial benign chronic pemphigus. *Arch Dermatol.* 1939;39:679–685.
18. Michel B. Hailey-Hailey disease (familial benign chronic pemphigus). *Arch Dermatol.* 1982;118:781–783.
19. Palmer DD, Perry HO. Benign familial benign chronic pemphigus. *Arch Dermatol.* 1962;86:493–502.
20. Bystryn JC. Immunofluorescence studies in transient acantholytic dermatosis (Grover's disease). *Am J Dermatopathol.* 1979;1:325–327.
21. Chalet M, Grover R, Ackerman AB. Transient acantholytic dermatosis. *Arch Dermatol.* 1977;113:431–435.
22. Grover RW. Transient acantholytic dermatosis. *Arch Dermatol.* 1970;101:426–434.
23. Hu CH, Michel B, Farber EM. Transient acantholytic dermatosis (Grover's disease). A skin disorder related to heat and sweating. *Arch Dermatol.* 1985;121:1439–1441.
24. Ackerman AB. Focal acantholytic dyskeratosis. *Arch Dermatol.* 1972;106:702–706.
25. Barr RJ, Globerman LM, Seeber FA. Transient neonatal pustular melanosis. *Int J Dermatol.* 1979;18:636–638.
26. Elpern DJ. Infantile acropustolosis and antecedent scabies. *J Am Acad Dermatol.* 1984;11:895–896.
27. Falanga V. Infantile acropustulosis with eosinophils (Ltr). *J Am Acad Dermatol.* 1985;13:826–828.
28. Jennings JL, Burrows WM. Infantile acropustulosis. *J Am Acad Dermatol.* 1983;9:733–738.
29. Hayden GF, Quackenbush K. Infantile acropustulosis: A "new" reticulopustular eruption of infants and children. *J Fam Pract* 1984;18:928–929, 932.
30. Lucky AW, McGuire JS. Infantile acropustulosis with eosinophilic pustulosis. *J Pediatr.* 1982;100:428.
31. Newton JA, Salisburg J, Marsden A, McGibbon DH. Acropustulosis of infancy. *Br J Dermatol.* 1986;115:735–739.
32. Vignon-Pennamen MD, Wallach D. Infantile acropustulosis: A clinicopathologic study of six cases. *Arch Dermatol.* 1986;122:1155–1160.
33. Ashly GR, Burgdorf WHC. Incontinentia pigmenti: Pigmentary changes independent of incontinence. *J Cutan Pathol.* 1987;14:284–250.
34. Burgess MC. Incontinentia pigmenti. *Br Dent J.* 1982;152:195–196.
35. Carney RG Jr. Incontinentia pigmenti: A world statistical analysis. *Arch Dermatol.* 1976;112:535–542.
36. Dahl MV, Matula G, Leonards R, et al. Incontinentia pigmenti and defective neutrophil chemotaxis. *Arch Dermatol.* 1975;111:1603–1605.
37. Eisenhaure, O'Brien J, Feingold CM. Incontinentia pigmenti. *Am J Dis Child.* 1985;139:711–712.
38. Emmerson RW, Wilson Jones E. Eosinophilic spongiosis in pemphigus: A report of an unusual case. *Arch Dermatol.* 1968;97:252–255.
39. Gordon H, Gordon W. Incontinentia pigmenti: Clinical and genetical studies of two familial cases. *Dermatologica.* 1970;140:150–168.
40. Hecht F, Hecht BK, Austin WJ. Incontinentia pigmenti in Arizona Indians, including transmission from mother to son inconsistent with the half chromatid mutation model. *Clin Genet.* 1982;21:293–296.
41. Jessen RT, VanEpps DE, Goodwin JS, Bowerman J. Incontinen-

tia pigmenti: Evidence for both neutrophil and lymphocyte dysfunction. *Arch Dermatol.* 1978;114:1182–1186.

42. Kelly TE, Rary JM, Young L. Incontinentia pigmenti: A chromosomal breakage syndrome. *J Hered.* 1976;67:171–172.

43. Lang PG Jr, Maize JC. Coexisting lichen planus and bullous pemphigoid or lichen planus pemphigoides? *J Am Acad Dermatol.* 1983;9:133–140.

44. Lenz W. Half chromatid mutations may explain incontinentia pigmenti in males. *Am J Hum Genet.* 1975;27:690–691.

45. Lever WF, Schaumburg-Lever G. *Histopathology of the Skin.* Philadelphia: JB Lippincott Co; 1983:83–85.

46. Person JR, Bishop GF. Is poikiloderma a graft-versus-host-like reaction? *Am J Dermatopathol.* 1984;6:71–72.

47. Matsuoka LY. Graft versus host disease. *J Am Acad Dermatol.* 1981;5:595–599.

48. Michel B, Sy EK. Labeled antibody studies, tissue-fixed immunoglobulins in lichen planus. In: Beutner EH, Chorzelski TP, Bean SF, Jordon RE, eds. *Immunopathology of the skin.* Stroudsburg, Penna: Dowden, Hutchinson & Ross; 1973:182–193.

49. Person JR. Incontinentia pigmenti: A failure of immune tolerance. *J Am Acad Dermatol.* 1985;13:120–124.

50. Ponsprasit P, Chittinand S. Lerchawnakul A, Charmsiriwat S. Incontinentia pigmenti, analysis of 18 cases. *J Med Assoc Thai.* 1985;68:630–637.

51. Sobel S, Miller R, Shatin H. Lichen planus pemphigoides: Immunofluorescence findings. *Arch Dermatol.* 1976;112:1280–1283.

52. Takematsu H, Terci T, Torinuki A, Tagami H. Incontinentia pigmenti: Eosinophil chemotactic activity of the crusted scales in the vesicobullous stage. *Br J Dermatol.* 1986;115:61–66.

53. Beutner EH, Chorzelski TP, Bean SF. *Immunopathology of the Skin.* 2nd ed. New York: John Wiley & Sons; 1979.

54. Beutner EH, Chorzelski TP, Kumar V. *Immunopathology of the Skin.* 3rd ed. New York: John Wiley & Sons; 1987.

55. Beutner EH, Chorzelski TP, Wilson RM, et al. IgA pemphigus foliaceous. A report of two cases and review of the literature. *J Am Acad Dermatol.* (in press)

56. Furtado TA. Histopathology of pemphigus foliaceous. *Arch Dermatol.* 1959;80:66–71.

57. Knight AG, Black MM, Delaney JJ. Eosinophilic spongiosis: Clinical, histologic and immunofluorescent correlation. *Clin Exp Dermatol.* 1976;1:141–153.

58. Lever WF. *Pemphigus and Pemphigoid.* Springfield, Ill: Charles C Thomas, 1965.

59. Maciejowska E, Jablonska S, Chorzelski T. Is pemphigus herpetiformis an entity? *Int J Dermatol.* 1987;26:571–577.

60. Sabolinski ML, Beutner EH, Krasny S, et al. Substrate specificity of anti-epithelial antibodies of pemphigus vulgaris and pemphigus foliaceous sera in immunofluorescence tests on monkey and guinea pig esophagus sections. *J Invest Dermatol.* 1987; 88:545–549.

61. American ML, Ahmed AR. Pemphigus erythematosus, Senear-Usher syndrome. *Int J Dermatol.* 1985;24:16–25.

62. Chorzelski T, Jablonska S, Blaszczyk M. Immunopathological investigation in the Senear-Usher syndrome (coexistence of pemphigus and lupus erythematosus). *Br J Dermatol.* 1968; 80:211–217.

63. Thorvaldsen J. Two cases of penicillamine-induced pemphigus erythematosus. *Dermatologica.* 1979;159:167–170.

CHAPTER 11
Subepidermal Bullous Disorders

Susan C. Parker and Martin M. Black

Subepidermal bullous disorders are a heterogeneous group characterized by separation of the epidermis and dermis to produce a vesicle or bulla. The split may occur at a number of levels, including through the basal cells, the lamina lucida, the lamina densa, the sublamina densa zone, and the upper part of the papillary dermis. The normal structure of the basement membrane zone (BMZ) is shown in Figure 11–1.

Classification of such a disparate group of diseases is difficult, but attempts have been made on the basis of either ultrastructural or histologic features. Braun-Falco[1] has devised four groups, based on probable mechanism of disjunction as assessed through electron microscopy:

1. Dermoepidermal disjunction by disintegration of basal cells (epidermolysis bullosa simplex)
2. Dermoepidermal disjunction by cleft formation between the dermal plasma membrane of basal cells and the electron microscopic basement membrane within the intermembranous space (epidermolysis bullosa hereditaria letalis, lichen planus, pemphigoid, erythema multiforme, suction blisters)
3. Dermoepidermal disjunction by disintegration of the connective tissue of the subjacent corium (epidermolysis bullosa dystrophica, porphyria cutanea tarda)
4. Excessive destruction of the dermoepidermal junction after initial dermal injury (dermatitis herpetiformis, erythema multiforme)

Some of these diseases are immunologically mediated, and it is now possible to classify them according to the ultrastructural localization of immunoreactants (Table 11–1).

Ackerman[2] classified subepidermal bullous disorders histologically, according to the nature and distribution of the inflammatory cell infiltrate. This classification was modified by Farmer[3] to include the presence or absence of epidermal necrosis or dyskeratosis (Table 11–2). The criteria for classification are not always unequivocal, however.

A. In an older lesion, the base of a subepidermal blister may regenerate, giving the appearance of an intraepidermal split.

B. An intraepidermal blister may burst through into the dermis, giving the appearance of a subepidermal lesion.
C. Secondary infection may occur, altering the histologic picture.
D. In older lesions, such changes as epidermal necrosis and the accumulation of eosinophils may occur and should not be used as diagnostic pointers.

Because of such potentially misleading changes, it is important to biopsy an early lesion, preferably a small intact vesicle. An elliptical scalpel biopsy that includes the whole lesion is preferred. However, it is not always possible, even with the utmost care, to make the correct diagnosis using light microscopy alone.[4] Immunofluorescence is mandatory for the immunologically mediated diseases, and sometimes immunoelectron microscopy also is required for precise localization of immunoreactants. Perilesional skin should be taken and snap frozen. This can be done by extending the ellipse biopsy above to include skin adjacent to the lesion. Fresh tissue is preferred for immunoelectron microscopy.

BULLOUS PEMPHIGOID

Clinical Features
Pemphigoid was first differentiated from pemphigus by Lever.[5] It is predominantly a disease of the elderly, although it may occur at any age. Males and females are affected equally, and there is no greater incidence in any racial group or HLA type.[6,7]

Pemphigoid is characterized clinically by large, tense bullae arising either on an erythematous base or from normal skin. These bullae may rupture, leaving denuded areas that, unlike similar lesions in pemphigus, show a tendency to heal spontaneously. They are often accompanied by erythematous lesions with a serpiginous edge and central clearing. There frequently is a preceding nonspecific, pruritic, erythematous, or urticarial eruption. Sites of predilection are the flexor surfaces of the limbs, the groins, axillae, and lower abdomen. Mucosal lesions are not a prominent

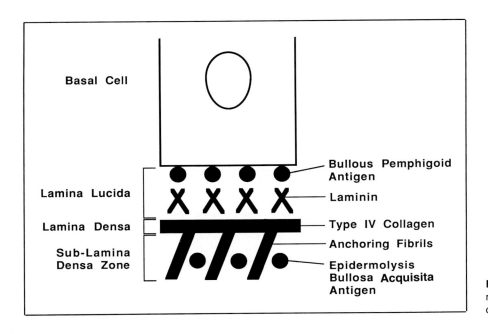

Figure 11–1. The epidermal basement membrane zone. Ultrastructural localization of immunoreactants.

TABLE 11–1. LOCALIZATION OF IMMUNOREACTANTS IN THE BULLOUS SKIN DISEASES

Lamina lucida	Sublamina densa	Dermal papillae
Bullous pemphigoid	Lupus erythematosus	Dermatitis herpetiformis
Cicatricial pemphigoid	Epidermolysis bullosa acquisita	
Herpes gestationis	Linear IgA dermatosis	
	Chronic bullous disease of childhood	

TABLE 11–2. CLASSIFICATION OF SUBEPIDERMAL BULLOUS DISEASES

	Blister Roof	
Inflammation	**Intact**	**Necrosis or Dyskeratosis**
Minimal	Epidermolysis bullosa (acqui- sita, junctional, dystrophic)	Toxic epidermal necrolysis
	Pemphigoid	Chemical or thermal burn
	Porphyria cutanea tarda	Autolysis
	Bullous amyloidosis	Coma blister
	Suction blister	Acute radiodermatitis
	Scleroderma	
Predominantly lymphocytes	Lupus erythematosus	Erythema multiforme
	Polymorphic light eruption	Toxic epidermal necrolysis
	Lichen planus	Fixed drug eruption
	Lichen sclerosus et atrophicus	Acute graft-versus-host disease
Predominantly neutrophils	Dermatitis herpetiformis	Leukocytoclastic vasculitis
	Lupus erythematosus	Septic emboli
	Chronic bullous dermatosis of childhood	
	Linear IgA dermatosis	
	Pemphigoid (rare)	
Predominantly eosinophils	Pemphigoid	Insect bites
	Herpes gestationis	
	Chronic bullous dermatosis of childhood	
	Drug eruption	
Predominantly mast cells	Bullous mastocytosis	

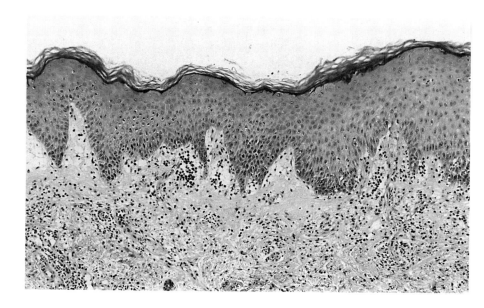

Figure 11–2. Bullous pemphigoid. An early lesion showing edema of the papillary dermis, many eosinophils and clefting at the dermoepidermal junction (H & E, ×150).

feature, but the oral mucosa may be affected. Treatment is with steroids and immunosuppressive agents. The prognosis is generally good, and eventual spontaneous remission can be expected.

Contrary to earlier opinion, there is probably no overall association between pemphigoid and internal malignancy, although it is still possible that people without circulating antibasement membrane antibodies may have a greater incidence of malignancy.[8–11]

Rarely, the disease may be localized, usually involving the legs. In such cases, a better response to treatment and a lower recurrence rate can be expected.[12] Other variants are the nodular prurigo form, the vesicular form (in which the blisters are small, tense, and sometimes grouped,[13] and the verrucous form (in which vegetating lesions are seen mainly in the axillae and groins.[14]

Histologic Features

Histologically, a pemphigoid lesion is a subepidermal blister with a variable inflammatory cell infiltrate. Pemphigoid has been subdivided into two distinct histologic types: cell-rich and cell-poor, according to the density of the inflammatory infiltrate.[2] However, it seems more likely that these differences represent two extremes of a continuous spectrum rather than distinct entities (Figs. 11–2, 11–3, 11–4, 11–5).

The blister cavity itself usually contains fibrin and eosinophils (Fig. 11–4) but also may contain some neutrophils. The dermal papillae at the base of the blister are widened and edematous (Fig. 11–3), and there is an upper dermal accumulation of inflammatory cells, chiefly eosinophils but also histiocytes, lymphocytes, and some neutrophils, particularly around the blood vessels. This infiltrate extends beyond the margins of the blister. Sometimes, there is a linear

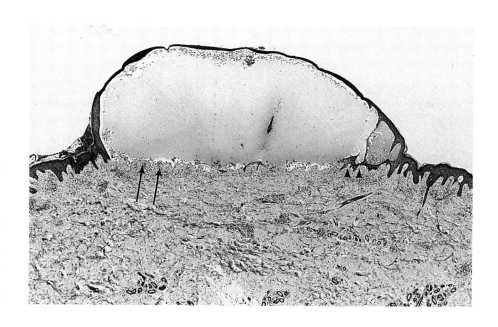

Figure 11–3. Bullous pemphigoid. This bulla has arisen on a nonerythematous base, and there is little inflammatory infiltrate. Dermal papillae at the base of the blister are widened and edematous (arrows). Regeneration of the basal layer has already begun at the right edge (arrowheads) (H & E, ×50).

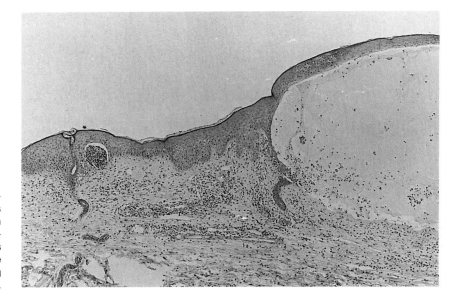

Figure 11–4. Bullous pemphigoid. A subepidermal bulla that has arisen on an erythematous base. There is an eosinophilic microabscess on the left and a moderate inflammatory infiltrate consisting chiefly of eosinophils. The papillary dermis is edematous. Epidermal regeneration at the edge of the blister has led to part of the blister being apparently intraepidermal in location (H & E, ×60).

band of eosinophils along the dermoepidermal junction. There may also be microabscesses at the tips of the dermal papillae at the blister margin that contain eosinophils (Figs. 11–4, 11–5). Rarely, however, the predominant cell type may be the neutrophil, and, therefore, pemphigoid cannot be distinguished absolutely from dermatitis herpetiformis by light microscopy alone. Immunofluorescence microscopy is mandatory.

The histologic structure varies with the age of the lesion. In early urticarial lesions without bulla formation, there is edema of the papillary dermis with a variable inflammatory cell infiltrate. Sometimes there are vacuoles at the dermoepidermal junction that later give rise to subepidermal clefts and then blisters (Fig. 11–2). Eosinophils are sometimes present in the epidermis, which may be spongiotic, presenting an appearance known as "eosinophilic spongiosis." This appearance was described originally as occurring in pemphigus, but it is now known to occur also in the early lesions of pemphigoid.[15,16] It is often accompanied by a peripheral blood eosinophilia.

In early lesions, the epidermis over the roof of the blister is intact. Regeneration of the epidermis over the floor of the blister soon begins, so that the lesion appears to have an intraepidermal location (Figs. 11–3, 11–4). Later, however, the epidermis becomes necrotic and may even disintegrate, eventually giving the appearance of a subcorneal blister. It is, therefore, particularly important that an early lesion be chosen for biopsy.

In blisters arising on normal-appearing skin, the inflammatory changes are much less marked and may be confused with some forms of epidermolysis bullosa or porphyria cutanea tarda (Fig. 11–3). In pemphigoid vegetans, there is,

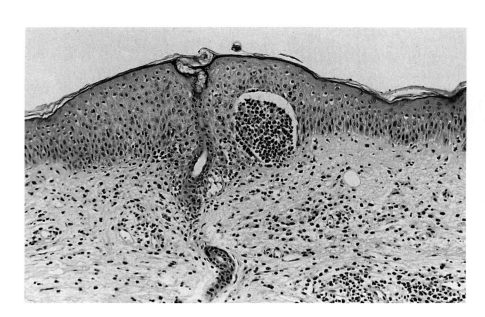

Figure 11–5. Bullous pemphigoid. This is a higher power view of the lesion in Figure 11–4, showing the papillary microabscess, which is identical to that seen in dermatitis herpetiformis except that the cells are chiefly eosinophils rather than neutrophils (H & E, ×150).

in addition, pseudoepitheliomatous hyperplasia of the epidermis.

Electron microscopic studies have revealed migration and degranulation of eosinophils with blister formation through the lamina lucida, fragmentation and destruction of the lamina densa, and damage to the basal cells.[17]

Immunopathology

Pemphigoid is an autoimmune disease in which antibodies are generated against the BMZ, specifically against the so-called bullous pemphigoid antigen, which is located in the lamina lucida. This antigen is found in the BMZ of all stratified squamous epithelia and also in the epithelia of the urethra, bladder, bronchi, and gallbladder.[18] It is synthesized by epithelial cells and has a molecular weight of about 220,000. It appears to be associated with the hemidesmosomes.[19,20]

In pemphigoid, immunoglobulins and complement are deposited in the lamina lucida and can be detected by immunoelectron microscopy.[21,22] In most cases, IgG and complement (C3) are deposited, although in 25% of cases, IgM or IgA is seen, and sometimes C3 appears alone. IgD or IgE deposition is very rare.[23,24] These reactants are seen as a linear band along the BMZ on immunofluorescence testing of uninvolved skin (Fig. 11–6). Over 70% of patients have circulating anti-BMZ antibodies, usually IgG and particularly IgG4.[25] The titer of these antibodies does not, in general, reflect disease activity, although it may in an individual patient. In skin cultures, bullous pemphigoid antibodies bind to the lamina lucida but alone do not cause blistering (in contrast to pemphigus antibodies). It appears that both complement and leukocytes, particularly eosinophils, are required.[26] Complement is fixed and activated via both classic and alternate pathways by the bullous pemphigoid antibodies. The anaphylatoxins produced attract a.) mast cells, which degranulate, releasing inflammatory mediators that, in turn, attract more eosinophils, and b.) some neutrophils, which release tissue-destructive enzymes. These enzymes damage the BMZ, resulting in blistering.

Differential Diagnosis

Pemphigus often can be differentiated clinically from bullous pemphigoid because of the flaccid blisters, positive Nikolsky sign, and prominence of mucosal involvement. Histologically, with pemphigus, there is an intraepidermal split with acantholysis.

Herpes gestationis is histologically identical and is distinguished on clinical and immunologic grounds.

Cicatricial pemphigoid differs from bullous pemphigoid in that it is a scarring process that affects principally mucous membranes. Patients usually do not have a circulating autoantibody, although they usually do have immunoreactants in the skin. Histologically, the two are very similar, although in cicatricial pemphigoid, fibrosis may be seen in older lesions.

Dermatitis herpetiformis usually can be distinguished by the preponderance of neutrophils in the lesions and

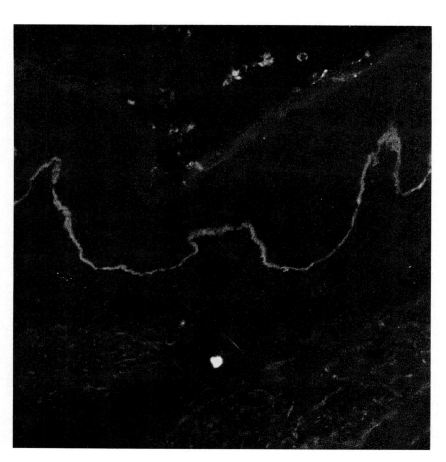

Figure 11–6. Bullous pemphigoid. Direct immunofluorescence showing a linear band of IgG deposited at the BMZ.

the large number of papillary microabscesses containing neutrophils. Bullae may be multilocular, sometimes even with acantholysis, and there often is fibrin deposition and leukocytoclasia in the dermal papillae. However, especially in older lesions, the eosinophils may predominate, and sometimes there may be fewer neutrophils than in lesions of bullous pemphigoid. In such cases, immunofluorescence is required to make a distinction.

Lesions of epidermolysis bullosa acquisita often are trauma-induced and heal with scarring and milia formation. They may be indistinguishable clinically and histologically from those of bullous pemphigoid. Direct immunofluorescence may fail to reveal a distinction. Fewer patients have circulating antibodies than with bullous pemphigoid; immunoelectron microscopy, however, will reveal sublamina densa deposits.

CICATRICIAL PEMPHIGOID

Clinical Features

Cicatricial pemphigoid (benign mucosal membrane pemphigoid, ocular pemphigoid) is a chronic disease characterized by blistering, principally of the mucous membranes, particularly the oral and ocular mucosae, which results in scarring.

Mouth lesions usually ulcerate and are characterized by the formation of adhesions and scars. The conjunctivae are inflamed, with eventual synechiae formation, entropion, corneal opacities, and sometimes blindness.[27] Because of the complication and also because operative intervention on the eye may precipitate the blindness and should therefore be avoided, early diagnosis of cicatricial pemphigoid is particularly important. Involvement of other mucous membranes can result in anal or vulval stenosis and laryngeal or esophageal stricture that, in rare cases, may be life threatening.

Skin lesions occur in up to 50% of cases. There may be a generalized bullous eruption similar to bullous pemphigoid or, more commonly, only a few bullae near a mucosal surface. There is a rare variant in which there are plaquelike, pigmented lesions with recurrent bullae on the head and neck[28] and usually no mucosal lesions. Cicatricial pemphigoid has a prolonged remitting and relapsing course. It occurs in the elderly, more commonly in females, but with no racial predominance.[29] Treatment with local steroid preparations may be sufficient. Alternatively, systemic steroids and immunosuppressants, such as azathioprine, may be necessary, although the response to these treatments is variable.

Histologic Features

In cicatricial pemphigoid, there is a subepidermal split with no acantholysis, although an intact blister usually is difficult to find. The inflammatory infiltrate often is more dense with less perivascular accentuation than in bullous pemphigoid.[29] This infiltrate consists of lymphocytes, eosinophils, occasional neutrophils, and, particularly in the mucosal areas, plasma cells. Dermal or submucosal scarring is the characteristic feature that differentiates cicatricial pemphigoid from bullous pemphigoid (Fig. 11–7). In some cases, however, particularly when eyes or mouth is affected alone,

histology is not diagnostic, and immunofluorescence is mandatory. Electron microscopy reveals an ultrastructure similar to that of bullous pemphigoid with a lamina lucida split. The basement membrane may be either intact or destroyed.

Immunopathology

Direct immunofluorescence of skin or mucous membranes usually shows linear deposition of immunoreactants along the BMZ—usually IgG and C3, sometimes IgM or IgA. Rarely C3 is found alone.[30] Circulating anti-BMZ antibodies are detected rarely and usually only with widespread skin disease. Immunoelectron microscopy has localized the immunoreactants to the lamina lucida, but there is some suggestion that the antigen involved is not identical to the bullous pemphigoid antigen.[31]

Differential Diagnosis

Pemphigus vulgaris is clinically unlike cicatricial pemphigoid in being painful, nonscarring, and slow to heal. It is histologically characterized by an intraepidermal split and acantholysis. Ulcerated lichen planus may clinically look similar to cicatricial pemphigoid in the mouth but is distinguishable by the characteristic lichenoid histology. Severe erythema multiforme, epidermolysis bullosa, or burns may, like cicatricial pemphigoid, result in scarring, but the history and the negative immunofluorescence should help to establish a diagnosis. Aphthous stomatitis is distinguishable by its negative immunofluorescence. In bullous pemphigoid, there are neither adhesions nor scarring, and circulating anti-BMZ antibodies usually are detectable.

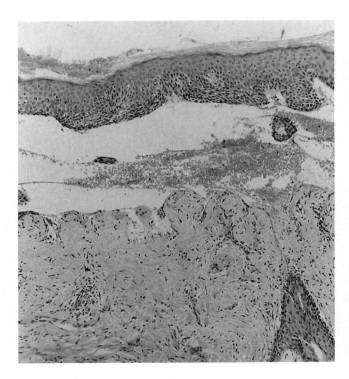

Figure 11–7. Cicatricial pemphigoid. A subepidermal separation is shown with marked scarring of the upper dermis and a sparse mononuclear cell infiltrate (H & E, ×150).

HERPES GESTATIONIS

Clinical Features

Herpes gestationis is a pruritic polymorphous bullous eruption that occurs in pregnancy and the puerperium, with an incidence of approximately 1 in 40,000 to 60,000 pregnancies. Rarely, it accompanies trophoblastic tumors.[32]

It is characterized by extensive erythema and subcutaneous edema, followed by the eruption of vesicles and then tense bullae. En cocade lesions are common. The eruption is frequently very similar to that of bullous pemphigoid. It often starts periumbilically and then spreads to the limbs so that the characteristic distribution is on the lower abdomen and thighs. The palms and soles are affected commonly. Mucous membrane lesions occur in about 20% of cases. A postpartum flare is common, but subsequently the disease usually remits, although prolonged courses have been reported. Flares may occur with menstruation and oral contraceptives. Rarely, a transient herpetiform eruption occurs in the infant.

Treatment with topical steroids rarely suffices, and systemic steroids often are required. Since the advent of steroid therapy, prognosis has improved significantly, and it now appears that there is only a slightly greater than normal infant mortality with this disease.[33]

Histologic Features

In areas of erythema and edema, a dermal perivascular infiltrate is seen, consisting of mononuclear cells and eosinophils (Fig. 11–8). Neutrophils are uncommon. There is marked papillary edema, sometimes leading to the formation of bulbous, teardrop-shaped papillae, which if sectioned to one side may give the appearance of an intraepidermal blister.[34] The epidermis may show eosinophilic spongiosis and intracellular edema. There may be focal necrosis of basal cells, some of which have the appearance of colloid bodies, as seen in lichen planus.[34] In bullous lesions, basal cell necrosis leads to subepidermal bulla for-

mation (Fig. 11–8), with a prominent inflammatory cell infiltrate within and around the bulla consisting mainly of eosinophils with much nuclear dust present.

Electron microscopy reveals severe damage to basal and sometimes also to squamous cells. The basement membrane is well preserved at the base of the bulla. Desmosomes and hemidesmosomes often are intact, as are anchoring fibrils. Most capillaries are well preserved, although a few endothelial cells may show vacuolar degeneration.[35,36]

Immunopathology

Direct immunofluorescence shows linear deposition of C3 in all patients and sometimes also IgG at the BMZ (in the lamina lucida).[32,37] Indirect immunofluorescence with standard techniques demonstrates an IgG C3 binding factor, the HG factor, in about 25% of cases.[38] This appears likely to be a secondary phenomenon. There is greater than normal incidence of HLA-DR3 and DR4 and also of antithyroid and anti-HLA antibodies, suggesting a generally increased immune responsiveness.[32] Current theory suggests that herpes gestationis is an autoimmune disease directed against chorioallantoic or trophoblastic (presumably paternally derived) antigens that cross-react with BMZ antigens. Hormonal modulation also appears to be important.

Differential Diagnosis

The clinical appearance of herpes gestationis is very similar to that of bullous pemphigoid, but the distribution of lesions in the latter is more varied, there is no hormonal effect, HLA typing is normal, and anti-BMZ antibodies usually are present. Histologically, the two are almost identical, but there are normally no necrotic basal cells in pemphigoid.

Polymorphic eruption of pregnancy, also known as pruritic urticarial papules and plaques of pregnancy, usually begins in the abdominal striae distensae, consists of vesicles rather than large bullae, and has negative immunofluorescence. With erythema multiforme, there is frank epidermal

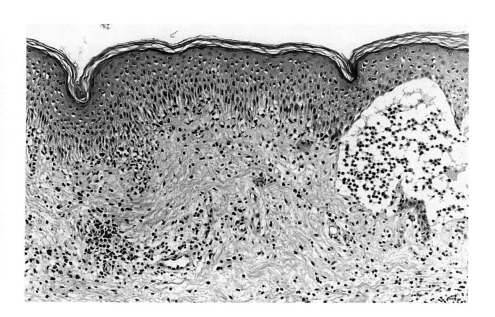

Figure 11–8. Herpes gestationis. An early lesion with an upper dermal infiltrate of mononuclear cells and eosinophils, particularly along the BMZ. There is vacuolization of basal cells on the left side, progressing to form a subepidermal blister on the right (H & E, ×150).

necrosis, there are very few eosinophils, and immuno-fluorescence is negative.

DERMATITIS HERPETIFORMIS

Clinical Features

Dermatitis herpetiformis is a chronic disease characterized by grouped vesicopapules on an erythematous base arranged symmetrically, usually on the scapulae, sacrum, and extensor surface of the arms and legs. It was first described by Duhring.[39] Pruritus is intense so that often only eroded lesions are present. Rarely, hemorrhagic vesicles are seen on the palms and soles. Mucosal lesions usually are absent, and there is no scarring. Dermatitis herpetiformis classically affects young adults but may be seen in any age group, including children. It usually is easily suppressed by dapsone, with pruritus disappearing within 24 hours.

The link with celiac disease was first reported by Marks et al.,[40] and it now appears that almost all (if not all) patients with dermatitis herpetiformis have an abnormality of the jejunal mucosa that may amount to full-blown celiac disease or may be revealed only as minor histologic changes detected on multiple biopsies.[41] Patients with dermatitis herpetiformis may have a greater risk of intestinal lymphoma, although this disease is so rare that the exact incidence is unknown. The severity of the skin lesions is not related to that of the gut lesions. The gut lesions always respond to a gluten-free diet, and there is at least a subgroup of dermatitis herpetiformis patients whose skin is helped or whose dapsone requirements are reduced by a gluten-free diet.[42] HLA-A1, B8, and DRW3 (which are in linkage disequilibrium) occur in about 80% of patients with celiac disease or dermatitis herpetiformis.[43] These patients are also more likely to have autoantibodies to thyroid and gastric mucosa.[44] Anti-BMZ antibodies are not usually found.[45] Antireticulin antibody (which cross-reacts with gliadin) is

found in about 20% of cases of dermatitis herpetiformis. More recently, both antigliadin and antiendomysial antibodies have been detected,[46] and they may play a role in pathogenesis.

Histologic Features

The most typical features are seen in early erythematous lesions without blistering (Fig. 11–9). Accumulation of neutrophils is seen at the tips of adjacent dermal papillae. These papillae increase in size, and microabscesses are formed that may contain a few eosinophils.[47] Dermoepidermal separation occurs with formation of the characteristic multilocular blister, which later forms a unilocular blister with papillary microabscesses often seen only at its edge (Fig. 11–10). Microabscesses probably are present in most cases of dermatitis herpetiformis.[48] There is edema, fibrin deposition, and basophilia of the collagen in the dermal papillae (Fig. 11–11), with gradual loss of the outline of the rete ridges.

The characteristic inflammatory infiltrate is seen in the upper dermis and consists mainly of neutrophils with some eosinophils. Disintegration of neutrophil nuclei produces significant quantities of nuclear dust. There is a superficial perivascular infiltrate of mononuclear cells as well as neutrophils and eosinophils. There may be vasculitis.[49]

The basal cells are sometimes necrotic in late lesions. Rarely, there are acantholytic keratinocytes singly or in groups at the base of the epidermis.[2] Electron microscopy reveals a structure very similar to that of cell-rich bullous pemphigoid, except that there are more neutrophils and marked fibrin deposition.[48]

Immunopathology

Immunofluorescence shows granular IgA deposition (usually dimeric) and sometimes also C3 in the dermal papillae of uninvolved skin (Fig. 11–12). Deposition of immunoreac-

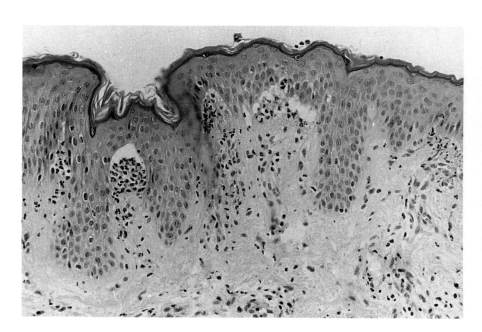

Figure 11–9. Dermatitis herpetiformis. An early lesion with neutrophil microabscess formation and clefting at the BMZ (H & E, ×230).

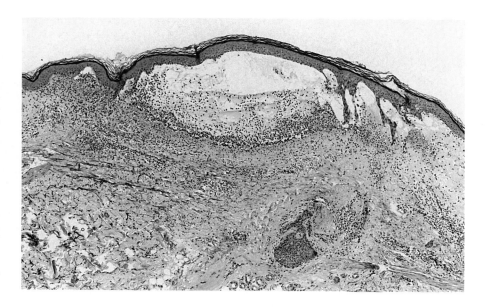

Figure 11–10. Dermatitis herpetiformis. A characteristic neutrophil microabscess is seen to the left of the blister. The blister itself contains neutrophils and fibrin, and its original multilocular nature is seen on the right, with the rete ridges that originally divided the blister clearly recognizable (H&E, ×50).

tants is associated with the bundles of dermal microfibrils[50] and is unaffected by treatment with dapsone but may disappear on a gluten-free diet.

Differential Diagnosis

A diagnosis of bullous pemphigoid is suggested if the number of eosinophils is great and there are no papillary microabscesses or fibrin deposition. This diagnosis can be confirmed by immunofluorescence. In linear IgA disease, also, multiple microabscesses do not appear, but there is extensive fibrin deposition, leukocytoclasis, and acantholysis. Again, immunofluorescence confirms the diagnosis.

LINEAR IgA DERMATOSIS

Clinical Features

Linear IgA dermatosis is characterized by a vesiculobullous eruption occurring after puberty. It previously was thought

to be a variant of dermatitis herpetiformis, but there are a number of distinguishing features. The lesions may be vesicular but are often large bullae. They tend to have an annular configuration and are distributed randomly. Indeed, they may clinically be more like bullous pemphigoid, and this has led to confusion in the past. Mucosal lesions are common and may scar.[51] Jejunal changes are rarely found, and there is no response to a gluten-free diet. HLA-B8 is found in less than half the cases.[52,53] The disease is initially responsive to sulfone but later tends to become resistant.

Histologic Features

Histologic features generally resemble dermatitis herpetiformis much more than bullous pemphigoid, although it is not always possible to make a definite differentiation on the basis of histology alone. There is a subepidermal blister with a moderate inflammatory cell infiltrate. These cells mainly are neutrophils rather than eosinophils. A linear

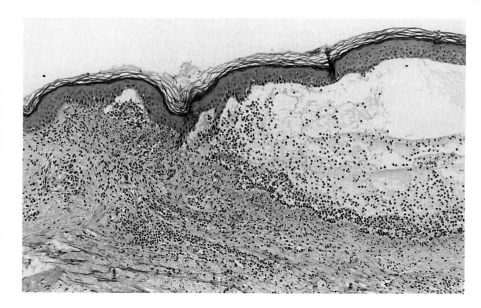

Figure 11–11. Dermatitis herpetiformis. A higher power view of the edge of the blister seen in Figure 11–10, showing the papillary microabscess and also fibrin deposition in the papillae. The predominant cell is the neutrophil (H & E, ×120).

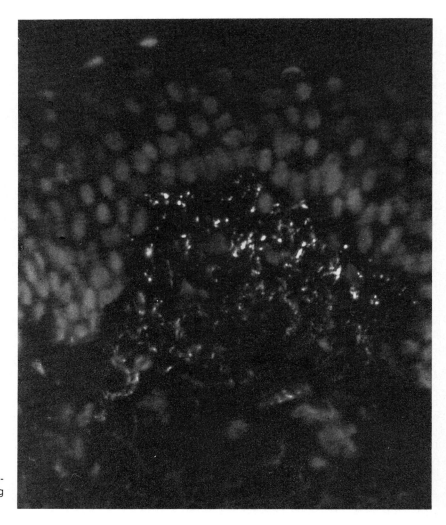

Figure 11–12. Dermatitis herpetiformis. Direct immunofluorescence on perilesional skin showing granular IgA deposition in the dermal papillae.

infiltrate of eosinophils along the basement membrane is not seen, whereas microabscesses, fibrin, and leukocytoclasis at the papillary tips often are present. Discrimination of linear IgA dermatosis from dermatitis herpetiformis depends on combined assessment of a number of features.[53,54] Extensive vacuolization and neutrophil infiltration of long sections of the BMZ or many rete tips with neutrophils in basal vacuoles favor a diagnosis of linear IgA dermatosis, whereas multiple microabscesses, extensive fibrin deposition, and leukocytoclasis at papillary tips and acantholysis favor a diagnosis of dermatitis herpetiformis.

Immunopathology

Immunofluorescence shows homogeneous linear IgA deposition at the basement membrane, which, with immunoelectron microscopy, can be localized to the lamina lucida or the sublamina densa zone in association with anchoring fibrils.[55,56] Circulating IgA anti-BMZ antibodies are found in less than 25% of patients.

Differential Diagnosis

A comparison of features of pemphigoid, dermatitis herpetiformis, and IgA dermatosis is given in Table 11–3.

CHRONIC BULLOUS DERMATOSIS OF CHILDHOOD

Clinical Features

Chronic bullous dermatosis of childhood is a bullous disorder that occurs in young children and is characterized by serpiginous plaques with peripheral bullae. It usually starts when the patient is under the age of 5. Tense bullae arise on a clear or normal base, often forming rosette-like lesions. Sites of predilection are the perioral area, the lower abdomen, genitalia, and thighs, but the eruption may be widespread. Mucosal lesions are common and may cause scarring.[57] There may or may not be pruritus. The disease usually remits within several years and is normally responsive to sulfone.[18] There is no gluten-sensitive enteropathy, but there is a strong association with HLA-B8.[59]

Histologic Features

Histologic study may reveal a nonspecific subepidermal bulla or a picture resembling dermatitis herpetiformis or bullous pemphigoid (Fig. 11–13.).

Immunopathology

Direct immunofluorescence shows linear IgA deposition in the vast majority of cases, occasionally accompanied by

IgM or fibrin. Immunoreactants have been variably reported as occurring in the lamina lucida or below the lamina densa.[60,61] Circulating anti-BMZ antibodies of the IgA class usually are present.[59] The precise relationship between adult linear IgA disease and chronic bullous dermatosis of childhood is still a matter of some dispute, although current evidence suggests a close link.[57]

Differential Diagnosis

Bullous pemphigoid and dermatitis herpetiformis rarely occur in childhood. These conditions are differentiated from chronic bullous dermatosis of childhood by immunofluorescence findings.

EPIDERMOLYSIS BULLOSA ACQUISITA

Clinical Features

Epidermolysis bullosa acquisita is a rare, chronic, nonhereditary disease classically presenting in adult life. Tense blisters occur predominantly on normal skin over joint surfaces, especially the hands and feet. Blisters often are trauma induced and heal with notable dystrophic scars and milia formation, thus mimicking porphyria cutanea tarda. Nails may be dystrophic. In rare cases, mucous membrane lesions are a severe problem, and the disease resembles cicatricial pemphigoid. Alternatively, there may be widespread blisters mimicking bullous pemphigoid.[62] Treatment with prednisolone or immunosuppressants is not usually successful. The disease has been associated with lymphoproliferative disease, Crohn's disease, ulcerative colitis, diabetes mellitus, and rheumatoid arthritis.

Histologic Features

Histology reveals a subepidermal blister with a sparse or moderate inflammatory infiltrate consisting of mononuclear cells, neutrophils, and eosinophils. These findings are not sufficient for diagnosis (Fig. 11–14).

Immunopathology

Immunofluorescence shows linear deposition of IgG and C3 (sometimes IgM or IgA) along the BMZ. A minority of

TABLE 11–3. COMPARISON OF PEMPHIGOID, DERMATITIS HERPETIFORMIS, AND IgA DERMATOSIS

	Bullous Pemphigoid	Dermatitis Herpetiformis	Linear IgA Dermatosis
Clinical features	Occurs predominantly in elderly patients	Occurs in any age group, but most frequently in young adults	
	Large tense blisters on normal or erythematous skin	Grouped papules and vesicles	Vesicular or bullous lesions
	Flexural surfaces of extremities, groin, axillae, lower abdomen	Symmetrical lesions	
		Elbows, buttocks, and interscalpular areas most commonly affected	
	Oral lesions present in 33%	Oral lesions rare	Oral lesions common
		Intensely pruritic	
		Associated with celiac disease	
		80% patients HLA-A1, B8, and DRW3	
Light microscopy	Subepidermal blister with intact roof	Subepidermal vesicle with intact roof	Subepidermal blister with intact roof
			Blister vacuolization may be present
	Blister cavity contains fibrin, serum, and inflammatory cells with many eosinophils	Lateral to blister, neutrophils accumulate in the dermal papillae to form abscesses	
	Widened, edematous dermal papillae; eosinophilic papillary dermal microabscesses occasionally seen		
	Upper dermal infiltrate composed of eosinophils admixed with eosinophils, neutrophils, and lymphocytes	Upper dermal infiltrate of neutrophils with occasional eosinophils and nuclear dust	Dermal infiltrate composed of neutrophils; papillary dermal microabscesses often present
Immunofluorescence	Linear deposition of IgG, IgM, and complement along BMZ	Granular IgA and occasionally C3 along BMZ	Linear deposition of IgA along BMZ
	Autoantibodies usually present in patient's serum	Circulating autoantibodies rarely detected	Circulating autoantibodies found in 25% of patients
Immunoelectron microscopy	Immunoglobulin and complement deposition in lamina lucida	Immunoglobulin deposition associated with dermal microfibrils	Immunoglobulin localized to lamina lucida or sub-lamina densa zone

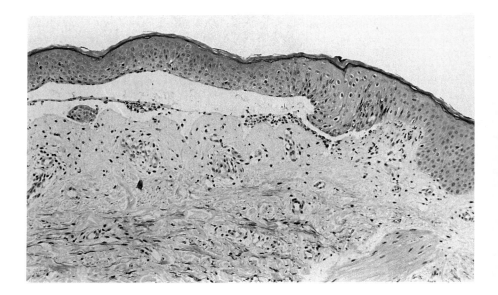

Figure 11–13. Chornic bullous dermatosis of childhood. The edge of a subepidermal bulla is shown. The predominant inflammatory cell is the neutrophil, as in dermatitis herpetiformis (H & E, ×150).

patients have circulating IgG anti-BMZ antibodies. Electron microscopy reveals electron-dense deposits below the lamina densa, through which blistering occurs. The number of anchoring fibrils is lower than normal. Immunoelectron microscopy shows that antibody deposition is localized to the areas below (but also occasionally within) the lamina densa.[63,64] The antigen against which these antibodies are directed has now been isolated and appears to be the carboxyl terminus of type VII procollagen.[65] It is synthesized by both keratinocytes and fibroblasts.[66,67]

Differential Diagnosis

Epidermolysis bullosa acquisita may be confused with the other primary bullous diseases. It can be differentiated on the basis of immunologic findings, particularly through electron microscopy.[62,63, 68] Porphyria cutanea tarda is excluded by porphyrin estimation.

ERYTHEMA MULTIFORME

Clinical Features

Erythema multiforme is common and occurs in patients of any age. As the name suggests, the clinical appearance is variable; sometimes there are red macules and urticated papules, occasionally progressing to vesicobullous lesions, which are not usually pruritic. The characteristic iris or target lesion forms when the center of a lesion becomes edematous and purpuric while the border remains pink. Such lesions are not always present. Rarely, a central bulla is surrounded by a halo of small vesicles (the Bateman iris lesion). Distribution is often acral but may be widespread.

Diagnosis is usually made clinically on the basis of appearance, but since this is so variable, confusion has arisen about the histology.[69] In severe forms of the disease (Stevens-Johnson syndrome), there is painful, life-threatening mucosal involvement (initially bullae, which rapidly ulcerate and then crust over) and widespread cutaneous involvement. It is principally the oral and ocular mucosae that are affected, and the advice of an ophthalmologist is essential to prevent serious sequelae. Anogenital involvement also is common. Esophageal and lung lesions are rare.

Erythema multiforme usually is self-limiting within a few weeks but may recur. Its cause is often unknown, although the disease may be traced to infection (herpes simplex or *Mycoplasma*), usually appearing 7 to 14 days later, or to drug ingestion (sulfonamides). A wide variety of other organisms and drugs has also been implicated on occasion. An immunologic basis has been postulated, and both cell-mediated and humoral factors have been implicated.[70]

Treatment may be specific (e.g., withdrawal of drug therapy) but is often supportive only. In Stevens-Johnson syndrome, prevention and treatment of secondary infection and careful maintenance of adequate fluid and calorie intake are important. Systemic steroids may be given.

Histologic Features

Although histologic findings vary, they usually enable a diagnosis to be made. In the dermis, there is papillary edema (which may be so severe as to lead to subepidermal vesiculation) and a mixed lymphohistiocytic perivascular infiltrate. A few eosinophils also may be present.[71] Endothelial cells are swollen, but there is no frank vasculitis, although there may be extravasation of red blood cells.[69]

Initial epidermal changes are spongiosis with vertical reorientation of keratinocytes and their nuclei, dyskeratosis of individual keratinocytes, and exocytosis of mononuclear cells (Fig. 11–15). In vesicular and bullous lesions (Fig. 11–16), changes are more pronounced, with vacuolization of the basal layer (which may lead to a subepidermal bulla) and a bandlike mononuclear infiltrate that obscures the dermoepidermal junction. Intraepidermal vesiculation may occur in coalescing necrotic foci, eventually leaving only the stratum corneum intact over a subcorneal blister. The lesions usually heal without scarring, but there are residual

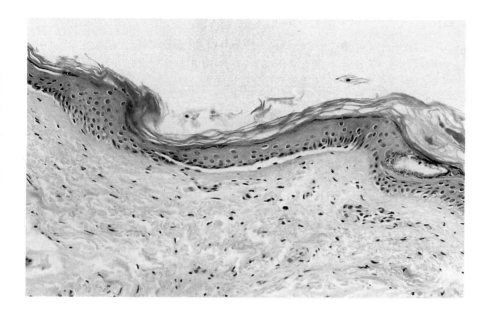

Figure 11–14. Epidermolysis acquisita. An early lesion demonstrating the characteristic subepidermal split and paucity of inflammatory infiltrate (H & E, ×230).

melanophages in the papillary dermis. Changes in the oral mucous membranes are similar.

Dyskeratosis and epidermal necrosis are generally thought to be the pathologic hallmarks of erythema multiforme. Ackerman et al.[72] also consider changes at the dermoepidermal junction to be necessary for the diagnosis, but this is not generally accepted. Some authors[73] subdivide erythema multiforme into epidermal, dermal, and dermoepidermal types according to the site of predominant histologic change, but it seems likely that there is a continuous spectrum of disease.

Immunopathology

Direct immunofluorescence is often positive, showing IgM or C3 deposited in cytoid bodies and sometimes perivascular C3 deposition or linear BMZ deposition or fibrinogen or C3.[74]

Differential Diagnosis

Clinically, erythema multiforme must be distinguished from a number of other diseases that also cause erythematous lesions, bullae, and mucosal ulcerations. Histologically, it must be distinguished from other subepidermal bullous diseases (in which dyskeratosis and epidermal necrosis do not usually occur) and graft-versus-host (GVH) disease (which is very similar but is characterized by satellite cell dyskeratosis and a paucity of dermal infiltrate). Confusion may arise also with lichenoid tissue reactions.

TOXIC EPIDERMAL NECROLYSIS

Clinical Features

Toxic epidermal necrolysis (TEN) is a rare, life-threatening condition in which there is initially painful erythema with

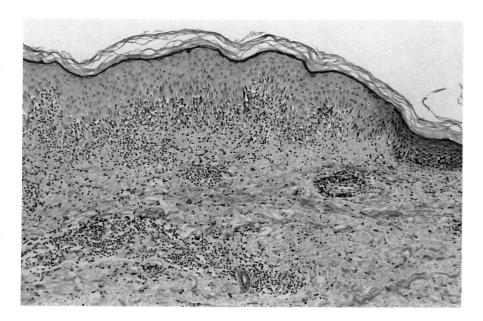

Figure 11–15. Erythema multiforme. An early lesion showing vacuolar alteration of the basal layer with a lymphohistiocytic infiltrate hugging the BMZ and also present around the blood vessels in the dermis. There is vertical reorientation of keratinocytes and exocytosis of mononuclear cells (H & E, ×120).

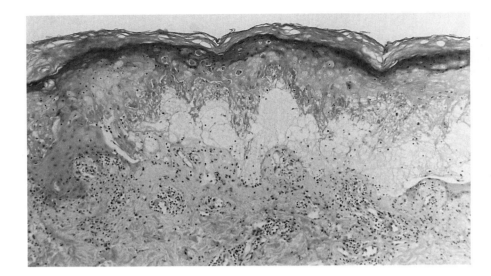

Figure 11–16. Erythema multiforme. A subepidermal bulla with marked necrosis of the epidermis showing hyalinization of individual keratinocytes. There is also papillary edema and a sparse mononuclear infiltrate (H & E, ×120).

bullae and then sheetlike exfoliation of the epidermis, clinically resembling a scald. Mucous membrane involvement is severe and usually scars. TEN may be idiopathic or related to drugs, viral infection, or GVH disease. There is a high mortality. Treatment is mainly supportive; there is disagreement over the role of corticosteroids.[75]

TEN is now separated from staphylococcal scalded skin syndrome (SSSS), which was formerly known as staphylococcal TEN. SSSS is mediated by a staphylococcal exotoxin and usually is indistinguishable clinically from TEN but occurs predominantly in children rather than adults (see Chapter 23).

Histologic Features

There is initially a vacuolization along the dermoepidermal junction, followed by dyskeratosis and epidermal necrosis eventually affecting the whole epidermis and resulting in subepidermal blister formation. There is minimal dermal inflammation. TEN is histologically indistinguishable from that form of erythema multiforme that principally affects the epidermis (Fig. 11–17).

Differential Diagnosis

TEN can be distinguished from SSSS, in which the level of split is not subepidermal but subgranular. Histologically, TEN is very similar to fixed bullous drug eruption but can be distinguished on the basis of the patient's history. Chemical or thermal burns are also distinguished primarily on the basis of history and by the extensive necrosis that accompanies them.

BULLOUS FIXED DRUG ERUPTION

Fixed drug eruptions are characterized by well-defined oval, erythematous, or violaceous plaques, sometimes with bulla formation, which occur in the same place each time the drug is given. Lesions heal with hyperpigmentation. Drugs commonly implicated include barbiturates, phenylbuta-

zone, phenolphthalein, sulfonamides, and tetracyclines.

Histologically, these lesions are similar to those of acute erythema multiforme, with epidermal necrosis and dyskeratotic keratinocytes, but usually there is very little inflammatory infiltrate in the dermis. In bullae, the split occurs subepidermally (Fig. 11–18). Repeated damage at the same site leads eventually to marked pigmentary incontinence, with large amounts of melanin in macrophages in the upper dermis.

BULLOUS LUPUS ERYTHEMATOSUS

Clinical Features

Bullous skin lesions are rare in lupus erythematosus. They occur almost exclusively in the systemic forms of the disease and usually appear to resemble one of the primary bullous skin diseases (bullous pemphigoid or dermatitis herpetiformis).[76,77] It is these lesions that are usually referred to as bullous lupus erythematosus, although occasionally bullae are due to severe liquefaction degeneration of the basal cells, to coincident drug-induced erythema multiforme, or to secondary infection. In order to make the diagnosis of bullous lupus erythematosus, it is first essential to establish the diagnosis of systemic lupus erythematosus by demonstration of four of the American Rheumatism Association criteria.[78]

The eruption of bullous lupus erythematosus usually is widespread, sometimes with nonscarring alopecia. There is little mucosal involvement. The disease is usually responsive to dapsone.[79]

Histologic Features

Histologic study reveals a subepidermal blister, usually with a neutrophilic infiltrate and microabscess formation. There may be a few eosinophils present. The histologic picture is often indistinguishable from that of dermatitis herpetiformis. However, there is more often a leukocytoclastic vasculi-

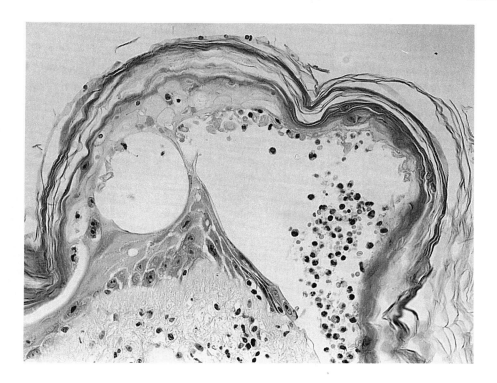

Figure 11–17. Toxic epidermal necrolysis. A subepidermal blister on the right and intraepidermal vesiculation on the left with marked epidermal necrosis and hyalinization of individual cells. There is a mixed inflammatory cell infiltrate (H & E, ×230).

tis with fibrin deposition and also mucin deposition.[2] Usually, there is no hydropic degeneration of the basal cells, although this may occur occasionally. Lupus erythematosus cells may be seen in the blister fluid.

Immunopathology

Direct immunofluorescence reveals a linear band of immunoglobulins (IgG, IgM, or IgA) and complement along the BMZ. This may be either a tubular band (more characteristic

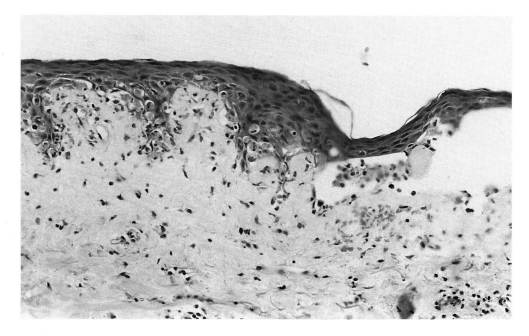

Figure 11–18. Bullous fixed drug eruption. A subepidermal split with a sparse mononuclear cell infiltrate and necrosis of the epidermis. These changes are indistinguishable from those of erythema multiforme. There is no pigmentary incontinence, since this is the first time the lesion has occurred (H & E, ×230).

of bullous pemphigoid) or a homogeneous band (more characteristic of systemic lupus erythematosus). Electron microscopy shows that the split occurs in the lamina lucida. Thus, neither the pattern of immunoreactants nor histology allows differentiation between bullous lupus erythematosus and a primary bullous disease occurring in association with systemic lupus erythematosus. Immunoelectron microscopy is required. A finding that the immunoreactants are localized below the lamina densa allows differentiation from bullous pemphigoid and dermatitis herpetiformis.[80] Circulating anti-BMZ antibodies usually are not detected, but there have been reports of detection of antibodies against the epidermolysis bullosa acquisita antigen.[81] It seems most likely that these antibodies are secondary to the lupus disease process and do not represent coexistence of epidermolysis bullosa acquisita and systemic lupus erythematosus.

Differential Diagnosis

Since bullous lupus erythematosus may be histologically indistinguishable from dermatitis herpetiformis, immunofluorescence and immunoelectron microscopy may be necessary to establish a definite diagnosis.

BULLOUS MASTOCYTOSIS

Clinical Features

Mastocytosis is the accumulation of mast cells in various organs of the body. There is a spectrum of disease ranging from benign to malignant and from limited cutaneous involvement to widespread systemic disease. Cutaneous disease may be classified according to the clinical appearance.

1. Mastocytoma
2. Multiple macular, papular, or nodular lesions
3. Telangiectasia macularis eruptive perstans
4. Diffuse mastocytosis

Bullous lesions are believed to occur when histamine release from large numbers of mast cells leads to edema, vesiculation, and eventually bulla formation. They consequently are seen usually in mastocytoma, papulonodular or diffuse disease and are rare in macular forms, where there may be very few mast cells present in the dermis.

In mastocytosis, bullae usually occur in children at birth or in infancy and are rare in adults. There are two probable reasons; first, infantile skin is more fragile and tends to blister more easily, and, second, infants are more likely to have diseases with large accumulations of metabolically active mast cells. Bullae usually occur on a preexisting lesion either spontaneously or after trauma. However, the underlying abnormality may not be clinically apparent, as in the cases of diffuse mastocytosis reported by Miller and Shapiro,[82] where the bullae appeared to be arising on normal skin.

The bullae are of variable size, tense, and filled with serous or serosanguineous fluid. Nikolsky's sign is negative. Darier's sign is positive, and, indeed, the urticated lesion so produced may subsequently blister. Distribution may be limited (usually to the legs) or widespread. Sometimes the bullae appear in crops and may precede episodes of flushing or histamine shock. They normally heal without scarring.

It usually is agreed that mastocytosis arising in childhood has a good prognosis,[83] but there has been some suggestion that bullous disease, if present at birth, has an

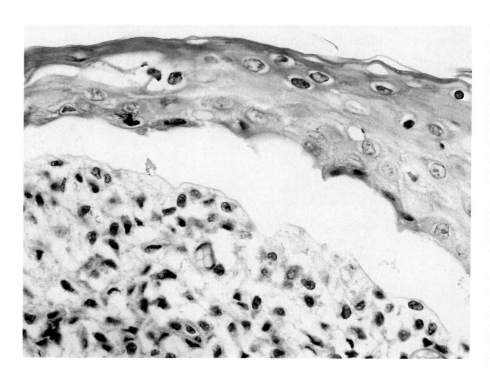

Figure 11–19. Bullous mastocytosis. This high-power view of a subepidermal blister shows clearly the accumulation of mast cells in the dermis (H & E, ×620).

ominous outlook.[84] Bullae are common in mastocytoma and usually remain confined to the lesion. Bullae usually settle within the first few years, although other signs of the disease may persist. The child's health usually is not impaired unless there are associated attacks of flushing. Antihistamines do not suppress bulla formation, although they help other symptoms. Disodium cromoglycate appears to be of great benefit.[85]

Histologic Features

Microscopy reveals a subepidermal blister with an underlying infiltrate of mast cells. An old lesion may start to regenerate and give rise to an apparent intraepidermal blister. In nodular forms of the disease and in mastocytoma, the mast cells are closely packed in tumorlike aggregates extending throughout the dermis and sometimes into the subcutis.[86] Morphology is characteristic, with a well-defined cell border, ample granular eosinophilic cytoplasm, and central oval nucleus with a clumped chromatin pattern and no nucleoli (Fig. 11–19). In the diffuse disease, there is a dense bandlike infiltrate of mast cells. The Grenz zone may be preserved. In both types, a few eosinophils usually are present. The increased pigment of the clinical lesions may be seen as increased melanin in the basal layer or as melanophages in the dermis. Metachromatic staining is used to confirm the diagnosis. The diagnosis also can be made by taking a smear from the base the base of a blister, which shows mast cells and sometimes also eosinophils.

Differential Diagnosis

Closely related in appearance are bullous impetigo, insect bites, or papular urticaria. Bullous mastocytosis is less likely to be confused with juvenile pemphigoid, epidermolysis bullosa simplex, incontinentia pigmenti, syphilis, erythema multiforme, acrodermatitis enteropathica, and bullous ichthyosiform erythroderma. Histologically, confusion may occur with histiocytosis X, but these cells have indented nuclei and foamy cytoplasm; electron microscopy is diagnostic. Nevertheless, it is important to confirm the diagnosis of mastocytosis by metachromatic staining.

REFERENCES

1. Braun-Falco O. The pathology of blister formation. In: Kopf AW, Andrade R, eds. *Year Book of Dermatology.* Chicago: Year Book Medical Publishers; 1969;16–22.
2. Ackerman AB. *Histologic Diagnosis of Inflammatory Skin Diseases: A Method by Pattern Analysis.* Philadelphia: Lea & Febiger; 1978.
3. Farmer ER. Subepidermal bullous diseases. *J Cutan Pathol.* 1985;12:316–321.
4. Black MM, Meyrick Thomas RH, Bhogal B. The value of immunofluorescence techniques in the diagnosis of bullous disorders: A review. *Clin Exp Dermatol.* 1983;8:337–353.
5. Lever WF. Pemphigus. *Medicine (Baltimore).* 1953;32:1–123.
6. Ahmed AR, Cohen E, Blumenson LE, et al. HLA in bullous pemphigoid. *Arch Dermatol.* 1977;113:1121.
7. Lever WF. *Pemphigus and Pemphigoid.* Springfield, Ill: Charles C Thomas; 1965.
8. Ahmed AR, Chu TM, Provost TT. Bullous pemphigoid. Clinical and serological evaluation for associated malignant neoplasms. *Arch Dermatol.* 1977;113:969.
9. Chlorzelski TP, Jablonska S, Maciejowska E, et al. Coexistence of malignancies with bullous pemphigoid. *Arch Dermatol.* 1978;114:964.
10. Hodge L, Marsden RA, Black MM, et al. Bullous pemphigoid: The frequency of mucosal involvement and concurrent malignancy related to indirect immunofluorescent findings. *Br J Dermatol.* 1981;105:65–69.
11. Stone SP, Schroeter AL. Bullous pemphigoid and associated malignant neoplasms. *Arch Dermatol.* 1975;111:991–994.
12. Person JR, Rogers RS, Perry HO. Localised pemphigoid. *Br J Dermatol.* 1976;95:531–534.
13. Bean SF, Michel B, Furey N. Vesicular pemphigoid. *Arch Dermatol.* 1976;112:1402–1404.
14. Winkelmann RK, Su WPD. Pemphigoid vegetans. *Arch Dermatol.* 1979;115:446–448.
15. Emmerson RW, Wilson Jones E. Eosinophilic spongiosis in pemphigus. *Arch Dermatol* 1968;97:252–257.
16. Crotty C, Pittelkow M, Muller SA. Eosinophilic spongiosis: A clinicopathological review of seventy-one cases. *J Am Acad Dermatol.* 1983;8:337–343.
17. Schaumburg-Lever G, Orfanos CE, Lever WF. Electron microscopic study of bullous pemphigoid. *Arch Dermatol.* 1972;106:662–667.
18. Beutner EH, Jordan RE, Chorzelski TP. The immunopathology of pemphigus and pemphigoid. *J Invest Dermatol.* 1968;51:63–80.
19. Mutasim DF, Takahashi Y, Labib RS, et al. A pool of bullous pemphigoid antigen(s) is intracellular and associated with the basal cell cytoskeleton-hemidesmosome complex. *J Invest Dermatol.* 1985;84:47–53.
20. Westgate GE, Weaver AC, Couchman JR. Bullous pemphigoid antigen localisation suggests an intracellular association with hemidesmosomes. *J Invest Dermatol.* 1985;84:218–224.
21. Holubar K, Wolff K, Konrad K, Beutner EH. Ultrastructural localisation of immunoglobulins in bullous pemphigoid skin. *J Invest Dermatol.* 1975;64:220–227.
22. Schaumburg-Lever G, Rule A, Schmidt-Ullrich B, Lever WF. Ultrastructural localisation of in vivo bound immunoglobulins in bullous pemphigoid—A preliminary report. *J Invest Dermatol.* 1975;64:47–49.
23. Ahmed AR, Maize JC, Provost TT. Bullous pemphigoid: Clinical and immunological follow-up after successful therapy. *Arch Dermatol.* 1977;113:1043–1046.
24. Jordan RE, Triftshauser CT, Schroeter AL. Direct immunofluorescent studies of pemphigus and bullous pemphigoid. *Arch Dermatol.* 1971;103:486–491.
25. Bird P, Friedman PF, Ling N, et al. Subclass distribution of IgG autoantibodies in bullous pemphigoid. *J Invest Dermatol.* 1986;86:21–25.
26. Gammon WR, Merritt CC, Lewis DM, Sams WM Jr, Carlo JR, Wheeler CE. An in vitro model of immune complex-mediated basement membrane zone separation caused by antibodies, leukocytes and complement. *J Invest Dermatol.* 1982;78:285–290.
27. Hardy KM, Perry HO, Pingree GC, Kirby TJ. Benign mucous membrane pemphigoid. *Arch Dermatol.* 1971;104:467–475.
28. Brunsting LA, Perry HO. Benign pemphigoid? A report of seven cases with chronic scarring herpetiform plaques about the head and neck. *Arch Dermatol.* 1957;75:489–501.
29. Person JR, Rogers RS. Bullous and cicatricial pemphigoid. *Mayo Clin Proc.* 1977;52:55–66.
30. Rogers RS, Perry HO, Bean SF, Jordon RE. Immunopathology of cicatricial pemphigoid: Studies of complement deposition. *J Invest Dermatol.* 1977;68:39–43.
31. Fine J, Neises GR, Katz SI. Immunofluorescence and immunoelectron microscopic studies in cicatricial pemphigoid. *J Invest Dermatol.* 1984;82:39–43.

32. Holmes RC, Black MM. Herpes gestationis. *Dermatol Clin.* 1983;1:195–203.

33. Holmes RC, Black MM. The foetal prognosis in pemphigoid gestationis (herpes gestationis). *Br J Dermatol.* 1984;110:67–72.

34. Hertz KC, Katz SI, Maize J, Ackerman AB. Herpes gestationis, a clinicopathologic study. *Arch Dermatol.* 1976;112:1543–1548.

35. Yaoita H, Gullino M, Katz SI. Herpes gestationis. Ultrastructure and ultrastructural localisation of in vivo-bound complement. *J Invest Dermatol.* 1976;66:383–388.

36. Schaumburg-Lever G, Saffold OE, Orfanos CE, Lever WF. Herpes gestationis, histology and ultrastructure. *Arch Dermatol.* 1973;107:888–892.

37. Holubar K, Konrad K, Stingl G. Detection by immunoelectron microscopy of immunoglobulin G deposits in skin of immunofluorescence negative herpes gestationis. *Br J Dermatol.* 1977;96:569–571.

38. Holmes RC, Black MM, Jurecka W, et al. Clues to the aetiology and pathogenesis of herpes gestationis. *Br J Dermatol.* 1983;109:131–139.

39. Duhring LA. Dermatitis herpetiformis. *JAMA* 1884;3:225–230.

40. Marks JM, Shuster S, Watson AJ. Small-bowel changes in dermatitis herpetiformis. *Lancet.* 1966;2:1280–1282.

41. Katz SI, Hall RH, Lawley TJ, et al. Dermatitis herpetiformis: The skin and the gut. *Ann Intern Med.* 1980;93:857–874.

42. Fry L, McMinn RMH, Cowan JD, Hoffbrand AV. Effect of gluten-free diet on dermatological, intestinal, and haematological manifestations of dermatitis herpetiformis. *Lancet.* 1968;1:557–561.

43. Seah PP, Fry L, Kearney JW, et al. A comparison of histocompatibility antigens in dermatitis herpetiformis and adult coeliac disease. *Br J Dermatol.* 1976;94:131–138.

44. Fraser N. Autoantibodies in dermatitis herpetiformis. *Br J Dermatol.* 1970;83:609–613.

45. Yaoita H, Katz SI. Circulating IgA anti-basement membrane zone antibodies in dermatitis herpetiformis. *J Invest Dermatol.* 1977;69:558–560.

46. Chorzelski TP, Beutner EH, Sulej J. IgA anti-endomysial antibody. A new immunological marker of dermatitis herpetiformis and coeliac disease. *Br J Dermatol.* 1984;111:395–402.

47. Pierard J, Whimster I. The histological diagnosis of dermatitis herpetiformis, bullous pemphigoid and erythema multiforme. *Br J Dermatol.* 1961;73:253–266.

48. Lever WF, Schaumberg-Lever G. *Histopathology of the Skin.* Philadelphia: JB Lippincott Co; 1983:120.

49. Connor BL, Marks R, Wilson Jones E. Dermatitis herpetiformis, histological discriminants. *St. John's Hos Derm Soc.* 1972;58:191–198.

50. Yaoita H, Katz SI. Immunoelectron microscopic localisation of IgA in skin of patients with dermatitis herpetiformis. *J Invest Dermatol.* 1976;67:502–506.

51. Leonard JN, Wright P, Williams DM, et al. The relationship between linear IgA disease and benign mucous membrane pemphigoid. *Br J Dermatol.* 1984;110:307–314.

52. Lawley TJ, Yancey KB. Dermatitis herpetiformis. *Dermatol Clin.* 1983;1:187–194.

53. Blenkinsopp WK, Fry L, Haffenden GP, Leonard JN. Histology of linear IgA disease, dermatitis herpetiformis and bullous pemphigoid. *Am J Dermatopathol.* 1983;5:547–554.

54. Smith SB, Harrist TJ, Murphy GF, et al. Linear IgA bullous dermatosis v. dermatitis herpetiformis. *Arch Dermatol.* 1984;120:324–328.

55. Yaoita H, Hertz KC, Katz SI. Dermatitis herpetiformis: Immunoelectron microscopic and ultrastructural studies of a patient with linear deposition of IgA. *J Invest Dermatol.* 1976;67:691–695.

56. Chorzelski TP, Jablonska S, Beutner EH, et al. Linear IgA bullous dermatosis. In: Beutner EH, Chorzelski TP, Bean SF, eds.

57. Wojnarowska F, Marsden RA, Bhogal B, Black MM. Chronic bullous disease of childhood, childhood cicatricial pemphigoid and linear IgA disease of adults. A comparative study demonstrating clinical and immunopathologic overlap. *J Am Acad Dermatol.* 1988;19:792–805.

58. Bean SF, Furey NL, Chorzelski TP, Jablonska S. Childhood form of linear IgA bullous dermatosis. In Beutner EH, Chorzelski TP, Bean SF, eds. *Immunopathology of the Skin.* 2nd ed. New York: John Wiley and Sons; 1979:320–323.

59. Marsden RA, McKee PH, Bhogal B, Black MM, Kennedy LA. A study of benign chronic bullous dermatosis of childhood and comparison with dermatitis herpetiformis and bullous pemphigoid occurring in childhood. *Clin Exp Dermatol.* 1980;5:159–172.

60. Horiguchi YH, Toda K, Okamoto H, Imamura S. Immunoelectron microscopic observations in a case of linear IgA bullous dermatosis of childhood. *J Am Acad Dermatol.* 1986;14:593–599.

61. Bhogal B, Wojnarowska F, Marsden RA, Das A, Black MM, McKee PH. Linear IgA bullous dermatosis of adults and children: An immunoelectron microscopic study. *Br J Dermatol.* 1987;117:289–296.

62. Gammon WR, Briggaman RA, Woodley DT, et al. Epidermolysis bullosa acquisita—A pemphigoid-like disease. *J Am Acad Dermatol.* 1984;11:820–832.

63. Yaoita H, Briggaman RA, Lawley RJ, Provost TT, Katz SI. Epidermolysis bullosa acquisita: Ultrastructural and immunological studies. *J Invest Dermatol.* 1981;76:288–292.

64. Nieboer C, Boorsma DM, Woerdeman MJ, Kalsbeek GL. Epidermolysis bullosa acquisita. *Br J Dermatol.* 1980;102:383–392.

65. Woodley DT, Burgeson RE, Lunstrum S et al. Epidermolysis Bullosa Acquisita Antigen is the Globular Carboxyl Terminus of Type VII Procollagen. *J Clin Invest* (1988) 81:683–687.

66. Stanley JR, Rubinstein N, Klaus-Kovtun V. EBA antigen is synthesised by both human keratinocytes and human dermal fibroblasts. *J Invest Dermatol.* 1985;85:542–545.

67. Woodley DT, Briggaman RA, Gammon WR, et al. EBA antigen, a major cutaneous basement membrane component, is synthesised by human dermafibroblasts and other cutaneous tissues. *J Invest Dermatol.* 1986;87:227–231.

68. Roenigk HH Jr, Ryan JG, Bergfeld WF. Epidermolysis bullosa acquisita: Report of three cases and review of all published cases. *Arch Dermatol.* 1971;103:1–10.

69. Huff JC, Weston WL, Tonnesen MG. Erythema multiforme: A critical review of characteristics, diagnostic criteria and causes. *J Am Acad Dermatol.* 1983;8:763–775.

70. Duvic M. Erythema multiforme. *Dermatol Clin.* 1983;1:217–230.

71. Bedi TR, Pinkus H. Histopathological spectrum of erythema multiforme. *Br J Dermatol.* 1976;95:243–250.

72. Ackerman AB, Penneys NS, Clark WH. Erythema multiforme exudativum: Distinctive pathological process. *Br J Dermatol.* 1971;554–566.

73. Orfanos CE, Schaumburg-Lever G, Lever WF. Dermal and epidermal types of erythema multiforme. *Arch Dermatol.* 1974;109:682–688.

74. Finan MC, Schroeter AL. Cutaneous immunofluorescence study of erythema multiforme: Correlation with light microscopic patterns and etiologic agents. *J Am Acad Dermatol.* 1984;10:497–506.

75. Lyell A. Toxic epidermal necrolysis (the scalded skin syndrome): A reappraisal. *Br J Dermatol.* 1979;100:69–86.

76. Penneys NS, Wiley HE. Herpetiform blisters in systemic lupus erythematosus. *Arch Dermatol.* 1979;115:1427–1428.

77. Kumar V, Binder WL, Schotland E, et al. Coexistence of bullous pemphigoid and systemic lupus erythematosus. *Arch Dermatol.* 114:1187–1190.

78. Camisa C, Sharma H. Vesiculobullous systemic lupus erythematosus. *J Am Acad Dermatol.* 1983;9:924–933.
79. Hall RP, Lawley TJ, Smith H, Katz SI. Bullous eruption of systemic lupus erythematosus. *Ann Intern Med.* 1982;97:165–170.
80. Olansky AO, Briggaman RA, Gammon WR, et al. Bullous systemic lupus erythematosus. *J Am Acad Dermatol.* 1982;7:511–520.
81. Barton DD, Fine J, Gammon WR, Sams WM. Bullous systemic lupus erythematosus: An unusual clinical course and detectable circulating autoantibodies to the epidermolysis bullosa acquisita antigen. *J Am Acad Dermatol.* 1986;15:369–373.

82. Miller RC, Shapiro LS. Bullous urticaria pigmentosa in infancy. *Arch Dermatol.* 1965;91:595–598.
83. Klaus SN, Winkelmann RK. Course of urticaria pigmentosa in children. *Arch Dermatol.* 1962;86:116–119.
84. Orkin M, Good RA, Clawson CC, et al. Bullous mastocytosis. *Arch Dermatol.* 1970;101:547–564.
85. Welch EA, Alper JC, Bogaars H, Farrell DS. Treatment of bullous mastocytosis with disodium cromoglycate. *J Am Acad Dermatol.* 1983;9:349–353.
86. Johnson WC, Helwig EB. Solitary mastocytosis. *Arch Dermatol.* 1961;84:148–157.

CHAPTER 12

Superficial Perivascular Dermatitis

John C. Maize and John S. Metcalf

Superficial perivascular dermatitis includes a number of diseases characterized by a variably dense inflammatory cell infiltrate predominantly around vessels of the superficial vascular plexus. Epidermal changes usually are not present.

APPROACH TO DIAGNOSIS

There are several diseases that, on scanning examination, show only an inflammatory cell infiltrate around the vessels of the upper dermis without alteration of the epidermis. In the majority of such cases, it is possible either to make a diagnosis on the basis of the histopathologic findings or to provide the clinician with a limited differential diagnosis from which the correct diagnosis can be arrived at by clinicopathologic correlation. There are four major factors to be considered when examining dermal inflammatory infiltrates: (1) the distribution of the infiltrate, (2) the composition of the infiltrate, (3) the density of the infiltrate, and (4) concomitant changes in the connective tissue of the papillary dermis.

First, it must be determined if the infiltrate is confined to the superficial vascular plexus. The superficial plexus lies in the uppermost reticular dermis just beneath the papillary dermis. A capillary loop arises from the plexus to supply each dermal papilla. Communicating vessels connect the superficial plexus and the deep vascular plexus. When an inflammatory process involves the superficial plexus, inflammatory cells may be seen around the horizontally oriented vessels of the superficial plexus, the vertically oriented capillaries in the dermal papilla, and, in some cases, the communicating vessels of the upper half of the reticular dermis. Unless the inflammatory process also involves the deep reticular dermis, it should be considered in the category of superficial perivascular dermatitis.

After the depth of distribution of the infiltrate is known, it must be determined whether the inflammatory cells are circumscribed around the vessels or also are found interstitially between the collagen bundles of the papillary and the superficial reticular dermis. In urticaria and urticarial reactions, the infiltrate is not just perivascular. The inflammatory cells, especially eosinophils, are found interposed between collagen bundles away from immediate perivascular space, whereas in most other inflammatory disorders affecting only the superficial vascular plexus, an interstitial component is lacking or only a few inflammatory cells are found away from the perivascular compartment. In superficial gyrate erythemas, the inflammatory cells usually are coalesced closely around the vessels.

Determination of the composition of the cellular infiltrate characterizes the nature of the process and thereby limits the diagnostic possibilities. Much progress has been made in recent years in determining the pathophysiology of inflammation, and an important rationale for morphologic differential diagnosis of superficial perivascular dermatitis is that each specific type of immunologic or nonimmunologic injury induces a consistent type of cellular response that depends on the chemical mediators released or produced in the tissue. For example, immune complex deposition activates complement, thereby generating neutrophil chemotaxins that result in a cellular infiltrate with a predominance of neutrophils, whereas delayed hypersensitivity reactions result in an infiltrate comprising predominantly lymphocytes and monocytes. There are four types of infiltrates: (1) lymphomonocytic, (2) mixed, with a predominance of eosinophils, (3) mixed, with a predominance of neutrophils, and (4) mast cell.

In regard to density of the cellular infiltrate, some conditions, such as urticaria or some cases of morbilliform drug eruption, are characterized by a sparse infiltrate that may not even be seen easily at scanning magnification, whereas others characteristically have a more dense inflammatory infiltrate that is readily apparent at low magnification.

The papillary dermal connective tissue should be examined to determine whether the process is chronic. Persistent inflammation usually results in fibroplasia, which is manifested by thickening of the papillary dermis, coarsening of the usually delicate collagen bundles, and an increase in fixed tissue cells, such as fibrocytes and mast cells. Evanescent conditions, for example, urticaria or morbilliform drug eruptions, never produce such connective tissue alterations, but a relatively long-lived condition, such as lichen planus, may leave residual connective tissue changes as evidence of previous inflammation at the site. Papillary dermal fibrosis often is present in postinflammatory pigmentary alteration.

Certain caveats must always be kept in mind. An important one is that all inflammatory processes evolve over time. For instance, a perivascular infiltrate in the papillary dermis precedes the development of spongiosis in allergic contact dermatitis. A biopsy specimen of an early edematous papule of allergic contact dermatitis may show only the picture of superficial perivascular dermatitis without detectable epidermal changes. This is but one example in which clinicopathologic correlation would be important in reconciling the histopathologic findings. If the clinical diagnosis or description does not correlate well with the histopathologic features, further investigation is warranted to resolve the disparity. This may include discussing the case with the clinician to clarify the nature of the clinical findings, cutting additional histologic sections to resolve a sampling problem, doing special stains to look for specific tissue changes or cell types, obtaining additional biopsy material for histologic study, or some combination of these.

LYMPHOCYTIC INFILTRATES

Of the superficial perivascular dermatitides, those diseases characterized by lymphomonocytic infiltrates are not easily distinguished from each other on a strictly morphologic basis. However, some general morphologic features, such as density of the infiltrate, presence of focal mild spongiosis, and identification of lymphocytes, sideropahges, or melanophages in the dermis, when combined with pertinent clinical data, frequently enable the examiner to narrow the differential diagnosis considerably.

POSTINFLAMMATORY PIGMENTARY ALTERATION

Clinical Features

Postinflammatory pigmentary alterations are hyper- or hypopigmented macules or patches that occur as the sequelae of previous inflammatory disorders. The clinical change is the result of pigment loss from the basal cells and melanocytes of the epidermis (pigment incontinence) stimulated by inflammation and uptake of this melanin by dermal melanophages. Although frequently there is no clinical or histologic clue to indicate the precise nature of the preceding disorder, in some cases, the clinical configuration and location of the lesion and the degree and pattern of the morphologic alterations are helpful.

Histologic Features

It is usually impossible to determine histologically whether the clinical appearance is one of hyper- or hypopigmentation. The histologic picture is a slight superficial perivascular dermatitis, the infiltrate consisting of lymphocytes and macrophages, some of the latter containing melanin pigment (Fig. 12–1). There frequently are no residual epidermal changes. At times, however, the preceding process is reflected in residual changes in the stratum corneum and alteration in the topography of the epidermis. There also

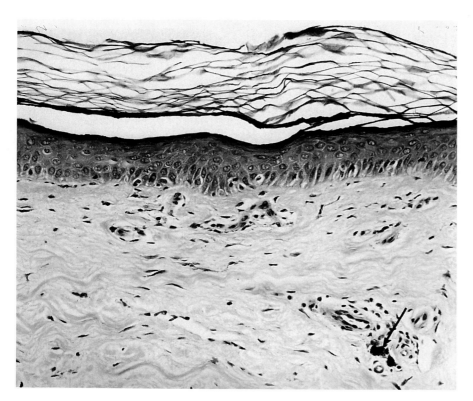

Figure 12–1. Postinflammatory pigmentary alteration. The epidermis is normal. There is a slight perivascular mononuclear infiltrate containing several melanophages (arrow) (H&E, ×200).

may be papillary dermal fibrosis. Thus, slight epidermal hyperplasia and an associated compact orthokeratotic horny layer might represent residua of a chronic spongiotic process. Where there is more pronounced dermal fibrosis or effacement of the epidermal rete ridges, a preceding interface dermatitis might be more likely. By correlating the histologic changes with the clinical pattern, it may be possible to reconstruct in the mind's eye the previous process. A diagnosis of postinflammatory pigmentary alteration following a fixed drug eruption might be suggested in a patient with a well-circumscribed patch of deep hyperpigmentation and histologic picture of a lymphomonocytic infiltrate and melanophages in a fibrotic papillary dermis. Photosensitizers, such as 5-methoxypsoralen (oil of bergamot), result in postinflammatory pigmentary alterations in a clinical pattern corresponding to the pattern of exposure to the substance.

Differential Diagnosis

The differential diagnosis includes vitiligo, such regressed melanocytic lesions as halo nevi and melanoma, and macular amyloidosis. The distinction from vitiligo is made by identification of melanocytes and pigment along the basal layer, facilitated by stains for melanin if necessary. Regressed melanocytic lesions generally show significant dermal fibrosis and frequently retain the overall topography of the neoplasm. The identification of amyloid in the papillary dermis distinguishes macular amyloidosis from postinflammatory pigmentary change.

SCHAMBERG'S DISEASE

Clinical Features

Schamberg's disease, a chronic pigmented purpuric eruption, is characterized clinically by red-brown macules and patches containing red to brown puncta, described as "Cayenne pepper spots."[1] The process develops most frequently in middle-aged men, usually involving the distal lower extremities and at times extending more proximally.

Histologic Features

The histologic appearance is that of a superficial perivascular dermatitis, frequently with no epidermal involvement but occasionally exhibiting focal parakeratosis and spongiosis (Fig. 12–2). The infiltrate is lymphomonocytic and contains siderophages if the biopsy was taken from a more chronic lesion. There is a variable degree of erythrocyte extravasation in the papillary dermis. However, no true vasculitis, in the sense of leukocytoclasis or destruction of blood vessel walls, can be identified at the light microscopic level.

Schamberg's disease is thought to be closely related to other pigmented purpuric eruptions, the clinical and morphologic patterns showing considerable overlap.[2,3] In this disease spectrum, Schamberg's disease histologically shows the least epidermal change and dermal fibrosis, with other pigmented purpuric dermatoses showing comparatively more interface change, a denser and more bandlike dermal infiltrate, and more dermal fibroplasia. The pathogenesis of the disorder has still not been explained satisfactorily although increased capillary fragility and delayed hypersensitivity have been implicated.[3,4] The identification of C3 and C1q in the walls of papillary dermal blood vessels has been noted by Iwatsuki et al.,[5] but it is uncertain whether it signifies a role for immune complexes or represents an event secondary to a cell-mediated process.

Differential Diagnosis

Stasis dermatitis is distinguished from Schamberg's disease by epidermal hyperplasia and sometimes ulceration, spongiosis, and the presence of thick-walled vessels in the superficial and deep dermis. Purpura annularis telangiectoides

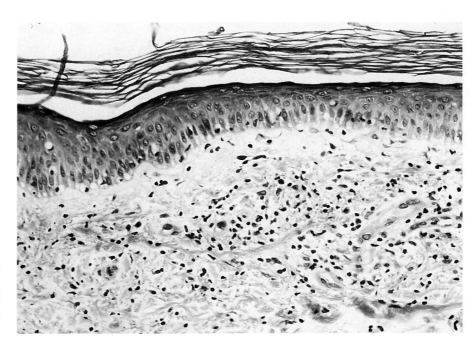

Figure 12–2. Schamberg's disease. Some mild interface changes are identified and also mild spongiosis. Erythrocytes are identified in the interstitium, and there is a perivascular lymphohistiocytic infiltrate. Siderophages may be found (H & E, ×40).

of Majocchi is histologically similar and must be distinguished clinically.

MORBILLIFORM DRUG ERUPTIONS

Clinical Features

Morbilliform drug eruptions are erythematous eruptions of macules and papules that usually have a symmetrical distribution. The upper body or extremities may be involved first, but the lesions frequently become widespread. There may be associated pruritus and mild temperature elevation in some patients. Although these eruptions may be caused by a wide variety of agents, morbilliform drug reactions to ampicillin have been documented most thoroughly. The process usually begins within 1 or 2 weeks of the onset of exposure but may occur even after the drug therapy has been discontinued.[6]

Histologic Features

A spectrum of epidermal changes may be seen in morbilliform drug eruptions, ranging from no identifiable epidermal changes to instances in which there is easily identifiable vacuolar alteration at the dermoepidermal junction. There is a mild perivascular infiltrate surrounding the vessels of the superficial plexus, which consists predominantly of lymphocytes. However, a few eosinophils or neutrophils may be seen (Fig. 12–3). Although the lesion has been described as a vasculitis, in our experience there is no evidence of vascular damage that can be seen in H & E-stained sections. However, there is evidence to suggest that, in some cases, antigen-antibody complexes form within vessel walls.[7] The formation of antiepithelial antibodies has been reported in morbilliform reactions to penicillin.[8]

Ultrastructurally, changes may be identified within the basal layer ranging from intercellular and intracellular edema to frank disruption of basal cells.[8]

Differential Diagnosis

The histologic differential diagnosis includes viral exanthems and tinea versicolor. The latter may, of course, be distinguished through identification of the organisms within the stratum corneum, at times facilitated by the use of special stains. It may be difficult histologically to distinguish morbilliform drug eruption from erythema multiforme, but in well-developed lesions of the latter, interface change is much more pronounced, and necrotic keratinocytes are prominent in the epidermis, with confluent areas of keratinocyte necrosis in many instances.

SUPERFICIAL GYRATE ERYTHEMA

Clinical Features

Gyrate erythemas have been subdivided by some authors into two varieties: those in which the inflammatory cell infiltrate surrounds the vessels of only the superficial vascular plexus (superficial gyrate erythema) and those in which the deep vascular plexus also is involved (deep gyrate erythema).[9,10] Of these, the former has the microscopic appearance of a superficial perivascular dermatitis.

Clinically, gyrate erythemas have been divided into nonspecific gyrate erythema, known to some as erythema annulare centrifugum, erythema marginatum rheumaticum, erythema chronicum migrans, and erythema gyratum repens. Of these, nonspecific gyrate erythema, erythema marginatum rheumaticum, and erythema gyratum repens may have the morphology of a superficial perivascular dermatitis. Erythema marginatum rheumaticum is distinguished from the other gyrate erythemas by the presence of neutrophils in the infiltrate and clinically by its association with rheumatic fever. The nonspecific form and erythema gyratum repens must be distinguished on clinical grounds, the latter being characterized by erythematous bands in a distinctive woodgrain pattern with scaling. There is a well-

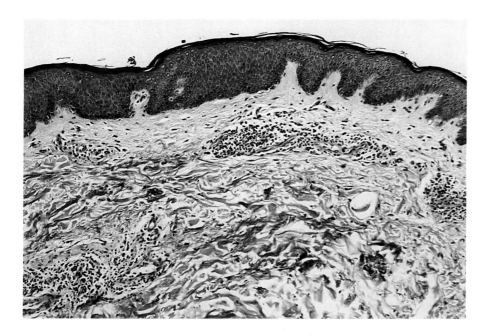

Figure 12–23. Morbilliform drug reaction. Although a few neutrophils and eosinophils may be seen in some instances, lymphocytes and monocytes are the most common cell types in the perivascular infiltrate (H & E, ×80).

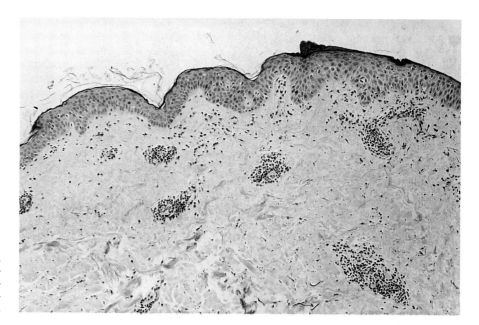

Figure 12–4. Superficial gyrate erythema. There is focal parakeratosis, and the adjacent epidermis shows mild spongiosis. Lymphocytes and histiocytes cluster around vessels of the superficial plexus (H & E, ×80).

documented association between this disease and systemic illness, usually malignancy.[11]

Histologic Features

Histologically, the nonspecific gyrate erythemas are characterized by a dermal infiltrate, predominantly lymphocytic, confined to the areas surrounding the vessels of the superficial plexus. The infiltrate is usually more dense than in other superficial perivascular dermatitides. If the biopsy includes the edge of the lesion, focal mild spongiosis and parakeratosis may be seen (Fig. 12–4). More centrally, in areas where the inflammation has subsided, postinflammatory pigmentary changes may be identified.

Differential Diagnosis

The tumid form of lupus erythematosus may resemble superficial gyrate erythemas. It can be distinguished, however, by the presence of abundant mucin in the reticular dermis.

MIXED INFILTRATES WITH EOSINOPHILS PROMINENT

Eosinophils contain a number of important, biologically potent substances in their granules, including eosinophil major basic protein, eosinophil peroxidase, eosinophil-derived neurotoxin, Charcot-Leyden crystal protein, and eosinophil cationic protein.[12] Eosinophils are important in host defense mechanisms against certain parasites. Experimental evidence indicates also that the protein products of eosinophils are released into the extracellular space and contribute to the increased vascular permeability in some cutaneous diseases associated with edema, such as urticaria.[12,13] Histamine is chemotactic for eosinophils, as are other mast cell-

derived factors, such as eosinophil chemotactic factor of anaphylaxis (ECF-A).[14,15]

URTICARIA

Clinical Features

Urticaria has been defined traditionally by its major clinical feature, the wheal. A wheal is a papule or plaque caused mostly by dermal edema that is transient in nature. A wheal may be the color of the surrounding skin, but most often it is pallid, with or without an erythematous halo around it. The papule or plaque often has a peau d'orange appearance on the surface and is usually irregular in contour, with pseudopodlike extensions at the periphery.

It has become apparent, however, as more has become known about inflammatory mechanisms, that wheals may be produced by several different inflammatory mediators released by different types of immunologic or pharmacologic reactions. Therefore, the wheal can be regarded as a clinical final common pathway that is not specific to any single mechanism or mediator. It is reasonable to expect that urticaria may have different histopathologic features depending on the inflammatory mechanism that led to its development. In one person, penicillin may produce an urticarial reaction via an IgE-dependent mechanism, whereas in another, the skin lesions are caused by a serum sickness-like reaction as the result of immune complexes that activate the complement system. The etiology of the hives in both instances is penicillin allergy, but the pathogenesis is different and the hives will look different histologically.

A thorough account of the clinical features, etiologic factors, and pathophysiology of urticaria is beyond the scope of this discussion, which focuses on different histologic pictures that may be seen in clinically typical urticaria, be it acute or chronic. Chronic urticaria should be thought of as recurrent acute urticaria. The wheals that occur in patients who have urticaria for weeks, months, or years come in crops and are evanescent, lasting only for a matter of hours. Wheals that last more than 24 hours should alert the clinician to the possibility of urticarial vasculitis.

Histologic Features

The usual urticarial wheal shows the following histologic features: (1) dermal edema indicated by dermal pallor and widening of the spaces between the collagen bundles, (2) dilatation of the small blood vessels of the superficial plexus,

and (3) a sparse, superficial perivascular and interstitial infiltrate consisting primarily of lymphocytes, and in most cases, a few eosinophils[16] (Fig. 12–5). Except for dilatation, the blood vessels show no abnormal alterations. In some cases, these changes affect not only the superficial but also the deep reticular dermis. This classic type of sparse-infiltrate lesion is typical of IgE-mediated urticaria.

Less commonly, there is a moderately dense perivascular infiltrate composed primarily of lymphocytes and eosinophils but sometimes also containing a few neutrophils (Fig. 12–6). Some cases show marked eosinophilic infiltrates with eosinophil degranulation.[16] Patients with the more dense

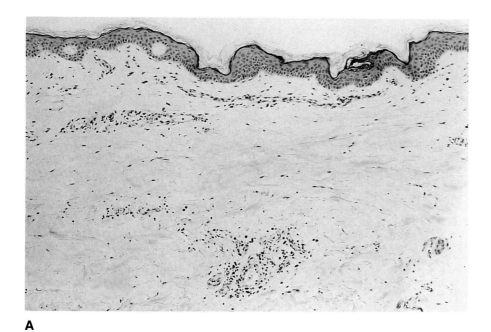

A

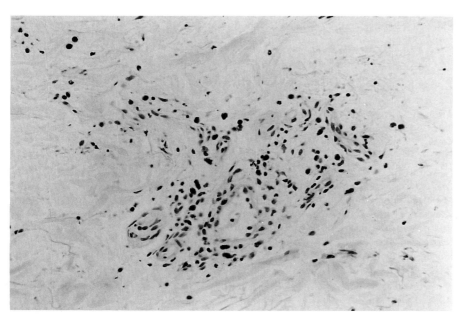

B

Figure 12–5. Urticaria. **A.** There is a sparse inflammatory cell infiltrate and interstitial edema (H & E, ×80). **B.** Perivascular infiltrate of lymphocytes and a few eosinophils around dilated vessels (H & E, ×200).

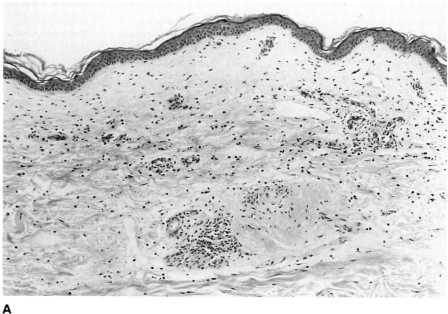

A

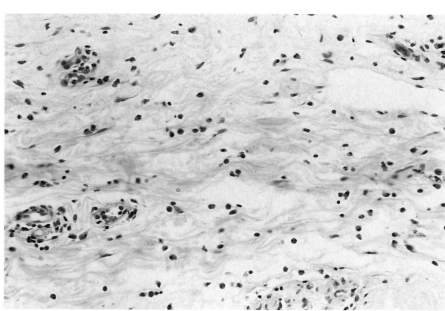

Figure 12–6. Dense-infiltrate urticaria. **A.** There is a moderately dense perivascular and interstitial infiltrate, interstitial edema and prominent vascular ectasia (H & E, ×80). **B.** Infiltrate consists of lympyocytes, eosinophils, and rare neutrophils (H & E, ×200).

B

cellular infiltrates are much more likely to have detectable circulating immune complexes than are patients with the usual sparse infiltrates, suggesting that the pathogenesis is different.[16,17] Furthermore, they are more likely to have longer-lasting wheals, some persisting for more than 24 hours. This group has clinical, immunopathologic, and histologic features intermediate between ordinary urticaria and urticarial vasculitis. Some patients have urticaria that shows an infiltrate with a predominance of neutrophils and a minor component of lymphocytes and eosinophils.[18] These cases differ from urticarial vasculitis in that there is no leukocytoclasia, fibrin deposition, or extravasation of red blood cells.

Patients with the denser infiltrates, whether they have infiltrates rich in eosinophils or neutrophils, have a high incidence of pressure urticaria.

PRURITIC URTICARIAL PAPULES AND PLAQUES OF PREGNANCY (PUPP)

Clinical Features
PUPP is a distinctive cutaneous eruption that occurs in the third trimester, most commonly in primagravidas.[19] The cause is unknown. The earliest lesions are minute erythema-

tous papules that enlarge and often coalesce to form urticarial plaques. Papulovesicles also may develop in some patients. The eruption usually begins on the abdomen, especially around the umbilicus, where it may be localized to striae distensae. Other body sites may be involved, but the face and mucous membranes usually are spared. There is no association of this condition with increased fetal wastage or birth defects. The eruption resolves spontaneously or at delivery and does not recur in subsequent pregnancies in most patients.

Histologic Features

The histology of PUPP is protean. In some cases, there is only a sparse superficial perivascular infiltrate of mononuclear cells, but occasional eosinophils are usually present also (Fig. 12–7).[20] Sometimes the infiltrate is interstitial as well as perivascular. Papillary dermal edema varies from moderate to undetectable. In some cases, focal spongiosis with or without parakeratosis also is present. Immunofluorescence studies are negative.[21] The urticarial papules of herpes gestationis have a similar infiltrate, but they usu-

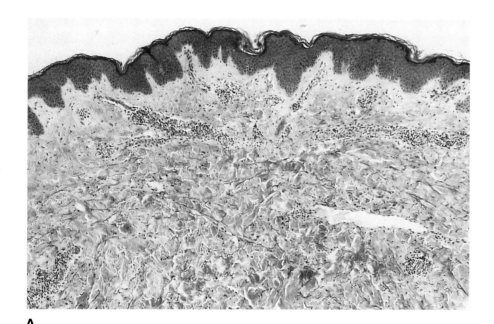

A

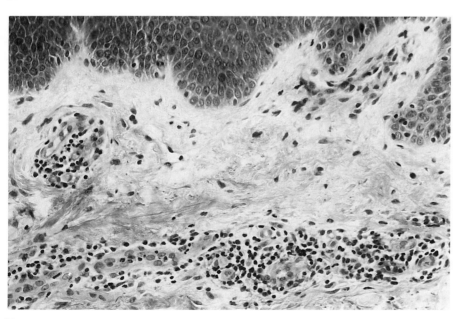

B

Figure 12–7. Pruritic urticarial papules and plaques of pregnancy. Urticarial lesion. **A.** Superficial perivascular inflammatory cell infiltrate, slight interstitial edema, and vascular ectasia (H & E, ×40). **B.** Infiltrate consists of lymphocytes and occasional eosinophils (H & E, ×200).

ally show much more marked papillary dermal edema, which expands some dermal papillae so that they may resemble a light bulb in profile, and they often demonstrate eosinophilic spongiosis and necrosis of some basal cells overlying the edematous papillae.

THE HYPEREOSINOPHILIC SYNDROME

Clinical Features

The idiopathic hypereosinophilic syndrome (HES) encompasses a spectrum of disease that ranges from a benign, self-limited condition to eosinophilic leukemia. HES is primarily a diagnosis of exclusion because there are many causes of eosinophilia. Criteria proposed for diagnosis include (1) persistent eosinophilia of greater than 1,500 eosinophils/mm^3 for longer than 6 months, or death associated with the signs and symptoms of HES before 6 months, (2) no evidence for parasitic, allergic, or other known causes of eosinophilia, and (3) presumptive signs and symptoms of parenchymal organ involvement.[22] Eosinophilic infiltrates may be found in many organs, including the heart, lungs, kidneys, gastrointestinal tract, and neurologic system.

Cutaneous involvement occurs in over one third of the cases.[22,23] The cutaneous lesions may be pruritic erythematous macules, papules, plaques, or nodules (some of which may ulcerate), or urticaria and angioedema.

Histologic Features

The histopathologic changes are not diagnostic and are comprised of mixed dermal perivascular infiltrate of mononuclear cells and eosinophils, sometimes with neutrophils or plasma cells. The papules and plaques may show spongiosis. The urticarial lesions show more prominent interstitial edema than the papules and are identical to the dense infiltrate type of wheal that may occur in chronic urticaria not associated with HES.

MIXED INFILTRATES WITH NEUTROPHILS PREDOMINANT

Superficial perivascular infiltrates showing a preponderance of neutrophils are rarely seen. When such an infiltrate is seen in the dermis, there are three pathogenetic mechanisms that should be suspected. Most physicians would suspect the possibility of infection. Erysipelas, however, usually involves the deep as well as the superficial plexus. Immune complex-mediated disease probably is the most common cause of such infiltrates. In the early urticarial papules of vasculitis, there may be only a superficial perivascular infiltrate of neutrophils without leukocytoclasia or fibrin deposition.[20] In leukocytoclastic vasculitis, the immune complexes affect primarily the postcapillary venules of the superficial plexus. A similar histologic picture has been noted as the earliest detectable histologic change in secondary syphilis, suggesting the possibility of immune complex-mediated vessel injury as the primary event in that disease.[24] Rarely, biopsies of patients with chronic urticaria may also show leukocytoclastic vasculitis. We have seen this pattern

mainly in patients with SLE who have either presented with or subsequently developed chronic urticaria, although the experience of some others is different.[18] Erythema marginatum and the evanescent urticarial lesions of Still's disease show an infiltrate of neutrophils; the pathogenesis of these lesions is not known, but they most likely are due to immune complexes also.

A third major pathogenetic mechanism to be considered is tissue injury from toxins injected by certain insects and other noxious organisms. (Cutaneous reactions to arthropod bites and stings are discussed in Chapter 30.) Erythropoietic protoporphyria (EPP) is a rare disease in which the excess protoporphyrin that is produced causes UVA-induced tissue injury. The solar urticaria seen in affected patients shows an infiltrate rich in neutrophils. The nature of the inflammatory mediators elaborated in the skin in EPP is not known.

ERYTHEMA MARGINATUM

Clinical Features

Erythema marginatum is one of the five major clinical criteria of Jones for diagnosis of rheumatic fever, the others being carditis, polyarthritis, chorea, and subcutaneous nodules.[25] It occurs in up to 18% of patients, especially those with active carditis.[26] Its incidence has decreased along with that of rheumatic fever. Dull red, flat or palpable, polycyclic or reticulated rings or ring segments occur in crops, particularly on the abdomen. They are nonpruritic and usually fade in a few hours but occasionally last 2 to 3 days. The lesions begin as erythematous macules or papules and spread centrifugally. They may recur for up to a few weeks.

Histologic Features

Histologically, the epidermis is normal. There is a superficial perivascular infiltrate of neutrophils and a few mononuclear cells (Fig. 12–8).[27] Small collections of neutrophils may be seen in the dermal papillae. Nuclear debris may sometimes be present, but absence of fibrin deposition in and around the small vessels and lack of red blood cell extravasation distinguish this neutrophilic vascular reaction from leukocytoclastic vasculitis.

EVANESCENT ERUPTION OF STILL'S DISEASE

Clinical Features

Still's disease (juvenile rheumatoid arthritis) is a type of chronic polyarthritis primarily affecting children that is associated with splenomegaly, lymphadenopathy, polyserositis, and intermittent fever. About one fourth of patients develop a characteristic eruption that may herald the disease.[28] The primary lesion is a salmon-pink macule that is often surrounded by a narrow zone of blanching. Annular lesions and papules also can occur. An important feature of the eruption is its evanescence, as it tends to appear in the evenings in association with high temperatures and then fade. It may be accentuated in areas of pressure and can be linear, suggesting a Koebner-like reaction. Peripheral

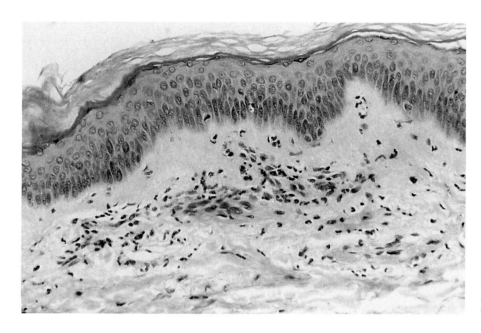

Figure 12–8. Erythema marginatum. There is a sparse superficial perivascular infiltrate of neutrophils, some of which show nuclear fragmentation (H & E, ×200).

leukocytosis of polymorphonuclear leukocytes is common. It has a median duration, on and off, of about 1 year.

Histologic Features

On histologic examination, there is dermal edema and a sparse superficial perivascular infiltrate of neutrophils and a few mononuclear cells.[28] The small vessels are dilated and may contain numerous neutrophils. There is no fibrin deposition or diapedesis of red blood cells, but some nuclear debris may be present.

ERYTHROPOIETIC PROTOPORPHYRIA

Clinical Features

Erythropoietic protoporphyria (EPP) is a dominantly inherited disorder in which there is decreased activity of the enzyme heme synthase, resulting in the accumulation of its substrate, protoporphyrin IX.[29] Elevated levels of protoporphyrin IX are found in red blood cells and in feces, but not in the urine. On exposure to sunlight, persons with EPP develop a burning or stinging sensation in the exposed skin that may be followed by erythema and edema. Sometimes, urticaria or vesicles may develop. Chronically exposed skin, especially on the dorsa of the hands, becomes thickened and leathery, and there may be superficial scarring.

Histologic Features

The major histologic feature of EPP, as of the other porphyrias that produce photosensitivity, is the formation of a rim of homogeneous, eosinophilic material around the capillaries and venules of the superficial vascular plexus (Fig. 12–9). This material is PAS-positive and diastase resistant.[30] Examinaiton of a specimen taken from erythematous edematous skin after exposure to sunlight shows a perivascular infiltrate of neutrophils, some mononuclear cells, and occa-

sional eosinophils.[31] This infiltrate is most prominent around the vessels of the superficial plexus but may extend into the reticular dermis. Some nuclear debris may be present, and there may be slight extravasation of RBCs. The presence of the homogeneous eosinophilic material around the walls of the blood vessels serves to distinguish EPP from leukocytoclastic vasculitis, in which there may be deposits of fibrin that are more fibrillary in appearance.

Immunopathology

Direct immunofluorescence has shown IgG, sometimes with IgM and C3, in and around blood vessels in the papillary dermis and, to a lesser extent, at the basement membrane zone.[30] Photoactivation of complement has been demonstrated in sera from patients with EPP after irradiation with 400 nm light in vitro,[32] thereby suggesting that the products of complement activation may play a role in the development of the skin lesions. Furthermore, injection of protoporphyrin into the skin of guinea pigs followed by 400 nm irradiation produces an infiltration of neutrophils in the dermis.[33]

MAST CELL INFILTRATES

URTICARIA PIGMENTOSA

Clinical Features

Urticaria pigmentosa is a disease complex with a broad clinical spectrum that ranges from childhood forms, which frequently involute spontaneously, to the adult forms, which rarely resolve. The cutaneous lesion may be a macule that is hyperpigmented or erythematous, a papule, or a tumor nodule. All have in common the characteristic wheal and flare when they are stroked or traumatized (Darier's sign).

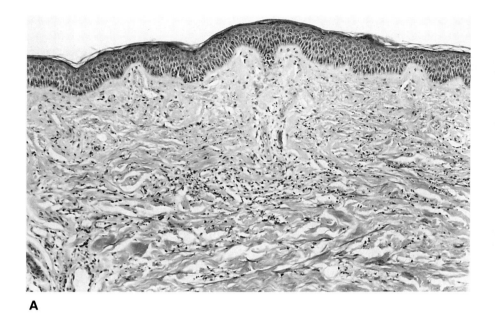

A

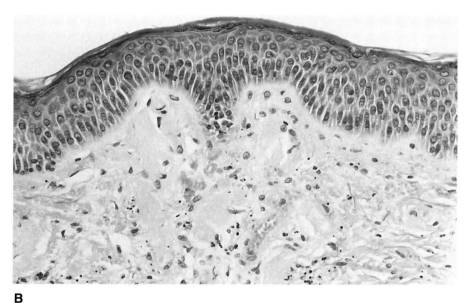

B

Figure 12–9. Erythropoietic protoporphyria. **A.** Superficial perivascular infiltrate of neutrophils and some mononuclear cells (H & E, ×80). **B.** Higher magnification showing homogeneous material around the vessels of the superficial plexus (H & E, ×200). **C.** High magnification showing vessel walls surrounded by fibrillar and homogeneous material and fragmentation of neutrophil nuclei (H & E, ×400).

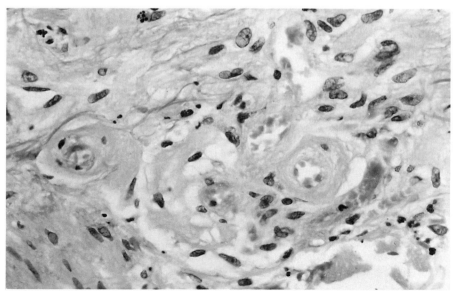

C

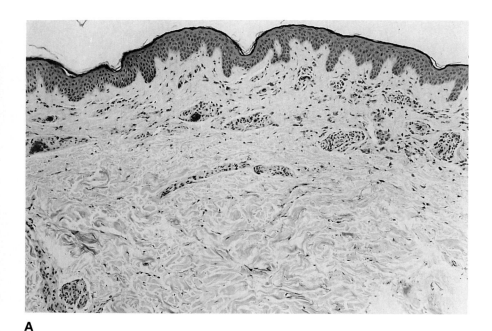

A

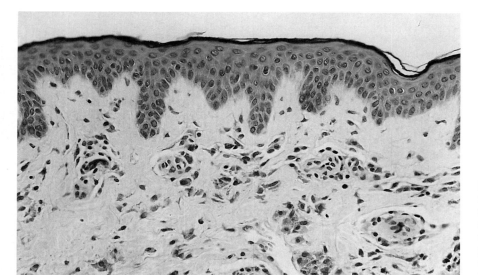

B

Figure 12–10. Mast cell disease, telangiectasia, macularis eruptiva perstans. **A.** At this magnification, the cellular infiltrate appears similar to that seen in inflammatory conditions (H & E, ×80). **B.** In this case, cytoplasmic mast cell granules can be identified even without the use of special stains. Frequently, however, special stains are necessary to identify the population of mast cells in a perivascular infiltrate (H & E, ×200).

Histologic Features

The histologic appearance of some forms, i.e., macular lesions seen in either the childhood or adult mast cell diseases and in telangiectasia macularis eruptiva perstans (TMEP), resembles that of superficial dermal perivascular infiltrates. An infiltrate predominantly of mast cells surrounds dilated vessels of the vascular plexus similar in distribution and density to that seen in the lymphomonocytic infiltrates described previously (Fig. 12–10A). Indeed, the mast cells may be difficult to distinguish from lymphocytes, histiocytes, or pericytes on H & E stained sections unless a dendritic outline or cytoplasmic granules can be discerned (Fig.

12–10B). Usually, however, special stains, such as the Giemsa, toluidine blue, or chloracetate esterase (Leder), are necessary in these more histologically subtle forms of mast cell proliferation to confirm that the infiltrate is predominantly of mast cells.

REFERENCES

1. Schamberg JF. A peculiar progressive pigmentary disease of the skin. *Br J Dermatol.* 1901;13:1–5.
2. Randall SJ, Kierland RR, Montgomery H. Pigmented purpuric eruptions. *AMA Arch Dermatol.* 1951;64:177–191.

3. Newton RC, Raimer SS. Pigmented purpuric eruptions. *Dermatol Clin.* 1985;3:165–169.

4. Klug H, Haustein UF. Ultrastructure of macrophage-lymphocyte interaction in purpura pigmentosa progressiva. *Dermatologica.* 1976;153:209–217.

5. Iwatsuki K, Tadahiro A, Tagami H, et al. Immunofluorescent study in purpura pigmentosa chronica. *Acta Derm Venereol. (Stockh).* 1980;60:341–345.

6. Fitzpatrick TB, Eisen AZ, et al. *Dermatology in General Medicine.* 2nd ed. New York: McGraw-Hill Book Company; 1979:562.

7. Fellner MJ. Adverse effects of drugs on skin. In: Helwig E, Mostofi FK, eds. *The Skin.* Williams & Wilkins; Baltimore: 1971:230–234.

8. Fellner MJ, and Prutkin L. Morbilliform eruptions caused by penicillin: A study of electron microscopy and immunologic tests. *J Invest Dermatol.* 1970;55:390–395.

9. Ackerman AB. *Histologic Diagnosis of Inflammatory Skin Diseases.* Philadelphia: Lea & Febiger; 1978:174–175.

10. Bressler GS, Jones RE Jr. Erythema annulare centrifugum. *J Am Acad Dermatol.* 1981;4:597–602.

11. White JW Jr. Gyrate erythema. *Dermatol Clin.* 1985;3:129–139.

12. Lieferman KM, Peters MS, and Gleich GJ. The eosinophil and cutaneous edema. *J Am Acad Dermatol.* 1986;15:513–517.

13. Peters MS, Schroeter AL, Kephart GM, and Gleich GJ. Localization of eosinophil granule major basic protein in chronic urticaria. *J Invest Dermatol.* 1983;81:39–43.

14. Clark RAF, Callin JL, Kaplan AD. The selective eosinophil chemotactic activity of histamine. *J Exp Med.* 1975;142:1462–1473.

15. Kay AB, Stechschulte DJ, Austen KF. An eosinophil leukocyte chemotactic factor of anaphylaxis. *J Exp Med.* 1971;113:602–613.

16. Monroe EW, Schulz CI, Maize JC, Jordan RE. Vasculitis in chronic urticaria: An immunopathologic study. *J Invest Dermatol.* 1981;76:103–107.

17. Jones RR, Bhogal B, Dash A, Schifferli J. Urticaria and vasculitis: A continuum of histological and immunopathological changes. *Br J Dermatol.* 1983;108:695–703.

18. Peters MS, Winkelmann RK. Neutrophilic urticaria. *Arch Dermatol.* 1984;120:1614A.

19. Yancey K, Hall R, Lawley T. Pruritic urticarial papules and plaques of pregnancy: Clinical experience in twenty-five patients. *J Am Acad Dermatol.* 1984;10:473–480.

20. Ackerman AB, Jones RE Jr. Making chronic nonspecific dermatitis specific: How to make precise diagnoses of superficial perivascular dermatitides devoid of epidermal involvement. *Am J Dermatopathol.* 1985;7:307–323.

21. Ahmed A, Kaplan R. Pruritic urticarial papules and plaques of pregnancy. *J Am Acad Dermatol.* 1981;4:679–681.

22. Kazmierowski JA, Chusid MJ, Parillo JE, Fauci AS, Wolf SM. Dermatologic manifestations of the hypereosinophilic syndrome. *Arch Dermatol.* 1978;114:531–535.

23. Chusid MJ, Dale DC, West BC, Wolff SM. The hypereosinophilic syndrome. *Medicine (Baltimore).* 1975;54:1–27.

24. McNeely MC, Jorizzo JL, Solomon AR Jr, et al. Cutaneous secondary syphilis: Preliminary immunohistopathological support for a role for immune complexes in lesion pathogenesis. *J Am Acad Dermatol.* 1986;14:564–71.

25. Jones TD. The diagnosis of rheumatic fever. *JAMA.* 1944;126:481–486.

26. Bywaters EGL. Skin manifestations of rheumatic disease. In: Fitzpatrick TB, Eisen AZ, Wolff K, et al, eds. *Dermatology in General Medicine.* 2nd ed. New York: McGraw-Hill Book Company; 1979:1316–1320.

27. Troyer C, Grossman ME, Silvers DN. Erythema marginatum in rheumatic fever: Early diagnosis by skin biopsy. *J Am Acad Dermatol.* 1983;8:724–728.

28. Isdale IC, Bywaters EGL. The rash of rheumatoid arthritis and Still's disease. *Q J Med.* 1956;99:377–387.

29. Elder GH. Metabolic abnormalities in the porphyrias. *Semin Dermatol.* 1986;5:88–98.

30. Epstein JH, Tufanelli DL, Epstein WL. Cutaneous changes in the porphyrias: A microscopic study. *Arch Dermatol.* 1973;107:689–698.

31. Ackerman AB. *Histologic Diagnosis of Inflammatory Skin Disease.* Philadelphia: Lea & Febiger; 1978:292–294.

32. Gigli I, Schothurst AA, Pathak M, Suter NA. Photoinhibition of the complement system in erythropoietic protoporphyria. *Clin Res.* 1974;22:418A.

33. Lim HM, Gigli I. Role of complement in porphyrin-induced photosensitivity. *J Invest Dermatol.* 1981;76:4–9.

SECTION III
Non-Infectious Predominantly Deep Inflammatory Diseases

CHAPTER 13
Vasculitis

Thomas G. Olsen

Vasculitis is a general term used to describe cutaneous and potentially systemic reaction patterns, microscopically characterized by inflammatory cells in vessel walls coexistent with varying degrees of endothelial cell and vessel wall necrosis. Affected vessels can be of any caliber, ranging in size from large arteries (giant cell arteritis) to small dermal capillaries and venules (leukocytoclastic vasculitis). The size of the involved vessel, the composition of the inflammatory infiltrate affecting the vessel, and the constellation of associated clinical signs and symptoms and laboratory findings allow for a more precise label of a vasculitic syndrome.

Most classifications of the vasculitides are derived from Zeek's original work in 1952, with subsequent modifications based on more precise histopathologic criteria and immunopathologic mechanisms[1-3] (Table 13–1). Several points of the classification deserve emphasis regarding nomenclature and incidence. The term "leukocytoclastic vasculitis" is preferred to describe the small vessel vasculitides because of convention and descriptive accuracy, namely, neutrophils and karyorrhectic debris—nuclear dust—in vessel walls. The designations hypersensitivity vasculitis, allergic angiitis, small vessel necrotizing vasculitis, nodular dermal allergids, and anaphylactoid purpura are synonymous with leukocytoclastic vasculitis but are not used in this text. The lymphocytic vasculitides, including Mucha-Habermann disease, certain drug hypersensitivities, pernio-chilblains, and pyoderma gangrenosum, are not classified herein because, although loosely fulfilling the definition of vasculitis, i.e., inflammation of vessels, there are few objective findings to substantiate a vasculitis process producing vessel damage. Moreover, although many authorities have used the term periarteritis nodosa to describe the leukocytoclastic vasculitis of small and medium-sized arteries, "periarteritis" implies a perivascular inflammatory process rather than a true vasculitis. Polyarteritis nodosa is a more suitable term and the one used in this chapter. Finally, the dermatopathologist should realize that the incidence of leukocytoclastic vasculitis is much greater than that of polyarteritis nodosa, the granulomatous vasculitides, and giant cell vasculitis. In 1 year, a busy dermatopathology service will review

30–50 cases of leukocytoclastic vasculitis, compared to 10 or less of the larger vessel and granulomatous vasculitides.

PATHOGENESIS

Experimental evidence has accumulated in the past two decades to support immune mechanisms for practically all the diseases and syndromes listed in Table 13–1.[4-6] This provides a linking theme and explains why there is considerable histologic and immunologic overlap among the various disease conditions. Cell-mediated immune mechanisms, the mast cell, and direct cellular cytotoxicity contribute to the pathogenesis of vasculitis, yet their role has been less well defined and requires further investigation.[2,7,8]

An immune complex pathogenesis for vasculitis follows the classic Arthus-type reaction.[2,9,10] With the host in a state of antigen excess, soluble antigen-antibody complexes form and circulate. In combination with vasoactive amine release from platelets and IgE-stimulated basophils, importantly allowing for gaps between endothelial cells, circulating immune complexes are deposited in vessel walls. The deposited immune complexes activate the complement system, with anaphylatoxins C3a and C5a serving as attractants for polymorphonuclear neutrophils and the degranulation of mast cells. Polymorphonuclear neutrophils release catalases and elastases, which are damaging to the various blood vessel components.

The clinical correlation to the vascular damage depends largely on the size of the vessel involved and the degree and intensity of the insult. The clinical spectrum of vasculitic lesions is broad and includes erythematous macules and papules, purpuric papules (palpable purpura), urticarial plaques, nodules, hemorrhagic nodules and plaques (Fig. 13–1), necrotic pustules, hemorrhagic bullae, and livedo reactions.

Identification of antigens responsible for the immune complex series of events has been reported by the use of immunofluorescent studies and indirectly through the use of epidemiologic data.[2] Hepatitis B antigen and group A

TABLE 13–1. CLASSIFICATION OF VASCULITIS

I. Leukocytoclastic vasculitis
  A. Leukocytoclastic vasculitis as major feature of syndrome
    1. Henoch-Schoenlein disease
    2. Essential mixed cryoglobulinemia
    3. Serum sickness
    4. Urticarial vasculitis
    5. Erythema elevatum diutinum
    6. Granuloma faciale
  B. Leukocytoclastic vasculitis from specific antigen exposure
    1. Infections
    2. Drugs
    3. Physical agents
  C. Leukocytoclastic vasculitis as variable and major/minor components of disease process
    1. Connective tissue diseases
    2. Malignancy
    3. Miscellaneous
    4. Idiopathic
II. Polyarteritis nodosa
  A. Systemic
  B. Cutaneous
III. Granulomatous vasculitis
  A. Allergic granulomatosis (Churg-Strauss disease)
  B. Wegener's granulomatosis
IV. Giant cell arteritis
  A. Temporal arteritis (cranial arteritis)
  B. Takayasu's disease
V. Miscellaneous

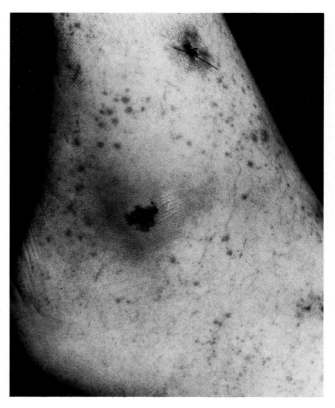

Figure 13–1. Purpuric papules and nodular ulcerative plaques in a patient with vasculitis, specifically, Wegener's granulomatosis. The combination of palpable purpura and hemorrhagic nodules and plaques is a reliable clinical indicator for a granulomatous vasculitis. (*Courtesy of Gary D. Palmer, MD.*)

streptococcal antigens have been found in association with their corresponding antibody and an ongoing vasculitic process.[11] Other microbial agents, drugs, toxins, hyposensitization antigens, and miscellaneous endogenous antigens, as might occur in connective tissue diseases and malignancies, have been implicated by association.

HISTOPATHOLOGIC CRITERIA OF VASCULITIS

The two major histologic criteria essential to the diagnosis of vasculitis, regardless of the size of the vessel involved, are damage to endothelial cells or vessel wall structures and infiltration of the vessel walls by inflammatory cells, most commonly neutrophils and lymphocytes, and also nuclear dust.[12–15] The presence of polymorphonuclear neutrophils is a less consistent finding of the two major criteria for vasculitis, especially as an acute lesion ages and in the larger vessel and granulomatous vasculitides, in which tissue macrophages (histiocytes) often dominate. However, because of the linking theme of immune complex deposition and complement activation, typifying the majority of vasculitic syndromes, one can expect to see polymorphonuclear neutrophils if the timing of the biopsy is appropriate. Mononuclear cells and eosinophils commonly are observed in the vasculitides but are less dominant and usually are noted in a perivascular or interstitial location.

Damage to the vessel wall is most commonly and conclusively manifest by fibrinoid deposits and fibrinoid necrosis of the vessel wall and related structures. This fibrinoid material, variously described as granular eosinophilic, amorphous, fibrillary, and hyalinlike, has been shown by electron microscopy and immunofluorescent studies to be a composite of fibrin and precipitated antigen-antibody complexes.[15] The presence of fibrinoid is indicative of vascular damage and the triggering of the clotting sequence and helps to establish the diagnosis of vasculitis.

Minor histologic criteria contributing to the microscopic diagnosis of vasculitis, and also a reflection of assault on the vascular structures, include endothelial swelling, hemorrhage in continuity with the involved vessel, thrombosis, epidermal necrosis with or without epidermal/subepidermal vesiculation, a mixed infiltrate including mononuclear cells and eosinophils, perivascular reparative fibroplasia in the older lesion, and rarely calcinosis and aneurysm formation.[12] Minor criteria are inconsistently observed in the vasculitides, and their importance is variable. For example, endothelial swelling is an objective feature of vasculitis and is often emphasized. However, this finding is very nonspecific, with similar changes found in various spongiotic and perivascular dermatoses, such as pityriasis rosea and capillaritis.

A definitive diagnosis of vasculitis generally can be established by the presence of one major criterion, particularly fibrinoid deposits and fibrinoid necrosis, and two or more minor microscopic findings (Table 13–2).

TABLE 13–2. HISTOPATHOLOGIC CRITERIA[a] FOR VASCULITIS

Major Criteria	Minor Criteria
1. Polymorphonuclear neutrophils and karyorrhectic debris (nuclear dust) in vessel walls	1. Endothelial cell swelling
2. Necrosis of endothelial cells and vessel walls with fibrin deposition	2. Hemorrhage in continuity with vessel
	3. Thrombosis
	4. Epidermal necrosis
	5. Epidermal and subepidermal vesicles
	6. Mixed infiltrate, including monocytes and eosinophils in an adventitial location
	7. Perivascular reparative fibroplasia
	8. Aneurysm formation
	9. Calcinosis

[a] One major criterion plus two or more minor criteria will establish the diagnosis of vasculitis.

APPROACH TO THE MICROSCOPIC DIAGNOSIS OF VASCULITIS

An approach to the microscopic diagnosis of vasculitis should include (1) an awareness of certain caveats in making the diagnosis of necrotizing vasculitis, (2) low power findings for suspected diagnosis, (3) application of major and minor criteria at higher powers, with attention given to the size of the vessel involved and infiltrate composition, and (4) the role of special stains and immunofluorescent procedures as adjuncts to the diagnosis of vasculitis.

The dermatopathologist, in addition to seeking a detailed clinical history to correlate with the pathologic findings, must be aware of several caveats when considering the diagnosis of vasculitis. These include the timing of the biopsy compared to the onset of the lesion, the depth and technique of the biopsy, i.e., punch vs excision, and an awareness of the need for step sectioning if a segmental process is likely.

Indicative of the dynamic series of events of immune complex clearance by the reticuloendothelial system, experimental studies have demonstrated that the microscopic diagnosis of vasculitis may be missed if the biopsy is taken more than 24 hours after the appearance of the lesion.[16,17] Moreover, a punch biopsy that does not include fat cannot be expected to rule out a vasculitis of small and medium-sized arteries because of the anatomic location in the panniculus. Ideally, a full-thickness excisional biopsy ensures the maximum opportunity for accurate diagnosis when considering small, medium, and large vessel vasculitis. Additionally, because certain vasculitides, namely, polyarteritis nodosa and giant cell arteritis, may involve only segments of a vessel, multiple sections may be required to identify the inflammatory vasculitic process.

Although low and intermediate power findings often are nonspecific in dermatopathology, they provide an important overview in establishing an accurate diagnosis. Low power clues to the microscopic diagnosis of vasculitis include extravasation of red blood cells, a background smudging of the dermis secondary to the accumulation of polymorphonuclear cells and karyorrhectic debris, and fibrin loops resulting from damaged vessel walls (Fig. 13–2). If any one of these findings is observed, the diagnosis of vasculitis should at least be suspected.

At higher powers, the diagnosis of vasculitis is confirmed or refuted by application of specific major and minor criteria as they pertain to the caliber size of the vessel involved (Fig. 13–3). Assessment of the cellular composition also is relevant, particularly as one considers both larger vessel and granulomatous vasculitides when there is a tendency for more direct vascular damage and lumen oblitera-

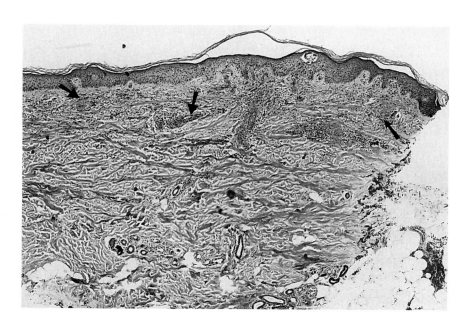

Figure 13–2. The diagnosis of vasculitis is suspected at this intermediate power view by the presence of fibrin loops (arrows) and a busy, smudged appearance of the pars papillaris.

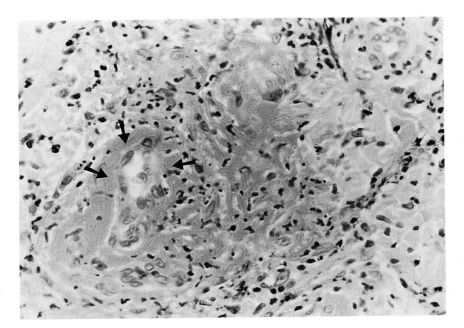

Figure 13–3. The diagnosis of vasculitis, leukocytoclastic type, is confirmed at higher powers by the presence of two major criteria: polymorphonuclear neutrophils invading vessel walls and fibrinoid material in the wall itself (arrow). Endothelial swelling and red blood cell extravasation also are noted. The involvement, confined to the superficial venules, with the infiltrate dominated by polymorphonuclear neutrophils, classifies this lesion in the leukocytoclastic vasculitis spectrum. Further subtyping depends on clinical and laboratory data.

tion with a monomorphous and mixed infiltrate (Figs. 13–4, 13–5).

The use of special stains is of minor importance in the microscopic diagnosis of vasculitis, but if they are used selectively, they may facilitate diagnosis. For example, a phosphotungsic hemotoxylin stain may assist in identification of fibrin in vessel walls by color contrast; it stains blue.[18] Microbial stains, a tissue gram stain (Brown-Brenn), an acid-fast stain, and a PAS stain occasionally may uncover rickettsial forms, leprae bacilli, and yeast forms in the septic vasculitides of Rocky Mountain spotted fever, Lucio's phenomenon of erythema nodosum leprosum, and systemic candidiasis, respectively. In certain small, medium, and large vessel vasculitides, where there may be compromise of both the internal and the elastic lamina, an elastic stain may highlight the damage. An elastic tissue stain also is helpful in distinguishing large venous structures that have only an external elastic lamina, whereas arterial structures have both an internal and an external elastic lamina, i.e., thrombophlebitis vs polyarteritis nodosa.

Direct immunoflourescent studies used to diagnose the smaller vessel vasculitides may add additional correlating data to the light microscopic findings. Biopsies should be taken from lesional or perilesional skin of early lesions. IgM, IgG, IgA, C3, and fibrin have all been observed in dermal blood vessels in several large series of patients with leukocytoclastic vasculitis.[19,20] Isolated IgA in vessel walls is fairly specific for Henoch-Schoenlein purpura, a subset of leukocytoclastic vasculitis.[21,22] Positive findings are less consistent in granulomatous and large vessel vasculitis. A negative immunofluorescent study does not exclude the diagnosis of vasculitis.

LEUKOCYTOCLASTIC VASCULITIS

The spectrum of etiologic cause in the leukocytoclastic grouping is broad, yet the histopathologic findings are similar. Only the small vessels of the skin and viscera are in-

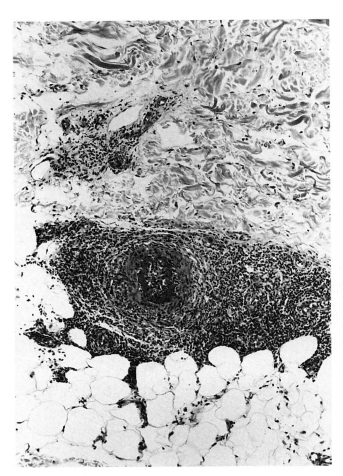

Figure 13–4. Fibrinoid necrosis of an arterial structure at the dermal–fat interface accompanied by polymorphonuclear neutrophils invading the vessel wall. Intimal compromise also is apparent. The size of the vessel, a medium-sized artery, and the relative monomorphous infiltrate, dominated by polymorphonuclear neutrophils, is most consistent with polyarteritis nodosa.

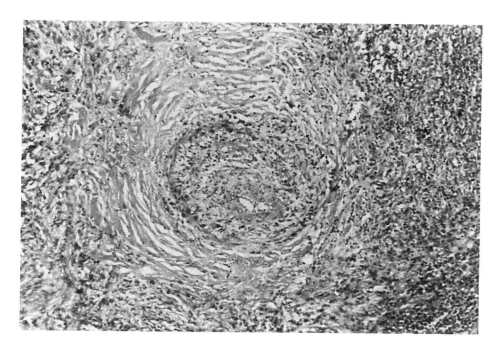

Figure 13–5. A mixed cellular infiltrate, dominated by tissue macrophages and a few giant cells, invades this vessel wall with associated fibrinoid material rimming the small luminal opening. The granulomatous infiltrate also extends to extravascular zones and includes eosinophils. The composition and distribution of the infiltrate, as well as the vessel size, would most accurately classify this lesion as allergic granulomatosis (Churg-Strauss).

volved. Specifically in the skin, postcapillary venules less than 0.1 mm in diameter are the primary target structure, with capillaries and arterioles affected to a lesser extent and, rarely, smaller muscular arteries.[3]

LEUKOCYTOCLASTIC VASCULITIS AS MAJOR FEATURE OF SYNDROME

HENOCH-SCHOENLEIN PURPURA

Clinical Features
Henoch-Schoenlein purpura is a distinctive syndrome of leukocytoclastic vasculitis, most common among the pediatric age group and clinically characterized by palpable purpura of the buttocks and lower extremity, abdominal pain,

arthralgias, and microscopic hematuria.[23,24] The onset of the skin lesions, as well as the other systemic complaints, is often preceded by several weeks by a streptococcal upper respiratory infection. Henoch-Schoenlein purpura is a self-limited disease, with resolution expected 6–16 weeks after the onset of symptomatology. The morbidity depends largely on the incidence of glomerulonephritis.

Histologic Features
Early lesions of Henoch-Schoenlein purpura are microscopically characterized by papillary dermal edema combined with a sparse infiltrate of polymorphonuclear neutrophils surrounding the superficial venules. Endothelial cells are swollen, but nuclear dust and red blood cell extravasation are minimally present (Fig. 13–6). As lesions become more

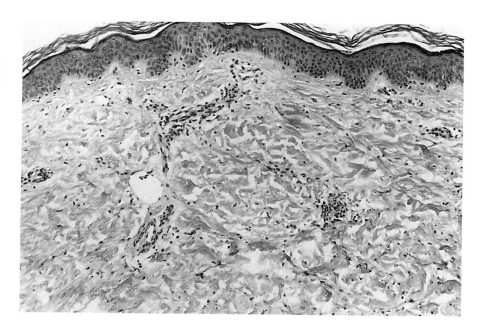

Figure 13–6. An early lesion of Henoch-Schoenlein purpura showing a perivascular mixed cellular infiltrate. Polymorphonuclear neutrophils are the dominant cell in the infiltrate, but nuclear dust is absent. Invasion of the vessel wall is at an early stage.

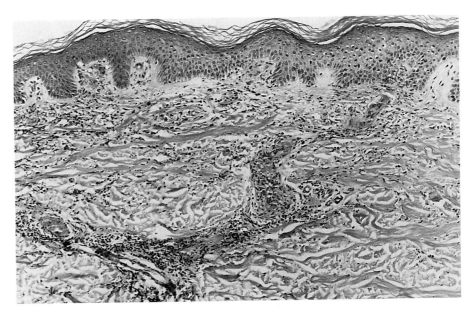

Figure 13–7. A fully developed lesion of Henoch-Schoenlein purpura, with extravasation of red blood cells, fibrinoid necrosis of venules, and polymorphonuclear neutrophils invading vessel walls.

papular and purpuric, the histologic correlates are increased numbers of polymorphonuclear neutrophils distinctly invading vessel walls, nuclear dust, erythrocyte extravasation, and fibrin in vessel walls (Fig. 13–7). These microscopic changes of Henoch-Schoenlein purpura most commonly involve the superficial vascular plexus, yet if there is widespread organ involvement, deeper vascular structures may be affected.[20]

If older lesions of Henoch-Schoenlein purpura are biopsied, the diagnosis of leukocytoclastic vasculitis is more difficult to make, since there is variable fibrin deposition in vessel walls, scant nuclear dust, and an inflammatory infiltrate that is more perivascular, with mononuclear cells dominating. Siderophages in the infiltrate and background reparative perivascular fibroplasia are expected in older lesions.

Differential Diagnosis

The microscopic findings in Henoch-Schoenlein purpura are not unique among the majority of disease conditions within the leukocytoclastic vasculitis classification. Diagnosis depends largely on the clinical and laboratory findings and the results of direct immunofluorescent studies. The presence of IgA, mostly as a single immunoglobulin in dermal and glomerular vessels, is fairly specific for Henoch-Schoenlein purpura.[25] The ability to find IgA in dermal vessels of patients with Henoch-Schoenlein purpura is closely correlated to biopsy of an early lesion.

ESSENTIAL MIXED CRYOGLOBULINEMIA

Clinical Features

Cryoglobulins are immunoglobulins that precipitate on exposure to cold. The syndrome of circulating cold-precipitable immunoglobulins (IgM, IgG) associated with fever, acral purpura, arthralgias, hepatosplenomegaly, lymphadenopathy, and glomerulonephritis is termed essential mixed cryoglobulinemia and is a second distinctive subset of leukocy-

toclastic vasculitis. Essential mixed cryoglobulinemia may be idiopathic, or there may be an association with connective tissue diseases (systemic lupus erythematosus and rheumatoid arthritis) or infections (hepatitis, fungal, bacterial).[26,27]

Histologic Features

Circulating cryoglobulins have the capacity to lodge in small vessel walls, particularly of the skin and kidney, triggering the complement cascade to produce an influx of polymorphonuclear neutrophils and vessel wall damage. The histologic findings of essential mixed cryoglobulinemia are indistinguishable from those of other small vessel vasculitides, with the exception that a PAS-positive, amorphous eosinophilic substance, representing precipitated cryoglobulins, often is observed in the lumina of vessels in the pars papillaris.[28]

Immunofluorescent studies show the presence of IgM, IgG, C3, and fibrin, within both vessel lumina and vessel walls, in patients with essential mixed cryoglobulinemia.[2]

Differential Diagnosis

The finding of cryoglobulin precipitates within blood vessel lumina, in association with other major and minor criteria of small vessel vasculitis, helps to establish the diagnosis of essential mixed cryoglobulinemia. The vascular plugging phenomenon is variable in Henoch-Schoenlein purpura, and cryoprecipitates are not found in the latter. Septic vasculitis can be excluded by the relative absence of nuclear dust and cryoglobulin precipitates. Disseminated intravascular coagulation affecting the skin is noninflammatory, with the superficial vessels plugged by fibrin rather than cryoglobulins.

Cryoglobulinemia can occur without vasculitis. This is commonly observed in type I cryoglobulinemia, where the cryoprecipitate is a homogeneous IgM alone or, rarely, IgG alone. This form of cryoglobulinemia normally is associated with lymphoma, leukemia, multiple myeloma, or Waldenstrom's macroglobulinemia.[29] Patients may manifest purpura and ulcers, but microscopically, there is vascular plugging without vasculitis.

SERUM SICKNESS

Clinical Features

Serum sickness is a leukocytoclastic vasculitis syndrome of morbilliform urticaria, fever, arthralgias-myalgias, and lymphadenopathy, occurring 7–10 days after a primary antigenic exposure or 2–4 days after a secondary exposure. Horse serum antithymocyte globulin (bone marrow failure), arthropod stings, drugs (penicillin and sulfa), and preceding infections (β-hemolytic streptococcus and hepatitis B) may be the inciting antigenic source for serum sickness. Serum sickness is a self-limited condition, and complete recovery is expected 10 or more days after the onset. Complications of peripheral neuritis and the Guillan-Barré syndrome are rare.

Histologic Features

Biopsies from patients with serum sickness show dermal edema combined with polymorphonuclear neutrophils infiltrating the superficial vessels and interstitial spaces. Fibrinoid changes of vessel walls are not dramatic but usually are demonstrable.[2] Red blood cell extravasations, deeper vessel involvement, and fibrin thrombi are rare when compared to the leukocytoclastic vasculitis of Henoch-Schoenlein purpura. In patients with bone marrow failure who are receiving horse antithymocyte globulin, the inflammatory infiltrate is perivascular and lymphohistiocytic. This may be related to the inability of these patients to generate polymorphonuclear neutrophils to the focus of inflammation, in addition to the blunting effect on the immune response while taking corticosteroids.[30]

IgM, IgA, IgE, C3, and fibrin can all be found in vessel walls of patients with serum sickness provided the biopsy is performed sufficiently early after the onset of a lesion.[30,31] The presence of IgG is variable.

Differential Diagnosis

The dominance of polymorphonuclear neutrophils, unaccompanied by extreme damage to the vessel walls, help to distinguish serum sickness from the majority of the syndromes in the leukocytoclastic grouping. The two exceptions are the early lesions of Henoch-Schoenlein purpura and urticarial vasculitis (hypocomplementemic vasculitis), in which the microscopic findings are practically identical to those of serum sickness. The clinical presentation and the laboratory findings differentiate serum sickness from Henoch-Schoenlein purpura and urticarial vasculitis.

URTICARIAL VASCULITIS (HYPOCOMPLEMENTEMIC VASCULITIS)

Clinical Features

First described in 1973, urticarial vasculitis is characterized by depressed complement levels (total complement and components of complement) in association with fixed burning urticaria, sometimes gyrate in form, arthralgias, abdominal pain, adenopathy, and, uncommonly, nephritis.[32] A small number of patients with urticarial vasculitis may develop a connective tissue disease, but generally the course is benign and episodic, lasting 6–18 months.[33,34]

Histologic Features

The microscopic criteria for leukocytoclastic urticaria are met in urticarial vasculitis by the presence of polymorphonuclear neutrophils and nuclear dust invading vessel walls and perivascular deposits of fibrin. Red blood cell extravasation is mild. The density of the mononuclear cells in the inflammatory infiltrate of urticarial vasculitis is distinctly less than in normocomplementemic forms of leukocytoclastic vasculitis.[34,35]

IgM, C3, and fibrin are observed consistently in vessel walls of biopsies taken from patients with urticarial vasculitis. IgG, IgM, and C3 have been found at the basement membrane in a granular pattern.[34]

Differential Diagnosis

A mixed cellular infiltrate lacking mononuclear cells and the mild red blood cell extravasation help to distinguish urticarial vasculitis from other leukocytoclastic vasculitic syndromes.[35] However, the microscopic findings of urticarial vasculitis and serum sickness are similar, requiring laboratory and clinical data to make the distinction. IgE-mediated urticaria can be distinguished from urticarial vasculitis, with the former having a perivascular nonnecrotizing lymphocytic infiltrate with an increased number of mast cells.[36]

ERYTHEMA ELEVATUM DIUTINUM

Clinical Features

Erythema elevatum diutinum is a chronic form of leukocytoclastic vasculitis clinically characterized by erythematous, purple, sometimes yellow, nodules and plaques having a predilection for acral extensor surfaces as well as the upper legs and buttocks.[37,38] Other organ systems characteristically are not involved in erythema elevatum diutinum, although some patients experience mild constitutional signs and symptoms. Before the onset of lesions, there is commonly an antecedent history of a streptococcal infection, and it has been theorized that this microbial antigen may be the source of immune complex formation.[37] The course of erythema elevatum diutinum is chronic, with the majority of cases resolving in a 5–10-year period.

Histologic Features

Epidermal changes are variable in erythema elevatum diutinum, ranging from necrosis to epithelial hyperplasia. The small vessels in the upper and middermis are invaded by polymorphonuclear neutrophils, nuclear dust, and a fair number of eosinophils.[38] Fibrinoid necrosis of vessel walls is common. As lesions age, the dermis exhibits fibrous repair, in combination with tufting of capillaries and ectasia of venules. During both the acute and chronic stages, one may observe tissue macrophages containing lipid (Fig. 13–8). This phenomenon of extracellular cholesterosis was thought to be specific for erythema elevatum diutinum in the past and to reflect a lipid disturbance. However, investigations have failed to substantiate this finding, since lipid probably represents a secondary event and lipid esters.[39]

Direct immunoflourescence studies on biopsies of pa-

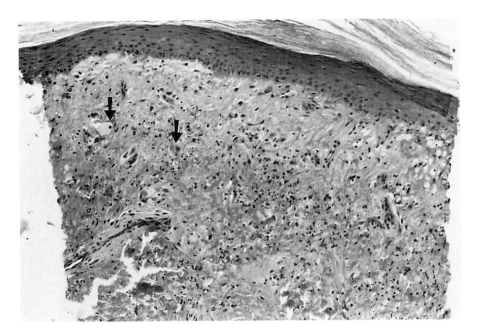

Figure 13–8. Polymorphonuclear neutrophils and nuclear dust in vessel walls and interstitial spaces in association with lipid-laden macrophages (arrows) suggest the diagnosis of erythema elevatum diutinum of the hypercellular cholesterolosis type.

tients with erythema elevatum diutinum has shown the presence of IgG, IgM, C3, and fibrin in the blood vessel walls.[37]

Differential Diagnosis

Both Sweet's syndrome and granuloma faciale should be considered in the microscopic differential diagnosis of erythema elevatum diutinum. Unlike erythema elevatum diutinum, Sweet's syndrome lacks the necessary vascular criteria for leukocytoclastic vasculitis. Although the inflammation of Sweet's syndrome generally is diffuse and intense and contains many polymorphonuclear neutrophils and nuclear debris, vessels are distinctly spared.

When compared to granuloma faciale, erythema eleva-

tum diutinum lacks a grenz zone and has more epidermal changes and fewer eosinophils. There are generally more nuclear dust and necrosis in erythema elevatum diutinum than in granuloma faciale.

GRANULOMA FACIALE

Clinical Features

Granuloma faciale is a cutaneous disease of middle age and is clinically characterized by dull red, brown-purple plaques most commonly located over the facial surface and upper extremities. Plaques typically have a smooth appearance, with prominent patulous follicular openings.[40] Granu-

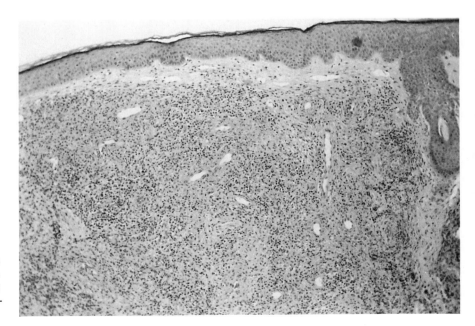

Figure 13–9. The characteristic grenz zone of granuloma faciale accompanied by a diffuse mixed inflammatory infiltrate, having an angiocentric focus and containing many eosinophils.

loma faciale has not been found to be unassociated with other systemic abnormalities.

Histologic Features

The epidermis is generally normal in patients with granuloma faciale. In the dermis, beneath a grenz zone of normal collagen, one most often observes a diffuse and nodular mixed cellular infiltrate having vascular foci. Closer examination reveals polymorphonuclear neutrophils, nuclear dust, eosinophils, and deposits of fibrin in dilated vessel walls and an admixture of extravasated red blood cells and tissue macrophages (Fig. 13–9). The predominant cell in the inflammatory infiltrate is the lymphocyte, but increased numbers of eosinophils also are observed.[41] Hemosiderin usually is present, often in macrophages.

Immunofluorescent studies have helped support the theory that granuloma faciale is a leukocytoclastic vasculitis, namely, deposits of IgG, IgM, IgA, C3, and fibrin in blood vessel walls and at the dermal–epidermal junction.[19,42]

Differential Diagnosis

The histologic findings of granuloma faciale must be differentiated from those of erythema elevatum diutinum and Sweet's syndrome. Sweet's syndrome is not a vasculitis, although the infiltrate can be dense and contain many polymorphonuclear neutrophils. Eosinophils are uncommon in Sweet's syndrome.

LEUKOCYTOCLASTIC VASCULITIS RELATED TO SPECIFIC ANTIGEN EXPOSURE AND AS A COMPONENT OF A DISEASE PROCESS

The histopathologic changes of leukocytoclastic vasculitis associated with a specific antigen exposure, such as infections (meningococcemia, gonococcemia, or infections with *Pseudomonas, Streptococcus, Staphylococcus, Streptococcus pneumoniae, Candida,* rickettsia, spirochetes, hepatitis B virus, varicella, herpes simplex, *Mycobacterium leprae*), drugs (penicillin, sulfa, tetracycline, disulfiram, thiazide, gold, allopurinol, phenytoin, quinidine), and physical agents (radiocontrast agents, photocopy material), or when leukocytoclastic vasculitis is a component part of a disease spectrum, as in connective tissue diseases (rheumatoid arthritis, lupus erythematosus, dermatomyositis, scleroderma, Sjögren's syndrome), malignancy (lymphoma, leukemia, myeloma), and miscellaneous diseases (inflammatory bowel disease, cystic fibrosis, otitis media) are indistinguishable from other disorders in the heterogeneous grouping, except for septic vasculitis and leukocytoclastic vasculitis occurring in aggressive connective tissue disease.

Lesions of septic vasculitis, most commonly chronic gonococcemia and meningococcemia, are clinically characterized by erythematous-purpuric macules and papules, few in number and asymmetrically distributed over acral parts. Progression to necrotic vesiculopustular lesions is common. Microscopically, septic vasculitides fulfill the criteria for leukocytoclastic vasculitis yet may show crossover pathogenic features of a Shwartzman reaction and immune complex disease.[43,44] The dermatopathologist should question an underlying etiology of sepsis if the following are observed: (1) vascular damage at both superficial and deep levels, (2) consistent presence of fibrin thrombi, but little fibrinoid necrosis of the vessel walls, (3) polymorphonuclear neutrophils invading vessel walls, but nuclear debris and eosinophils rare, and (4) necrotic epithelium often related to intraepidermal vesicles and pustules (Fig. 13–10).[2,43,44] Special stains may reveal organisms in vessel walls if the process is acute compared to the low incidence of organisms in chronic sepsis.

Leukocytoclastic vasculitis is most commonly associated with the connective tissue diseases, lupus erythematosus and rheumatoid arthritis.[3] Clinical lesions are typically ulcerative, with a distribution over the distal extremities.[45,46] A background livedo reticularis is common.

Microscopically, unlike the majority of the other syndromes within this heterogeneous group of leukocytoclastic vasculitides, lupus vasculitis and rheumatoid vasculitis tend to be both superficial and deep processes, with a potential to involve larger vessels (Fig. 13–11).[2,45] The inflammatory infiltrate may be lymphocytic and decreased in lupus vasculitis when compared to typical leukocytoclastic vasculitis lesions, but fibrinoid is more apparent. The histologic changes in this setting may closely resemble polyarteritis

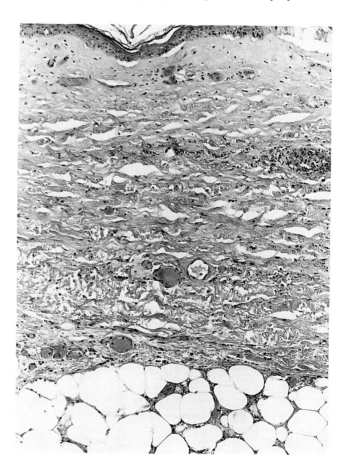

Figure 13–10. Septic vasculitis of gonococcemia. Note the criteria for leukocytoclastic vasculitis; however, there is a dominance of fibrin thrombi as well as early necrosis of the epidermis and sparse nuclear dust.

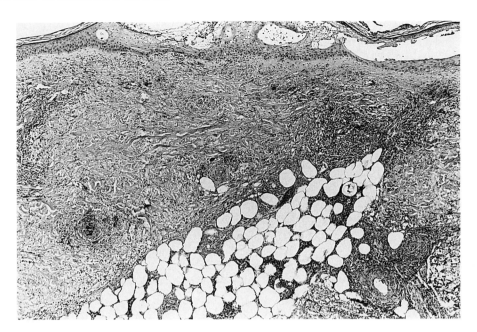

Figure 13–11. Rheumatoid vasculitis. Note the deeper vessel involvement, which often can be correlated with more severe and widespread vasculitis. The epidermal necrosis is secondary to the vascular insult.

nodosa, especially if a larger vessel is involved, so that serologic and immunopathologic evaluation may be necessary to separate the two disorders.

In instances when a specific syndrome for leukocytoclastic vasculitis or an antigenic source is not obvious, the name "idiopathic leukocytoclastic vasculitis" is used. This is not uncommon, yet the clinician is obligated to pursue systemic involvement. The microscopic findings of idiopathic leukocytoclastic vasculitis are not unique among the leukocytoclastic vasculitis conditions.

POLYARTERITIS NODOSA

Clinical Features
Polyarteritis nodosa is a multisystem, segmental vasculitis most often affecting the bifurcations of small and medium-sized arteries, with overlapping involvement of arterioles and adjacent veins.[1] Dermal venules are spared.[3] Hepatitis B antigenemia can be found in approximately 30% of patients with systemic polyarteritis nodosa and is thought to represent a major antigenic source for immune complex formation.[47,48]

Patients with systemic polyarteritis nodosa are characteristically males (2:1), who have malaise, fever, arthralgias, hypertension, glomerulonephritis, abdominal pain, and mononeuritis multiplex. Vasculitis involving other systems may produce seizures, testicular or ovarian pain, pericarditis, and even myocardial infarction. Distinctly not part of the vasculitis of polyarteritis nodosa are lung involvement (pulmonary artery), eosinophilia, and a history of allergy.[2,49]

The skin lesions of systemic polyarteritis nodosa occur in only 5–15% of cases and consist of skin-colored erythematous nodules, often pulsatile, and following the anatomic course of involved arteries, in addition to ulcerations, and livedo reticularis.[49]

Untreated, the prognosis of systemic polyarteritis no-

dosa is poor, with patients dying of renal failure and abdominal complications.

Cutaneous polyarteritis nodosa is a subset of polyarteritis nodosa, with similar skin lesions to the systemic form but with essentially no significant involvement of other organ systems. The course is typified by the intermittent appearance of skin lesions and the tendency for patients occasionally to have associated fever, arthralgias, and, rarely, mononeuritis multiplex or periosteal involvement.[50]

Histologic Features
Biopsies of skin lesions of patients with systemic or cutaneous polyarteritis nodosa yield a panarteritis of small and medium-sized arteries at the dermal–fat interface. Polymorphonuclear neutrophils invade vessel walls and adventitial zones, producing fibrinoid necrosis and intimal thickening (Fig. 13–4). Thrombus formation with infarction of the surrounding tissue is commonplace as the intima narrows and is obliterated. Mononuclear cells infiltrate the vessels in the subacute and chronic stages of polyarteritis nodosa, but discrete granuloma formation, vascularly and extravascularly, is absent.[1,2,49,50] Eosinophils are rare in lesions of polyarteritis nodosa. The smaller blood vessels in the dermis usually are surrounded by a lymphocytic infiltrate of intermediate intensity, but there is minimal histologic evidence for necrotizing vasculitis.

A focal panniculitis may be observed in the immediate vicinity of the inflamed blood vessel in polyarteritis nodosa, but diffuse granulomatous panniculitis does not occur.[15] Aneurysmal dilatations, approximating 0.5–1.0 cm, along the course of an involved larger vessel in polyarteritis nodosa may be seen in the classic form of the disease, but these dilatations are observed rarely in cutaneous lesions of polyarteritis nodosa.[49]

IgM, C3, and fibrin may be observed in affected blood vessels in polyarteritis nodosa, as may smaller papillary dermal and uninvolved vascular structures.[50] This finding is suggestive that immune complex deposition may be associated as an etiology. The histologic selective event of a large vessel vasculitis may be related to immune complex size, the differences in intravascular hydrostatic pressures, and the relative blood flow turbulence.

Differential Diagnosis

The granulomatous vasculitides, superficial thrombophlebitis, and nodular vasculitis should all be considered in the differential diagnosis of polyarteritis nodosa. Whereas vessel size is roughly equivalent when comparing the vasculitis of polyarteritis nodosa and the granulomatous vasculitides, tissue macrophages invading vessel walls and granuloma formation, vascularly and extravascularly, are not observed in polyarteritis nodosa. They are the dominant features in the granulomatous vasculitides.

Superficial thrombophlebitis may resemble polyarteritis nodosa because of a large inflamed vascular structure, but the vessel involved in superficial thrombophlebitis is distinctly a vein characterized by a tortuous lumen and lacking an internal elastic lamina.

Polyarteritis nodosa, when compared to nodular vasculitis, lacks an associated diffuse granulomatous panniculitis and tends to involve a single vascular structure compared to a more widespread vascular involvement of nodular vasculitis.

GRANULOMATOUS VASCULITIS

Allergic granulomatosis (Churg-Strauss disease) and Wegener's granulomatosis are pathologically classified as granulomatous vasculitides because of a mixed cellular infiltrate dominated by tissue macrophages and a variable number of giant cells in both vascular and extravascular locations.[3] More specifically, allergic granulomatosis and Wegener's granulomatosis manifest the phenomenon of palisaded, allergic granuloma formation, a pathologic marker within the broader spectrum of pathergic granulomatosis,[51–54] pathergy being any lesion caused by an altered state of immune reactivity of blood tissue.[55]

Microscopically, palisaded, allergic granulomas consist of a central focus of necrosis and pyknotic inflammatory cells surrounded by a mantle of tissue macrophages and giant cells, with a peripheral zone of altered connective tissue and loose inflammation (Fig. 13–12). Although it is fairly characteristic for allergic granulomatosis and Wegener's granulomatosis, in an extravascular location, the phenomenon of palisaded, allergic granuloma formation also has been observed in vasculitis associated with lymphoproliferative disease, necrotizing vasculitis of sarcoidosis, lymphomatoid granulomatosis, and in lupus erythematosus, rheumatoid arthritis, and bacterial endocarditis.[51–53]

Giant cell arteritis also may be considered a granulomatous vasculitis by the dominance of tissue macrophages and giant cells in vessel walls. However, giant cell arteritis is classified separately because it is so dominated by large arterial involvement, without palisaded, allergic granuloma formation.

When vasculitis is identified as allergic granulomatosis or Wegener's granulomatosis, there is a tendency to involve a polymorphous grouping of blood vessels (capillaries, venules, arterioles, and veins) when compared to the rather specific venulitis of leukocytoclastic vasculitis and the small and medium-sized arterial concentration of polyarteritis nodosa.[3]

ALLERGIC GRANULOMATOSIS (CHURG-STRAUSS DISEASE)

Clinical Features

Although some authorities believe that allergic granulomatosis is a subset of polyarteritis nodosa with pulmonary involvement, there are sufficient distinctive clinicopatho-

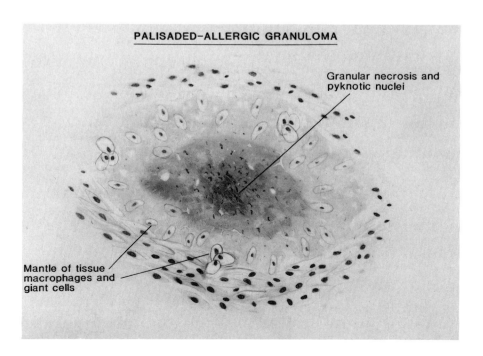

PALISADED–ALLERGIC GRANULOMA

Granular necrosis and pyknotic nuclei

Mantle of tissue macrophages and giant cells

Figure 13–12. A schematic representation of a palisaded, allergic granuloma within the microscopic spectrum of pathergic granulomatosis, having a central focus of necrosis, usually pyknotic neutrophils admixed with necrotic connective tissue, surrounded by a mantle of tissue macrophages and giant cells. This microscopic lesion may be correlated to an ongoing systemic vasculitis.

logic criteria to warrant a separate classification for allergic granulomatosis.[53,54] For example, although both polyarteritis nodosa and allergic granulomatosis may be considered systemic vasculitides of small and medium-sized arteries, the pulmonary and airway features of allergic granulomatosis, namely, asthma, nasal polyps, and rhinitis, dominate the clinical picture and rarely are found in polyarteritis nodosa. Moreover, unlike polyarteritis nodosa, patients with allergic granulomatosis characteristically have prominent tissue and peripheral blood eosinophilia and have little tendency to hypertension and renal disease.[56]

Cutaneous lesions of allergic granulomatosis occur in two thirds of patients and consist of painful dermal and subcutaneous nodules, having little tendency to ulceration. Ecchymotic plaques, livedo reticularis, and, rarely, erythema multiforme-like lesions also have been reported.[54]

Untreated allergic granulomatosis has high morbidity and mortality; however, with immunosuppressive therapy, the prognosis is favorable.

Histologic Features
The vasculitis of allergic granulomatosis involves small and medium-sized arteries, yet there is a distinctive tendency for vessel damage to extend to veins, arterioles, capillaries, and venules. Biopsies from early lesions may yield a polymorphonuclear neutrophilic infiltrate and nuclear dust within vessel walls, but this is rare. Rather, the infiltrate is predominantly lymphohistiocytic with an admixture of giant cells and a variable number of eosinophils (Fig. 13–5). This mixed granulomatous infiltrate of the vessel wall, commonly accompanied by fibrinoid necrosis, vessel narrowing, and thrombosis, also may appear extravascularly in both a diffuse and a well-organized arrangement. Frequently, palisaded, allergic granulomas are observed in the extravascular spaces and are composed of fibrin, altered collagen, and debris within the central zone, with a surrounding accumulation of histiocytes, epithelioid cells, and giant cells.[52–54]

Differential Diagnosis
Polyarteritis nodosa, Wegener's granulomatosis, various necrobiotic granulomas, and sarcoidal vasculitis must all be included in the differential diagnosis of allergic granulomatosis. Unlike polyarteritis nodosa, allergic granulomatosis involves a more polymorphous grouping of vessels and is dominated by tissue macrophages and eosinophils. Importantly, and contrasting with polyarteritis nodosa, allergic granulomatosis characteristically reveals a diffuse form of extravascular granulomatous inflammation in addition to the frequently observed localized palisaded, allergic granuloma. The distinction from Wegener's granulomatosis is more difficult, yet lesions of allergic granulomatosis tend to have more eosinophils, less necrotizing inflammation involving the blood vessels and extravascular spaces, and less of a liquefactive necrotic center within the palisaded, allergic granulomas. Although well-organized granulomas are observed in allergic granulomatosis, often vascularly and extravascularly, they do not conform to the epithelioid granulomas of sarcoid and the rare sarcoid vasculitis. The palisaded granuloma of a rheumatoid nodule may be analogous to the palisaded, allergic granuloma of allergic granulo-

matosis, but the central zone of the rheumatoid nodule is purely fibrin, and there is no ongoing vasculitis.

WEGENER'S GRANULOMATOSIS

Clinical Features
Wegener's granulomatosis is a disease of uncertain etiology, characterized by necrotizing granulomas of the lung and upper airway, a multisystem vasculitis of medium small arteries as well as capillaries, venules, and arterioles, and a glomerulitis.[57–59] Patients with Wegener's granulomatosis are typically middle-aged males who have various combinations of constitutional signs and symptoms: sinusitis, otitis media, cavitary and nodular infiltrates of the lung, cough, hemoptysis, proteinuria, hematuria, and red blood cell casts. A limited form of Wegener's granulomatosis has been described in which symptomatology is limited to lungs, sparing the upper airways and kidneys, and associated with a good prognosis.[60] Although the clinical feature of Wegener's granulomatosis overlap with those of allergic granulomatosis, important distinguishing features are the low incidence of asthma and tissue and blood eosinophilia in Wegener's granulomatosis and the rare presence of cutaneous ulcers in allergic granulomatosis.

The cutaneous manifestations of Wegener's granulomatosis include erythematous-purpuric papules, vesicles, subcutaneous nodules, ecchymotic plaques, nodulo-ulcerative lesions, and frank ulceration.[61,62] Necrotizing ulcers of the mucosa and skin, remaining localized for months to years in untreated cases and having the potential for extreme mutilation, are fairly characteristic of Wegener's granulomatosis and have been characterized as the protracted superficial phenomenon.[52] Skin lesions may be observed in 40–50% of patients with Wegener's granulomatosis during the course of their disease, yet the cutaneous findings are the presenting complaint in only 10–13% of reported cases.

Untreated, a high percentage of patients with Wegener's granulomatosis routinely died from renal failure and infection. Immunosuppressive therapy has completely altered this dismal prognosis, and remissions are now achieved in approximately 90% of patients.[59]

Histologic Features
The typical microscopic features of Wegener's granulomatosis, in the skin and other organs, affecting vascular and extravascular tissues are small foci of granular and fibrinoid necrosis, palisaded, allergic granulomas, giant cells, and vasculitis.[52,58] The first change in a lesion of Wegener's granulomatosis is typically extravascular foci of granular necrosis, with an admixture of epithelioid cells and giant cells, with little tendency to form palisaded structures. This process may be poorly contained, so that large areas of serpentine necrosis course throughout the dermis. As lesions evolve, tissue macrophages may form a mantle around zones of acellular necrotic collagen, i.e., palisaded, allergic granuloma (Fig. 13–13). Sometimes, nuclear dust may be observed within these foci, and in these instances, the relationship of the karyorrhectic debris to a preexisting vascular structure is uncertain. Giant cells are common in the zones of diffuse and focal mixed inflammation (Fig. 13–14).

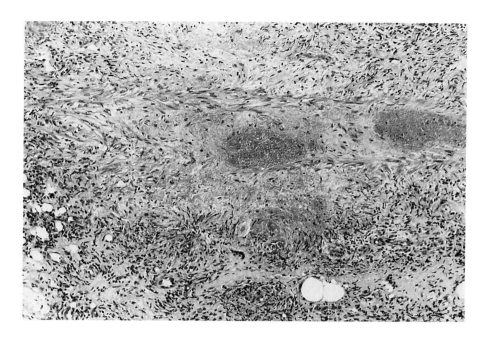

Figure 13–13. A palisaded, allergic granuloma composed of two foci of granular necrotic collagen and pyknotic nuclei surrounded by tissue macrophages and a smattering of lymphocytes.

The identical spectrum of microscopic changes also may involve the walls of larger dermal blood vessels and those in the fat, thus fulfilling various major and minor criteria for the diagnosis of vasculitis. Damage to the vessel wall is evidenced by fibrinoid deposits as well as intimal compromise and thrombosis. Inflammatory cells in the vessel walls are a mixture of polymorphonuclear neutrophils, nuclear dust, and often many tissue macrophages and giant cells. Eosinophils are uncommon.

The definitive diagnosis of Wegener's granulomatosis depends on the combination of extravascular necrotizing granulomas and vasculitis. Although one cannot minimize the vasculitic changes, they may be absent.[52] In these uncertain circumstances, an elastic tissue stain may add diagnostic yield, since vascular remnants may be observed. A deep biopsy avoids the potential pitfall of observing only nonspecific findings of granulation tissue and inflammation.

Immunofluorescent studies performed on skin lesions of Wegener's granulomatosis have inconsistently yielded granular deposits of IgM, C3, and fibrin in vessel walls.[63] The significance of these findings is ambiguous.

Differential Diagnosis
The differential diagnosis of Wegener's granulomatosis includes allergic granulomatosis, tuberculosis, rheumatoid nodule, lymphomatoid granulomatosis, and the vasculitis

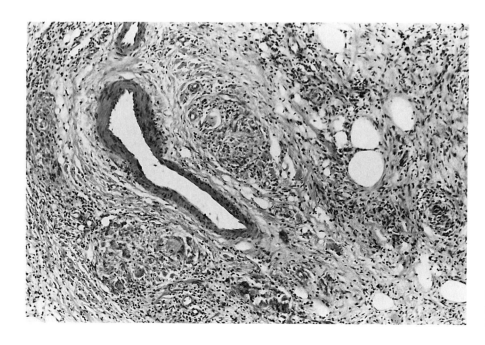

Figure 13–14. Vascular proliferations accompanied by diffuse granulomatous inflammation and many giant cells.

of sarcoidosis. The most difficult differentiation is Wegener's granulomatosis vs allergic granulomatosis, since both entities show microscopic changes of diffuse granulomatous inflammation, focal zones of palisaded, allergic granulomas, and vasculitis involving structures of different caliber. Nevertheless, tissue eosinophilia is rarely observed in Wegener's granulomatosis, whereas this cell is not uncommon in the infiltrate in Churg-Strauss disease. The granulomatous necrosis that occurs in Wegener's granulomatosis tends to be more liquefactive and poorly circumscribed than that in Churg-Strauss disease. Finally, clinical presentation is often helpful in distinguishing Wegener's granulomatosis from Churg-Strauss disease.

Tuberculosis can be excluded by special stains and cultures of tissue. Moreover, the granulomas of tuberculosis begin with the accumulation of histiocytes and evolve to foci of caseation necrosis. The opposite occurs in Wegener's granulomatosis, as liquefactive necrosis is followed by cellular accumulations of tissue macrophages.

The lack of major and minor criteria for vasculitis in rheumatoid nodule would tend to exclude this entity. In addition, the central zone of necrosis in a rheumatoid nodule is dry and most commonly composed of fibrin, whereas the central palisaded zones in Wegener's granulomatosis are more necrotic and liquefactive.

Lymphomatoid granulomatosis, an entity showing overlapping clinical pathologic features to Wegener's granulomatosis, is identified by the presence of atypical mononuclear cells in the granulomatous infiltrate in both vascular and extravascular locations.[64] This atypia is not observed in Wegener's granulomatosis, and the lymphocyte is not a dominant cell.

Although a granulomatous vasculitis may appear rarely as a part of the microscopic spectrum of sarcoidosis, purulent necrotic zones and palisaded granulomas are not observed.

GIANT CELL ARTERITIS

Although there have been isolated reports of the giant cell arteritides involving medium and small-sized arteries of the skin and subcutaneous tissue, both temporal and arteritis (cranial arteritis) and Takayasu's arteritis characteristically spare the skin and subcutaneous tissue, affecting large arteries of the carotid and aortic tributaries, respectively.[2,3]

TEMPORAL ARTERITIS (CRANIAL ARTERITIS)

Temporal arteritis is an uncommon, large vessel vasculitis of elderly Caucasian females. Patients have fever, headache, polymyalgia rheumatica, anemia, and an increased erythrocyte sedimentation rate. Visual impairment and total blindness may be complications from vasculitis involving the retinal artery.[65]

Scalp necrosis and ulceration are the two most commonly observed cutaneous lesions of temporal arteritis, and when they occur, there is a high correlation to visual loss. Palpable purpura, ecchymoses, and scalp bullae also may be part of the cutaneous spectrum of temporal arteritis.[66]

The prognosis of temporal arteritis is generally favorable, although mortality approximates 12% and usually is related to a coronary thrombosis or cerebrovascular accident.

TAKAYASU'S DISEASE

Clinical Features

Takayasu's disease is less common than temporal arteritis and is mostly restricted to young Oriental females. Systemic signs and symptoms can be related to the involved vessels and include hypertension, cardiac failure, syncopal episodes, pulseless extremities, anemia, and an increased-erythrocyte sedimentation rate.[67,68] The course of the disease is variable, but generally prognosis is poor and is associated with a high mortality from congestive heart failure or cerebral vascular accident.

Histologic Features

The histopathology of temporal arteritis and Takayasu's disease is similar, with a few exceptions. Biopsies from patients with temporal arteritis and Takayasu's disease show similar histopathologic features characterized by a segmental panarteritis of large arteries. An excisional biopsy should be performed over a painful segment of the artery, with the arterial segment being at least 3 cm long. Technical preparation should include multiple sections in both a transverse and a longitudinal orientation.[69]

The most prominent microscopic changes in temporal arteritis and Takayasu's arteritis are intimal proliferation and fibrosis, coupled with fibrous replacement of the media and destruction of the internal elastic lamina. Necrosis of the adventitial portion of the vascular unit also occurs and often is associated with fibrinoid degeneration. A mixed inflammatory infiltrate invades the vessel wall in the acute phase, dominated by polymorphonuclear neutrophils and a smattering of eosinophils, lymphocytes, and plasmacytoid cells. As lesions evolve, tissue macrophages and giant cells replace the acute phase reactants (Fig. 13–15). The giant cell reaction has been linked to a host response to damaged and fragmented elastic lamina.[2,65]

Whereas giant cells are a dominant feature of temporal arteritis, they are fewer in number in Takayasu's disease.[65,68] Also, in Takayasu's disease, there is more of a tendency for thrombosis and fibrosis of the vessel wall than in temporal arteritis.

Extracellular granular deposits of IgM adjacent to the internal elastic lamina have been reported in patients with temporal arteritis. However, these findings have been challenged by a study that was able to demonstrate only intracellular (plasma cells and macrophages) immunoglobulins (IgA, IgM, IgG), a nonspecific finding observed in a broad range of inflammatory processes.[70] The conflicting data raise the question of whether there is a primary deposition of immune complexes in the vessel walls or their presence is secondary to diffusion from the lumen to the site of injury.[71]

Differential Diagnosis

A differential diagnosis of temporal arteritis and Takayasu's arteritis should include polyarteritis nodosa and Wegener's granulomatosis. An important distinction between temporal arteritis or Takayasu's arteritis and polyarteritis nodosa is

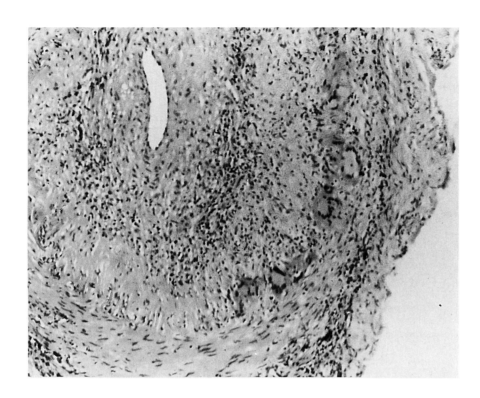

Figure 13–15. Large artery with intimal thickening and fibrosis. A rim of giant cells and focal fibrin deposition is at the interface of the media and adventitia.

the lack of intravascular granuloma formation, specifically the lack of consistent giant cell formation in polyarteritis nodosa. Lesions of polyarteritis nodosa only rarely involve large arteries.

Wegener's granulomatosis, in contrast to temporal arteritis or Takayasu's arteritis, does not affect large arteries, and its granulomatous features are more suppurative and necrotizing and include extravascular and vascular tissue.

MISCELLANEOUS ENTITIES

A number of disease conditions have been described in which the microscopic features loosely fulfill the criteria for vasculitis (Table 13–3). Whether these entities are finally classified within the spectrum of vasculitis depends largely on the accumulation and interpretation of additional histologic and immunopathologic data.

TABLE 13–3. DISEASES WITH UNCERTAIN RELATIONSHIP TO VASCULITIS

Disease	Histology	Conclusion
Pyoderma gangrenosum[72]	Lymphocytes in perivascular location as well as in vessel walls; fibrinoid necrosis variable; leukocytoclasis rare	Not a vasculitis by accepted criteria; lymphocytic inflammation secondary to exogenous or endogenous antigen
Pityriasis lichenoides et varioliformis acuta (Mucha-Habermann disease)	Endothelial cell hyperplasia, hemorrhage, and lymphocytes in vessel walls in superficial and deep dermis; interface necrosis; fibrinoid necrosis and polymorphonuclear neutrophils involving vessels rare	Not a vasculitis by accepted criteria
Chilblains (pernio)[73]	Papillary dermal edema; lymphocytes in vessel walls in superficial and deep dermis	Not a vasculitis by accepted criteria
Kawasaki disease (infantile polyarteritis nodosa)[74]	Panvasculitis of major coronary arteries with intimal thickening and thrombosis (2% of cases)	Vasculitis of medium-sized arteries with predilection for coronary arteries; histopathologic features of infantile polyarteritis nodosa identical to Kawasaki disease
Malignant atrophic papulosis (Degos' disease)[75,76]	Cone-shaped zone of acellular necrosis of dermis; thrombosed vessel at the base of infarct without inflammation	Cutaneous infarct of uncertain etiology
Pustular necrotizing vasculitis[77]	Leukocytoclastic vasculitis of dermal vessels with associated necrotic pustule of epidermis	Leukocytoclastic vasculitis but ? distinct entity, i.e., pustules described in leukocytoclastic vasculitis

continued

TABLE 13–3. DISEASES WITH UNCERTAIN RELATIONSHIP TO VASCULITIS (Continued)

Disease	Histology	Conclusion
Intestinal bypass syndrome[78]	Polymorphonuclear neutrophils and nuclear dust in vessel walls without much fibrinoid necrosis; positive immunoglobulins and complement by immunofluorescence	Leukocytoclastic vasculitis secondary to stasis of bacterial antigens
Livedo vasculitis (atrophie blanche)[79]	Dilated and thrombosed vessels in middermis with perivascular mixed infiltrate dominated by mononuclear cells; no nuclear dust or fibrinoid necrosis	Primary vasospastic disorder with secondary thrombosis and perivascular inflammation
Osler's nodes and Janeway lesions[15,80]	Similar histopathologic findings as septic vasculitis	Leukocytoclastic vasculitis secondary to small septic emboli
Thromboangiitis obliterans (Buerger's disease)[81]	Intense mixed inflammation with thromboses mainly of arteries and veins	Not a vasculitis but an occlusive peripheral vascular disease of uncertain etiology
Behcet's syndrome[82]	Nonspecific granulation tissue; thrombophlebitis; rarely, polymorphonuclear neutrophils and nuclear dust invading small venules	Not a vasculitis; probable delayed hypersensitivity reaction to unknown antigen
Disseminated intravascular coagulation (DIC)[83]	Thrombi in small vessels with little inflammatory infiltrate	Consumption coagulopathy, not a vasculitis
Lucio's phenomenon	Dense, diffuse infiltrate of foamy histiocytes associated with polymorphonuclear netrophils invading vessel walls and fibrinoid necrosis	A leukocytoclastic vasculitis in an immunologically compromised host
Nodular vasculitis[14,15]	Mixed inflammatory cells in vessel walls with focal fibrinoid necrosis; associated severe lobular panniculitis	A vasculitis (granulomatous), but dominant feature is a lobular panniculitis
Early granuloma annulare and necrobiosis lipoidica[84,85]	Nuclear debris and a necrotic vessel as center for palisaded granuloma—rarely	Vasculitic changes in small percentage of cases
IgE-mediated urticaria[36]	Edema and mononuclear infiltrate around superficial venules; polymorphonuclear neutrophils sparse; mast cells increased	Nonnecrotizing perivascular inflammation
Scleroderma[86]	Rarely segmental mixed inflammation in vessel walls; endothelial cytotoxicity	Not a vasculitis; small percentage of cases may show vasculitis-like changes
Lethal midline granuloma[87]	Diffuse granulomatous inflammation involving the structures of the nasal septum and turbinates	Not a vasculitis; hypersensitivity reaction of uncertain etiology; ? relationship to lymphomatoid granulomatosis
Lymphomatoid granulomatosis[64]	Angiocentric concentration of mononuclear cells, some atypical, with evolution to lymphoma in small percentage of cases.	Not a vasculitis; hypersensitivity reaction of uncertain etiology

REFERENCES

1. Zeek PM. Periarteritis nodosa: A critical review. *Am J Clin Pathol.* 1952;22:777–790.
2. Fauci AS, Haynes BF, Katz P. The spectrum of vasculitis: Clinical, pathologic, immunologic, and therapeutic considerations. *Ann Intern Med.* 1978;89:660–676.
3. Gilliam JN, Smiley JD. Cutaneous necrotizing vasculitis and related disorders. *Ann Allergy.* 1976;37:328–339.
4. Sams WM Jr, Thorne EG, Small P, et al. Leukocytoclastic vasculitis. *Arch Dermatol.* 1976;112:219.
5. Cochrane CG. Mechanisms involved in the deposition of immune complexes in tissues. *J Exp Med.* 1971;134:75s–89s.
6. Prince AM, Trepo C. Role of immune complexes involving SH antigen in pathogenesis of chronic active hepatitis and polyarteritis nodosa. *Lancet* 1971;1:1309–1312.
7. Waksman BH. Delayed (cellular) hypersensitivity. In: Samter M, ed. *Immunological Diseases*, I. Boston: Little, Brown & Co; 1971:220.
8. Epstein WL. Granulomatous hypersensitivity. *Prog Allergy.* 1967;11:36–88.
9. Cochrane CG, Weigle WO, Dixon FJ. The role of polymorpho-
nuclear leukocytes in the initiation and cessation of the Arthus vasculitis. *J Exp Med.* 1959;110:481–494.
10. Cochrane CG, Dixon FJ. Antigen-antibody complex-induced diseases. In: Miescher FA, Muller-Eberhard HJ, eds. *Textbook of Immunology.* New York: Grune & Stratton; 1976:137.
11. Sams WM Jr. Vasculitis. In Thiers BH, Dobson RL, eds. *Pathogenesis of Skin Disease.* New York: Churchill Livingstone; 1986:215.
12. Cox AJ. Pathologic changes in hypersensitivity angiitis. In Helwig EB, Mostofi FK, eds. *The Skin.* Baltimore: Williams & Wilkins: 1971:279–292.
13. Lever WF, Schaumburg-Lever G. *Histopathology of the Skin.* 6th ed. Philadelphia: JB Lippincott Co; 1983.
14. Mehregan AH. *Pinkus' Guide to Dermatohistopathology.* 4th ed. E. Norwalk, Conn: Appleton-Century-Crofts; 1986.
15. Ackerman AB. *Histologic Diagnosis of Inflammatory Skin Diseases.* Philadelphia: Lea & Febiger; 1978.
16. Braverman IM, Yen A. Demonstration of immune complexes in spontaneous and histamine-induced lesions and in normal skin of patients with leukocytoclastic angiitis. *J Invest Dermatol.* 1975;64:105–112.
17. Gower RG, Sams WM Jr, Thorne EG, et al. Leukocytoclastic

vasculitis: Sequential appearance of immunoreactants and cellular changes in serial biopsies. *J Invest Dermatol*. 1977;69:477–484.

18. Luna LG, ed. *Manual of Histologic Staining Methods of the Armed Forces Institute of Pathology*. 3rd ed. New York: McGraw-Hill; 1968.

19. Schroeter AL, Copeman PWM, Jordon RE, et al. Immunofluorescence of cutaneous vasculitis associated with systemic disease. *Arch Dermatol*. 1971;104:254–259.

20. Sanchez NP, Van Hale HM, Su WPD: Clinical and histopathologic spectrum of necrotizing vasculitis. Report of findings in 101 cases. *Arch Dermatol*. 1985;121:220–224.

21. Giangiacomo J, Toai C. Dermal and glomerular deposition of IgA in anaphylactoid purpura. *Am J Dis Child*. 1977;131:981–983.

22. Levinsky RJ, Barratt TM. IgA immune complexes in Henoch-Schoenlein purpura. *Lancet*. 1979;2:1100–1103.

23. Allen DM, Diamond LK, Howell DA. Anaphylactoid purpura in children (Schoenlein-Henoch syndrome). *Am J Dis Child*. 1960;99:833–854.

24. Cream JJ, Gumpel JM, Peachy RD. Schoenlein-Henoch purpura in the adult: A study of 77 adults with anaphylactoid or Schonlein-Henoch purpura. *Q J Med*. 1970;39:461–484.

25. Faille-Kuyper EH de la, Kater L, Koviker CJ, et al. IgA-deposits in cutaneous blood vessel walls and mesangium in Henoch-Schoenlein syndrome. *Lancet*. 1973;1:892–893.

26. Meltzer M, Franklin EC: Cryoglobulinemia—A study of twenty-nine patients: I. IgG and IgM cryoglobulins and factors affecting cryoprecipitability. *Am J Med*. 1966;40:828–836.

27. Ellis FA. The cutaneous manifestations of cryoglobulinemia. *Arch Dermatol*. 1964;89:690–697.

28. Nir MA, Piak AI, Schreibman S, et al. Mixed IgG-IgM cryoglobulinemia with follicular pustular purpura. *Arch Dermatol*. 1974;109:539–542.

29. Kyle RA, Gleich GJ, Bayrd ED, et al. Benign hypergammaglobulinemic purpura of Waldenstrom. *Medicine (Baltimore)*. 1971;50:113–138.

30. Lawley TJ, Bielory L, Gascon P, Yancey KB, Young NS, Frank MM. A prospective clinical and immunologic analysis of patients with serum sickness. *N Engl J Med*. 1984;311:1407–1413.

31. Bielory L, Yancey KB, Young NS, Frank MM, Lawley TJ. Cutaneous manifestations of serum sickness in patients receiving antithymocyte globulin. *Am Acad Dermatol*. 1985;13:411–417.

32. McDuffie FC, Sams WM Jr, Maldonado JE, et al. Hypocomplementemia with cutaneous vasculitis and arthritis: Possible immune complex syndrome. *Mayo Clin Proc*. 1973;48:340–348.

33. Monroe EW. Urticarial vasculitis: An updated review. *J Am Acad Dermatol*. 1981;5:88–95.

34. Sanchez NP, Winkelmann, Schroeter AL, et al. The clinical and histopathologic spectrums of urticarial vasculitis: Study of forty cases. *J Am Acad Dermatol*. 1982;7:599–605.

35. Soter NA, Mihm Mc Jr, Gigli I, et al. Two distinct cellular patterns in cutaneous necrotizing angiitis. *J Invest Dermatol*. 1976;66:344–350.

36. Natbony SF, Phillips M, Elias JM, et al. Histologic studies of chronic idiopathic urticaria. *J Allergy Clin Immunol*. 1983;71:177–183.

37. Cream JJ, Levine GM, Calnan DD. Erythema elevatum diutinum. *Br J Dermatol*. 1971;84:393–399.

38. Katz SI, Gallin JI, Hertz KC, et al. Erythema elevatum diutinum. *Medicine (Baltimore)*. 1977;56:443–455.

39. Wolf HH, Scherer R, Maciejewski W, et al. Erythema elevatum diutinum: I. Electron microscopy of a case with extracellular cholesterolosis. *Arch Dermatol Res*. 1978;261:7–16.

40. Johnson WC, Higdon RS, Helwig EB: Granuloma faciale. *Arch Dermatol*. 1959;79:42–52.

41. Pedace FJ, Perry HO: Granuloma faciale: A clinical and histopathological review. *Arch Dermatol*. 1966;94:387–395.

42. Nieboer C, Kalsbeek GL. Immunofluorescence studies in granuloma eosinophilia faciale. *J Cutan Pathol*. 1978;5:68–75.

43. Shapiro L, Teisch JA, Brownstein MH. Dermatohistopathology of chronic gonococcal sepsis. *Arch Dermatol*. 1973;107:403–406.

44. Sotto MN, Langer B, Hoshino-Shimizu S, de Brito T. Pathogenesis of cutaneous lesions in acute meningococcemia in humans: Light, immunofluorescent, and electron microscopic studies of skin biopsy specimens. *J Infect Dis*. 1976;135:506–514.

45. Braverman IM. *Skin Signs of Systemic Disease*. 2nd ed. Philadelphia: WB Saunders; 1981.

46. Scott DGI, Bacon PA, Tribe CR. Systemic rheumatoid vasculitis: A clinical and laboratory study of 50 cases. *Medicine (Baltimore)*. 1981;60:288–297.

47. Gocke DJ, Hsu K, Morgan C, et al. Vasculitis in association with Australia antigen. *J Exp Med*. 1976;134:330s–336s.

48. Sergent JS, Lockshin MD, Christian CL, et al. Vasculitis with hepatitis B antigenemia: Long-term observations in nine patients. *Medicine (Baltimore)*. 1976;55:1–18.

49. Cohen RD, Conn DL, Ilstrup DM. Clinical features, prognosis, and response to treatment in polyarteritis. *Mayo Clin Proc*. 1980;55:146–155.

50. Diaz-Perez JL, Winkelmann RK. Cutaneous periarteritis nodosa. *Arch Dermatol*. 1974;110:407–414.

51. Churg J, Strauss L. Allergic granulomatosis, allergic angiitis, and periarteritis nodosa. *Am J Pathol*. 1951;27:277–301.

52. Fienberg R. The protracted superficial phenomenon inpathergic (Wegener's) granulomatosis. *Hum Pathol*. 1981;12:458–467.

53. Dicken C-H, Winkelmann RK. The Churg-Strauss granuloma. Cutaneous necrotizing palisading granuloma in vasculitis syndromes. *Arch Pathol Lab Med*. 1978;102:576–580.

54. Crotty CP, DeRemee RA, Winkelmann RK. Cutaneous clinicopathologic correlation of allergic granulomatous. *J Am Acad Dermatol*. 1981;5:571–581.

55. Fienberg R. Pathergic granulomatosis (editorial). *Am J Med*. 1955;19:829–830.

56. Lanham JG, Elkon KB, Pusey CD, Hughes GR. Systemic vasculitis with asthma and eosinophilia: A clinical approach to the Churg-Strauss syndrome. *Medicine (Baltimore)*. 1984;63:65–81.

57. Wegener F. Uber eine eigenartige rhinogene Granulomatose mit besonderer Beteiligung des Arteriensystems und der Nieren. *Beitr A Pathol Anat*. 1939;102:36–68.

58. Godman GC, Churg J. Wegener's granulomatosis: Pathology and review of the literature. *Arch Pathol*. 1954;58:533–553.

59. Fauci AS, Haynes BF, Katz P, Wolff SM. Wegener's granulomatosis: Prospective clinical and therapeutic experience with 85 patients for 21 years. *Ann Intern Med*. 1983;98:76–85.

60. Cassan SM, Coles DT, Harrison EG, Jr. The concept of limited forms of Wegener's granulomatosis. *Am J Med*. 1970;49:366–374.

61. Reed WB, Jensen AK, Konwaler BE, et al. The cutaneous manifestations in Wegener's granulomatosis. *Acta Derm Venereol (Stockh)*. 1963;43:250–262.

62. Hu CH, O'Laughlin S, Winkelmann RK. Cutaneous manifestations of Wegener's granulomatosis. *Arch Dermatol*. 1977;113:175–182.

63. Shillitoe EJ, Lehner T, Lessof MH, Harrison DFN. Immunological features of Wegener's granulomatosis. *Lancet*. 1974;1:281–284.

64. Liebow AA, Carrington CRB, Friedman PJ. Lymphomatoid granulomatosis. *Hum Pathol*. 1972;3:457–558.

65. Fairchild P, Ryguold O, Oydestese B. Temporal arteritis and polymyalgic rheumatica. Clinical and biopsy findings. *Ann Intern Med*. 1972;77:845–852.

66. Braum EW, Sams WM Jr, Payne RR. Giant cell arteritis: A systemic disease with rare cutaneous manifestations. *J Am Acad Dermatol*. 1982;6:1081–1088.

67. Nakas K, Nutani H, Miyahara M, et al. Takayasu's arteritis.

Clinical report of eighty-four cases and immunological studies of seven cases. *Circulation*. 1967;35:1141–1155.

68. Ishikawa K. Natural history and classification of occlusive thromboaortopathy (Takayasu's disease). *Circulation*. 1978;57:27–35.

69. Klein RG, Campbell RJ, Hunder GG, et al. Skin lesions in temporal arteritis. *Mayo Clin Proc*. 1976;51:504–510.

70. Liang GC, Simkin PA, Mannik M. Immunoglobulins in temporal arteritis: An immunofluorescent study. *Ann Intern Med*. 1974;81:19–24.

71. Gallagher P, Jones K. Immunohistochemical findings in cranial arteritis. *Arthritis Rheum*. 1982;25:75–79.

72. Su WPD, Schroeter AL, Perry HO, et al. Histopathologic and immunopathologic study of pyoderma gangrenosum. *J Cut Pathol*. 1986;13:323–330.

73. Wall LM, Smith NP. Perniosis: A histopathologic review. *J Clin Exp Dermatol*. 1981;6:263–267.

74. Landing BH, Larsen EJ. Are infantile periarteritis nodosa with coronary artery involvement and fatal mucocutaneous lymph node syndrome the same? Comparison of 20 patients from North America with patients from Hawaii and Japan. *Pediatrics*. 1977;59:651–652.

75. Degos R. Malignant atrophic papulosis. *Br J Dermatol*. 1979;100:21–35.

76. Su DWP, Schroeter AL, Lee DA, et al. Clinical and histologic findings in Degos' syndrome (malignant atrophic papulosis). *Cutis*. 1985;35:131–137.

77. Diaz LA, Provost TT, Tomasi TB. Pustular necrotizing angiitis. *Arch Dermatol*. 1973;108:114–118.

78. Goldman JA, Casey HL, Davidson ED, et al. Vasculitis associated with intestinal bypass surgery. *Arch Dermatol*. 1979;115:725–727.

79. Millstone LM, Braverman IM, Lucky P, et al. Classification and therapy of atrophie blanche. *Arch Dermatol*. 1983;119:963–969.

80. Alpert JS, Krous HF, Dalen JE, et al. Pathogenesis of Osler's nodes. *Ann Intern Med*. 1976;85:471–743.

81. Shionoya S, Ban I, Nakata Y, et al. Diagnosis, pathology, and treatment of Buerger's disease. *Surgery*. 1974;75:695–700.

82. O'Duffy JD, Carney JA, Deodhar S. Behcet's disease. Report of 10 cases, three with new manifestations. *Ann Intern Med*. 1971;75:561–570.

83. Colman RW, Minna JD, Robboy SJ. Disseminated intravascular coagulation: A dermatologic disease. *Int J Dermatol*. 1977;16:47–55.

84. Dahl MV, Ullman S, Goltz RW. Vasculitis in granuloma annulare. *Arch Dermatol*. 1977;113:463–467.

85. Ullman S, Dahl MV. Necrobiosis lipoidica. *Arch Dermatol*. 1977;113:1671–1673.

86. Fleischmajer R, Perlish JS. Capillary alterations in scleroderma. *J Am Acad Dermatol*. 1980;2:161–170.

87. Crissman JD. Midline malignant reticulosis and lymphomatoid granulomatosis. *Arch Pathol*. 1979;103:561–564.

CHAPTER 14
Superficial and Deep Infiltrates of the Skin

Antoinette F. Hood

The histologic category of superficial and deep perivascular inflammatory reaction pattern encompasses a large number of widely divergent dermatologic disorders. An attempt to impose a semblance of structure to this group of disorders is shown in Table 14–1. This classification is neither inclusive nor failproof, but it does provide an organized approach to a difficult diagnostic problem. Many of the diseases listed in Table 14–1 are discussed in depth elsewhere in this book and are dealt with in only a cursory manner in this chapter.

DEEP FIGURATE OR GYRATE ERYTHEMAS

A recent review on the subject of persistent figurate erythemas suggests a classification based on morphology and histologic findings (Table 14–2).[1] In general, the figurate erythemas are histologically characterized by a mild to moderately intense, predominantly mononuclear cell perivascular infiltrate that may be present in only the upper dermis or may extend into the deep reticular dermis. Epidermal changes, including parakeratotic scale, intercellular edema, and spongiotic microvesicle formation, are seen in association with an infiltrate confined to the superficial dermis.

ERYTHEMA ANNULARE CENTRIFUGUM

Clinical Features
Erythema annulare centrifugum (EAC) is a cutaneous disease of unknown etiology that may occur in any age group. The majority of EAC cases are idiopathic. However, there are known associations with dermatophytosis, other infections, and, rarely, internal malignancy. The typical lesion of EAC begins as an erythematous papule that extends peripherally and fades centrally to form an annular, gyrate, circinate lesion. The inner edge of the advancing border is often scaly and occasionally vesicular. One or many lesions may be present, and they may be asymptomatic or mildly pruritic. An individual lesion lasts for days to weeks.[2]

Histologic Features
The superficial form of EAC shows a moderately intense lymphohistiocytic infiltrate densely arranged around vessels in the papillary and upper reticular dermis. The term "coat sleeve infiltrate" has been used to describe localization and density of the inflammation. A few eosinophils may be present; extravasation of erythrocytes is associated with endothelial cell swelling. Epidermal changes consist of intercellular edema, spongiotic microvesicle formation, exocytosis of lymphocytes, and focal parakeratotic scale. The deep form of EAC has no epidermal changes and shows a moderately intense superficial and deep perivascular, occasionally periappendageal, lymphocytic infiltrate (Figs. 14–1, 14–2).

The histologic differential diagnosis for superficial EAC includes erythema multiforme, pityriasis lichenoides et varioliformis acuta, light-induced eruptions, and drug eruptions. The first two entities characteristically have prominent dyskeratosis. The presence of prominent papillary dermal edema may help distinguish a light eruption from EAC. Drug eruptions often, but not inevitably, have numerous eosinophils in the infiltrate.

ERYTHEMA GYRATUM REPENS

Clinical Features
This distinctive and rare dermatologic entity occurs exclusively in middle-aged and elderly individuals and is characterized by a widespread eruption most often compared to the appearance of a knotty wood grain pattern. The lesions are elevated, erythematous, circinate, or serpiginous bands or concentric rings involving most of the skin surface. In almost all reported cases of erythema gyratum repens, the eruption is associated with an internal malignancy, and it often clears with successful treatment of the tumor.

Histologic Features
Biopsies from lesions of erythema gyratum repens show a superficial perivascular infiltrate, papillary dermal edema, and epidermal changes similar to those described for erythema annulare centrifugum.

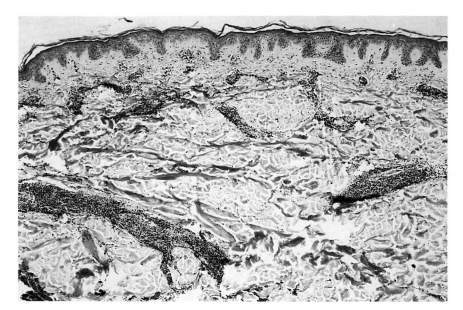

Figure 14–1. Erythema annulare centrifugum, deep form. There is a prominent superficial and deep perivascular mononuclear cell infiltrate with a characteristic coat sleeve or tubular pattern in the reticular dermis. The epidermis appears relatively normal (H&E, ×60).

TABLE 14–1. CLASSIFICATION OF SUPERFICIAL AND DEEP PERIVASCULAR INFILTRATES OF THE SKIN

I. Superficial and deep perivascular infiltrates without significant epidermal change
  A. Lymphocytes predominate
    1. Deep figurate erythema
    2. Lymphocytic infiltrate of the skin (Jessner-Kanof)
    3. Polymorphous light eruption
    4. Lupus erythematosus
    5. Indeterminate leprosy
  B. Neutrophils predominate
    1. Acute febrile neutrophilic dermatosis
    2. Cellulitis
    3. Vasculitis
  C. Eosinophils predominate
    1. Eosinophilic cellulitis
  D. Mixed infiltrate
    1. Urticaria and angioedema

II. Superficial and deep perivascular infiltrates with epidermal change
  A. Interface dermatitis
    1. Lupus erythematosus
    2. Pityriasis lichenoides et varioliformis acuta
    3. Lymphomatoid papulosis
    4. Secondary syphilis
  B. Spongiotic dermatitis
    1. Arthropod bite reaction
    2. Stasis dermatitis
    3. Papulovesicular light eruption
  C. Psorisiform dermatitis
    1. Secondary syphilis
    2. Mycosis fungoides
    3. Anthropod bite reaction

TABLE 14–2. PERSISTENT FIGURATE ERYTHEMAS

Disease	Histologic Features
Erythema annulare centrifugum	Superficial infiltrate
Erythema gyratum repens	Epidermis usually involved
Erythema annulare centrifugum	Superficial and deep infiltrate
Erythema chronicum migrans	Epidermis usually not involved

Modified from Lambert et al.[1]

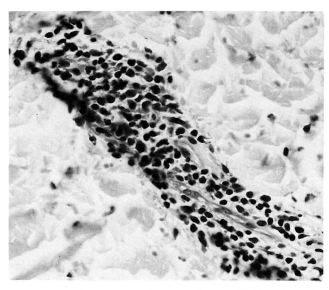

Figure 14–2. Erythema annulare centrifugum. Tight perivascular lymphocytic infiltrate (H&E, ×450).

ERYTHEMA CHRONICUM MIGRANS

Clinical Features

Erythema chronicum migrans is a characteristic cutaneous eruption associated with a tick bite, and, at least when associated with Lyme disease, it is due to infection with a spirochete, *Borrelia burgdorferi*. The eruption, which may occur days to months after a tick bite, begins as an erythematous macule or papule that expands peripherally to form a variably sized annular lesion. The border may be flat or raised but is usually neither scaly or vesicular (in contradistinction to EAC). The central area may show hemorrhage, vesiculation, or necrosis. Erythema chronicum migrans has been described in association with Lyme disease, and in many of these cases, spirochetes have been demonstrated in skin lesions.[3] Systemic symptoms in Lyme disease include malaise, fatigue, transient myalgias, and arthralgias. Untreated patients with Lyme disease may develop recurrent cutaneous lesions, as well as cardiac, joint, or neurologic involvement.

Histologic Features

Biopsies taken from the periphery and the center of a lesion of erythema chronicum migrans show notably different histologic features. The advancing border shows a normal epidermis and a moderately intense perivascular and interstitial superficial and deep infiltrate composed of lymphocytes, histiocytic cells, and plasma cells.[4,5] The center of the lesion shows variable epidermal changes, including ananthosis, and intercellular edema. In the upper dermis there is edema, vascular ectasia, fibrin deposition, nuclear debris, and hemorrhage. Throughout the dermis there is a predominantly perivascular infiltrate composed of lymphocytes, histiocytic cells, and eosinophils. Warthin Starry stains or darkfield examination of tissue may demonstrate spirochetes, but they are not numerous in tissue.

LYMPHOCYTIC INFILTRATE OF THE SKIN (JESSNER-KANOF)

Clinical Features

This entity typically shows asymptomatic well-demarcated, smooth, red to red-brown, firm papules, plaques, or nodules on the face or upper trunk. An annular or circinate appearance may occur as an individual lesion expands peripherally or as a plaque develops central clearing.[6] Patients with the disorder exhibit no evidence of systemic disease or of a connective tissue disease, such as lupus erythematosus.

Histologic Features

The epidermis is either normal or slightly flattened, and there is often mild edema of the papillary dermis. Within the reticular dermis there is a dense, circumscribed aggregate of mononuclear cells arranged around blood vessels and appendages (Fig. 14–3). Most of the inflammatory cells are small lymphocytes, but there may be an admixture of histiocytic cells and occasional plasma cells.[7] The presence of glycosaminoglycans (mucin) in the reticular dermis is described by most authors.[8,9] Fibroplasia may be seen in association with the glycosaminoglycan deposition.[9]

Differential Diagnosis

Histologically, it may be impossible to differentiate lymphocytic infiltrate of the skin from lupus erythematosus. Patients suspected of having this disorder should be evaluated

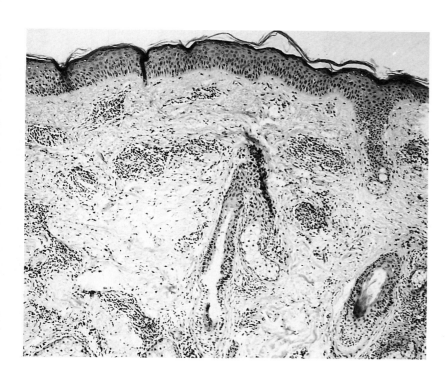

Figure 14–3. Lymphocytic infiltrate. A moderately intense perivascular and a mild periappendageal mononuclear cell infiltrate (H&E, ×95).

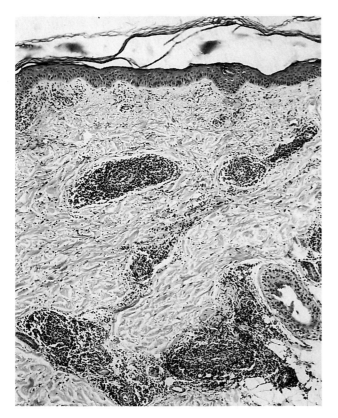

Figure 14–4. Polymorphous light eruption. Intense superficial and deep perivascular infiltrate (H&E, ×145).

initially and periodically with serologic and immunofluorescence studies to rule out connective tissue disorder.

POLYMORPHOUS LIGHT ERUPTION

Clinical Features

Polymorphous light eruption (PMLE) is an acquired disorder characterized by an acute inflammatory reaction in the skin to ultraviolet radiation. The skin lesions occur in areas exposed to sunlight hours to a few days after exposure and may be accompanied by a burning sensation or pruritus. The eruption, which spontaneously improves in 2–10 days, often is recurrent, particularly in the spring and early summer. Patients with PMLE exhibit neither clinical nor serologic evidence of systemic disease, specifically lupus erythematosus.

The adjective "polymorphous" refers to the varying morphologic patterns described in this disorder, which range from small papules to large plaques, vesicles to prurigo-like lesions. An individual, however, tends to have a constant morphologic pattern. As a result of this wide morphologic diversity, the nosology of the disorder is confusing.[10–12]

The clinical heterogeneity of PMLE is reflected by the divergent action spectra reported by different investigators. Although most studies implicate UVB wavelengths of 290–320 nm as the cause of PMLE,[13] experimental reproduction of skin lesions has been induced by UVA (320–410 nm).[14]

Histologic Features

Because of the clinical diversity of the lesions, the histologic findings in PMLE also are diverse. The single unifying feature is the presence of a moderate to intense perivascular infiltrate (Fig. 14–4). Other findings correlate with the morphologic appearance of the lesion.

The papular form of the disease shows a mild to moderately intense mononuclear cell infiltrate in the upper dermis, occasionally accompanied by extravasation of erythrocytes and foci of neutrophilic infiltrate with nuclear debris. Edema of the dermis and endothelial cell swelling are regularly observed.[15] Mild epidermal changes include intercellular edema, focal dyskeratotic cells, and slight vacuolar alteration of the basal layer (Figs. 14–5, 14–6). In one study, direct immunofluorescence showed fibrin deposition in and between vessels but no immunoglobulin or complement deposition. Immunohistochemical studies showed an increase in Langerhans cells (OKT6) in the epidermis.[15]

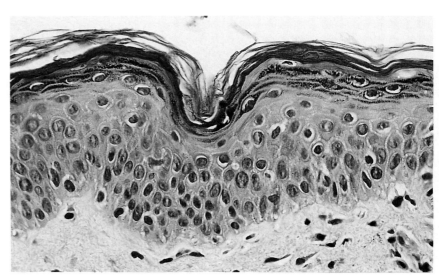

Figure 14–5. Polymorphous light eruption, papular variant, showing variability in epidermal changes. **A.** Mild basal vacuolization. (Continued.)

A

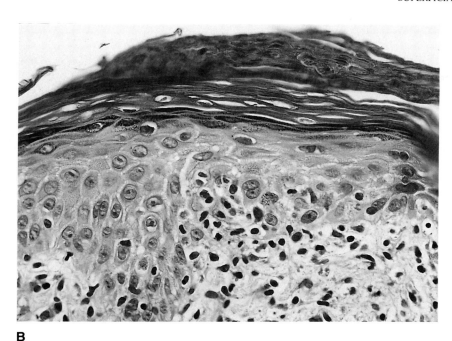

B

Figure 14–5. (Continued). **B.** Focal parakeratosis, exocytosis of mononuclear cells, and basal vacuolization (H&E, ×475).

Plaque-type PMLE shows less epidermal change, mild to moderate edema of the upper dermis, and a bandlike mononuclear cell infiltrate.[14]

The papulovesicular form of PMLE shows a combination of findings, including intraepidermal spongiotic microvesicles, marked subepidermal edema, extravasation of erythrocytes, and either a bandlike or perivascular mixed infiltrate in the dermis[16] (Figs. 14–7, 14–8).

The eczematous form as expected, shows parakeratosis, acanthosis, occasional dyskeratosis, and variable inter-cellular edema. As with other forms of PMLE, a perivascular infiltrate is present throughout the dermis.

Differential Diagnosis

These histologic changes, although characteristic, are far from diagnostic, and although many authors stress the histologic similarity to lupus erythematosus, in our experience, the histologic differential diagnosis more commonly includes allergic contact dermatitis, photoallergic dermatitis

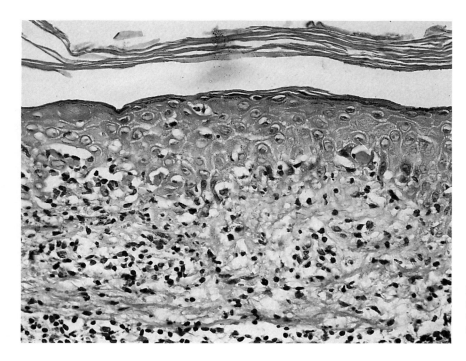

Figure 14–6. Polymorphous light reaction, papular variant. Prominent epidermal changes consisting of basal vacuolization, dyskeratosis, and exocytosis of mononuclear cells. (H&E, ×300).

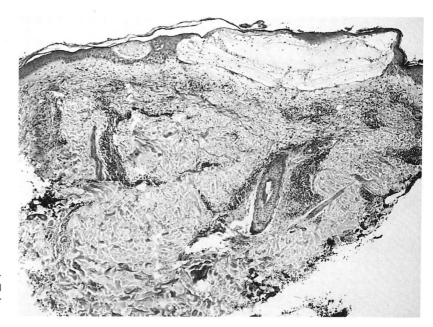

Figure 14–7. Polymorphous light eruption, papulo-vesicular variant. Intraepidermal and subepidermal bullae plus intense superficial and deep perivascular infiltrate. (H&E, ×8.5).

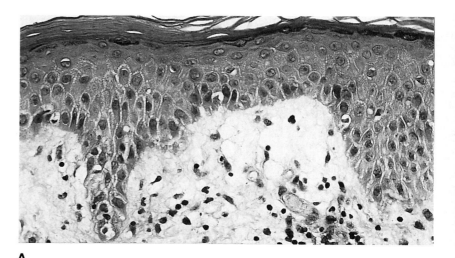

A

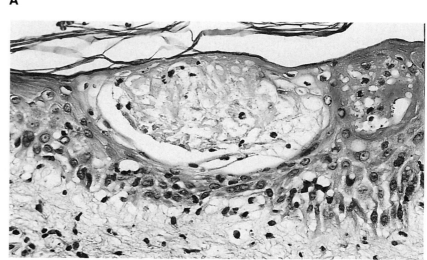

Figure 14–8. Polymorphous light eruption, vesicular variant. **A.** Prominent papillary dermal edema and basal vacuolization. **B.** Intraepidermal vesicle and basal vacuolization (H&E, ×280).

B

and erythema multiforme. Careful clinical histologic correlation is necessary to establish the diagnosis in most cases.

LUPUS ERYTHEMATOSUS

Clinical Features

The clinical and histologic manifestations of cutaneous lupus erythematosus are discussed in detail in Chapter 9. As noted previously, the histologic findings in lupus erythematosus differ markedly according to the subset of the disease, the morphology of the lesion, and the age of the lesion.[17] One constant histologic feature, however, is a perivascular mononuclear cell infiltrate that usually extends into the reticular dermis (Fig. 14–9).[18] The infiltrate, composed predominantly of lymphocytes admixed with a few histiocytic cells, is of variable intensity.[19] Periappendageal (perifollicular and perieccrine) infiltrate is common and often prominent.

The inflammatory cells occasionally extend between vessels and appendages and may assume a bandlike infiltrate in the upper dermis. Extension into the panniculus may be seen. Extravasation of erythrocytes adjacent to blood vessels is a common finding, but frank vasculitis (lymphocytic or leukocytoclastic) is uncommon. Deposition of glycosaminoglycans, specifically hyaluronic acid, is seen frequently in the reticular dermis. Epidermal changes may be absent or mild, consisting merely of vacuolar changes along the basal layer. More pronounced epidermal changes consist of orthohyperkeratosis, occasional focal parakeratosis, epidermal atrophy alternating with acanthosis, dyskeratosis, squamatization of the basal layer, and basement membrane thickening (best detected with the periodic acid-Schiff stain). In mature discoid lesions, there may be dilated appendageal ostia filled with keratin.

Differential Diagnosis

The histologic differential diagnosis includes lymphocytic infiltrate of Jessner and PMLE.

INDETERMINATE LEPROSY

Clinical Features

Leprosy is discussed in detail in Chapter 26. The indeterminate stage of disease caused by *Mycobacterium leprae* may consist of one or more scattered, small, ill-defined macular areas that are pink or hypopigmented. There are no demonstrable changes in tactile sensitivity, sweating, or hair growth. The lesions may resolve spontaneously, remain stationary, or develop signs of one of the determined, or defined, stages of leprosy.

Histologic Features

Histologically, biopsies taken from lesions classified as indeterminate leprosy will show a mild superficial and deep perivascular infiltrate that is also characteristically present around cutaneous nerves and adnexae[20,21] (Fig. 14–10). Acid-fast stains reveal a few organisms in the dermis or in the nerves. The presence of perineural inflammation in a patient who might be at risk for leprosy is a strong indication to order acid-fast stains, especially the Fite stain.

ACUTE FEBRILE NEUTROPHILIC DERMATOSIS

Clinical Features

In 1964, Sweet described eight patients with distinctive clinical and histologic findings, including (1) fever, (2) leukocytosis, (3) tender red lesions on the face, neck, and extremities,

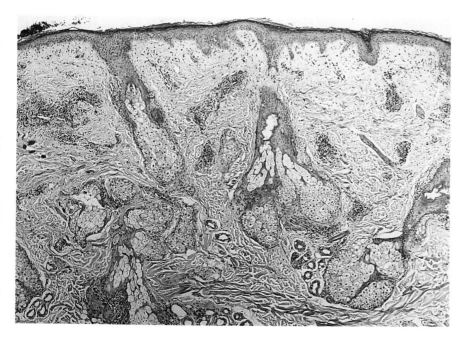

Figure 14–9. Lupus erythematosus. A moderately intense superficial and deep perivascular and periappendageal infiltrate (H&E, ×45).

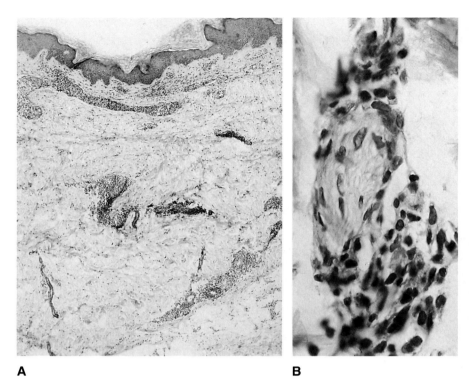

Figure 14–10. Indeterminate leprosy. **A.** Low power magnification showing mild superficial and deep perivascular and perineural infiltrate (H&E, ×60). **B.** Perineural lymphohistiocytic infiltrate (H&E, ×575).

A   **B**

(4) rapid response to corticosteroid administration, and (5) a dermal infiltrate with a predominance of neutrophils.[22,23] The entity was originally described as occurring in association with an upper respiratory tract infection. However, subsequent numerous reports have associated Sweet's syndrome with myeloproliferative disorders, leukemia, and, rarely, solid tumors.[24–26]

The lesions in Sweet's disease are typically red to plum colored, raised, indurated, tender nodules or plaques with an uneven surface. Central clearing may occur and result in annular or arcuate patterns. Occasionally, vesicles or papules appear on the surface of the lesions. The lesions usually are multiple but may occur singly. Resolution often is accompanied by desquamation and hyperpigmentation, but never scarring.

Histologic Features
Biopsy specimens taken from idiopathic Sweet's syndrome and from lesions associated with malignancy show similar histopathologic changes. The epidermis usually is normal but may be slightly acanthotic in older lesions. Minor focal epidermal changes, including parakeratosis, intercellular edema, and exocytosis of neutrophils, occur. Papillary dermal edema occasionally is quite severe, and subepidermal bulla formation may occur.[24,27]

In the reticular dermis there is a dense nodular, patchy, or bandlike infiltrate composed predominantly of mature neutrophils admixed with lymphocytes and eosinophils. Leukocytoclasis and extravasation of erythrocytes are common, but other features of vasculitis, such as fibrin deposition or vessel wall damage, are specifically absent. The infiltrate usually is most prominent in the upper reticular dermis but may extend throughout the dermis and even

involve subcutaneous tissue. There is separation of collagen fibers by the inflammatory infiltrate as well as focal fragmentation and basophilic degeneration of the fibers. Special stains for microorganisms are always negative.

Differential Diagnosis
The lack of true leukocytoclastic vasculitis separates acute febrile neutrophilic dermatosis from erythema elevatum diutinum and hypersensitivity angiitis. It may be difficult to differentiate Sweet's syndrome from pyoderma gangrenosum histologically. Indeed, some authors have suggested that the two entities are related and are part of the spectrum of a single disease.[28] Leukocytoclasis usually is not seen in cellulitis; the diagnosis of infection usually is confirmed by special stains or culture.

CELLULITIS

Clinical Features
Cellulitis is an acute inflammatory process of the skin, particularly the deep reticular dermis and subcutaneous tissues. The lesions are characteristically erythematous, edematous, and warm to the touch. Borders often are indistinct.

Histologic Features
Biopsies from lesions of cellulitis show a mild to moderately intense perivascular and interstitial infiltrate composed of neutrophils and lymphocytes, with occasional eosinophils and plasma cells. Focal aggregates of neutrophils may produce microscopic abscesses. There may be extravasation of erythrocytes. Dermal blood vessels usually are ectatic, and edema of the reticular dermis may be prominent.

Special stains for organisms usually are positive, but microorganisms may be few in number. Examination of multiple, appropriately stained sections often is necessary to confirm the infectious etiology. Cellulitis in the immunocompromised host may be produced by mycobacteria or fungi, and this should be taken into account when ordering special stains.

EOSINOPHILIC CELLULITIS

Clinical Features

This disorder is discussed in Chapter 15. Patients with eosinophilic cellulitis (Wells' syndrome) typically have recurrent erythematous, edematous, annular, or circinate infiltrated plaques. In the early stage of the disease, the lesions may resemble cellulitis, but older lesions become indurated and often resemble morphea. Blistering may occur, and peripheral eosinophilia is a common finding.[29]

Histologic Features

The epidermis usually is normal but may be separated from the edematous dermis in bullous lesions. In the dermis there is a perivascular and interstitial infiltrate composed of eosinophils admixed with lymphocytes and histiocytes. Focal areas of amorphous or granular eosinophilic material known as "flame figures" may be present.[29–31] Flame figures are not specific for eosinophilic cellulitis but may be seen also in arthropod bite reactions, pemphigoid, and dermatophyte infection. These entities usually are easily separated from Wells' syndrome by the presence of epidermal changes, subepidermal vacuoles or blister formation, and the presence of fungal organisms in the stratum corneum or hair follicle. Immunoflourescent studies may be necessary to definitively rule out pemphigoid.

URTICARIA AND ANGIOEDEMA

Clinical Features

Urticaria are transient, circumscribed, erythematous areas of edema that are usually pruritic. The term "angioedema" implies extension of the edema into the deep dermis and subcutaneous tissue. Urticaria and angioedema may occur anywhere on the skin surface, individually or concurrently. Individual lesions tend to last less than 24 hours but may recur episodically for long periods of time.

Urticaria and angioedema commonly are classified as immunologically mediated, nonimmunologically mediated, and idiopathic. Immunologically mediated, IgE-dependent urticaria may be associated with an atopic diathesis, specific antigen sensitivity to foods, drugs, arthropod venom, and pollens, or physical stimuli, such as pressure, cold, light, or heat. Complement-mediated urticaria is seen in association with serum sickness, reactions to blood products, necrotizing vasculitis, hereditary angioedema, and acquired angioedema with lymphoma.

Nonimmunologic urticaria may be produced by the direct effect of a drug on the mast cell and basophil or as a presumed abnormality of arachidonic acid metabolism. Drugs implicated in the production of nonimmunologically mediated urticaria include the opiates, antibiotics (poly-myxin B), curare, radiocontrast media, aspirin, and nonsteroidal anti-inflammatory agents.

Histologic Features

Typical IgE-mediated urticaria is characterized histologically by a superficial, sparse to moderately intense lymphohistiocytic and eosinophilic infiltrate with variable dermal edema[32] (Figs. 14–11, 14–12). In some giant urticaria, angioedema, and pressure-induced urticaria, the infiltrate may be quite intense and be prominent in the deep reticular dermis and subcutaneous tissue[33] (Fig. 14–12). This may give the infiltrate a somewhat bottom-heavy appearance when viewed microscopically at a low power. This deep perivascular infiltrate is composed of lymphocytes and eosinophils, with occasional neutrophils and mast cells (Fig. 14–12). Vascular ectasia and dermal edema are both characteristically present. Vasculitis is seen only rarely in chronic idiopathic urticaria, complement-mediated urticaria, and some of the physical urticarias.[34]

PITYRIASIS LICHENOIDES ET VARIOLIFORMIS ACUTA

Clinical Features

Pityriasis lichenoides et varioliformis acuta (PLEVA) is an uncommon disorder of unknown etiology that occurs in adolescents and young adults. The disease is characterized

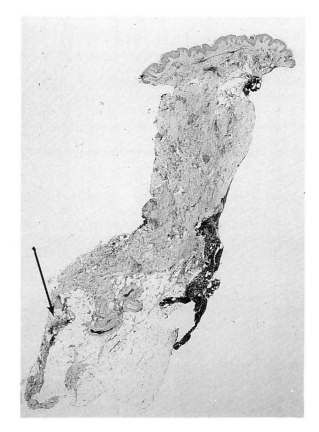

Figure 14–11. Urticaria and angioedema. Mild superficial and deep (arrow) perivascular infiltrate and dermal edema (H&E, ×9.5).

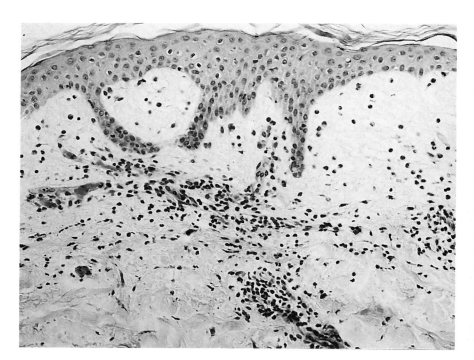

Figure 14–12. Urticaria and angioedema. Prominent papillary dermal edema and a moderately intense perivascular mixed infiltrate (H&E, ×110).

by recurrent crops of lesions that begin as flesh-colored to erythematous papules and rapidly evolve into vesicles, hemorrhagic lesions, and crusted ulcerations. Resolution of an individual lesion is accompanied by hyperpigmentation, hypopigmentation, and varioliform scarring. Resolution of an individual lesion occurs within a few weeks, but new lesions may continue to erupt for many months or even years. The most frequently involved areas are the trunk and flexor aspects of the proximal extremities, but the eruption may be generalized. Although usually asymptomatic, occasionally, patients describe a burning or pruritic sensation associated with the rash. Systemic symptoms are exceedingly rare.

The relationship between PLEVA and pityriasis lichenoides chronica is not clear, but there have been cases reported of the acute form progressing clinically and histologically into the more chronic disease. Some authors consider PLEVA and pityriasis lichenoides chronica to be variants of the same disease.[35]

Histologic Features
The histopathologic findings in PLEVA are distinctive but cover a wide spectrum and depend on the clinical stage at which the biopsy specimen is obtained.[35] A constant finding, however, is a superficial and deep perivascular infiltrate (Fig. 14–13). Epidermal changes include focal parakeratosis, focal epidermal necrosis, dyskeratosis, and basilar vacuolar changes. Necrosis may be extensive, and ulceration may occur. Exocytosis of lymphocytes and erythrocytes into the epidermis is seen frequently (Fig. 14–14). The lymphocytes occasionally aggregate to form microabscesses. Unlike the Pautrier microabscesses seen in mycosis

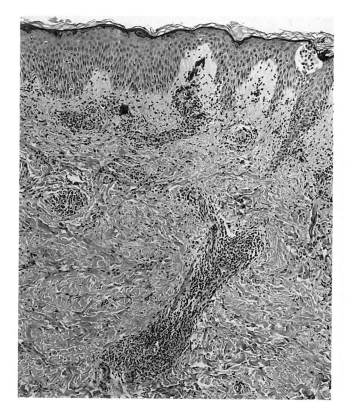

Figure 14–13. Pityriasis lichenoides et varioliformis acuta. Intraepidermal microabscess, exocytosis, papillary dermal edema, and a moderately intense perivascular infiltrate, with endothelial cell swelling and luminal obliteration (H&E, ×85).

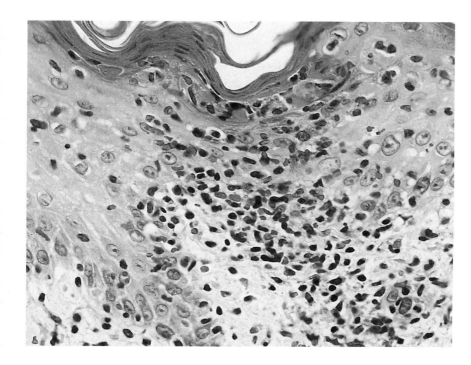

Figure 14–14. Pityriasis lichenoides et varioliformis acuta. Dyskeratosis, exocytosis of lymphocytes, and diapedesis of erythrocytes (H&E, ×440).

fungoides, the intraepidermal microabscesses in PLEVA contain cytologically normal lymphocytes[36] (Fig. 14–15).

Subepidermal microvesicles may be seen in association with severe vacuolar alteration. Dermal edema is usually mild. There is an intense perivascular infiltrate that is most prominent in the upper dermis but also extends into the deep reticular dermis. The infiltrate is composed predominantly of mononuclear cells, but there is a variable admixture of neutrophils. Endothelial cell swelling and prolifera-

tion and dermal hemorrhage are commonly seen. Sclerosis of the dermis is present in older lesions.

Differential Diagnosis
The histologic differential diagnosis includes pityriasis rosea, insect bite reaction, syphilis, PMLE, and lymphomatoid papulosis. Pityriasis rosea, especially the clinically inflammatory subset, may be difficult, and occasionally impossible, to distinguish histologically from PLEVA. Pityriasis

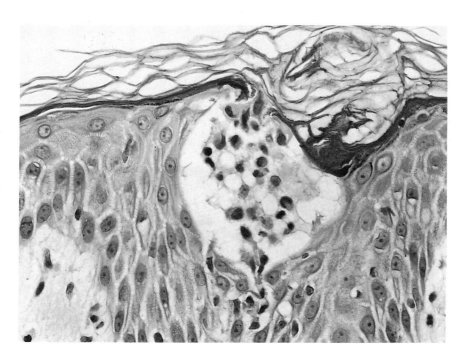

Figure 14–15. Pityriasis lichenoides et varioliformis acuta. Intraepidermal microabscess filled with normal appearing mononuclear cells (H&E, ×440).

rosea typically has less epidermal necrosis and dyskeratosis, epidermal spongiosis with small intraepidermal spongiotic microvesicles often located in the upper half of the epidermis, and a more superficially located dermal infiltrate. Insect bite reaction is characterized by more pronounced dermal edema and the presence of eosinophils in the infiltrate. Secondary syphilis usually can be distinguished from PLEVA by the presence of plasma cells in the infiltrate; the diagnosis may be confirmed by demonstrating *Treponema pallidum* with a silver stain. PMLE has less dyskeratosis and epidermal necrosis than PLEVA and may show striking dermal edema. Lymphomatoid papulosis is distinguished by the presence of numerous large atypical mononuclear cells in the dermal infiltrate.

LYMPHOMATOID PAPULOSIS

Clinical Features

This disorder was originally defined by Macaulay in 1968 as a clinically benign, histologically malignant, self-healing eruption.[37,38] Clinically, many cases of lymphomatoid papulosis resemble pityriasis lichenoides. Crops of papules develop that often vesiculate, become hemorrhagic and crusted, and spontaneously resolve in a few weeks with or without a residual scar. A second subset of patients develops nodules, sometimes quite large (several centimeters in diameter), which often become necrotic or ulcerated. The lesions occur anywhere on the body and often are generalized. Mild pruritus may accompany the eruption. Clinically, lymphomatoid papulosis differs from PLEVA by its later onset in life (fourth decade versus third decade), female predominance, and longer duration (years instead of months).

Although characteristically clinically benign, up to 10% of cases reported in the literature as lymphomatoid papulosis developed lymphoreticular malignant neoplasms.[39] It

has been argued that these malignant cases were initially misdiagnosed as lymphomatoid papulosis. However, recent immunophenotypic and immunogenotypic evidence has been offered supporting the belief that lymphomatoid papulosis belongs in the spectrum of T cell lymphomas.[40,41]

Histologic Features

Epidermal changes are variable and depend on the stage of development of the lesion. Early papular lesions may show only a mild exocytosis of mononuclear cells. Later lesions, however, will show more extensive epidermotropism, intercellular and intracellular edema, dyskeratosis, and necrosis with overlying crust formation.

Within the dermis, there is a wedge-shaped triangular infiltrate with the apex pointed to the subcutis[42] or a superficial and deep perivascular infiltrate (Fig. 14–16). The infiltrate is perivascular and interstitial and even may assume a bandlike appearance in the upper dermis. The infiltrate is composed of large and small lymphocytes admixed with occasional plasma cells, eosinophils, and neutrophils. Characteristic large atypical mononuclear cells are scattered throughout the infiltrate. These cells may be hyperchromatic (chunks of coal), kidney-shaped, or binucleated resembling Reed-Sternberg cells.[43] The abnormal cells may be localized to the dermis or may be present also within the epidermis. Dermal hemorrhage is common.

SECONDARY SYPHILIS

Clinical Features

The clinical features and histopathology of secondary syphilis are described with greater detail in Chapter 27 but, for the sake of completeness, are discussed briefly here. The skin lesions of secondary syphilis are very variable and include macular, papular, papulosquamous, follicular,

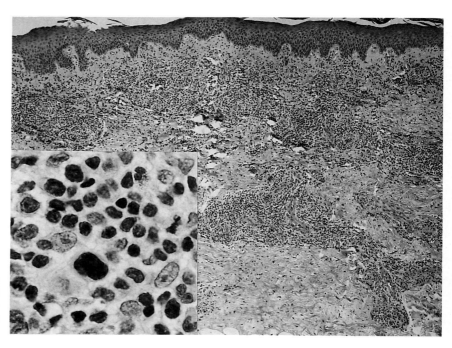

Figure 14–16. Lymphomatoid papulosis. Dense perivascular and interstitial infiltrate composed of lymphocytes, histiocytic cells, and bizarre hyperchromatic, large, atypical mononuclear cells (H&E, ×55, inset ×750).

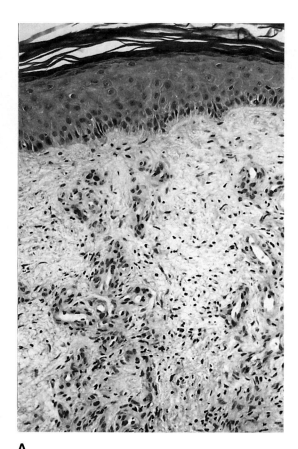
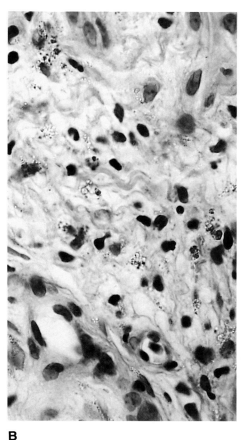

Figure 14–17. Stasis dermatitis. In addition to a variably intense superficial and deep perivascular mononuclear cell infiltrate, there is vascular proliferation, fibroplasia, and hemosiderin deposition (H&E, A ×150, B ×725).

A   **B**

pustular, and nodular varieties. The diagnosis is confirmed by serologic tests. Rapid resolution of disease occurs following administration of appropriate antimicrobial therapy. Atypical clinical patterns and response to therapy may occur in immunocompromised individuals.

Histologic Features

Epidermal changes are quite variable. Parakeratotic scale, often focal, is common. Some lesions are characterized by interface dermatitis changes, such as basal vacuolization, exocytosis of lymphocytes, and dyskeratosis. Other lesions may have marked acanthosis, often in a psorisiform pattern, with associated intercellular edema and exocytosis of mononuclear cells.[44] The dermal infiltrate also is variable in intensity, pattern, and composition, but typically, there is a moderately intense superficial and deep perivascular infiltrate composed of lymphocytes, histiocytic cells, plasma cells, and occasional eosinophils. Plasma cells are characteristically, but not invariably, present. The presence of numerous plasma cells in a dermal infiltrate is strongly suggestive of syphilis, although the relative paucity of plasma cells does not rule out the diagnosis.[45,46] Scattered large atypical cells also have been described. Epithelioid cell granulomas admixed with plasma cells may be prominent or focally present. Endothelial cell swelling, hypertrophy, and vessel proliferation may be prominent.

STASIS DERMATITIS

Clinical Features

Stasis dermatitis occurs on the lower legs of people with chronic venous insufficiency. The lesions occur most commonly over the region of the medial malleolus and are characterized by hyperpigmentation and scaliness.

Histologic Features

The overlying epidermis may be normal, acanthotic, or atrophic, with mild to moderate intercellular edema and hyperkeratosis. In the reticular dermis, there is a moderate to intense perivascular lymphohistiocytic infiltrate that may extend into the subcutaneous tissue. Vascular ectasia and vessel proliferation are usually prominent, and vessel walls often are thickened. Dermal hemorrhage, hemosiderin deposition, and dermal fibrosis usually are present (Fig. 14–17).

REFERENCES

1. Lambert WC, Reed K, Arndt K. Erythema perstans: The persistent figurate erythemas. *J Am Acad Dermatol.* (in press).
2. Harrison, PV. The annular erythemas. *Int J Dermatol.* 1979;18:282–290.
3. Berger BW, Kaplan MH, Rothberg IR, Barbour AG. Isolation and characterization of the Lyme disease spirochete from the

skin of patients with erythema chronicum migrans. *J Am Acad Dermatol.* 1985;13:444–449.

4. Berger BW, Clemmensen OJ, Ackerman AB. Lyme disease is a spirochetosis. A review of the disease and evidence for its cause. *Am J Dermatopathol.* 1983;5:111–124.

5. Berger BW. Erythema chronicum migrans of Lyme disease. *Arch Dermatol.* 1984;120:1017–1021.

6. Jessner M, Kanof NB. Lymphocytic infiltration of the skin. *Arch Dermatol Syph.* 1953;68:447–449.

7. Cerio R, MacDonald DM. Benign cutaneous lymphoid infiltrates. *J Cutan Pathol.* 1985;12:442–452.

8. Gottlieb B, Winkelmann, RK. Lymphocytic infiltrate of skin. *Arch Dermatol.* 1962;86:106–113.

9. Clark WH, Mihm MC Jr, Reed RJ, Ainsworth AM. The lymphocytic infiltrates of the skin. *Hum Pathol.* 1974;5:25–43.

10. Epstein JH. Polymorphous light eruption. *J Am Acad Dermatol.* 1980;3:329–343.

11. Lamb JH, Shelmire B, Cooper Z, Morgan RJ, Keaty C. Solar dermatitis. *Arch Dermatol Syph.* 1950;60:1–27.

12. Elpern DJ, Morison WL, Hood AF. Papulovesicular light eruption. A defined subset of polymorphous light eruption. *Arch Dermatol.* 1985;121:1286–1288.

13. Frain-Bell W, Dickson A, Herd J, Sturrock I., et al. The action spectrum in polymorphic light eruption. *Br J Dermatol.* 1973;89:243–249.

14. Hölzle E, Plewig G, Hofman C, Roser-Maass E. Polymorphous light eruption: Experimental reproduction of skin lesions. *J Am Acad Dermatol.* 1982;7:111–125.

15. Muhlbauer JE, Bahn AK, Harrist TJ, Bernhard JD, Mihm MC Jr. Papular polymorphic light eruption: An immunoperoxidase study using monoclonal antibodies. *Br J Dermatol.* 1983;108:153–162.

16. Hood AF, Elpern DJ, Morison WL. Histopathologic findings in papulovesicular light eruption. *J Cutan Pathol.* 1986;13:13–21.

17. Hood AF. Pathology of lupus erythematosus. *Adv Dermatol.* 1987;2:153–170.

18. Clark WH, Reed RJ, Mihm MC Jr. Lupus erythematosus: Histopathology of cutaneous lesions. *Hum Pathol.* 1973;4:157–163.

19. Winkelmann RK. Spectrum of lupus erythematosus. *J Cutan Pathol.* 1979;6:457–462.

20. Ridley SD. *Skin Biopsy in Leprosy.* 2nd ed. Basel: Ciba-Geigy; 1985.

21. Liv TC, Yen LZ, YE GYK, Dung GL. Histology of indeterminate leprosy. *Int J Lepr.* 1982;50:172–176.

22. Sweet RD. An acute febrile neutrophilic dermatosis. *Br J Dermatol.* 1964;76:349–356.

23. Sweet RD. Further observations on acute febrile neutrophilic dermatosis. *Br J Dermatol.* 1968;80:800–805.

24. Cooper PH, Innes DJ Jr, Greer KE. Acute febrile neutrophilic dermatosis (Sweet's syndrome) and myeloproliferative disorders. *Cancer.* 1983;51:1518–1526.

25. Shapiro L, Baraf CS, Richheimer LL. Sweet's syndrome (acute febrile neutrophilic dermatosis): Report of a case. *Arch Dermatol.* 1971;103:81.

26. Krolikowski FJ, Reuter K, Shultis EW. Acute neutrophilic dermatosis (Sweet's syndrome) associated with lymphoma. *Hum Pathol.* 1985;16:520–522.

27. Su WP, Liu H-NH. Diagnostic criteria for Sweet's syndrome. *Cutis.* 1986;38:167–170.

28. Caughman W, Stern R, Haynes H. Neutrophilic dermatosis of myeloproliferative disorders: Atypical forms of pyoderma gangrenosum and Sweet's syndrome associated with myeloproliferative disorders. *J Am Acad Dermatol.* 1983;9:751–758.

29. Wells GC, Smith NP. Eosinophilic cellulitis. *Br J Dermatol.* 1979;100:101–109.

30. Schorr WF, Tauscheck AL, Dickson KB, Melski JW. Eosinophilic cellulitis (Well's syndrome): Histologic and clinical features in arthropod bite reactions. *J Am Acad Dermatol.* 1984;11:1043–1049.

31. Stern JB, Sobel HJ, Rotchford JP. Well's syndrome: Is there collagen damage in the flame figures? *J Cutan Pathol.* 1984;11:501–550.

32. Natbony SF, Phillips ME, Elias JM, et al. Histologic studies of chronic idiopathic urticaria. *J Allergy Clin Immunol.* 1983;71:177–183.

33. Czarnetzki BM, Meentken J, Kolde G, et al. Morphology of the cellular infiltrate in delayed pressure urticaria. *J Am Acad Dermatol.* 1985;12:253–259.

34. Monroe EW, Schultz CI, Maize JC, et al. Vasculitis in chronic urticaria: An immunopathologic study. *J Invest Dermatol.* 1981;76:103–107.

35. Marks R, Black M, Wilson-Jones E. Pityriasis lichenoides. A reappraisal. *Br J Dermatol.* 1972;86:215–222.

36. Hood AF, Mark EJ. Histopathologic diagnosis of pityriasis lichenoides et varioliformis acuta and its clinical correlation. *Arch Dermatol.* 1982;118:478–482.

37. Macaulay WL. Lymphomatoid papulosis: A continuing self-healing eruption, clinically benign—histologically malignant. *Arch Dermatol.* 1968;97:23–30.

38. Macaulay WL. Lymphomatoid papulosis. *Int J Dermatol.* 1978;17:204–212.

39. Sina B, Burnett JW. Lymphomatoid papulosis. Case reports and literature review. *Arch Dermatol.* 1983;119:189–197.

40. Weiss LM, Wood GS, Trela M, Warnke RA, Sklar J. Clonal T cell populations in lymphomatoid papulosis: Evidence for a lymphoproliferative origin for a clinically benign disease. *N Engl J Med.* 1986;315:475–479.

41. Wood GS, Strickler JG, Deneau DG, Egbert B, Warnke RA. Lymphomatoid papulosis expresses immunophenotypes associated with T cell lymphoma but not inflammation. *J Am Acad Dermatol.* 1986;15:444–458.

42. Black MM, Wilson-Jones E. "Lymphomatoid" pityriasis lichenoides: A variant with histological features simulating a lymphoma. *Br J Dermatol.* 1972;86:329–347.

43. Valentino LA, Helwig EB. Lymphomatoid papulosis. *Arch Pathol.* 1975;96:409–416.

44. Jeerapaet P, Ackerman AB. Histologic patterns of secondary syphilis. *Arch Dermatol.* 1973;107:373–377.

45. Abell E, Marks R, Wilson-Jones E. Secondary syphilis: A clinicopathologic review. *Br J Dermatol.* 1975;93:53–61.

46. Alessi E, Innocenti M, Ragusa G. Secondary syphilis. Clinical morphology and histopathology. *Am J Dermatopathol.* 1983;5:11–17.

CHAPTER 15
Nodular or Diffuse Infiltrates

Kenneth J. Friedman

This chapter examines the clinical and histopathologic features of the cutaneous diseases that may present a predominant pattern of nodular or diffuse infiltration of the dermis, with or without involvement of the epidermis or subcutis. For ease of diagnosis, the subject headings are organized according to the predominant cell type involved, including the lymphocyte, eosinophil, mast cell, neutrophil, and histiocyte–monocyte–macrophage. Disorders involving the neutrophil or histiocyte as the predominant infiltrating cell type are mentioned only briefly, since they are discussed primarily elsewhere.

PREDOMINANTLY LYMPHOCYTIC INFILTRATION

PSEUDOLYMPHOMA

Pseudolymphoma is a heterogeneous group of benign dermatoses that simulate malignant lymphoma both histologically and clinically. The variety of terms historically applied to cutaneous pseudolymphoma include Spiegler-Fendt sarcoid, lymphocytoma cutis, lymphadenosis benigna cutis, cutaneous lymphoid hyperplasia, and cutaneous lymphoplasia. This variety of terms reflects the morphologic diversity of cutaneous pseudolymphoma as well as the general lack of knowledge about the stimuli for these reaction patterns in the skin. Even after careful histologic and immunohistochemical study, a number of lymphoid infiltrative processes will not be clearly defined as benign or malignant. Establishment of the true nature of this type of indeterminate lymphoid infiltrate requires clinical data, workup, and long-term follow-up.

Clinical Features
Cutaneous pseudolymphoma has been reported following trauma, tattoos, arthropod assaults, injection of arthropod venom, antigen hyposensitization injections, vaccinations,

herpes zoster infection, and acupuncture.[1–8] In most cases, no initiating event is evident.

A pseudolymphoma syndrome that may mimic malignant lymphoma clinically and histopathologically has been produced by the hydantoins, including phenytoin (Dilantin). This syndrome is characterized by fever, eosinophilia, arthralgia, lymphadenopathy, hepatosplenomegaly, and a generalized maculopapular skin eruption.[9,10] The development of cutaneous nodules has been reported in one patient.[11] In addition, a reversible pseudomycosis fungoides syndrome following hydantoin administration has been reported.[12]

Cutaneous pseudolymphoma occurs most frequently in a localized distribution as plaques, papules, nodules, or, rarely, miliary lesions. A solitary nodule measuring up to 4 cm in diameter is the most common presentation.[8] Disseminated forms may occur rarely.[13] Typically, the lesions occur on exposed areas of the body, with a predilection for the face and neck. Other common sites are the extremities, areola, vulva, and scrotum. The lesions have a doughy to firm consistency and may be skin-colored, red, or violaceous. Lesions secondary to arthropod assault may be associated with ulceration and pruritus. Lesions may often undergo spontaneous resolution. Some lesions may persist for months to years, and persistence or recurrence is most often associated with the disseminated form.[13,14] Persistent pseudolymphoma may precede the development of malignant lymphoma.[15]

Histologic Features
A dense nodular to diffuse infiltrate is present. The infiltrate is top-heavy, favoring the upper half of the dermis over the lower dermis and subcutis (Fig. 15–1), although diffuse dermal involvement and extension into the subcutis can be seen[14] (Fig. 15–2). The infiltrate may assume a preferential perivascular location, particularly at its periphery, and is generally separated from the epidermis by a narrow grenz zone of normal collagen. If the epidermis is involved, it displays hyperplasia or disruption in the form of hyper-

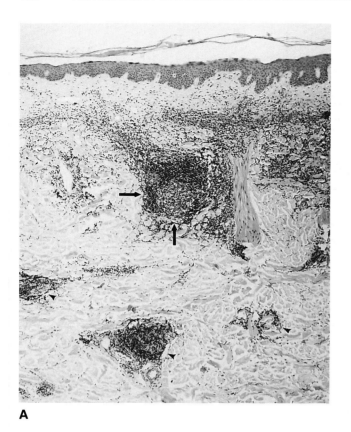

A

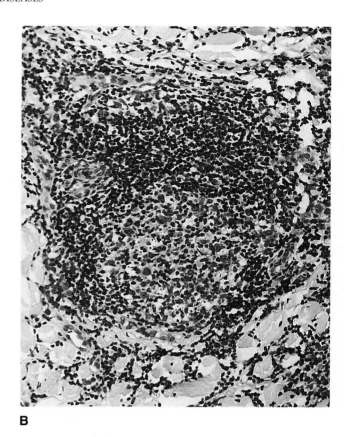

B

Figure 15–1. Pseudolymphoma. **A.** Top-heavy lymphocytic infiltrate with germinal center formation (arrows) and distinct perivascular pattern (arrowheads) (H&E, ×45). **B.** Germinal center surrounded by cuff of mature small lymphocytes (H&E, ×110).

keratosis, parakeratosis, dyskeratosis, spongiosis, and basal vacuolar damage.

In most cases, the infiltrate is dominated by small, mature lymphocytes with a scattered number of large lymphocytes with large pale-staining or vesicular nuclei containing one or two small nucleoli[8] (Fig. 15–3). These large cells rarely may occur as the dominant cell type. Scattered atypical mononuclear cells may be present; however, these cells should constitute a minority in the infiltrate. Scattered large macrophages, referred to as tingible-body macrophages, may be seen containing fragmented basophilic nuclear and cytoplasm fragments of degenerated lymphoid cells. In addition, there may be admixtures of plasma cells, eosinophils, mast cells, neutrophils, and scattered giant cells. Small clusters of plasma cells may be found admixed with other types of lymphoid cells.

Persistent reactions to arthropod assault may show marked epidermal hyperplasia or ulceration and generally are rich in eosinophils and plasma cells. However, these reactions may consist of only large and small lymphocytes (Figs. 15–4, 15–5). Retained mouth parts rarely may be found associated with foreign body giant cell reactions.

Only in a minority of cases will well-formed germinal centers be present[8] (Figs. 15–1B, 15–3). These must be distinguished from follicle formation in nodular lymphoma; the distinguishing features are summarized in Table 15–1. Although numerous mitoses may be present within the germi-

nal centers, mitoses are rare outside the germinal centers. Proliferation of capillaries at all dermal levels as well as endothelial swelling are common findings. The presence of single rows of lymphocytes migrating between collagen bundles (the Indian file sign) is more often associated with malignant lymphoid infiltrates; however, this feature may be seen as a minor pattern in pseudolymphoma.[14]

The nodular skin lesions of hydantoin-induced pseudolymphoma demonstrate aggregates of large lymphocytes suggestive of malignant lymphoma.[11] Subcutaneous lympyh nodes may show reactive hyperplasia or may suggest lymphoma. In pseudomycosis fungoides syndrome, the dermis shows infiltration with atypical mononuclear cells with clefted cerebriform nuclei.[12] The overlying epidermis may be hyperplastic, with intraepidermal mononuclear cell nests similar to Pautrier's microabscesses.

Differential Diagnosis

The most important and often the most difficult step in evaluating a dense dermal lymphocytic infiltrate is the differentiation of a benign infiltrate from malignant lymphoma. All of the histologic criteria summarized in Table 15–2 should be used in making this often difficult assessment. However, it must be stressed that the most consistent histopathologic criteria for extranodal lymphoma are cellular monomorphism and cellular atypia.

Lesions rich in plasma cells must be differentiated from

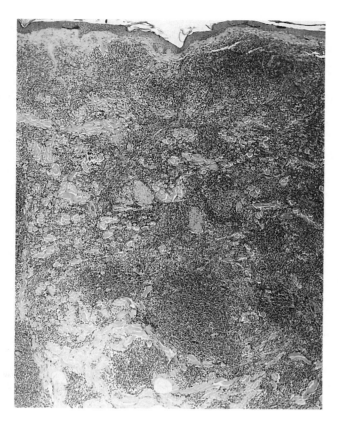

Figure 15–2. Pseudolymphoma. Usually dense lymphocytic infiltrate extending well into deep dermis, overlapping with architectural pattern of malignant lymphoma (H&E, ×40).

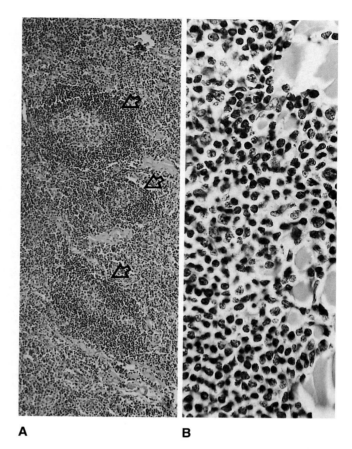

A   **B**

Figure 15–3. Pseudolymphoma. **A.** Dense diffuse infiltrate with germinal center formation (arrows) (H&E, ×55). **B.** Predominantly small mature lymphocytes with scattered large lymphocytes (H&E, ×450).

plasmacytoma. Plasmacytoma will display sheets of plasma and plasmacytoid cells, with only a minor admixture of other cell types. Diffuse small cell (well-differentiated lymphocytic) lymphoma, which only rarely involves the skin,[16] must be differentiated from pseudolymphomas in which predominantly small mature lymphocytes dominate without germinal center formation or admixtures of other cell types. Immunohistochemistry may be useful. Lymphocytic infiltration of the skin (Jessner) displays a patchy perivascular and sometimes periappendageal infiltrate of predominantly small lymphocytes.[17,18] This generally can be distinguished from the dense nodular to diffuse pattern of infiltration characteristic of pseudolymphoma.

Immunohistochemical studies of cutaneous pseudolymphoma have shown mixed infiltrates of B cells with polyclonal light chains, T cells, Langerhans cells, and HLA-DR-positive dendritic cells.[19] A predominance of polyclonal B cells is generally present.[20] The T cell population is composed of either equal populations of helper and suppressor cells or a predominance of helper cells. Germinal centers display immunologic features similar to those in reactive lymph nodes, including follicular dendritic cells.[21] These findings contrast with those of malignant lymphoma of B cell type in which a monoclonal light chain B cell phenotype is found. The immunohistochemical profile of cutaneous T cell lymphoma is more diverse. Neoplastic cutaneous T cell infiltrates usually can be distinguished from benign T

cell infiltrates by the presence of one T cell subset to the exclusion of others.[22] However, mixtures of T cell types have been found in some cases of mycosis fungoides,[23,24] lessening the application of immunostaining toward recognizing a malignant T cell population. No universally accepted cell surface markers of clonality for T cells have been identified. DNA hybridization techniques have been used to analyze the gene arrangement encoding the T cell antigen receptor and to identify clonality in T cell lymphoproliferative disorders.[25,26] This technique is a powerful tool in evaluating for T cell monoclonality.

EXTRAMEDULLARY PLASMACYTOMA

Clinical Features

Skin involvement in extramedullary plasmacytoma is rare. The upper respiratory tract mucosa is the site of predilection. Multiple metastatic lesions may occur. The primary or solitary cutaneous plasmacytoma in the absence of multiple myeloma is extremely rare.[27] Long-term observation of cutaneous extramedullary plasmacytoma is essential because the lesions may antedate the development of multiple myeloma by many years. The tumors may remain limited to

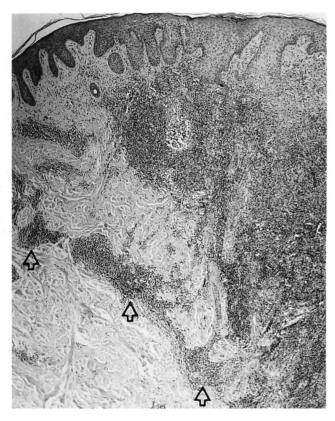

Figure 15–4. Pseudolymphoma. Persistent arthropod assault reaction; irregular acanthosis and a dense diffuse infiltrate with a perivascular arrangement peripherally (arrows) (H&E, ×55).

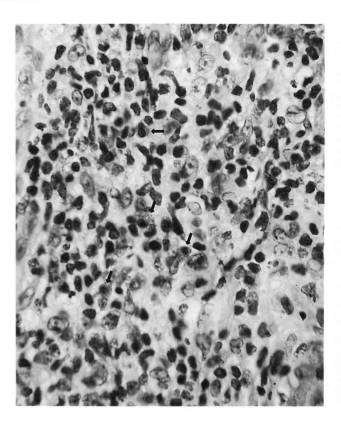

Figure 15–5. Pseudolymphoma. Persistent arthropod assault reaction; polymorphous infiltrate with large and small lymphocytes and scattered eosinophils (arrows) (H&E, ×450).

the skin or may give rise to metastases to soft tissues, lymph node, or bone.[28] Skin involvement in multiple myeloma is discussed in Chapter 56.

Histologic Features

Large nodular aggregates to sheets of plasma cells are present, with varying degrees of atypia, mitotic activity, and maturity (Fig. 15–6). These cells are characterized by their eccentric nuclei and clumped chromatin.

Differential Diagnosis

Poorly differentiated (anaplastic) plasmacytoma merges with B cell lymphoma, highgrade, immunoblastic type. Anaplastic plasmacytoma also may be confused with small cell carcinoma, melanoma, granulocytic sarcoma (chloroma), and mast cell disease. Giemsa and chloroacetate esterase (Leder) stain will help to identify mast cells and myeloid cells (chloroma), respectively, and will not label plasma cells. Immunohistochemical markers for plasma cells, such as immunoglobulins and panleukocyte antigens, and markers of tumors of nonplasma cell origin, such as S100 protein, neuron-specific enolase, and cytokeratins, will aid in the differential diagnosis. Low grade, well-differentiated extramedullary plasmacytomas must be distinguished from reactive plasma cell aggregates. The presence of intracytoplasmic or intranuclear immunoglobulin inclusions

TABLE 15–1. DISCRIMINATING FEATURES BETWEEN REACTIVE GERMINAL CENTERS AND FOLLICLES IN NODULAR LYMPHOMA

Reactive Germinal Centers	Follicles in Nodular Lymphoma
1. May vary in size and shape	1. More regular in size and shape
2. May be numerous, but not crowded back to back	2. Crowded back to back
3. Well-developed paracortical mantle zone	3. No well-developed paracortical mantle zone
4. Mixtures of small and large cells and cleaved and noncleaved cells with polarization (large cells in center; smaller, more mature cells at periphery)	4. One or two cell types with no polarization
5. Tingible body macrophages (large, pale-staining macrophages containing phagocytosed basophilic nuclear and cytoplasmic debris) with starry sky appearance	5. No tingible body macrophages
6. Variable numbers of mitoses	6. Variable numbers of mitoses

TABLE 15–2. DISCRIMINATING FEATURES BETWEEN BENIGN AND MALIGNANT CUTANEOUS LYMPHOID INFILTRATES

Benign	Malignant
1. Architectural pattern Predominantly superficial and perivascular (top heavy); no predominantly deep involvement; no prominent single cell infiltration between collagen bundles	1. Architectural pattern Diffuse, expansive, full-thickness, or predominantly deep involvement without perivascular preference (bottom heavy); fat may be involved; cells are interposed in single columns between collagen bundles (Indian file sign)
2. Recognizable as an organized immune response May be variably sized germinal centers (follicles) and mixtures of cell groups (plasma cells, neutrophils, mast cells); vascular proliferation is prominent; granulomas or multinucleate giant cells may be present	2. No features of an organized immune response No germinal centers (reactive germinal centers must be distinguished from follicles in nodular lymphoma; see Table 15–1); no mixtures of cell groups; vascular proliferation not prominent *Exception:* Foreign body giant cell reactions to ruptured hair follicles may be seen in malignant lymphoma
3. Epidermal reaction Grenz zone is common; if involved, the epidermis shows disruption: hyperkeratosis, parakeratosis, dyskeratosis, spongiosis, basal vacuolar damage; may be epidermal hyperplasia	3. No epidermal reaction Grenz zone is present in B cell lymphoma; no hyperplasia *Exception:* T cell lymphomas often show epidermotrophism, but epidermis shows little reaction to the infiltration
4. Cellular constituency Heterogeneous, polymorphous; may be lymphocytes, plasma cells, eosinophils, neutrophils; if only lymphocytes are present, they appear as predominantly mature small lymphocytes	4. Cellular constituency Homogeneous, monomorphous; if more than one cell type, the combinations are those recognized by lymphoma classification systems, such as small cleaved and large lymphocytes *Exception:* Cutaneous T cell lymphomas may contain mixtures of cell types (i.e., eosinophils, lymphocytes, plasma cells)
5. Cytology Cytologic maturity; if large and mitotically active cells are present, they correspond to benign functional cell types; mitoses not abundant outside of germinal centers	5. Cytology Atypical to bizarre forms not within the limits of activated elements (hyperchromatism, atypical mitoses, notable nuclear membrane complexity); mitoses may be numerous *Exception:* Well-differentiated lymphoma consists of small cytologically mature lymphocytes
6. Immunohistochemistry Mixed infiltrate of polyclonal B cells, T helper cells, T suppressor cells, and dendritic cells	6. Immunohistochemistry B cell lymphoma: monoclonal light chain; T cell lymphoma: variable, but generally one T cell subset to the exclusion of others

(Dutcher bodies) favors neoplasia.[29] These inclusions are enhanced by PAS staining. Admixtures of other cell types favor an inflammatory process. Immunohistochemistry will demonstrate polyclonal light chains in reactive infiltrates and monoclonal light chain expression in true plasmacytoma.[29]

Dense infiltrates of lymphoid cells with differentiation toward plasma cells may be found within the dermis or subcutis of the plaques or nodules that infrequently occur in Waldenstrom's macroglobulinemia.[30] Intranuclear immunoglobulin inclusions may be present.

ANGIOLYMPHOID HYPERPLASIA WITH EOSINOPHILS

This term represents a poorly understood, ill-defined spectrum of vascular tumorlike lesions of the skin. It is included in this section because of the inflammatory component of the lesion, which may be both dense and diffuse, dominating or obscuring the vascular component. A number of designations, including Kimura's disease, pseudopyogenic granuloma, papular angioplasia, inflammatory angiomatous nodule, and histiocytoid hemangioma, have been proposed.

Clinical Features

Lesions may be solitary or multiple and commonly involve the scalp, face, or ears but are occasionally seen at other sites.[31] The lesions appear as light pink to red-brown papules, nodules, or plaques, 0.2–8.0 cm in diameter. Lesions may involve the dermis, the subcutis, or both. The disease is benign, and excision is usually curative, although clinical recurrence has been reported in up to one third of patients.[31] No metastases have been documented. Trauma has been associated in some patients. Lesions are most common in the third and fourth decades of life, and 70% of patients are female.[32] Significant blood eosinophilia is rare. The oriental form is characterized by younger age of onset, male predominance, and more frequent significant blood eosinophilia.[32]

Histologic Features

There are two major components: an anomalous vascular proliferation and an inflammatory infiltrate. Each component has a considerable spectrum of expression in different tumors or in different zones within a single lesion. The process usually involves the dermis but may be entirely subcutaneous. The vascular component comprises thick- and thin-walled vessels, immature small vascular lumina within endothelial aggregates, and open, anastomosing, cleftlike and sinusoidal vascular channels (Fig. 15–7). The

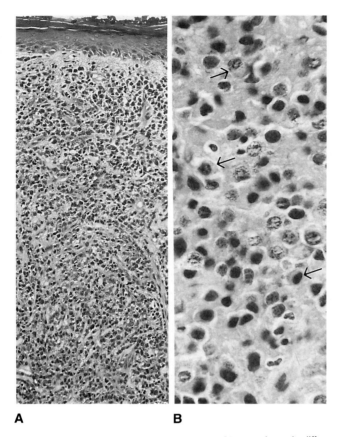

A   **B**

Figure 15–6. Cutaneous plasmacytoma. **A.** Sheets of poorly differentiated cells fill the dermis (H&E, ×125). **B.** Poorly differentiated cells with scattered plasmacytoid cells (arrows) (H&E, ×450).

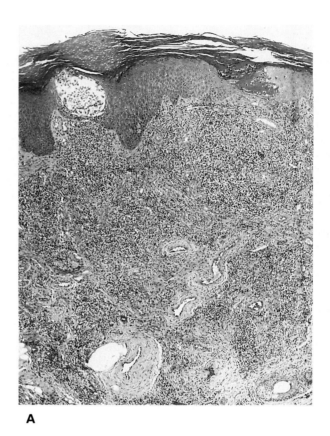

A

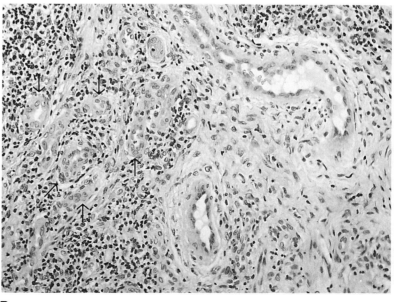

Figure 15–7. Angiolymphoid hyperplasia with eosinophils. **A.** Dense diffuse dermal inflammatory process with vascular proliferation comprising variably sized thick and thin-walled vessels. (H&E, ×45). **B.** Larger thick-walled vessels on left; smaller more immature vessels with endothelial aggregates (arrows) and inflammatory infiltrate on right (H&E, ×225).

B

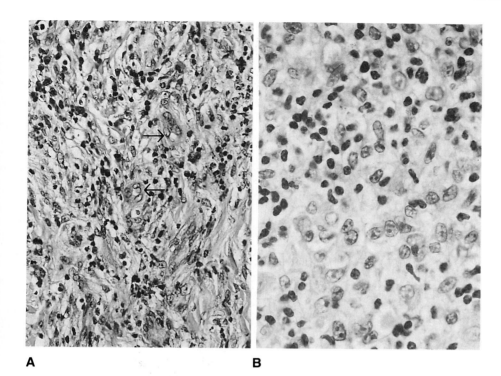

Figure 15–8. Angiolymphoid hyperplasia with eosinophils. **A.** Endothelial aggregates with occasional lumen formation (arrows) and infiltrate rich in lymphocytes, eosinophils, (H&E, ×620). **B.** Small mature lymphocytes admixed with large vesicular endothelial cells (H&E, ×425).

thick-walled vessels may demonstrate an elastic lamina.[33] The endothelial cells within the endothelial cell aggregates and within some of the larger vessels are plump, often histiocytoid, with large vesicular nuclei and rare mitoses (Fig. 15–8). Arteriovenous malformations and intravascular endothelial hyperplasia may be seen.[31] Some lesions are dominated by endothelial cell aggregates, others by large vessel proliferation.

A diffuse inflammatory infiltrate of variable intensity surrounds and infiltrates between the proliferative vascular component. The infiltrate usually is dominated by small and large lymphocytes and eosinophils, with moderate numbers of mast cells and plasma cells. Eosinophils may be few to absent.[34] Germinal center (follicle) formation may be present. The surrounding stroma is both fibrous and myxoid and may contain red cell extravasation and hemosiderin.

The ultrastructure of the histiocytoid endothelial cell demonstrates overlapping characteristics of histiocytes, smooth muscle, and endothelial cells.[34–37]

Immunoperoxidase staining for lysozyme, a histiocytic marker, have been uniformly negative. Factor VIII antigen, an endothelial cell marker, has been identified in the cells lining the large vessels and to a lesser extent in the cells within the endothelial aggregates.[31] These findings suggest proliferation of a stimulated subpopulation of endothelial cells.

Differential Diagnosis

The differential diagnosis includes benign vascular tumors, reactive inflammatory infiltrates, and angiosarcoma. Angiolymphoid hyperplasia with eosinophils can be distinguished by its anomalous vascular hyperplasia with endothelial cell proliferation and lymphocytic infiltration, most often dominated by eosinophils. Unlike angiosarcoma, frank anaplasia of the endothelial cell component and dense sarcomatous proliferation of plump spindled endothelial cells are not found.

ANGIOIMMUNOBLASTIC LYMPHADENOPATHY

Clinical Features

Angioimmunoblastic lymphadenopathy (AILD) is a lymphoproliferative disease occurring in elderly patients and is characterized by generalized lymphadenopathy and hepatosplenomegaly. Many patients also have anemia and hypergammaglobulinemia.[38] Involvement of the skin occurs in about 40% of patients, typically as a generalized maculopapular eruption. Some of the cutaneous manifestations have been attributed to drug reactions.[39] The development of large plaques or nodules has been reported.[40] AILD may be associated with or may evolve into malignant lymphoma, usually of the diffuse, large cell, immunoblastic type.

Histologic Features

Lymphocytic periadnexal and perivascular infiltrates admixed with plasma cells and occasional large immunoblastic mononuclear cells are found. Rarely, a more specific infiltrate of predominantly plasma cells, plasmacytoid cells, and immunoblasts is seen. Vascular proliferation may be present. In reports of plaque and nodule formation, a diffuse monomorphous round cell infiltrate with rare mitoses was found in some biopsies, with nonnecrotizing granulomatous inflammation present in others.[39] The cutaneous findings generally are poorly developed and nondiagnostic but can be suggestive of AILD.

CASTLEMAN'S SUPERFICIAL PSEUDOTUMOR (SUBCUTANEOUS ANGIOFOLLICULAR LYMPHOID HYPERPLASIA)

Clinical Features

Castleman's disease (giant lymph node hyperplasia) is a lymphoproliferative disorder characterized by lymph node hyperplasia, occurring most often as a solitary mediastinal lesion. Multiple lesions as well as occurrence in other locations have been reported. It may occur rarely as an isolated subcutaneous mass in a number of body sites.[41] The evolution is favorable in most cases, and surgical excision ensures recovery.

Histologic Features

Two morphologic variants exist.[42] In the more frequent hyaline vascular variant, concentrically whorled small follicles are present, surrounded by a zone of concentrically arranged (onion skin) small lymphocytes that may obscure the follicular centers. The interfollicular area contains an extensive proliferation of capillaries.

In the rarer plasma cell variant, large, hyperplastic follicular centers are present associated with a highly vascular interfollicular zone rich in plasma cells.

Differential Diagnosis

The lesion must be distinguished from eosinophil-poor angiolymphoid hyperplasia with eosinophils (ALHE). The characteristic vascular proliferation and endothelial cell hyperplasia present in ALHE will distinguish it from the subcutaneous form of Castleman's disease.

PREDOMINANTLY EOSINOPHILIC INFILTRATION

EOSINOPHILIC CELLULITIS (WELLS' SYNDROME)

Clinical Features

The disorder typically occurs as painful or pruritic, erythematous, annular or circinate, edematous plaques resembling cellulitis or urticaria.[43] Lesions may be single or multiple, and blisters may be associated with early lesions. Lesions may persist for weeks, and as they age, they become more firm and blue-green to gray and occasionally resemble morphea. New eruptions are common, however, and the total course rarely may last for years. Sites of predilection are the extremities, buttocks, and trunk. Blood eosinophilia ranging from 2–48% is present in most cases. Eosinophilic cellulitis probably represents a distinctive hypersensitivity reaction pattern secondary to a variety of trigger stimuli, including arthropod assault, parasite infection, dermatophyte infection, atopy, carcinoma, rheumatoid arthritis, and drugs.[43–47] Histologic features of eosinophilic cellulitis have been described associated with various inflammatory dermatoses, including erythema chronicum migrans,[45] bullous pemphigoid, and eczematous dermatitis.[43]

Histologic Features

In early lesions, the dermis is edematous, with a diffuse, often massive, infiltrate of eosinophils admixed with large histiocytic cells separating collagen bundles (Fig. 15–9). The infiltrate is most often concentrated in the deep dermis,

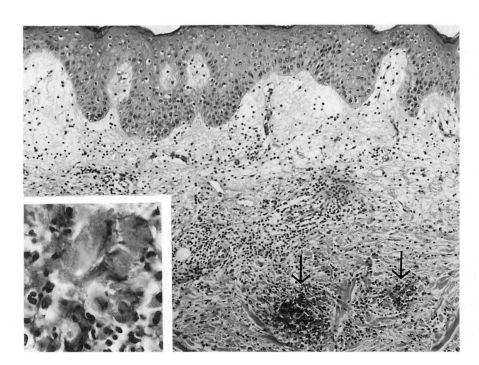

Figure 15–9. Eosinophilic cellulitis. Diffuse infiltrate within reticular dermis associated with papillary dermal edema. Flame figures are present (arrows) (H&E, ×85). **Inset.** Degenerated collagen bundles associated with eosinophilic granules and intact eosinophils (H&E, ×400).

with possible involvement of subcutis, fascia, and skeletal muscle. Panniculitis with massive eosinophilia may be seen.[48] Extreme edema of the papillary dermis may be associated with spongiosis, intraepidermal vesicle formation, or subepidermal bullae. A prominent perivascular component can be seen in addition to the diffuse infiltration. Eosinophils may be found migrating through vessel walls, associated with endothelial cell hypertrophy, focal deposits of fibrin, and red cell extravasation. However, no necrotizing vasculitis is found.

Eosinophilic granular material adheres to collagen fibers, creating the flame figures characteristic of eosinophilic cellulitis (Fig. 15–10). These altered foci of collagen are closely bordered by intact eosinophils or histiocytes, including foreign body type giant cells. Electron microscopic study of the flame figures has demonstrated nondegenerated collagen bundles coated with free eosinophil granules.[49] Flame figures are absent in some cases.[43] As the lesions age, eosinophils decrease in number, and granulomatous features become better developed. The persisting histiocytes and giant cells are present both grouped and scattered diffusely between collagen bundles. Sometimes they are associated with flame figures or with zones of altered collagen that appears similar to that seen in granuloma annulare.

Differential Diagnosis

The absence of both necrotizing vasculitis and large zones of fibroid necrosis helps to distinguish eosinophilic cellulitis from allergic granulomatosis of Churg and Strauss. Infiltrates of histiocytosis X may be rich in eosinophils, but histiocytosis X, unlike eosinophilic cellulitis, displays a predominance of large cells displaying the characteristic features of Langerhans cells.

HYPEREOSINOPHILIC SYNDROME

Clinical Features

Hypereosinophilic syndrome shares some features with eosinophilic cellulitis, and it is, therefore, included in this section. In contrast to eosinophilic cellulitis, hypereosinophilic syndrome is a systemic disorder characterized by organ infiltration by eosinophils associated with hepatosplenomegaly, as well as cardiovascular, pulmonary, neurologic, and dermatologic abnormalities.[50] It is a continuum of disease, with eosinophilic leukemia at one end and asymptomatic patients with skin lesions and heart disease at the other end. One third to one half of patients across the entire spectrum of the disease develop skin lesions.[50,51] Skin involvement consists of a pruritic erythematous maculopapular eruption over the trunk and extremities or urticaria and angioedema of the face and extremities.

Histologic Features

A variable perivascular or periappendageal infiltrate of lymphocytes and eosinophils is present within the dermis and subcutis. Neutrophils and plasma cells may be present. The dense, diffuse infiltrate with flame figures that characterizes eosinophilic cellulitis is not found.

PREDOMINANTLY MAST CELL INFILTRATION

MASTOCYTOSIS

Clinical Features

Diffuse mast cell infiltrates can be associated with cases of urticaria pigmentosa or systemic mast cell disease in

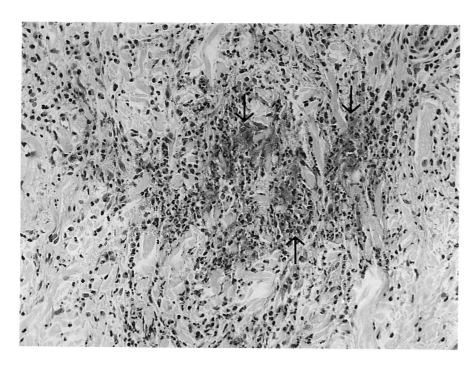

Figure 15–10. Eosinophilic cellulitis. Massive dermal eosinophilic infiltrate with flame figures (arrows) (H&E, ×230).

which either a solitary large nodule or multiple nodules or plaques are present.

Solitary mastocytosis (mastocytoma) accounts for approximately 10% of total cases[52] of mastocytosis. It is observed at birth or within the first month of life but has been reported in adults.[53] The most common location is the dorsal hand, but it can occur anywhere. The solitary mastocytoma is considered the most benign form of mastocytosis, and in most cases, there is spontaneous resolution. Only rarely has progression to widespread urticaria pigmentosa been reported.[54]

Histologic Features

The histopathology of solitary mastocytosis cannot be distinguished from an equivalent plaque or nodular lesion from a patient with urticaria pigmentosa or systemic mastocytosis with multiple lesions.

A dense diffuse infiltrate of oval, round, cuboidal, or elongated spindle cells with granular eosinophilic cytoplasm is found predominantly in the upper dermis but often involves the entire dermis with extension into the subcutis (Figs. 15–11, 15–12). The cytoplasmic granules stain metachromatically with toluidine blue, deep blue with alcian blue, and red-purple with the Giemsa satin (Fig. 15–13). Nuclei are central to eccentrically positioned and are relatively uniform in size and shape. Eosinophils may be present in small numbers. The epidermis may be normal or display acanthosis, ulceration, or bulla formation.

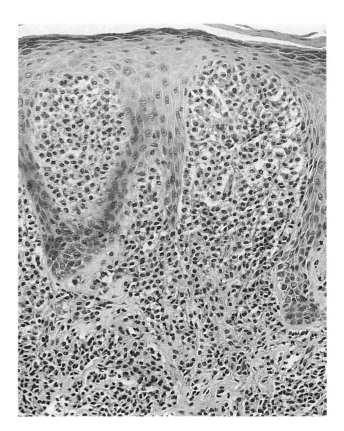

Figure 15–12. Mastocytoma. Predominantly superficial dermal infiltrate of round cells simulating a nevocellular nevus (H&E, ×220).

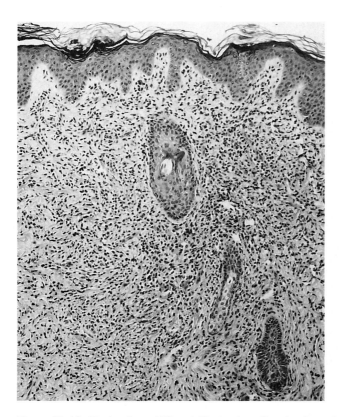

Figure 15–11. Mastocytoma. Diffuse infiltrate of small oval and round spindle cells (H&E, ×110).

Differential Diagnosis

The differential diagnosis includes lymphoma, plasmacytoma, histiocytosis X, and nevocellular nevus. Unlike histiocytosis X, the cells of mastocytosis share no tendency to invade the epidermis; they do not display nesting, junctional activity, or melanin production as expected in a nevus. The demonstration of the characteristic metachromatic granules rules out other infiltrative processes.

PREDOMINANTLY NEUTROPHILIC INFILTRATION

The differential diagnosis of diffuse predominantly neutrophilic infiltrates includes cellulitis, acute febrile neutrophilic dermatosis (Sweet's syndrome), bowel bypass syndrome, erythema elevatum diutinum, granuloma faciale, and leukocytoclastic vasculitis.

PREDOMINANTLY HISTIOCYTIC INFILTRATION

The differential diagnosis of diffuse predominantly histiocytic infiltrates is broad and includes xanthoma, xanthogranuloma, reticulohistiocytosis, histiocytoma, malakopla-

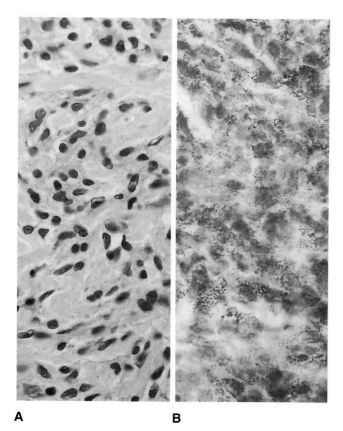

A　　　　　　**B**

Figure 15–13. Mastocytoma. **A.** Round, oval, and spindle mast cells with some degree of cytoplasmic granularity (H&E, ×550). **B.** Metachromatic cytoplasmic granules demonstrated with Giemsa stain (×550).

kia, histiocytosis X, regressing atypical histiocytosis, and malignant histiocytosis.

REFERENCES

1. Anderson BL, Brandrup F, Petri J. Lymphocytoma cutis: A pseudomalignancy treated with penicillin. *Acrta Derm Venereol (Stockh)*. 1986;66:213–219.
2. Blumental G, Okun MR, Ponitch JA. Pseudolymphomatous reaction to tattoos. *J Am Acad Dermatol*. 1982;6:485–488.
3. Barr-Nea L, Sandbank M, Ishay J. Pseudolymphoma of skin induced by oriental hornet venom. *Experientia*. 1926;32:1564–1565.
4. Bernstein H, Shupack J, Ackerman AB. Cutaneous pseudolymphoma resulting from antigen injections. *Arch Dermatol*. 1974;110:756–757.
5. Gross PR. Benign lymphoid hyperplasia (lymphocytoma cutis). *Arch Dermatol*. 1971;103:347–349.
6. Sanchez JL, Mendez JA, Palacio R. Cutaneous pseudolymphoma at the site of resolving herpes zoster. *Arch Dermatol*. 1981;117:377.
7. Bork K. Multiple lymphocytoma cutis following acupuncture. *Hautarzt*. 1983;34:496–499.
8. Mach KW, Wilgram GF. Characteristic histopathology of cutaneous lymphoplasia (lymphocytoma). *Arch Dermatol*. 1966; 94:26–32.
9. Saltzstein SL, Ackerman LV. Lymphadenopathy induced by anticonvulsant drugs and mimicking clinically and pathologically malignant lymphomas. *Cancer*. 1959;12:164–182.
10. Gams RA, Neal JA, Conrad FD. Hydantoin-induced pseudolymphoma. *Ann Intern Med*. 1968;69:557–568.
11. Adams JD. Localized cutaneous pseudolymphoma associated with phenytoin therapy: A case report. *Aust J Dermatol*. 1981;22:28–29.
12. Rosenthal CJ, Noguera CA, Coppola A, Kapelner SN. Pseudolymphoma with mycosis fungoides manifestations, hyperresponsiveness to diphenylhydantoin, and lymphocyte disregulation. *Cancer*. 1982;49:2305–2314.
13. Gilkes JH, Monro DD. Lymphocytoma cutis. *Br J Clin Pract*. 1974;28:157–162.
14. Caro WA, Helwig EB. Cutaneous lymphoid hyperplasia. *Cancer*. 1969;24:487–502.
15. Shelley WB, Wood MG, Wilson JF, Goodman R. Premalignant lymphoid hyperplasia. *Arch Dermatol*. 1981;117:500–503.
16. Burke JS, Hoppe RT, Cibull ML, Dorfman RF. Cutaneous malignant lymphoma: A pathologic study of 50 cases with clinical analysis of 37. *Cancer*. 1981;47:300–310.
17. Wantzin GL, Hou-Jensen K, Nielsen M, et al. Cutaneous lymphocytomas: Clinical and histologic aspects. *Acta Derm Venereol (Stock)*. 1982;62:119–124.
18. Clark WH, Mihm MC, Reed RJ, Ainsworth AM. The lymphocytic infiltrates of the skin. *Hum Pathol*. 1974;5:25–43.
19. Ralfkiaer E, Wantzin GL, Mason DY, et al. Characterization of benign cutaneous lymphocytic infiltrates by monoclonal antibodies. *Br J Dermatol*. 1984;111:635–645.
20. Hale HM, Winkelmann RK. Nodular lymphoid disease of the head and neck: Lymphocytoma cutis, benign lymphocytic infiltrate of Jessner, and their distinction from malignant lymphoma. *J Am Acad Dermatol*. 1985;12:455–461.
21. Wirt DP, Grogan TM, Jolley CS, et al. The immunoarchitecture of cutaneous pseudolymphoma. *Hum Pathol*. 1985;16:492–510.
22. Payne CM, Grogan TM, Lynch PJ. An ultrastructural morphometric and immunohistochemical study of cutaneous lymphomas and benign lymphocytic infiltrates of the skin. *Arch Dermatol*. 1986;122:1139–1153.
23. Tosca AD, Varelzidis AG, Economidan J, Stratigos JD. Mycosis fungoides: Evaluation of immunohistochemical criteria for the early diagnosis of the disease and differentiation between stages. *J Am Acad Dermatol*. 1986;15:237–245.
24. Buechner SA, Winkelmann RK, Banks PM. T cells and T cell subsets in mycosis fungoides and parapsoriasis. *Arch Dermatol*. 1984;120:897–905.
25. Minden MD, Toyonaga B, Ha K, et al. Somatic rearrangement of T cell antigen receptor gene in human T cell malignancies. *Proc Natl Acad Sci USA*. 1985;82:1224–1227.
26. Waldmann TA, Davis MM, Bongiovanni KF, Korsmeyer SJ. Rearrangements of genes for the antigen receptor on T cell as markers of lineage and clonality in human lymphoid neoplasms. *N Engl J Med*. 1985;313:776–783.
27. LaPerriere RJ, Wolf JE, Gellin GA. Primary cutaneous plasmacytoma. *Arch Dermatol*. 1973;107:99–102.
28. Mikhail GR, Spindler AC, Kelly AP. Malignant plasmacytoma cutis. *Arch Dermatol*. 1970;101:59–62.
29. Banks PM. Lymphoid neoplasms of the skin. In: Wick MR, ed. *Pathology of Unusual Malignant Cutaneous Tumors*. New York: Marcel Dekker; 1985:332–335.
30. Mascaro JM, Montserrat E, Estrach T, et al. Specific cutaneous manifestations of Waldenstrom's macroglobulinemia. A report of two cases. *Br J Dermatol*. 1982;106:217–222.
31. Olsen TG, Helwig EB. Angiolymphoid hyperplasia with eosinophilia. A clinicopathologic study of 116 patients. *J Am Acad Dermatol*. 1985;12:781–796.

32. Henry PG, Burnett JW. Angiolymphoid hyperplasia with eosinophilia. *Arch Dermatol.* 1978;114:1168–1172.

33. Moesner J, Palleson R, Sorensen B. Angiolymphoid hyperplasia with eosinophilia (Kimura's disease). *Arch Dermatol.* 1981;117:650–563.

34. Burrall BA, Barr RJ, King DF. Cutaneous histiocytoid hemangioma. *Arch Dermatol.* 1982;118:166–170.

35. Waldo E, Sidhu GS, Stahl R, Zolla-Pazners. Histiocytoid hemangioma with features of angiolymphoid hyperplasia and Kaposi's sarcoma. *Am J Dermatopathol.* 1983;5:525–538.

36. Castro C, Winkelmann RK. Angiolymphoid hyperplasia with eosinophils in the skin. *Cancer.* 1974;34:1696–1705.

37. Eady RAJ, Wilson-Jones E. Pseudopyogenic granuloma: Enzyme histochemical and ultrastructural study. *Hum Pathol.* 1977;8:653–668.

38. Nathwani BN, Winberg CD, Bearman RM. Angioimmunoblastic lymphadenopathy with dysproteinemia and its progression to malignant lymphoma. In: Jaffe ES, ed. *Surgical Pathology of the Lymph Nodes and Related Organs.* Philadelphia: WB Saunders; 1985:57–85.

39. Matloff RB, Neiman RS. Angioimmunoblastic lymphadenopathy. *Arch Dermatol.* 1978;114:92–94.

40. Frizzera G, Moran EM, Rappaport H. Angioimmunoblastic lymphadenopathy: Diagnosis and clinical course. *Am J Med.* 1975;59:803–817.

41. Grossin M, Crickx B, Aitken G, et al. Subcutaneous forms of the Castleman's benign lymphoma. *Ann Dermatol Venereol.* 1985;112:497–506.

42. Keller AR, Hochholzer L, Castleman B. Hyaline-vascular and plasma cell types of giant lymph node hyperplasia of the mediastinum and other locations. *Cancer.* 1972;29:670–683.

43. Wells GC, Smith NP. Eosinophilic cellulitis. *Br J Dermatol.* 1979;100:101–109.

44. Fisher GB, Greer KE, Cooper PH. Eosinophilic cellulitis (Wells' syndrome). *Int J Dermatol.* 1985;24:101–107.

45. Schorr WF, Tauscheck AL, Dickson KB, Melski JW. Eosinophilic cellulitis (Wells' syndrome): Histologic and clinical features in arthropod bite reactions. *J Am Acad Dermatol.* 1984;11:1043–1049.

46. Van der Hoogenband HM. Eosinophilic cellulitis as a result of onchocerciasis. *Clin Exp Dermatol.* 1973;8:405–408.

47. Spigel GT, Winkelmann RK. Wells' syndrome: Recurrent granulomatous dermatitis with eosinophilia. *Arch Dermatol.* 1979;115:611–613.

48. Winkelmann RK, Frigas E. Eosinophilic panniculitis: A clinicopathologic study. *J Cutan Pathol.* 1986;13:1–12.

49. Stern JB, Sobel HJ, Rotchford JP. Wells' syndrome: Is there collagen damage in the flame figures? *J Cutan Pathol.* 1984;11:501–505.

50. Kazmierowski JA, Chusid MJ, Parrillo JE, et al. Dermatologic manifestations of the hypereosinophilic syndrome. *Arch Dermatol.* 1978;114:531–535.

51. Chusid MJ, Dale DC, West BC, et al. The hypereosinophilic syndrome: Analysis of fourteen cases with review of the literature. *Medicine* (Baltimore). 1975;54:1–27.

52. Johnson WC, Helwig EB. Solitary mastocytosis (urticaria pigmentosa). *Arch Dermatol.* 1961;84:148–157.

53. Caplan RM. The natural course of urticaria pigmentosa: Analysis and follow-up of 112 cases. *Arch Dermatol.* 1963;87:56–67.

54. Lantis SH, Koblenzer PJ. Solitary mast cell tumor: Progression to disseminated urticaria pigmentosa in a Negro infant. *Arch Dermatol.* 1969;99:60–63.

CHAPTER 16

Predominantly Mononuclear Cell Granulomas

Clifton R. White, Jr.

Granulomatous dermatitis may be defined simply as an inflammatory process in the skin in which the preponderant inflammatory cells are histiocytes. An exception to this definition is the presence of multinucleated histiocytes (giant cells), which may be few in number but connote granulomatous inflammation as well. Accordingly, an extremely diverse group of diseases is characterized during their evolution by granulomatous inflammation. For example, numerous cutaneous infections, such as tuberculosis in its many manifestations, leprosy, leishmaniasis, syphilis, and many deep fungal infections, as well as numerous noninfectious conditions, including sarcoidosis, rosacea, halogenodermas, and foreign body reactions, may be classified as granulomatous dermatitis. Not surprisingly, the histology of granulomatous diseases is as varied as the provoking factors but falls generally into two major microscopic categories:[1] nodular collections of histiocytes filling portions of but not the entire dermis (Fig. 16–1) and more diffusely scattered granulomatous inflammation involving most or all of the dermis (Fig. 16–2). Nodular granulomatous infiltrates are frequently, although not always, composed entirely of histiocytes and lymphocytes and, hence, may be termed predominantly mononuclear cell granulomas. In contrast, diffuse granulomatous inflammation often is characterized by histiocytes intermixed with other inflammatory cells (neutrophils, eosinophils) and may be termed mixed cell granulomas (Chapter 17).

Other histologic features also help distinguish these two patterns. Many mononuclear cell granulomas are composed of epithelioid histiocytes, so named because when viewed through the microscope, their close proximity to one another, their recognizable cytoplasm, and their indistinct cell borders impart an epithelial quality to these mesenchymally derived inflammatory cells (Fig. 16–3). Accumulations of epithelioid histiocytes are called tubercles, which may or may not develop central necrosis (Fig. 16–4). In contrast, mixed cell granulomas frequently are accompanied by pseudoepitheliomatous hyperplasia with diffuse histiocytic infiltrates, rather than epithelioid tubercles.

Typically, cutaneous granulomatous diseases are char-

acterized either by mononuclear granulomas (nodular pattern), such as sarcoid and its mimics, several forms of tuberculosis, palisaded granulomatous diseases (granuloma annulare, necrobiosis lipoidica), and some stages of foreign body reactions or by mixed cell granulomas (diffuse pattern), as in numerous deep fungal and atypical mycobacterial diseases, halogenodermas, and some foreign body reactions as well.[1] The terms granuloma and granulomatous inflammation are interchangeable, although granuloma often implies closely aggregated epithelioid histiocytes (tubercles, or mononuclear granulomas), whereas granulomatous inflammation may refer also to cells dispersed through the dermis.

Multinucleated histiocytes (giant cells), common generally in granulomatous dermatitis, are of three histologic types. Although none is diagnostic of any specific disease, some conditions usually are characterized by one or another of the three types. The most common giant cell is the foreign body type, without particular geometric orientation of its multiple nuclei (Fig 16–5). Langhans giant cells have wreath-like, or annular, arrangements of nuclei (Fig. 16–6). Finally, Touton multinucleated histiocytes also have circularly arranged nuclei but with amphophilic, slightly granular cytoplasm centrally and paler, foamy cytoplasm peripheral to the nuclear wreath (Fig. 16–7). Some multinucleated histiocytes may show characteristics of several "classic" giant cells, further evidence of their nonspecificity (Figure 16–8).

SARCOIDOSIS

Clinical Features

Sarcoidosis is a systemic granulomatous disease with variable cutaneous manifestations.[2] Although it was described by Sir Jonathan Hutchinson in 1875,[3] Caesar Boeck first coined the term "multiple benign sarkoid" in 1899.[4] Commonly, chronic cutaneous sarcoid consists of orangish brown or red papules or plaques that occasionally may have an annular configuration.[5-7] Lesions involving the nose, cheeks, and ears have been termed lupus pernio.

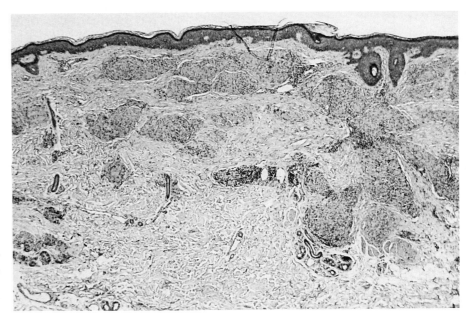

Figure 16–1. Predominantly mononuclear cell granuloma, or nodular granulomatous dermatitis. Scanning power of numerous epithelioid cell tubercles scattered throughout the dermis in sarcoidosis (H&E, ×25).

Less frequent manifestations include lichenoid papules,[8,9] erythroderma,[10,11] and ichthyosiform,[12,13] ulcerating,[14] or hypopigmented[15] lesions. Sarcoidosis also may involve the subcutaneous fat alone, as described by Darier and Rousey,[16–19] or in conjunction with dermal nodules.[11]

Another presentation is subacute, transient sarcoidosis characterized by erythema nodosum associated with hilar adenopathy, fever, migrating polyarthritis, and acute iritis. The course is typically short-lived, with spontaneous resolution.[5,20]

Histologic Features

In sarcoidosis, noncaseating tubercles composed of large, plump epithelioid histiocytes are found throughout the der-mis and, at times, the subcutaneous fat (Fig. 16–9).[21] The tubercles are variously sized, may contain occasional multinucleated cells (usually Langhans type), and typically have scant lymphocytes at their peripheries (naked tubercle) (Fig. 16–10). Occasionally, small areas of coagulation necrosis or fibrin may be present in the centers of some tubercles. Infrequently, cytoplasmic inclusions, such as asteroid and Schaumann bodies, may be present, although neither is specific for sarcoidosis. Asteroid bodies are stellate eosinophilic inclusions (Fig. 16–11), and Schaumann bodies are round to oval, laminated, calcified inclusions.

Not all cases of sarcoidosis show naked tubercles. Rather, a range exists within the histologic spectrum of sarcoidosis from the characteristic tubercles without sur-

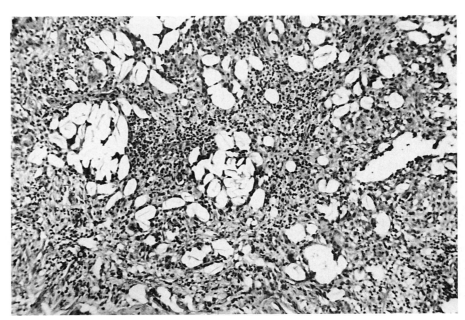

Figure 16–2. Mixed cell granuloma, or diffuse granulomatous dermatitis. Low power shows the entire dermis filled with histiocytes, lymphocytes, and neutrophils as well as cornified cells from a ruptured follicular cyst (H&E, ×63).

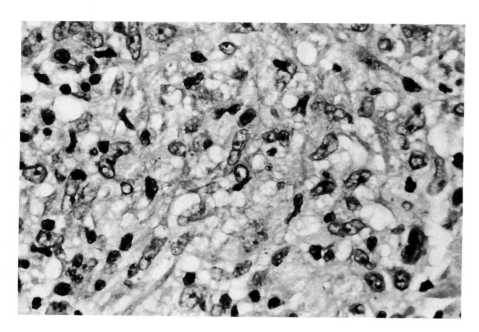

Figure 16–3. Epithelioid histiocytes with scattered lymphocytes. The histiocytes have large, pale nuclei and indistinct cytoplasmic boundaries, giving them an epithelial appearance (H&E, ×400).

rounding lymphocytic inflammation to unusual cases with dense lymphocytic and plasmocytic infiltrates around and within the nodular histiocytic aggregates. In addition, it should be emphasized that sarcoidosis is a diagnosis of exclusion. Great care should be taken when dealing with sarcoidal inflammation to identify other potential histologic mimics, such as zirconium,[22] beryllium, or silica granulomas. In the case of zirconium and beryllium, careful attention to historical review, as well as special laboratory techniques (histochemical, microincineration, or spectrophotometric), may be required to identify the causative agents. Alternatively, examination with polarizing lenses may reveal doubly refractile particles of silica,[23] usually a result of traumatic implantation (glass, sand, gravel), which

cause granulomas indistinguishable from sarcoidosis. Special stains for acid-fast, fungal, protozoan, and spirochetal organisms as well as culture of involved tissue should be obtained to identify or eliminate possible infectious causes.[24] Other clinical or laboratory investigations, including radiographic and ophthalmologic screens and skin tests (Kveim), may be necessary to substantiate the diagnosis of sarcoidosis.

Differential Diagnosis

As aforementioned, the light microscopic changes seen in systemic beryllium, zirconium, and silica granulomas are indistinguishable from sarcoidosis.

Certain infections, including tuberculoid leprosy and

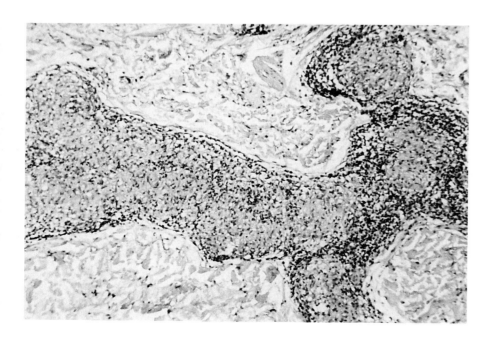

Figure 16–4. Tubercles composed of epithelioid histiocytes with few scattered lymphocytes ("naked" tubercle, characteristic of sarcoidosis) (H&E, ×63).

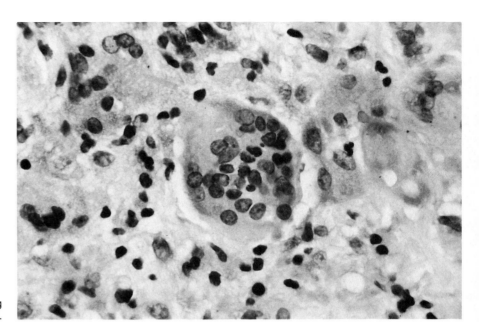

Figure 16–5. Foreign body giant cell, lacking geometric distribution of nuclei (H&E, ×400).

lupus vulgaris, also may closely resemble cutaneous sarcoidosis. In tuberculoid leprosy, crucial clues to diagnosis include inflammation within and around peripheral nerves (where acid-fast *Mycobacterium leprae* occasionally may be demonstrated with special stains), elongated tubercles (reflecting nerve involvement), and denser collections of lymphocytes and plasma cells around the tubercles. Histologic features, including caseation necrosis within the central portion of tubercles, denser collections of peripheral lymphocytes, and frequent epidermal changes, such as ulceration or hyperplasia (at times, pseudoepitheliomatous), characterize lupus vulgaris and usually allow distinction from sarcoidosis.

Depending on the clinical history and symptoms accompanying the skin lesions, Crohn's disease, cheilitis granulomatosa, and granulomatous rosacea must be included in the differential diagnosis.

BERYLLIUM AND ZIRCONIUM GRANULOMAS

Clinical Features

Cutaneous berylliosis occurs at sites of lacerations from beryllium-containing fluorescent light bulbs, as well as at beryllium patch test sites in sensitized individuals.[25,26] Zirconium granulomas typically occur in the axillae of sensi-

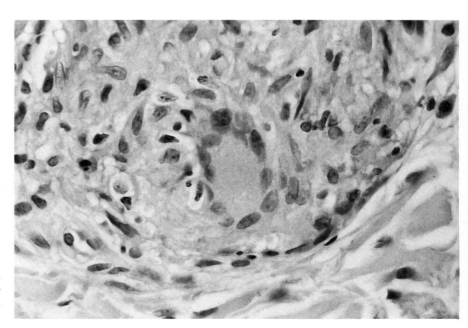

Figure 16–6. Langhans multinucleated histiocyte (giant cell) with characteristic annular configuration of nuclei and granular cytoplasm (H&E, ×400).

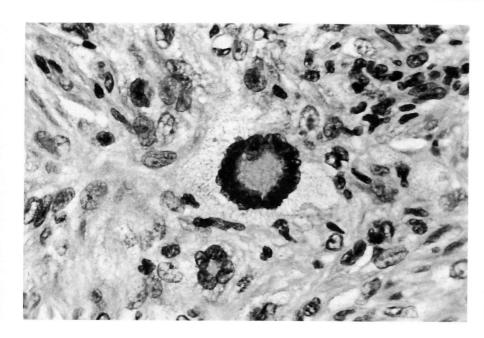

Figure 16–7. Touton giant cell with circularly arranged nuclei, central amphophilic cytoplasm, and peripheral foamy cytoplasm (or a "two-tone" giant cell) (H&E, ×400).

tized patients using zirconium-containing deodorants or elsewhere from poison ivy remedies.[22,27,28]

Histologic Features

Both beryllium and zirconium granulomas show large, epithelioid cell, mononuclear granulomas, with few peripheral lymphocytes, identical to the changes seen in sarcoidosis. In some cases, localized berylliosis may show tubercles with prominent central necrosis,[29] more closely simulating cutaneous tuberculosis. In both zirconium and beryllium granulomas, the metallic particles are not visualized by polarized light but may be demonstrated by spectrographic analysis.[30]

Differential Diagnosis
See sarcoidosis.

CHEILITIS GRANULOMATOSA

Clinical Features
Cheilitis granulomatosa (Miescher-Melkersson-Rosenthal syndrome) was described by Melkersson in 1928 as facial palsy associated with swelling of the lip. In 1930, Rosenthal expanded the syndrome to include lingua plicata (scrotal tongue) and genetic factors.[31] Patients with cheilitis granulo-

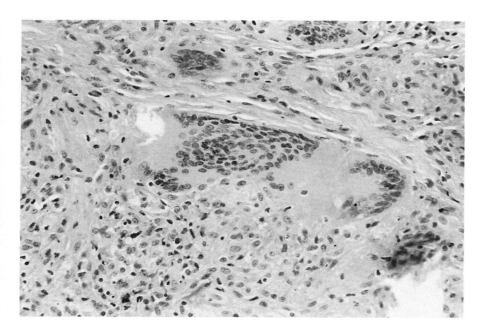

Figure 16–8. Enormous multinucleated histiocyte with numerous nuclei, with foreign body appearance centrally and arcuate Langhans appearance at right end (H&E, ×250).

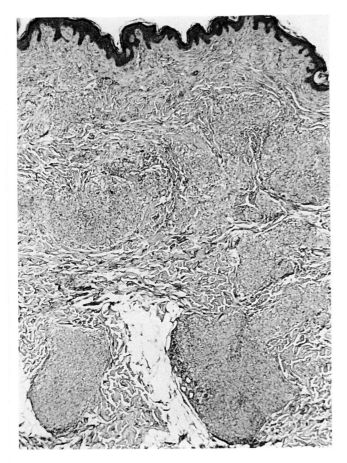

Figure 16–9. Sarcoidosis. Numerous epithelioid tubercles with few peripheral lymphocytes ("naked" tubercles). Note involvement of both dermis and subcutaneous fat (H&E, ×25).

matosa develop intermittent, recurrent labial edema as well as swelling of the central face, including the forehead, eyelids, chin, cheeks, and tongue.[32,33] After recurrent attacks, the swelling may persist and become firm. Facial paralysis occurs in about one third of patients and may precede or succeed the facial edema. Other cranial nerves may be involved, including the olfactory, auditory, glossopharyngeal, and hypopharyngeal.

Histologic Features
In lip or skin biopsies, there are epithelioid tubercles without surrounding lymphocytes (sarcoidal or naked tubercles), as well as perivascular mononuclear cell infiltrates of lymphocytes and plasma cells.[34,35] The infiltrate may be deeply extending, involving muscle.[36] Lymph nodes may be involved and show the same histologic features as the skin. A genital counterpart to cheilitis granulomatosa has been described.[37]

Differential Diagnosis
Although the individual tubercles of cheilitis granulomatosa may be indistinguishable from sarcoidosis, the characteristic clinical features and unusual anatomic location of the former usually allow differentiation between the diseases. The other entities discussed in this chapter, such as granulomatous rosacea, foreign body granuloma, Crohn's disease, and infectious granulomas, must be considered in the differential diagnosis.

CROHN'S DISEASE (REGIONAL ENTERITIS)

Historical and Clinical Features
Crohn's disease, first described in 1932,[38] is characterized by segmental granulomatous inflammation of the intestinal tract[39] and frequently involves cutaneous tissues as well.

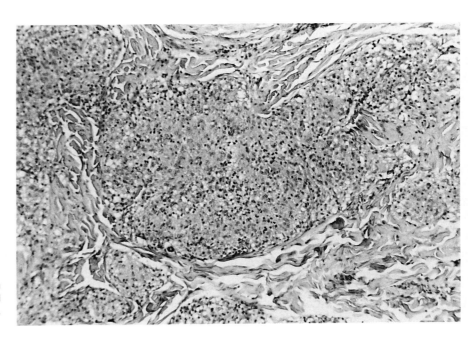

Figure 16–10. Sarcoidosis. Tubercles with occasional lymphocytes scattered around and within the histiocyte collections (H&E, ×63).

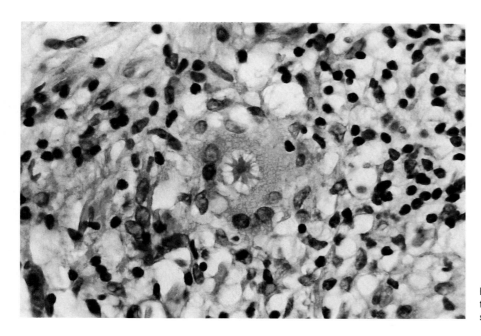

Figure 16–11. Asteroid body within the cytoplasm of a multinucleated histiocyte in sarcoidosis (H&E, ×400).

Perianal lesions, which may extend to adjacent perineum, buttocks, or abdomen, may consist of ulcers, fissures, sinus tracts, or vegetating lesions.[40] Abdominal surgical sites, such as laparotomy scars, colostomies, and ileostomies, also may be sites of Crohn's inflammation. Rarely, skin involvement distant from the perirectal area occurs, such as in retroauricular sites[41] or extremities.[42-44] Oral ulcerations,[45,46] cheilitis,[47] and erythema nodosum also may occur.

Histologic Features

The cutaneous perianal and oral lesions of Crohn's disease consist of nodular, noncaseating epithelioid tubercles with surrounding lymphocytes.[42] The histopathologic changes are the same as those seen in intestinal lesions.

In some erythema nodosum lesions, vasculitis may be present, characterized by fibrin deposition, occlusion, and inflammation, which may be granulomatous.[48,49]

Differential Diagnosis

The histologic picture of cutaneous Crohn's disease is, at times, indistinguishable from other tuberculoid diseases, including lupus vulgaris. Central necrosis in tubercles in the latter is a helpful distinguishing clue. Cutaneous lesions of Crohn's disease may have striking similarity to sarcoidosis, although denser lymphocytic collections in the former may help in differentiation. Zirconium and beryllium granulomas, foreign body granulomas, and infectious granulomas must also be considered in the histologic differential diagnosis.

GRANULOMATOUS ROSACEA

Among the varied histologic changes seen in rosacea, one typical but less common pattern is epithelioid tubercles formed in response to follicular injury and rupture. The

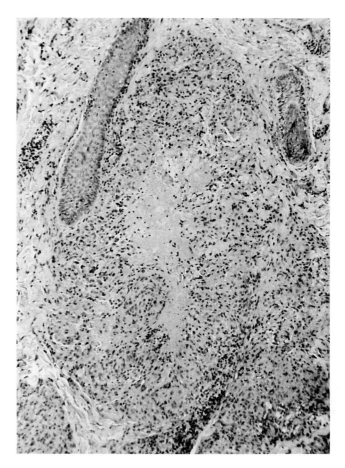

Figure 16–12. Granulomatous rosacea. Epithelioid tubercle is between two vellus follicles of the face. Note central necrosis, giving a striking resemblance to cutaneous tuberculosis; hence, the synonym, lupus miliaris disseminatus faciei (H&E, ×63).

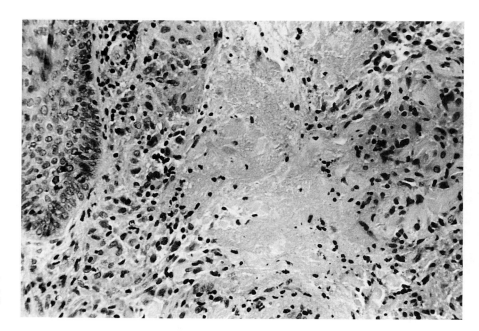

Figure 16–13. Granulomatous rosacea. Higher power showing epithelioid tubercle, central necrosis, and scattered lymphocytes adjacent to vellus follicle (H&E, ×250).

tubercles often may have central necrosis and peripheral lymphocytes showing striking similarity to some forms of cutaneous tuberculosis (tuberculoid pattern).[50,51] This histologic similarity has resulted in a plethora of synonyms for granulomatous rosacea (micropapular tuberculid, tuberculid-like rosacea, rosacea-like tuberculid, lupus miliaris disseminatus faciei). Although the histologic changes of granulomatous rosacea are not distinguishable from cutaneous tuberculosis, often the histiocytic collections in rosacea are juxtaposed between, beneath, or near vellus follicles of the face (Figs. 16–12, 16–13). The granulomatous inflammation is almost certainly a response to follicular contents, such as cornified cells, sebum, or *Demodex*, released from the damaged adnexae.[50] Other aspects of rosacea are covered in Chapter 58.

FOREIGN BODY GRANULOMAS

At one point in their evolution, inflammatory reactions to ruptured follicular cysts in nonrosacea conditions as well as reactions to other types of foreign bodies may be almost purely granulomatous, such as those simulating sarcoidosis (e.g., due to silicates). More frequently, however, foreign body reactions are mixed in character, including neutrophils, eosinophils, or plasma cells (Chapter 17).

MONONUCLEAR GRANULOMAS CAUSED BY INFECTIOUS AGENTS

A number of diseases characterized by mononuclear granulomas are caused by infectious agents. These include cutaneous tuberculosis (lupus vulgaris, scrofuloderma), tuberculoid leprosy, chronic cutaneous leishmaniasis, and late secondary and tertiary syphilis. Each may have nodular epithelioid tubercles with dense accumulations of sur-

rounding lymphocytes and plasma cells. Each of these diseases is characterized by predominantly mononuclear granulomas.

REFERENCES

1. Ackerman AB. *Histologic Diagnosis of Inflammatory Skin Diseases.* Philadelphia: Lea & Febiger; 1978.
2. Izumi T. Sarcoidosis. *Clin Dermatol.* 1986;4:1–170.
3. Hutchinson J. Illustrations of clinical surgery. *N Engl J Med.* 1936;214:346–352.
4. Boeck C. Multiple benign sarcoid of the skin. *J Cutan Genitourin Dis.* 1899;17:543.
5. Umbert P, Winkelmann RK. Granuloma annulare and sarcoidosis. *Br J Dermatol.* 1977;97:481–486.
6. Veien NK. Cutaneous sarcoidosis treated with levamisole. *Dermatologica.* 1977;154:185–189.
7. Hanno R, Needelman A, Eiferman RA, et al. Cutaneous sarcoidal granulomas and the development of systemic sarcoidosis. *Arch Dermatol.* 1981;117:203–207.
8. Brunner MJ, Robin M. Lichen scrofulosorum-like lesions associated with sarcoidosis. *Arch Dermatol Syph.* 1949;60:1212–1214.
9. Nozaki T. Sarcoidosis with lichenoid type eruption. *Jpn J Dermatol.* 1972;82:47–54.
10. Morrison JGL. Sarcoidosis in a child, presenting as an erythroderma with keratotic spines and palmar pits. *Br J Dermatol.* 1976;95:93–97.
11. Lever WF, Freiman DG. Sarcoidosis: A report of a case with erythrodermic lesions, subcutaneous nodes and asteroid inclusion bodies in giant cells. *Arch Dermatol Syph.* 1948;57:639–654.
12. Kauh YC, Goody HE, Luscombe HA. Ichthyosiform sarcoidosis. *Arch Dermatol.* 1978;114:100–101.
13. Kelly AP. Ichthyosiform sarcoid. *Arch Dermatol.* 1978;114:1551–1552.
14. Saxe N, Benatar SR, Bok L, Gordon W. Sarcoidosis with leg ulcers and annular facial lesions. *Arch Dermatol.* 1984;120:93–96.
15. Clayton R, Breathnach A, Martin B, Feiwel M. Hypopigmented sarcoidosis in the Negro. *Br J Dermatol.* 1977;96:119–125.

16. Darier J, Rousey G. Des sarcoids sous-cutaneous. *Arch Med Exp Anat Pathol.* 1906;18:1–50.
17. Vainsencher D, Winkelmann RK. Subcutaneous sarcoidosis. *Arch Dermatol.* 1984;120:1028–1031.
18. Clayton R, Wood PL. Subcutaneous nodular sarcoid. *Dermatologica.* 1974;149:51–54.
19. Gross MD, Andriacci F, Gordon R, et al. Nodular subcutaneous sarcoidosis. *Arch Dermatol.* 1977;113:1442–1443.
20. James DG, Siltzbach LE, Sharma OP, et al. A tale of two cities. A comparison of sarcoidosis in London and New York. *Arch Intern Med.* 1969;123:187–191.
21. Barrie HJ, Bogoch A. The natural history of the sarcoid granuloma. *Am J Pathol.* 1953;29:451–469.
22. Shelley WB, Hurley HJ. The allergic origin of zirconium deodorant granulomas. *Br J Dermatol.* 1958;70:75–101.
23. Terzakis TA, Shustak SR, Stock EG. Talc granuloma identified by x-ray microanalysis. *JAMA.* 1978;239:2371–2372.
24. Gibson LE, Winkelmann RK. The diagnosis and differential diagnosis of cutaneous sarcoidosis. *Clin Dermatol.* 1986;4:62–74.
25. Sneddon IB. Berylliosis: A case report. *Br J Med.* 1955;1:1448.
26. Epstein WL. Metal-induced granulomatous hypersensitivity in man. *Adv Biol Skin.* 1971;11:313–335.
27. Shelley WB, Hurley HJ. Experimental evidence for an allergic basis for granuloma formation in man. *Nature.* 1957;180:1060.
28. Epstein WL. Granulomatous hypersensitivity. *Prog Allergy.* 1967;11:36–88.
29. Neave HJ, Frank SB, Tolmach J. Cutaneous granulomas following laceration by fluorescent light bulbs. *Arch Dermatol Syph.* 1950;61:401–406.
30. Boler GR. Granulomas from topical zirconium in poison ivy dermatitis. *Arch Dermatol.* 1965;91:145–148.
31. Hornseien OP. *Curr Probl Dermatol.* 1973;5:117–120.
32. Layman CW. Cheilitis granulomatosa and Melkersson-Rosenthal syndrome. *Arch Dermatol.* 1963;83:112–118.
33. Cerimele D, Serri F. Cheilitis granulomatosa. *Arch Dermatol.* 1965;92:695–696.
34. Rhodes EL, Stirling GA. Granulomatous cheilitis. *Arch Dermatol.* 1965;92:40–44.
35. Kintchkoff D, James R. Cheilitis granulomatosa. *Arch Dermatol.* 1978;114:1203–1206.
36. White IR, Souteryrand P, MacDonald DM. Granulomatous cheilitis (Miescher). *Clin Exp Dermatol.* 1981;6:391–397.
37. Westermark P, Henriksson TG. Granulomatous inflammation of the vulva and penis, a genital counterpart to cheilitis granulomatosa. *Dermatologica.* 1979;158:269–274.
38. Crohn BB, Gingburg L, Oppenheimer GD. Regional ileitis; pathologic and clinical entity. *JAMA.* 1932;99:1323–1329.
39. Crohn BB, Yarnis H. *Regional Ileitis.* 2nd ed. New York: Grune & Stratton; 1958.
40. McCallum DI, KiniMont PDC. Dermatologic manifestations of Crohn's disease. *Br J Dermatol.* 1968;80:1–8.
41. McCallum DI, Gray WM. Metastatic Crohn's disease. *Br J Dermatol.* 1976;95:551–554.
42. Witkowski JA, Parish LC, Lewis JE. Crohn's disease, noncaseating granulomas on the legs. *Acta Derm Venereol (Stockh).* 1977;57:181–183.
43. Levine N, Bangert J. Cutaneous granulomatosis in Crohn's disease. *Arch Dermatol.* 1982;118:1006–1009.
44. Liebermann TR, Greene JF Jr. Transient subcutaneous granulomatosis of the upper extremities in Crohn's disease. *Am J Gastroenterol.* 1979;72:89–90.
45. Croft CB, Wilkinson AR. Ulceration of the mouth, pharynx, and larynx. *Br J Surg.* 1972;59:249–252.
46. Taylor VE, Smith CJ. Oral manifestations of Crohn's disease without demonstrable gastrointestinal lesions. *Oral Surg.* 1975;39:58–66.
47. Carr M. Granulomatous cheilitis in Crohn's disease. *Br Med J.* 1974;4:636.
48. Verbov J, Stansfeld AG. Cutaneous polyarteritis nodosa and Crohn's disease. *Trans St John's Hosp Dermatol Soc.* 1972;58:261–268.
49. Burgdorf W, Orkin M. Granulomatous perivasculitis in Crohn's disease. *Arch Dermatol.* 1981;117:674–675.
50. Ecker RI, Winkelmann RK. *Demodex* granuloma. *Arch Dermatol.* 1979;115:343–344.
51. Erlach E, Gebhart W, Niebauer G. Zuer pathogenese der granulomatosen rosacea. *Z Hautkr.* 1976;51:459–464.

CHAPTER 17
Mixed Cell Granulomas

Clifton R. White, Jr.

Mixed cell granulomas are inflammatory infiltrates characterized by the presence of histiocytes, preponderant in some areas, mixed with other inflammatory cells (neutrophils, eosinophils, lymphocytes, plasma cells). Predominantly mononuclear cell vs mixed cell granulomas have rather distinct histologic patterns when viewed at scanning power. As a general rule, whereas mononuclear granulomas are typically nodular, mixed cell granulomas usually fill large portions or all of the dermis and thus are termed diffuse. As with other granulomatous processes, mixed cell granulomas characterize diverse diseases, including cutaneous reactions to foreign material and excessive halogen ingestion, deep fungal and atypical mycobacterial infections, and xan-

thomas and related diseases (Fig. 17–1). Foreign body reactions are exceptional in that virtually any granulomatous inflammatory pattern (mononuclear or mixed, nodular or diffuse) may develop (Figs. 17–2, 17–3, 17–4). Similar generalizations apply to granulomatous reactions to infectious agents, particularly deep fungi and mycobacteria. Sound practice, then, when interpreting any biopsy with granulomatous features is to always:

1. Polarize the tissue in search of foreign material
2. Obtain special stains for fungal and acid-fast organisms, particularly when the diagnosis is in question

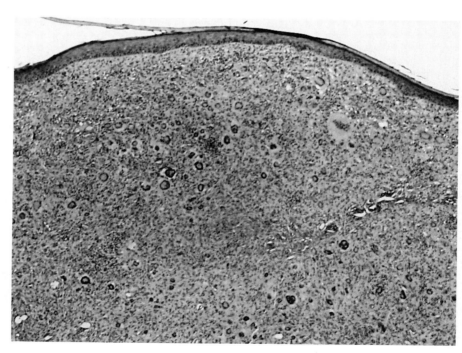

Figure 17–1. Mixed cell granuloma. At scanning power, the entire dermis is filled with histiocytes, many of them multinucleated (Touton giant cells), as well as lymphocytes, plasma cells, and eosinophils in xanthogranuloma (H&E, ×25).

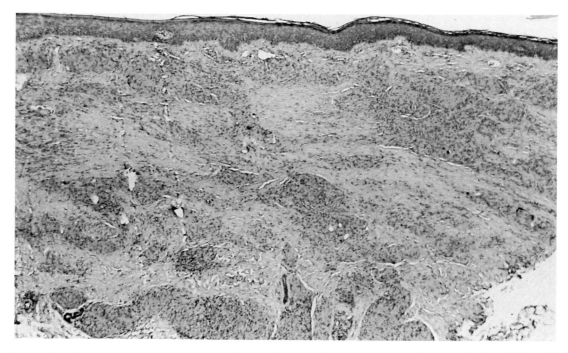

Figure 17–2. Foreign body granuloma due to silica. Striking sarcoidal pattern at scanning magnification (H&E, ×25).

FOREIGN BODY GRANULOMAS

Clinical Features

Foreign body granulomas are among the most common granulomas that occur in the skin.[1,2] Although frequently they are caused by inoculation or abrasion, the most common stimulus is the response to ruptured follicular cysts or inflamed follicular units. Although cornified cells and other cyst contents within intact epithelial structures are inert, rupture of the follicular structures with spewing of the contents into the dermis invariably provokes a characteristic, dense, mixed cell granulomatous reaction. The corresponding clinical picture is that of a reddened, swollen, painful, and, at times, draining cyst. Such lesions typify

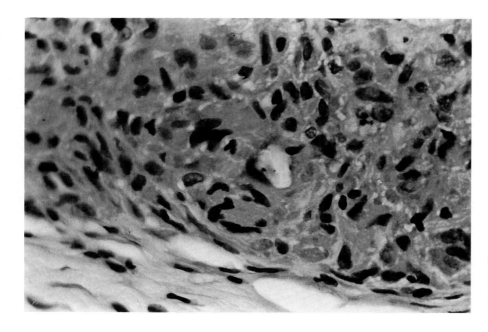

Figure 17–3. Foreign body granuloma. Higher power of Fig. 17–2 shows epithelioid histiocytes, a few giant cells, and a small fragment of silica (glass) within the vacuole (H&E, ×400).

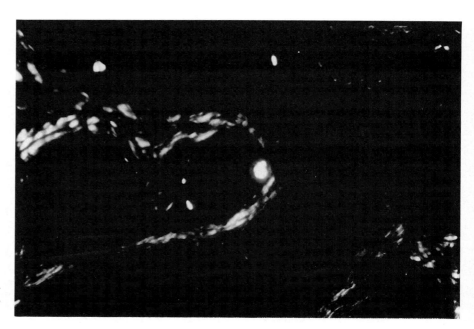

Figure 17–4. Foreign body granuloma. Polarization of Fig. 17–2 shows brightly illuminated particles of silica (×250).

a variety of follicular diseases, such as acne vulgaris, rosacea, hidradenitis suppurativa, and nodular solar elastosis with cysts and comedones (Favre-Racouchot).

Other foreign bodies, such as tattoos,[3–7] paraffin,[8] silicone,[9–11] sutures, insect bites, gravel, dirt, lead pencils, thorns, splinters, cactus spines,[12,13] silica,[14–18] and sea urchin spines,[19] may cause a similar mixed cell granulomatous inflammatory pattern. Foreign material in these cases frequently may be visualized by polarization. Other reported causes of foreign body granulomas include vaccinations[20] and pollen grains.[21]

Histologic Features

Certain foreign substances cause characteristic nodular granulomatous reactions (Chapter 16), including silica, zirconium, and beryllium. In contrast, most reactions to foreign material, such as follicular cyst contents (from a ruptured cyst or follicle) including cornified cells and sebum, are diffuse and mixed in character, consisting of neutrophils, occasionally eosinophils and plasma cells, and histiocytes, including foreign body type giant cells, and lymphocytes.

The inflammatory reaction to ruptured cysts varies in appearance with time. Initially, edema surrounds increased numbers of small blood vessels and extravasated erythrocytes, with neutrophils, lymphocytes, and histiocytes giving a granulation tissue appearance. Later, greater numbers of histiocytes, including giant cells, appear as do numerous neutrophils, resulting in suppurative granulomatous inflammation (Figs. 17–5, 17–6). Still later, the infiltrate may be almost purely histiocytic (granulomatous). Eventually, fibroblasts and fibrosis are the only residua of the inflammatory reaction. Often, as the inflammatory reaction progresses, the entire cyst epithelium disappears, presumably phagocytized by inflammatory cells, so that the only clue to diagnosis may be a few flakes of cornified cells, often within the cytoplasm of multinucleated giant cells (Fig. 17–7). Although the nature of the foreign material may

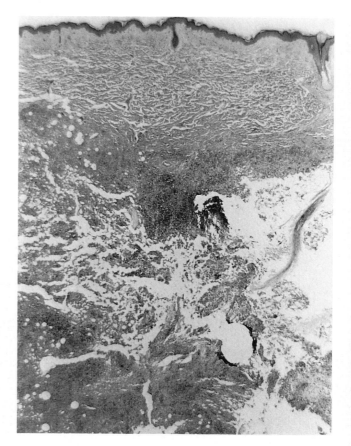

Figure 17–5. Ruptured follicular cyst with diffuse mixed cell granulomatous and suppurative dermatitis. At low power, most of the dermis and subcutaneous fat are filled with histiocytes, including many giant cells, neutrophils, and lymphocytes, with edema. Note the laminated cornified cells (cyst contents) to the right, the only remaining clue that a ruptured cyst provoked this inflammatory response (H&E, ×25).

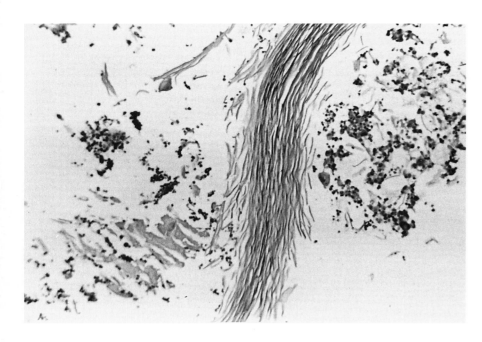

Figure 17–6. Cyst contents. Higher power of Figure 17–5 shows laminated cornified cells, characteristic contents of a follicular cyst of the infundibular type (epidermoid cyst), surrounded by histiocytes and neutrophils. The epithelial cyst lining is no longer present in these sections (H&E, ×160).

vary, the histologic pattern of mixed cell granulomatous inflammation is a common response.

Differential Diagnosis

In the skin, the most common cause of diffuse, mixed cell granulomatous inflammation involving neutrophils and histiocytes (suppurative, granulomatous inflammation) is the response to ruptured follicular cysts or inflamed follicles. Halogenodermas also are characterized by diffuse neutrophil infiltrates, epidermal abscesses and epidermal hyperplasia, but few histiocytes. Deep fungal and atypical mycobacterial diseases should be considered with any suppurative granulomatous dermatitis. Clinical history,

special stains, and cultures usually allow distinction from foreign body reactions.

HALOGEN ERUPTIONS

Clinical Features

Ingestion of halogenated substances, mainly iodides, bromides, and fluorides, will cause marked cutaneous changes in predisposed individuals. Excessive bromide and iodide intake results in pustular, vegetating plaques called bromoderma and iododerma.[22–26] Iododerma is typically less vegetating and softer than bromoderma, may ulcerate, and may

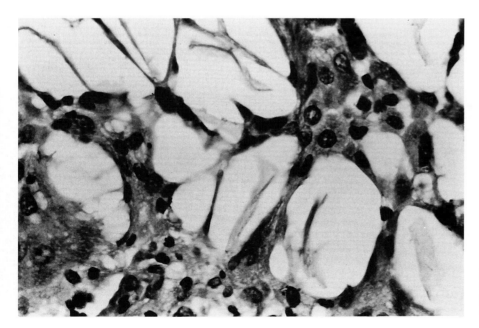

Figure 17–7. Thin cornified cells of cyst within cytoplasm of histiocytes, subtle but incontrovertible proof of a ruptured follicular cyst or structure (H&E, ×400).

be associated with fever, further simulating infectious processes (e.g., North American blastomycosis). Iododerma may be precipitated or exacerbated by ingestion of iodine-containing radiographic substances.

Frequent topical application of a fluoride gel to the teeth to prevent caries during radiation therapy to the face has resulted in fluoroderma. These lesions consist of papules and nodules on the face and neck.[27]

Histologic Features

Although halogenodermas are included under mixed cell granulomas, the histologic picture is not prominently granulomatous because the lesions lack a preponderance of histiocytes. The characteristic features include a dense, diffuse, mixed infiltrate with numerous neutrophils, histiocytes, lymphocytes and occasional atypical mononuclear cells, eosinophils, and extravasated erythrocytes with marked edema. Nuclear dust often is present,[23] although fibrin deposition, thrombosis, and other signs of vasculitis are not. The histologic reflection of the vegetating clinical lesions is papillomatosis with marked epidermal hyperplasia, which may be pseudoepitheliomatous. Often, collections of neutrophils and eosinophils (microabscesses) are present in the hyperplastic epidermis accompanied by necrotic keratinocytes. Follicular pustules are seen in the early lesions of iododerma and bromoderma.

Fluoroderma has similar, although less pronounced, findings to iododerma and bromoderma, including a mixed infiltrate of neutrophils, eosinophils, lymphocytes, and histiocytes as well as epidermal hyperplasia with microabscesses.[27]

Differential Diagnosis

Both the clinical and histologic features of iododerma and bromoderma are similar to those of some deep fungal infections, such as North American blastomycosis. The diffuse mixed granulomatous inflammation with pseudoepitheliomatous hyperplasia containing abscesses are found in each instance. However, in blastomycosis, yeast cells usually are readily identified, and numerous multinucleated histiocytes are present, allowing differentiation. Pemphigus vegetans similarly shows epidermal hyperplasia containing abscesses of neutrophils and eosinophils but also shows acantholysis, which may be extensive, and lacks the dense, diffuse dermal infiltrate seen in halogenodermas.

MIXED CELL GRANULOMAS CAUSED BY INFECTIOUS AGENTS (DEEP FUNGAL INFECTIONS AND ATYPICAL MYCOBACTERIAL INFECTIONS)

Clinical Features

Many deep fungal infections involving the skin are characterized by clinically elevated, vegetating, or verrucous plaques, often studded with pustules. Some of the causative organisms are listed in Table 17–1. Atypical mycobacterial infections may cause similar lesions.

TABLE 17–1. DEEP FUNGAL SPECIES CHARACTERIZED BY MIXED CELL GRANULOMAS

Actinomycosis
Chromoblastomycosis
Coccidioidomycosis
Cryptococcosis
Histoplasmosis
North and South American blastomycosis
Sporotrichosis

From Epstein.[28]

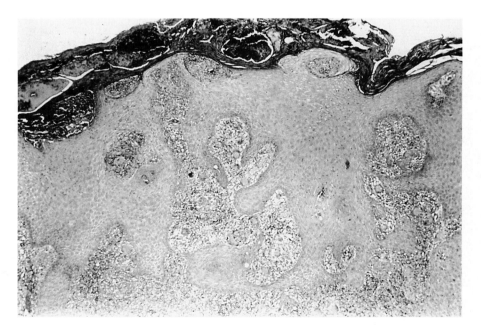

Figure 17–8. Chromomycosis. Scanning magnification shows marked pseudoepitheliomatous hyperplasia with dense, diffuse mixed cell granulomatous inflammation consisting predominantly of histiocytes and neutrophils (suppurative granulomatous dermatitis) (H&E, ×64).

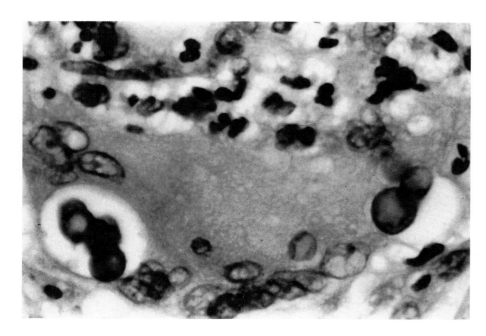

Figure 17–9. Chromomycosis. Higher power of Figure 17–8 of several pigmented spores of chromomycosis within a large multinucleated histiocyte with surrounding neutrophils (H&E, ×400).

Histologic Features

The histologic counterparts to the vegetating plaques in these infectious dermatitides are pseudoepitheliomatous hyperplasia with diffuse mixed cell granulomatous inflammation consisting of histiocytes, usually with numerous foreign body or Langhans giant cells, lymphocytes, neutrophils, eosinophils, and plasma cells (Fig. 17–8). Frequently, neutrophils are present in accumulations, as are histiocytes, giving a predominantly suppurative granulomatous inflammatory infiltrate. Often, deep fungal organisms may be seen with routine stains, surrounded by neutrophils or within the cytoplasm of multinucleated histiocytes (Fig. 17–9). Atypical mycobacterial organisms require special stains, such as the Fite-Faraco or Ziehl-Neelsen for visualization. Special stains also may be used to further characterize fungi, including PAS with prior diastase digestion or silver stains, such as Gomori-metnenamine silver.

Acknowledgment

I would like to express my appreciation to Jennifer Parnell for her invaluable assistance in the preparation of this manuscript.

REFERENCES

1. Epstein WL. Foreign body granulomas. In: Boros DL, Yosida T, eds. *Basic and Clinical Aspects of Granulomatous Diseases.* Amsterdam: Elsevier/North Holland; 1980:181–197.
2. Epstein WL. Chemical-induced granulomas. In Fitzpatrick TB, ed. *Dermatology in General Medicine.* 2nd ed. New York: McGraw-Hill; 1979:1590–1598.
3. Madden JF. Reactions in tattoos. *Arch Dermatol Syph.* 1939;40:256–262.
4. Beerman H, Lane RAG. Tattoo. *Am J Med Sci.* 1954;227:444–465.
5. Goldstein N. Special issue on tattoos. *J Dermatol Surg Oncol.* 1979;5:848.
6. Bjornberg A. Allergic reaction to cobalt in light blue tattoo markings. *Acta Derm Venereol (Stockh).* 1961;41:259–263.
7. Weidman AI, Andrader R, Franks AG. Sarcoidosis reactions to light in yellow tattoos from cadmium sulfide. *Arch Dermatol.* 1966;94:320–325.
8. Oertel YC, Johnson FB. Sclerosing lipogranuloma of male genitalia. *Arch Pathol Lab Med.* 1977;101:321–326.
9. Winer LH, Sternberg TH, Lehman R, et al. Tissue reactions to injected silicone liquids. *Arch Dermatol.* 1964;90:588–593.
10. Boo-Chai K. The complications of augmentation mammoplasty by silicone injection. *Br J Plast Surg.* 1969;22:281–285.
11. Hausner RJ, Schoen FJ, Pierson KK. Foreign body reaction to silicone gel in axillary lymph nodes after an augmentation mammoplasty. *Plast Reconstr Surg.* 1978;62:381–384.
12. Schreiber MM, Shapiro SI, Berry CZ. Cactus granuloma of the skin. *Arch Dermatol.* 1971;104:374–379.
13. Winer LH, Zaclenga RH. Cactus granulomas of the skin. *Arch Dermatol.* 1955;72:566–569.
14. Shattock SG. Pseudotuberculoma silicoticum of the lip. *Proc R Soc Med.* 1916;10:6–19.
15. Epstein E. Silica granulomas of the skin. *Arch Dermatol.* 1955;71:24–35.
16. Rank BK, Hicks JD, Lovie M. Pseudotuberculoma granulosum siliconicum. *Br J Plast Surg.* 1972;25:42–48.
17. Eskeland G, Langmark F, Husby G. Silica granuloma of the skin and subcutaneous tissue. *Acta Pathol Microbial Scand [Suppl].* 1974;248:69–73.
18. Kuchemann K, Holm R. Unusual silica granulomas of the skin with massive involvement of axillary lymph nodes. *Pathol Res Pract.* 1979;164:198–204.
19. Cooper P, Wakefield MC. A sarcoid reaction to injury by sea urchin spines. *J Pathol.* 1974;112:33–36.
20. Slater DW. Aluminum hydroxide granulomas. *Br J Dermatol.* 1982;107:103–108.
21. Schwartz DA, Baker RD. Pollen grain granuloma: A new clinicopathologic entity. *Hum Pathol.* 1986;17:856–857.
22. Jones LE, Pariser H, Murray PF. Recurrent iododerma. *Arch Dermatol.* 1958;78:353–358.
23. Rosenburg FR, Einbinder J, Walzer RA, et al. Vegetating iododerma. *Arch Dermatol.* 1972;105:900–905.

24. Kincaid MC, Green WR, Hoover RE, et al. Iododerma of the conjunctiva and skin. *Ophthalmology.* 1981;88:1216–1220.

25. Hollander L, Fetterman GH. Fatal iododerma. *Arch Dermatol Syph.* 1936;34:228–241.

26. Goldberg HK. Iodism with severe ocular involvement. *Am J Ophthalmol.* 1939;22:65–68.

27. Blasik LG, Spencer SK. Fluoroderma. *Arch Dermatol.* 1979;115:1334–1335.

28. Epstein WL. Granulomatous inflammation in skin. In: Ioachin HL, ed. *Pathology of Granulomas.* New York: Raven Press; 1983;21–59.

CHAPTER 18
Palisading Granulomas

Robert M. Taylor

Palisading granulomas are areas of connective tissue alteration surrounded by radially aligned fibroblasts and histiocytes. They are characterized by collagenous degeneration (called, in the past, necrobiosis), with or without extracellular deposition of fibrin, glycosaminoglycans, or lipid. This collagenous degeneration may range from slight basophilia, swelling, and distortion of collagen fibers to total dissolution.[1–4] Blood vessels in and around areas of collagen alteration may appear relatively normal, or they may exhibit significant alteration; elastic fibers in these areas may be preserved or destroyed.[4,5] In extreme cases, this alteration or degeneration may lead to the total destruction of all connective tissue elements, resulting in a tissue void that must be refilled by adjacent living tissue. Whether the degeneration of tissue in palisading granulomas is a primary event or is secondary to vascular changes is a debatable issue, which is discussed for particular diagnostic entities, as appropriate. Immune cell populations and reactants are also discussed for various types of palisading granulomas.

Palisading granulomas classically have included granuloma annulare, necrobiosis lipoidica, rheumatoid nodule, and rheumatic fever nodule. Annular elastolytic granuloma, or actinic granuloma, is included in this chapter even though elastolysis appears to be the primary event. Granuloma multiforme,[6] although similar to granuloma annulare, is found primarily in central Africa and is not discussed.

GRANULOMA ANNULARE

Clinical Features
Granuloma annulare (GA) is a benign, self-limited disease of unknown origin. It has been reported to occur after trauma,[7] sun exposure,[7] insect bites,[8] and herpes zoster infection,[8–10] among others. Clinical variants of GA include localized,[7] generalized[11] (including a perforating variant[12]), subcutaneous,[13–16] perforating,[17–18] and an erythema multiforme or erythema annulare centrificum type.[19]

The exact cause of GA is unknown. Possible causes include acute vasculitis in necrobiotic areas[20–22] and circulat-ing immune complexes.[23] Some studies have favored a cell-mediated immune pathogenesis, having detected activated T helper lymphocytes,[24] cytokine production,[25] and the abnormal release of monocyte-derived lysozyme in and around areas of altered collagen.[24–26] Others have contended that the connective tissue change is primary and the other changes (e.g., vasculopathy and immunoreactant deposition) are secondary.[27]

Histologic Features
The primary focus of disease in GA is upper to midreticular dermis. Less commonly, the subcutis is involved. Except in the rare perforating variants of GA,[17] the epidermis generally appears normal. Foci of collagen degeneration take two forms: (1) complete collagenous alteration with a peripheral palisade of fibroblasts and histiocytes and (2) ill-defined, incomplete, piecemeal collagenous alteration without a peripheral palisade of histiocytes and fibroblasts. Both forms may be seen in the same specimen.[4] The palisading form has a well-defined, cell-poor dermal focus of collagen degeneration (Fig. 18–1). The dermal changes are characterized by indistinct basophilic collagen fibers and diminished numbers of cell nuclei. Histiocytes and fibroblasts are aligned in a palisade, or picket fence, fashion around the altered collagen (Fig. 18–2). Peripheral to the zone of dermal change there is often a superficial, or superficial and deep, perivascular lymphocytic infiltrate. Although collagenous degeneration may appear complete, elastic fibers may be present (Fig. 18–3).[5] Uncommonly, multinucleate giant cells surround the degenerating collagen, mingling with the pali-sading fibroblasts and histiocytes. This feature is more often seen in necrobiosis lipoidica. In the second form, incomplete piecemeal alteration of collagen predominates (Fig. 18–4). Small indistinct foci of collagen fiber alteration appear side by side with normal collagen. Abundant fibroblasts and histiocytes mingling with beaded, basophilic collagen fibers may be the only clue to diagnosis. Invariably, there is minimal to moderate perivascular lymphocytic infiltrate peripheral to the necrobiotic areas. Infrequently, epithelioid cell aggregates are present within the centers of collagen

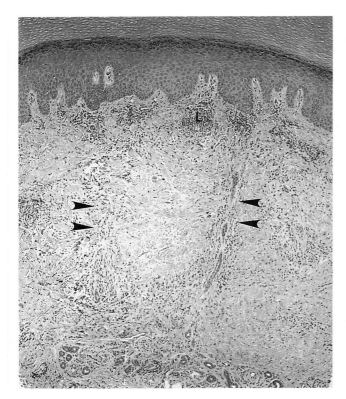

Figure 18–1. Superficial and middermal granuloma annulare exhibiting a central, cell-poor, necrobiotic palisading granuloma (arrowheads). There is a perivascular lymphohistiocytic infiltrate (L) peripheral to the zone of collagenous necrobiosis. (H&E, ×60.)

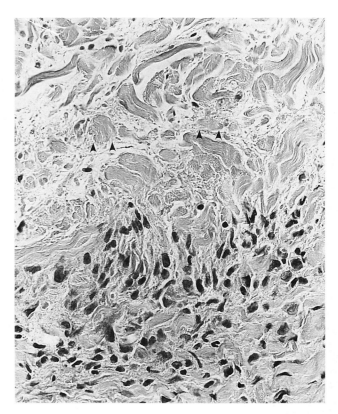

Figure 18–2. Higher power of granuloma annulare in Figure 1. Histiocytes and fibroblasts are arranged in a palisade alignment around indistinct, basophilic collagen fibers (arrowheads), which appear separated from one another by a granular-appearing clear space. (H&E, ×370.)

degeneration.[28,29] Eosinophils may be present around blood vessels or areas of degeneration,[29] and plasma cells are uncommon.[4] Recent immunological[20–23] and light microscopic[23,30] studies have found evidence of acute leukocytoclastic vasculitis in GA. In most cases, however, the vascular pathology is minimal and consists primarily of endothelial cell swelling.[29,31]

In both types of GA, minimal to marked glycosaminoglycan (hyaluronic acid) deposition is seen in areas of collagen degeneration (Fig. 18–5). Hyaluronic acid is best demonstrated with special stains, such as colloidal iron, with and without hyaluronidase, and alcian-blue, pH 2.4.[4,31,32] In addition, minimal amounts of extracellular lipid have been found within and around areas of collagen degeneration.[31,32] In the rare perforating variant of GA, altered collagen is extruded through the epidermis[17,33] or follicles[18] or, simply, through a central epidermal ulcer (Figs. 18–6, 18–7).[34]

In subcutaneous GA (pseudorheumatoid nodule),[15,16] there are large areas of collagenous eosinophilic degeneration entirely within the subcutis or deep dermis–subcutis (Fig. 18–8). As in dermal GA, there are palisading areas with more alcian blue-positive glycosaminoglycans than normal,[35] but these foci appear more eosinophilic and fibrinoid than those seen in dermal GA.[13–16,36]

Differential Diagnosis

The differential diagnosis includes necrobiosis lipoidica, rheumatoid nodule, and rheumatic fever nodule (Table 18–1). Other diseases that may simulate the dermal palisading variant of GA include localized beryllium granuloma,[37] primary inoculation cat-scratch disease,[38] and lupus miliaris disseminatus faciei.[39] In contrast to GA, all of these diseases exhibit marked necrosis of dermal collagen and elastic fibers secondary to a granulomatous process but no stromal deposition of glycosaminoglycans.

NECROBIOSIS LIPOIDICA

Clinical Features

Necrobiosis lipoidica (NL) is a granulomatous disease usually occurring as yellow, indurated, atrophic, sclerotic plaques on the lower extremities.[1] Approximately 75% of patients are women and 66% are diabetic. However, NL is a complication in only 0.39 of patients with diabetes mellitus.[40,41] NL may appear elsewhere (e.g., calves, thighs, hands, feet, scalp) as papules, nodules, or plaques with or without atrophy.[40,41] A rare transfollicular elimination variant occurs clinically as follicular comedo-like plugs.[42]

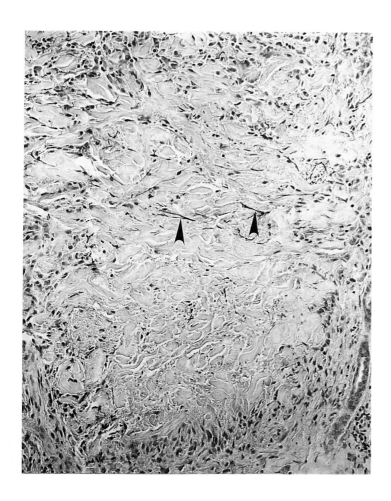

Figure 18–3. Palisading necrobiotic granuloma annulare demonstrating preservation of elastic fibers (arrowheads) within the zone of altered collagen. (Acid orcein and Giemsa, ×148.)

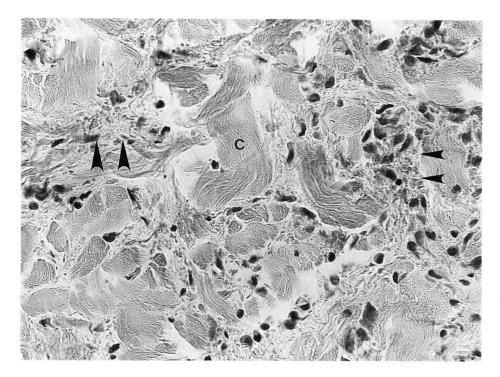

Figure 18–4. Granuloma annulare demonstrating incomplete piecemeal altered collagen. Increased numbers of fibroblasts and histiocytes surround beaded, basophilic collagen fibers (arrowheads), which are adjacent to normal-appearing collagen fibers (C). (H&E, ×370.)

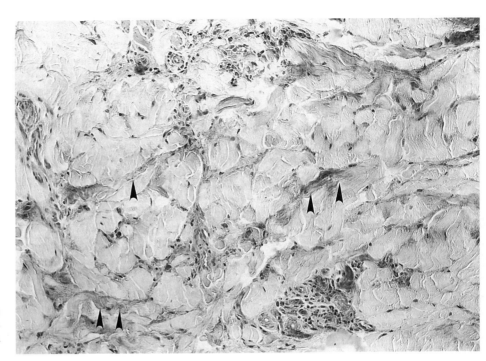

Figure 18–5. Abundant hyaluronic acid (arrowheads) is present between collagen fibers in a focal area of granuloma annulare. (Colloidal iron, ×148.)

The pathogenesis of NL is something of an enigma. It is not known whether the collagen alteration seen in NL is secondary to microangiopathy or causes the observed vascular changes. Since frank diabetes mellitus is seen in the majority of patients with NL, some authors have assumed that the microangiopathy is diabetic in origin.[40–43]

These findings, however, do not explain the 33% of patients with NL who do not histologically exhibit vessel changes.[44] Others have proposed that the vascular abnormalities in NL are secondary to increased platelet aggregation via elevated plasma levels of α_2-macroglobulin and factor VIII-related antigen.[14] Immune complex vasculitis also has been

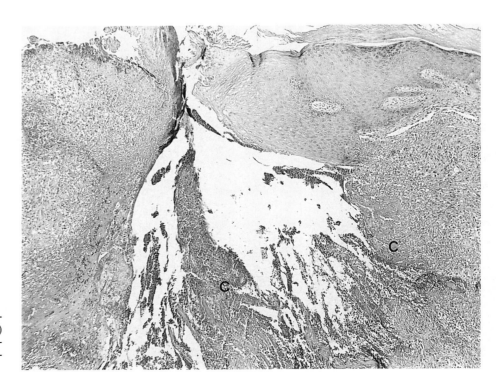

Figure 18–6. Ulcerative perforating granuloma annulare. Necrotic collagen (C) surrounded by acute and chronic inflammation is extruded through a central epidermal ulceration. (H&E, ×48.)

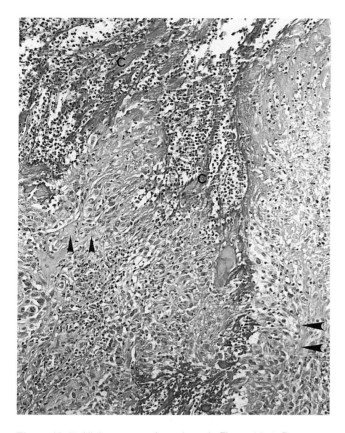

Figure 18–7. Higher power of specimen in Figure 18–6. Degenerating collagen (C) is extruded superiorly (small arrowheads) into the ulcer base, and laterally and inferiorly altered collagen is surrounded by fibroblasts, histiocytes, and flocculent material (large arrowheads). (H&E, ×148.)

suggested because IgM and C_3 are present in and around dermal blood vessels in approximately 50% of NL patients.[45]

Histologic Features

In NL, the entire dermis is affected, with little dermal collagen being spared. Extension to the subcutis is not unusual. Under scanning magnification, large, indistinct, elongate foci of collagen degeneration appear, creating a sandwich-like effect between zones of degenerated and sclerotic collagen (Fig. 18–9). Palisading granulomas, when present, are usually less distinct and frequently surrounded by an inflammatory infiltrate of lymphocytes, histiocytes, plasma cells, multinucleate foreign body giant cells, and epithelioid cells (Fig. 18–10). Within areas of dermal sclerosis, cutaneous adnexae frequently are atrophic or absent, and the collagen bundles appear eosinophilic, hyalinized, and thickened. Elastic fibers are present to a variable degree, although they may be totally absent in areas of sclerosis (Fig. 18–11). Inflammatory changes may occur, ranging from a mild to moderately granulomatous reaction, as outlined previously, to a predominantly granulomatous sarcoidal tissue reaction (Fig. 18–12). NL sarcoidal tissue reactions have been noted most frequently in the scalp.[46,47] Although the inflammatory changes are seen throughout the dermis, most are in the mid- and deep dermis with extension into the subcutis (Fig. 18–9). The depth of collagen alteration may coincide with the greater involvement of blood vessels in the mid- and deep dermis. Both large and small caliber vessels may show intimal proliferation, with PAS-positive, diastase-resistant thickening and sclerosis of the muscular arterioles and arteries.[31] Perivascular adventitial fibrosis frequently is present, with varying degrees of luminal narrowing or obliteration. If sufficiently granulomatous, the vascular alterations may take on the appearance of a

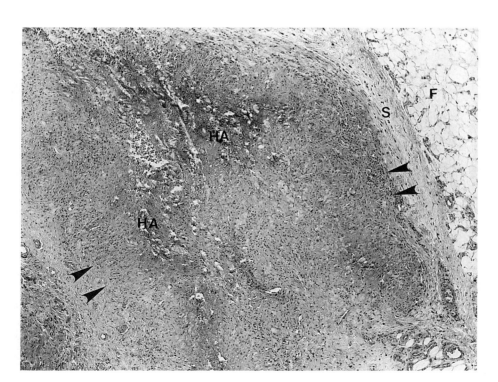

Figure 18–8. Subcutaneous palisading granuloma annulare. A peripheral palisade of fibroblasts and histiocytes (arrowheads) surrounds a central area of degenerating collagen and colloidal iron-positive glycosaminoglycans (hyaluronic acid). Thickened fibrotic fat lobule septae surround the area of inflammation. HA, hyaluronic acid; F, fat lobule; S, fat lobule septum. (Colloidal iron, ×60.)

TABLE 18–1. COMPARATIVE HISTOLOGY OF THE CLASSIC PALISADING GRANULOMAS

Disease	Location of Palisading Granuloma	Pattern of Change	Constituent Cellular Components		Constituent Extracellular Components		
			Inflammatory	Vascular	GAGs[a]	Fibrin	Lipid
Granuloma annulare	Upper and midreticular dermis; uncommonly, subcutis (pseudorheumatoid nodule); rarely epidermis (perforating variant)	Two types: 1. Palisading granuloma with complete collagen degeneration 2. Small incomplete piecemeal collagen alteration, without palisading granuloma; fibrosis uncommon	Histiocytes, lymphocytes, occasional eosinophils, rarely giant cells; tuberculoid, sarcoid tissue reaction rare	Perivascular mononuclear cell infiltrate Acute vasculitis in early lesions postulated	Often present	Generally absent	Minimal to absent
Necrobiosis lipoidica	Entire dermis with extension to subcutis	Large, indistinct elongate areas of collagen degenerating; palisading granulomas may be less distinct; fibrosis common	Histiocytes, lymphocytes, plasma cells, giant cells; tuberculoid sarcoid tissue reaction common	Intimal proliferation, PAS + medial thickening and advential fibrosis; granulomatous vasculitis may be present	Minimal to absent	Often present	Present
Rheumatoid nodule	Subcutis; the deep dermis may be involved	Zonal foci of lamellated fibrinous collagen degeneration surrounded by a palisade of inflammatory cells; fibrosis common	Histiocytes, lymphocytes, plasma cells, occasional giant cells; tuberculoid sarcoid tissue reaction is rare	Capillary proliferation peripherally, fibrinoid necrosis of vessels centrally; acute vasculitis in early lesions postulated	Generally absent	Present	Often present as small droplets
Rheumatic fever nodule	Subcutis	Areas of latticelike fibrinoid change; palisading granuloma poorly defined; fibrosis present but not marked	Neutrophils, histiocytes, lymphocytes	Thick-walled vessels in fibrinoid areas	May be present	Present	May be present

[a] Glycosaminoglycans

granulomatous vasculitis (Fig. 18–13). In fact, it has been suggested that NL is an evolving process, beginning in the acute phase as a necrotizing vasculitis, progressing to a subacute phase of granulomatous vasculitis, and ultimately resolving as an area of dense sclerosis.[48] This hypothesis is supported by the finding of cutaneous immunoreactants (IgM, C$_3$) within cutaneous blood vessels, which suggests an immune complex vasculitis.[45] This hypothesis does not, however, account for the fact that vascular changes are minimal or absent in NL biopsied at sites other than the legs.[49]

Stromal glycosaminoglycans (hyaluronic acid) may be present but not usually to the degree seen in granuloma annulare.[32,44,48] Dermal fibrin and PAS-positive diastase-resistant material often are present, as are extracellular lipids in the areas of altered dermis, thereby imparting a yellow color often seen in established lesions.[48]

Differential Diagnosis

The differential diagnosis includes the classic palisading granulomas (Table 18–1). The granulomatous variant of annular elastolytic granuloma (actinic granuloma) can be very similar to the sarcoidal variant of NL[50] and is discussed below. Also included in the differential diagnosis are sar-

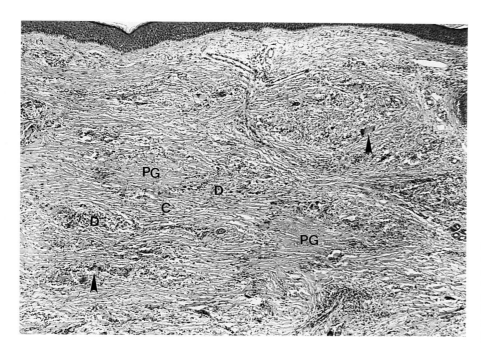

Figure 18–9. Necrobiosis lipoidica. Large, elongate zones of indistinct collagen degeneration (D) alternate with sclerotic collagen (C), creating a sandwichlike effect within the dermis. Multinucleate giant cells (arrowheads) and chronic inflammation surround the degenerated collagen. PG, palisading granuloma. (H&E, ×54.)

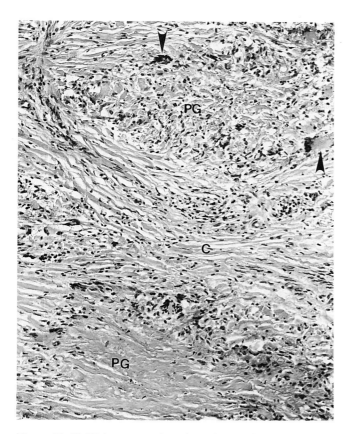

Figure 18–10. Higher power view of specimen in Figure 18–9. Two foci of necrobiotic palisading granulomas (PG) sandwiching an area of collagen sclerosis (C). Multinucleate giant cells (arrowheads) and chronic inflammation are present peripheral to the areas of collagen alteration. (H&E, ×136.)

coidosis and the allergic foreign body granulomas of silica[51,52] and zirconium,[53,54] which can be very similar to granulomatous NL. Nonetheless, the presence of collagenous degeneration and extracellular lipids in the dermis favors the diagnosis of NL. Refractile silica crystals seen in polarized light distinguish silica allergic granuloma from NL.

RHEUMATOID NODULE

Clinical Features
Palpable rheumatoid nodules occur in about 20% of patients with rheumatoid arthritis.[55] Although they are most common on the extensor surface of the forearms, rheumatoid nodules also may occur on other areas, such as the dorsal surface of the hands, the knees, and the scapulae.[55] The nodules are firm, range from millimeters to several centimeters in size, and tend to ulcerate, particularly over pressure areas (sacrum, buttocks, heels).[55,56] Perforating rheumatoid nodules have been described in a patient with rheumatoid arthritis, although the mechanism is not clear.[57] Subcutaneous necrobiotic nodules with a predilection for bony prominences of extremities have been described in children. These nodules were similar histologically to rheumatoid nodules, but the patients were seronegative or did not exhibit clinical findings of rheumatoid arthritis.[14–16,36] These lesions have been termed "pseudorheumatoid" or "rheumatoidlike" nodules.[15,16] Some authors believe that, in children and most adults, it is best to regard subcutaneous necrobiotic nodules as granuloma annulare.[15,16,36,58–60]

The pathogenesis of true rheumatoid nodules seems by many to be related to severe rheumatoid arthritis, high titer rheumatoid factor, and rheumatoid vasculitis.[61–63] Vas-

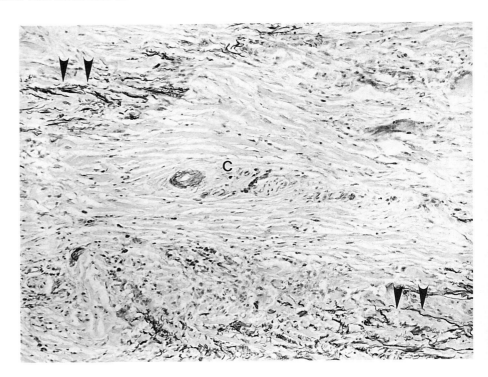

Figure 18–11. Necrobiosis lipoidica. Elastic fibers are absent in areas of collagen sclerosis (C) but present within the surrounding dermis (arrowheads). (Acid orcein and Giemsa, ×136.)

culitis in rheumatoid nodules has been demonstrated by light and immunofluorescent microscopy.[62–66] In the opinion of some authors, rheumatoid nodules may be the consequence of immune complex disease.[67]

Histologic Features

The pertinent histopathologic features of rheumatoid nodule are primarily in the subcutis or deep dermis.[4,48,68] Generally, the epidermis is normal unless traumatic ulceration over pressure points or perforation occurs.[55–57] Low-power

pattern analysis of rheumatoid nodules reveals large, discrete, fibrinous foci of degenerated collagen within the subcutis or deep dermis surrounded by fibrosis (Fig. 18–14).

The earliest changes seen in a rheumatoid nodule are endothelial cell proliferation, neoangiogenesis, thickening of capillary, venular, and arteriolar walls, increasing numbers of lymphocytes and histiocytes, and fibrosis.[4,69–70] Subsequently, fibrinoid necrosis appears in the thickened vessel walls, apparently spreading to adjacent tissues.[4] Some authors think that the early histology of a rheumatoid nodule

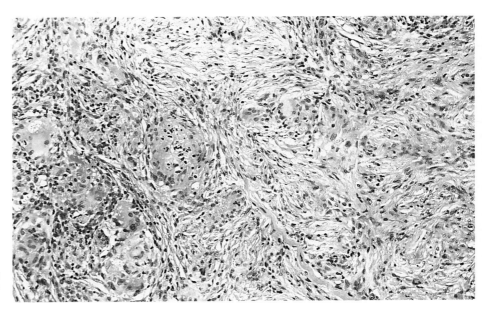

Figure 18–12. Dermal sarcoidal tissue reaction in an area of necrobiosis lipoidica. (H&E, ×136.)

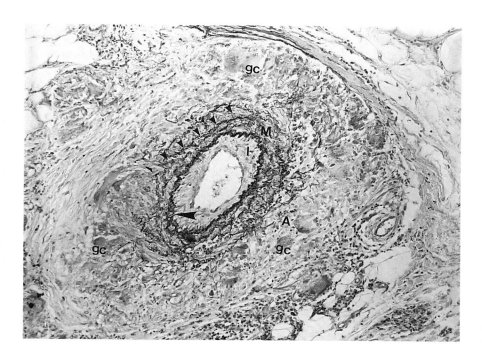

Figure 18–13. Necrobiosis lipoidica. Subcutaneous muscular artery exhibiting marked intimal hyperplasia and fibrosis, thickening of the internal elastic lamina (large arrowheads), medial fibrosis with fragmentation of the external elastic lamina (small arrowheads), and marked granulomatous inflammation with fibrosis of the adventitia. I, intima; M, media; A, adventitia; gc, giant cells. (Acid orcein and Giemsa, ×136.)

is an acute vasculitis.[4,56,61–66] This hypothesis is supported by the fact that rheumatoid nodules are seen in association with severe rheumatoid arthritis, high-titer rheumatoid factor, and rheumatoid vasculitis.[61–63] Regardless of pathogenesis, the resultant histology is a well-developed rheumatoid nodule with distinctive zonal foci of lamellated fibrinous degeneration, surrounding which is a palisaded array of lymphocytes, histiocytes, and fibroblasts (Fig. 18–14). Pe-

ripherally, there is stromal fibrosis, vascular proliferation, and scattered lymphocytes and plasma cells.[66,68,70,71] Staining for lipid frequently reveals small droplets in necrobiotic centers as well as intra- and extracellular lipid in the peripheral palisade zone.[58] Glycosaminoglycan deposition is usually negligible.[36] Eventually, with burnout of the process, there is dense fibrosis with a pink festooned scar the only remaining hint of a previous palisade process (Fig. 18–15).

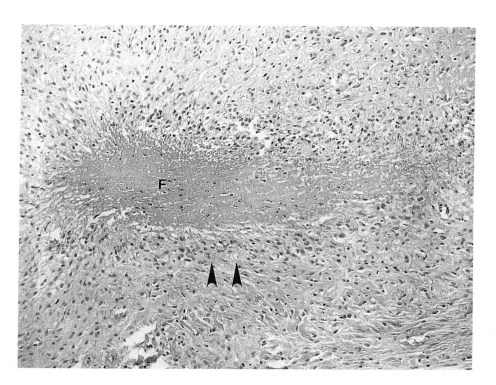

Figure 18–14. Rheumatoid nodule. A large fibrinous focus (F) of subcutaneous collagen is surrounded by a peripheral palisade of fibroblasts and histiocytes (arrowheads). There is marked stromal fibrosis present peripheral to the palisading granuloma. (H&E, ×136.)

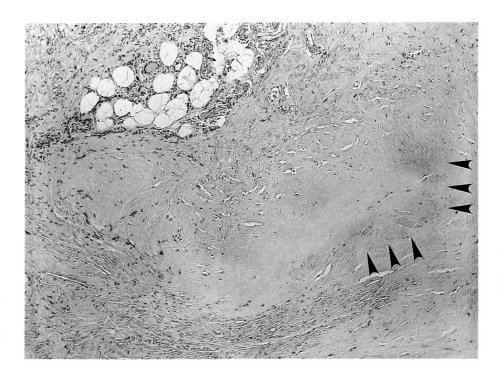

Figure 18–15. A pink, festooned scar (arrowheads) is all that remains of a subcutaneous rheumatoid nodule. Remnants of fat cells are seen in the upper left corner. (H&E, ×54.)

NODULES ASSOCIATED WITH RHEUMATIC FEVER AND JUVENILE RHEUMATOID ARTHRITIS

Clinical Features

Subcutaneous nodules have been found to occur in 34% of patients with rheumatic fever.[63] Once thought to be a rarity, rheumatic fever appears to be undergoing a resurgence in certain parts of the United States.[72] Rheumatic fever nodules are small (2 to 5 mm), multiple, and have a tendency to occur over bony prominences (knuckles, olecranon processes, humoral epicondyles, and occiput).[63]

Histologic Features

Histologically, the subcutaneous rheumatic fever nodule has a central area of latticelike fibrinoid change within which are groups of thick-walled vessels, neutrophils, and sparse numbers of lymphocytes. There generally is not a well-defined palisading of histiocytes and fibrocytes around the central fibrinous area, and there is generally much less peripheral fibrosis surrounding the nodule.[4,63,68]

Histologically, the subcutaneous nodules found in patients with chronic juvenile polyarthritis (Still's disease) resemble rheumatic fever nodules more than rheumatoid nodules.[63] In the opinion of some authors, however, the histologic difference between rheumatoid nodules and rheumatic fever nodules is only a reflection of the age of the lesion biopsied. Early lesions of rheumatoid nodules have an appearance similar to rheumatic fever nodules, but rheumatoid nodules generally are not biopsied until late in their development, when the histology appears different from rheumatic fever nodules.[4,69]

Differential Diagnosis

Differential diagnosis includes the classic palisading granuloma (Table 18–1) as well as epithelioid sarcoma[73,74] and localized beryllium granuloma.[37] In epithelioid sarcoma, there are pleomorphic epithelioid and spindle-shaped cells with prominent mitoses and eosinophilic cytoplasm that palisade around a zone of altered collagen. Such nuclear pleomorphism is not seen in rheumatoid nodules. Localized beryllium granuloma, unlike rheumatoid nodule, often involves epithelioid cell granulomas within the dermis and subcutis as well as prominent foci of eosinophilic hyalinized necrosis of stroma.[37]

ANNULAR ELASTOLYTIC GRANULOMA

Clinical Features

Clinically, annular elastolytic granuloma appears as small pink papules that expand to form centrally hypopigmented, 1 to 6 cm annular plaques with raised borders (annuli) that measure 2 to 5 mm in width.[75,76] The patient is typically past his third decade; favored sites include the neck, face, chest, and arms.[75,76]

The pathogenesis of annular elastolytic granuloma is unknown, but there is some evidence to indicate that the giant cell granulomas are a cell-mediated immune response modulated by a predominance of T helper lymphocytes.[77]

Histologic Features

A radial three-zone biopsy of a clinical lesion should be taken that includes noninvolved skin, annulus (raised border), and centrally located involved skin.[75] Histologic examination of the annulus reveals a pattern of predominantly upper and middermal inflammatory reaction composed of numerous multinucleated giant cells, histiocytes, lymphocytes, and epithelioid cells (Fig. 18–16). The multinucleate giant cells may contain cytoplasmic fragments of basophilic, degenerate elastic fibers (elastolysis) (Fig. 18–17) and may

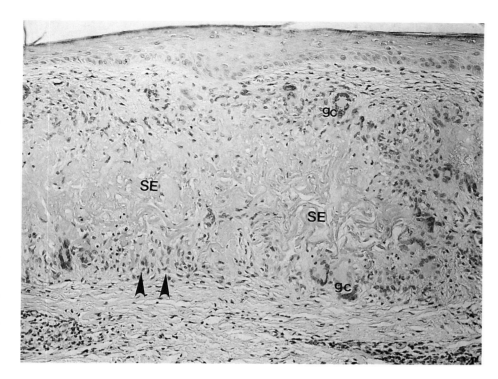

Figure 18–16. Annular elastolytic granuloma (actinic granuloma). A central dermal focus of basophilic solar elastosis (SE) is surrounded by a peripheral palisade of multinucleate giant cells (gc), fibroblasts, and histiocytes (arrowheads). The epidermis is flattened, and there is a chronic perivascular inflammatory cell infiltrate immediately below the elastolytic granuloma. (H&E, ×136.)

surround typical foci of elastosis in a palisade fashion (Fig. 18–16).[50] Often, however, the elastolytic giant cells are mixed with other inflammatory cells within a dermal focus that may contain moderate to minimal numbers of elastic fibers.[50,76,78] Central to the annulus, the elastic fibers appear to be absent, and peripheral to the annulus (noninvolved skin), there is moderate elastosis. Asteroid bodies, if pres-

ent, may stain with acid orcein.[49,50] The epidermis may be normal or exhibit actinic change, such as mild keratinocytic atypia, and flattening of the rete ridge pattern. There is no deposition of lipid, fibrin, or glycosaminoglycans in the affected dermis, nor is there any apparent alteration of collagen.[76,78]

Similar disease entities have been described under a

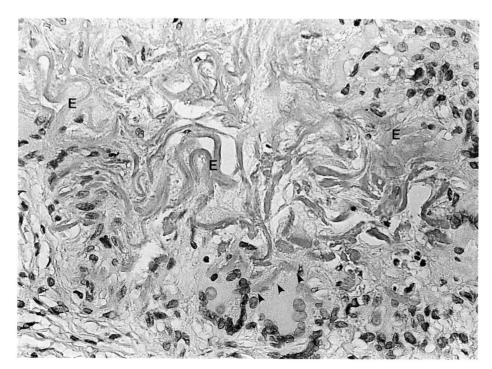

Figure 18–17. Higher power of specimen Figure 16. Deeply basophilic thickened elastic fibers (E) are surrounded by multinucleate giant cells and histiocytes. Note an intracytoplasmic elastic fiber (arrowheads) within one giant cell. (H&E, ×340.)

variety of names: atypical annular necrobiosis lipoidica,[49,79] Miescher's granuloma,[80] actinic granuloma,[50,75,77] and granuloma annulare in sun-exposed skin.[4,81] Although some authors believe that these entities should be placed under a single category,[76] some subtle histologic differences do exist. With the exception of O'Brien,[50] no one has given any attention to actinic elastotic damage of dermal blood vessels and its postulated relationship to the development of actinic granuloma. In O'Brien's view, actinic granuloma has four main histologic patterns: giant cell, necrobiotic (vascular), histiocytic, and sarcoidal.[50] In the giant cell type of actinic granuloma (Figs. 18–16, 18–17), actinic exposure leads to an intense process of focal elastolysis, resulting in a multinucleated giant cell elastolytic response. The histologic pattern depends on the degree of actinically induced vasculopathy, which in turn depends on (1) the size of blood vessels involved, (2) acuteness or chronicity of vascular blockage, and (3) vascular collateralization. In this variant, there is an irregular dermal focus of altered collagen surrounded by large numbers of histiocytes and some giant cells. Actinic vascular change can sometimes be seen adjacent to the areas of degenerated collagen and is characterized by elastotic damage to the internal elastic lamina with variable degrees of thickening and luminal narrowing. The histocytic variant of actinic elastolytic granuloma may be the same pathogenically as the giant cell type except that, for unknown reasons, histiocytes predominate. Patients with the frankly sarcoidal type of annular elastolytic granuloma may have a unique susceptibility to elastolytic inflammation, which leads to epithelioid giant cell formation.

There is no uniform agreement whether the entity actinic granuloma exists or whether all of the different but similar diseases described should be categorized under one heading: annular elastolytic granuloma. Mehregan et al. prefer the term Miescher's granuloma of the face because in their series of patients there was no palisading process. Therefore, they reasoned, this entity should not be classified with the palisading granulomas.[80] However, Hanke et al. disagree with the idea of using Miescher's name for conditions that are not clinically like necrobiosis lipoidica (yellow, atrophic, telangiectatic), since Miescher's original description was of lesions on the lower legs of nondiabetics.[76] Furthermore, Hanke et al.[76] believe that since previous published photographs described as necrobiosis lipoidica of the scalp and face[79] and Miescher's granuloma of the face[80] did not show solar elastosis, the inclusion of these cases under a general category of actinic granuloma was inappropriate.[76] O'Brien disputed this interpretation of the published photomicrographs by Hanke et al. and emphasized the need for a controlled hematoxylin and eosin stain to better define the different phases of actinic elastotic damage.[50] Finally, some authors do not agree with the designation of actinic granuloma as a disease sui generis because (1) the presence of elastotic material within giant cells is not specific for any entity and can be seen incidentally in any granulomatous process, (2) absence of elastotic material in areas of active and healed granulomatous inflammation is not specific, and (3) there is not a consistent association between solar elastosis and granulomatous inflammation of the skin.[81]

Annular elastolytic giant cell granuloma probably best describes the clinicopathologic entity discussed, since by definition, there are dermal multinucleate giant cells with or without asteroid bodies, histiocytes, lymphocytes, scattered epithelioid giant cells, elastolysis, negligible dermal collagen alteration, and absence of lipid and mucin.[76] This working definition seems to exclude most cases of granuloma annulare, necrobiosis lipoidica, and sarcoidosis. The relationship of actinic vascular change and actinic granulomatous change[50] is an interesting and provocative concept and deserves further serious study.

Differential Diagnosis

The differential diagnosis includes granuloma annulare, necrobiosis lipoidica, and sarcoidosis. Unlike annular elastolytic granuloma, necrobiosis lipoidica and granuloma annulare exhibit characteristic well-defined areas of collagen degeneration (Table 18–1). Also, extracellular deposition of glycosaminoglycans, fibrin, or lipid generally seen in either necrobiosis lipoidica or granuloma annulare are not seen in annular elastolytic granuloma. In contrast to most cases of annular elastolytic granuloma, sarcoidosis exhibits numerous epithelioid granulomas at varying depths throughout the dermis with occasional involvement of the subcutis.

Acknowledgment

The author gratefully acknowledges the expert photographic assistance of Milton D. Tudahl, Sr., Director of Photographic Services, Francis Scott Key Medical Center, Baltimore, Maryland.

REFERENCES

1. Freinkel RK, Freinkel N. Cutaneous manifestations of endocrine disorders. In: Fitzpatrick TB, Eisen AZ, Wolff K, et al. eds. *Dermatology in General Medicine.* 3rd ed. New York: McGraw-Hill Book Co; 1987:2077–2078.
2. Hood AF, Kwan TH, Burnes DC, et al. *Primer of Dermatopathology.* Boston: Little, Brown and Co; 1984:29.
3. Ackerman AB. *Histologic Diagnosis of Inflammatory Skin Diseases.* Philadelphia: Lea & Febiger; 1978:145.
4. Johnson WC. Necrobiotic granulomas. *J Cutan Pathol.* 1984; 12:289–299.
5. Mehregan AH. *Pinkus' Guide to Dermatohistopathology.* 4th ed. Norwalk, CT: Appleton-Century-Crofts; 1986:292.
6. Allenby CF, Wilson Jones E. Granuloma multiforme. *Trans St Johns Hosp Dermatol Soc.* 1969; 64:88–89.
7. Muhlbauer JE. Granuloma annulare. *J Am Acad Dermatol.* 1980; 3:217–230.
8. Moyer DG. Papular granuloma annulare. *Arch Dermatol.* 1964; 89:41–45.
9. Friedman SJ, Fox BJ, Albert HL. Granuloma annulare arising in herpes zoster scars. *J Am Acad Dermatol.* 1986; 14:764–770.
10. Shideler SJ, Richards M. Granuloma annulare arising after herpes zoster. *J Am Acad Dermatol.* 1986; 15:1049–1050.
11. Eng AM. Erythematous generalized granuloma annulare. *Arch Dermatol.* 1979; 115:1210–1211.
12. Izum AK. Generalized perforating granuloma annulare. *Arch Dermatol.* 1973; 108:708–709.
13. Rubin M, Lynch FW. Subcutaneous granuloma annulare. *Arch Dermatol Syph.* 1966; 93:416–420.

14. Draheim JH, Johnson LC, Helwig EB. A clinico-pathological analysis of "rheumatoid" nodules occurring in 54 children. *Am J Pathol.* 1959; 35:678.

15. Taranta A. Occurrence of rheumatic-like subcutaneous nodules without evidence of joint or heart disease. *N Engl J Med.* 1962; 2667:13–16.

16. Mesara BW, Brady GL, Oberman HA. Pseudorheumatoid subcutaneous nodules. *Am J Clin Pathol.* 1966; 45:684–691.

17. Owens DW, Freeman RG. Perforating granuloma annulare. *Arch Dermatol.* 1971; 103:64–67.

18. Bordach HG. Granuloma annulare with transfollicular perforation. *J Cutan Pathol.* 1977; 4:99–104.

19. Brown GR. Target lesions in granuloma annulare. *Arch Dermatol.* 1972; 105:928.

20. Dahl MV, Ullman S, Goltz RW. Vasculitis in granuloma annulare. *Arch Dermatol.* 1977; 113:463–467.

21. Umbert P, Winkelmann RK. Granuloma annulare: Direct immunofluorescence study. *Br J Dermatol.* 1976; 95:487–492.

22. Thyresson HN, Doyle JA, Winkelmann RK. Granuloma annulare. Histopathologic and direct immunofluorescence study. *Acta Derm Venereol (Stockh).* 1980; 60:261–263.

23. Dahl MV, Cherney KJ. Circulating immune complexes in granuloma annulare. *Clin Res.* 1979; 27:712A. Abstract.

24. Buechner SA. Identification of T-cell subpopulations in granuloma annulare. *Arch Dermatol.* 1983; 119:125–128.

25. Modlin RL, Howritz DA, Jordan RR, et al. Immunopathologic demonstration of T lymphocyte populations and interleukin 2 in granuloma annulare. *Pediatr Dermatol.* 1984; 2:26–30.

26. Padilla RS, Holguin T, Burgdorf WH. Serum lysosyme in patients with localized and generalized granuloma annulare. *Arch Dermatol.* 1985; 121:624–625.

27. Wolf HH, Maciejewski W. The ultrastructure of granuloma annulare. *Arch Dermatol Res.* 1977; 259:225–234.

28. Umbert P, Winkelmann RK. Histologic ultrastructural, and histochemical studies of granuloma annulare. *Arch Dermatol.* 1977; 113:1681–1686.

29. Silverman RA, Rabinowitz AD. Eosinophils in the cellular infiltrate of granuloma annulare. *J Cutan Pathol.* 1985; 12:13–17.

30. Ackerman AB. *Histologic Diagnosis of Inflammatory Skin Diseases.* Philadelphia: Lea & Febiger; 1978:349, 416–421.

31. Wood MG, Beerman H. Necrobiosis lipoidica, granuloma annulare and rheumatoid nodule. *J Invest Dermatol.* 1960; 34:139–147.

32. Gray HR, Graham JH, Johnson WC. Necrobiosis lipoidica: A histopathological and histochemical study. *J Invest Dermatol.* 1965; 44:369–380.

33. Duncan WC, Smith JD, Knox JM. Generalized perforating granuloma annulare. *Arch Dermatol.* 1973; 108:570–572.

34. Delaney SC, Gold TJ, Leppard B. Disseminated perforating granuloma annulare. *Br J Dermatol.* 1973; 89:523–526.

35. Patterson JW. Rheumatoid nodule versus subcutaneous granuloma annulare—A histologic and histochemical study. *J Cutan Pathol.* 1986; 13:458. Abstract.

36. Beatty EC Jr. Rheumatic-like nodule occurring in nonrheumatic children. *Arch Pathol.* 1959; 68:154–159.

37. Neave HJ, Frank SB, Tolmach J. Cutaneous granulomas following laceration by fluorescent light bulbs. *Arch Dermatol Syph.* 1950; 61:401–406.

38. Johnson WT, Helwig EB. Cat-scratch disease. Histopathologic changes in the skin. *Arch Dermatol.* 1969; 100:148–154.

39. Mehregan AH. *Pinkus' Guide to Dermatohistopathology.* 4th ed. Norwalk, CT: Appleton-Century-Crofts; 1986:291.

40. Cunliffe WJ. Necrobiotic disorders. In: Rock A, Wilkinson DS, Ebling FJG, et al., eds. *Textbook of Dermatology.* 4th ed. Oxford: Blackwell Scientific Publications; 1986:1687–1697.

41. Muller SA, Winkelmann RK. Necrobiosis lipoidica diabeticorum. *Arch Dermatol.* 1966; 93:272–281.

42. Parra CA. Transepithelial elimination in necrobiosis lipoidica. *Br J Dermatol.* 1977; 96:83–86.

43. Bauer MF, Hirsch P, Bullock WK, et al. Necrobiosis lipoidica diabeticorum. A cutaneous manifestation of diabetic microangiopathy. *Arch Dermatol.* 1984; 90:558–566.

44. Muller SA, Winkelmann RK. Necrobiosis lipoidica diabeticorum. *Arch Dermatol.* 1966; 94:1–10.

45. Ullman S, Dahl MV. Necrobiosis lipoidica. *Arch Dermatol.* 1977; 113:1671–1673.

46. Mehregan AH, Pinkus H. Necrobiosis lipoidica with sarcoid reaction. *Arch Dermatol.* 1961; 83:143–145.

47. Williams RM. Necrobiosis lipoidica diabeticorum with alopecia showing sarcoid-like reaction. *Arch Dermatol.* 1959; 79:366–368.

48. Ackerman AB. *Histologic Diagnosis of Inflammatory Skin Diseases.* Philadelphia: Lea & Febiger; 1978:424–431.

49. Dowling GB, Wilson Jones E. Atypical (annular) necrobiosis lipoidica of the face and scalp. *Dermatologica.* 1967; 135:11–26.

50. O'Brien JP. Actinic granuloma: The expanding significance: An analysis of its origin in elastotic ("aging") skin and a definition of necrobiotic (vascular), histocytic and sarcoid variants. *Int J Dermatol.* 1985; 24:473–490.

51. Arzt L. Foreign body granulomas and Boeck's sarcoid. *J Invest Dermatol.* 1955; 24:155–166.

52. Epstein WL, Skahen JR, Krasnobrod H. The organized epithelioid cell granuloma: Definition of allergic (zirconium) from colloidal (silica) types. *Am J Pathol.* 1963; 43:391–405.

53. Epstein WL, Skahen JR, Krasnobrod H. Granulomatous hypersensitivity to zirconium: Localization of allergen in tissue and its role in formation of epithelioid cells. *J Invest Dermatol.* 1962; 38:223–232.

54. Epstein WL, Allen JR. Granulomatous hypersensitivity after use of zirconium-containing poison oak lotions. *JAMA.* 1964; 190:940–942.

55. Rowell NR. Lupus erythematosus, scleroderma, and dermatomyositis. The "collagen" or "connective-tissue" diseases. In: Rook A, Wilkinson DS, Ebling FJG, et al. eds. *Textbook of Dermatology.* 4th ed. Oxford: Blackwell Scientific Publications; 1986:1386–1388.

56. Sibbitt WL, Williams RC Jr. Cutaneous manifestations of rheumatoid arthritis. *Int J Dermatol.* 1982; 21:563–572.

57. Horn RT, Detlef KG. Perforating rheumatoid nodule. *Arch Dermatol.* 1982; 118:696–697.

58. Lever WF, Schaumburg-Lever G. *Histopathology of the Skin.* 6th ed. Philadelphia: JB Lippincott Co; 1983:234–241.

59. Kossard S, Goellner JR, Su WPD. Subcutaneous necrobiotic granulomas of the scalp. *J Am Acad Dermatol.* 1980; 3:180–185.

60. Lowney ED, Simons HM. Rheumatoid nodules of the skin. *Arch Dermatol.* 1963; 88:853–858.

61. Gordon DA, Stein JL, Broden I. The extraarticular features of rheumatoid arthritis. A systemic analysis of 127 cases. *Am J Med.* 1973; 54:445–452.

62. Rapoport RJ, Kozin F, Mackel SE, et al. Cutaneous vascular immunofluorescence in rheumatoid arthritis. A correlation with circulating immune complexes and vasculitis. *Am J Med.* 1980; 68:325–331.

63. Bywaters EGL. Skin manifestations of rheumatic disease. In: Fitzpatrick TB, Eisen AZ, Wolff K, et al. eds. *Dermatology in General Medicine.* 3rd ed. New York: McGraw-Hill Book Co; 1987:1859–1870.

64. Kulka JP. The pathogenesis of rheumatoid arthritis. *J Chronic Dis.* 1959; 10:388–402.

65. Munthe E, Natvig JB. Characterization of the IgG complexes in eluates from rheumatoid tissue. *J Clin Exp Med.* 1971; 8:249–262.

66. Sokologg L, McCluskey RT, Bunim JJ. Vascularity of the early subcutaneous nodule of rheumatoid arthritis. *Arch Pathol Lab Med.* 1953; 55:475–495.

67. Rasker JJ, Kuipers FC. Are rheumatoid nodules caused by vasculitis? A study of 13 early cases. *Ann Rheum Dis.* 1983; 42:384–388.

68. Hood AF, Kwan TH, Burnes DC, et al. *Primer of Dermatopathology.* Boston: Little, Brown and Co; 1984: 207–212.

69. Bennet GA, Zeller JW, Bauer W. Subcutaneous nodules of rheumatoid arthritis and rheumatic fever. *Arch Pathol.* 1940; 30:70–89.

70. Collins DH. The subcutaneous nodule of rheumatoid arthritis. *J Pathol Bacteriol.* 1937; 45:97–115.

71. Watt TL, Bauman RR. Pseudoxanthomatous rheumatoid nodules. *Arch Dermatol.* 1967; 95:156–160.

72. Veasy LG, Wiedmeier SE, Orsmond GS. Resurgence of acute rheumatic fever in the intermountain area of the United States. *N Engl J Med.* 1987; 316:421–427.

73. Enzinger FM. Epithelioid sarcoma. A sarcoma simulating a granuloma or carcinoma. *Cancer.* 1970; 26:1029–1041.

74. Heenan PJ, Quirk CJ, Papadmitriou JM. Epithelioid sarcoma. A diagnostic problem. *Am J Dermatopathol.* 1986; 8:95–104.

75. O'Brien JP. Actinic granuloma. An annular connective tissue disorder affecting sun and heat-damaged (elastotic) skin. *Arch Dermatol.* 1975; 111:460–466.

76. Hanke WC, Balin PL, Roenigk HH Jr. Annular elastolytic giant cell granuloma. A clinicopathologic study of five cases and a review of similar entities. *J Am Acad Dermatol.* 1979; 1:413–421.

77. McGrae JD Jr. Actinic granuloma. A clinical, histopathologic, and immunocytochemical study. *Arch Dermatol.* 1986; 122:43–47.

78. Schwartz TH, Lindlbauer R, Gschnait F. Annular elastolytic giant cell granuloma. *J Cutan Pathol.* 1983; 10:321–326.

79. Wilson-Jones E. Necrobiosis lipoidica presenting on the face and scalp. *Trans St Johns Hosp Dermatol Soc.* 1971; 57:203–220.

80. Mehregan AH, Altman J. Miescher's granuloma of the face. *Arch Dermatol.* 1973; 107:62–64.

81. Ragaz A, Ackerman AB. Is actinic granuloma a specific condition? *Am J Dermatopathol.* 1979; 1:43–50.

CHAPTER 19
Histiocytic and Langerhans Cell Reactions

Margot S. Peters

The cutaneous diseases that may be classified as histiocytic and Langerhans cell reactions exhibit a heterogeneous spectrum of histopathologic changes characterized by variation in three main features—histiocytes, foam cells, and mixed inflammatory cells. These entities (Table 19–1) thus may be classified as xanthohistiocytic proliferations and subdivided into Langerhans cell and non-Langerhans cell (or non-X) histiocytoses. In certain diseases, the histologic picture is diagnostic. More commonly, the presence of one or more of the three features enables one only to place the entity within this broad category of reactions rather than to make a specific diagnosis.

This chapter reviews the structural and functional characteristics of normal histiocytes and Langerhans cells as well as the clinical and histologic features of the cutaneous syndromes that are characterized by proliferation of these cells. The overlap in histologic features between the different entities classified as histiocytic and Langerhans cell reactions emphasizes the importance of considering clinical, histologic, ultrastructural, enzymatic, and immunocytochemical properties in arriving at a specific diagnosis.

STRUCTURE AND FUNCTION

The mononuclear phagocyte system (MPS) includes a functionally and morphologically similar group of cells derived directly or indirectly from bone marrow stem cells.[1-9] These cells are widely distributed in the body and are named according to location—for example, alveolar macrophages in lung, and monocytes in peripheral blood. Mononuclear phagocytes appear to develop from a line of monoblasts, promonocytes, and eventually mature monocytes. The terms "histiocyte" and "macrophage" often are used interchangeably. Basset et al.[1] described histiocytes as "fasting" cells and macrophages as cells that have used their phagocytic capacity and contain ingested material. Although there has been some debate concerning the precise definition of the histiocyte, it is generally accepted that histiocytes represent MPS cells that are located in connective tissue.

The ultrastructural features of mononuclear phagocytes are shared by all cells of this system but are most developed in mature cells. An MPS cell is 10 to 25 μm in diameter, contains an indented or kidney-shaped nucleus with dispersed chromatin and a single nucleolus, and has a nucleus/cytoplasm ratio of less than 1. The cytoplasm is rich in mitochondria, smooth and rough endoplasmic reticulum, and Golgi apparatus. The characteristic cytoplasmic organelles are lysosomes and micropinocytotic vesicles. Lysosomes are pleomorphic and usually numerous, although the number present in a given cell may vary. Lysosomes with ingested particles are phagosomes. The plasma membrane of MPS cells contains numerous irregular folds. With pathologic changes, variations in morphology occur, such as the appearance of lipid inclusions or formation of multinucleated giant cells by membrane fusion.

One of the main functions of mononuclear phagocytes is elimination of particles by phagocytosis (uptake of material larger than 1 μm) or pinocytosis. Macrophages are capable of both immune phagocytosis mediated by surface receptors for complement and the Fc fragment of IgG and nonimmune phagocytosis of nonopsonized particles. Macropinocytosis is the uptake, into vacuoles, of particles 0.1 to 1.0 μm; micropinocytosis involves vacuoles smaller than 0.1 μm. Ingested materials are digested mainly by lysosomal acid hydrolases present in copious amounts within the lysosomes. All cells of the MPS are capable of adherence to glass.

MPS cells serve an important function in the induction phase of T cell activation, via expression of immune response gene products and elaboration of secretory mediators. Recognition of antigens by T lymphocytes requires uptake and processing by accessory cells, that is, specialized macrophages. MPS cells exhibit Ia/HLA-DR/major histocompatibility-linked antigens, produce interleukin 1 (IL-1, lymphocyte-activating factor), and are able to process and present antigen to T cells. T cells activated by mononuclear phagocytes elaborate lymphokines, which in turn may cause

TABLE 19–1. CUTANEOUS HISTIOCYTIC AND LANGERHANS CELL REACTIONS

Histiocytosis X[a]

Xanthoma

Xanthoma disseminatum

Papular xanthoma

Juvenile xanthogranuloma

Necrobiotic xanthogranuloma

Multicentric reticulohistiocytosis

Generalized eruptive histiocytoma

Congenital or infantile self-healing reticulohistiocytosis[a]

Benign cephalic histiocytosis

Progressive nodular histiocytoma

Sinus histiocytosis with massive lymphadenopathy

Malignant histiocytosis

[a] Langerhans granules are observed by electron microscopy.

further stimulation of macrophages. MPS cells produce mediators that influence afferent and efferent limbs of immunologic responses as well as nonimmunologic inflammatory reactions. The soluble products of MPS cells—monokines—include neutral proteases, complement components, prostaglandins, and interferon. Mononuclear phagocytes are also capable of direct cytotoxicity.

The group of dendritic histiocytes includes Langerhans cells, cutaneous indeterminate cells, paracortical interdigitating cells, and follicular dendritic cells.[2,6,7] In addition to their distinction by the presence of dendritic processes, these cells have other functional and structural properties that separate them from macrophages. In comparison with nondendritic macrophages, dendritic cells have greater accessory cell function, minimal phagocytic activity, fewer cytoplasmic organelles associated with phagocytosis, and lower levels of lysosomal enzymes.[8] Dendritic cells of skin and lymphoid tissues have been referred to as antigen-presenting cells.[5]

Interdigitating cells are located in the T cell zones (paracortex) of lymph nodes and tonsils and in the periarteriolar lymphoid sheaths of the spleen. They are usually surrounded by T helper cells. Follicular dendritic cells are seen in association with B cells in germinal centers and mantles of lymphoid follicles.

The Langerhans cell (LC) was described by Paul Langerhans in 1868, when he recognized a population of dendritic epidermal cells that stained with gold chloride.[5] As discussed in Chapter 1, LCs are found in skin and also in other stratified squamous epithelia, such as mouth, oropharynx, esophagus, vagina, and cervix, and they also have been identified in lymph nodes and thymus.[8] LCs are derived from bone marrow and constitute 2% to 8% of all epidermal cells.[4] They are located mainly in the suprabasilar portions of the epidermis but have dendritic processes extending around keratinocytes and into the granular layer. LCs are approximately 12 μm in diameter.[10] In 1961, Birbeck noted rod-shaped cytoplasmic granules with a vesicle at one end, which have since been nicknamed "tennis racquet" granules and also are referred to as Birbeck or Langerhans granules. They are pathognomonic for these cells. The gran-

ules are variable in length (190 to 360 nm) but relatively constant in width (33 nm).[10] The three main ultrastructural criteria for LC are clear cytoplasm, lobulated nucleus, and the characteristic granules[5] (Figs. 19–1, 19–2). The cells do not contain desmosomes or tonofilaments. Like nondendritic macrophages, LCs contain mitochondria, lysosomes, endoplasmic reticulum, and Golgi apparatus. LCs also contain other cytoplasmic bodies that are not unique to this type of cell, including trilaminar membranous loops (wormlike or comma-shaped bodies).

Cutaneous indeterminate cells and LCs exhibit similar morphologic characteristics and surface markers, but because indeterminate cells lack Birbeck granules, it has been postulated that they may represent LC precursors.[8] LCs, indeterminate cells, and dendritic cells of lymphoid tissues share with nondendritic MPS cells the presence of surface receptors for the Fc fragment of IgG and for complement.

LCs appear to play a critical role in the induction phase of cutaneous delayed-type hypersensitivity reactions, that is, allergic contact dermatitis.[4] The importance of LCs in contact sensitivity is supported by the presence of these cells apposed to lymphocytes in skin sensitized with dinitrochlorobenzene.[11] LCs stimulate antigen-specific T cell proliferation in vitro as well as allogeneic and syngeneic T cell activation in mixed leukocyte reactions.[5] LCs produce Il-1 and thus influence T cell proliferation in vivo. In experimental animals, depletion of cutaneous LCs followed by topical application of a contact allergen results in antigen-specific tolerance rather than sensitivity. LCs are responsible for uptake and processing of antigen so that, in conjunction with a major histocompatibility locus, the antigen may be recognized by T cells. By a similar mechanism, these cells probably play an important role in immune defense against tumors and infections. Keratinocytes, LCs, epidermotropic T lymphocytes, and lymph nodes have been considered to represent the system of so-called skin-associated lymphoid tissues (SALT) that mediate immunologic surveillance.[4]

SPECIAL STAINS: ENZYME HISTOCHEMISTRY, IMMUNOCYTOCHEMISTRY

Recognition of the staining properties of dendritic and nondendritic mononuclear phagocytes is important in the detection of these cells in normal tissues and in tissues from patients with cutaneous diseases characterized by proliferation of LCs and non-X histiocytes.

LCs cannot be visualized by routine light microscopy. They are distinguished from other epidermal cells by reactivity with gold chloride stain and by membrane ATPase activity[5,12] (Fig. 19–3). However, indeterminate cells, dendritic lymphoid cells, and nondendritic macrophages also exhibit ATPase activity.[7] Expression of HLA-A,B,C, or HLA-DR antigens is not specific for LCs.[8,12] Although antibody to S100 protein does not appear to stain nondendritic histiocytes, it does stain indeterminate cells and various other cell types, including melanocytes.[13,14] LCs are vimentin-positive, as are other mesenchymal cells or tissue.[15]

T6 antigen is a major histocompatibility complex class

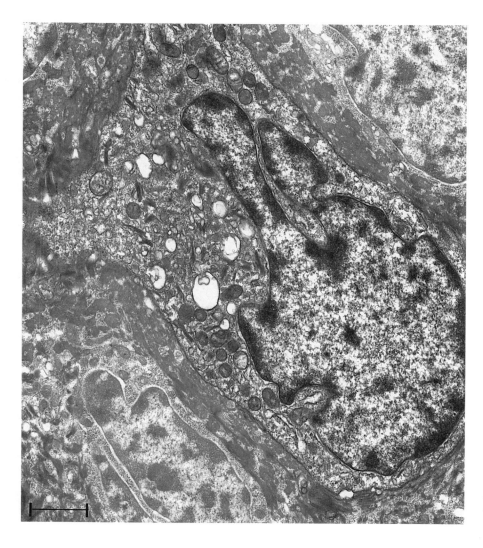

Figure 19–1. Langerhans cells. Electron micrograph, illustrating the indented nucleus and scattered organelles. (Scale bar = 1 μm, H&E ×13,200.)

I antigen structurally different from HLA-A,B,C.[5] Studies of thymocyte development have shown that at an intermediate stage these cells react with antibodies to T6, T4, and T5 but lose T6 reactivity with subsequent maturation. Anti-T6 (OKT6/Leu-6) reacts with 70% of cortical thymocytes (but not peripheral T cells), intraepidermal and lymph node LCs, and cutaneous indeterminate cells. T6, HLA-A,B,C, and M241 glycoproteins are β_2-microglobulin-associated proteins found on the LC membranes. T6 appears to be the most specific light microscopic marker for LCs.[5,6,8] HLA-A,B,C is also present on keratinocytes as well as on nondendritic macrophages, and M241 is also detected on endothelial cells.[5,8,12] The suggestion that indeterminate cells are precursors of LCs is further supported by the staining of both types of cells with antibody to T6.[6]

Nondendritic histiocytes and macrophages are negative for T6 and S100 protein.[7–9] However, they contain nonspecific esterase, acid phosphatase, lysozyme, and α_1-antitrypsin activities.[7] Leu-M1 antigen is present on the majority of peripheral blood monocytes and granulocytes as well as histiocytes, and thus it is of limited value in identifying tissue histiocytes.[16] Leu-M3 and Mac-1 are produced by LCs and nondendritic histiocytes.[4,8,9] The enzyme activities and antigenic markers of histiocytic and LCs are summarized in Table 19–2.

Immunostaining, particularly for T6 and S100 protein, has facilitated analysis of alterations in the LC population in various cutaneous diseases, including lupus erythematosus, psoriasis, alopecia areata, papilloma virus infections, lichen planus, atopic dermatitis, basal cell carcinoma, and cutaneous T cell lymphomas.[12,17–26] It is difficult to draw conclusions concerning mechanisms of disease from such studies, but these preliminary morphologic data provide evidence that LCs play a role in a broad spectrum of cutaneous diseases.

HISTIOCYTOSIS X

Clinical Features

"Histiocytosis X" is the traditional and most commonly used term applied to a clinically heterogeneous group of diseases that result from proliferation of Langerhans type histiocytes.[10,27–38] Histiocytosis X has been referred to also

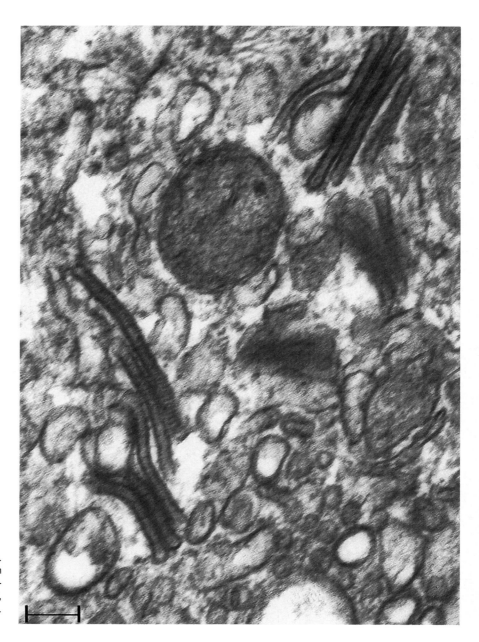

Figure 19–2. Langerhans cell granules. Higher magnification of the cytoplasm shown in Figure 19–1, demonstrating the characteristic rods, sometimes with vesicle at one end, that are pathognomonic for Langerhans cells. (Scale bar = 0.1 μm, H&E, ×137,000.)

as type II histiocytosis, LC granulomatosis, and nonlipid reticuloendotheliosis.[10] The clinical variants were initially described by Letterer in 1924, Siwe in 1933, Hand in 1893, Schüller in 1915, and Christian in 1919.[39-43] In 1953, Lichtenstein[44] coined the term "histiocytosis X" to denote that the entities previously described and referred to as Letterer-Siwe disease, Hand-Schüller-Christian disease, and eosinophilic granuloma all are variants of the same syndrome of unknown cause. Although its cause is not known, histiocytosis X is generally considered to represent a nonneoplastic proliferation of histiocytes, probably due to a disorder of immune function. One estimate of the incidence of histiocytosis X cites 0.6 case per year per 10[6] white children under age 15 years, compared with 42.1 cases of leukemia in the same age group.[10] The disease occurs more commonly in males.

Letterer-Siwe disease is characterized by fever, lymphadenopathy, hepatosplenomegaly, draining otitis media, pulmonary involvement, cutaneous eruption, anemia, and thrombocytopenia. It generally is seen in children less than age 2 years, but rare cases do occur in adults.[28,33] Cutaneous lesions, present in virtually all patients, appear as seborrhea-like dermatitis involving the scalp, perineum, and axillae or as red-brown purpuric papules and nodules, or in both forms.

Hand-Schüller-Christian disease, occurring typically in children ages 2 to 6 years, traditionally has been referred to as the triad of exophthalmos, diabetes insipidus, and bony involvement of the skull. However, all three features are not usually seen synchronously in the same patient.[29] This is a more chronic progressive form of histiocytosis X, in contrast to Letterer-Siwe disease, which represents

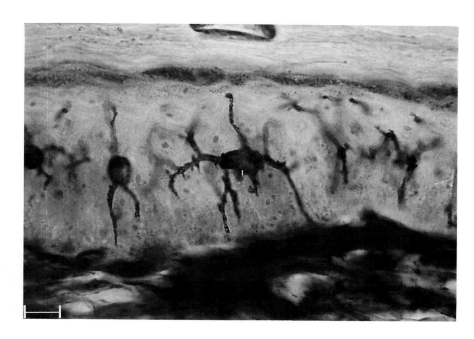

Figure 19–3. Dendritic epidermal cells. Normal skin stained for ATPase shows cells with long dendritic processes occupying mid-dermis. (Scale bar = 10 μm, H&E, ×860.)

acute fulminant disseminated and rapidly progressive multisystem histiocytosis X.

Eosinophilic granuloma, affecting children and young adults, was initially described as synonymous with a solitary bone lesion but may occur as isolated involvement of an-

TABLE 19–2. STAINING PROPERTIES OF DENDRITIC AND NONDENDRITIC HISTIOCYTES

Stain Method	Langerhans Cells	Nondendritic Histiocytes/ Monocytes/ Macrophages
HLA-A,B,C	+	+
HLA-DR	+	+
ATPase	+	+
Fc receptor for IgG	+	+
C3 receptor	+	+
T6	+	−
S100 protein	+	−
Lysozyme	−	+
α_1-Antitrypsin	−	+
Leu-M3	+	+
Leu-3 (T4)	Variable +	Weak +
Leu-M1	−	+
Acid phosphatase	−/weak	+
5′-Nucleotidase	−	Weak +
Alkaline phosphatase	−	−
Chloroacetate esterase	−	−
α-Naphthyl acetate esterase	+/weak	+
β-Glucuronidase	−	Weak +
Mac-1,2,3	+	+
Common leukocyte antigen	+	+

Data from references 6-9, 15, 16.

other organ, commonly lymph nodes. Such lesions are sometimes referred to as benign localized histiocytosis X because of their limited extent and generally good prognosis.

Overlap in clinical features among these three syndromes may make classification as Letterer-Siwe, Hand-Schüller-Christian, or eosinophilic granuloma difficult. However, staging according to extent of disease has prognostic significance.[27,35,36] The prognosis with histiocytosis X is related to the extent of multisystem disease, the type of organ(s) involved, and the presence of organ dysfunction. The outcome is worse in patients under age 2 years, probably reflecting a high percentage of patients with systemic disease in this age group.

Cutaneous involvement is common (more than 80%) and usually extensive in Letterer-Siwe type, common (30%) but less extensive in Hand-Schüller-Christian type, and rare in eosinophilic granuloma. Winkelmann[30] classified the skin lesions of histiocytosis X into five types: (1) diffuse papular scaling eruption, (2) petechial–purpuric lesions, (3) granulomatous ulcerative lesions, (4) xanthomatous lesions, and (5) bronzing of the skin. Infants typically have crops of brown scaling papules on the scalp, face, neck, and trunk, with or without associated vesicles, pustules, or erosions. Lesions may show hemorrhage, ulceration, crusting, or surrounding petechiae or purpura. Intertriginous involvement is common. Purpura rarely may be the only presenting skin lesion; it usually is associated with thrombocytopenia, anemia, and visceral involvement. Oral involvement, including gingivitis, ulceration, or hemorrhage, may be seen.

Cutaneous involvement usually is less florid, less destructive, and more chronic in the Hand-Schüller-Christian type of disease. Again, lesions usually appear as brown to red maculopapules, with or without hemorrhage and crust. Nodules also may be present. Oral lesions have been noted in more than 50% of cases, and perianal or genital lesions are common.

Eosinophilic granuloma is defined as localized disease. However, because the clinical features of the three types of histiocytosis X may overlap, one may see cutaneous lesions in a patient whose main problem is that of localized eosinophilic granuloma of the bone or whose clinical picture is more consistent with Hand-Schüller-Christian disease. Localized eosinophilic granuloma occurring as an ulcerative lesion of the skin or oral mucosa, such as palate, has been reported. Xanthomatous lesions of histiocytosis X are rare but have been emphasized by Altman and Winkelmann.[31]

Lymph nodes may be involved in histiocytosis X with or without apparent involvement of other organs. Histiocytosis X may resemble malignant lymphoma clinically and, in rare cases, may be associated with lymphoma or leukemia.[45,46] Lymphoma and histiocytosis X occurring together in the same lymph node have been described in patients with both Hodgkin's and non-Hodgkin's lymphoma. In most of such cases reported to date, the lymphadenopathy was due to lymphoma, and histiocytosis X was an incidental finding. Involvement of the thymus[47] along with other organs may be seen as part of the presentation of histiocytosis X or may be found incidentally, as in a patient who underwent thymectomy for myasthenia gravis.[48]

Histologic Features

The constant histologic feature that defines all forms of histiocytosis X is a proliferation of histiocytes that have abundant pale eosinophilic cytoplasm with indistinct cell borders, a folded, indented, kidney-shaped nucleus with finely dispersed chromatin, and small inconspicuous nucleoli.[30,36,38,49–51] There may be a wide variation in the presence of other histologic features, including inflammatory infiltrate and stromal changes, depending on the age and type of lesion. Attempts at categorizing the morphologic variants into distinct patterns corresponding to increasing maturity of the lesion have led to descriptions of proliferative, granulomatous, and xanthomatous histologic subtypes.[38,49] However, just as there is overlap in the clinical presentation, the variations in histologic features also make specific classification difficult. More than one pattern may be seen in the same patient.

Early lesions often show the proliferative pattern. Skin biopsy shows multiple plump histiocytes filling the superficial dermis, atrophy and disruption of overlying epidermis by histiocytes crowding the papillary dermis, and intraepidermal collections of histiocytes in a pagetoid pattern or resembling Pautrier's microabscess (Fig. 19–4). The histiocytes occupying the papillary dermis often are separated by an edematous background and focal hemorrhage. They are more densely packed in the reticular dermis (Fig. 19–5). Although there generally is infiltration of both the papillary and the superficial reticular dermis, the papillary dermal involvement is characteristic of early histiocytosis X. The infiltrate may appear bandlike. At scanning magnification, histiocytes appear relatively uniform, but at higher magnification, the cells show moderate variation in size and shape, and sometimes mitotic figures are apparent. The early lesions consist of almost pure populations of histiocytes (Fig. 19–6) with or without a minor component of other cells such as eosinophils, lymphocytes, and foam cells. Large histiocytes may invade dermal vessels. Necrosis also may be seen in the early stage but is more commonly observed in bone than in skin lesions.[36] In the granulomatous pattern, there is more extensive dermal involvement with histiocytes and varying mixtures of eosinophils, neutrophils, plasma cells, lymphocytes, and multinucleated giant cells of the foreign body or Touton type. The typical

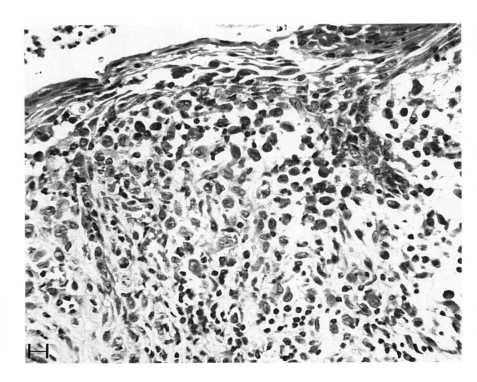

Figure 19–4. Histiocytosis X. Typical proliferative-stage lesion consisting of papillary dermal infiltration with histiocytes on an edematous background and disruption of epidermis by exocytosis of histiocytes. (Scale bar = 10 μm, H&E, ×400.)

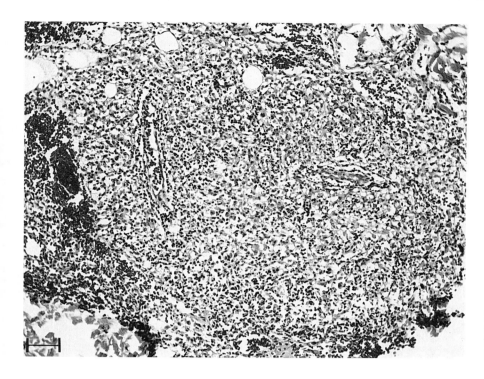

Figure 19–5. Histiocytosis X. Deep dermis contains focal hemorrhage and a dense infiltrate of histiocytes mixed with lymphocytes. (Scale bar = 50 μm, H&E, ×160.)

xanthomatous pattern consists of numerous foam cells along with histiocytes, eosinophils, and multinucleated giant cells.

Attempts at using histopathologic criteria to judge prognosis have been unsuccessful. Risdall et al.[51] evaluated 51 patients with histiocytosis X, including 17 with osseous involvement alone and 34 with multisystem disease. Eosinophils were present in 92% of patients, multinucleated giant cells in 84%, lymphocytes in 75%, necrosis in 61%, neutrophils in 49%, and foamy histiocytes in 29%. Fibrosis was rare. No one histologic feature appeared to correlate with clinical outcome.

Special Stains and Ultrastructure

Histiocytosis X cells and normal nondendritic histiocytes stain similarly for acid phosphatase and nonspecific esterase

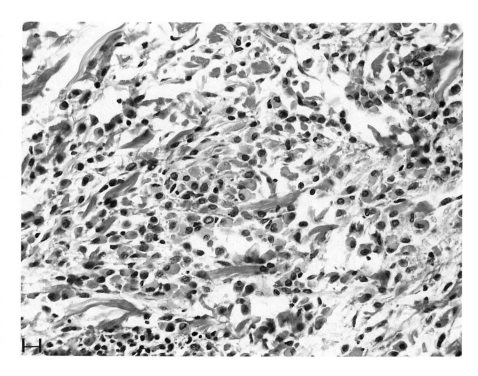

Figure 19–6. Histiocytosis X. This section shows an almost pure infiltrate of histiocytes on an edematous background. (Scale bar = 10 μm, H&E, ×400.)

TABLE 19–3. S100 PROTEIN IN CUTANEOUS HISTIOCYTIC DISEASES

Present in
Histiocytosis X
Congenital self-healing reticulohistiocytosis
Sinus histiocytosis with massive lymphadenopathy

Absent in
Papular xanthoma
Xanthoma disseminatum
Multicentric reticulohistiocytosis
Generalized eruptive histiocytoma
Juvenile xanthogranuloma
Benign cephalic histiocytosis
Necrobiotic xanthogranuloma
Progressive nodular histiocytoma
Malignant histiocytosis

activities.[7,50] Stains for lysozyme and α_1-antitrypsin are negative. In contrast to the infiltrate in most non-X histiocytoses, histiocytosis X cells are positive for S100 protein[13,52] (Table 19–3). Antibody to T6 stains histiocytosis X cells (Figs. 19–7, 19–8), normal LCs and indeterminate cells, 70% of cortical thymocytes, MOLT-4 (T cell leukemia line), and a neuroblastoma cell line[53] (Table 19–4). T6 generally is considered to be superior to S100 protein for detecting Langerhans-type histiocytes because of the wide range of cells and tumors that contain S100 protein. Antibody to T4 also stains histiocytosis X cells, but normal nondendritic histiocytes and LCs are negative or variably positive.[8,53]

The most specific evidence in favor of the diagnosis of histiocytosis X is the ultrastructural finding of Langerhans-type cytoplasmic granules in the histiocytes.[54] However, one should keep in mind that there is a wide variation in the number of histiocytes containing Langerhans granules. Mierau et al.[55] found Langerhans granules in 2% to 79% of histiocytes in their cases of histiocytosis X. An unproductive search for Langerhans granules by electron microscopy does not absolutely exclude histiocytosis X, particularly in the granulomatous and xanthomatous variants. Although Langerhans granules are characteristic for histiocytosis X, comma-shaped cytoplasmic bodies also may be observed.[54]

Differential Diagnosis

The main problem in differential diagnosis is that of histiocytosis X vs the non-X type of histiocytoses. This is a problem less often with the typical proliferative lesions showing a relatively monomorphous infiltrate, but it is more difficult with granulomatous or xanthomatous types. The varying proportions of histiocytes, eosinophils, lymphocytes, foam cells, and fibrosis may make specific diagnosis difficult. Juvenile xanthogranuloma may present an early monomorphous picture with paucity of Touton giant cells. Similarly, Touton giant cells may be numerous, although not the predominant cell type, in some cases of histiocytosis X. Xanthoma disseminatum containing Touton giant cells and numerous foam cells also may resemble histiocytosis X. Relatively monomorphous types of non-X histiocytoses, such as generalized eruptive histiocytoma, should be included in the differential diagnosis. Because of the prognostic importance of distinguishing X from non-X histiocytic infiltrates, it is best to use a battery of immunocytochemical stains and electron microscopy to verify the diagnosis in cases lacking typical clinical and histologic features.

XANTHOMAS

Clinical Features

Cutaneous xanthomas consist of infiltrates of lipid-containing histiocytes, called foam cells, located in dermis or

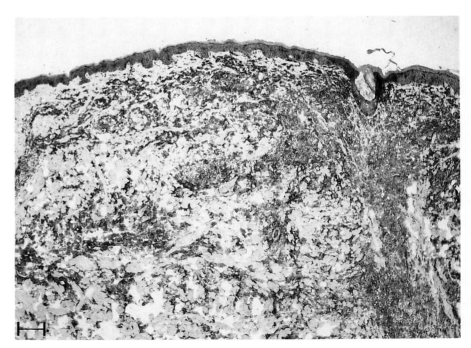

Figure 19–7. Histiocytosis X. Application of antibody to T6 (OKT6) results in staining of most cells throughout the dermal infiltrate. (Scale bar = 0.1 mm, H&E, ×64.)

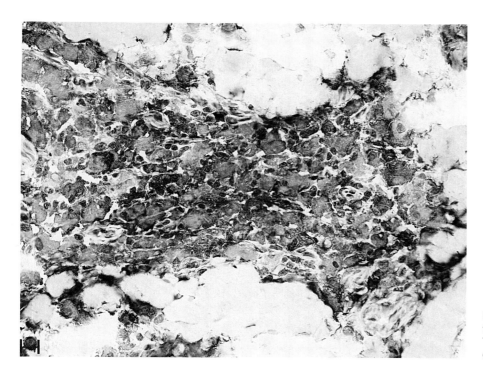

Figure 19–8. Histiocytosis X. Higher magnification of another section exposed to anti-T6 shows staining of a cluster of plump histiocytes. (Scale bar = 10 μm, H&E, ×400.)

TABLE 19–4. CELLS CONTAINING T6 MARKER (OKT6/LEU-6)

Langerhans cells
Indeterminate cells
70% of cortical thymocytes
Histiocytosis X
MOLT-4 (T cell leukemia line)
Neuroblastoma cell line

tendon.[56] A large amount of the lipid content of xanthomas originates from the plasma, and the lesions may vary in size along with variations in serum lipoprotein levels. This is particularly true in the eruptive and tuberous xanthomas. Experiments by Parker et al.[57] have provided data to suggest that lipoproteins infiltrate the walls of dermal capillaries and subsequently are phagocytized by dermal histiocytes that then become foam cells. The lipids contained in xanthomas most often are cholesterol or cholesterol esters but also may be triglycerides or other sterols.[56] Abnormal lipoprotein metabolism has been classified into five types based on electrophoresis: type I, hyperchylomicronemia; type IIa, increase in β-lipoprotein (LDL) level; type IIb, increase in β- and pre-β-lipoprotein (VLDL) levels; type III, increase in indeterminant density lipoprotein (IDL) (remnant lipoprotein); type IV, increase in pre-β-lipoprotein; type V, excess chylomicrons and pre-β-lipoprotein. Abnormal lipid metabolism may be due to primary genetic hyperlipoproteinemia or to secondary abnormalities in lipid metabolism related to various underlying diseases, such as pancreatitis, diabetes, renal disease, hypothyroidism, and cholestatic liver disease.

Eruptive xanthomas occur as 1-mm to 4-mm, yellow to red papules occurring in crops primarily over the extensor surfaces of the extremities and over the buttocks. They may be seen in primary disorders of lipid metabolism (particularly types I, IV, and V), in association with diabetes, pancreatitis, myxedema, or nephrotic syndrome, or caused by a drug (such as 13-*cis*-retinoic acid, estrogen, or corticosteroid). Tuberous xanthomas consist of variably sized yellow to red nodules usually located on the extensor aspects of the elbows and knees, on the buttocks, and on the dorsal surface of the hands over the joints. They are typical in broad β-lipoprotein disease and associated with xanthoma striatum palmaris. Tendinous xanthomas develop in tendons, ligaments, and fascia as deep, smooth, firm nodules most frequently located in extensor tendons of the hands, knees, and elbows and in Achilles tendon in association with hyper-β-lipoproteinemia. Both tendinous and tuberous xanthomas may be seen in normolipemic patients.

Xanthelasmas are the most common type of xanthoma seen in type IIa disease. However, patients with xanthelasmas usually have normal lipid profiles. These lesions involve the inner canthi of the eyelids; rarely, other sites are affected.

Plane xanthomas appear as flat or minimally palpable, yellow-orange plaques with a predilection for the folds or palmar creases. These may be seen in type IIa or III hyperlipoproteinemia or in patients without lipid abnormalities. There have been multiple reports of so-called diffuse normolipemic plane xanthoma[58–62] manifested as large "lemon-yellow" macular lesions.[58] In the series of Altman and Winkelmann,[58] xanthelasmas of the eyelids occurred before or simultaneously with the development of plane xanthomas on the neck, trunk, and extremities. The main significance of diffuse plane xanthoma is its association with systemic disease. Malignancies of the reticuloendothelial system, particularly multiple myeloma and leukemias, have been noted in many cases. Xanthoma associated with myeloma also has been observed in a hyperlipemic patient.[60] Normolipemic xanthoma may be associated with cryoglobulinemia.[61] Hu and Winkelmann[62] reported a case of diffuse normolipemic plane xanthoma, IgG λ monoclonal gammopathy, hypernephroma, and acquired C1 esterase inhibitor deficiency associated with low total hemolytic complement, C1, and C4 levels.

Histologic Features

Xanthomas are characterized by foam cells. These cells have a pale fine granular but mostly clear cytoplasm with a high cytoplasm/nucleus ratio. The nuclei are usually single and inconspicuous. Xanthelasmas generally show the picture of superficial dermal infiltration with variably sized collections of foamy histiocytes and a paucity or absence of inflammatory cells. There usually is no fibrosis, even in late lesions. In addition to numerous foamy histiocytes, eruptive xanthomas also may contain numerous lymphocytes, histiocytes, and neutrophils, particularly in the early stage. Tuberous and tendinous xanthomas also may contain a mixture of foam cells and inflammatory cells. Mature tendinous and tuberous xanthomas predominantly contain foam cells (Fig. 19–9), whereas old lesions may show extensive fibrosis (Fig. 19–10). Plane xanthomas are characterized by clusters of large foam cells with single, round, central nuclei. These foam cells are located in perivascular clusters (Fig. 19–11), as well as diffusely in the dermis.[58] There usually is a minor component of neutrophils and lymphocytes. Foreign body and Touton type giant cells are absent.

Special Stains and Ultrastructure

The foam cells usually are so characteristic that special stains are not necessary. Their lipid-containing cytoplasm stains with scarlet red, Sudan red, or Sudan black. Electron microscopic study shows that in tuberous xanthoma the foam cells predominantly contain large non-membrane-bound lipid droplets. Lesser quantities of lipid appear as electron-lucent cholesterol crystals or electron-dense ceroid granules.[63] Eruptive xanthomas show lipid droplets in the intercellular spaces of dermal capillary walls and lipid phagocytized by macrophages in the vicinity of the capillaries. These macrophages contain non-membrane-bound lipid droplets, numerous lysosomes, and myelin figures.[64] In plane xanthomas, histiocytes contain numerous intracytoplasmic lipid vacuoles, lysosomes, and myelin figures.[65,66] The perivascular arrangement of foamy histiocytes, particularly in generalized plane xanthoma and xanthelasma, has been emphasized.[65] Vacuoles have been observed in pericytes and occasionally in endothelial cells. Crystalline cleft-like spaces have been seen in histiocytes and extracellularly, probably representing cholesterol.[65]

Differential Diagnosis

Relatively pure collections of foam cells seldom create a problem in diagnosis. However, in old lesions, particularly of tuberous xanthoma, the mixture of fibrosis and inflammatory cells may resemble a late stage of several histiocytoses. Varying and sometimes large numbers of foam cells may be seen in juvenile xanthogranuloma, xanthoma disseminatum, necrobiotic xanthogranuloma, and histiocytosis X.

XANTHOMA DISSEMINATUM

Clinical Features

Although the first case of xanthoma disseminatum was probably reported by Grafe in 1867, this term is credited to the article by Montgomery and Osterberg published

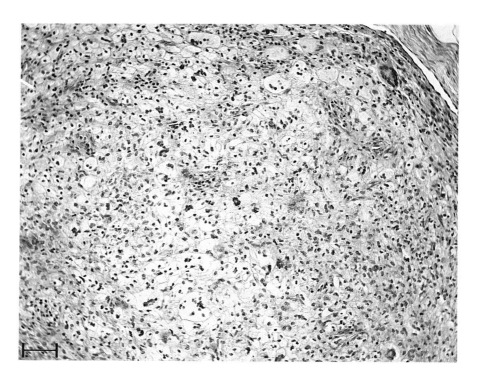

Figure 19–9. Tuberous xanthoma. The predominant cell type is the foam cell in this well-developed lesion. (Scale bar = 50 μm, H&E, ×160.)

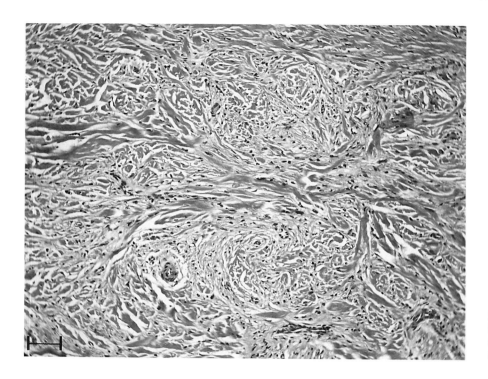

Figure 19–10. Tuberous xanthoma. This old lesion contains extensive fibrosis and lacks the characteristic foam cells. (Scale bar = 50 μm, H&E, ×160.)

in 1938; the disease is also termed "Montgomery's syndrome."[67–69] Patients have numerous inflammatory redbrown papules and xanthomatous plaques symmetrically involving the trunk, face, and proximal extremities. Lesions preferentially involve flexural or intertriginous surfaces, such as axillae, groin, neck, and antecubital and popliteal fossae, and have a tendency to become confluent in these areas. The coalescence of lesions in the folds may have a verrucous appearance. Eyelids, conjunctivae, lips, pharynx, and larynx also may be involved by red to yellow plaques. In the review by Altman and Winkelmann,[68] mucous membrane lesions were noted in almost 40% of patients, sometimes associated with dyspnea or dysphagia. The lesions may have a benign chronic course or may involute over many years.

These patients are normolipemic. The presence of dia-

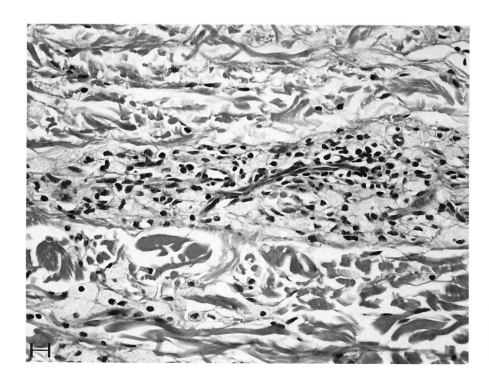

Figure 19–11. Diffuse normolipemic plane xanthoma. This section illustrates the typical perivascular collection of foam cells; a few lymphocytes also are present. (Scale bar = 10 μm, H&E, ×400.)

betes insipidus in approximately 40% of patients has led to confusion of xanthoma disseminatum with histiocytosis X.[68] However, in contrast to histiocytosis X, xanthoma disseminatum generally is a disease of adults, bone lesions and exophthalmos are not present, and xanthoma disseminatum is associated with a much better prognosis.

Histologic Features

Early lesions of xanthoma disseminatum are characterized by dermal infiltration of large, mature-appearing histiocytes with abundant eosinophilic cytoplasm, foam cells, and an inflammatory cell infiltrate mainly of lymphocytes and neutrophils with occasional eosinophils.[68] There may be slight atrophy of the overlying epidermis and increased pigmentation of the basal layer. Numerous Touton giant cells are present; foreign body type giant cells are uncommon. Mature lesions are dominated by foam cells. The cellular infiltrate in xanthoma disseminatum involves superficial and middermis but may extend into underlying tissue.

Special Stains and Ultrastructure

The presence of numerous lipid-laden histiocytes is verified by staining with Sudan IV.[68] Iron has been noted in histiocytes and giant cells as well as extracellularly within the dermis. Ultrastructural study has shown numerous lipid droplets.[29] Electron-dense membrane-bound phagosomes, myeloid bodies, crystals, and macrophages containing elastic fibers also have been observed.[29,70] Most investigators have not observed Langerhans granules in lesions of xanthoma disseminatum.[29,70,71]

Differential Diagnosis

Xanthoma disseminatum is a non-X type of histiocytosis. It differs from papular xanthoma by the presence of inflammatory cells in addition to histiocytes. It may be more readily confused histologically with a tuberous xanthoma than with the true histiocytoses because of the presence of numerous foam cells, although a foam cell component may be seen in histiocytosis X and in several non-X histiocytoses. Xanthoma disseminatum also may be confused with juvenile xanthogranuloma because of the striking presence of Touton giant cells as well as histiocytes, foam cells, lymphocytes, and neutrophils in both entities. However, juvenile xanthogranuloma usually contains many foreign body type giant cells and eosinophils, which are sparse or absent in xanthoma disseminatum. Electron microscopy or immunocytochemistry may be used to rule out histiocytosis X.

JUVENILE XANTHOGRANULOMA

Clinical Features

Juvenile xanthogranuloma, named by Senear and Caro in 1936, was initially described by MacDonagh in 1912 under the name "nevoxanthoendothelioma." Although most commonly seen in children, the lesions also occur in adults.[29,38,69,72,73] Seventy-five percent of cases appear in the first 9 months of life, and in 30%, the lesions are present at birth. Gianotti classified the lesions into two types: a small nodular form and a large nodular form.[29,38] Small nodular lesions begin as 2-mm to 5-mm papules or nodules that evolve from erythematous to yellow. In this subtype,

patients usually have numerous lesions, sometimes more than 100, in a generalized distribution but predominantly over the upper body. Nodular lesions may be present on the epibulbar portion of the iris. The large nodular type usually occurs as less than a dozen lesions usually on the head and trunk. The nodules are 10 to 20 mm in diameter, translucent, erythematous, and telangiectatic. In contrast to the small nodular type, the large nodular type is associated with multiple extracutaneous xanthogranulomas of lung, colon, kidney, bone, pericardium, testes, ovaries, and, occasionally, mucous membranes. Cutaneous and systemic lesions spontaneously involute in 3 to 6 years. Central nervous system lesions recently have been reported in juvenile xanthogranulomas.[74] There is an association of xanthogranuloma with neurofibromatosis and particularly with café au lait spots.[72]

Histologic Features

Early lesions show a relatively monomorphous dermal infiltrate of non-X histiocytes (Fig. 19–12). With time, xanthomatization, inflammation, and fibrosis develop.[69] The typical mature lesion is composed of histiocytes, foam cells, eosinophils, lymphocytes, plasma cells, and neutrophils.[69,72] Foreign body and Touton giant cells are often distributed in the upper portion of the dermis and at the border of the infiltrate (Fig. 19–13). The cellular infiltrate is dense and associated with overlying epidermal atrophy. Old lesions contain fibrosis.

Special Stains and Ultrastructure

Special stains for lipid are positive, and those for iron are negative.[69] Antibody to S100 protein does not stain histiocytes in juvenile xanthogranuloma. By electron microscopy, histiocytes have been observed to contain dense and multivesicular bodies, myeloid bodies, numerous non-membrane-limited fat droplets, and occasional comma-shaped bodies.[29] Langerhans granules have not been identified.

Differential Diagnosis

Although Touton giant cells may be seen in histiocytosis X, they are an inconstant feature. Histiocytosis X may be differentiated from juvenile xanthogranuloma by electron microscopy and immunocytochemistry. Differential diagnosis of juvenile xanthogranuloma and xanthoma disseminatum was reviewed in the preceding section. Benign cephalic histiocytosis and generalized eruptive histiocytoma do not contain foam cells or giant cells. Papular xanthoma lacks a pure histiocytic phase and does not show the inflammatory infiltrate of mature juvenile xanthogranuloma.

PAPULAR XANTHOMA

Clinical Features

Winkelmann's descriptions of papular xanthoma emphasized a distinction from xanthoma disseminatum.[37,69] This syndrome occurs in normolipemic adults and consists of multiple, generalized, 2-mm to 15-mm discrete, round, papular and nodular lesions of the skin and, rarely, mucosa. Cutaneous lesions generally involve the face and trunk. In contrast to xanthoma disseminatum, papular xanthoma lesions are not red-brown in color and do not form confluent plaques.

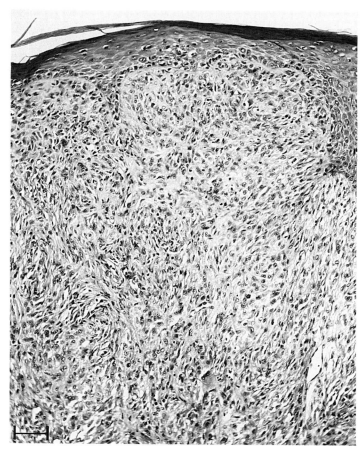

Figure 19–12. Juvenile xanthogranuloma. The papillary superficial and midreticular dermis are filled with a relatively monomorphous collection of histiocytes; other inflammatory cells are rare. (Scale bar = 50 μm, H&E, ×180.)

Histologic Features

Lesions of papular xanthoma are composed predominantly of foam cells and Touton giant cells, without a mixed inflammatory infiltrate or a pure histiocytic stage.[37,69] Sanchez et al.[75] noted a paucity of histiocytes, lymphocytes, and eosinophils in their case. The relative absence of inflammatory cells is the most characteristic feature of papular xanthoma and distinguishes this entity from xanthoma disseminatum, with which it is most often confused.

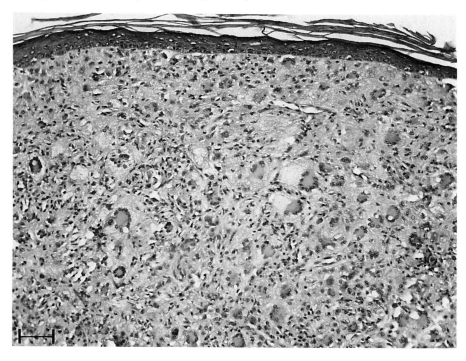

Figure 19–13. Juvenile xanthogranuloma. Characteristic histologic picture of histiocytes and Touton giant cells without intraepidermal involvement. (Scale bar = 50 μm, H&E, ×150.)

Special Stains and Ultrastructure

Cytoplasmic vacuoles are negative on periodic acid-Schiff staining.[37,75] Hemosiderin granules have been seen in the cytoplasm of foam cells as well as extracellularly.[75] Lysozyme is variably present.[75] Stain for S100 protein is negative.[29,75]

Ultrastructural study[75] has shown that the foam cells have characteristics of macrophages. Fat droplets do not contain a limiting membrane and are electron dense. There are numerous cytoplasmic dense bodies with a single limiting membrane. Membrane-bound laminated bodies, up to 0.6 μm, are noted in most cells. Myelin figures and secondary lysosomes also have been observed. Langerhans granules and comma-shaped bodies have not been noted.[37,75]

Differential Diagnosis

The lack of inflammatory cells distinguishes papular xanthoma from juvenile xanthogranuloma as well as xanthoma disseminatum. Generalized eruptive histiocytosis, reticulohistiocytosis, progressive nodular histiocytoma, and histiocytosis X have a prominent histiocytic infiltrate and, hence, should not be confused with papular xanthoma.

NECROBIOTIC XANTHOGRANULOMA

Clinical Features

In 1980, Kossard and Winkelmann[76] described eight patients with granulomatous xanthomas and paraproteinemia or lymphoproliferative disease. The "xanthomas" were located in the periorbital region as well as on the trunk and consisted of ulcerative nodules and plaques up to 10 cm in diameter. In 1984 Robertson and Winkelmann[77] reported 16 cases with emphasis on the ophthalmic abnormalities and the destructive quality of the xanthogranulomatous inflamma-

tion. On review, previously reported cases of "atypical necrobiosis lipoidica," xanthoma disseminatum, or "atypical reticulohistiocytosis" have been considered to fit the syndrome of necrobiotic xanthogranuloma. In the series of Finan and Winkelmann,[78] approximately 60% of the patients were female and 40% were male. The mean age at onset of skin lesions was 53 years. Twenty of the 22 patients had serum protein abnormalities; 16 patients had IgG type monoclonal gammopathy. Other associated findings included cryoglobulinemia, multiple myeloma, chronic lymphocytic leukemia, urticaria, and angioedema with decreased C1 esterase inhibitor level. The typical clinical appearance consists of violaceous to red to orange or yellow papules, nodules, and plaques 0.3 to 20 cm in diameter, with ulceration of lesions in approximately half the patients. The lesions most often involve periorbital skin (usually in a bilateral and symmetric distribution); less frequently, the trunk, nonperiorbital face region, and extremities are affected. In all reported cases, the patients had multiple lesions.

Histologic Features

The typical histologic picture includes granulomatous masses containing histiocytes, lymphocytes, and numerous giant cells of both Touton and foreign body types involving deep dermis or subcutaneous fat.[76,78] Other major features include broad areas of altered collagen, also known as hyaline necrobiosis, many foamy histiocytes, lymphoid nodules with or without germinal centers, plasma cells, and cholesterol clefts (Figs. 19–14, 19–15, 19–16). In most cases, these features extend from middermis well into the panniculus, with prominent panniculitis.

Special Stains and Ultrastructure

Periodic acid-Schiff-positive, diastase-resistant granules

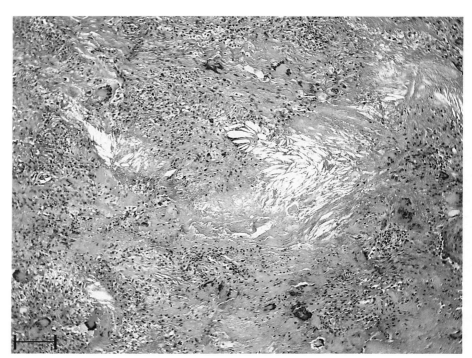

Figure 19–14. Necrobiotic xanthogranuloma. There is extensive hyaline necrobiosis with cholesterol clefts among dense granulomatous inflammation. (Scale bar = 0.1 mm, H&E, ×125.)

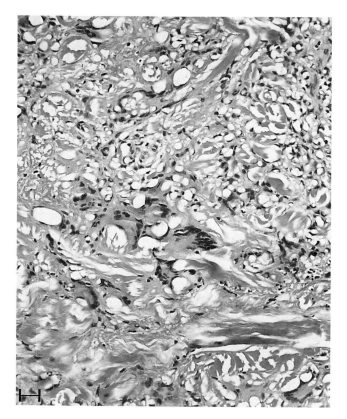

Figure 19–15. Necrobiotic xanthogranuloma. Higher magnification of a necrobiotic granuloma shows vacuolated histiocytes and multiple, somewhat bizarre-shaped multinucleated giant cells. (Scale bar = 20 μm, H&E, ×230.)

may be seen in giant cells and histiocytes.[78] Elastic tissue stains show that these fibers are greatly decreased in areas of altered collagen. Alcian blue staining shows glycosaminoglycans to be absent or sparse. Oil red O and Sudan IV show focal lipid droplets in giant cells and histiocytes. Stain for S100 protein is negative.[78] Direct immunofluorescence has shown vascular staining in the mid- and deep dermis for IgM, C3, or fibrinogen. Electron microscopic study has demonstrated the presence of multilaminar bodies but no Langerhans granules.[76]

Differential Diagnosis

The broad differential diagnosis is illustrated by the diagnoses given to patients with necrobiotic xanthogranuloma before recognition of this syndrome, which included necrobiosis lipoidica diabeticorum, granuloma annulare, foreign body type granuloma, granulomatous panniculitis, xanthoma tuberosum, xanthoma disseminatum, and reticulohistiocytoma. Necrobiotic xanthogranuloma is most often mistaken for necrobiosis lipoidica. However, the granulomatous infiltrate is more massive in necrobiotic xanthogranuloma and shows more numerous and bizarre-shaped giant cells. In addition, necrobiosis lipoidica has more extensive lipid deposition, lymphoid nodules are absent, and cholesterol clefts are rare.

MULTICENTRIC RETICULOHISTIOCYTOSIS

Clinical Features

The first description of a case of multicentric reticulohistiocytosis was by Weber and Freudenthal in 1937,[79] but the name was proposed by Goltz and Laymon in 1954.[80] The syndrome is characterized by cutaneous nodules associated

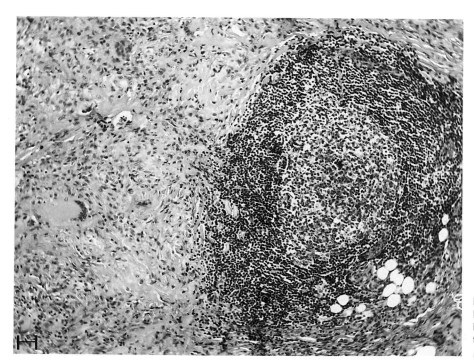

Figure 19–16. Necrobiotic xanthogranuloma. Lymphoid nodule with germinal-center-like structure embedded in the granulomatous inflammatory mass. (Scale bar = 50 μm, H&E, ×160.)

with polyarthritis.[81–85] Skin lesions may occur before, after, or with the onset of the polyarthritis. The syndrome is more common in women, mean age at onset is in the fourth decade, and the mean duration of disease activity is 8 years. Arthritis and rapidly progressive articular destruction most frequently involve the interphalangeal joints, leading to a characteristic accordion or opera glass deformity, followed in frequency by shoulders, knees, wrists, and other sites. Cutaneous lesions are 0.5-cm to 2-cm scattered or coalescent flesh-colored to dark red-brown papules and nodules, typically arising on the head and hands. Lesions on the hands usually are in a periarticular distribution. Forearms, elbows, neck, and trunk also may show papules and nodules. Lesions are present on the oral or nasal mucosa in over half the patients.[83] Pruritus has been noted by at least 25% of patients. Lesions may vary in size, along with variation in joint symptoms. Approximately one third of these patients have xanthelasmas.[83,84] Underlying malignancy has been documented in at least 25% of the patients, and thyroid disease in 15%.[82] Hypercholesterolemia, of uncertain significance, has been noted in a third of the patients.

Histologic Features

Multicentric reticulohistiocytosis and reticulohistiocytic granuloma have similar histologic pictures.[37,81,82,84] Early lesions are composed of lymphocytes surrounding histiocytes. Mature lesions show a dense infiltrate, sometimes well demarcated but not encapsulated, of giant multinucleated or mononucleated cells 50 to 100 μm in diameter occupying the superficial, mid-, and sometimes deep dermis (Figs. 19–17, 19–18). The multinucleated cells may contain up to 20 nuclei. These giant cells have a pale, fine, granular (ground glass) eosinophilic cytoplasm that also may contain vacuoles. There are numerous histiocytes and lymphocytes. Plasma cells are present in variable numbers, and eosinophils are a minor component. The epidermis may show thinning over the infiltrate. There may be a perivascular distribution of histiocytes, lymphocytes, and plasma cells. In some cases, capillary dilatation and proliferation are prominent. The typical picture dominated by the characteristic giant cells may not always be seen. Giant cells may make up a small percentage of the infiltrate or even be absent.[84] Lesions often are associated with proliferation of fibroblasts and fibrosis so that the giant cells appear to be embedded in a fibrous stroma (Fig. 19–19).

Special Stains and Ultrastructure

The cytoplasm of the giant cells is periodic acid-Schiff positive and diastase resistant.[81,84] Lipid stains are variably positive. Reticulum stains have shown fine and thick fibers around individual giant cells. Stains for acid phosphatase, nonspecific esterase, and lysozyme are positive.[81] Stains for α_1-antitrypsin and S100 protein are negative.[13]

Electron microscopy[29,86,87] has shown numerous, small, electron-dense cytoplasmic granules, 50 to 500 nm in diameter. The granules are membrane limited, generally ovoid to spherical or, less often, rod-shaped, and show a lucent zone (halo) between membrane and dense matrix.[86] These granules are found mainly near the Golgi apparatus. Acid phosphatase activity has been shown to correspond to the electron-dense granules.[86] Approximately 40% of the histiocytes contain pleomorphic cytoplasmic inclusions of membranes and vesicles.[29] Histiocytes that do not contain these inclusions may show evidence of collagen phagocytosis, which may be responsible for the presence of myelin bodies.[88] Langerhans granules are absent.

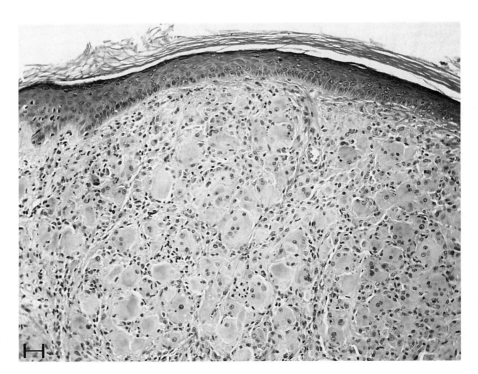

Figure 19–17. Reticulohistiocytoma. This lesion consists almost entirely of giant histiocytes packing the dermis, with slight thinning of the overlying epidermis. (Scale bar = 50 μm, H&E, ×160.)

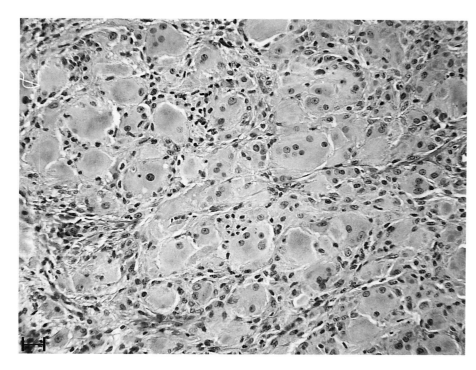

Figure 19–18. Reticulohistiocytoma. Higher magnification of the section shown in Figure 19–17 demonstrates the copious ground glass cytoplasm of the multinucleated histiocytes and paucity of intervening lymphocytes. (Scale bar = 20 μm, H&E, ×250.)

Differential Diagnosis

In mature lesions with abundant giant cells, the histologic diagnosis usually is not difficult. Cases showing a paucity of giant cells and prominent fibroblastic proliferation may be confused with granuloma annulare or the fibrotic stage of a xanthoma. Absence of foam cells in reticulohistiocytoma should facilitate differentiation from xanthoma, juvenile xanthogranuloma, papular xanthoma, and xanthoma disseminatum. However, that the first case was described as "nodular nondiabetic cutaneous xanthomatosis with hypercholesterolemia and atypical histologic features" should indicate that confusion with xanthoma may occur. Eruptive histiocytoma also lacks foam cells but consists of a more uniform population of histiocytes without giant cells.

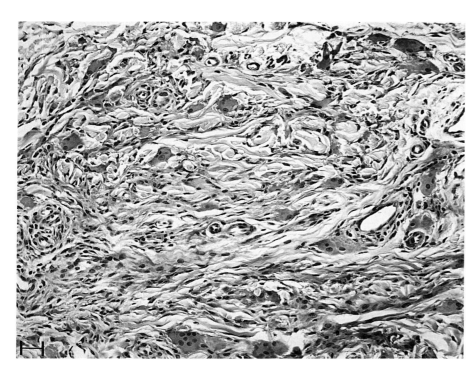

Figure 19–19. Reticulohistiocytoma. In contrast to the typical histologic picture illustrated in Figures 19–17 and 19–18, this section shows a few giant cells, dermal fibrosis, and focal vascular proliferation. (Scale bar = 20 μm, H&E, ×250.)

GENERALIZED ERUPTIVE HISTIOCYTOMA

Clinical Features

In 1963, Winkelmann and Muller[89] described three adult patients with a disseminated benign papular histiocytic syndrome that they termed "generalized eruptive histiocytoma." These patients had progressive crops of multiple asymptomatic disseminated symmetric papules involving the trunk and proximal extremities.[89–92] The lesions are 2-mm to 10-mm flesh-colored to dark blue-red papules lacking grouping or coalescence. They develop into brown macules as they age and involute. There may be hundreds or even thousands of discrete papules involving the skin, but mucous membranes are rarely involved. There is no visceral involvement. The disease tends to persist for several years before spontaneously involuting. Winkelmann[37] has postulated that generalized eruptive histiocytoma may represent a primitive form of other types of non-X histiocytosis.

Histologic Features

Generalized eruptive histiocytoma is characterized by a monomorphous dense infiltrate of histiocytes occupying the superficial and middermis.[89,93] The cells contain abundant pale cytoplasm with poorly defined borders and nuclei with scant chromatin.[29,93] Lymphocytes may be observed; however, there are no giant cells or foam cells. There are no connective tissue or vascular alterations.

Special Stains and Ultrastructure

Stains for lipid, mucopolysaccharide, iron, and S100 protein are negative.[29,89,90] Enzyme histochemistry has shown moderate amounts of acid phosphatase uniformly distributed, copious nonspecific esterase, nucleoside triphosphatase, and leucine aminopeptidase. By electron microscopy, generalized eruptive histiocytoma characteristically shows many dense bodies and regular laminated bodies in the cytoplasm.[29,93] Comma-shaped and myeloid bodies also have been observed, but Langerhans granules are absent.[29,93]

Differential Diagnosis

Generalized eruptive histiocytoma may be distinguished from multicentric reticulohistiocytosis and progressive nodular histiocytoma by its lack of multinucleated giant cells and paucity of lymphocytes. Absence of foam cells helps to exclude juvenile xanthogranuloma, xanthoma disseminatum, and papular xanthoma. Stain for S100 protein or electron microscopy may be used to rule out histiocytosis X.

CONGENITAL OR INFANTILE SELF-HEALING RETICULOHISTIOCYTOSIS

Clinical Features

Self-healing reticulohistiocytosis, described by Hashimoto and Pritzker in 1973,[94] usually is present at birth or may develop in early infancy.[95–97] Typically, the patient has multiple disseminated, firm, asymptomatic, elevated, dark red to blue cutaneous nodules. The lesions tend to grow and become more numerous during the first weeks of life and later develop an overlying brown crust. They involute spon-

taneously in 3 weeks to $3\frac{1}{2}$ months. There are no mucosal lesions. There is only one report of a patient with systemic abnormalities.[95] This child's neutropenia, lymphocytosis, and hepatomegaly resolved within 1 month after onset. A solitary form of self-healing reticulohistiocytosis, also occurring at birth, has been described[98] in four neonates, each of whom had a rapidly growing ulcerated nodule, up to 2.5 cm in diameter, on the temple, foot, hand, or inguinal area.

Histologic Features

The histologic features are similar to those of reticulohistiocytomas seen in adults.[94,96] The large histiocytes show copious ground glass eosinophilic cytoplasm and indented nuclei. Some cells exhibit foamy cytoplasm. Both mononucleated and multinucleated histiocytes are present. The infiltrate may involve superficial, mid-, and deep dermis. When papillary dermis is involved, there may be histiocytes infiltrating epidermis, with associated ulceration. Lymphocytes and eosinophils usually are mixed in with the histiocytic infiltrate. Increased thin and thick reticulum fibers are located around large histiocytes.

Special Stains and Ultrastructure

The histiocytes in this entity contain periodic acid-Schiff-positive, diastase-resistant inclusions.[94,96] Antibody to S100 protein stains approximately 20% of the histiocytes.[96] One case was positive for lysozyme.[98] The most characteristic organelles are dense bodies.[94] Approximately 10% to 25% of the cells contain Langerhans granules,[94,96] and the giant histiocytes usually are marked by dense bodies and regularly laminated bodies. Langerhans granules and regularly laminated bodies often are seen together in the same cell. Comma-shaped bodies and octopus-like bodies also have been observed.[96]

Differential Diagnosis

Self-healing reticulohistiocytosis resembles reticulohistiocytoma by virtue of its periodic acid-Schiff-positive cytoplasm and the presence of an increased number of reticulum fibers around large histiocytes. It lacks the Touton giant cells and foam cells of juvenile xanthogranuloma. Both histiocytosis X and self-healing reticulohistiocytosis exhibit Langerhans granules on electron microscopy, whereas benign cephalic histiocytosis does not and also lacks the intraepidermal involvement. It has been postulated that congenital self-healing reticulohistiocytosis may represent a reactive histiocytosis that could be considered a benign form of histiocytosis X.[95] However, self-healing reticulohistiocytosis develops at a much earlier age, has only nodular lesions without papules or erosions, lacks the intertriginous predilection of histiocytosis X, and rapidly involutes without recurrence.

BENIGN CEPHALIC HISTIOCYTOSIS

Clinical Features

Benign cephalic histiocytosis was first described in 1971 by Gianotti et al.[99] under the name "histiocytosis with intracytoplasmic worm-like bodies," as distinguished by ultrastructural study. Because other histiocytic diseases may also contain so-called wormlike or comma-like cytoplasmic structures, Gianotti et al. later proposed the term "benign cephalic histiocytosis."[29,38,100] Over a dozen children with this disease have been studied by these and other authors.[100,101] It is found with almost equal frequency in boys and girls, with mean age at onset of 13.5 months (range 5 to 34 months). From a few to more than 100, raised, round or oval, pink and brown to yellow, 2-m to 8-mm papules usually develop on the face (with preferential localization to the eyelids, forehead, and cheeks) as well as neck and ears. Over many months, new lesions develop. Although the face is most often involved early and is a characteristic location, the trunk or extremities may be affected later. Mucosa, palms, and soles are spared. Lesions exhibit partial spontaneous regression within 8 months to 4 years after onset, without residual scarring. There are no associated systemic abnormalities.

Histologic Features
The infiltrate is usually well demarcated and located in the superficial dermis, closely apposed to the epidermis.[100] There is atrophy of overlying epidermis and intraepidermal infiltration of histiocytes. The infiltrate is composed predominantly of histiocytes with indistinct pale glassy cytoplasm and pleomorphic nuclei containing sparse chromatin. There is a paucity of eosinophils. Individual or clustered lymphocytes are seen, particularly in new lesions, and few giant cells usually are present in older lesions.

Special Stains and Ultrastructure
The histiocytes do not stain for lipid or mucopolysaccharide. They are positive for Leu-M3 and OKM1 but do not stain with antibodies to S100 protein or T6.[29,100] They contain copious smooth and rough endoplasmic reticulum, mitochondria, lysosomes, phagosomes, and 70-nm filaments.[100] Numerous coated vesicles, 500 to 1500 nm, are most characteristic. Comma-shaped bodies are present in only 5% to 30% of the histiocytes. The comma-shaped bodies are composed of two electron-dense membranes 60 nm wide, separated by a relatively less electron-dense 80-nm space. Langerhans granules, fatty droplets, and regular laminated bodies have not been observed.

Differential Diagnosis
Although the comma-shaped bodies were initially considered to be characteristic of benign cephalic histiocytosis, they are found also in sinus histiocytosis with massive lymphadenopathy, histiocytosis X, congenital self-healing reticulohistiocytosis, juvenile xanthogranuloma, and generalized eruptive histiocytoma.[29] In contrast to histiocytosis X, in benign cephalic histiocytosis S100 protein and T6 are absent. Lesions of juvenile xanthogranuloma usually have foam cells and multinucleated Touton and foreign body type giant cells, although the early monomorphous variant may resemble benign cephalic histiocytosis. The entity that most closely resembles benign cephalic histiocytosis histologically is generalized eruptive histiocytoma, in that both are predominantly composed of non-X histiocytes with a minor component of lymphocytes and eosinophils but no foam cells. However, these entities may be distinguished by electron microscopy. Generalized eruptive histiocytoma

lacks the coated vesicles that are so numerous in benign cephalic histiocytosis.

PROGRESSIVE NODULAR HISTIOCYTOMA

Clinical Features
In 1978, Taunton et al.[102] introduced the term "progressive nodular histiocytoma" in their report on a 9-year-old girl who had a history of multiple cutaneous lesions, previously thought to represent xanthomas, for 3 years. She had numerous papules and nodules involving the skin and mucous membranes. Conjunctival and laryngeal mucosae contained multiple, smooth, round, pedunculated, yellow-brown lesions. There were "hundreds" of lesions asymmetrically involving her face, trunk, and extremities, with two morphologic patterns: (1) early 0.4-cm to 0.75-cm yellow-orange papules that enlarged to form firm pedunculated yellow-brown 1-cm to 5-cm lesions, and (2) violaceous papules evolving into 1-cm to 5-cm deep nodules with telangiectasias. Large lesions became necrotic over pressure sites. It is the presence of the two clinically distinct lesions that separates progressive nodular histiocytoma from other non-X histiocytoses.[103] In the original case of Taunton et al. the patient also had hepatosplenomegaly and apparent involvement of the Achilles tendon. Burgdorf et al.[103] subsequently described a similar cutaneous syndrome in an adult.

Histologic Features
There are two histologic patterns associated with early superficial lesions and later deep dermal nodules, respectively.[102,103] Early lesions show a dermal aggregate of large, pale, foamy histiocytes, with dilated vessels throughout the cellular infiltrate. There is overlying epidermal atrophy and lateral epidermal collarettes. Deep dermal nodules consist of a dense cellular nonencapsulated mass of small histiocytes, with numerous multinucleated giant cells and overlying atrophic epidermis.

Special Stains and Ultrastructure
Sudan black and oil red O stains show lipid in histiocytes in early and late lesions.[102,103] Fat droplets also may be present extracellularly. Mucin and elastic fibers are absent in the nodules. Iron has been demonstrated within the nodules and in the subepidermal zone. Histiocytes do not stain for lysozyme.[103]

Electron microscopic examination[103] has shown cytoplasm with abundant endoplasmic reticulum, Golgi apparatus, mitochondria, and numerous membrane-bound, electron-dense lysosomes 70 to 360 nm in diameter. Vacuolated lipid material, 2000 to 3000 nm, with myelin-like figures and remnants of granules also has been noted. Langerhans granules have not been observed.

Differential Diagnosis
The clinical presentation is more readily distinguished from that of the other xanthohistiocytic diseases than is the histologic pattern. Because of the variation in proportion of histiocytes, giant cells, foam cells, and fibrosis in the group of non-X histiocytoses and normolipemic xanthomas, there tend to be more similarities than differences among these

entities. No single histologic feature is unique to progressive nodular histiocytoma. Burgdorf et al.[103] emphasized a fibro-histiocytic quality similar to dermatofibroma.

SINUS HISTIOCYTOSIS WITH MASSIVE LYMPHADENOPATHY

Clinical Features

In 1969, Rosai and Dorfman[104] coined the term "sinus histio-cytosis with massive lymphadenopathy" in a report of four cases of a benign clinical syndrome characterized by massive lymphadenopathy, particularly of the cervical nodes, as well as fever, leukocytosis, and hypergammaglobuline-mia.[105–108] The erythrocyte sedimentation rate is increased in most patients.[105] Subsequent studies by these and other investigators have shown that extranodal lesions occur in approximately 30% of the patients with this disease. Approximately 80% of the patients present before age 20 years, and the male/female ratio is 2:1.[106–108] Although the cause is unknown, association with immunologic abnormal-ities suggests that sinus histiocytosis with massive lymph-adenopathy may represent a disorder of immune func-tion.[109] An infectious cause also has been proposed.

Multiple extranodal sites may be involved, including the upper respiratory tract, orbit, skin, viscera, bones, and nervous system. Approximately 10% of the patients have skin involvement.[106–108] Cutaneous lesions include solitary or multiple papules or nodules up to 4 cm in diameter, often with a xanthomatous appearance.

Histologic Features

Histologic examination of enlarged lymph nodes shows dilated subcapsular and medullary sinuses stuffed with his-tiocytes. Many of these histiocytes appear foamy or vacuo-lated. Lymphophagocytosis (emperipolesis) by histiocytes is a characteristic feature. Medullary cords between dilated sinuses are packed with plasma cells. There is also capsular and pericapsular fibrosis.

Cutaneous lesions consist of dermal infiltration with histiocytes, plasma cells, and lymphocytes.[107] The infiltrate is dense and well defined but not encapsulated, and it may extend into the fat. There is no subepidermal Grenz zone. Increased vascularity with plump endothelial cells and fibrosis is variable. The histiocytes contain large vesic-ular nuclei, small single nucleoli, abundant pale acidophilic cytoplasm, and indistinct, spidery cell borders. Multinu-cleated histiocytes, foamy histiocytes, and clusters of foamy histiocytes resembling Touton giant cells may be seen. As in lymph nodes, lymphophagocytosis by histiocytes occurs in the skin lesions. Although the histiocytic infiltrate domi-nates the histologic picture, lymphocytes, plasma cells, and neutrophils also are present. Eosinophils are rare, and ex-travasation of erythrocytes is uncommon. Apparent separa-tion of clusters of histiocytes from other inflammatory cells in spaces suggestive of lymph vessels has been observed in some cases.

Special Stains and Ultrastructure

Periodic acid-Schiff stains the glycogen granules in the cyto-plasm of histiocytes.[108] There is minimal neutral fat in these cells, as demonstrated by oil red O staining. Histiocytes contain many phagosomes, and clusters of comma-shaped bodies have been observed.[29]

Differential Diagnosis

Of the xanthohistiocytic diseases, juvenile xanthogranu-loma has the greatest similarity to sinus histiocytosis with massive lymphadenopathy—because of the multinucleated foamy cells that resemble Touton giant cells. Other entities that have been listed in the differential diagnosis include xanthoma, Tangier disease, histiocytosis X, reticulohistiocy-toma, leprosy, and Hodgkin's disease.[107] The presence of many plasma cells and lymphophagocytosis in sinus histio-cytosis with massive lymphadenopathy helps to exclude most of these other entities.

MALIGNANT HISTIOCYTOSIS

Clinical Features

Histiocytic medullary reticulosis was described by Scott and Robb-Smith in 1939,[110] and the term "malignant histiocyto-sis" was coined by Rappaport in 1966 for "a systemic pro-gressive invasive proliferation of morphologically atypical histiocytes."[111] The patients have fever, pancytopenia, jaundice, hepatosplenomegaly, and lymphadenopathy. The course is rapidly progressive, with death in less than 1 year in most cases.[111–114] The terms "true histiocytic lym-phoma" and "malignant histiocytosis" often are used syn-onymously to refer to malignancy of the mononuclear phagocyte system.[113] However, the former refers to local-ized tumor masses that subsequently may disseminate, and the latter refers to involvement throughout the reticuloen-dothelial system.

True histiocytic lymphoma and malignant histiocytosis are seen mainly in adults but have been reported in children and adolescents.[112,113] Approximately half of the patients have extranodal lesions, most commonly involving skin, bone, or gastrointestinal tract.[113] In malignant histiocytosis, the skin is involved in 10% to 20% of patients.[114,115] Cutane-ous lesions involving the trunk or extremities may be single or multiple, red-brown or bluish red, hemorrhagic papules, nodules, or plaques, with or without ulceration.[113–117] Ten-der, ulcerated subcutaneous nodules are characteristic. Gin-gival involvement is uncommon, in contrast to acute mono-cytic leukemia. Patients with malignant histiocytosis generally have more widespread cutaneous lesions than do patients with so-called true histiocytic lymphoma.

Histologic Features

The diagnosis of malignant histiocytosis or histiocytic lym-phoma is based on finding true histiocytic cells with malig-nant cytologic features.[112,113] The infiltrate is dominated by noncohesive histiocytes that usually are large (up to 50 μm in diameter) and have abundant pale eosinophilic or amphophilic cytoplasm with vacuolization. Nuclei are large, vesicular, pleomorphic, and multilobulated, with fine granular to reticulated chromatin and prominent nucleoli. Mitotic figures are numerous. Wright-stained touch prepa-rations may help in evaluating the cytologic features.[113] A characteristic finding in malignant histiocytosis is phagocy-

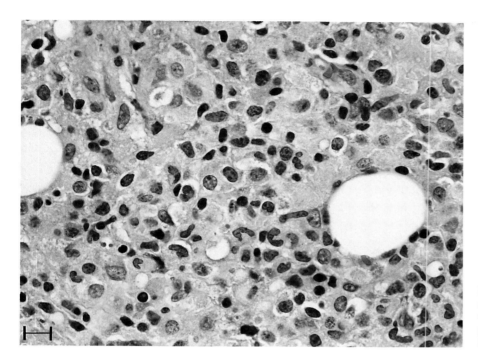

Figure 19–20. Malignant histiocytosis. A dense infiltrate of plump histiocytes mixed with a few inflammatory cells involves the panniculus in this case. (Scale bar = 10 μm, H&E, ×620.) (From ref. 117.)

tosis of erythrocytes, and sometimes leukocytes or platelets, by the malignant histiocytes.

Several histologic patterns are seen on biopsy of cutaneous lesions.[112–115,117–119] In general, there is relative sparing of the papillary dermis, and epidermis usually is not affected. Perivascular and periappendageal histiocytic infiltration of mid- and sometimes deep dermis forms a common pattern similar to that seen in leukemia cutis. There may be a minor component of lymphocytes and plasma cells and occasional multinucleated or giant cells. Eosinophils are variable in number and may be numerous in some cases. A massive diffuse infiltrate of histiocytes (Fig. 19–20) may occupy the superficial and deep dermis and extend into fat, infiltrating between connective tissue bundles. Predominant involvement of the panniculus and lower dermis also may be seen. Such cases are usually associated with necrosis and hemorrhage in subcutaneous tissue and deep dermis. Cytophagia is characteristic but not specific for malignant histiocytosis.

Special Stains and Ultrastructure

A battery of special stains should be performed to confirm the true histiocytic nature of the infiltrate.[113,117,118,120] Nonspecific esterase (particularly α-naphthyl butyrate esterase), acid phosphatase, and β-glucuronidase activities may be demonstrated. Alkaline phosphatase and chloroacetate esterase activities are absent. T cells show focal punctate or perinuclear activity of acid phosphatase compared with diffuse staining in histiocytes. Stains for lysozyme, α_1-antitrypsin, and α_1-antichymotrypsin are variably positive.[120] Stain for S100 protein is negative. Stains for HLA-DR, Leu-M1, and Leu-M2 are positive; however, the Leu-M1 marker is found also in Hodgkin's disease. The histiocytic nature is confirmed by ultrastructural study demonstrating the presence of phagolysosomes and primary lysosomal granules.

Differential Diagnosis

Peripheral T cell lymphomas, particularly the large cell type, may be confused with malignant histiocytosis or histiocytic lymphoma. However, T cell lymphomas show greater chromatin clumping, inconspicuous nucleoli, and generally smaller cells. The absence of epidermotropism also favors the diagnosis of malignant histiocytosis over cutaneous T cell lymphoma. Enzyme and immunocytochemical stains usually are necessary to exclude lymphoma or leukemia cutis. Distinction from acute monocytic leukemia may not be possible. Various benign syndromes characterized by histiocytic proliferation with erythrophagocytosis should be excluded by their bland cytologic features. Nonhistiocytic lymphoma may show erythrophagocytosis. However, the phagocytizing cells appear benign cytologically, whereas the lymphoid cells show atypia. Sinus histiocytosis with massive lymphadenopathy is characterized by lymphophagocytosis rather than erythrophagocytosis and contains a more consistent plasma cell infiltrate. Histiocytosis X generally involves superficial dermis and epidermis, and S100 protein is present.

REFERENCES

1. Basset F, Nezelof C, Ferrans VJ. The histiocytoses. *Pathol Annu.* 1983;18 Part 2:27–78.
2. van Furth R. Mononuclear phagocytes of the skin and other organs. *G Ital Dermatol Venereol.* 1980;115:7–20.
3. Claudy AL, Schmitt D. The monocyte-macrophage system in man: contribution to its identification by immuno-electron-microscopic techniques. *G Ital Dermatol Venereol.* 1980;115:43–49.
4. Breathnach SM, Katz SI. Cell-mediated immunity in cutaneous disease. *Hum Pathol.* 1986;17:161–167.

5. Murphy GF. Cell membrane glycoproteins and Langerhans cells. *Hum Pathol.* 1985;16:103–112.

6. Weiss LM, Beckstead JH, Warnke RA, Wood GS. Leu-6-expressing cells in lymph nodes: dendritic cells phenotypically similar to interdigitating cells. *Hum Pathol.* 1986;17:179–184.

7. Turner RR, Wood GS, Beckstead HJ, et al. Histiocytic malignancies: morphologic, immunologic, and enzymatic heterogeneity. *Am J Surg Pathol.* 1984;8:485–500.

8. Wood GS, Turner RR, Shiurba RA, et al. Human dendritic cells and macrophages: in situ immunophenotypic definition of subsets that exhibit specific morphologic and microenvironmental characteristics. *Am J Pathol.* 1985;119:73–82.

9. Murphy GF, Messadi D, Fonferko E, Hancock WW. Phenotypic transformation of macrophages to Langerhans cells in the skin. *Am J Pathol.* 1986;123:401–406.

10. Favara BE, McCarthy RC, Mierau GW. Histiocytosis X. *Hum Pathol.* 1983;14:663–676.

11. Silberberg I, Baer RL, Rosenthal SA. The role of Langerhans cells in allergic contact hypersensitivity. A review of findings in man and guinea pigs. *J Invest Dermatol.* 1976;66:210–217.

12. Drijkoningen M, De Wolf-Peeters C, van den Oord JJ, et al. Expression of HLA-DR and T6 antigens on keratinocytes and dendritic cells: a comparative immunohistochemical study. *Arch Pathol Lab Med.* 1986;110:321–325.

13. Wood GS, Hu C-H, Beckstead JH, et al. The indeterminate cell proliferative disorder: report of a case manifesting as an unusual cutaneous histiocytosis. *J Dermatol Surg Oncol.* 1985;11:1111–1119.

14. Takahashi K, Isobe T, Ohtsuki Y, et al. Immunohistochemical localization and distribution of S100 proteins in the human lymphoreticular system. *Am J Pathol* 1984;116:497–503.

15. Schaumburg-Lever G. Immunoenzyme techniques in dermatopathology. *Int J Dermatol.* 1986;25:217–223.

16. Wieczorek R, Burke JS, Knowles DM II. Leu-M1 antigen expression in T-cell neoplasia. *Am J Pathol.* 1985;121:374–380.

17. Bergroth V, Konttinen YT, Johansson E. Langerhans cells in SLE skin: a role in lymphocyte migration and activation in situ. *Scand J Rheumatol.* 1985; 14:411–416.

18. Kohchiyama A, Hatamochi A, Ueki H. Increased number of OKT6-positive dendritic cells in the hair follicles of patients with alopecia areata. *Dermatologica.* 1985;171:327–331.

19. Zachary CB, Allen MH, MacDonald DM. In situ quantification of T-lymphocyte subsets and Langerhans cells in the inflammatory infiltrate of atopic eczema. *Br J Dermatol.* 1985;112:149–156.

20. Sloberg K, Jonsson R, Jontell M. Assessment of Langerhans' cells in oral lichen planus using monoclonal antibodies. *J Oral Pathol.* 1984;13:516–524.

21. Oguchi M, Komura J, Tagami H, Ofuji S. Ultrastructural studies of spontaneously regressing plane warts: Langerhans cells show marked activation. *Arch Dermatol Res.* 1981;271:55–61.

22. Murphy GF, Krusinksi PA, Myzak LA, Ershler WB. Local immune response in basal cell carcinoma: characterization by transmission electron microscopy and monoclonal anti-T6 antibody. *J Am Acad Dermatol.* 1983;8:477–485.

23. Berti E, Cavicchini S, Cusini M, et al. Heterogeneity of dermal OKT6+ cells in inflammatory and neoplastic skin diseases. *J Am Acad Dermatol.* 1985;12:507–514.

24. Haftek M, Faure M, Schmitt D, Thivolet J. Langerhans cells in skin from patients with psoriasis: quantitative and qualitative study of T6 and HLA-DR antigen-expressing cells and changes with aromatic retinoid administration. *J Invest Dermatol.* 1983;81:10–14.

25. Chu A, Berger CL, Kung P, Edelson RL. In situ identification of Langerhans cells in the dermal infiltrate of cutaneous T cell lymphoma. *J Am Acad Dermatol.* 1982;6:350–354.

26. McMillan EM, Beman K, Wasik R, Everett MA. Demonstration of OKT 6-reactive cells in mycosis fungoides. *J Am Acad Dermatol.* 1982;6:880–887.

27. Lahey ME. Prognostic factors in histiocytosis X. *Am J Pediatr Hematol Oncol.* 1981;3:57–60.

28. Esterly NB, Maurer HS, Gonzalez-Crussi F. Histiocytosis X: a seven-year experience at a children's hospital. *J Am Acad Dermatol.* 1985;13:481–496.

29. Gianotti F, Caputo R. Histiocytic syndromes: a review. *J Am Acad Dermatol.* 1985;13:383–404.

30. Winkelmann RK. The skin in histiocytosis X. *Mayo Clin Proc.* 1969;44:535–548.

31. Altman J, Winkelmann RK. Xanthomatous cutaneous lesions of histiocytosis X. *Arch Dermatol.* 1963;87:164–170.

32. Colby TV, Lombard C. Histiocytosis X in the lung. *Hum Pathol.* 1983;14:847–856.

33. Lipton JM. The pathogenesis, diagnosis, and treatment of histiocytosis syndromes. *Pediatr Dermatol.* 1983;1:112–120.

34. Roper SS, Spraker MK. Cutaneous histiocytosis syndromes. *Pediatr Dermatol.* 1985;3:19–30.

35. Pritchard J. Histiocytosis X: natural history and management in childhood. *Clin Exp Dermatol.* 1979;4:421–433.

36. Nezelof C, Frileux-Herbet F, Cronier-Sachot J. Disseminated histiocytosis X: analysis of prognostic factors based on a retrospective study of 50 cases. *Cancer.* 1979;44:1824–1838.

37. Winkelmann RK. Adult histiocytic skin disease. *G Ital Dermatol Venereol.* 1980;115:67–76.

38. Gianotti F. Cutaneous proliferative histiocytoses in children. *G Ital Dermatol Venereol.* 1980;115:59–66.

39. Letterer E. Aleukämische Retikulose. (Ein Beitrag zu den proliferativen Erkrankungen des Retikuloendothelialapparates.) *Frankfurt Z Pathol.* 1924;30:377–394.

40. Siwe SA. Die Reticuloendotheliose—ein neues Krankheitsbild unter den Hepatosplenomegalien. *Z Kinderheilk.* 1933;55:212–247.

41. Hand A Jr. Polyuria and tuberculosis. *Arch Pediatr.* 1893; 10:673–675.

42. Schüller A. Über eigenartige Schädeldefekte im Jugendalter. *Fortschr Geb Rontgenstr.* 1915;23:12–18.

43. Christian HA. Defects in membraneous bones, exophthalmos, and diabetes insipidus: an unusual syndrome of dyspituitarism; a clinical study. In: *Contributions to Medical and Biological Research.* New York: Paul B. Hoeber; 1919;1:390–401.

44. Lichtenstein L. Histiocytosis X: integration of eosinophilic granuloma of bone, ''Letterer-Siwe disease,'' and ''Schüller-Christian disease'' as related manifestations of a single nosologic entity. *Arch Pathol.* 1953;56:84–102.

45. Neumann MP, Frizzera G. The coexistence of Langerhans' cell granulomatosis and malignant lymphoma may take different forms: report of seven cases with a review of the literature. *Hum Pathol.* 1985;17:1060–1065.

46. Burns BF, Colby TV, Dorfman RF. Langerhans' cell granulomatosis (histiocytosis X) associated with malignant lymphomas. *Am J Surg Pathol.* 1983;7:529–533.

47. Siegal GP, Dehner LP, Rosai J. Histiocytosis X (Langerhans' cell granulomatosis) of the thymus: a clinicopathologic study of four childhood cases. *Am J Surg Pathol.* 1985;9:117–124.

48. Bramwell NH, Burns BF. Histiocytosis X of the thymus in association with myasthenia gravis. *Am J Clin Pathol.* 1986;86:224–227.

49. Bonvalet D, Civatte J. Histiocytosis histopathology. *G Ital Dermatol Venereol.* 1980;115:51–58.

50. Gebhart W, Knobler R, Niebauer G. Langerhans cells in histiocytosis X. *G Ital Dermatol Venereol.* 1980;115:121–128.

51. Risdall RJ, Dehner LP, Duray P, et al. Histiocytosis X (Langerhans' cell histiocytosis): prognostic role of histopathology. *Arch Pathol Lab Med.* 1983;107:59–63.

52. Rowden G, Connelly EM, Winkelmann RK. Cutaneous histio-

cytosis X: the presence of S100 protein and its use in diagnosis. *Arch Dermatol.* 1983;119:553–559.

53. Murphy GF, Harrist TJ, Bhan AK, Mihm MC Jr. Distribution of cell surface antigens in histiocytosis X cells: quantitative immunoelectron microscopy using monoclonal antibodies. *Lab Invest.* 1983;48:90–97.

54. Caputo R, Gianotti F. Cytoplasmic markers ultrastructural features in histiocytic proliferations of the skin. *G Ital Dermatol Venereol.* 1980;115:107–120.

55. Mierau GW, Favara BE, Brenman JM. Electron microscopy in histiocytosis X. *Ultrastruct Pathol.* 1982;3:137–142.

56. Parker F. Xanthomas and hyperlipidemias. *J Am Acad Dermatol.* 1985;13:1–30.

57. Parker F, Bagdade JD, Odland GF, Bierman EL. Evidence for the chylomicron origin of lipids accumulating in diabetic eruptive xanthomas: a correlative lipid biochemical, histochemical and electron microscopic study. *J Clin Invest.* 1970;49:2172–2187.

58. Altman J, Winkelmann RK. Diffuse normolipemic plane xanthoma: generalized xanthelasma. *Arch Dermatol.* 1962;85:633–640.

59. Lynch PJ, Winkelmann RK. Generalized plane xanthoma and systemic disease. *Arch Dermatol.* 1966;93:639–646.

60. Marien KJC, Smeenk G. Plane xanthomata associated with multiple myeloma and hyperlipoproteinaemia. *Br J Dermatol.* 1975;93:407–415.

61. Feiwel M. Xanthomatosis in cryoglobulinaemia and other paraproteinaemias, with report of a case. *Br J Dermatol.* 1968;80:719–729.

62. Hu C-H, Winkelmann RK. Unusual normolipidemic cutaneous xanthomatosis: a comparison of two cases illustrating the differential diagnosis. *Acta Derm Venereol (Stockh).* 1977;57:421–429.

63. Bulkley BH, Buja LM, Ferrans VJ, et al. Tuberous xanthoma in homozygous type II hyperlipoproteinaemia: a histologic, histochemical, and electron microscopical study. *Arch Pathol.* 1975;99:293–300.

64. Parker F, Odland GF. Electron microscopic similarities between experimental xanthomas and human eruptive xanthomas. *J Invest Dermatol.* 1969;52:136–147.

65. Ferrando J, Bombi JA. Ultrastructural aspects of normolipidemic xanthomatosis. *Arch Dermatol Res.* 1979;266:143–159.

66. Zemel H, Deeken J, Asel N, Packer J. The ultrastructural features of normolipemic plane xanthoma. *Arch Pathol.* 1970;89:111–117.

67. Montgomery H, Osterberg AE. Xanthomatosis; correlation of clinical, histopathologic and chemical studies of cutaneous xanthoma. *Arch Dermatol Syphilol.* 1938;37:373–401.

68. Altman J, Winkelmann RK. Xanthoma disseminatum. *Arch Dermatol.* 1962;86:582–596.

69. Winkelmann RK. Cutaneous syndromes of non-X histiocytosis: a review of the macrophage-histiocyte diseases of the skin. *Arch Dermatol.* 1981;117:667–672.

70. Kumakiri M, Sudoh M, Miura Y. Xanthoma disseminatum: report of a case, with histological and ultrastructural studies of skin lesions. *J Am Acad Dermatol.* 1981;4:291–299.

71. Sonnex TS, Ryan TJ, Dawber RPR. Progressive xanthoma disseminatum. *Br J Dermatol.* 1981;105(Suppl 19):79–81.

72. Guinnepain MT, Puissant A. Juvenile xanthogranuloma. *G Ital Dermatol Venereol.* 1980;115:101–105.

73. Webster SB, Reister HC, Harman LE Jr. Juvenile xanthogranuloma with extracutaneous lesions: a case report and review of the literature. *Arch Dermatol.* 1966;93:71–76.

74. Flach DB, Winkelmann RK. Juvenile xanthogranuloma with central nervous system lesions. *J Am Acad Dermatol.* 1986;14:405–411.

75. Sanchez RL, Raimer SS, Peltier F, Swedo J. Papular xanthoma:
a clinical, histologic, and ultrastructural study. *Arch Dermatol.* 1985;121:626–631.

76. Kossard S, Winkelmann RK. Necrobiotic xanthogranuloma with paraproteinemia. *J Am Acad Dermatol.* 1980;3:257–270.

77. Robertson DM, Winkelmann RK. Ophthalmic features of necrobiotic xanthogranuloma with paraproteinemia. *Am J Ophthalmol.* 1984;97:173–183.

78. Finan MC, Winkelmann RK. Necrobiotic xanthogranuloma with paraproteinemia: a review of 22 cases. *Medicine.* 1986;65:376–388.

79. Weber FP, Freudenthal W. Nodular non-diabetic cutaneous xanthomatosis with hypercholesterolaemia and atypical histological features. *Proc R Soc Med.* 1937;30:522–526.

80. Goltz RW, Laymon CW. Multicentric reticulohistiocytosis of the skin and synovia: reticulohistiocytoma or ganglioneuroma. *Arch Dermatol.* 1954;69:717–731.

81. Heathcote JG, Guenther LC, Wallace AC. Multicentric reticulohistiocytosis: a report of a case and a review of the pathology. *Pathology.* 1985;17:601–608.

82. Lesher JL Jr, Allen BS. Multicentric reticulohistiocytosis. *J Am Acad Dermatol.* 1984;11:713–723.

83. Barrow MV, Holubar K. Multicentric reticulohistiocytosis: a review of 33 patients. *Medicine.* 1969;48:287–305.

84. Belaïch S. Multicentric reticulohistiocytosis. *G Ital Dermatol Venereol.* 1980;115:77–82.

85. Nunnink JC, Krusinksi PA, Yates JW. Multicentric reticulohistiocytosis and cancer: a case report and review of the literature. *Med Pediatr Oncol.* 1985;13:273–279.

86. Tani M, Hori K, Nakanishi T, et al. Multicentric reticulohistiocytosis: electron microscopic and ultracytochemical studies. *Arch Dermatol.* 1981;117:495–499.

87. Coode PE, Ridgway H, Jones DB. Multicentric reticulohistiocytosis: report of two cases with ultrastructure, tissue culture and immunology studies. *Clin Exp Dermatol.* 1980;5:281–293.

88. Caputo R, Alessi E, Berti E. Collagen phagocytosis in multicentric reticulohistiocytosis. *J Invest Dermatol.* 1981;76:342–346.

89. Winkelmann RK, Muller SA. Generalized eruptive histiocytoma: a benign papular histiocytic reticulosis. *Arch Dermatol.* 1963;88:586–595.

90. Muller SA, Wolff K, Winkelmann RK. Generalized eruptic histiocytoma: enzyme histochemistry and electron microscopy. *Arch Dermatol.* 1967;96:11–17.

91. Sohi AS, Tiwari VD, Subramanian CSV, Chakraborty M. Generalized eruptive histiocytoma: a case report with a review of the literature. *Dermatologica.* 1979;159:471–475.

92. Pegum JS. Generalized eruptive histiocytoma. *Proc R Soc Med.* 1973;66:1175–1176.

93. Caputo R, Alessi E, Allegra F. Generalized eruptive histiocytoma: a clinical, histologic, and ultrastructural study. *Arch Dermatol.* 1981;117:216–221.

94. Hashimoto K, Pritzker MS. Electron microscopic study of reticulohistiocytoma: an unusual case of congenital, self-healing reticulohistiocytosis. *Arch Dermatol.* 1973;107:263–270.

95. Hashimoto K, Griffin D, Kohsbaki M. Self-healing reticulohistiocytosis: a clinical, histologic, and ultrastructural study of the fourth case in the literature. *Cancer.* 1982;49:331–337.

96. Hashimoto K, Takahashi S, Lee RG, Krull EA. Congenital self-healing reticulohistiocytosis: report of the seventh case with histochemical and ultrastructural studies. *J Am Acad Dermatol.* 1984;11:447–454.

97. Kapila PK, Grant-Kels JM, Allred C, et al. Congenital, spontaneously regressing histiocytosis: case report and review of the literature. *Pediatr Dermatol.* 1985;2:312–317.

98. Berger TG, Lane AT, Headington JT, et al. A solitary variant of congenital self-healing reticulohistiocytosis: solitary Hashimoto-Pritzker disease. *Pediatr Dermatol.* 1986;3:230–236.

99. Gianotti F, Caputo R, Ermacora E. Singulière "histiocytose

infantile àcellules avec particules vermiformes intracytoplasmiques." *Bull Soc Fr Dermatol Syphilgr.* 1971;78:232–233.

100. Gianotti F, Caputo R, Ermacora E, Gianni E. Benign cephalic histiocytosis. *Arch Dermatol.* 1986;122:1038–1043.

101. Eisenberg EL, Bronson DM, Barsky S. Benign cephalic histiocytosis: a case report and ultrastructural study. *J Am Acad Dermatol.* 1985;12:328–331.

102. Taunton OD, Yeshurun D, Jarratt M. Progressive nodular histiocytoma. *Arch Dermatol.* 1978;114:1505–1508.

103. Burgdorf WHC, Kusch SL, Nix TE Jr, Pitha J. Progressive nodular histiocytoma. *Arch Dermatol.* 1981;117:644–649.

104. Rosai J, Dorfman RF. Sinus histiocytosis with massive lymphadenopathy: a newly recognized benign clinicopathological entity. *Arch Pathol.* 1969;87:63–70.

105. Rosai J, Dorfman RF. Sinus histiocytosis with massive lymphadenopathy: a pseudolymphomatous benign disorder; analysis of 34 cases. *Cancer.* 1972;30:1174–1188.

106. Sanchez R, Rosai J, Dorfman RF. Sinus histiocytosis with massive lymphadenopathy: an analysis of 113 cases with special emphasis on extranodal manifestations. *Lab Invest.* 1977;36:349–350. Abstract.

107. Thawerani H, Sanchez RL, Rosai J, Dorfman RF. The cutaneous manifestations of sinus histiocytosis with massive lymphadenopathy. *Arch Dermatol.* 1978;114:191–197.

108. Schweitzer VG, Bobier GD. Sinus histiocytosis with massive cervical lymphadenopathy: case report and literature review. *Ann Otol Rhinol Laryngol.* 1986;95:331–335.

109. Foucar E, Rosai J, Dorfman RF, Eyman JM. Immunologic abnormalities and their significance in sinus histiocytosis with massive lymphadenopathy. *Am J Clin Pathol.* 1984;82:515–525.

110. Scott RB, Robb-Smith AHT. Histiocytic medullary reticulosis. *Lancet.* 1939;2:194–198.

111. Rappaport H. Tumors of the hematopoietic system. In: *Atlas of Tumor Pathology.* Fascicle 8. Washington, DC: Armed Forces Institute of Pathology; 1966:49–63.

112. Warnke RA, Kim H, Dorfman RF. Malignant histiocytosis (histiocytic medullary reticulosis). I. Clinicopathologic study of 29 cases. *Cancer.* 1975;35:215–230.

113. Jaffe ES. Malignant histiocytosis and true histiocytic lymphomas. *Major Probl Pathol.* 1985;16:381–411.

114. Bernengo MG. Histiocytic medullary reticulosis. *G Ital Dermatol Venereol.* 1980;115:83–90.

115. Kerl H, Hödl S. Cutaneous manifestations of malignant histiocytosis (histiocytic medullary reticulosis). *G Ital Dermatol Venereol.* 1986;115:155–157.

116. Dodd HJ, Stansfeld AG, Chambers TJ. Cutaneous malignant histiocytosis—a clinicopathological review of five cases. *Br J Dermatol.* 1985;113:455–461.

117. Wick MR, Sanchez NP, Crotty CP, Winkelmann RK. Cutaneous malignant histiocytosis: a clinical and histopathologic study of eight cases, with immunohistochemical analysis. *J Am Acad Dermatol.* 1983;8:50–62.

118. Ducatman BS, Wick MR, Morgan TW, et al. Malignant histiocytosis: a clinical, histologic, and immunohistochemical study of 20 cases. *Hum Pathol.* 1984;15:368–377.

119. Liao KT, Rosai J, Daneshbod K. Malignant histiocytosis with cutaneous involvement and eosinophilia. *Am J Clin Pathol.* 1972;57:438–448.

120. Roholl PJM, Kleyne J, Pijpers HW, van Unnik JAM. Comparative immunohistochemical investigation of markers for malignant histiocytes. *Hum Pathol.* 1985;16:763–771.

CHAPTER 20
Sclerosing Disorders

Robert M. Taylor

Cutaneous sclerosis is a clinically palpable hardening or induration of the skin. It may be circumscribed, as in morphea, or diffuse, as in progressive systemic sclerosis (PSS). Microscopically, the defining feature is sclerosis of collagen, irrespective of whether the disease is primary in origin (PSS) or secondary (sclerodermoid porphyria cutanea tarda). The sclerosing disorders discussed in this chapter can be classified arbitrarily as autoimmune (PSS, morphea, lichen sclerosis et atrophicus), reparative (keloid, hypertrophic scar), iatrogenic (radiodermatitis, bleomycin and pentazocine sclerosis), occupational (acroosteolysis), and idiopathic (atrophoderma). Many other disorders not discussed here might appropriately be included in these categories, and there are other sclerosing disorders that lie outside this classification scheme, such as genodermatoses (Winchester syndrome, pachydermoperiostosis) and metabolic disorders (necrobiosis lipoidica and porphyria cutaneous tarda).

PROGRESSIVE SYSTEMIC SCLEROSIS

Clinical Features

Progressive systemic sclerosis (PSS) is a disease of unknown cause characterized by sclerosing changes in the skin, lungs, kidneys, and other organ systems.[1] In the skin, PSS progresses in three stages[2]: nonpitting edema of the extremities, trunk, and face, induration, and atrophic, sclerotic, bound-down skin.[3] The disease is four times more common in women than in men; its average annual incidence is 2.7 new patients per million population.[3]

The immunopathogenesis of PSS can be studied from three perspectives: (1) vascular changes, (2) changes in humoral and cell-mediated immunity, and (3) aberrant fibroblast function.[1] Perivascular inflammation in early PSS may be the result of a factor or factors (possibly lymphokines) cytotoxic for endothelial cells.[4–7] Alternately, vascular damage may be the result of circulating immune complexes deposited in vascular walls.[8] Cell-mediated immunity is also thought to play a role in PSS in that most of the perivas-

cular mononuclear cells of early PSS are macrophages and T lymphocytes.[1] It is known that macrophages attract fibroblasts and induce them to increase collagen production.[3,9] Studies have also shown a relatively high ratio of T helper to T suppressor lymphocytes in peripheral blood.[9–12] An increase in T helper lymphocyte activity may lead to (1) increased autoantibody production by B lymphocytes, (2) increased effector T lymphocyte function, and (3) increased production of cytokines, which may influence fibroblasts to increase collagen production.[1,3,11] Although collagen production is high in PSS, so is its urinary excretion.[1] Paradoxically, the collagenase content of PSS skin is low.[13] Investigators have speculated that other protease systems exist for collagen breakdown.[1] Since the thickness of PSS skin and its collagen content are greater than normal, however,[1,2] it was postulated that the abnormal hydroxylation and glycosylation of propetides, which occur during the formation of tropocollagen in PSS, may adversely affect the negative feedback system in collagen production, resulting in increased collagen deposition.[1]

Histologic Features

The primary location of disease in PSS is the dermis and subcutis. Epidermal involvement, if any, occurs predominantly in the late stages.[14,15] A recent study compared epidermal thickness in the abnormal and normal skin of a PSS patient and found it normal in both sites.[16]

In early PSS, a superficial and deep lymphocytic infiltrate is seen around blood vessels and eccrine coils as well as in the subcutis.[17] At this stage, vascular changes are minimal.[16] As lesions progress to the tumid or inflammatory stage, particularly in the fingers, there is an increase in lymphocytes, fibroblasts, fixed tissue macrophages, eosinophils, and plasma cells around and between blood vessels.[18,19] Over time, the inflammatory infiltrate diminishes or disappears, fibroblast numbers decrease, and there is progressive swelling, thickening, and ultimately hyalinization of horizontally oriented dermal collagen, predominantly in the lower two thirds of the dermis and in the subcutis.[14,17,20] The dermal appendages, first the dermal

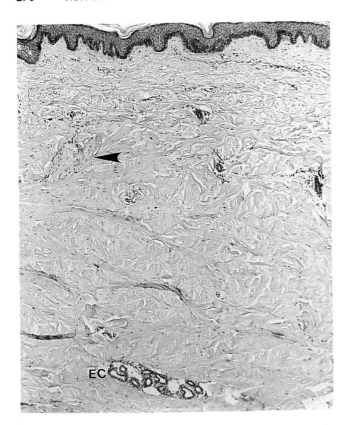

Figure 20–1. Progressive systemic sclerosis, late stage. Within the subcutis and lower two thirds of the dermis are densely packed, horizontally oriented, hyalinized bundles of dermal collagen that entrap eccrine sweat coils (EC). With the exception of a residual arrectores pilorum muscle (large arrowhead), cutaneous adnexae are absent. The epidermis appears normal. (H&E, ×62.)

sweat coils and then the pilosebaceous units progressively atrophy.[21] Gradually, as thickened collagen bundles form at the dermal–subcutaneous junction, the dermal and subcutaneous sweat coils become entrapped, and, ultimately, most adnexal structures are lost (Figs. 20–1, 20–2).[14] Dermal elastic fibers, however, are usually preserved in PSS (and morphea), in contrast to other sclerosing disorders, such as keloid and hypertrophic scar.[19,21] In the late stages of PSS, vascular changes are more prominent. There is intimal proliferation with subsequent thickening and hyalinization of vessel walls, with or without luminal obliteration.[3,22] Increased glycosaminoglycans (chondroitin sulfate, dermatan sulfate, and hyaluronic acid) have been found within the dermis, although their significance is uncertain.[23–25] Possibly, increased glycosaminoglycans have a chemotactic as well as a mitogenic effect on immune inflammatory cells.[1] Hyaluronic acid also has been detected in thickened blood vessel walls.[14]

Microscopic findings in the late or end-stage of PSS include markedly thickened, densely packed, horizontally oriented collagen bundles that replace normal dermis and subcutis. There are also fewer fibroblasts and almost no appendageal structures (Figs. 20–1, 20–2). There may be epidermal atrophy and dermal–subcutaneous dystrophic calcification.[14–15,17]

Differential Diagnosis

The differential diagnosis includes many sclerosing disorders, but only some of the more important entities are discussed. The inflammatory infiltrate in morphea is much more intense and tends to last longer than PSS. Also, although the epidermis may be of normal thickness in both PSS and morphea, in morphea, it can also be abnormally thick.[16] Unlike PSS, sclerodermoid porphyria cutanea tarda may have residual dermal PAS positivity within blood ves-

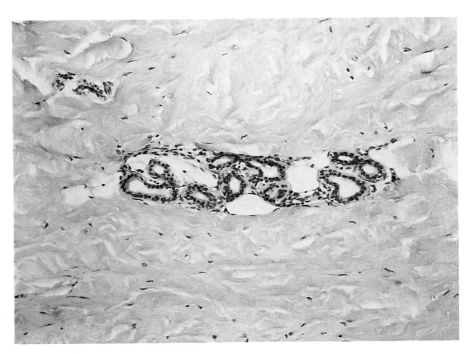

Figure 20–2. Higher power of Figure 20–1. Eccrine sweat coils are encased by dense hyalinized, sclerotic dermal collagen. (H&E, ×156.)

sels and interstitial dermis,[26] and sclerodermoid GVH generally shows residual epidermal hyperkeratosis, atrophy, dyskeratotic epidermal cells, and vacuolation at the epidermal basilar layer.[27] If the characteristic epidermal changes are absent, however, it may be very difficult to differentiate between the late stage of PSS and sclerodermoid GVH.[28,29] In lichen sclerosus et atrophicus (LSA), sclerodermoid changes do occur. However, in most instances, LSA exhibits epidermal atrophy with hyperkeratosis, appendageal ostial plugging, basal cell layer vacuolation, and homogenization of upper dermal collagen. In contrast to PSS, radiodermatitis shows many bizarre appearing fibroblasts within the dermis. Although scleredema and PSS may appear similar, there is generally no homogenization and hyalinization of dermal collagen bundles in scleredema. One ultrastructural study found that the collagen bundles of scleredema were larger in diameter than those of PSS.[29] Finally, unlike PSS, hypertrophic or keloidal scars exhibit loss of elastic fibers, increased cellularity of the dermis with vertical orientation of blood vessels (hypertrophic scar), and peculiar compact, thick eosinophilic collagen bundles haphazardly arranged in the dermis (keloid).

MORPHEA

Clinical Features

Often called "localized scleroderma," morphea is a cutaneous sclerosing disorder with four clinical presentations: localized, generalized, guttate, and linear.[3] Morphea affects women three times more often than men, is more common in Caucasians than blacks, and in 75% of the cases has an onset between the second and fifth decades.[3] Linear scleroderma, however, generally occurs before age 40, often within the first two decades of life.[3]

Although its cause is unknown, morphea is thought to have an immunologic basis because (1) it is known to coexist with other autoimmune diseases (PSS,[30] systemic lupus erythematosus,[31,32] and dermatomyositis[33]), (2) antinuclear antibodies are found in many morphea patients (15–72%, depending on the substrate used),[34] and (3) in linear scleroderma, there are multiple serologic abnormalities, including antinuclear antibodies, rheumatoid factor, and antibodies to single-stranded DNA.[34]

Histologic Features

In an established lesion of morphea, the primary focus of pathology is in the lower two thirds of the dermis and subcutis where there are (1) swelling of collagen bundles, (2) loss of the three-dimensional orientation of collagen fibers, (3) a moderately intense infiltrate of mononuclear cells, especially at the dermal–subcutaneous interface, (4) new collagen production oriented parallel to the epidermis, and (5) prominent inflammation and early fibrosis of fat lobule septae (Figs. 20–3, 20–4).[15,22,35] In addition, there is mild vascular ectasia with variable degrees of initial hyperplasia and medial edema (Fig. 20–4). The epidermis may be abnormally thick,[16] or it may be normal. As the lesion ages, dermal cellularity decreases and hyalinization and homogenization of collagen bundles oriented parallel to the surface epidermis increase. The eccrine coils become

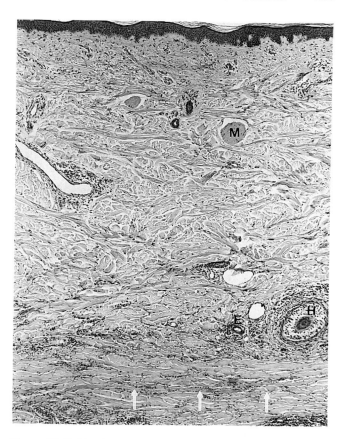

Figure 20–3. Morphea. In the lower dermis and subcutis there is a dense mononuclear cell inflammatory infiltrate around and between blood vessels and around appendages. New collagen production is oriented parallel to the epidermis (arrows), and there is profound atrophy of cutaneous adnexae. The epidermis appears relatively normal. H, hair follicle; E, eccrine duct; M, arrectores pilorum muscle. (H&E, ×62.)

entrapped in dense collagen, and, as the subcutis becomes more sclerotic, the eccrine glands appear to be located in the midreticular dermis. Along with atrophic changes of the sweat coils, the other dermal appendages also atrophy to the extent that, in the late stage, they may be entirely absent. Cutaneous blood vessels gradually decrease, possibly because of progressive fibrosis of vascular walls and luminal obliteration.[35] The dermal elastic tissue, however, is preserved (Fig. 20–5). In cases of linear scleroderma, the sclerosis may extend to fascia and muscle.[3,30] Rarely, subepidermal bullae have been reported in localized or generalized morphea,[36–38] possibly as a result of lymphatic blockage in the area of sclerosis[36] or simple trauma.[38]

Recently, the term morphea profunda (MP) has been introduced to describe the condition of patients with deep, bound-down sclerotic plaques or diffuse zones of sclerosis who have microscopic thickening and hyalinization not only in the deep dermis and subcutis but also in fascia and muscle.[39] The inflammatory infiltrate in MP is predominantly lymphocytic, with some plasma cells and histiocytes, and there is greater involvement of the panniculus than in the usual lesions of morphea.[39] A similar histologic pic-

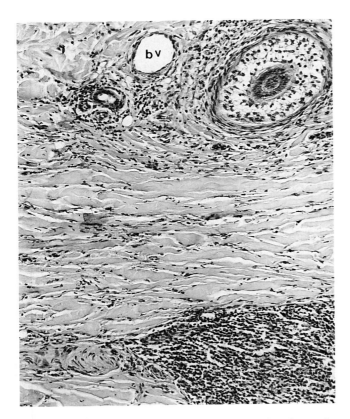

Figure 20–4. Higher power of Figure 20–3, showing a periappenda-geal, perivascular, and interstitial mononuclear cell inflammatory infil-trate parallel to surface epidermis. One ectatic blood vessel (bv) exhibits mild intimal hyperplasia and edema of its wall. (H&E, ×156.)

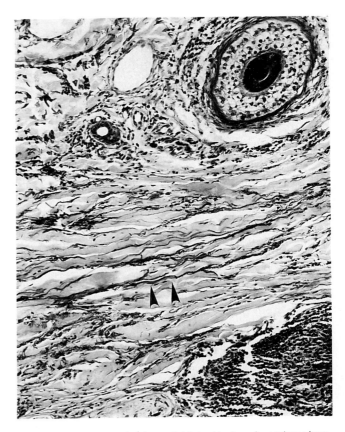

Figure 20–5. Elastic stain of an established lesion of morphea show-ing preservation of elastic fibers (arrowheads) within active areas of inflammation and new collagen production. (Acid orcein and Giemsa, ×156.)

ture is seen in the fascia and to a lesser degree in muscle. Tissue eosinophils are not present in significant numbers in most cases.[39] The upper and middermis generally appear normal, and normal numbers of sweat glands are present, but sebaceous glands and hair follicles usually are diminished in number and size.[39] Some authors consider MP to be but one variant in the disease spectrum of morphea, especially since some of their patients displayed typical morphea lesions elsewhere.[38–40]

Differential Diagnosis
For the distinction of morphea from PSS, sclerodermoid porphyria cutanea tarda, sclerodermoid GVH disease, lichen sclerosus et atrophicus, late-stage radiodermatitis, and scar, see the discussion of differential diagnosis for PSS. One additional entity should be considered: eosinophilic fasciitis, which was originally described by Shulman as an unusual scleroderma-like syndrome.[41] The term "eosinophilic fasciitis" was coined by Rodnan et al. in 1975.[42] In the cases described by Shulman[43,44] and by Rodnan et al., there was inflammation and fibrosis of the subcutis and underlying fascia as well as peripheral blood eosinophilia. The fascia appeared thickened and showed moderate to marked numbers of lymphocytes, plasma cells, and eosinophils. In Schulman's patients, there apparently were no

histologic findings of classic cutaneous scleroderma or myositis.[43,44] Some studies of this disorder have shown tissue eosinophilia or myositis,[45] whereas others have shown neither.[46] In some cases, there was inflammation of the fascia only, and the dermis, subcutis, and muscle appeared normal.[47] Over time, a number of authors have taken the view that eosinophilic fasciitis should be considered a variant of morphea or diffuse scleroderma,[17,18,38,48,49] partly because eosinophilic fasciitis shares some features with generalized morphea, such as inflammation and fibrosis of fascia, blood eosinophilia, and hypergammaglobulinemia,[17] and partly because one instance of eosinophilic fasciitis progressed to diffuse scleroderma.[49] There also has been one report of eosinophilic fasciitis in association with morphea and systemic sclerosis.[50] No consensus has been reached, however, about the relationship between eosinophilic fasciitis and scleroderma.

LICHEN SCLEROSUS ET ATROPHICUS

Clinical Features
Lichen sclerosus et atrophicus (LSA) is an uncommon disease that occurs more often in women than in men. It is characterized by white to pink, polygonal, hyperkeratotic

papules, which coalesce to white atrophic plaques.[51] LSA primarily affects the genitalia, although extragenital lesions may occur in females (about 20%) and, rarely, in males.[51] Although primarily a disease of adults, it also can occur in children.[52] LSA of the vulvar region is also known as kraurosis vulvae, and on the glans penis it is called balanitis xerotica obliterans. Squamous cell carcinoma arises in LSA of the vulva in about 3 to 4% of patients but is rare in males.[51,53,54]

The cause of LSA is unknown, but some evidence favors an autoimmune pathogenesis. Recent studies have found in LSA patients increased organ-specific antibodies, including, in women, thyroid microsomal, parietal cell, and intrinsic factor antibodies[55] and, in men, smooth muscle and parietal cell antibodies.[56] Autoimmune-related disorders also are more common in these patients: thyroid disease and pernicious anemia in females[55] and vitiligo and alopecia areata in males.[57] There are some data to indicate that LSA may somehow be related to a partial deficiency of plasma testosterone and elevated levels of androstenedione.[58]

Histologic Features

The histopathologic features of established but active lesions of LSA include pronounced epidermal orthokeratotic hyperkeratosis, atrophy, and basal cell layer vacuolation, which often results in dermal–epidermal clefting (Fig. 20–6).[14,19,59–60] Orthokeratotic horny plugging of cutaneous follicular and sweat duct ostia also is present. There are striking edema and homogenization of collagen in the upper dermis, beneath which is a focal perivascular or band-like mononuclear cell infiltrate often including plasma cells (Figs. 20–6, 20–7).[14,29,59–60] Within the homogenized zone of dermal collagen, there is vascular ectasia, loss of elastic fibers, and increased deposition of glycosaminogly-

cans.[14,19,59–61] If the epidermal basilar vacuolation and papillary dermal edema are severe, dermal–epidermal separation with bulla formation occurs (Fig. 20–8).[61,62]

In older lesions, the epidermis becomes more squamotized because of basal cell layer dropout. On mucosal surfaces there may be areas of atrophy that alternate with hyperplasia, with or without basilar squamotization. Orthokeratotic plugging is present in cutaneous appendageal ostia, and the previously edematous homogenized papillary dermis is gradually replaced by sclerotic collagen.[14,19,59,60] Frequently, there is a focal, patchy mononuclear cell infiltrate in the upper dermis. Areas of mucosal epithelial hyperplasia may merge into frank atypia and, over long periods, invasive squamous cell carcinoma.[53,54,63,64] There is no record of LSA of cutaneous surfaces other than anogenital progressing to squamous cell carcinoma.[14]

Differential Diagnosis

Differential diagnosis in LSA includes lupus erythematosus, chronic radiodermatitis, and morphea. Lupus erythematosus may be similar to LSA, but the dermal infiltrate is more lichenoid and there generally is thickening of the epidermal basement membrane in lupus erythematosus.[14] Also, the inflammatory infiltrate in lupus erythematosus is generally both superficial and deep, and dermal deposition of hyaluronia and may be seen throughout the dermis. Unlike LSA, radiodermatitis generally involves the deeper dermis and shows bizarre dermal radiation fibroblasts. There is disagreement over whether LSA and morphea are distinct entities or simply different stages of the same disease.[61] LSA has classically been distinguished from morphea by (1) an atrophic epidermis with hydropic basilar degeneration and cornified ostial appendageal plugging, (2) an edematous, homogenized papillary dermis that later becomes

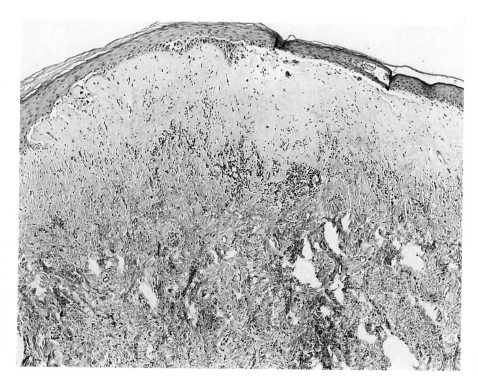

Figure 20–6. Lichen sclerosis et atrophicus (vulva). The epidermis is atrophic, and there is pronounced epidermal basilar layer vacuolation with clefting. There are pronounced edema and homogenization of the papillary dermis, directly beneath which is a bandlike zone of mononuclear cells. The reticular dermis appears unremarkable. (H&E, ×62.)

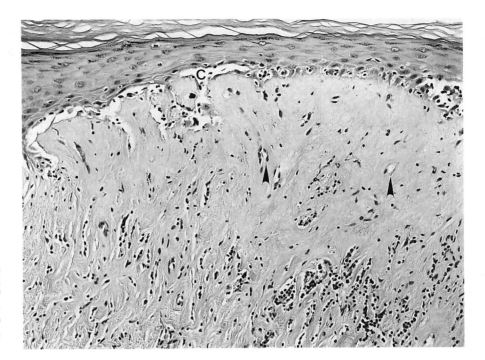

Figure 20–7. Higher power of Figure 20–6. Atrophy of the epidermis with prominent hydropic change in the basilar layer results in cleft formation (C). There is pronounced homogenized edema with early sclerosis of the papillary dermis. Capillary vascular ectasia (arrowheads) is also present within the zone of papillary dermal edema. (H&E, ×156.)

sclerotized, with relative loss of elastic fibers, and (3) a relatively normal reticular dermis and subcutis.[61] In morphea, however, the epidermis and papillary dermis usually are normal, but the reticular dermis and subcutis show increasingly sclerotic changes, with a moderate inflammatory interstitial mononuclear infiltrate and relative preservation of dermal elastic tissue. However, according to some authors, in addition to the usual deeper dermal and subcutaneous sclerosing changes, morphea also can show initial ostial appendageal cornification, epidermal atrophy (but no vacuolation), and papillary dermal edema similar to LSA (Fig. 20–9).[61] Other authors contend that morphea and LSA may coexist in the same patient and even in the same lesion.[65,66]

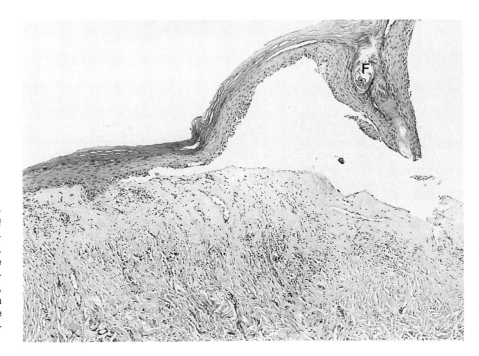

Figure 20–8. Bullous LSA. Dermal–epidermal separation with subepidermal bulla. If epidermal basilar hydropic change and papillary dermal edema are sufficiently severe, a bulla may form. The other features include (1) epidermal compact lamellar orthokeratotic hyperkeratosis, (2) epidermal atrophy, (3) papillary dermal homogenized edema and vascular ectasia, and (4) a band-like mononuclear cell infiltrate. A cornified follicular plug (F) is present. (H&E, ×62.)

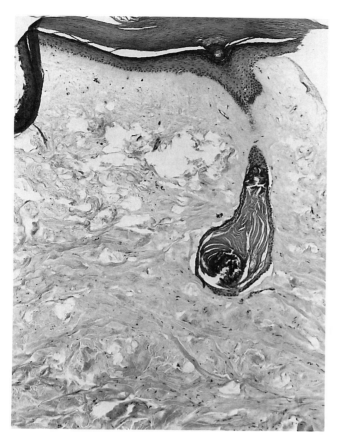

Figure 20–9. Punch biopsy showing features of LSA and morphea. There is compact orthokeratotic hyperkeratosis and atrophy of the epidermis with underlying papillary dermal homogenized edema and early sclerosis (LSA). There is cornified plugging of a hair follicle. Hydropic change of the epidermal basilar layer is noticeably absent, however. The deep dermis and subcutis are replaced by dense eosinophilic hyalinized bundles of sclerotic collagen arranged somewhat parallel to the surface epidermis (morphea). There is artifactual separation of the upper dermis. (H&E, ×62.)

WOUND HEALING

Clinical Features

Keloids and hypertrophic scars are aberrations of wound healing; that is, they are manifestations of an abnormal connective tissue response. Clinically, they are raised, red, firm, pruritic or tender growths that become more flesh-colored or hyperpigmented as they age.[67] They occur most frequently in patients between the ages of 10 and 30, although they may be seen in those of any age.[67] Keloids are seen equally in either sex and tend to be more common in blacks and darkly pigmented races.[68] They frequently are found on areas of the body where skin tension is the greatest: upper back, shoulders, chest, and upper arms. Keloids differ from hypertrophic scars by their extension beyond their site of origin and their clinical persistence (hypertrophic scars tend to involute over 1 to 2 years).[67–69]

The cause of keloids is unknown, although there is some speculation that trauma, skin tension, and hormones

play a role.[67,69] There is some evidence that mast cells play a role in the pathogenesis of both hypertrophic scars and keloids through the extracellular release of cytoplasmic granules containing histamine, heparin, and acid hydrolases.[70] Histamine, for example, has been shown to increase the amount of soluble collagen by competitively inhibiting the collagen cross-linking enzyme, lysyl oxidase.[70] Through some unknown mechanism, this inhibition apparently interferes with a chemotactic feedback mechanism[70] and increases collagen synthesis. Histamine may also accelerate collagen formation in fibroblasts.[71]

Histologic Features

Early tissue repair in keloid and hypertrophic scars[67,69] is similar to the initial inflammatory phase of wound healing[72]: there is an influx of neutrophils and blood monocytes into the cutaneous wound; the monocytes subsequently convert to tissue macrophages. It is in the second, or granulation tissue, phase of wound healing that hypertrophic scars and keloids grow awry. During this early phase of keloid and scar formation, there is exaggerated fibroplasia and angiogenesis, with formation of nodular, compact vascular proliferations surrounded by fibroblasts.[67,69] Electron microscopy reveals variably increased numbers of myofibroblasts in the active stages of keloid and hypertrophic scar formation.[73,74] Myofibroblast proliferation also is seen in the granulation tissue phase of normal wound healing.[72] As the lesions age, the growth becomes less vascular and more collagenous, with whorl-like or nodular compact thickened collagen fibers of variable size.[69,75] At this stage, the microvasculature tends to be arranged peripherally to the aggregates of dense collagen bundles.[69,75] In the developing hypertrophic scar, there is an increase in extracellular glycosaminoglycans, most of which is chondroitin-4-sulfate (chondroitin sulfate A).[76] When the hypertrophic scar is well formed it has a characteristic histologic picture: (1) abundant dermal fibroblasts and dermal collagen fibers are oriented somewhat parallel or perpendicular to the surface epidermis, (2) numerous dermal blood vessels are oriented perpendicular to the surface epidermis, and (3) cutaneous adnexae are few or nonexistent (Figs. 20–10, 20–11). Unlike keloids, hypertrophic scars tend to mature with time, and there are fewer fibroblasts and capillaries, less nodularity and thickening of collagen bundles, and fewer elastic fibers.[75] Well-formed keloids rarely involute.[69] The mature keloid exhibits a characteristic histology: (1) nodular, whorled eosinophilic collagen bundles that tend to persist indefinitely, (2) few cutaneous adnexae, and (3) few elastic fibers (Figs. 20–12, 20–13). Rarely, calcification may occur in keloids.[77] In both keloids and hypertrophic scars, compression of the papillary dermis by the expansile fibroplasia of the reticular dermis may flatten the epidermal rete ridge pattern (Figs. 20–10, 20–12). The inflammatory infiltrate in well-established hypertrophic scars and keloids is composed of perivascular mast cells, plasma cells, and lymphocytes.[67,78]

Differential Diagnosis

The differential diagnosis of hypertrophic scars and keloids includes morphea, PSS, connective tissue nevus, dermatofibroma, and fibromatoses. None of the first four entities

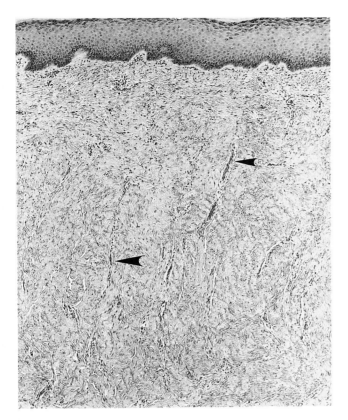

Figure 20–10. Hypertrophic scar. There are increased numbers of dermal fibroblasts and dermal collagen bundles oriented vertically or parallel to the surface epidermis. Increased numbers of dermal blood vessels (arrowheads) also appear to course upward, perpendicular to the overlying epidermis. Cutaneous adnexae are noticeably absent. (H&E, ×62.)

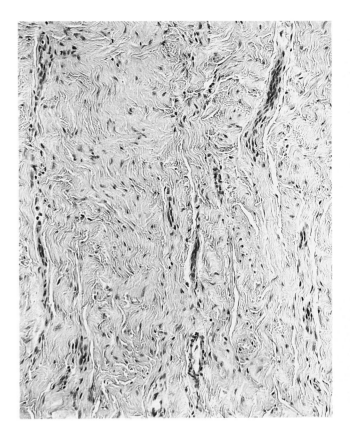

Figure 20–11. Higher power of Figure 20–10 showing the increased numbers of dermal fibroblasts and vertically oriented dermal collagen fibers and blood vessels. (H&E, ×156.)

in the differential diagnosis exhibits the nodular, whorled, thickened eosinophilic collagen bundles of a keloid. Also, none of the first four entities exhibits the combination of dermal hypercellularity, vertical orientation of blood vessels, or marked collagen fiber parallelism of a hypertrophic scar. In addition, elastic fibers, which are relatively scarce in keloids and hypertrophic scars, generally appear in normal numbers in morphea and PSS. In connective tissue nevus, their quantity may be normal or abnormally high or low. Fibromatoses may be difficult to distinguish from keloids or hypertrophic scars histologically, although fibromatoses tend to be much more cellular and have distinctive features, which depend on the variant.[14] Finally, there is a rare entity called "nodular (keloidal) scleroderma," in which patients at risk may develop keloids within sclerodermatous skin.[79] Nonetheless, there are typical histologic features of scleroderma/morphea to help distinguish keloids from keloidal scleroderma.[79]

RADIODERMATITIS

Clinical Features
Several forms of ionizing radiation may affect the skin so as to produce radiodermatitis: x- and γ-radiation (especially

at the orthovoltage level below 1 Mev) and particulate radiation, such as electrons (β-radiation) and neutrons.[80] In the past, most ionizing skin reactions occurred at the orthovoltage level (90–100 Kev), but today much less radiation dermatitis is seen because of the use of deeper penetrating megavoltage (2–4 Mev).[80] Radiodermatitis is usually divided into two clinical categories: acute (early) and chronic (late).[80,81] These categories are delineated best for x- and γ-radiation and less completely for particulate radiation.[80] In acute radiodermatitis, after an initial threshold dose of ionizing radiation has been exceeded, a diphasic or triphasic response is seen.[81] In the first phase, there is a progressive, reactive erythema secondary to release of histamine or serotonin.[81,82] This response occurs within 24 hours of exposure, lasts 2 to 6 days, and may result in vesiculation.[81–83] The second or delayed erythema phase occurs 7 to 9 days after irradiation. Occasionally, a third phase of erythema develops 6 to 7 weeks after radiation, resulting in hyperpigmentation.[81,82] Acute ulceration secondary to high radiation doses may be seen at any time, beginning after 2 weeks. However, this is much less common today than in previous years because of changes in radiation dosimetry.[80]

In chronic radiodermatitis, the skin appears atrophic and telangiectatic. The condition first becomes noticeable

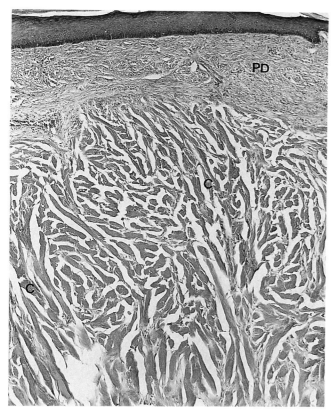

Figure 20–12. Keloid. In the lower two thirds of the dermis are prominent thickened, nodular, whorled eosinophilic collagen bundles (C), which stand in relief against the overlying widened fibrotic papillary dermis (PD). The epidermal rete ridge pattern is flattened by the expansile fibroplasia of the underlying dermis. (H&E, ×62.)

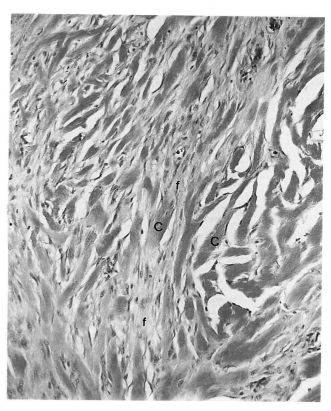

Figure 20–13. Higher power of Figure 20–12 demonstrating thickened eosinophilic collagen bundles (C) within a background of fibrotic collagen fibers (F). (H&E, ×156.)

within weeks or months after ionizing radiation therapy and is fully developed within 2 years or longer.[82,83] If orthovoltage radiation is employed, radionecrosis may occur approximately 1 year after treatment. It usually appears over high-density structures, such as bone or cartilage (e.g., lower legs, nose), and is most often precipitated by trauma or infection.[83] One complication of megavoltage radiation therapy is deep subcutaneous fibrosis, which can occur months after therapy and last for years.[84] As a late sequela to radiation therapy, skin cancers may develop within the treated sites. Basal cell and squamous cell carcinoma are the most common, but other tumors may also occur, including sebaceous and sweat gland carcinomas, sarcomas, and even malignant melanomas.[80,81]

Histologic Features

In radiodermatitis, the primary location of the pathology, depending on the age of the lesion, is epidermal, dermal, and subcutaneous.[80–85] If the less penetrating (electron beam) β-radiation has been given, subcutaneous fibrosis may not occur.[80–85]

In acute radiation dermatitis, there is ballooning degeneration of epidermal cells, with variable degrees of nuclear pyknosis and dyskeratosis, basal cell layer hydropic change, and lower epidermal spongiosis.[80,86,87] Dermal changes include (1) cellular degenerative changes in hair follicles, sebaceous glands, and sweat glands, (2) upper dermal edema, (3) upper dermal vascular ectasia and endothelial edema, and (4) frequent lower-dermal arteriolar fibrinous thrombosis.[80,81,86,87] The interstitial dermal inflammatory infiltrate changes over time: neutrophils are seen early, followed by macrophages, eosinophils, plasma cells, and lymphocytes.[80] Stromal fibrin frequently is present,[80] and there is variable pyknosis of fibroblasts and histiocytes.[86] If the total dose is 40 Gy or higher, there may be subepidermal bulla formation, epidermal ulceration, and a histologic picture similar to a second-degree burn.[80] In the healing stage of acute radiation dermatitis, there is epidermal atrophy with orthokeratotic and parakeratotic hyperkeratosis, epidermal hypermelanization, vascular ectasia, appendageal atrophy, and fragmentation with clumping of dermal collagen.[80–82]

In chronic or late-stage radiodermatitis, epidermal changes include (1) orthokeratotic and parakeratotic hyperkeratosis, (2) areas of atrophy alternating with acanthosis, (3) keratinocytic edema and homogenization with dyskeratosis and variable degrees of nuclear atypia, and (4) hypermelanization and vacuolation of the basal layer (Figs. 20–14, 20–15).[14,80,86] Epidermal ulceration may occur secondary to a number of causes: atrophy, trauma, infection

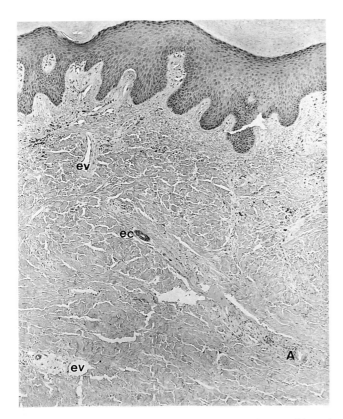

Figure 20–14. Chronic radiodermatitis. There is moderate epidermal acanthosis with orthokeratotic- and parakeratotic hyperkeratosis. Dermal collagen appears thickened, and sclerotic and cutaneous adnexae are absent or atrophic. There is dermal vascular ectasia with prominent luminal endothelial cell nuclei and thickened arterioles. ev, ectatic venules; ec, eccrine coil; and A, thickened arteriol exhibiting myointimal proliferation. (H&E, ×61.)

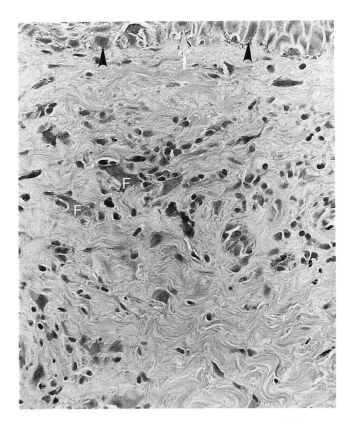

Figure 20–15. Chronic radiodermatitis. The epidermis exhibits spongiosis, focal dyskeratosis (white arrow), keratinocytic nuclear atypia (black arrowheads), and basilar layer vacuolation. Dermal fibroblasts exhibit large pleomorphic, hyperchromatic nuclei (F) and basophilic, flocculated cytoplasm (radiation fibroblasts). (H&E, ×380.)

(Fig. 20–16). The underlying dermal collagen appears swollen and homogenized and exhibits varying degrees of eosinophilia. As the lesion ages, the collagen bundles thicken and appear sclerotic and rigid (Fig. 20–17).[80] Fibroblast nuclei are large, pleomorphic, and hyperchromatic and are surrounded by abundant, flocculated cytoplasm (radiation fibroblasts) (Figs. 20–15, 20–18). Vascular changes are prominent and may include (Fig. 20–14): (1) upper dermal vascular ectasia with or without hyperchromasia of endothelial cell nuclei and subendothelial vacuolar change, (2) decreased numbers of capillaries in the upper dermis, (3) deeper dermal arteriolar and arterial myointimal proliferation, with occasional luminal narrowing and thrombosis, and (4) rare instances of vascular wall fibrinous necrosis.[14,80,81,86–88] Pilar structures frequently are absent, residual arrectores pilorum muscles frequently are present, and sweat ducts and glands may be present but show differing degrees of atrophy (Fig. 20–14, 20–17).[14,81,86–88] Fibrosis of the subcutis occurs especially after megavoltage therapy.[14,80,84] The intensity and composition of the dermal inflammatory infiltrate is quite variable, consisting of upper dermal melanophages and siderophages[80] and, in the absence of epidermal ulceration, small to insignificant numbers of dermal lymphocytes, plasma cells, and histiocytes (Fig. 20–15).[80,88] Dermal elastic fibers may be abundant or scarce.[80] Fibrinous material frequently is seen at the dermal–epidermal junction as well as within the dermis.[80,88]

Differential Diagnosis

The differential diagnosis includes PSS, morphea, lichen sclerosus et atrophicus, lupus erythematosus, and scar. Although these entities have end-stage dermal fibrosis in common, they do not exhibit the atypical dermal fibroblasts and hyperchromatic vascular endothelial cell nuclei seen in radiation dermatitis.

BLEOMYCIN SCLEROSIS

Clinical Features

Systemic bleomycin-induced cutaneous fibrosis appears as infiltrated plaques, nodules, and bands with concomitant acrocyanosis, acrosclerosis, and patchy, sometimes flagellated erythema and hyperpigmentation.[89–92] The sclerosis may sometimes disappear when administration of the drug is stopped.[90]

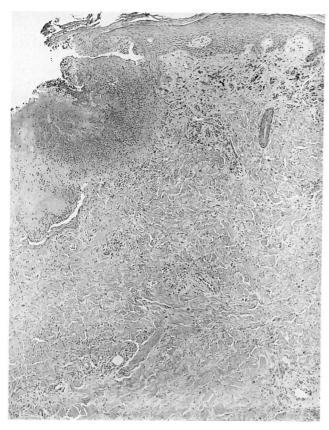

Figure 20–16. Dermal–epidermal ulceration with acute and chronic inflammation in an area of chronic radiodermatitis. (H&E, ×61.)

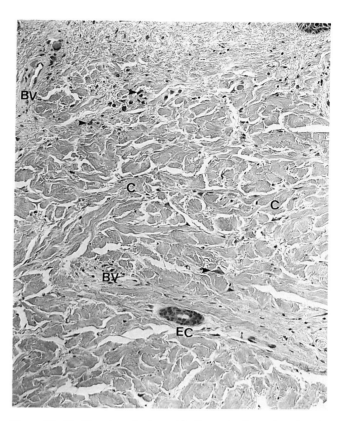

Figure 20–17. Chronic radiodermatitis. Dermal collagen bundles (C) appear thickened and sclerotic. Large radiation fibroblasts (arrowheads) are seen scattered throughout the dermis, and prominent endothelial cell nuclei are seen in blood vascular lumina (bv). EC, eccrine coil. (H&E, ×152.)

Histologic Features

Histologically indurated lesions secondary to bleomycin therapy appear as dense, homogenized, sclerotic collagen involving the entire dermis and resulting in collagenous entrapment of cutaneous adnexae.[89] The epidermal pigmentary changes seem to be secondary to increased melanization of the basal cell layer,[93,94] possibly as a result of increased localized melanogenesis.[93] In one case report, lesions of linear plaquelike erythema developed subsequent to a course of multiple-agent chemotherapy including bleomycin. The rash apparently resolved with postinflammatory hyperpigmentation after withdrawal of bleomycin only.[92] The histologic features of the erythematous plaque were similar to those of fixed drug eruption, including epidermal acanthosis, hydropic basilar layer change, dermal melanophage activity, and a dense superficial and middermal perivascular lymphohistiocytic infiltrate.[92]

PENTAZOCINE SCLEROSIS

Clinical Features

In pentazocine-induced sclerosis, there is woody induration of the skin and subcutaneous tissue at the sites of injection.[95–97] Ulceration, cellulitis, phlebitis, fibrous my-

opathy, and, ultimately, limb contractures have been reported to occur after pentazocine use.[96,97]

Histologic Features

Histologically, all layers of the skin may be involved.[95–97] There is epidermal necrosis with or without dermal necrosis, moderate to marked perivascular, periadnexal, and interstitial dermal and subcutaneous mononuclear cell inflammatory infiltrate, and areas of lobular fat degeneration.[95,96] There are numerous dermal and subcutaneous giant cells, which exhibit clear-space clefting of their cytoplasm.[95] The fibrotic dermis becomes increasingly thickened, with concomitant widening of fat lobule septae.[95–97] There may be deep dermal or subcutaneous vascular wall thickening and thrombosis (endarteritis).[95–97] Ultimately, there is severe extensive sclerodermoid change in the dermis-subcutis and a reduction in elastic fibers.[14] Various mechanisms have been proposed for this tissue destruction. One study proposed that myonecrosis is secondary to vasoconstriction or occlusion, ischemia, and tissue necrosis.[96] Another hypothesized that pentazocine-induced vasoconstriction complicates diabetic vasculopathy and thus leads to ischemia and tissue necrosis.[97] This latter study found a high percentage (65%) of patients wth pentazocine-induced sclerosis who gave a personal or family history of diabetes mellitus.[97]

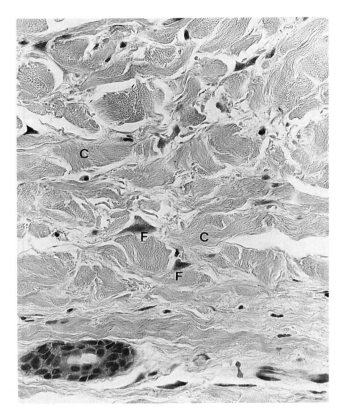

Figure 20–18. Higher power of Figure 20–17 showing thickened sclerotic collagen bundles (C) surrounding a remnant of an eccrine duct (lower left corner). Prominent radiation fibroblasts (F) are seen throughout the field. (H&E, ×380.)

OCCUPATIONAL ACROOSTEOLYSIS

Occupational acroosteolysis secondary to polyvinylchloride exposure consists of a triad of clinical findings: Raynaud's phenomenon, sclerodermatous skin changes, and lytic le-

sions of bone (mostly the upper extremities and especially the phalanges).[98] Other abnormalities include hepatosplenomegaly, thrombocytopenia, and hepatic angiosarcoma.[98]

The focus of histopathology is primarily in the dermis, where there is homogenization and thickening of haphazard configurations of eosinophilic collagen bundles.[99,100] Other findings include (1) a predominantly lymphohistiocytic perivascular inflammatory infiltrate, (2) occasional dermal vascular intimal fibrosis and medial hypertrophy, (3) thickening and fragmentation of elastic fibers, (4) variable dermal edema, and (5) normal-appearing epidermis and epidermal appendages.[99,100]

ATROPHODERMA OF PASINI AND PIERINI

Clinical Features

Atrophoderma of Pasini and Pierini is considered by some to be an atrophic variant of morphea,[14,17,19,101–103] whereas others beieve it is a distinct entity.[104,105] Clinically, the lesions are smooth, gray-brown to blue-brown, depressed patches of skin ranging in size from 1 to 10 cm and exhibiting a cliff-drop border that is thought to be an optical effect of the slate gray discoloration.[17,101] The eventual development of sclerodermatous change within atrophodermatous skin has been noted.[101]

Histologic Features

Microscopically, atrophoderma can be considered one of the "invisible dermatoses" unless adjacent normal skin is submitted with the specimen.[106] Because the primary focus of pathology is dermal and the dermal thickness at times can be difficult to judge without reference to normal skin, the atrophy of atrophoderma can be easily overlooked, especially if the dermal inflammatory component is minimal. Compared with normal skin, however, there may be 25 to 75% thinning of the affected dermis. Therefore a full-thickness excision of normal and abnormal skin, including fat, should be taken perpendicular to the edge of the lesion.[106]

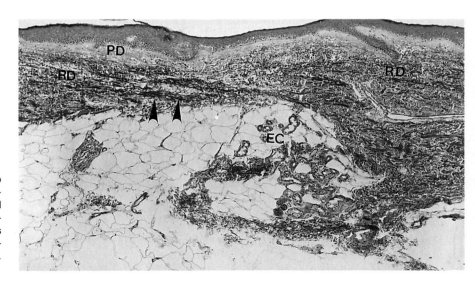

Figure 20–19. Atrophoderma. Compared to normal dermis on the right, the affected dermis is markedly reduced in thickness and exhibits a mild degree of sclerosis (arrowheads). The epidermis and papillary dermis appear relatively normal. PD, papillary dermis; RD, reticular dermis; EC, eccrine coils. (H&E, ×64.)

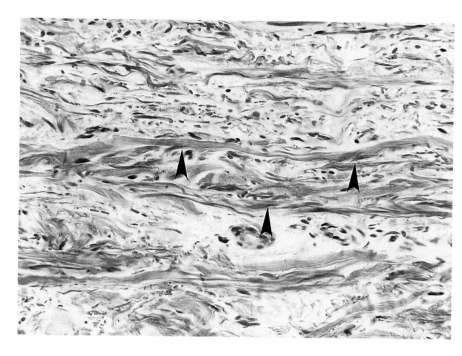

Figure 20–20. Higher power of Figure 20–19. Mild compression and thickening of dermal collagen (arrowheads) oriented parallel to surface epidermis. (H&E, ×380.)

In the early lesions of atrophoderma, there is focal minimal thickening of collagen bundles, with minimal scattered mononuclear cell infiltrates.[14] As the lesion ages, dermal collagen bundles become more tightly packed and may show homogenization and hyalinization of the collagen fibers (Figs. 20–19, 20–20).[14,103] The epidermis and subcutis usually appear normal (Fig. 20–19).

Differential Diagnosis

The differential diagnosis includes scar and morphea. Neither keloid nor hypertrophic scar exhibits the marked thinning of the dermis seen in atrophoderma. Also, atrophoderma does not show the thickened, hyalinized, eosinophilic collagen bundles of a keloid or the striking vertical orientation of blood vessels seen in hypertrophic scar. Some consider atrophoderma to be a variant of morphea,[14,17,19,101–103] even though the clinical presentation of atrophoderma is different. In atrophoderma the lesions are gray-brown to bluish brown, depressed patches of skin exhibiting a cliff-drop appearance, whereas in morphea, the lesions appear as smooth, indurated plaques with ivory centers and violaceous borders. Those who consider atrophoderma as a variant of morphea do so because of reported cases of atrophoderma and morphea appearing simultaneously[103] or subsequent to one another[102] in the same patient and because of cases in which morphea has actually transformed into atrophoderma.[17] Others argue, less convincingly, that atrophoderma is a separate disease from morphea, since atrophy precedes sclerosis in atrophoderma, whereas sclerosis precedes atrophy in morphea.[105] Atrophoderma seems to be, at least, related to morphea in the sense that both are in the spectrum of sclerosing disorders.

Acknowledgments

The author gratefully acknowledges the expert photographic assistance of Milton B. Tudahl, Sr., Director of Photographic Services, Francis Scott Key Medical Center, Baltimore, Maryland.

REFERENCES

1. Haustein UF, Herrmann K, Bohme HJ. Pathogenesis of progressive systemic sclerosis. *Int J Dermatol.* 1986;25:286–293. Review.
2. Rodnan GP, Lipinski E, Luksick J. Skin thickness and collagen content in progressive systemic sclerosis and localized scleroderma. *Arthritis Rheum.* 1979;22:130–140.
3. Eisen AZ, Uitto JJ, Bauer AB. Scleroderma. In: Fitzpatrick TB, Eisen AZ, Wolff K, et al., ed. *Dermatology in General Medicine.* 3rd ed, New York: McGraw-Hill Book Co; 1987:1841–1852.
4. Kahalen MB, Sherer GK, Leroy EC. Endothelial injury in scleroderma. *J Exp Med.* 1979;149:1326–1335.
5. Shanahan WR, Korn JH. Cytotoxic activity of sera from scleroderma and other connective tissue diseases: lack of cellular and disease specificity. *Arthritis Rheum.* 1982;25:1391–1395.
6. Cohen S, Johanson AR, Hurd E. Cytotoxicity of sera from patients with scleroderma. *Arthritis Rheum.* 1983;26:170–178.
7. Penning CA, Cunningham J, French MAH, et al. Antibody-dependent cellular cytotoxicity of human vascular endothelium in systemic sclerosis. *Clin Exp Immunol.* 1984;57:548–550.
8. Lapenus D, Rodnan GP, Cavallo T. Immunopathology of the renal vascular lesion of progressive systemic sclerosis (scleroderma). *Am J Pathol.* 1978;91:243–258.
9. Duncan MR, Perlish JS, Fleischmajer R. Lymphokine/monokine inhibition of fibroblast proliferation and collagen production. A role in progressive systemic sclerosis (PSS). *J Invest Dermatol.* 1984;83:377–384.
10. Gupta S, Malaviya AN, Rajagopalan P, et al. Subsets of human T lymphocytes: imbalance of T-cell population in patients with progressive systemic sclerosis. *Clin Exp Immunol.* 1979;38:342–348.
11. Krakauer RS, Sundeen J, Sauder DN, et al. Abnormalities of immunoregulation in progressive systemic sclerosis. Evidence of excess helper-cell function and altered B-cell function. *Arch Dermatol.* 1981;117:80–82.

12. Inoshita T, Whiteside TL, Rodnan GP, et al. Abnormalities of T lymphocyte subsets in patients with progressive systemic sclerosis (PSS, scleroderma). *J Lab Clin Med.* 1981; 97:264–277.

13. Brady AH. Collagenase in scleroderma. *J Clin Invest.* 1975;56:1175–1180.

14. Young EM Jr, Barr RJ. Sclerosing dermatoses. *J Cutan Pathol.* 1985;12:426–441.

15. O'Leary PA, Montgomery H, Ragsdale WE. Dermatohistopathology of various types of scleroderma. *Arch Dermatol.* 1957;75:78–87. Review.

16. Morley SM, Gaylarde PM, Sarkany I. Epidermal thickness in systemic sclerosis and morphea. *Clin Exp Dermatol.* 1985;10:51–57.

17. Lever WF, Schaumburg-Lever G. *Histopathology of the Skin.* 6th ed. Philadelphia: JB Lippincott Co; 1983:461–467.

18. Fleischmajer R, Perlish JS, Reeves JR. Cellular infiltrates in scleroderma skin. *Arthritis Rheum.* 1977;20:975–984.

19. Ackerman AB. *Histologic Diagnosis of Inflammatory Skin Diseases.* Philadelphia: Lea & Febiger; 1978:760–767.

20. Fleischmajer R, Damiano V, Nedwich A. Alteration of subcutaneous tissue in systemic scleroderma. *Arch Dermatol.* 1972;105:59–66.

21. Mehregan AH. *Pinkus' Guide to Dermatohistopathology.* 4th ed. Norwalk, CT: Appleton-Century-Crofts; 1986:313–314.

22. Hood AF, Kwan TH, Burns DC, et al. *Primer of Dermatopathology.* Boston: Little, Brown and Co; 1984:252–253.

23. Fleischmajer R, Perlish JS. Glycosaminoglycans in scleroderma and scleredema. *J Invest Dermatol.* 1972;58:129–132.

24. Kitabatake M, Ishikawa H, Maeda H. Immunohistochemical demonstration of proteoglycans in the skin of patients with systemic sclerosis. *Br J Dermatol.* 1983;108:257–262.

25. Buckingham RB, Pince RK, Rodnan GP. Progressive systemic sclerosis (PSS, scleroderma) dermal fibroblasts synthesize increased amounts of glycosaminoglycan. *J Lab Clin Med.* 1983;659–669.

26. Epstein JH, Tuffanelli DL, Epstein WL. Cutaneous changes in the porphyrias. *Arch Dermatol.* 1973;107:689–698.

27. Hood AF, Soter NA, Rappaport J, et al. Graft-versus-host reaction. Cutaneous manifestations following bone marrow transplantation. *Arch Dermatol.* 1977;113:1087–1091.

28. Shulman HM, Sale GE, Lernere KG, et al. Chronic cutaneous graft-versus-host disease in man. *Am J Pathol.* 1978;91:545–570.

29. Spielvogel RL, Goltz RW, Kersey JH. Scleroderma-like changes in chronic graft-versus-host disease. *Arch Dermatol.* 1977;113:1424–1428.

30. Christianson HB, Dorsey CS, O'Leary PA, et al. Localized scleroderma: a clinical study of 235 cases. *Arch Dermatol.* 1956;74:629–639.

31. Mitchell AJ, Rusin LJ, Diaz LA. Circumscribed scleroderma with immunologic evidence of systemic lupus erythematosus. *Arch Dermatol.* 1980;116:69–73.

32. Mackel SE, Kozin F, Ryan LM, et al. Concurrent linear scleroderma and systemic lupus erythematosus: a report of two cases. *J Invest Dermatol.* 1979;73:368–372.

33. Woo TY, Rasmusen JE. Juvenile linear scleroderma associated with serologic abnormalities. *Arch Dermatol.* 1985;121:1403–1405.

34. Falanga V, Medsger TA, Reichlin M. High titers of antibodies to single-stranded DNA in linear scleroderma. *Arch Dermatol.* 1985;121:345–347.

35. Fleischmajer R, Nedwich A. Generalized morphea. I. Histology of the dermis and subcutaneous tissue. *Arch Dermatol.* 1972;106:509–514.

36. Templeton HJ. Localized scleroderma with bullae. *Arch Dermatol Syphilol.* 1941;43:361–365.

37. Synkowski DR, Lobitz WC Jr, Provost TT. Bullous scleroderma. *Arch Dermatol.* 1981;117:135–137.

38. Su DWP, Greene SL. Bullous morphea profunde. *Am J Dermatopathol.* 1986;8:144–147.

39. Su DWP, Person JR. Morphea profunda. A new concept and a histologic study of 23 cases. *Am J Dermatopathol.* 1981;3:251–260.

40. Person JR, Su DWP. Subcutaneous morphea. A clinical study of sixteen cases. *Br J Dermatol.* 1979;100:371–380.

41. Shulman LE. Diffuse fasciitis with hypergammaglobulenemia and eosinophilia: a new syndrome? 1974; *J Rheumatol.* 1(Suppl 1):46. Abstract.

42. Rodnan GP, DiBartolomeo AG, Medsger TA Jr, et al. Eosinophilic fasciitis—report on seven cases of a newly recognized sclerodema-like syndrome. *Arthritis Rheum.* 1975;18:422–423.

43. Shulman LE. Diffuse fasciitis with eosinophilia: a new syndrome? 443A, 1975. Abstract.

44. Shulman LE. Diffuse fasciitis with eosinophilia: a new syndrome? *Trans Assoc Am Phys.* 1975;88:70–85.

45. Gray RG, Poppo MJ. Eosinophilic fasciitis: a scleroderma-like illness. *JAMA.* 1977;237:529–530.

46. Krauser RE, Tuthill RJ. Eosinophilic fasciitis. *Arch Dermatol.* 1977;113:1092–1093.

47. Torres VM, George WM. Diffuse eosinophilic fasciitis. A new syndrome or variant of scleroderma? *Arch Dermatol.* 1977;113:1591–1593.

48. Ackermann AB. *Histologic Diagnosis of Inflammatory Skin Disease.* Philadelphia: Lea & Febiger; 1978:285–287.

49. Jarratt M, Bybee JD, Ramsdell W. Eosinophilic fasciitis: an early variant of scleroderma. *J Am Acad Dermatol.* 1979;1:221–226.

50. Coyle HE, Chapman RS. Eosinophilic fasciitis (Shulman syndrome) in association with morphea and systemic sclerosis. *Acta Derm Venereol (Stockh).* 1980;60:181–182.

51. Rowell NR. Lupus erythematosus, scleroderma and dermatomyositis. The "collagen" or "connective-tissue" diseases. In Rook A, Wilkinson DS, Ebling FJG, et al. eds. *Textbook of Dermatology.* 4th ed. Oxford: Blackwell Scientific Publications; 1986:1368–1374.

52. Chalmers RJG, Burton PA, Bennett RF. Lichen sclerosus et atrophicus. A common and distinctive phimosis in boys. *Arch Dermatol.* 1984;120:1025–1027.

53. Hart WR, Norris HJ, Helwig EB. Relation of lichen sclerosis et atrophicus of the vulva to the development of carcinoma. *Obstet Gynecol.* 1975;45:369–377.

54. Wallace HJ. Lichen sclerosis et atrophicus. *Trans St Johns Hosp Dermatol Soc.* 1971;57:9–30.

55. Harrington CI, Dunsmore IR. An investigation into the incidence of autoimmune disorders in patients with lichen sclerosus et atrophicus. *Br J Dermatol.* 1981;104:563–566.

56. Thomas RHM, Ridley CM, Black MM. The association of lichen sclerosus et atrophicus and autoimmune related disease in males. *Br J Dermatol.* 1983;109:661–664.

57. Harrington CI, Gelsthorpe K. The association between lichen sclerosus et atrophicus and HLA-B40. *Br J Dermatol.* 1981;104:561–562.

58. Friedrich EG, Kalra PS. Serum levels of sex hormone in vulvar lichen sclerosus and the effect of topical testosterone. *N Engl J Med.* 1984;310:488–492.

59. Bergfeld WF, Lesowitz SA. Lichen sclerosus et atrophicus. *Arch Dermatol.* 1970;101:247–248.

60. Hood AF, Kwan TH, Burnes DC, et al. *Primer of Dermatopathology.* Boston: Little, Brown and Co; 1984:104.

61. Patterson JAK, Ackerman AB. Lichen sclerosus et atrophicus is not related to morphea. A clinical and histologic study of 24 patients in whom both conditions were reputed to be present simultaneously. *Am J Dermatopathol.* 1984;6:323–335.

62. Gottschalk HR, Cooper ZK. Lichen sclerosus et atrophicus with bullous lesions and extensive involvement. *Arch Dermatol.* 19xx;55:433.

63. Eng AM, Jacobs RA. Lichen sclerosus et atrophicus and squamous cell carcinoma alterations of the vulva. *J Am Acad Dermatol.* 1982;6:378–388.

64. Sanchez NP, Mihm MC. Reactive and neoplastic epithelial alterations of the vulva. *J Am Acad Dermatol.* 1982;6:378–388.

65. Goltz R, Pinkus H, Winkelmann RK, et al. Questions to the editorial board and other authorities. *Am J Dermatopathol.* 1980;2:283–286.

66. Connelly MG, Winkelmann RK. Coexistence of lichen sclerosus, morphea, and lichen planus. *J Am Acad Dermatol.* 1985;12:844–851.

67. Murray JC, Pollack SV, Pinnell SR. Keloids: a review. *J Am Acad Dermatol.* 1981;4:461–470.

68. Ketchum LD, Cohen IK, Masters FW. Hypertrophic scars and keloids. A collective review. *Plast Reconstr Surg.* 1974; 53:140–154.

69. Murray JC, Pollack SV, Pinnell SR. Keloids and hypertrophic scars. *Clin Dermatol.* 1984;2:121–133.

70. Smith CJ, Smith JC, Finn MC. The possible role of mast cells (allergy) in the production of keloid and hypertrophic scarring. *JBCR,* 1987;8:126–131.

71. Sandberg N. Accelerated collagen formation and histamine. *Nature.* 1962;194:183.

72. Clark RAF. Cutaneous tissue repair: basic biologic considerations. *J Am Acad Dermatol.* 1980;3:50–57.

73. James WD, Besanceney CD, Odom RB. The ultrastructure of a keloid. *J Am Acad Dermatol.* 1980;3:50–57.

74. Bauer PS, Barratt G, Linares HA, et al. Wound contractions, scar contractions, and myofibroblasts. *J Trauma.* 1978;18:8–22.

75. Linares HA, Larson DL. Early differential diagnosis between hypertrophic and nonhypertrophic healing. *J Invest Dermatol.* 1972;62:512–516.

76. Kischer CW, Shetlar MR. Collagen and mucopolysaccharides in the hypertrophic scar. *Connect Tissue Res.* 1974;2:205–213.

77. Redmond WJ, Baker SR. Keloidal calcification. *Arch Dermatol.* 1983;119:270–272.

78. Mancini RF, Quaife JV. Histogenesis of experimentally produced keloids. *J Invest Dermatol.* 1962;38:143–150.

79. James WD, Berger TG, Butler DF, et al. Nodular (keloidal) scleroderma. *J Am Acad Dermatol.* 1984;11:1111–1114.

80. Fajardo LF, Berthrong M. Radiation injury in surgical pathology. Part III. Salivary glands, pancreas, and skin. *Am J Surg Pathol.* 1981;5:279–296.

81. Goldschmidt H, Sherwin WK. Reactions to ionizing radiation. *J Am Acad Dermatol.* 1980;3:551–579.

82. Malkinson FD, Wiskemann A. Some principles of radiobiology and the effects of ionizing radiation on skin. In: Fitzpatrick TB, Eisen AZ, Wolf K, et al., eds. *Dermatology in General Medicine.* 3rd ed. New York: McGraw-Hill Book Co; 1987:1431–1440.

83. Spittle MF. Ionizing radiation. In: Rook A, Wilkinson DS, Ebling FJG, et al., eds. *Textbook in Dermatology.* 4th ed. Oxford: Blackwell Scientific Publications; 1986:652–656.

84. James WD, Odom RB. Late subcutaneous fibrosis following mega voltage radiotherapy. *J Am Acad Dermatol.* 1980;3:616–618.

85. Price NM. Radiation dermatitis following electron beam therapy. *Arch Dermatol.* 1978;114:63–66.

86. Hood AF, Kwan TH, Burns DC, et al., eds. *Primer of Dermatopathology.* Boston: Little, Brown, and Co; 1984:155.

87. Lever WF, Schaumburg-Lever G. *Histopathology of the Skin.* 6th ed. Philadelphia: JB Lippincott Co; 1983:214–215.

88. Ackerman AB. *Histologic Diagnosis of Inflammatory Skin Diseases.* Philadelphia: Lea & Febiger; 1978:201–202.

89. Cohen IS, Mosher MB, O'Keefe EJ, et al. Cutaneous toxicity of bleomycin therapy. *Arch Dermatol.* 1973;107:553–555.

90. DeBast C, Moriame N, Wanet J. Bleomycin in mycosis fungoides and reticulum cell lymphoma. *Arch Dermatol.* 1973;104:508–512.

91. Haustein UF, Ziegler V. Environmentally induced systemic sclerosis-like disorders. *Int J Dermatol.* 1985;24:147–151.

92. Lindae ML, Hu CH, Nickoloff BJ. Pruritic erythematous linear plaques on the neck and back. *Arch Dermatol.* 1987;123:393–398.

93. Bronner AK, Hood AF. Cutaneous complications of chemotherapeutic agents. *J Am Acad Dermatol.* 1983;9:645–663.

94. Fernandez-Obregon AC, Hogan KP, Bibro MK. Flagellate pigmentation from intrapleural bleomycin. A light microscopy and electron beam microscopy study. *J Am Acad Dermatol.* 1985;13:464–468.

95. Parks DL, Perry HO, Muller SA. Cutaneous complications of pentazocine injections. *Arch Dermatol.* 1971;104:231–235.

96. Padilla RS, Becker LE, Hoffman H, et al. Cutaneous and venous complications of pentazocine abuse. *Arch Dermatol.* 1979;115:975–977.

97. Palestine RF, Millns JL, Spigel GT, et al. Skin manifestations of pentazocine abuse. *J Am Acad Dermatol.* 1980;2:47–55.

98. Emmett EA. Occupational dermatoses and disorders due to chemical agents. In: Fitzpatrick TB, Eisen AZ, Wolff K, et al., eds. *Dermatology in General Medicine.* 3rd ed. New York: McGraw-Hill Book Co; 1987:1578–1579.

99. Markowitz SS, McDonald CZ, Fethiere W, et al. Occupational acroosteolysis. *Arch Dermatol.* 1972;106:219–223.

100. Myerson LB, Meier GC. Cutaneous lesions in acroosteolysis. *Arch Dermatol.* 1972;106:224–227.

101. Burton JL, Ebling FJG. Disorders of connective tissue. In: Rook A, Wilkinson DS, Ebling FJG, et al., eds. *Textbook of Dermatology.* 4th ed. Oxford: Blackwell Scientific Publications; 1986:1809–1810.

102. Kee CE, Brothers WS, New W. Idiopathic atrophoderma of Pasini and Pierini with coexistent morphea. *Arch Dermatol.* 1960;82:100–103.

103. Miller RF. Idiopathic atrophoderma. *Arch Dermatol.* 1965; 92:653–660.

104. Canizares O, Sachs PM, Jaimovich, et al. Idiopathic atrophoderma of Pasini and Pierini. *Arch Dermatol.* 1958;77:42–60.

105. Weiner M. Idiopathic atrophoderma of Pasini and Pierini. *Arch Dermatol.* 1965;92:737–738.

106. Brownstein MH, Rabinowitz AD. The invisible dermatoses. *J Am Acad Dermatol.* 1983;8:579–588.

CHAPTER 21
Panniculitis

James W. Patterson

Panniculitis represents one of the most difficult areas in the field of dermatopathology. Although the subcutaneous fat is structurally a rather simple organ, this tissue responds to inflammation and injury in a limited variety of ways. In part, as a result of these limitations, the classification and terminology of the panniculitides has been confusing. New understanding of pathophysiology has resulted in the reclassification of some disorders and the introduction of new ones. Furthermore, a number of disorders located primarily in the dermis (e.g., necrobiosis lipoidica), around adnexae (e.g., deep forms of folliculitis), or in deeper fascial structures (e.g., eosinophilic fasciitis) also extend into the subcutaneous fat, thereby adding considerably to the diagnostic difficulties. Despite the obvious drawbacks, histologic pattern analysis is still the major method of diagnosing the panniculitides and will probably remain so until better understanding of mechanisms of disease permits the use of more precise methods.

The types of panniculitis are listed in Table 21–1. Two forms of large vessel vasculitis, polyarteritis nodosa and superficial migratory thrombophlebitis, are discussed in detail in Chapter 13 and are not considered here. Other disorders, including connective tissue diseases, necrobiotic granulomas, and sarcoidosis, also are considered elsewhere. Only their relevance to the diagnosis of panniculitis is discussed in this chapter.

SEPTAL PANNICULITIS

ERYTHEMA NODOSUM

Clinical Features
This disorder consists of an eruption of erythematous, tender nodules often bilaterally over the pretibial region, but occasionally occurring elsewhere. It is usually a short-lived condition, lasting only a few weeks, but a more chronic form also occurs. Erythema nodosum is considered to be a hypersensitivity response to a number of inciting factors,

TABLE 21–1. TYPES OF PANNICULITIS

I. Septal panniculitis
  A. Erythema nodosum
  B. Subacute nodular migratory panniculitis

II. Large vessel vasculitis
  A. Polyarteritis nodosa
  B. Superficial migratory thrombophlebitis
  C. Nodular vasculitis (erythema induratum)

III. Lobular and mixed panniculitides
  A. With needle-shaped clefts in the subcutaneous fat
    1. Sclerema neonatorum
    2. Subcutaneous fat necrosis of the newborn
    3. Poststeroid panniculitis
  B. Pancreatic (enzymic) fat necrosis
  C. Traumatic panniculitis
    1. Cold injury
    2. Therapeutic agents
    3. Sclerosing lipogranuloma
    4. Blunt trauma
  D. Weber-Christian disease
  E. α_1-Antitrypsin deficiency panniculitis
  F. Lupus erythematosus panniculitis (lupus profundus)
  G. Lipodystrophy

IV. Malignancy and panniculitis
  A. Malignant infiltrates
  B. Cytophagic histiocytic panniculitis

V. Other disorders occurring as panniculitis
  A. Infectious panniculitis
  B. Noninfectious granulomas
  C. Panniculitis associated with connective tissue diseases

including streptococcal infection, tuberculosis, deep mycoses, such drugs as oral contraceptives, and inflammatory disorders, such as sarcoidosis and ulcerative colitis.

Histologic Features
The classic presentation is an acute septal panniculitis (Fig. 21–1), with neutrophils predominating in early lesions.[1,2] Vasculitis has been described by some authors,[2,3] but

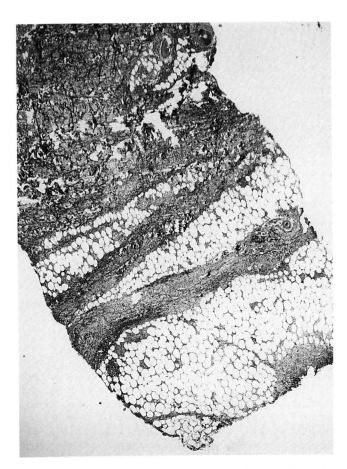

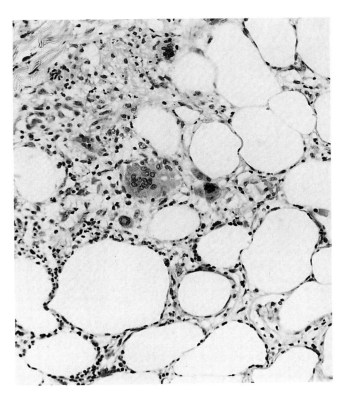

Figure 21–2. Erythema nodosum. Lesion of somewhat longer duration, showing multinucleated giant cells. Note lacelike infiltration of fat lobule. (H&E, ×100.)

Figure 21–1. Erythema nodosum. Low power view showing acute inflammation and septal thickening. Note, however, that there is some spillover of inflammation into fat lobules. (H&E, ×25.)

changes usually are limited to perivascular inflammation, vessel wall thickening, and swollen endothelium. Hemorrhage often is prominent. Lesions of somewhat longer duration contain mostly lymphocytes. Inflammatory cells frequently extend into fat lobules, producing a lacelike infiltrative pattern (Fig. 21–2). Fat necrosis with microcyst and foam cell formation also may occur.[2–4] With resolution, thickened, sometimes hyalinized septa and diminished sizes of fat lobules may result.[4]

Lesions of longer duration show a granulomatous histology, including foreign body giant cells (Fig. 21–3). A characteristic feature is the microgranulomatous focus of Miescher[5]—a collection of histiocytes within the septa that at first surrounds collagen bundles but later is arrayed around cleftlike spaces (Figs. 21–3, 21–4). These cells may act as collagenoclasts.[3] Miescher's granulomas have been considered pathognomonic of erythema nodosum, but similar structures have been reported in panniculitis associated with Sweet's syndrome.[5]

Lesions meeting all the clinical criteria for erythema nodosum have shown histologic features differing from this classic picture. Atypical histologic variants included an eo-

sinophilic panniculitis[6] and panniculitis with cellular infiltration of lobules and relative sparing of the septa.[7] The lobules may be the site of small, focal, Miescher-like granulomas or of massive granulomatous infiltration, without caseous necrosis. These variants considerably expand the range of histologic features that are acceptable for erythema nodosum. Immunofluorescent studies are usually negative,[8] arguing against an immune complex etiology for this condition.

Differential Diagnosis

The classic septal panniculitis of erythema nodosum can be distinguished from most other primary forms of panniculitis. Early scleroderma also occurs with a lymphocytic septal panniculitis, but the extent of hyalinization and fibrosis within the subcutis and lower dermis points to a diagnosis of scleroderma. As the histologic pattern becomes progressively more lobular, erythema nodosum can resemble several other entities. In nodular vasculitis, careful search usually reveals an arteritis or venulitis. Caseation sometimes is observed in nodular vasculitis but is not a feature of erythema nodosum. Acute neutrophilic inflammation with lobular extension can resemble forms of infective panniculitis. Cases with lobular granulomatous nodules surrounded by lymphocytes may resemble sarcoidosis, but this is a distinctly unusual picture for erythema nodosum. Eosinophilic panniculitis can occur in a wide variety of inflammatory disorders that are not primary panniculitides.[6]

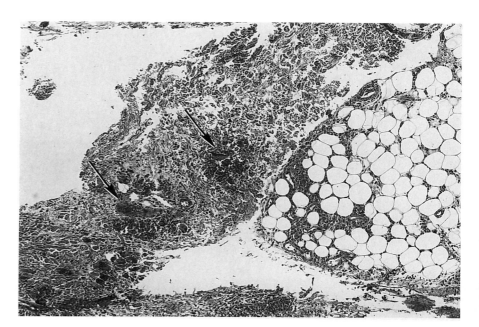

Figure 21–3. Erythema nodosum. Within the septum, there are multiple aggregates of epithelioid and giant cells (arrows), constituting microgranulomatous foci of Miescher. (H&E, ×40.)

SUBACUTE NODULAR MIGRATORY PANNICULITIS

Clinical Features

This condition was first described in 1954 by Bäfverstedt, who recognized its distinctive features while classifying it together with erythema nodosum.[9] In 1956, Vilanova and Pinol Aguade suggested that it might represent a distinct entity. Over the years, Bäfverstedt's opinion has become the prevailing one, and most authors now regard acute and chronic erythema nodosum and subacute nodular migratory panniculitis as variants of the same disease process.[7]

Subacute nodular migratory panniculitis is a nodular, frequently unilateral erythema of the lower legs seen most often in women of middle age. Lesions enlarge by peripheral extension and confluence to form sharply demarcated, asymptomatic plaques with central clearing.[10,11] Lesions may last from 4 months to several years. Suspected underlying causes have included streptococcal infection, pregnancy, and sarcoidosis.[12]

Histologic Features

Like erythema nodosum, subacute nodular migratory panniculitis is chiefly a septal process. Within the interlobular

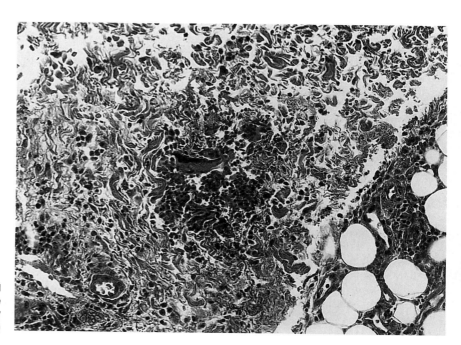

Figure 21–4. Erythema nodosum. Epithelioid and giant cells are arrayed around cleftlike spaces, which suggests that these cells may be functioning as collagenoclasts. (H&E, ×100.)

septa there are capillary proliferation and granulomatous inflammation. Capillary proliferation often is pronounced, resulting in a spiral configuration of the vessels,[10] with swelling and proliferation of endothelium. Fibroblasts, histiocytes, and lymphocytes infiltrate the septa but do not involve the vessels, and evidence of true vasculitis is absent. Numerous extravasated erythrocytes are sometimes observed. Small granulomas of the septa described by Vilanova and Pinol Aguade are probably examples of Miescher's microgranulomas.[10] Lobular inflammation usually is confined to the periphery, adjacent to involved septa. Connective tissue changes include edema and fragmentation of collagen bundles, fibrinoid change, and fibrosis.[10] In later stages, there may be septal sclerosis and a few persistent giant cells.

Differential Diagnosis

The differential diagnosis is similar to that for erythema nodosum in its chronic, granulomatous form. Scleroderma panniculitis is not granulomatous and lacks the peculiar vascular changes of subacute nodular migratory panniculitis. Vasculitis involving a medium-sized artery or vein is the essential feature of nodular vasculitis and is not present in subacute nodular migratory panniculitis. The relative lack of a lobular infiltrate also separates this disorder from lupus panniculitis.

LARGE VESSEL VASCULITIS

NODULAR VASCULITIS (ERYTHEMA INDURATUM)

Clinical Features

Erythema induratum, first described by Bazin in 1861,[13] is an eruption of red, indurated plaques on the lateral and lower portions of the legs, especially in women. The calf of the leg seems to be a favored site. Lesions of longer duration become dusky, soften in the center, and sometimes ulcerate. The disorder may be recurrent and persistent.

Erythema induratum has long been associated with tuberculosis and is regarded by some as a tuberculid rather than a direct infection by *Mycobacterium tuberculosis*. Over the years, it has become apparent that a similar eruption with identical histopathologic features occurs in the absence of tuberculosis. This condition, termed "nodular vasculitis," may be idiopathic or possibly associated with bacterial infection. There is evidence that both conditions are caused by an immune complex-mediated vasculitis.[14] The current trend is to refer to all lesions with these clinical and microscopic features as nodular vasculitis, although some prefer the term "erythema induratum" for those cases associated with tuberculosis.

Histologic Features

The essential microscopic feature is a vasculitis of a subcutaneous artery or vein, manifested by inflammatory cell infiltration of vessel walls, endothelial swelling, luminal obliteration, and sometimes fibrosis (Fig. 21–5). Multiple microscopic sections often are necessary to demonstrate the vasculitis. The affected vessel is found in the center of an area of lobular panniculitis.[15,16] At an early stage, the lobular infiltrate is neutrophilic, and there may be extensive fat necrosis. Lesions of longer duration show lymphocytic or granulomatous inflammation of the lobules (Fig. 21–6). Lymphocytic infiltration may take the form of nodular masses. Granulomas include many foreign body giant cells and can be distributed around muscular vessels.[7] Caseation may be prominent within focal granulomatous areas and is sometimes massive, in both tuberculous and nontuberculous types.[7] However, caseous necrosis is absent in over one half of cases.[17]

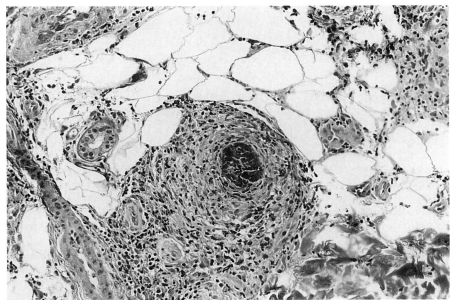

Figure 21–5. Nodular vasculitis. Near the center of an area of lobular panniculitis, a small artery shows changes of vasculitis and thrombosis. (H&E, ×100.)

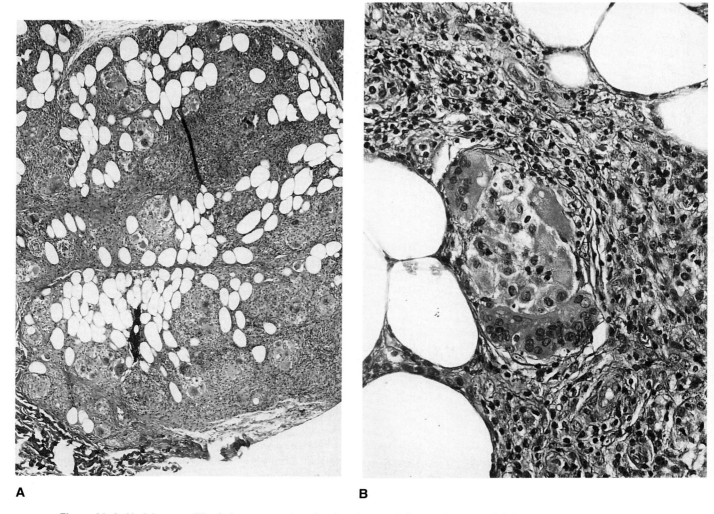

A

B

Figure 21–6. Nodular vasculitis. **A.** Low power view showing characteristic granulomatous, lobular panniculitis. **B.** Higher power magnification of the infiltrate, showing focal granuloma (A. H&E, ×25; B., ×250.)

Differential Diagnosis

Erythema nodosum and subacute nodular migratory panniculitis are predominantly septal rather than lobular panniculitides. Neither true vasculitis nor caseation is observed in these disorders. Polyarteritis nodosa and superficial thrombophlebitis also are forms of vasculitis, but extension of inflammatory changes outside of the immediate vicinity of a vessel often is limited. Cases with lymphoid aggregates may resemble lupus panniculitis. However, granulomas are not a prominent feature of lupus panniculitis. Hyalinized septae and occasional pools of mucin are other features of lupus panniculitis, and the overlying epidermis and dermis may show features of discoid lupus erythematosus or poikiloderma atrophicans vasculare. True infective panniculitis, including mycobacterial infection, lacks the vasculitis of muscular subcutaneous vessels, and organisms often can be demonstrated with special stains.

LOBULAR AND MIXED PANNICULITIDES

NEEDLE-SHAPED CLEFTS IN SUBCUTANEOUS FAT

Three forms of panniculitis in infancy and childhood are characterized by needle-shaped clefts within lipocytes: sclerema neonatorum, subcutaneous fat necrosis of the newborn, and poststeroid panniculitis. Neonatal fat is characterized by an increased ratio of saturated to unsaturated fatty acids, resulting in higher melting and solidification points for stored fat. It has been suggested that this and other possible defects in the metabolism of fat predispose the subcutis to crystal formation, fat necrosis, and inflammation when subjected to stresses, such as vascular compro-

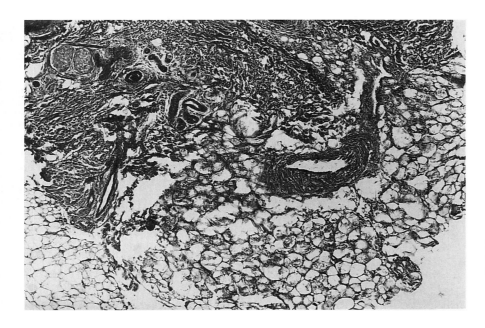

Figure 21–7. Sclerema neonatorum. Somewhat thickened fibrous bands can be seen extending into the subcutis. Even at low power, needle-shaped clefts can be seen within lipocytes. Note the relative absence of inflammation. (H&E, ×40.)

mise, mechanical pressure,[18] trauma (hypothermia), poor nutrition, or infection.[19]

Sclerema Neonatorum

Clinical Features
This condition arises in premature infants and consists of extensive hardening of the subcutaneous fat during the first few weeks of life. Typically the skin is cold, rigid, and boardlike. Affected infants are hypothermic, with diminished pulse and respiratory rates, and early death is the usual result. Exposure to cold with peripheral vasocon-

striction around the time of birth has been suspected as a precipitating cause.

Histologic Features
The epidermis and dermis are normal. There are broad intersecting fibrous septa and large lipocytes (Fig. 21–7) that contain needle-shaped clefts (Fig. 21–8). The latter are believed to represent crystals of triglyceride that dissolved during processing. Although a diffuse, lobular panniculitis has been described, usually the degree of inflammation is slight. In later stages of the disease, fibrosis and calcification can be observed.

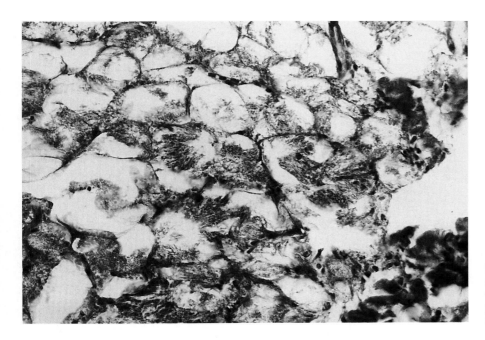

Figure 21–8. Sclerema neonatorum. Needle-shaped clefts within lipocytes, believed to represent triglyceride dissolved out during processing. Inflammation is not observed. (H&E, ×250.)

Differential Diagnosis

The lack of inflammation in this disease distinguishes it from subcutaneous fat necrosis of the newborn or poststeroid panniculitis, which typically show significant lobular panniculitis. Ordinary cold panniculitis lacks the needle-shaped clefts within lipocytes and also has a greater degree of inflammation.

Subcutaneous Fat Necrosis of the Newborn

Clinical Features

In this condition, multiple mobile, firm subcutaneous nodules or plaques develop in infants 2 to 3 weeks after birth,[20] although onset may be delayed for weeks or months.[19] Complications can include thrombocytopenia, cachexia, infection, and hypercalcemia.[21] Deaths have occurred,[19] but usually the prognosis is favorable, with spontaneous resolution taking place in a few weeks to several months. The frequent location of these lesions in areas such as the buttocks and shoulders suggests that mechanical pressure may bring about lesions in subcutaneous tissue that is already metabolically abnormal.[18]

Histologic Features

Subcutaneous fat necrosis of the newborn is a lobular panniculitis. The infiltrate is at first neutrophilic and later becomes granulomatous, showing fat necrosis and foam cell formation with accumulations of lymphocytes and multinucleated giant cells. The septa also may be involved.[19] The characteristic features are needle-shaped clefts within lipocytes and sometimes in giant cells (Fig. 21–9).[22] However, otherwise typical cases have been reported in which these crystals were not observed.[19,21] Occasional features are calcifications within and between lipocytes[18,20,21] and hemorrhages secondary to thrombocytopenia. Healing with fibrosis is the rule.

Differential Diagnosis

The combination of granulomatous, lobular panniculitis and crystal formation within lipocytes points to a diagnosis of subcutaneous fat necrosis of the newborn. Sclerema neonatorum seldom has significant degrees of inflammation, and the broad fibrous septae of the latter disorder are characteristic. Poststeroid panniculitis closely resembles subcutaneous fat necrosis of the newborn and requires clinical data for differentiation. Cases of subcutaneous fat necrosis without needle-shaped crystals are difficult to distinguish from other granulomatous lobular panniculitides, particularly cold panniculitis, which may have a similar pathogenesis.[18–20] However, cases without crystal formation would seem to be in the minority.

Poststeroid Panniculitis

Clinical Features

This disorder is a rare complication of rapid corticosteroid withdrawal in children being treated for rheumatic fever or other conditions. Within a month after corticosteroid withdrawal, subcutaneous nodules develop that range from 0.5 to 4.0 cm in diameter. The condition resolves spontaneously. Paradoxically, resolution is hastened when corticosteroids are readministered.[23,24]

Histologic Features

Poststeroid panniculitis is a patchy lobular panniculitis featuring infiltration of the fat by lymphocytes, macrophages, and foreign body giant cells. Foam cells are prominent, and crystals are observed within lipocytes. The subcutaneous vessels are spared by this process.

Differential Diagnosis

The findings are identical to those of subcutaneous fat necrosis of the newborn, and clinical data are needed for differen-

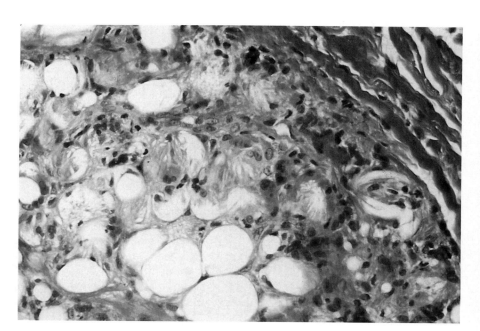

Figure 21–9. Subcutaneous fat necrosis of the newborn. Needle-shaped clefts are observed within lipocytes and in giant cells. Significant inflammatory component serves to differentiate this condition from sclerema neonatorum. Poststeroid panniculitis has the same histologic features. (H&E, ×250.)

tiation. The presence of a significant patchy, lobular panniculitis with foam cell formation is distinct from the usually infiltrate-poor sclerema neonatorum.

PANCREATIC (ENZYMIC) FAT NECROSIS

Clinical Features

Subcutaneous nodules may develop in association with acute pancreatitis, with pancreatic carcinoma (either adenocarcinoma or acinar cell carcinoma), and occasionally with pancreatic pseudocysts or traumatic pancreatitis.[25,26] Their occurrence is characteristic if uncommon, with a reported incidence in pancreatic disease ranging from 0.33% to 2%.[26,27] Erythematous nodules typically develop on the legs but can develop elsewhere. Other signs and symptoms include fever, abdominal pain, arthritis, ascites, or pleural effusion. Typical skin lesions occasionally develop in the absence of overt pancreatic disease.[25,26]

This panniculitis is believed to result from the effects of amylase, lipase, or a variety of other enzymes[25] on visceral and subcutaneous fat. These enzymes are released into the lymphatic or vascular circulation and escape into the fat, where lipolytic enzymes hydrolyze fat to form free fatty acids and glycerol.[22,25–28] This sets in motion the chain of events responsible for the classic histologic changes. Amylase and lipase activities have been detected in skin lesions,[28] but there is also some evidence for an immune-mediated pathogenesis for this disorder.[29]

Histologic Features

The epidermis and dermis are normal except for a nonspecific perivascular infiltrate composed of mononucleated cells. In the subcutis there is an initial neutrophilic, lobular panniculitis that even in early stages shows fat necrosis with liquefaction and microcyst formation.[28] Fat cells lose their nuclei and develop thick, shadowy walls (ghost cells) (Fig. 21–10), and saponification of fat by calcium salts results

in deposition of granular or homogeneous basophilic material[22,25,30,31] (Fig. 21–11). Other inflammatory cells, including mononucleated cells, eosinophils, and occasional giant cells, may be present and sometimes encroach on the septa.[2] Macrophages ingest lipid and occasionally also engage in erythrophagocytosis.[28] Healing lesions demonstrate fibrosis and atrophy.

Differential Diagnosis

The presence of fat necrosis as an early microscopic change, together with the formation of shadow cells and calcium soaps, strongly suggests pancreatic or enzymic fat necrosis. Lesions without calcification or well-developed shadow cells can resemble other lobular panniculitides. The lack of frank vasculitis of medium-sized vessels distinguishes pancreatic fat necrosis from nodular vasculitis, and polarization microscopy and special stains are useful in ruling out some forms of traumatic or factitial panniculitis. In other cases, clinical or laboratory data, including serum or urinary amylase/lipase levels, are essential for clarifying the diagnosis.

TRAUMATIC PANNICULITIS

The term "traumatic panniculitis" has been chosen to refer to any inflammatory process in the subcutis resulting from external injury, be it accidental, purposeful, or the manifestation of an underlying psychiatric disturbance.

Cold Panniculitis

Clinical Features

In this disorder, various forms of cold injury rapidly induce the formation of tender erythematous plaques and subcutaneous nodules. This form of panniculitis is particularly common in children and is perhaps related to the altered composition of fat in this age group.[18–20,32] Such injury can occur

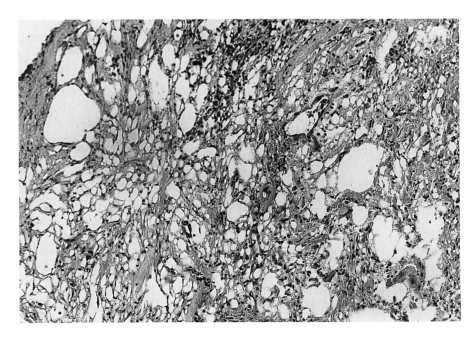

Figure 21–10. Pancreatic fat necrosis. There are acute inflammation, fat necrosis with microcyst formation, and lipocytes with thickened, shadowy walls. (H&E, ×140.)

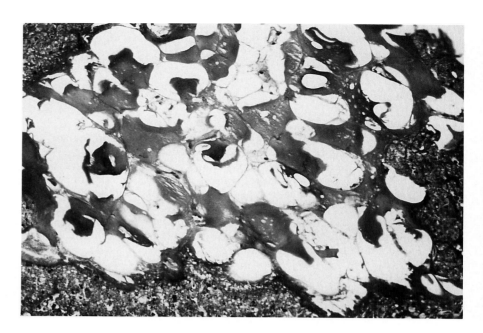

Figure 21–11. Pancreatic fat necrosis. Homogeneous, basophilic material resulting from saponification of fat by calcium salts. (H&E, ×250.)

about the time of birth,[18,20] after hypothermic cardiac surgery,[19] or even after sucking on popsicles.[33] Lesions can be reproduced by applying an ice cube to the skin; this sensitivity apparently diminishes as the child matures.[32] Cold injury also has been implicated in panniculitis of other age groups, e.g., young women who are equestrians.[32]

Histologic Features

There is inflammation chiefly located in the region of the dermal–subcutaneous junction, with diminished changes in the deeper subcutis.[32] Cells include lymphocytes, neutrophils, and foamy macrophages. There may be scattered epithelioid and giant cells, but granulomas tend not to be well formed or prominent.[19,32] Inflammation may be both lobular and septal and tends to surround vessels, sweat coils, and neurovascular plexuses.[32] Frank vasculitis is not observed, although there is some swelling of venular walls. There is mild to moderate fat cell necrosis with microcyst formation. Mucin deposits occasionally are identified.

Differential Diagnosis

The absence of needle-shaped clefts in lipocytes and localization of inflammation to the more superficial subcutis help to distinguish these cases from classic subcutaneous fat necrosis of the newborn, although cold injury may play a role in the latter disorder as well.

Therapeutic Agents

An incredible variety of substances has been instilled or injected into the skin, with panniculitis as a result. These may be introduced accidentally, purposely, or iatrogenically. Substances associated with factitial panniculitis include milk, feces, camphor, silicones, and several types of oils (mineral oil or paraffin, cottonseed oil, sesame oil).[34] Drugs or therapeutic agents have included phytonadione (vitamin K_1),[35] morphine, tetanus antitoxoid, pentazocine,[34]

and povidone.[36] Several forms of traumatic panniculitis have been found to accompany distinctive clinicopathologic conditions.

Therapeutic Agents

Clinical Features

A syndrome of subcutaneous sclerosis, fasciitis, and eosinophilia following injections of phytonadione (vitamin K_1) is known as "Texier's disease." The clinical picture includes erythematous, sclerotic plaques of the lower trunk in the distribution of a cowboy gunbelt and holster.[35] Complications of pentazocine injections include sclerosis, ulceration, and hyperpigmentation. A high percentage of individuals with this syndrome have evidence of psychiatric illness, diabetes mellitus, or some connection with the medical profession.[37] Meperidine abuse also causes panniculitis, although it is not as deforming as that associated with pentazocine. Multiple subcutaneous calcifications can be identified on x-ray study of the lesions.[34] Intramuscular injection of povidone, a plasma expander and dispersing agent, can produce subcutaneous nodules, flu-like symptoms, and occasional pulmonary and arthritic symptoms.[36]

Histologic Features

Infection-induced panniculitis often shows a central nidus of subcutaneous inflammation (Fig. 21–12). Both phytonadione and pentazocine produce marked dermal and subcutaneous sclerosis. Phytonadione is accompanied by dermal–subcutaneous sclerosis and an infiltrate of lymphocytes and mast cells.[35] In pentazocine abuse, there are dermal and subcutaneous fibrosis, fat necrosis with foam cell formation, large, lipid-containing vacuoles with a Swiss cheese appearance, small vessel thrombosis, and endarteritis.[37] Meperidine panniculitis shows patchy septal and lobular involvement, with a mixture of acute inflammation, focal necrosis, fibroblast–macrophage reaction, and fibrosis. Massive gran-

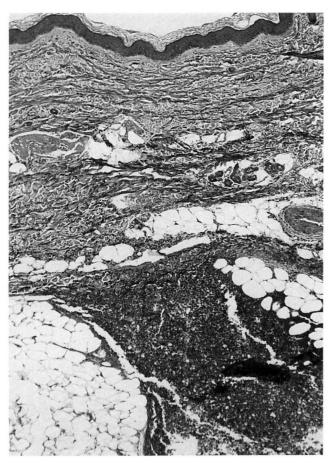

Figure 21–12. Traumatic panniculitis. Central nidus of acute inflammation in the subcutis resulting from injection of a foreign substance. Ruptured follicles and cysts produce a similar picture, but fragments of epithelium usually can be found in the vicinity. (H&E, ×25.)

uloma formation and vasculitis are not observed.[34] Birefringent material can be observed with polarization microscopy. Povidone panniculitis shows the usual changes of panniculitis, with focal hemorrhage and necrosis. Polarization microscopy is negative, but gray-blue material within macrophages can be seen on hematoxylin and eosin-stained sections. This material also can be identified with special stains, such as Congo red and chlorazol-fast pink.[36] Eosinophilic panniculitis has been observed following injections in emotionally labile, narcotic-dependent patients.[6]

Differential Diagnosis

Panniculitis caused by injectable substances usually can be distinguished from primary panniculitides by such findings as coexistent dermal involvement, presence of foreign material identified by routine methods, polarization microscopy or special stains, and subcutaneous calcifications seen on x-ray study. Distinction among injectable substances in the absence of identifiable material may be impossible without an accurate clinical history. On purely microscopic grounds, sclerosing forms due to phytonadione or pentazocine may resemble scleroderma. On electron microscopy, involved fascia from patients receiving phytonadione fails to show the 40-Angstrom microfibrils seen in scleroderma.[35] Furthermore, the ulcerations, large lipid vacuoles, and thrombotic changes seen in pentazocine abuse are not features of scleroderma.

Sclerosing Lipogranuloma

Clinical Features

This term was introduced in 1950 to describe a localized reactive process after tissue injury. Since then, it has become identified with lesions of the genital region believed to be caused by injection of oils.[38] The classic patient is a male over 40 years of age with erythema, swelling, and nodular thickening of the genital region or buttocks, sometimes with enlarged inguinal lymph nodes. Patients routinely deny self-administered injections, but there is a frequent history of psychiatric disturbances, trauma, operations, or local infections. There is a possibility that topical therapy can produce these lesions in some cases.[39] It is generally considered that sclerosing lipogranuloma is the same disorder as paraffinoma, which results from the injection of paraffin for cosmetic purposes[38,40] and is closely related to silicone granulomas following injection of impure, nonmedical grade liquid silicones. Similar lesions result from instillation of oils following grease gun injury.[41]

Histologic Features

There is a granulomatous lobular panniculitis accompanied by marked fibrosis (Fig. 21–13). There may be nodular aggregates of lymphocytes, plasma cells, and eosinophils as well as macrophages and giant cells. Numerous round, oval, or needle-shaped vacuoles of varying sizes are observed in the dermis and subcutis (Figs. 21–14, 21–15), surrounded by fibrous tissue or occasionally by giant cells.[38] The vacuoles stain positively with oil-red-O and Sudan black but negatively with the silver bromide or osmium tetroxide methods. This is because exogenous oils, such as mineral oil (paraffin), are fully saturated lipids, and only unsaturated lipids can reduce compounds such as silver bromide and osmium tetroxide to form a black reaction product.[41] There may be intimal proliferation of larger vessels, leading to occlusion. In addition, lesions of grease gun granulomas may show pseudoepitheliomatous hyperplasia of the overlying epidermis.[41]

Differential Diagnosis

The presence of large vacuoles in the dermis and subcutis strongly suggests deposition of oils from an exogenous source. The needle-shaped clefts of sclerema neonatorum and related diseases are much smaller, often only the size of a single lipocyte or within giant cells. Similarly, the microcysts in other forms of panniculitis are smaller and confined to the subcutis. Special stains for saturated lipids can be performed on frozen sections. Roentgenographic studies sometimes are helpful in distinguishing lipogranulomas from silicone reactions: lipogranulomas are radiolucent, whereas silicone granulomas are radiopaque.[40] Paraffin in nonprocessed tissue can be identified by infrared spectrophotometry.[41] Finally, vacuolated lesions from the genital region must be distinguished from adenomatoid tumor, sclerosing liposarcoma, and lymphangioma.[38]

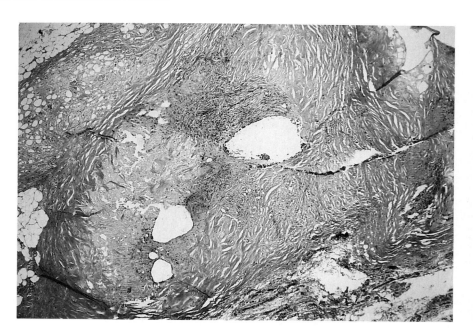

Figure 21–13. Sclerosing lipogranuloma. Hyalinization and fibrosis of the subcutis. Several large vacuoles representing lipid deposits are identified. (H&E, ×25.)

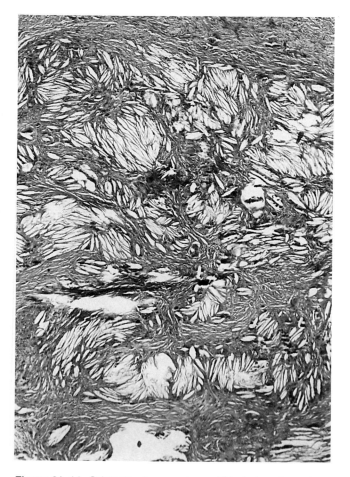

Figure 21–14. Sclerosing lipogranuloma. This lesion shows large needle-shaped clefts and fibrosis. The clefts are much larger than those observed in sclerema neonatorum and subcutaneous fat necrosis of the newborn. (H&E, ×25.)

Lesions Due to Blunt Trauma

Clinical Features

Blunt trauma also is capable of producing panniculitis. Such trauma can be accidental or the result of an assault (e.g., child abuse) or a symptom of an underlying psychiatric disturbance. Two clinical syndromes in this category are Secretan's syndrome, a traumatic edema of the dorsum of the hand, and l'oedeme bleu, a factitial edema due to forearm trauma.[42] Disorders of this type tend to be chronic and recurrent, occurring in individuals with passive, evasive personalities.

Histologic Features

Lesions caused by repeated blunt trauma show organizing hematomas, but there are also focal granulomas with deposition of mucopolysaccharides and iron pigment. The latter changes may result from breakdown of lipids and pigments from erythrocyte membranes.[42]

Differential Diagnosis

The presence of organizing hematomas with deposition of iron pigments suggests blunt trauma and requires clinical evaluation of the possible causes.

WEBER-CHRISTIAN DISEASE

Clinical Features

Of all disorders of the subcutaneous fat, none has created greater controversy and misunderstanding than Weber-Christian disease.

There were early reports of a syndrome consisting of recurrent subcutaneous nodules, with or without fever, and followed by depressions of the skin on involution. In

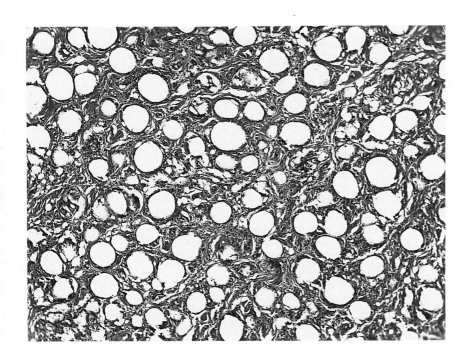

Figure 21–15. Grease gun granuloma. Cystic spaces representing deposits of exogenous lipid. (H&E, ×80.) (*From ref. 41.*)

1925, Weber reported a woman with relapsing nonsuppurative nodular panniculitis.[43] Three years later, Christian reported a similar case associated with fever and constitutional symptoms.[44] The disorder later became known as "relapsing febrile nonsuppurative panniculitis" or "Weber-Christian disease."[45] Subsequent experience has led some authors to discard the "nonsuppurative" modifier.[46]

In recent years, as greater understanding of the pathogenesis of disease has led to the discovery of new forms of panniculitis, there has been a corresponding decrease in reports of Weber-Christian disease. Cases that might have been considered Weber-Christian disease have now been classified as factitial panniculitis,[34,42] lupus profundus, pancreatic (enzymic) fat necrosis, α_1-antitrypsin-deficient panniculitis,[28] connective tissue panniculitis,[47] or cytophagic histiocytic panniculitis.[48] As a result of this evolutionary process, Weber-Christian disease appears to be a fading and ill-defined concept.[28]

There remains a group of patients with relapsing subcutaneous nodules, fever, variable inflammation of the perivisceral fat with systemic symptoms, and a sometimes fatal outcome,[46,49] with no clear explanation of the cause. This ever-shrinking group could perhaps be labeled "Weber-Christian disease" until further investigations reveal the true etiology.

Histologic Features

Classically, Weber-Christian disease is divided into three stages. The first, or acute, stage consists of a neutrophilic lobular panniculitis. This acute stage is seen uncommonly in cases meeting the criteria for Weber-Christian disease.[34] This is followed by a second stage in which there are necrosis of fat cells with microcyst formation and ingestion of lipid by macrophages to form foam cells. The third stage consists of fibrosis, resulting in depression of the overlying skin.

It will be noted that these are nonspecific changes that are encountered to some degree in most forms of panniculitis.

Differential Diagnosis

A microscopic diagnosis of Weber-Christian disease probably should never be made in the absence of a firm clinical history, and even then, "findings consistent with" should probably be added to the diagnosis. This is so because the microscopic features are entirely nonspecific. A diagnosis of Weber-Christian disease should merely signal the beginning of an investigation into the true cause of the disorder.

α_1-ANTITRYPSIN DEFICIENCY PANNICULITIS

Clinical Features

In recent years, several reports have described a Weber-Christian-like syndrome associated with severe α_1-antitrypsin deficiency.[49–52] These patients have multiple, painful, subcutaneous nodules on the trunk and extremities. Lesions may become fluctuant, ulcerate, and drain.[49,52] Patients with this disorder have the PiZZ phenotype and show absent α_1 globulin on serum protein electrophoresis. It has been proposed that once an inflammatory process has been initiated,[53] the absence of α_1-antitrypsin permits unchecked endothelial cell damage[52] and increased inflammatory cell activity,[51] thereby potentiating tissue injury.

Histologic Features

The histopathologic changes include a lobular panniculitis with a mixture of inflammatory cell types, including neutrophils, lymphocytes, and macrophages.[53] Focal fat cell degeneration and lipophage formation also are observed.[50] A lymphocytic vasculitis, consisting of vessel wall invasion and mucin deposition in vessel walls, has been observed in deep dermal and subcutaneous venules.[50,51]

Differential Diagnosis

The microscopic features closely resemble those described for Weber-Christian disease and other lobular panniculitides, such as nodular vasculitis and connective tissue panniculitis. However, not all patients with a Weber-Christian-like syndrome have α_1-antitrypsin deficiency.[52] Since the histopathology is relatively nonspecific, diagnosis requires a high index of suspicion as well as serologic and phenotypic studies. It should be realized that other factors (e.g., histoplasmosis in one patient) may trigger panniculitis in these predisposed individuals.[53]

LUPUS ERYTHEMATOSUS PANNICULITIS (LUPUS PROFUNDUS)

Clinical Features

Inflammation of the subcutaneous fat associated with lupus erythematosus was recognized as early as 1883 by Kaposi.[54] In recent years, it has become apparent that lupus panniculitis has reasonably distinctive histopathologic features that enable an accurate diagnosis in most instances.

Lupus panniculitis occurs most frequently in middle-aged women[47,55] as discrete, erythematous or flesh-colored, variably tender subcutaneous nodules with a predilection for the face, upper outer arms, shoulders, and trunk.[55–57] Trauma is a frequent initiating factor.[57] It is most commonly associated with discoid lupus erythematosus[56] but can occur in systemic disease as well.[57] Lupus panniculitis can precede, accompany, or follow the establishment of a diagnosis of lupus erythematosus.[47]

Histologic Features

The overlying epidermis and upper dermis may appear normal or show the characteristic changes of discoid lupus erythematosus or poikiloderma atrophicans vasculare.[55] There is a lymphocytic, lobular panniculitis that ranges from sparse[58] or patchy[55] to heavy.[56] A patchy perivascular lymphocytic infiltrate usually is observed. In addition, vessels of all calibers show varying degrees of endothelial cell hyperplasia, vessel wall thickening, fibrinoid deposition, and thrombosis, suggesting a lymphocytic vasculitis.[55,56] Associated with, and perhaps a consequence of, these vascular changes is hyalinization around vessels and sweat glands and within fat lobules and connective tissue septa (Fig. 21–16). Deposition of mucin may be insignificant[55] or pronounced, forming "pools of mucin" that stain positively with alcian blue and other mucin stains.[56] A striking feature is the appearance of nodular aggregates of lymphocytes that may be surrounded by plasma cells. These aggregates

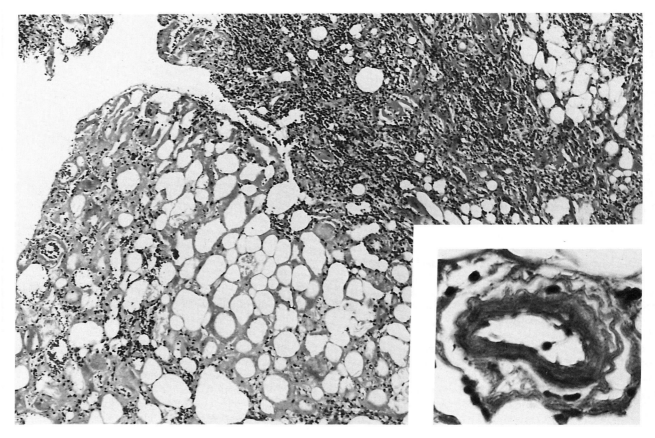

Figure 21–16. Lupus erythematosus panniculitis. There is both a septal and a lobular panniculitis. Note perivascular inflammation and hyalinization of septa extending into lobules. Inset. Hyalinized vessel in subcutis. (H&E, ×375, inset: H&E, ×60.)

tend to be located in the periphery of the lobules adjacent to the septa,[55] and they sometimes have the appearance of lymphoid follicles.[59] Calcium deposition often is observed in the dermis and subcutis. Less common changes include focal granulomas within the septa.[55] However, granulomatous inflammation usually is not a prominent feature.

Immunofluorescent studies frequently show deposition of immunoglobulins and complement along the overlying dermal–epidermal junction, around hair follicles,[55,56] and occasionally in deep dermal vessels.[57]

Differential Diagnosis

The combination of lymphocytic lobular panniculitis, lymphocytic vasculitis, hyalinization of the subcutis, and nodular lymphoid aggregates strongly suggests lupus panniculitis, even in the absence of overlying epidermal changes. Less fully developed changes can resemble other forms of panniculitis, especially those associated with other connective tissue diseases. Lymphoid follicles occasionally are observed in erythema nodosum, erythema induratum, and morphea.[59,60] Other forms of panniculitis also can occur in patients with lupus erythematosus, including erythema nodosum,[55] thrombophlebitis,[61] and pancreatic (enzymic) fat necrosis.[27]

LIPODYSTROPHY (LIPOATROPHY)

Clinical Features

The atrophic changes of lipodystrophy occur in a variety of clinical settings. These have been reviewed in several publications.[47,62] Total lipodystrophy represents a congenital or acquired complete loss of adipose tissue associated with carbohydrate intolerance, hyperlipidemia, and hepatomegaly. Partial lipodystrophy is a symmetrical loss of adipose tissue involving the face, arms, and upper trunk. It may progress in a cephalocaudal direction. The typical patient is a female child who may have numerous other abnormalities, including mesangocapillary glomerulonephritis, diabetes, hirsutism, and hyperlipidemia. The most familiar form of localized lipodystrophy results from injections of corticosteroids or insulin. There are also localized forms associated with connective tissue disease, as well as annular varieties that encircle the ankles or abdomen.[63]

Lipodystrophy has been described as a "reversal of embryogenesis"[3] because of the resemblance of affected tissue to embryonic fat. In many cases, no significant inflammatory infiltrate is observed. However, scattered reports have described an associated lobular panniculitis. Evidence that inflammation may play a role derives from studies of partial lipodystrophy, in which there is activation of the alternative complement pathway and C3-splitting activity in serum.[47,64] Recent studies indicate that a dichotomy exists, at least in the case of localized lipodystrophy: one group of patients shows simple involution of fat, whereas another group shows inflammatory changes along with serologic and direct immunofluorescent evidence of connective tissue disease.[65]

Histologic Features

The features of lipodystrophy include decreased sizes of fat lobules (Fig. 21–17) and formation of lipocytes of variable

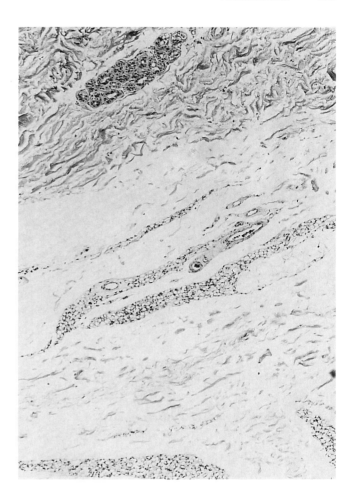

Figure 21–17. Lipodystrophy. Note the dramatic decrease in size of fat lobules. In this case of localized lipodystrophy, no inflammation was noted. (H&E, ×40.)

sizes with irregular cell membranes. There is a pale myxomatous or hyalinized background stroma containing numerous capillaries (Fig. 21–18). The overall appearance is suggestive of fetal fat.[3,65] Biopsies obtained at an early stage sometimes show a lymphocytic lobular panniculitis that is at first diffuse and later focal in distribution.[62] Admixtures of macrophages, focal fat necrosis, and foreign body giant cells sometimes are observed.[62,63] Inflammatory changes are more likely to be observed in cases associated with connective tissue disease,[62] in semicircular lipodystrophy,[63] and perhaps in cases with associated complement activation.

Differential Diagnosis

The changes of lipodystrophy differ from those usually seen in late stages of panniculitis and are specific enough to allow diagosis based on histologic features alone. Precise subtyping of lipodystrophy usually requires correlation with clinical data. Localized cases showing a lymphocytic lobular infiltrate may represent forms of connective tissue disease, and some of these may show deposits of immunoglobulin or complement along the basement membrane zone or in

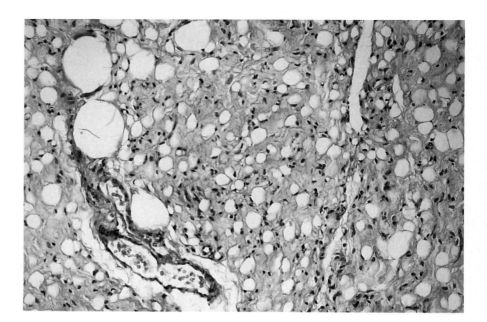

Figure 21–18. Lipodystrophy. This case resulted from local corticosteroid injection. Note the small lipocytes of varying sizes, myxoid appearance of stroma, and prominence of small capillaries. (H&E, ×100.)

vessel walls.[65] Localized lipodystrophy has been observed to accompany morphea and lichen sclerosis et atrophicus.[47]

MALIGNANCY AND PANNICULITIS

MALIGNANT INFILTRATES

Infiltration by malignant cells, either from metastasis or direct extension from an underlying focus, can produce a picture resembling panniculitis. When the associated malig-

nancy is relatively well differentiated, histologic recognition is seldom a problem, but poorly differentiated carcinomas, lymphomas, multiple myeloma, and leukemia at first glance may resemble inflammatory infiltrates. Admixtures of true inflammatory cells and such changes as fat necrosis and fibrosis may add to the diagnostic difficulty. Clinical history may be crucial in such cases.

Helpful histologic clues to the diagnosis of malignancy include the presence of a monomorphous cell population (Fig. 21–19), relatively minor fatty and connective tissue alterations out of proportion to the density of the infiltrate, a tendency for malignant cells to infiltrate between collagen

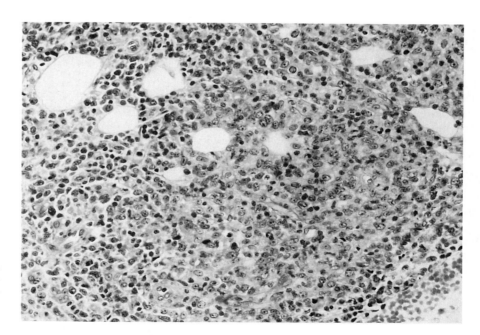

Figure 21–19. Malignant infiltration: in this case, a poorly differentiated lymphoma. Almost all the cells are lymphoid, and there is marked nuclear pleomorphism. (H&E, ×160.)

bundles in the dermis and into periadnexal connective tissue sheaths,[66] and evidence of cytologic atypia, including bizarre nuclei and mitotic figures. Tissue imprints permit more detailed cytologic study.[67] Finally, enzyme histochemistry, marker studies using immunoperoxidase methodology, and electron microscopy can add to diagnostic precision.

CYTOPHAGIC HISTIOCYTIC PANNICULITIS

Clinical Features
In recent years, there have been reports of a systemic disorder that features panniculitis composed of benign-appearing cytophagic histiocytes. Patients have a chronic illness consisting of fever, panniculitis, hepatosplenomegaly, liver failure, and a terminal hemorrhagic diathesis.[48,68] An association with B cell[69] and T cell[49] lymphomas has been described.

Histologic Features
There is a lobular panniculitis associated with fat necrosis, edema, and hemorrhage. The infiltrate may include lymphocytes, neutrophils, and plasma cells,[48] but the most striking feature is the infiltration of large numbers of benign-appearing histiocytes engaged in erythrophagocytosis and leukophagocytosis.[48,68,70] These cells have oval or reniform nuclei with homogeneous chromatin and occasional prominent nucleoli. The cytoplasm may be so filled with nuclear debris that these histiocytes have a beanbag appearance (Fig. 21–20).[68] These cells stain positively for lysozyme and occasionally for α_1-antitrypsin.[70] Langerhans cell granules have not been observed on ultrastructural study.[48] Autopsy has revealed similar infiltrating cells in other organs, such as the liver, spleen, bone marrow, myocardium, and lung.[48,68]

Differential Diagnosis
The microscopic appearance of this disorder is quite distinctive. Erythrophagocytosis occasionally is observed in other benign and malignant conditions,[49] but seldom if ever to the degree seen in cytophagic histiocytic panniculitis. Some clinical and histologic similarities to malignant histiocytosis suggest that cytophagic panniculitis may be a variant of that disorder.[70] However, differences from malignant histiocytosis include the benign appearance of the histiocytes, the primary involvement of subcutaneous fat, and the chronic clinical course of cytophagic panniculitis.[48]

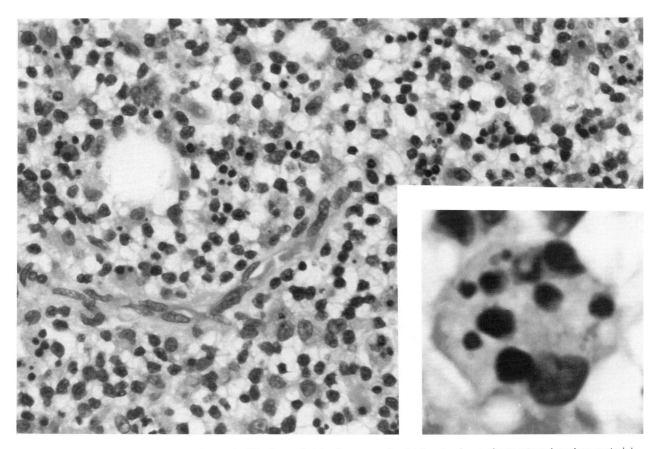

Figure 21–20. Cytophagic histiocytic panniculitis. Large but benign-appearing histiocytes have phagocytosed nuclear material, producing a characteristic beanbag appearance. Inset. High-power magnification of a beanbag cell. (H&E, ×250; inset, H&E, ×1500.)

OTHER DISORDERS OCCURRING AS PANNICULITIS

INFECTIOUS PANNICULITIS

A wide array of infectious diseases can occur as panniculitis. These range from localized processes to manifestations of septicemia and frequently are observed in patients who are immunocompromised or on chronic corticosteroid therapy. Histologic features are dependent to a large extent on the type of infecting organism. Cellulitis and necrotizing fasciitis caused by bacteria frequently show dermal–subcutaneous edema, dilated lymphatics, and a mixed infiltrate including neutrophils, thrombosis, and fat necrosis.[71] Atypical mycobacteria produce a panniculitis that features infiltration of lymphocytes, focal collections of neutrophils, fat necrosis,[72] and focal or diffuse granulomatous inflammation (Fig. 21–21). Eosinophilic panniculitis may accompany several parasitic diseases.[6]

The diagnosis of infective panniculitis requires a high index of suspicion and a thorough history. Special stains and culture studies are essential for diagnosis.

NONINFECTIOUS GRANULOMAS

Disorders associated with granulomatous inflammation, including ruptured hair follicles and cysts, necrobiosis lipoidica, granuloma annulare, and sarcoidosis, can extend into and at times primarily involve the subcutaneous fat. Generally, these conditions maintain their characteristic histopathologic features. Often the center of gravity of non-infectious granulomas will lie in the dermis rather than the subcutis. Microscopic features that are helpful in diagnosing these disorders include the presence of fragments of epithelium, keratin, or hair (ruptured follicles and cysts), broad zones of necrobiosis with layered granulomas and plasma cells (necrobiosis lipoidica), palisaded histiocytes surrounding areas of mucinous necrobiosis (subcutaneous granuloma annulare), and noncaseating granulomas within septa and lobules (sarcoidosis).[73,74]

PANNICULITIS ASSOCIATED WITH CONNECTIVE TISSUE DISEASES

In addition to lupus erythematosus, dermatomyositis, localized and systemic scleroderma, and eosinophilic fasciitis can produce subcutaneous inflammation. Dermatomyositis shows a nonspecific perivascular and lobular infiltrate composed of plasma cells, lymphocytes, and macrophages.[75] Morphea in early stages shows a septal panniculitis composed of lymphocytes, plasma cells, and histiocytes; lymphoid follicles sometimes are observed. Later, the subcutis is replaced by hyalinized connective tissue. Systemic scleroderma has similar features but often to a lesser degree, and lymphoid follicles are not observed.[60] Most of the inflammatory changes in eosinophilic fasciitis take place in the fascia, but within the subcutis, there may be fat necrosis adjacent to the fascia,[76] infiltration by lymphocytes and plasma cells, and thickening of the septa.[77,78]

Winkelmann has described a form of panniculitis associated with connective tissue disease that does not fit clearly into one of the above categories. These patients develop subcutaneous nodules on the back, shoulders, and legs and have serologic findings that include positive antinuclear antibody and antibody to an extractable nuclear antigen that is neither Smith antigen nor ribonucleoprotein.[47,79] Histologic changes include a heavy lymphohistiocytic lobular panniculitis associated with caseous necrosis. Septa are spared, and vasculitis is not observed. Further studies will be necessary to determine if these cases represent a unique

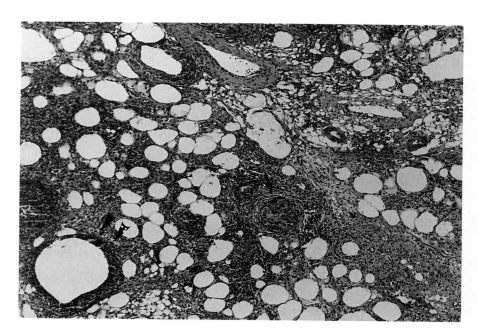

Figure 21–21. Infective panniculitis. The histologic features are not entirely specific, but note the presence of small focal granulomas (arrow) and vacuolar spaces surrounded by neutrophils (arrowheads). (H&E, ×100.)

disease entity or a transitory phase of one of the established connective tissue disorders.

REFERENCES

1. Pinkus H, Mehregan AH. *A Guide to Dermatohistopathology.* New York: Appleton-Century-Crofts; 1976:235–242.
2. Förström L, Winkelmann RK. Acute panniculitis: a clinical and histopathologic study of 34 cases. *Arch Dermatol.* 1977;113:909–917.
3. Reed RJ, Clark WH, Mihm MC. Disorders of the panniculus adiposus. *Hum Pathol.* 1973;4:219–229.
4. Ackerman AB. *Histologic Diagnosis of Inflammatory Skin Diseases.* Philadelphia: JB Lippincott; 1975:225–238.
5. Blaustein A, Moreno A, Noguera J, et al. Septal granulomatous panniculitis in Sweet's syndrome: report of two cases. *Arch Dermatol.* 1985;121:785–788.
6. Winkelmann RK, Frigas E. Eosinophilic panniculitis: a clinico-pathologic study. *J Cutan Pathol.* 1986;13:1–12.
7. Förström L, Winkelmann RK. Granulomatous panniculitis in erythema nodosum. *Arch Dermatol.* 1975;111:335–340.
8. Niemi K-M, Förström L, Hannuksela M, et al. Nodules on the legs. *Acta Dermatovenereol (Stockh).* 1977;57:145–154.
9. Bäfverstedt B. Erythema nodosum migrans. *Acta Dermatovenereol (Stockh).* 1954;34:181–193.
10. Vilanova X, Pinol Aguade J. Subacute nodular migratory panniculitis. *Br J Dermatol* 1959;71:45–50.
11. Perry HO, Winkelmann RK. Subacute nodular migratory panniculitis. *Arch Dermatol.* 1964;89:170–179.
12. Rostas A, Lowe D, Smout MS. Erythema nodosum migrans in a young woman. *Arch Dermatol.* 1980;116:325–326.
13. Bazin E. *Lecons Theoriques et Cliniques sur la Scrofule.* 2nd ed. Paris; 1861:146.
14. Parish WE, Rhodes EL. Bacterial antigens and aggregated gamma globulin in lesions of nodular vasculitis. *Br J Dermatol.* 1967;79:131–141.
15. Eberhartinger C. Das Problem des Erythema induratum Bazin. *Arch Klin Exp Dermatol.* 1963;217:196–254.
16. Schneider W, Undeutsch W. Vasculitiden des subcutanen Fettgewebes. *Arch Klin Exp Dermatol.* 1965;221:600–610.
17. Andersen S, La C. Erythema induratum (Bazin) treated with isoniazid. *Acta Dermatovenereol (Stockh).* 1970;50:65–68.
18. Chen TH, Shewmake SW, Hansen DD, et al. Subcutaneous fat necrosis of the newborn. *Arch Dermatol.* 1981;117:36–37.
19. Silverman AK, Michels EH, Rasmussen JE. Subcutaneous fat necrosis in an infant, occurring after hypothermic cardiac surgery: case report and analysis of etiological factors. *J Am Acad Dermatol.* 1986;15:331–336.
20. Moreno-Gimenez JC, Hernandez-Aguado I, Arguisjuela MT, et al. Subcutaneous fat necrosis of the newborn. *J Cutan Pathol.* 1983;10:277–280.
21. Thomsen RJ. Subcutaneous fat necrosis of the newborn and idiopathic hypercalcemia. *Arch Dermatol.* 1980;116:1155–1158.
22. Levine N, Lazarus GS. Subcutaneous fat necrosis after paracentesis: report of a case in a patient with acute pancreatitis. *Arch Dermatol.* 1976;112:993–994.
23. Roenigk HH Jr, Haserick JR, Arundell FD. Poststeroid panniculitis. *Arch Dermatol.* 1964;90:387–391.
24. Smith RT, Good RA. Sequellae of prednisone treatment of acute rheumatic fever. *Clin Res Proc.* 1956;4:156–157.
25. Bennett RG, Petrozzi JW. Nodular subcutaneous fat necrosis: a manifestation of silent pancreatitis. *Arch Dermatol.* 1975;111:896–898.
26. Goldman MP. Ascites, gastrointestinal bleeding, and leg nodules (off-center fold). *Arch Dermatol.* 1985;121:673–678.

27. Simons-Ling N, Schachner L, Penneys N, et al. Childhood systemic lupus erythematosus: associated with pancreatitis, subcutaneous fat necrosis, and calcinosis cutis. *Arch Dermatol.* 1983;119:491–494.
28. Förström L, Winkelmann RK. Acute, generalized panniculitis with amylase and lipase in skin. *Arch Dermatol.* 1975;111:497–502.
29. Potts DE, Mass MF, Iseman MD. Syndrome of pancreatic disease, subcutaneous fat necrosis, and polyserositis: case report and review of literature. *Am J Med.* 1975;58:417–423.
30. Hughes PSH, Apisarnthanarax P, Mullins JF. Subcutaneous fat necrosis associated with pancreatic disease. *Arch Dermatol.* 1975;111:506–510.
31. Niemi K-M. Panniculitis of the legs with urate crystal deposition: report of a case. *Arch Dermatol.* 1977;113:655–656.
32. Beacham BF, Cooper PH, Buchanan CS, et al. Equestrian cold panniculitis in women. *Arch Dermatol.* 1980;116:1025–1027.
33. Epstein EH Jr, Oren MF. Popsicle panniculitis. *N Engl J Med.* 1970;282:966–967.
34. Förström L, Winkelmann RK. Factitial panniculitis. *Arch Dermatol.* 1974;110:747–750.
35. Janin-Mercier A, Mosser C, Souteyrand P, et al. Subcutaneous sclerosis with fasciitis and eosinophilia after phytonadione injections. *Arch Dermatol.* 1985;121:1421–1423.
36. Kossard S, Ecker RI, Dicken CH. Povidone panniculitis: polyvinylpyrrolidone panniculitis. *Arch Dermatol.* 1980;116:704–706.
37. Palestine RF, Millns JL, Spigel GT, et al. Skin manifestations of pentazocine abuse. *J Am Acad Dermatol.* 1980;2:47–55.
38. Oertel YC, Johnson FB. Sclerosing lipogranuloma of the male genitalia: review of 23 cases. *Arch Pathol Lab Med.* 1977;101:321–326.
39. Foucar E, Downing DT, Gerber WL. Sclerosing lipogranuloma of the male genitalia containing vitamin E: a comparison with classical "paraffinoma." *J Am Acad Dermatol.* 1983;9:103–110.
40. Claudy A, Garcier F, Schmidt D. Sclerosing lipogranuloma of the male genitalia: ultrastructural study. *Br J Dermatol.* 1981;105:451–456.
41. Henrichs WD, Helwig EB. Grease gun granulomas. *Mil Med.* 1986;151:78–82.
42. Winkelmann RK, Barker SM. Factitial traumatic panniculitis. *J Am Acad Dermatol.* 1985;13:988–994.
43. Weber FP. A case of relapsing nonsuppurative nodular panniculitis showing phagocytosis of subcutaneous fat cells by macrophages. *Br J Dermatol Syphilol.* 1925;37:301–311.
44. Christian HA. Relapsing febrile nodular nonsuppurative panniculitis. *Arch Intern Med.* 1928;42:338–351.
45. Brill IC. Relapsing febrile nodular nonsuppurative panniculitis (Weber-Christian disease). In: *Medical Papers Dedicated to Henry Asbury Christian.* Baltimore: Waverly Press; 1936:694–704.
46. Arndt KA. Case Records of the Massachusetts General Hospital. *N Engl J Med.* 1982;306:1035–1043.
47. Winkelmann RK. Panniculitis in connective tissue disease. *Arch Dermatol.* 1983;119:336–344.
48. Crotty CP, Winkelmann RK. Cytophagic histiocytic panniculitis with fever, cytopenia, liver failure, and terminal hemorrhagic diathesis. *J Am Acad Dermatol.* 1981;4:181–194.
49. Aronson I, West DP, Variakojis D, et al. Fatal panniculitis. *J Am Acad Dermatol.* 1985;12:535–551.
50. Bleumink E, Klokke HA. Protease inhibitor deficiencies in a patient with Weber-Christian panniculitis. *Arch Dermatol.* 1984;120:936–940.
51. Breit SN, Clark P, Robinson JP, et al. Familial occurrence of alpha-1-antitrypsin deficiency and Weber-Christian disease. *Arch Dermatol.* 1983;119:198–202.
52. Rubinstein HM, Jaffer AM, Kudrua JC, et al. Alpha-1-antitrypsin deficiency with severe panniculitis: report of two cases. *Ann Intern Med.* 1977;86:742–744.

53. Pottage JC Jr, Trenholme GM, Aronson IK, et al. Panniculitis associated with histoplasmosis and alpha-1 antitrypsin deficiency. *Am J Med*. 1983;75:150–153.

54. Staff, University of Michigan. Lupus erythematosus profundus (Transactions of Michigan Dermatological Society. *Arch Dermatol*. 1974;109:583–584.

55. Sanchez NP, Peters MS, Winkelmann RK. The histopathology of lupus erythematosus panniculitis. *J Am Acad Dermatol*. 1981;5:673–680.

56. Izumi AK, Takiguchi P. Lupus erythematosus panniculitis. *Arch Dermatol*. 1983;119:61–64.

57. Tuffanelli DL. Lupus erythematosus. *J Am Acad Dermatol*. 1981;4:127–142.

58. Fountain RB. Lupus erythematosus profundus. *Br J Dermatol*. 1968;80:571–579.

59. Harris RF, Duncan SC, Esker RI, et al. Lymphoid follicles in subcutaneous inflammatory disease. *Arch Dermatol*. 1979;115:442–443.

60. Fleischmajer R, Nedwich A. Generalized morphea. I. Histology of the dermis and subcutaneous tissue. *Arch Dermatol*. 1972;106:509–514.

61. Peck B, Hoffman GS, Franck WA. Thrombophlebitis in systemic lupus erythematosus. *JAMA*. 1978;240:1728–1730.

62. Peters MS, Winkelmann RK. Localized lipoatrophy (atrophic connective tissue disease panniculitis). *Arch Dermatol*. 1980;116:1363–1368.

63. Makino K, Inoue T, Shimeo S. Lipodystrophia centrifugalis abdominalis infantilis. *Arch Dermatol*. 1972;106:899–900.

64. Sissons JP, West RJ, Fallows J, et al. Complement abnormalities of lipodystrophy. *N Engl J Med*. 1976;294:461–465.

65. Peters MS, Winkelmann RK. The histopathology of localized lipoatrophy. *Arch Dermatol*. 1984;120:1614. Abstract.

66. Sumaya CV, Baber S, Reed RJ. Erythema nodosum-like lesions of leukemia. *Arch Dermatol*. 1974;110:415–418.

67. King DT, Sun NCJ, Barr RJ. Touch preparations in diagnosis of skin disorders. *Arch Dermatol*. 1979;115:1034. Letter.

68. Willis SM, Opal SM, Fitzpatrick JE. Cytophagic histiocytic panniculitis: systemic histiocytosis presenting as chronic, nonhealing ulcerative skin lesions. *Arch Dermatol*. 1985;121:910–913.

69. Peters MS, Winkelmann RK. Cytophagic panniculitis and B cell lymphoma. *J Am Acad Dermatol*. 1985;13:882–885.

70. Baron DR, Davis BR, Pomeranz JR, et al. Cytophagic histiocytic panniculitis: a variant of malignant histiocytosis. *Cancer*. 1985;55:2538–2542.

71. Koehn GG. Necrotizing fasciitis. *Arch Dermatol*. 1979;1124:581–583.

72. Sanderson TL, Moskowitz L, Hensley GT, et al. Disseminated *Mycobacterium avium-intracellulare* infection appearing as a panniculitis. *Arch Pathol Lab Med*. 1982;106:112–114.

73. Gross MD, Andriacchi F, Gordon R, et al. Nodular subcutaneous sarcoidosis. *Arch Dermatol*. 1977;113:1442–1443.

74. Kroll JJ, Shapiro L, Koplon BS, et al. Subcutaneous sarcoidosis with calcification. *Arch Dermatol*. 1972;106:894–895.

75. Raimer SS, Solomon AR, Daniels JC. Polymyositis presenting with panniculitis. *J Am Acad Dermatol*. 1985;13:366–369.

76. Krauser RE, Tuthill RJ. Eosinophilic fasciitis. *Arch Dermatol*. 1977;113:1092–1093.

77. Botet MV, Sanchez JL. The fascia in systemic scleroderma. *J Am Acad Dermatol*. 1980;3:36–42.

78. Jarratt M, Bybee JD, Ramsdell W. Eosinophilic fasciitis: an early variant of scleroderma. *J Am Acad Dermatol*. 1979;1:221–226.

79. Winkelmann RK, Padilha-Goncalves A. Connective tissue panniculitis. *Arch Dermatol*. 1980;116:291–294.

SECTION IV
Infections and Infestations

CHAPTER 22
Viral Infections

Antoinette F. Hood

Cutaneous changes may be prominent clinical manifestations in human viral infections. Viruses are obligate intracellular parasites, and primary changes associated with infection occur intracellularly. The histopathologic changes occurring in the skin with viral infection vary tremendously from nonspecific to pathognomonic. There are, in some infections, sufficiently characteristic inclusion bodies or consistent cytologic and histologic findings to provide the dermatopathologist a high degree of diagnostic accuracy.[1] For the sake of organization and simplification, in this chapter cutaneous viral infections have been divided into those with relatively characteristic or specific histologic changes and those with less specific histopathologic findings (Table 22–1).

HERPESVIRUS INFECTIONS

The herpesviruses infecting humans include herpes varicella-zoster virus, herpes simplex virus, cytomegalovirus, and Epstein-Barr virus. All are double-stranded DNA viruses with similar ultrastructural features. Herpesviruses have an affinity for cells of ectodermal origin and replicate in the cell nucleus. Although frequently producing localized, self-limited disease, herpesviruses (1) may produce latent infections and (2) may disseminate and kill individuals who are immunodeficient or immunocompromised.[2] A characteristic histologic feature of herpesvirus infection is the presence of the Cowdry type A intranuclear inclusion, formed by coalesced viral nucleoplasm. These acidophilic inclusions are approximately half the diameter of the infected nucleus and are surrounded by a clear zone, or halo.

HERPES VARICELLA-ZOSTER VIRUS

Clinical Features
The herpes varicella-zoster (HVZ) virus, spread by droplet inhalation or direct contact is highly contagious, producing varicella (chickenpox) in nonimmune individuals and zoster (shingles) in persons previously exposed. The primary le-

sion in both infections is a discrete erythematous papule that rapidly becomes a tense clear vesicle. Within a short period of time, the vesicle becomes cloudy and umbilicated, then ruptures and develops a crust. Lesions in varicella begin on the trunk and spread centrifugally to the face and extremities. Unless secondary bacterial infections or excoriations occur, varicella usually heals without scarring. Lesions in zoster are confined to one or more contiguous dermatomes, where vesicles often become confluent and hemorrhagic. Zoster is almost always a painful eruption, and healing frequently is accompanied by scarring.

Histologic Features
The lesions of varicella and zoster are not distinguishable with routine light microscopy.[3] Infected keratinocytes initially undergo ballooning degeneration, characterized by enlargement of an individual cell with pale, vacuolated cytoplasm. Reticular degeneration occurs when cells become greatly distended with fluid, and cells rupture, forming a vesicle with residual cell walls. The loss of intercellular bridges also occurs, resulting in acantholysis. Multinucleated giant cells form by aggregation and fusion of adjacent infected epithelial cells (Fig. 22–1).

Nuclei exhibit margination of chromatin and contain inclusion bodies. Intranuclear inclusion bodies progress from being large, homogeneous, and basophilic to being small, demarcated, acidophilic bodies separated from the basophilic marginated chromatin at the nuclear membrane by a clear halo (Fig. 22–1). Characteristic cytopathic changes may be prominent in pilosebaceous and other adnexal structures, especially in older lesions. Swollen endothelial cells and fibroblasts may also contain intranuclear inclusions.

Mature lesions show a unilocular or multilobular intraepidermal vesicle containing proteinaceous material, loose acantholytic infected keratinocytes, and a few inflammatory cells. Late lesions show epidermal necrosis that may extend through the basal cell layer, giving the appearance of a subepidermal bulla (Fig. 22–1).

Dermal changes include papillary dermal edema and vessel ectasia. There is a variably intense patchy dermal

TABLE 22–1. VIRAL INFECTIONS GROUPED BY HISTOLOGIC FINDINGS

I. Cutaneous viral infections with characteristic histopathologic findings.
   A. Herpesvirus infections
     1. Herpes varicella-zoster
     2. Herpes simplex, types 1 and 2
     3. Cytomegalovirus
   B. Human papillomavirus infections
     1. Warts
     2. Bowenoid papulosis
     3. Verrucous carcinoma
     4. Epidermodysplasia verruciformis
   C. Molluscum contagiosum
   D. Milker's nodules
   E. Smallpox and vaccinia
II. Viral infections with less specific histopathologic changes.
   A. Hand-foot-and-mouth disease
   B. Measles
   C. Orf
   D. Papular acrodermatitis of childhood
   E. Generic viral exanthem, i.e., infectious mononucleosis

infiltrate composed of mononuclear cells admixed with neutrophils that may extend into deep reticular dermis. Inflammation may be sparse to absent in the immunocompromised individual.

Leukocytoclastic vasculitis occasionally is present, particularly in the reticular dermis. Perineural inflammation may be prominent, especially in herpes zoster infections.

Differential Diagnosis
Ballooning degeneration of keratinocytes may be seen in other viral infections, including smallpox, vaccinia, warts, and orf. Herpesvirus (simplex, varicella-zoster) infections can be distinguished from the vesicular lesions caused by poxviruses (smallpox, vaccinia) or enteroviruses (echo viruses, Coxsackie viruses) by the presence of multinucleated giant cells and intranuclear inclusion bodies.

HERPES SIMPLEX VIRUS

Clinical Features
Herpes simplex virus is an enveloped DNA containing neutrotropic virus responsible for the cause of a common infection spread by droplet infection and direct contact. There are two major antigenic types of human herpesvirus: type 1, which causes labial lesions, and type 2, which is generally associated with genital infection. Primary infection occurs in individuals with no previous exposure and is characterized by a variably severe acute gingivostomatitis or vesicular genital eruption. During the primary infection, the virus invades the nerve endings of the mucous membrane or skin, ascends within axons, and produces a latent infection in the spinal ganglion that may persist for life. Reactivation of the latent virus results in recurrent grouped vesicles. When the vesicles rupture, an erosion forms, and the lesion heals slowly over a period of 7 to 10 days without scarring. Atypical clinical manifestations of localized herpes simplex virus infections, as well as dissemination, may occur in immunocompromised hosts.[4]

Histologic Features
The histologic changes seen in primary and recurrent herpes simplex virus infections are similar to those described for herpes varicella-zoster lesions.

CYTOMEGALOVIRUS INFECTION

Clinical Features
Cutaneous manifestations of cytomegalovirus (CMV) infections include a macular and papular exanthem and localized mucocutaneous ulcerations that are usually genital or perineal. Petechiae secondary to vasculitis or thrombocytopenia, vesiculobullous lesions, and urticarial lesions also have

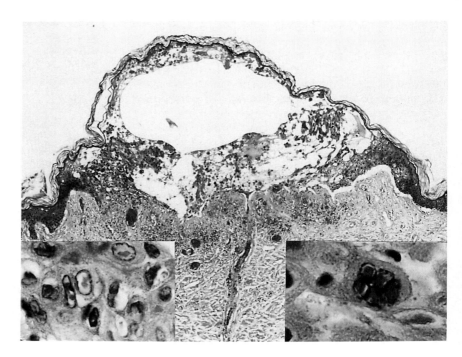

Figure 22–1. Herpesvirus infection. Intraepidermal vesicle with destruction of the basal cell layer, producing an apparent subepidermal bulla. Infected keratinocytes with intranuclear homogeneous eosinophilic inclusions (left). Multinucleated giant cell (right). (H&E, ×55; left inset, ×650; right inset, ×775.)

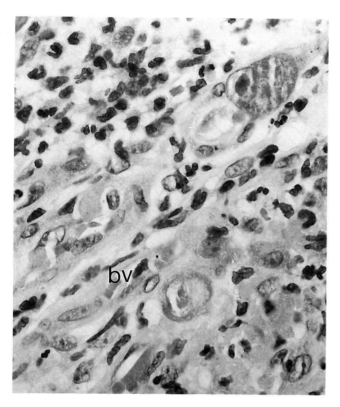

Figure 22–2. Cytomegalovirus infection. Cells in and around dermal blood vessel (bv) exhibit characteristic cytomegaly, smudged cytoplasm, and prominent large eosinophilic intranuclear inclusion surrounded by a perinuclear halo. (H&E, ×750.)

intranuclear inclusion bodies containing viral material form. The inclusion consists of large, round, sharply outlined eosinophilic or amphophilic body (Fig. 22–2). The inclusion is surrounded by a clear space, or halo, that may contain delicate strands of eosinophilic material radiating from the inclusion to the nuclear chromatin. The nucleus itself is enlarged, and the chromatin is marginated. The nucleolus also is often prominent and marginated.

In addition to cytomegaly, the infected cell may be irregular in shape, with smudgy cytoplasm. Intracytoplasmic inclusion bodies appear late and are not present in all cells. The intracytoplasmic inclusion appears as one or more small, rounded, amphophilic to basophilic granular masses in the perinuclear region. There is no surrounding peri-inclusion halo. The intracytoplasmic inclusion may stain positively with periodic acid-Schiff.

PAPILLOMAVIRUS INFECTIONS

WARTS

Clinical Features

Warts, or verrucae, are mucocutaneous intraepithelial tumors induced by human papillomaviruses (HPV), which are DNA-containing viruses. Morphologically, four basic types of human warts can be distinguished: the common wart (verruca vulgaris), the plantar wart (verruca plantaris), the flat wart (verruca plana), and the genital wart (condyloma acuminatum).

Using sensitive DNA-hybridization techniques, investigators have identified over 40 types of HPV. Each type generally is body site specific. Although most warts are entirely benign, a few have been found in association with mucocutaneous malignancies (Table 22–2).

Histologic Features

Common histologic features in all warts include hyperkeratosis and acanthosis with papillomatosis[9] (Fig. 22–3). Vertically oriented columns of parakeratosis often are seen. In the upper epidermis, koilocyte formation occurs. A koilocyte is an enlarged keratinocyte containing an eccentric pyknotic nucleus surrounded by a wide clear halo. Intracy-

been described. Although CMV is ubiquitous and the prevalence of seropositivity in normal adults is high, both the localized and widespread forms of the disease occur almost exclusively in immunocompromised individuals.[5,6]

Histologic Features

The most commonly infected cells in the skin are the endothelial cells lining small dermal blood vessels. Less frequently, histiocytic cells, eccrine glands, and keratinocytes are affected.[7,8] Initially, an infected cell enlarges, and the nucleus becomes prominent. Subsequently, characteristic

TABLE 22–2. HUMAN PAPILLOMAVIRUS (HPV)-ASSOCIATED LESIONS

HPV Type	Clinical Lesions	Oncogenic Potential
1, 2, 4	Palmar, plantar, common mosiac, oral, and anogenital warts	None described
3, 10	Flat warts in normal individuals and patients with epidermodysplasia verruciformis	HPV-10 has been found in rare cervical and vulvar squamous cell carcinomas
5, 8, 9	Macular lesions in epidermodysplasia verruciformis, warts in immunosuppressed patients	Found in some squamous cell carcinomas
6, 11, 16, 18	Anogenital and laryngeal warts, cervical condylomata, conjunctival papillomas	Urogenital dysplasias and carcinomas
7	Butcher's warts	None described
13	Oral focal epithelial hyperplasia	None described

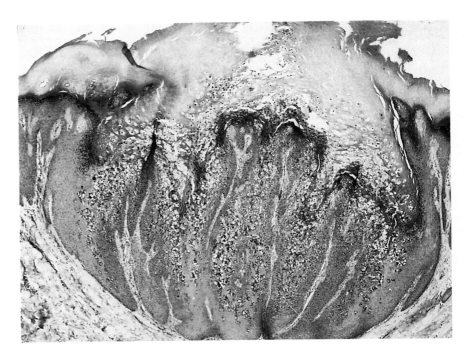

Figure 22–3. Verruca vulgaris. Cup-shaped lesion with orthohyperkeratosis, parakeratosis, and papillomatosis. (H&E, ×85.)

toplasmic basophilic or eosinophilic hyalinized masses probably representing degenerated keratohyaline material are pushed peripherally by the vacuole or halo. Viral intranuclear inclusion bodies usually are few in number and difficult to visualize (Fig. 22–4). They appear as small, spherical, deeply eosinophilic to basophilic nucleolus-like structures.

In the papillary dermis, the vessels are dilated, elongated, and tortuous. A patchy perivascular mononuclear cell infiltrate is commonly present. Characteristic histologic variations may be seen. *Flat warts* exhibit basketweave orthohyperkeratosis, no parakeratosis, and less acanthosis. Koilocytes are abundant and form so-called bird's eye cells (Fig. 22–5). The nuclear chromatin is dense, and the nucleolus frequently is prominent. *Anogenital warts* have an exophytic growth pattern with acanthosis and lobular rounded papillomatosis (Fig. 22–6). Parakeratosis often is diffuse. There are clusters of vacuolated koilocytes, some with sickle-shaped nuclei pushed to the margin of the cells. Dermal edema is prominent, as is vessel ectasia and proliferation.

BOWENOID PAPULOSIS

This disorder is characterized by the development of multiple, flesh-colored or hyperpigmented papules, nodules, or plaques on or near the genitalia of young men and women and is caused by HPV types 16 and 18.[10,11] The lesions often are clinically thought to be warts, seborrheic keratoses, or nevi.[12,13] Histologically, the lesions show variable hyperkeratosis, parakeratosis, and irregular acanthosis. There are scattered cytologically atypical keratinocytes but other-

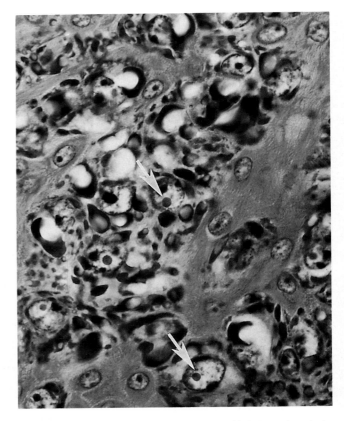

Figure 22–4. Verruca vulgaris. Koilocytes with intranuclear inclusions (arrows). (H&E, ×575.)

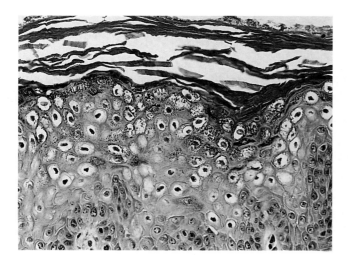

Figure 22–5. Flat wart (verruca plana). Basketweave orthohyperkeratotic scale, prominent koilocytes, or bird's eye cells, with pyknotic nuclei and condensed keratohyaline granules. (H&E, ×320.)

wise orderly epithelial maturation. Koilocytes are present. Mitoses, often in the same stage of development, are present focally. Bowenoid papulosis differs from Bowen's disease and erythroplasia of Queyrat by a lesser degree of atypia.[14]

The term "vulvar intraepithelial neoplasia (VIN)" has replaced bowenoid papulosis in the gynecologic literature.

VERRUCOUS CARCINOMA

Synonyms for this HPV-induced low-grade squamous cell carcinoma include carcinoma cuniculatum and giant condyloma of Buschke and Lowenstein. The disorder is discussed also in Chapter 43. The lesions, which occur on the plantar surface of the feet and genitalia, are slow growing, bulky, exophytic, ulcerated tumors with surface crypts and sinuses. Histologically, the tumor is characterized by a proliferation of well-differentiated keratinizing squamous epithelium that deeply invades the dermis. Intraepidermal microabscesses are frequent. Mitotic figures may be numerous, but cytologic atypia is mild or focal.[15,16]

EPIDERMODYSPLASIA VERRUCIFORMIS

Epidermodysplasia verruciformis is a rare heritable disease characterized by papillomavirus-induced macular and papular skin lesions that may transform to in situ and invasive squamous cell carcinomas.

Histologic features include basketweave hyperkeratosis, mild acanthosis, and pale vacuolated cells in the upper

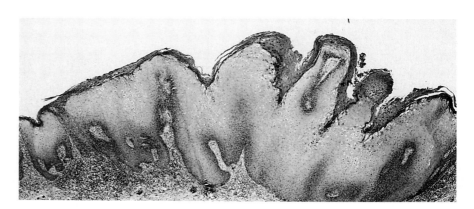

A

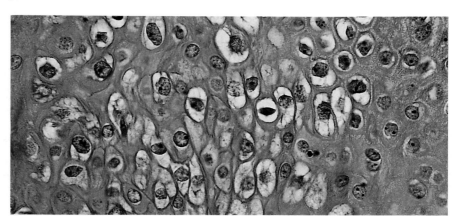

Figure 22–6. Anogenital wart (condyloma acuminatum). Diffuse parakeratosis, marked papillomatosis, and koilocytes in upper epidermis. (H&E, **A,** ×65; **B,** ×270.)

B

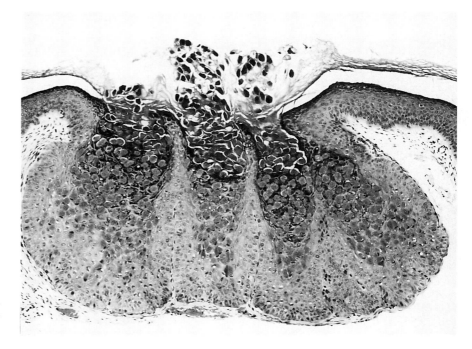

Figure 22–7. Molluscum contagiosum. Low-power view of typical lobular cup-shaped lesion. (H&E, ×95.)

stratum malpighili. The nuclei may be pyknotic and surrounded by clear halos. Cytoplasm of an affected cell occasionally stains pale bluish and may look foamy.

MOLLUSCUM CONTAGIOSUM

Clinical Features
Molluscum contagiosum is a common viral skin disease caused by a large DNA poxvirus. The infection, which is spread by direct contact or fomite, frequently is seen in children, adolescents, and immunocompromised patients, particularly individuals with acquired immunodeficiency syndrome (AIDS). A fully developed lesion is a pearly, flesh colored, dome-shaped, firm papule with a small central umbilication.

Histologic Features
There is a lobular hyperplasia of epithelium with downward growth, resulting in a cup-shaped lesion (Fig. 22–7). The basal cell layer appears normal, but the infected keratinocytes of the stratum malpighii become enlarged and acquire intracytoplasmic inclusions. These inclusions, known as molluscum bodies or Henderson-Patterson bodies, contain viral particles (Fig. 22–8). They are initially eosinophilic and somewhat granular. As the inclusions enlarge, the keratinocyte nucleus is displaced laterally and ultimately becomes flattened against the cell wall. With time, the inclusions become more amphophilic to basophilic, and the mature inclusion is basophilic and granular.

MILKER'S NODULES

Clinical Features
Milker's nodules is a benign skin disease caused by paravaccina virus, a poxvirus that is endemic to many cattle herds.

Human lesions consist of one to four nodules on the hand or forearms of cattle handlers.

Histologic Features
There is hyperkeratosis, parakeratosis, acanthosis, and marked elongation of the rete ridges. Early lesions show

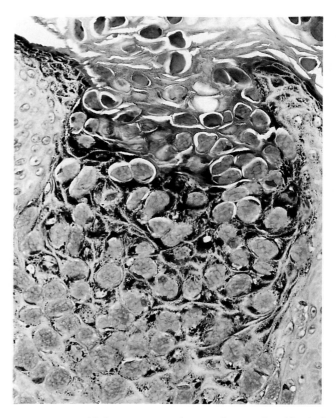

Figure 22–8. Molluscum contagiosum. Progressive histologic changes in Henderson-Patterson inclusion bodies throughout the epidermis. (H&E, ×270.)

ballooned cells with intracytoplasmic and intranuclear inclusions.[16a] Late lesions display reticular degeneration and intraepidermal vesiculation. Dermal changes include marked vessel proliferation and patchy to dense, diffuse dermal inflammation. The infiltrate is composed predominantly of lymphocytes admixed with histiocytic cells and eosinophils.

SMALLPOX AND VACCINIA

Clinical Features

There have been no cases of smallpox anywhere in the world since 1977, and discussion of this entity is for historical and comparative purposes only. This frequently fatal infection is characterized by a prodromal illness, a generalized centrifugal rash with rapidly successive papules, vesicles, pustules, umbilication, and crusting. Vaccinia, a complication of vaccination against smallpox, may be caused by abnormal viral replication or altered reactivity to viral component.

Histologic Features

Reticular degeneration, prominent in the early stage of vesiculation, produces intraepidermal multilocular vesicles. There are few ballooned cells and no multinucleated cells. Eosinophilic intracytoplasmic inclusion bodies (Guarnieri bodies) are characteristic but are present only early in vesicle formation. A fully developed inclusion is variable in size, round to oval, granular, eosinophilic, and paranuclear and is surrounded by a clear halo that enlarges to surround the entire nucleus. Intranuclear inclusions are neither constant nor conspicuous in cells containing intracytoplasmic inclusions. The presence of Guarnieri bodies differentiates smallpox infection from herpesvirus infection.

HAND-FOOT-AND-MOUTH DISEASE

Clinical Features

Hand-foot-and-mouth disease (HFMD) is a distinctive clinical syndrome caused by an enterovirus that is clinically manifested by characteristic lesions in the mouth and on the extremities. Epidemics and individual cases have been reported from around the world. The epidemic disease usually is associated with Coxsackie A_{16} virus or enterovirus 71. Sporadic cases have been reported in association with Coxsackie A_5, A_9, A_{10}, B_2, and B_5.

The most frequent finding of the disease is ulcerative oral lesions on the tongue, hard palate, and buccal mucosa. The cutaneous lesions appear together with or shortly after the oral lesions. They may vary in number from a few to over 100. The dorsal surfaces and sides of the fingers, hands, toes, and feet are most often involved. Each lesion begins as an erythematous macule or papule, in the center of which arises a gray, round to oval vesicle. Because the lesions often run in or parallel to the skin lines, they may be described as linear. They crust after a few days and gradually disappear over the course of 7 to 10 days.

Maculopapular erythematous lesions also have been described in association with the more typical lesions of HFMD in infants. This eruption occurs principally on the buttocks but occasionally is generalized.[17]

Histologic Features

The characteristic cutaneous lesion is an intraepidermal vesicle containing neutrophils, mononuclear cells, and proteinaceous eosinophilic material. As the lesion ages, there may be focal loss of the basal cell layer, resulting in a subepidermal bulla. The roof of the blister is often necrotic with discrete eosinophilic dyskeratotic and acantholytic epidermal cells. The epidermis immediately adjacent to the vesicle exhibits intercellular and intracellular edema (Fig. 22–9). Eosinophilic intranuclear inclusions have been described.[18] The dermis beneath a vesicle is edematous and contains a perivascular polymorphous infiltrate composed of lymphocytes and neutrophils. The lack of multinucleated giant cells and viral inclusion bodies differentiates this infection from herpesvirus infection.

Intracytoplasmic particles in a crystalline array characteristic of Coxsackie virus have been observed with electron microscopy.

MEASLES

Clinical Features

Measles, caused by an RNA paramyxovirus, is less commonly seen in the United States since the advent and distribution of live attenuated measles virus vaccine in 1963. Nevertheless, cases of typical and atypical measles still are reported. Typical measles is characterized by a 3- to 4-day prodrome of cough, conjunctivitis, and coryza. Subsequently, Koplik's spots and the characteristic papular exanthem appear. Atypical measles occurs in people who received killed measles virus vaccine and subsequently were exposed to and infected with natural measles. These individuals may have urticarial, vesicular, and petechial rashes, swollen hands and feet, severe pneumonia, and fever.

Histologic Features

Necrosis of epidermal and, occasionally, adnexal keratinocytes may be seen. Intranuclear inclusions are seen only rarely in the skin. Dermal edema and vessel proliferation may be accompanied by a leukocytic and lymphocytic perivascular infiltrate.

ORF (ECTHYMA CONTAGIOSUM)

Clinical Features

This disease, caused by a member of the poxvirus group, is endemic among sheep and goats and can be transmitted to humans. The disease in humans generally manifests itself as nodules on exposed areas. Individual lesions evolve through six clinical stages, each lasting approximately 6 days. The second, or target, stage has the most specific

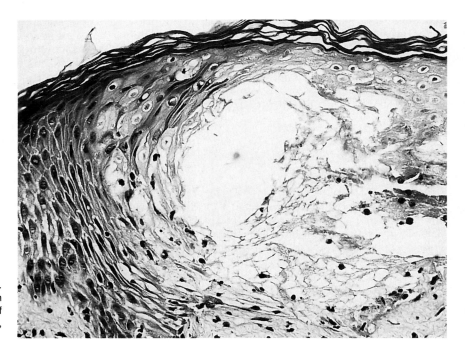

Figure 22–9. Hand-foot-and-mouth disease. Lateral border of an intraepidermal vesicle with intercellar and intracellar edema. The roof of the vesicle appears focally necrotic. (H&E, ×175.)

morphology and histopathologic changes. The entire disease, which is accompanied by regional lymphadenopathy, resolves spontaneously in approximately 5 weeks.

Histologic Features

There are no histologic descriptions of the papular stage in humans. In the target stage, acanthosis is first noted. Intranuclear and intracytoplasmic inclusions are present in superficial vacuolated keratinocytes corresponding to the clinically apparent white ring. Inclusions are also present in endothelial cells of the upper dermis. There is a dense dermal infiltrate composed of mononuclear cells. Central ulceration is characteristic of the acute stage. During this phase, reticular degeneration and intraepidermal microvesicle formation are prominent, and there is loss of follicle epithelium. In the regenerative stage, there is regeneration of the epidermis. Acanthosis and papillomatosis are prominent in the papillomatous stage. The acanthotic epidermis

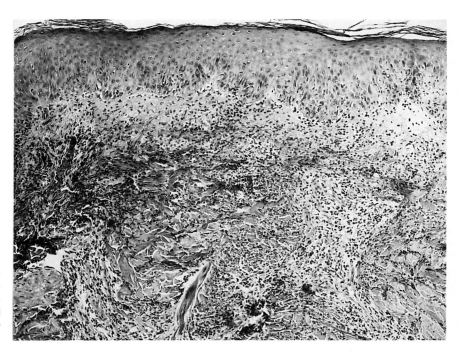

Figure 22–10. Papular acrodermatitis of childhood. Mild acanthosis, spongiosis, and intraepidermal microvesicle formation as well as a moderately intense perivascular and interstitial mononuclear cell infiltrate. (Original magnification ×85.)

becomes flatter and the dermal inflammation subsides in the final regressive phase.

PAPULAR ACRODERMATITIS OF CHILDHOOD (GIANOTTI-CROSTI SYNDROME)

Clinical Features
Papular acrodermatitis of childhood is a fairly common infectious disease characterized by asymptomatic papules on the face, buttocks, and limbs. Lesions last up to 3 weeks. Originally associated with hepatitis B virus, it has now been described in association with other viral infections.[19]

Histologic Features
Focal parakeratosis, spongiosis, and mild acanthosis are present as well as a moderately intense superficial perivascular and interstitial mononuclear cell infiltrate (Fig. 22–10). Although the histology of the lesions appears to be nonspecific, clinical–pathologic correlation may provide accurate diagnosis in these cases.

GENERIC EXANTHEM (INFECTIOUS MONONUCLEOSIS)

Clinical Features
The rash associated with infectious mononucleosis is used as an example of how many viral exanthems present clinically and histologically. It is an acute, self-limited disease caused by the Epstein-Barr virus characterized by fever, generalized lymphadenopathy, pharyngitis, and lymphocytosis with atypical lymphocytes. A rash occurs in up to 19% of infected persons and is described as being erythematous, macular, papular, or morbilliform. There is an appreciably higher incidence of skin rashes in patients given ampicillin.

Histologic Features
There are no distinctive histologic changes described for the rash associated with infectious mononucleosis or with many morbilliform viral exanthems. What is usually seen is vacuolar alteration of the basal layer, occasional dyskeratotic cells, and a sparse lymphohistiocytic perivascular or bandlike interface infiltrate.

Differential Diagnosis
The differential diagnosis for these histologic changes includes drug eruption and acute lupus erythematosus. The presence of eosinophils points toward a drug-induced eruption; the presence of the infiltrate throughout the reticular dermis or about appendages favors the diagnosis of lupus erythematosus.

REFERENCES

1. Strano AJ. Light microscopy of selected viral disease (morphology of viral inclusion bodies). *Pathol Annu.* 1976;11:53–75.
2. Kapan AS. *The Herpes Viruses.* New York: Academic, 1973.
3. McSorley J, Shapiro L, Brownstein MH, Hsu K. Simplex and varicella-zoster: Comparative cases. *Int J Dermatol.* 1974;13:69–75.
4. Corey L, Spear PG. Infections with herpes simplex viruses. *N Engl J Med.* 1986;314:686–691;749–757.
5. Ho M, ed. *Cytomegalovirus, Biology and Infection.* New York: Plenum; 1982.
6. Swanson S, Feldman PS. Cytomegalovirus infection initially diagnosed by skin biopsy. *Am J Clin Pathol.* 1987;8:113–116.
7. Parisier RJ. Histologically specific skin lesions in disseminated cytomegalovirus infection. *J Am Acad Dermatol.* 1983;9:937–946.
8. Walker JD, Chesney TMcC. Cytomegalovirus infection of the skin. *Am J Dermatopathol.* 1982;4:263–284.
9. Gross G, Pfister H, Hagedorn M, Gissmann L. Correlation between human papillomavirus (HPV) type and histology of warts. *J Invest Dermatol.* 1982;78:160–164.
10. Gross G, Hagedorn M, Ikenberg H, et al. Bowenoid papulosis. Presence of human papillomavirus (HPV) structural antigens and of HPV16-related DNA sequences. *Arch Dermatol.* 1985;121:858–863.
11. Guillet GY, Braun L, Masser, Aftimos J, Geniaux M, Texier L. Bowenoid papulosis. Demonstration of human papillomavirus (HPV) with anti-HPV immune serum. *Arch Dermatol.* 1984;120:514–516.
12. Wade TR, Kopf AW, Ackerman AB. Bowenoid papulosis of the penis. *Cancer.* 1978;42:1890–1903.
13. Wade TR, Kopf AW, Ackerman AB. Bowenoid papulosis of the genitalia. *Arch Dermatol.* 1979;115:306–308.
14. Patterson JW, Kao GF, Graham JH, Helwig EB. Bowenoid papulosis. A clinicopathologic study with ultrastructural observations. *Cancer.* 1986;57:823–836.
15. Kao GF, Graham JH, Helwig EB. Carcinoma cuniculatum (verrucous carcinoma of the skin). *Cancer.* 1982;49:2395-2403.
16. Prioleau PG, Santa Cruz DJ, Meyer JS, Bauer WC. Verrucous carcinoma. A light and microscopic, autoradiographic and immunofluorescence study. *Cancer.* 1980;45:2849–2857.
16a. Leavell UW Jr, Phillips IA. Milker's nodules: pathogenesis, tissue culture, electron microscopy, and calf innoculation. *Arch Dermatol.* 1975; 11:1307–1311.
17. Higgins PG, Warin RP. Hand, foot, and mouth disease: a clinically recognizable virus infection seen mainly in children. *Clin Pediatr.* 1967;6:373–376.
18. Kimura A, Abe N, Nakato T. Light and electron microscopic study of skin lesions of patients with the hand, foot, and mouth disease. *Tohoku J Exp Med.* 1977,122:237–247.
19. Gianotti F. Papular acrodermatitis of childhood and other papulovesicular acro-located syndromes. *Br J Dermatol.* 1979;100:49–59. Review.

CHAPTER 23
Bacterial Infections of the Skin

Gilles Landman and Antoinette F. Hood

In most pathology textbooks, chapters on infectious agents involving the skin are organized by etiologic agent (e.g., gram-positive infections, gram-negative infections) or by site of involvement (e.g., superficial, deep). This chapter is organized somewhat differently, with an emphasis on whether or not the histologic reaction pattern associated with a particular infection has specific and characteristic features (Table 23–1). At the end of the chapter, there is a brief discussion about cutaneous infections in immunocompromised individuals, an important subject that is briefly alluded to in other chapters in this book.

DISEASES WITH CHARACTERISTIC HISTOPATHOLOGY

ACTINOMYCETOMAS

Included under this heading are members of the family of Actinomycetes comprising the genera *Actinomyces, Arachnia, Nocardia, Actinomadura,* and *Streptomyces.* Initially classified as fungi, the bacterial origin of these organisms is now well established. Characteristically, these gram-positive bacilli tend to form chains or filaments. In this section, we discuss the two major diseases involving the skin, actinomycosis and mycetomas.

Actinomycosis

Clinical Features
Actinomycosis is a chronic, suppurative infection with three major clinical presentations: cervicofacial, thoracic, and abdominal. Disseminated disease and localized disease not included in the more common locations make up a smaller percentage of cases. Actinomycosis may be caused by any of the species *Actinomyces,* which are members of the normal flora of the mouth and gastrointestinal tract. This fact may

account for why more than half of the cases of actinomycosis are located in the cervicofacial region.

Cervicofacial actinomycosis typically occurs on the lower jaw as a discrete, painless mass or a diffuse swelling with overlying skin discoloration. Contiguous spread of the organisms within tissue results in the formation of inflammatory masses that develop central abscesses and subsequent interconnecting sinus tracts. *Actinomyces* have the capacity to invade periosteum and to produce osteomyelitis. Extension of the cervicofacial disease or aspiration of the organism may result in pulmonary infection. Abdominal infection usually follows traumatic rupture of the intestinal tract.

Histologic Features
The earliest lesions histologically resemble acute cellulitis with a diffuse dermal infiltrate of neutrophils. As the lesions evolve, there is a granulomatous suppurative dermal inflammation. Multinucleated giant cells and histiocytic cells surround microabscesses that contain masses of organisms referred to as sulfur granules. The granulomatous reaction is, in turn, surrounded by marked dermal fibrosis. Vascular proliferation is minimal.

Sulfur granules are sparse in number but, when present, are found within the microabscesses. These granules, which appear as round to oval bodies up to 300 μm in diameter, are composed of clumped colonies of bacteria with peripherally radiating, often club-shaped filaments (Fig. 23–1). The organisms are gram positive and are lightly acid fast; older filaments may take up silver stains.[1]

Mycetomas

A mycetoma is a chronic subcutaneous infection caused by one of several actinomycetes within the genera *Actinomadura, Arachnia, Nocardia,* and *Streptomyces.* These organisms are ubiquitous soil saprophytes more commonly found in subtropical and tropical regions. Mycetoma also may be caused by fungal pathogens.

TABLE 23–1. BACTERIAL INFECTIONS OF THE SKIN

Diseases with characteristic or specific histologic patterns
    Actinomycetomas
    Bartonellosis
    Botryomycosis
    Cat-scratch disease
    Chancroid
    Impetigo
        Staphylococcal scalded skin syndrome
        Toxic shock syndrome
    Rhinoscleroma
    Tularemia
Diseases with nonspecific histologic patterns
    Cutaneous anthrax
    Cellulitis
    Erythrasma
    Granuloma inguinale
    Septicemia
        Gonococcemia
        Meningococcemia
        Ecthyma gangrenosum

Clinical Features

Following traumatic inoculation of the skin, a painless subcutaneous nodule appears, gradually enlarges, and subsequently ulcerates. Satellite lesions may form that are connected to the primary site of infection by sinus tracts. Pus and exudate containing granules may be expressed from the sinus tracts.[2–4] Although any area of the body surface may become infected, exposed areas, such as the extremities, are most frequently involved. If the infection is allowed to progress without treatment, destruction of underlying muscle and bone occurs and may produce significant deformity.

Histologic Features

The histologic appearance of mycetoma is similar to that described for actinomycosis. There are extensive areas of dermal and subcutaneous fibrosis, granulomatous inflammation, and microabscesses containing granules. Skin fistulas and sinus tracts are composed of microabscesses and granulation tissue. The microorganisms in mycetoma are gram positive and faintly positive with acid-fast stains. Appropriate stains should be performed to rule out fungal infection (eumycetomas).

BARTONELLOSIS

This infectious disease is caused by *Bartonella bacilliformis*, which is transmitted to humans by the sandfly, *Phlebotomus verrucarum*. Bartonellosis occurs almost exclusively in South America, predominantly in Peru, Colombia, and Equador. The disease occurs in two stages: the first is known as Oroya fever or Carrión's disease and is characterized by an acute febrile hemolytic anemia. The second stage, called verruga peruana, is characterized by the appearance of hemangiomatous skin lesions.

Clinical Features

Approximately 3 weeks after being bitten by an infected sandfly, the patient develops sudden onset of fever, chills, and anemia. In this early phase of the disease, smears of peripheral blood will show small coccobacilli within erythrocytes. Phagocytosis of parasitized erythrocytes results in anemia and subsequent hepatosplenomegaly.[5,6] After a quiescent period of 3 to 6 months, the eruptive cutaneous phase begins, which occurs in one of three forms: (1) a miliary form, characterized by multiple superficial violaceous hemangioma-like papules diffusely distributed over

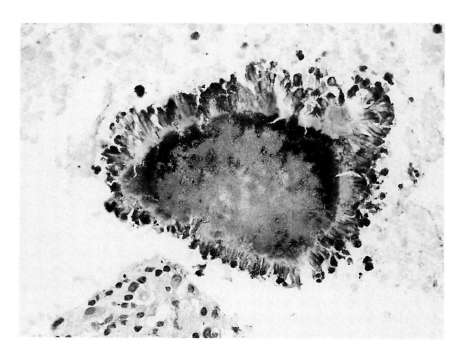

Figure 23–1. Actinomycosis. Sulfur granule showing stellate radiations (Splendore-Hoeppli phenomenon) surrounding a granular core with numerous clumps of bacteria. (PAS, ×320.)

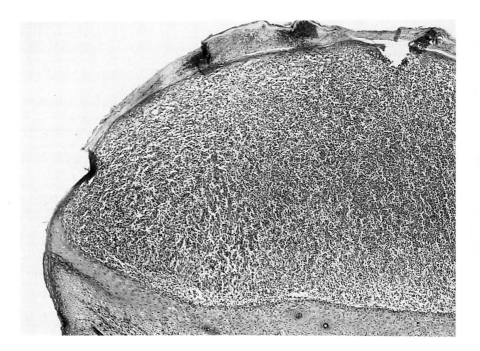

Figure 23–2. Bartonellosis. Dome-shaped nodule with marked vascular proliferation. (H&E, ×80.)

the skin surface, (2) a nodular form, with a small number of nodules located predominantly on the extensor surfaces of the extremities, and (3) a mular form, typified by one or more large, deep, ulcerated lesions.[6]

Histologic Features

The early papular lesions are polypoid with flattening of the overlying epidermis. In the dermis, there is a multifocal proliferation of capillaries, producing a lobular vascular appearance (Fig. 23–2). The surrounding stroma is edematous and infiltrated by neutrophils, lymphocytes, mast cells, and plasma cells. The proliferating endothelial cells either may form open vascular channels, similar to those seen in pyogenic granuloma, or they may remain as solid cords or aggregates of cells with frequent mitoses (Fig. 23–3). Between the vessels there are so-called verruca cells, with abundant eosinophilic cytoplasm and large oval or spindled nuclei containing granular chromatin and delicate nuclear membranes.[5] The verruca cells stain positively with antibodies against factor VIII-related antigen and *Ulex europeus*. End-stage lesions show extensive dermal necrosis and dermal lymphoid hyperplasia.

The coccobacilli are found in the stroma around blood vessels, but organisms are few in number and are difficult

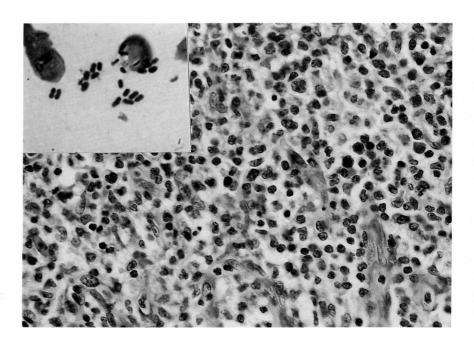

Figure 23–3. Bartonellosis. Higher magnification of Figure 23–2, showing marked vascular proliferation and endothelial cell swelling. (H&E, ×420.) **Inset:** Blood smear of bartonellosis in the acute phase. Note the coccobacilli in small clusters. (Giemsa, ×1250.)

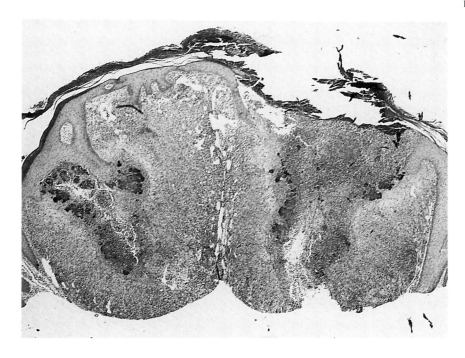

Figure 23–4. Botryomycosis. Multilobulated ulcerated nodule with sinus tracts lined by dark clumps of bacteria. (H&E, ×22.)

to find with the light microscope. Electron microscopic examination may be necessary to demonstrate *B. bacilliformis* in extracellular spaces adjacent to blood vessels. The differential diagnosis for this disorder includes hemangioma, pyogenic granuloma, Kaposi's sarcoma, and the cat-scratch disease as seen in immunodeficient patients.

BOTRYOMYCOSIS

Clinical Features
Botryomycosis is a rare chronic bacterial infection caused by staphylococci.[7] Lesions may occur in various organs, including the skin, liver, and bone. Cutaneous lesions typically consist of small tender erythematous nodules with draining sinuses.[8]

Histologic Features
The epidermis shows marked acanthosis with parakeratosis and focal spongiosis. In the dermis, there is a proliferation of vessels and a mixed inflammatory infiltrate composed of neutrophils and mononuclear cells (Fig. 23–4). Within this infiltrate, there are granules composed of tightly clustered or clumped gram-positive bacteria (Fig. 23–5). The granules are sometimes surrounded by an amorphous eosinophilic material creating what is called the "Splendore-Hoeppli phenomenon." This amorphous coating, which is PAS positive, often has lateral projections giving the granule a radiating appearance similar to that seen in actinomycotic granules.[8]

CAT-SCRATCH DISEASE

Cat-scratch disease is a benign, self-limiting illness characterized by regional lymphadenopathy and a history of contact with cats. A variant of this disease, epithelioid angioma-

tosis, has been described recently in patients with acquired immunodeficiency disease (AIDS).[9] Identification of the causative organism, a gram-negative coccobacillus, has been achieved through special staining techniques.[10]

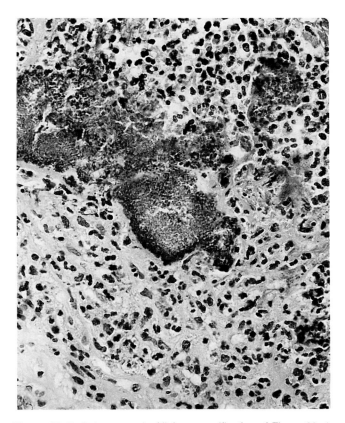

Figure 23–5. Botryomycosis. Higher magnification of Figure 23–4, showing the granular aspect of the bacterial colonies. (H&E, ×425.)

Clinical Features

The primary skin lesion occurs at the site of a cat scratch and is followed by fever and regional lymphadenopathy. The primary lesion usually is a solitary erythematous papule or multiple papules along a cat scratch. The lesion may subsequently become violaceous, scaly, or pustular. It heals without scarring. AIDS patients develop papular and nodular hemagioma-like skin lesions that clinically resemble Kaposi's sarcoma or dermatofibromas. These lesions regress after therapy with antibiotics. A history of contact with cats may be obtained.

Histologic Features

In the primary skin lesion, there are variable epidermal changes, including pseudoepitheliomatous hyperplasia, necrosis, and occasionally ulceration. Focal areas of altered (necrobiotic) and necrotic granular dermal collagen are surrounded by histiocytic cells, which may be aligned in a palisading arrangement. Multinucleated giant cells frequently are present. The cuff of histiocytic cells is, in turn, surrounded by a zone of lymphocytes. Eosinophils and nuclear debris may be seen in adjacent stroma.[11] Similar histologic changes are present in affected lymph nodes.

The vascular lesions seen in AIDS patients are characterized by a proliferation of endothelial cell-lined vascular spaces embedded in edematous stroma. The stroma contains variable nuclear dust, plasma cells, extravasated erythrocytes, and occasionally amorphous eosinophilic material around vessels.[12]

Pleomorphic organisms may be demonstrated in skin lesions and lymph nodes with the Warthin-Starry stain. The organisms have the structure of gram-negative rods when viewed with electron microscopy. Immunoperoxidase staining, using antisera raised in rabbits against cultured cat-scratch disease bacillus shows a positive reaction with the bacterium.[9]

Differential Diagnosis

The primary skin lesion of cat-scratch disease at low power resembles noninfectious palisading granulomas, such as necrobiosis lipoidica and rheumatoid nodule, and infectious granulomas associated with fungal, bacterial, and mycobacterial disease. Clinicopathologic correlation and special stains may be helpful in differentiating these processes from cat-scratch disease.

CHANCROID

Chancroid, also known as soft chancre, is a venereal disease caused by *Haemophilus ducreyi*. More prevalent in young men, the disease is seen in Africa, Central and South America, and less commonly in the United States.

Clinical Features

Following exposure and an incubation period of 2 to 5 days, a small painful papule appears in the genital area and rapidly becomes supurative and ulcerated. Characteristically, the ulcer is round to oval, with irregular edges, and is surrounded by hyperemia. Autoinoculation may result in small satellite lesions. Unilateral or bilateral inguinal lymphadenopathy may be prominent, and suppuration or rupture of nodes may occur.

Histologic Features

The epidermis adjacent to the ulceration is often acanthotic. Three distinct zones of inflammation are seen beneath the ulcer: (1) the surface of the ulceration is covered by neutrophils admixed with necrotic collagen, extravasated erythrocytes, and fibrin, (2) beneath the neutrophil-rich zone, there is an area of prominent vascular proliferation with endothelial cell swelling, occasional luminal occlusion, and even focal thrombosis, and (3) the deepest zone is characterized

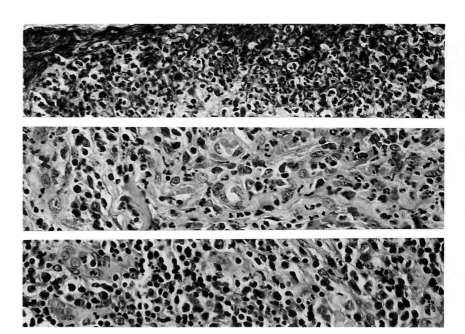

Figure 23–6. Chancroid. Composite of the three distinct zones found in chancroid. At the top (base of the ulcer), there is neutrophilic infiltrate and necrotic tissue; the middle section is characterized by marked vascular proliferation; the bottom zone shows a dense plasma cell infiltrate. (H&E, ×320.)

by an intense plasma cell and lymphocyte infiltration (Fig. 23–6). This zonal inflammation is quite typical and diagnostic of chancroid,[13,14] but further substantiation may be provided by demonstrating clusters of gram-negative bacilli arranged in short parallel chains between and within neutrophils near the surface of the ulcer.[15] The Giemsa stain also may be helpful in identifying organisms.[16] "Railroad tracks" or "school of fish" patterns of bacterial alignment are more typically observed in gram-stained swabs of the ulcer.

IMPETIGO, STAPHYLOCOCCAL SCALDED SKIN SYNDROME, AND TOXIC SHOCK SYNDROME

Clinical Features

Impetigo is a superficial infection of the skin caused by streptococci or staphylococci. The nonbullous form of impetigo occurs more commonly among preschool and school children, whereas the bullous form is seen more frequently in newborns and young children.[17,18]

Nonbullous impetigo is characterized by the appearance of transient, thin-walled vesicles on an erythematous base that rapidly rupture and form thick yellow-brown, honey-colored crusts. Initially appearing on exposed areas, such as the face and extremities, primary lesions tend to coalesce and spread to other parts of the body by autoinoculation. Nonbullous impetigo is caused by the introduction of group A β-hemolytic streptococcus into superficial abrasions or otherwise altered skin. *Staphylococcus aureus* also is frequently cultured from nonbullous impetigo lesions but is believed to be a secondary invader and not the primary cause of the disease. Predisposing conditions to the development of impetigo include insect bites, atopic dermatitis, eczematous dermatitis, and maceration of the skin. Bullous impetigo is caused by *S. aureus* and is clinically characterized by a thin-walled, flaccid blister, 1 to 3 cm in diameter, that appears on normal skin. The bullae, which are initially clear, rupture and form thin, light brown, varnishlike crusts.

Two associated cutaneous syndromes may follow staphylococcal impetigo or other localized staphylococcal infections: staphylococcal scalded skin syndrome (SSSS) and toxic shock syndrome (TSS). Both syndromes represent a response to the extracellular hematogenous dissemination of epidermolytic or exfoliative toxins produced by *S. aureus*, resulting in widespread erythema and desquamation of the skin.[19–22]

Histologic Features

Nonbullous and bullous impetigo have similar histopathologic features characterized by a subcorneal bulla filled with polymorphonuclear neutrophils and cellular debris. Spongiosis, neutrophilic exocytosis, and focal spongiotic microabscesses often are present lateral to the bulla (Fig. 23–7). Large blisters often contain a few acantholytic keratinocytes. Tissue Gram stains may reveal gram-positive cocci within the bullae, but the absence of bacteria does not preclude the diagnosis of impetigo. The dermis usually displays mild vascular ectasia and a mild perivascular lymphocytic infiltrate.

Lesions associated with SSSS show acantholysis at the level of the granular layer (Fig. 23–8). There is no agreement in the literature as to whether the primary site of damage is the desmosome or the interdesmosome cell region. However, it is generally accepted that the staphylococcal exfoliatin is not cytotoxic but rather affects cell adhesion.[23,24] Bacteria are neither observed in nor cultured from the lesions.

Histologic features of the TSS include foci of epidermal spongiosis containing neutrophils, necrotic keratinocytes (scattered individually or clustered), a perivascular and interstitial dermal infiltrate composed of mononuclear cells admixed with neutrophils, and occasional eosinophils. Intraepidermal microabscesses and extravasated erythrocytes also may be present.[25]

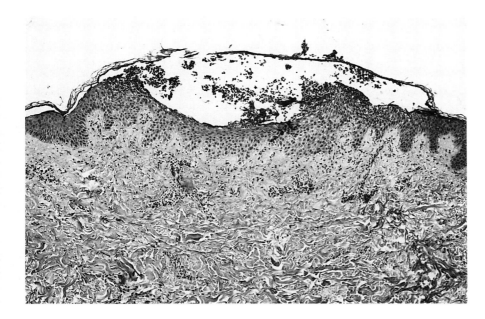

Figure 23–7. Impetigo. Subcorneal bulla filled with numerous neutrophils. Note spongiotic microabscesses within the epidermis. (H&E, ×16.)

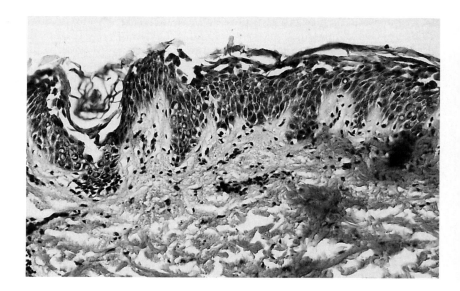

Figure 23–8. Staphylococcal scalded skin syndrome. Mild acantholysis of the granular cell layer. (H&E, ×120.)

Differential Diagnosis

Pustular psoriasis, subcorneal pustular dermatosis, superficial *Candida* infections, and pemphigus foliaceus must be differentiated histologically from lesions of impetigo. Pustular psoriasis may show psoriasiform hyperplasia at the base of or lateral to the spongiotic pustule. However, these features are not always present, and it is sometimes extremely difficult if not impossible to differentiate the two entities. Subcorneal pustular dermatosis usually shows collections of neutrophils above the granular layer, occasional acantholytic cells, mild epidermal spongiosis, mild dermal edema, and a few perivascular lymphocytes. Especially in older lesions, it may not be possible to differentiate these two diseases histologically. Organisms are usually present in *Candida* pustules and may be demonstrated with the PAS or methenamine silver stains. Lesions of pemphigus foliaceus characteristically exhibit more acantholytic keratinocytes within the subcorneal cleft of pustule than are present in impetigo lesions. Clinical–pathologic correlation and immunofluorescence findings are important adjuncts in establishing the diagnosis of pemphigus.

RHINOSCLEROMA

Rhinoscleroma, caused by *Klebsiella rhinoscleromatis* is a chronic disease usually involving the oral mucosa, upper respiratory mucosa, and skin. The disease is endemic in Africa, Asia, and Latin America.

Clinical Features

Three clinical stages are described: (1) a catarrhal or exudative stage, characterized by crusting and nasal discharge, (2) a granulomatous or proliferative stage, with papules and granulomatous lesions involving the nose, pharynx, larynx, trachea, or bronchi, and (3) a cicatrization stage with marked scarring and deformity.[26,27]

Histologic Features

In the granulomatous phase, the histopathologic picture is quite characteristic and consists of a granulomatous infiltrate rich in plasma cells, with numerous Russell bodies and Mickulicz cells.[26–28] Russell bodies appear as homogeneous eosinophilic material (immunoglobulin deposits) within the plasma cell. Mickulicz cells are large, pale, foamy, histiocytic cells containing clumps of encapsulated bacilli. The organisms can be seen in routinely stained sections but are better visualized as gram-negative organisms with the tissue gram stain. Staining of paraffin-embedded tissues with anti-*Klebsiella* antibodies may also be helpful.[29] In the late stages of the disease, the histologic findings are less specific and consist of marked fibrosis.

TULAREMIA

Tularemia is a zoonotic endemic disease that is caused by *Francisella tularensis*. Humans become infected through broken skin when handling infected animals, such as rabbits and rodents, by ingesting contaminated food and water, or by being bitten by infected arthropods, such as ticks, deerflies, or mosquitoes.[30,31]

Clinical Features

The most common form of tularemia is the ulceroglandular form, which begins as a small erythematous papule at the site of inoculation. The papule evolves into a nodule, which subsequently ulcerates. Regional lymph nodes enlarge and may even suppurate and drain. The patient then develops generalized lymphadenopathy, fever, chills, headache, cough, and myalgias.

Histologic Features

The epidermis adjacent to the central ulceration is acanthotic. Three zones of inflammation are characteristically present in active lesions. The central zone is composed of necrotic eosinophilic and granular dermis, neutrophil nuclear remnants, and extravasated erythrocytes. The intermediate zone consists of epithelioid and giant multinucleated histiocytic cells. The outer zone is made up of lymphocytes, histiocytic cells, plasma cells and erythrocytes. This histologic reaction pattern is also present in lymph nodes.[31] Organisms are rarely identified in biopsy specimens. In older lesions, zonal inflammation is replaced by epithelioid granulomas resembling sarcoidosis.

Differential Diagnosis

Necrotizing and suppurative reactions surrounded by granulomatous inflammation may be seen in cat-scratch disease, sporotrichosis, and lymphogranuloma venereum. The presence of extravasated erythrocytes may help to distinguish tularemia from the other entities, but these diseases cannot always be differentiated histologically.

DISEASES WITH NONSPECIFIC HISTOPATHOLOGY

CUTANEOUS ANTHRAX

A zoonotic disease caused by *Bacillus anthracis,* anthrax is occasionally transmitted to humans when they come in contact with hair, wool, or carcasses of infected animals.

Clinical Features

Lesions are typically found in friction areas, such as the neck, as well as around the lips and the eyes. There are two major clinical presentations: (1) the dry form, which begins as an erythematous papule, enlarges, forms vesicles, becomes hemorrhagic, and finally forms a black necrotic eschar, and (2) the edematous form, which is characterized by intense fluid extravasation and a vasospastic phenomenon.[32] The skin lesions are usually solitary and are not painful. Tender lymphadenopathy commonly occurs.

Histologic Features

There is extensive epidermal necrosis and ulceration. The surface of the ulcer is covered with fibrinopurulent membrane containing bacilli. The epidermis surrounding the ulceration may show intercellular edema, intraepidermal microvesicle formation, and infiltration by neutrophils. The papillary dermis is widened by intense edema and vasodilatation. Collagen bundles in the reticular dermis are separated by edema, hemorrhage, and marked neutrophilic infiltration. Notable abscess formation does not occur. The infiltrate extends to the subcutaneous fat. Organisms are present not only in the region of the central ulceration but also in the dermis. The bacilli are gram-positive rods, 3 to 5 μm in size, which are found free in the interstitium, not within neutrophils or macrophages.[33]

CELLULITIS AND ERYSIPELAS

Cellulitis is a deep-seated infection of the subcutaneous tissue and skin, with an accompanying ascending lymphangitis and involvement of regional lymph nodes. It is usually caused by *Streptococcus pyogenes* or *S. aureus.* Noncholera vibrio organisms also have been described as etiologic agents.[34] Edema (hypostatic, lymphatic, or renal), chronic

ulcers and minor abrasions are the usual predisposing conditions for the development of cellulitis.

Erysipelas is a specific form of superficial cellulitis, a rapidly spreading infection of the skin, usually due to group A β-hemolytic streptococcus but occasionally caused by other bacteria, such as group B streptococci or *S. aureus.*[35]

Clinical Features

Cellulitis is characterized by intense hyperemia, edema, and infiltration of the skin and subcutaneous tissue. The margins of the lesion are usually poorly demarcated and not raised. Regional lymphangitis and tender lymphadenopathy are frequent findings.

Erysipelas usually occurs on the face of infants and older adults. The lesions are more superficial than those of cellulitis and may be distinguished clinically from cellulitis by a sharp, well-demarcated serpiginous border.

Histologic Features

Cellulitis and erysipelas share similar histologic features. Vasodilatation and marked edema result in separation of collagen fibers in the dermis and the subcutaneous septae. A diffuse infiltration of neutrophils percolates between collagen bundles and extends deep into the fat. Dermal hemorrhage, subepidermal vesicle formation, and epidermal ulceration may occur in very severe cases. Dermal microabscess formation and small areas of necrosis are not uncommon. The Brown-Brenn or other tissue gram stain demonstrates gram-positive bacteria in most cases. Gram-negative bacteria may be seen in immunocompromised patients.[36]

ERYTHRASMA

Clinical Features

This superficial, usually asymptomatic disease is caused by a diphteroid organism, *Corynebacterium minutissimum.* The lesions are well demarcated, round to oval patches and plaques with fine scale involving intertriginous areas, including the toe webs, axillae, groin, and inframammary regions. The lesions are initially erythematous and may become reddish brown. Examination with a Wood's light (UVA, 365 nm) reveals a coral red fluorescence.

Histologic Features

The subtle histologic changes in erythrasma are restricted to the stratum corneum, where there are hyperkeratosis and mild separation of the cornified cells.[37] Gram-positive rods or filaments are present between the cells of the stratum corneum and rarely within keratinocytes. These findings have been well documented by electron microscopic studies.[38] The lower epidermis and the dermis do not show specific histologic changes.

GRANULOMA INGUINALE

Also known as donovanosis or granuloma venereum, granuloma inguinale is a sexually transmitted, mildly contagious disease. Caused by the gram-negative bacillus, *Calymmato-*

bacterium granulomatis, the disease is more common in tropical and subtropical climates but occasionally occurs in temperate zones.

Clinical Features

After an incubation period of approximately 15 days, a firm papule or nodule appears that rapidly becomes ulcerated. Lesions occur most frequently in the genital, inguinal, and perianal areas. The typical ulcer is variable in size and has a beefy red, friable surface. Less common presentations include hypertrophic or verrucous lesions, necrotic lesions with extensive genital destruction, and a sclerotic form of the disease.[39,40]

Histologic Features

Lateral to the ulcer, the epidermis exhibits acanthosis and occasionally pseudoepitheliomatous hyperplasia (Fig. 23–9). Neutrophils predominate on the surface of the ulcer. Throughout the dermis, extending into subcutaneous tissue, there is a dense infiltrate of plasma cells and histiocytic cells, admixed with lymphocytes and scattered or clustered neutrophils.[41] In the upper part of the lesion, there are variable numbers of large histiocytic cells, 25 to 90 μm in diameter, with large cytoplasmic vacuoles.[42,43] These histiocytic cytoplasmic vacuoles contain darkly staining inclusions, known as Donovan bodies (Fig. 23–10). Better visualized with Giemsa or a silver stain, such as the Warthin

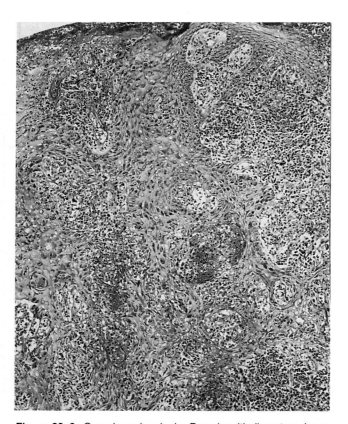

Figure 23–9. Granuloma inguinale. Pseudoepitheliomatous hyperplasia surrounded by a dense mixed infiltrate. (H&E, ×90.)

Starry stain, these inclusions are made up of 10 to 20 rod-shaped bacilli.[44] Rarely, one can find bacilli within neutrophils. Vascular proliferation and ectasia, with endothelial cell proliferation, are usually quite prominent.

Differential Diagnosis

Donovanosis must be differentiated from chancroid. Granuloma inguinale does not have the zonal inflammatory pattern of chancroid. Plasma cells and vascular proliferation occur evenly throughout the lesions, and the characteristic Donovan bodies are easily visualized with special stains. Histologic differentiation from squamous cell carcinoma may be difficult, especially if organisms are not readily identified.

SEPTICEMIA

Skin involvement may occur as a sequela of septicemia. Typically, lesions are limited in number and appear as erythematous papules. Despite the wide variety of organisms capable of producing sepsis, the histopathologic findings in the skin are similar in the majority of cases. The minor differences in clinical and histopathologic patterns seen in gonococcemia, meningococcemia, and ecthyma gangrenosum are discussed.

Gonococcemia

Sepsis associated with *Neisseria gonorrhoeae* infection frequently results in malaise, fever, arthritis, and skin lesions. Tender macules, papules, vesicopustules, and hemorrhagic bullae all have been described in gonococcemia.[45–47]

Histologic Features

Epidermal changes vary with the age of the lesion. Infiltration by neutrophils occurs in early lesions. Intraepidermal micropustules, subepidermal bullae, and frank necrosis of the epidermis occur in older lesion (Figs. 23–11, 23–12). Fibrin deposition, focal vessel thrombosis, endothelial cell necrosis, and a perivascular neutrophilic infiltrate with nuclear debris (dust) and hemorrhage are seen.[46,48] A moderately intense interstitial mononuclear cell infiltrate also is present. Gram-negative diplococci are only occasionally found within the lesions.[45–49]

Differential Diagnosis

The lesions of gonococcemia are histologically similar to those of leukocytoclastic vasculitis. However, the vessel thrombosis, profuse hemorrhage, interstitial mononuclear infiltrate, and involvement of deep vascular plexuses present in lesions of gonococcemia are exceedingly rare in leukocytoclastic vasculitis.

Meningococcemia

Meningococcemia, caused by *Neisseria menigitidis,* is accompanied by skin lesions, including petechiae, hemorrhagic papules, purpura, and ecchymoses.

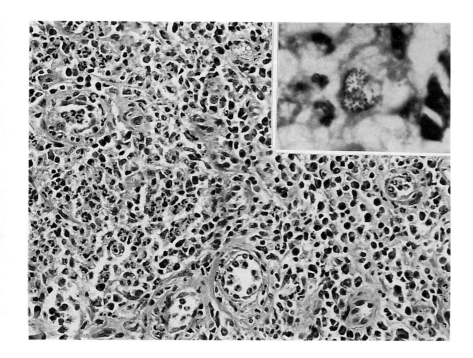

Figure 23–10. Granuloma inguinale. Higher magnification of Figure 23–9, with plasma cell infiltrate and focal microabscesses. (H&E, ×290.) **Inset.** Donovan body. Numerous bacilli within macrophage. (Giemsa, ×1150.)

Histologic Features

There is extensive vascular damage with prominent endothelial swelling and fibrin thromboses. A marked extravasation of erythrocytes and a neutrophilic infiltrate are found around affected vessels. Epidermal necrosis and subepidermal blisters are common. Gram-negative bacteria may be found within neutrophils and endothelial cells. Immunofluorescence shows IgG, IgM, IgA, complement, and fibrinogen deposition within the vessel walls, confirming that this reaction is immune-complex medicated.[50]

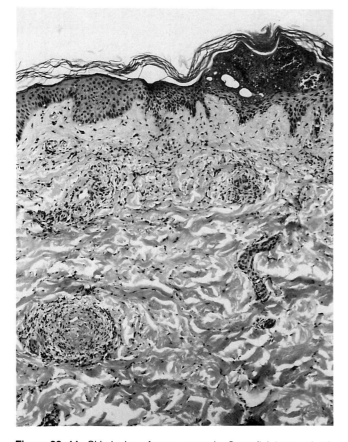

Figure 23–11. Skin lesion of gonococcemia. Superficial area of epidermal necrosis, with a moderately intense perivascular mixed infiltrate and vessel thrombosis. (H&E, ×95.)

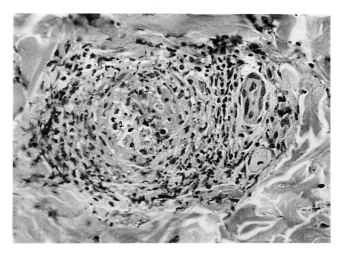

Figure 23–12. Skin lesion of gonococcemia. Vessel with fibrin thrombus, necrosis of the wall, and a surrounding polymorphonuclear infiltrate. (H&E, ×320.)

Ecthyma Gangrenosum

Ecthyma gangrenosum is a cutaneous manifestation of systemic infection caused by *Pseudomonas aeruginosa* and is usually seen in immunocompromised patients. Lesions evolve from an erythematous macule to a pustule, eventually forming a necrotic ulcer and black eschar, surrounded by an erythematous halo. Lesions are found more commonly in the perineum and the gluteal regions and on the extremities.

Histologic Features
Adjacent to an ulcer, the epidermis is necrotic and separated from the dermis. Throughout the dermis, extending into subcutaneous tissue, there are extensive tissue necrosis and inflammation. The inflammatory infiltrate is polymorphous, with neutrophils and histiocytic cells predominating over lymphocytes. Gram-negative bacilli may be identified with the gram stain and are more often found in the adventitia or medial layer of blood vessels. Neutrophils may be sparse to absent in patients with marked neutropenia.[51]

INFECTION IN THE IMMUNOCOMPROMISED HOST

An alteration in immunologic status may result from hereditary dysfunction, administration of drugs, malignancy, or infection. Examples of hereditary disorders include severe combined immunodeficiency disease, Wiscott-Aldrich syndrome, and ataxia–telangiectasia. Chemotherapeutic agents used in the treatment of various malignancies and other immunosuppressive agents used for inflammatory diseases and in organ transplant recipients, as well as systemic steroids, are responsible for iatrogenically induced immunodeficiency. Malignances, especially lymphoproliferative diseases, may result in impaired immunologic status. Systemic infections with such organisms as *Mycobacterium tuberculosis* and human immunodeficiency virus (HIV) may produce profound suppression of the immunologic system. Regardless of the etiology, altered immunity is associated with increased susceptibility to bacterial septicemia and systemic infection with fungi, yeast, and viruses.

Skin Infections in Immunocompromised Individuals

Wolfson et al.[52] have proposed a classification for skin infections occurring in immunocompromised individuals.

Typical Primary Skin Infection
These are commonplace infections that may occur also in immunocompetent persons. Examples include cellulitis, folliculitis, and wound infection. Cellulitis is commonly caused by group A streptococci and *S. aureus*. However, unusual causes of infection occur, such as gram-negative cellulitis in neutropenic patients or mycobacterial and fungal cellulitis in diseases affecting cell-mediated immunity.

Unusually Widespread Cutaneous Infection
Organisms that usually produce localized or trivial infections in immunologically intact persons may cause extensive disease in immunocompromised patients. Human papillomavirus infection occurs commonly after organ transplantation and is occasionally extensive and debilitating.[53] Localized herpesvirus infection may occur in unusual forms and may persist for a long period of time if not diagnosed and treated appropriately.[54] Superficial fungal infections with dermatophytes, yeast, and pityrosporon or superficial bacterial infections may be much more extensive and may provide a potential portal for life-threatening systemic infection.[55–59]

Opportunistic Primary Skin Infections
Impairment of the normal immunologic defense mechanisms allows organisms that are usually not virulent to invade and produce significant localized or disseminated disease. Examples of opportunistic organisms producing primary skin infections include atypical mycobacteria,[59] saprophytic fungi,[60] and protothecosis.[61]

Disseminated Systemic Infection Metastatic to Skin
Hematogenous spread of infection may be initially manifested as skin lesions. Gram-negative bacteria, such as *Pseudomonas aeruginosa* and *Escherichia coli*, often produce sepsis with cutaneous lesions in leukemia patients undergoing chemotherapy, but gram-positive bacteria, such as *Staphylococcus* and *Corynebacterium*,[62] also have been reported in this setting. Disseminated infection metastatic to the skin may be caused by fungi that cause systemic disease, such as *Histoplasma capsulatum*,[63] *Cryptococcus neoformans*,[64,65] *Nocardia*,[66] *Aspergillus sp*, and *Mucoraceae*, among others.

Finally, it should be noted that an increasing number of complex infections caused by two or more organisms have been reported in immunodeficient patients.[67,68] A histopathologist who receives a skin biopsy specimen from an immunocompromised individual should probably assume an infectious etiology until proven otherwise. The intensity and composition of the inflammatory infiltrate present in cutaneous infections in this population vary immensely, with the typical finding being less inflammation than normally seen. In order to assess accurately the role of infectious agents in the pathogenesis of a lesion, it is imperative that a panel of special stains, including immunoperoxidase when available, be applied to identify bacteria, fungi, mycobacteria, and viruses.

REFERENCES

1. Bennhoff DF. Actinomycosis: diagnostic and therapeutic considerations and a review of 32 cases. *Laryngoscope.* 1984;94:1198–1217.
2. Kamalam A, Thambiah AS. A clinico-pathological study of actinomycotic mycetomas caused by *Actinomadura madurae* and *Actinomadura pelletierii*. *Mycopathologia.* 1987;97:151–163.
3. Landau Z, Feld S, Frumkin A, Resnitzky P. *Nocardia brasiliensis* skin infections. *Isr J Med Sci.* 1986;22:397–399.
4. Kalb RE, Kaplan MH, Grossman ME. Cutaneous nocardiosis. Case reports and review. *J Am Acad Dermatol.* 1985;13:125–133.
5. Arias-Stella J, Lieberman PH, Erlandson RA, Arias-Stella J Jr.

Histology, immunohistochemistry, and ultrastructure of the verruga in Carrion's disease. *Am J Surg Pathol.* 1986;10:595–610.

6. Arias-Stella J, Lieberman PH, Garcia-Caceres U, Erlandson RA, Kruger H, Arias-Stella J Jr. Verruga peruana mimicking malignant neoplasms. *Am J Dermatopathol.* 1987;9:279–291.

7. Brunken RC, Lichon-Chao N, van den Broek H. Immunologic abnormalitis in botryomycosis. *J Am Acad Dermatol.* 1983;9:428–434.

8. Binford CH, Dooley JR. Botryomycosis. In: Binford CH, Connor DH, eds. *Pathology of Tropical and Extraordinary Diseases.* Washington, DC: Armed Forces Institute of Pathology; 1979:561.

9. LeBoit PE, Berger TG, Egbert BM, et al. Epithelioid haemangioma-like vascular proliferation in AIDS: manifestation of cat scratch disease bacillus infection? *Lancet.* 1988;1:960–963.

10. Wear DJ, Margileth AM, Hadfield TL, Fischer GW, Schlogel CJ, King FM. Cat scratch disease: a bacterial infection. *Science.* 1983;221:1403–1405.

11. Johnson WT, Helwig EB. Cat-scratch disease. Histopathologic changes in the skin. *Arch Dermatol.* 1969;100:148–154.

12. Knobler EH, Silvers DN, Fine KC, Lefkowitch JH, Grossman ME. Unique vascular skin lesions associated with human immunodeficiency virus. *JAMA.* 1988;260:524–527.

13. Margolis RJ, Hood AF, Chancroid: diagnosis and treatment. *J Am Acad Dermatol.* 1982;6:493–499.

14. Sheldon WH, Heyman A. Studies on chancroid. Observations on the histology with an evaluation of biopsy as a diagnostic procedure. *Am J Pathol.* 1946;32:415–425.

15. Heyman A, Beeson PB, Sheldon WH. Diagnosis of chancroid. The relative efficiency of biopsies, cultures, smears, autoinoculations and skin tests. *JAMA.* 1945;129:935–938.

16. Freinkel AL. Histological aspects of sexually transmitted genital lesions. *Histopathology.* 1987;11:819–831.

17. Ferrieri P, Dajani AS, Wannamaker LW, Chapman SS. Natural history of impetigo. Site sequence of acquisition and familial patterns of spread of cutaneous streptococci. *J Clin Invest.* 1972;51:2851–2862.

18. Dajani AS, Ferrieri P, Wannamaker LW. Natural history of impetigo. Etiologic agents and bacterial interactions. *J Clin Invest.* 1972;51:2863–2871.

19. Elias PM, Levy SW. Bullous impetigo. Occurrence of localized scalded skin syndrome in an adult. *Arch Dermatol.* 1976;112:856–858.

20. Melish ME, Glagow LA, Turner MD. The staphylococcal scalded-skin syndrome: isolation and partial characterization of the exfoliative toxin. *J Infect Dis.* 1972;125:129–140.

21. Wuepper KD, Dimond RL, Knutson DD. Studies of the mechanism of epidermal injury by a staphylococcal epidermolytic toxin. *J Invest Dermatol.* 1975;65:191–200.

22. Fritsch P, Elias P, Varga J. The fate of staphylococcal exfolatin in newborn and adult mice. *Br J Dermatol.* 1976;95:275–284.

23. Elias PM, Fritsch P, Epstein EH Jr. Staphylococcal scalded skin syndrome. Clinical features, pathogenesis, and recent microbiological and biochemical developments. *Arch Dermatol.* 1977;113:207–219.

24. Dimond RL, Wolff HH, Braun-Falco O. The staphylococcal scalded skin syndrome. An experimental histochemical and electron microscopic study. *Br J Dermatol.* 1977;96:483–492.

25. Hurwitz RM, Ackerman AB. Cutaneous pathology of the toxic shock syndrome. *Am J Dermatopathol.* 1985;7:563–578.

26. Hyams VJ. Rhinoscleroma. In: Binford CH, Connor DH, eds. *Pathology of Tropical and Extraordinary Diseases.* Washington, DC: Armed Forces Institute of Pathology; 1979:187–189.

27. Tapia A. Rhinoscleroma: a naso-oral dermatosis. *Cutis.* 1987;40:101–103.

28. Lever WF, Schaumburg-Lever G. *Histopathology of the Skin.* Philadelphia: JB Lippincott Co; 1983:290–314.

29. Altmann G, Ostfeld E, Zohar S, Theodor E. Rhinoscleroma. *Isr J Med Sci.* 1977;13:62–64.

30. Young LS, Bicknell DS, Archer BG, et al. Tularemia epidemic: Vermont, 1968. Forty-seven cases linked to contact with muskrats. *N Engl J Med.* 1969;23:1253–1260.

31. Evans ME, Gregory DW, Schaffner W, McGee ZA. Tularemia: a 30-year experience with 88 cases. *Medicine.* 1985;64:251–269.

32. Dutz W, Kohout-Dutz E. Anthrax. *Int J Dermatol.* 1981;20:203–206.

33. Lebowich RJ, McKillip BG, Conboy JR. Cutaneous anthrax. A pathologic study with clinical correlation. *Am J Clin Pathol.* 1943;13:505–515.

34. Limpert GH, Peacock JE. Soft tissue infections due to noncholera vibrios. *Am Family Physician.* 1988;37:193–198.

35. Finch R. Skin and soft-tissue infections. *Lancet.* 1988;1:164–167.

36. Meislin HW. Pathogen identification of abscesses and cellulitis. *Ann Emerg Med.* 1986;15:329–332.

37. Sarkany I, Taplin D, Blank H. Incidence and bacteriology of erythrasma. *Arch Dermatol.* 1962;85:578–582.

38. Montes LF, Black SH, McBride ME. Bacterial invasion of the stratum corneum in erythrasma. Ultrastructural evidence for a keratolytic action exerted by *Corynebacterium minutissimum.* *J Invest Dermatol.* 1967;49:474–485.

39. Sehgal VN, Shyamprasad AL. Donovanosis. Current concepts. *Int J Dermatol.* 1986;25:8–16.

40. Rosen T, Tschen JA, Ransdell W, Moore J, Markham B. Granuloma inguinale. *J Am Acad Dermatol.* 1984;11:433–437.

41. Sehgal VN, Shyamprasad AL, Beohar PC. The histopathological diagnosis of donovanosis. *Br J Vener Dis.* 1984;60:45–47.

42. Pund ER, Greenblatt RB. Specific histology of granuloma inguinale. *Arch Pathol.* 1937;23:224–229.

43. Dodson RF, Fritz GS, Winthroupe RH Jr, et al. Donovanosis: a morphologic study. *J Invest Dermatol.* 1974;62:611–614.

44. Davis CM, Collins C. Granuloma inguinale: an ultrastructural study of *Calymmatobacterium granulomatis.* *J Invest Dermatol.* 1969;53:315–321.

45. Abu-Nassar H, Hill N, Fred HL, Yow EM. Cutaneous manifestations of gonococcemia. A review of 14 cases. *Arch Intern Med.* 1963;112:731–737.

46. Ackerman AB, Miller RC, Shapiro L. Gonococcemia and its cutaneous manifestations. *Arch Dermatol.* 1965;91:227–232.

47. Ackerman AB. Hemorrhagic bullae in gonococcemia. *N Engl J Med.* 1970;282:793–794.

48. Shapiro L, Teisch JA, Brownstein MH. Dermatohistopathology of chronic gonococcal sepsis. *Arch Dermatol.* 1973;107:403–406.

49. Kahn G, Danielsson D. Septic gonococcal dermatitis. Demonstration of gonococci and gonococcal antigens in skin lesions by immunofluorescence. *Arch Dermatol.* 1969;99:421–425.

50. Sotto MN, Lnager B, Hoshino-Shimizu S, de Brito T. Pathogenesis of cutaneous lesions in acute meningococcemia in humans: light, immunofluorescent, and electron microscopic studies of skin biopsy specimens. *J Infect Dis.* 1976;133:506–514.

51. Greene SL, Su WP, Muller SA. Ecthyma grangrenosum: report of clinical, histopathologic, and bacteriologic aspects of eight cases. *J Am Acad Dermatol.* 1984;11:781–787.

52. Wolfson JS, Sober AJ, Rubin RH: Dermatologic manifestations of infections in immunocompromised patients. *Medicine.* 1985;64:115–133.

53. Spencer ES, Anderson HK. Viral infections in renal allograft recipients treated with long-term immunosuppression. *Br Med J.* 1979;2:829–830.

54. Shneidman DW, Barr RJ, Graham JH. Chronic cutaneous herpes simplex. *JAMA.* 1979;241:592–595.

55. Ray TL. Fungal infections in the immunocompromised host. *Med Clin North Am.* 1980;64:955–968.

56. Flick MR, Cluff LE. *Pseudomonas* bacteriemia: review of 108 cases. *Am J Med.* 60:501–508.

57. Spiers ASD. *Pseudomonas* septicemia following superficial infection. *Br Med J*. 1974;4:770.

58. El Baze P, Thyss A, Caldani C, Juhlin L, Schneider M, Ortonee J-P. *Pseudomonas aeruginosa* 0–11 folliculitis. Development into ecthyma gangrenosum in immunosuppressed patients. *Arch Dermatol*. 1985;121:873–876.

59. Hirsh FS, Saffold OE. *Mycobacterium kansasii* infection with dermatologic manifestations. *Arch Dermatol*. 1976;112:706–710.

60. Weitzman I. Saprophytic molds as agents of cutaneous and subcutaneous infection in the immunocompromised host. *Arch Dermatol*. 1986;122:1161–1168.

61. Wolfe ID, Sacks HG, Samoroden CS, Robinson HM. Cutaneous protothecosis in a patient receiving immunosuppressive therapy. *Arch Dermatol*. 1976;112:829–832.

62. Jerdan MS, Shapiro RS, Smith NB, Virshup DM, Hood AF. Cutaneous manifestations of *Corynebacterium* group JK sepsis. *J Am Acad Dermatol*. 1987;16:444–447.

63. Kalter DC, Tschen JA, Klema M. Maculopapular rash in a patient with acquired immunodeficiency syndrome. *Arch Dermatol*. 1985;121:1455–1460.

64. Schupbach CW, Wheeler CE, Briggaman RA, Warner NA, Kanof EP. Cutaneous manifestations of disseminated cryptococcosis. *Arch Dermatol*. 1976;112:1734–1740.

65. Rico MJ, Penneys NS. Cutaneous cryptococcosis resembling molluscum contagiosum in a patient with AIDS. *Arch Dermatol*. 1985;121:901–902.

66. Boudoulas O, Camisa C. *Nocardia asteroides* infection with dissemination to skin and joints. *Arch Dermatol*. 1985;121:898–900.

67. Boudreau S, Hines HC, Hood AF. Dermal abscesses with *Staphylococcus aureus*, cytomegalovirus and acid-fast bacilli in a patient with acquired immunodeficiency syndrome (AIDS). *J Cutan Pathol*. 1988;15:53–57.

68. Kwan TH, Kaufman HW. Acid-fast bacilli with cytomegalovirus and herpes virus inclusions in the skin of an AIDS patient. *Am J Clin Pathol*. 1986;85:236–238.

CHAPTER 24
Rickettsial Infections

Myles S. Jerdan

Named after the American physician, H. T. Ricketts, who first recognized rickettsiae as the cause of spotted fever and typhus,[1] the rickettsiae are of interest not only because of the diseases they cause but also because they are one of the simplest of bacterial forms. Once thought to be a transitional form between bacteria and viruses, they are now recognized as prokaryotes with structural characteristics of gram-negative bacilli.

Rickettsiae are distinguished from other bacteria because of their small size, obligate intracellular parasitism, and, with the exception of Q fever, transmission by arthropods. Although the rickettsiae are dependent on the host for essential metabolites, they do have limited metabolic activity. Like other bacteria, they possess a cell structure and they multiply by transverse binary fission. They also resemble bacteria by containing both RNA and DNA.

Several groups of rickettsiae are pathogenic for humans: the spotted fever group, the typhus group, the scrub typhus group, and a miscellaneous group that includes the organisms responsible for Q fever and trench fever. The first three groups are classified according to commonality in growth and metablism, fine structure, and pathogenic properties, as well as differences in size, intracellular location, extracellular behavior, antigenic composition, and pathologic lesions. For similar reasons, the rickettsiae causing Q fever and trench fever have been segregated and classified as *Coxiella burnetii* and *Rochalimaea quintana*, respectively (Table 24–1).

A developmental cycle has never been established for rickettsiae. Although rickettsiae in logarithmic growth phase are typically rod-shaped and those in the stationary phase are coccoid or filamentous, this pleomorphism is not believed to represent a developmental cycle.

ROCKY MOUNTAIN SPOTTED FEVER

Between 1906 and 1909, the causative organism for Rocky Mountain spotted fever (RMSF) was isolated from patients in Missoula, Montana, by Ricketts.[1] After identifying the organism in ticks, he also showed animal transmissibility.[1] A thorough discussion of the rich history of RMSF and the other rickettsial diseases has been written by Woodward.[2]

Clinical Features
The etiologic agent of RMSF, *Rickettsia rickettsii*, is a parasite of several species of ticks, the most prominent of which are *Dermacentor andersoni,* the western wood tick, and *Dermacentor variabilis,* the eastern dog tick. The rickettsia is passed from one generation of ticks to another and does not appear to have an adverse effect on the host. It is transmitted to humans by the bite of an infected tick.[3] Humans are incidentally involved, since the disease is primarily an infection of the tick and secondarily of small animals.[4]

Although the organism was originally endemic in the Rocky Mountain region during the first half of the century,[5] today the majority of RMSF cases occur in two areas, the south Atlantic and the west South Central regions.[4] However, cases are widely distributed in the United States and have occurred in metropolitan areas.[5] Interestingly, it has been suggested that RMSF be called Western Hemisphere or New World spotted fever because the rickettsial diseases of humans related to spotted fever and transmitted by ticks are of worldwide distribution, and their clinical and pathologic manifestations are sufficiently close for them to be considered variants of the same disease.[3] For example, RMSF is virtually identical to Sao Paulo fever, Colombian spotted fever, fiebre maculosa, fiebre petequial, and the fiebre manchada of Mexico.[3]

After an incubation period of 2 to 12 days, symptoms of RMSF begin suddenly or gradually. Once established, the infection tends to progress steadily, reaching a peak of severity some 7 to 14 days after onset.[6] Patients who die generally have been ill for more than 1 week.[4,7]

The features of RMSF often are absent in atypical or early cases. A rash is present in only half of the patients during the first 3 days, and it never develops in between 9 and 16% of patients.[7,8] Furthermore, in one recent study,

TABLE 24–1. HUMAN RICKETTSIAL DISEASES WITH CUTANEOUS LESIONS

Disease	Etiologic Agent	Transmission
Spotted fever group		
Rocky Mountain	*Rickettsia rickettsii*	Tick bite
Rickettsialpox	*Rickettsia akari*	Mite bite
Boutonneuse fever	*Rickettsia conorii*	Tick bite
North Asian tick	*Rickettsia sibirica*	Tick bite
Queensland tick	*Rickettsia australis*	Tick bite
Typhus group		
Epidemic typhus	*Rickettsia prowazekii*	Louse feces
Brill-Zinsser	*Rickettsia prowazekii*	
Flying Squirrel	*Rickettsia prowazekii*	Ectoparasite of flying squirrel
Murine typhus	*Rickettsia typhi*	Rat flea feces
Scrub typhus group	*Rickettsia tsutsugamushi*	Mite bite

the full triad of fever, rash, and history of tick exposure was identified in only 3% of patients.

When the classic rash is observed, it appears initially as macules, papules, or petechia on the ankles, feet, wrists, and hands. The eruption spreads centripetally to involve the entire body, including the palms and soles, within 24 to 39 hours.[9] This differs from the centrifugal spread of the cutaneous eruption associated with typhus infection. Edema of the patient's face or extremities also may be seen in RMSF. The clinical differential diagnosis of RMSF includes measles, meningococcemia, other rickettsial diseases, typhoid fever, and drug eruption.

Routine laboratory tests generally are not diagnostic. However, early in the course of the disease, an elevated white cell count with increased band forms (characteristic of RMSF and atypical for acute viral infections) and a low platelet count[7,10] may be observed.

Despite antibiotic therapy, mortality from RMSF in the United States has remained at 3 to 6% of identified cases.[4,6]

Histologic Features

After spreading in the bloodstream, rickettsiae penetrate endothelial and vascular smooth muscle cells in virtually all organ systems,[9,11] where they proliferate within the cytoplasm and nuclei.[3,9,12] Wolbach described the classic histologic features of RMSF[13] and typhus.[12] Subsequent studies attributed the nature and evolution of the rash, cutaneous necrosis, and possible gangrene to localized vasculitis resulting from multiplication of rickettsiae within infected cells of the microvasculature.

In all involved organ systems, including the dermis, vasculitis is manifested by swollen or necrotic endothelial cells and infiltration of the vessel walls by the mononuclear cells. Occasionally, a few polymorphonuclear leukocytes

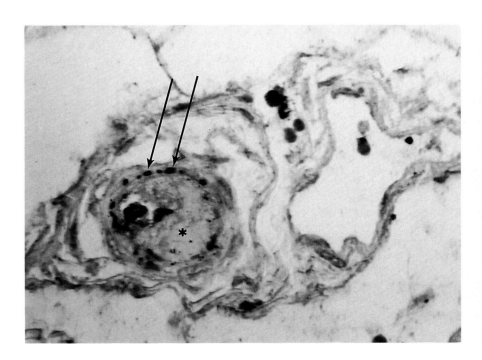

Figure 24–1. Indirect immunoperoxidase stain using hyperimmune anti-*R. rickettsii* serum demonstrates organisms within blood vessel walls (arrows) and luminal occlusion by a microthrombus. (×750.) (Courtesy of J. Stephen Dumler, MD)

are noted. The intramural vascular damage and infection by rickettsiae may result in extravasation of erythrocytes and both nonocclusive and occlusive microthrombi (Fig. 24–1).[9,11] Perivascular accumulations of mononuclear cells are an additional characteristic feature. Rickettsiae may stain bluish purple with Giemsa stain and are weakly gram negative. However, no stain differentiates rickettsiae from other bacteria.

Vascular perturbations are directly responsible for the cutaneous manifestations, as well as interstitial pneumonia, interstitial myocarditis, meningoencephalomyelitis, hepatic portal triaditis, and interstitial nephritis.[9,11] The mechanism causing the endovasculitis and capillary permeability typical of rickettsial infections is not known. Recent in vitro studies of endothelial cells infected with *R. rickettsii* have demonstrated ultrastructural evidence of damage to intracellular membranes, specifically, the rough-surfaced endoplasmic reticulum.[14] It remains to be proven whether the endothelial cell damage is due to a direct action by *R. rickettsii*, a localized cellular immune response, or possibly generation of free radicals or phospholipase A.[14]

OTHER DIAGNOSTIC TESTS

Cell Culture

Isolation of rickettsiae by culture is technically quite difficult, requiring inoculation of infected whole blood into guinea pigs, mice, or eggs and, therefore, is of limited usefulness in diagnosis.

Immunofluorescence

Direct immunofluorescence has proven to be a useful diagnostic aid when performed on fresh frozen tissue sections or tissue touch preparations early in the course of the disease.[15,16] Demonstration of specific microbial antigens by direct immunofluorescence remains the only definitive means available for early rapid diagnosis of RMSF before positive serologic reactions can be obtained.

Serologic Methods

Serologic tests have been the major method for making the diagnosis of RMSF. However, these tests are rarely positive early in the course of the illness, and they are relatively nonspecific and insensitive. The most commonly used serologic test, the Weil-Felix test, is based on the fact the rickettsiae and *Proteus vulgaris* share certain common antigens. The Weil-Felix test measures cross-reacting antibodies that agglutinate *P. vulgaris* strains OX19 or OX2. Weil-Felix agglutinins usually become elevated at 10 to 14 days after onset of symptoms but may take longer. Consequently, their use in diagnosis is diminished.

The complement-fixation test for RMSF is very specific for the spotted fever group of organisms, but it does not become positive until the second or possibly as late as the sixth week after onset of disease. Although newer, more specific and more sensitive tests are being developed, including microagglutination, microimmunofluorescence, and indirect hemagglutination techniques, a rapid diagnostic test that will improve on immunofluorescence testing of skin biopsies is still needed.

REFERENCES

1. Ricketts HT. The study of "Rocky Mountain spotted fever" (tick fever) by means of animal innoculations: a preliminary communication. *JAMA.* 1906;47:33–36.
2. Woodward TE. A historical account of the rickettsial diseases with a discussion of unsolved problems. *J Infect Dis.* 1973;127:583–594.
3. Riley HD. *Rickettsial Disease and Rocky Mountain Spotted Fever.* Part I. Chicago: Year Book; 1981:4–45.
4. Rocky Mountain Spotted Fever—United States, 1986. *MMWR.* 1987:314–315.
5. Salgo MP, Telzak EE, Currie B, et al. A focus of Rocky Mountain spotted fever within New York City. *N Engl J Med.* 1988;318:1345–348.
6. Durack DT. Rus in Urbe. Spotted fever comes to town. *N Engl J Med.* 1988;318:314–315.
7. Wilfert CM, MacCormack JN, Kleeman K, et al. Epidemiology of Rocky Mountain spotted fever as determined by active surveillance. *J Infect Dis.* 1984;150:480–488.
8. Helmick CG, Bernard KW, D'Angelo LJ. Rocky Mountain spotted fever: clinical, laboratory, and epidemiological features of 262 cases. *J Infect Dis.* 1984;150:480–488.
9. Lillie RD. The pathology of Rocky Mountain spotted fever. *NIH Bull.* 1941;177:1–10.
10. Koneti RA, Schapira M, Clements ML, et al. A prospective study of platelets and plasma proteolytic systems during the early stages of Rocky mountain spotted fever. *N Engl J Med.* 1988;318:1021–1028.
11. Walker DH, Mattern WD. Rickettsial vasculitis. *Am Heart J.* 1980;100:896–906.
12. Wolbach SB, Todd JL, Palfrey FW. Pathology of typhus in man. In: *Etiology and Pathology of Typhus,* the main report of the Typhus Research Commission of the League of Red Cross Societies of Poland. Cambridge: Harvard University Press; 1922:152–256.
13. Wolbach SR. Studies on Rocky Mountain spotted fever. *J Med Res.* 1919;41:1–197.
14. Silverman DJ. *Rickettsia rickettsii*-induced cellular injury of human vascular endothelium in vitro. Infect Immun. 1984;44:545–553.
15. Woodward TE, Pedersen ED, Oster CN, et al. Prompt confirmation of Rocky Mountain spotted fever: identification of rickettsiae in skin tissues. *J Infect Dis.* 1976;134:297–301.
16. Walker DH, Cain BG, Olmstead PM. Laboratory diagnosis of Rocky Mountain spotted fever by immunofluorescent demonstration of *Rickettsia rickettsii* in cutaneous lesions. *Am J Clin Pathol.* 1978;69:619.

CHAPTER 25
Chlamydial Infections

Myles S. Jerdan

Chlamydia are obligate intracellular parasites that are the causative agent for a diverse group of infections in humans and animals. More closely resembling bacteria than viruses, they differ from the latter by virtue of the following important characteristics: (1) they contain both DNA and RNA, (2) they multiply by binary fission, (3) they possess a cell envelope similar to that of gram-negative bacteria, (4) they contain ribosomes, (5) they possess limited but definite metabolic systems, and (6) they are susceptible to antimicrobial agents.[1] Although the gram stain is variable or negative, *Chlamydia* can be regarded as gram-negative bacteria because they are surrounded by a trilaminar envelope similar to other gram-negative bacteria.[1]

The taxonomy of *Chlamydia* has been confusing, in part because of a basic misconception regarding its name. Inclusions of the trachoma agent in infected ocular material were first observed by Halverstaedter and von Prowazek in 1907. They were thought to represent protozoans, and the name Chlamydozoacease was conferred to these "mantled animals."[2] Thus, the name *Chlamydia* (a cloak) is a misnomer, stemming from a basic misconception.[2]

Once it became clear that Chlamydiaceae could be distinguished from the other group of intracellular bacteria, the rickettsiae, by virtue of their inability to synthesize compounds for energy storage and use, by their lack of cytochromes and other components of the respiratory electron chain, and by their developmental cycle, they were moved from the order Rickettsiales and a new order, Chlamydiales, was established.[2]

The name was retained because of precedence in international rules for bacterial nomenclature. It consisted of one family, Chlamydiaceae, and one genus, *Chlamydia*. The genus *Chlamydia* is divided into two species, *Chlamydia trachomatis* and *Chlamydia psittaci*,[3] based on antigenic composition (group and specific cell wall antigen), colony morphology, intracellular inclusion, sulfonamide sensitivity, extent of DNA homology, and disease production.[1]

On the basis of biologic behavior and serology, two distinct groups of *C. trachomatis* can be identified. The group responsible for the sexually transmitted disease, lympho-granuloma venereum (the LGV group), has three serotypes, L1, L2, and L3.[3] It is generally more invasive than members of the other group, perhaps related to greater avidity for host cell receptors.[4] Unlike other chlamydiae, LGV immunotypes invade submucosal tissue and enter lymphatic vessels[5] (Table 25–1).

The second group of *C. trachomatis* comprises 12 serotypes and produces a variety of ocular and genital tract infections. They are referred to as the trachoma–inclusion conjunctivitis (TRIC) agents. The bacteria causing nongonococcal urethritis and inclusion conjunctivitis are caused by serotypes D–K[3] (Table 25–1).

LYMPHOGRANULOMA VENEREUM

Historical Background
Although LGV probably was mentioned in ancient medical texts[6] and described by John Hunter in 1786,[4] it was not until 1913 that Durand, Nicolas, and Favre recognized it as a distinct venereal disease.[7] The Frei skin test was introduced in 1925 and facilitated more specific identification of LGV infection. The causative agent was transmitted to animals in 1937 by Hellerstrom and Wassen, and Findlay isolated the agent from mice in 1933. Serologic tests followed shortly thereafter.[6]

Clinical Features
Of the 3 to 4 million Americans suffering from chlamydial infections each year, LGV is relatively uncommon, with less than 500 cases reported annually in the United States.[8] LGV is a venereal disease that is more common in tropical and semitropical countries. It is known variously as tropical or climatic bubo, strumous bubo, Nicolas-Favre disease, Frei's disease, poradenitis, fourth venereal disease, fifth venereal disease, and sixth venereal disease, lymphopathia venereum, and lymphogranuloma inguinale.[5,9] It is predominantly a disease of lymphatic and anogenital tissue, and it is characterized by three stages.[5]

After a variable incubation period of between 5 and

TABLE 25–1. HUMAN CHLAMYDIAL DISEASES

Species	Predominant Serotypes	Disease
Chlamydia trachomatis	L1, L2, L3	Lymphogranuloma venereum
Chlamydia trachomatis	A, B, Ba, C	Trachoma
Chlamydia trachomatis	D-K	Inclusion conjunctivitis Nongonorrheal urethritis Proctitis, pharyngitis, cervicitis, arthritis, epididymitis
Chlamydia psittaci		Ornithosis (psittacosis)

TABLE 25–2. CLINICAL FEATURES AND COMPLICATIONS OF LYMPHOGRANULOMA VENEREUM

Clinical Manifestations	Complications
Primary manifestations	
Vesicle, papule or ulcer	Regional lymphadenopathy Meningitis (rare)
Nongonococcal urethritis, endocervicitis	Urethral stricture, fistula, salpingitis, and parametritis
Secondary manifestations	
Inguinal syndrome	Local abscesses, sinus tracts, fistulas, ulcerations, elephantiasis
Anorectal syndrome	Rectal stricture, local abscesses, fistulas, ulcerations, elephantiasis (esthiomene)
Generalized	Lymphadenopathy, hepatosplenomegaly, erythema multiforme, erythema nodosum, polyarthritis, ulcerations

21 days, the first stage is manifested by evolution of the primary lesion, which can be a papule, a herpetiform lesion, a shallow ulcer or erosion, nonspecific urethritis,[3,6] or, less commonly, balanitis and nodular ulcerations. The most common form is the herpetiform ulcer. The primary lesion often goes unnoticed or never develops fully. It is painless.[6]

The second stage, which may last from days to weeks, is heralded by a significant systemic component and trophism for lymphoid tissue.[4] Unlike most other chlamydial infections, involvement of the lymphoid tissue rather than epithelial surfaces is the preferential pathologic event.[5] Consequently, inguinal lymphadenopathy follows, which is a constant finding in men (resulting in a positive groove sign due to inguinal lymphadenopathy on either side of Poupart's ligament) and a variable feature of infected women. Proctitis is a common feature in women owing to the preferred iliac and anorectal lymph drainage as compared to the inguinal drainage in men.[9] Proctocolitis has been observed frequently in homosexual men.[10] Involved lymph nodes are initially firm but subsequently suppurate and form draining sinuses. If left untreated, the lymphadenopathy often subsides in 2 to 3 months.

The long-term sequelae occur during the third stage, when fibrosis leads to lymphatic obstruction. This results in tertiary manifestations, which include elephantiasis of the genital region, rectal strictures, and hypertrophic ulceration of the pudenda, which is referred to as *esthiomene* in females (Greek for "eating away"). In addition, fistulas may develop that can result in rectovaginal fistulas in females, causing what has been referred to as the watering can perineum and rectal stricture[4] (Table 25–2).

Histologic Features
Early investigators thought that the pathologic features of LGV were distinct and were the same in the primary lesion, the bubonulus (a large, tender lymphangial nodule), and inguinal lymph nodes.[11] Furthermore, the histologic features of LGV were believed to be sufficiently distinct to permit differentiations of LGV from other venereal infections.[11] Today, histologic features of the primary lesions are considered nonspecific, and lymph node biopsies are considered relatively specific if the characteristic stellate microabscesses are identified.[9]

The primary lesion is a papule or vesicle (either intraepidermal or subepidermal), the histologic features of which

are nondiagnostic. Similarly, the shallow ulcer that usually follows generally is not specific for LGV. The surface of the ulcer is bathed in exudate composed of fibrin, cellular debris, and occasional neutrophils, and the ulcer base is surrounded by a mixed cellular infiltrate composed predominantly of large mononuclear cells with an admixture of occasional neutrophils. The mononuclear cells often proliferate to form solid granulomas.[11] Although some authors have described endothelial swelling and reactive connective tissue, in addition to a mixed inflammatory response,[12] others have noted no significant endothelial proliferation or thrombosis.[11] Rather, vessel occlusion seemed to occur as a result of compression by mononuclear cells within the granulomas. This resulted in necrosis and small abscesses within the granulomas.[11]

Edema and fibroblastic proliferation with prominent and dilated lymphatics have been observed at the periphery of the lesion,[11] and plasma cells tend to be increased toward the periphery of the lesion.[11] The adjacent skin may show pseudoepitheliomatous hyperplasia.[13,14] Should chlamydial inclusions be observed in phagocytes by Giemsa stain, the otherwise nonspecific nature of the cutaneous lesions takes on added significance.[15] Giemsa stain, which can be used on tissue sections and conjunctival smears, demonstrates purple staining of the elementary bodies in contrast to the blue of the host cell cytoplasm; the larger, noninfective reticulate body type intracytoplasmic cell inclusions stain blue. Fully formed, mature inclusions are compact perinuclear masses that stain dark purple. The Giemsa stain is relatively tedious to perform and has poor sensitivity and specificity.

Initially, the lymph node shows a nonspecific reactive hyperplasia and permeation of the tissue, primarily the cortex, by mononuclear cells. Subsequently, small granulomas form associated with necrosis of their centers, which form small abscesses. Coalescence of these minute abscesses eventuates in the characteristic irregular, elongated stellate abscess.[11,13,16] (Fig. 25–1). This is characterized by a rim of granulomatous reaction composed of epithelioid histiocytes admixed with occasional Langhans or foreign body

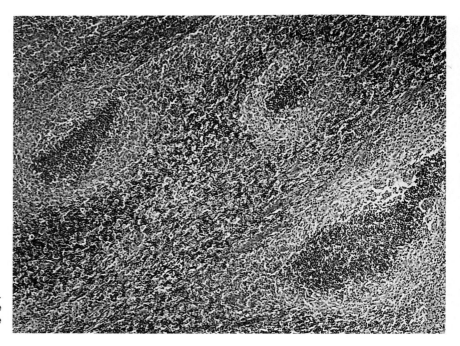

Figure 25–1. Lymphogranuloma venereum. Lymph node with several characteristic stellate abscesses. (H&E, ×80.) (*Courtesy of George Lupton, MD.*)

giant cells around the center of the abscesses.[11,16] Surrounding the granulomatous reaction is an intense infiltrate composed of plasma cells and lymphocytes. The great dominance of plasma cells has been emphasized by some authors.[16] The uninvolved portions of the lymph node show large follicles with prominent and active germinal centers.[11] Although these stellate abscesses, consisting of focal areas of suppuration surrounded by a granulomatous wall, are distinctive, they are not pathognomonic of LGV, since similar abscesses can be seen in such disease as cat-scratch fever, certain fungal infections, and occasionally tularemia.[15,17]

Giemsa stain or immunofluorescent technique occasionally will show inclusion bodies within the phagocytes. Gamna described cytoplasmic inclusions, 1 to 4 μm in size, in mononuclear cells from lymph nodes in patients with LGV.[9,18] Several investigators have identified these Gamna bodies and considered them to be of diagnostic value.[9] These inclusions stain blue with Giemsa stain and may be similar in appearance to initial bodies, but according to one study, they represent phagocytized cellular debris.[11]

OTHER DIAGNOSTIC TESTS

Cell Culture

Isolation of *C. trachomatis* in cell culture remains the most sensitive and specific test for identifying the agent. Consequently, when it is available and cost efficient, it is the diagnostic method of choice.[19] However, since *C. trachomatis* is an obligate intracellular pathogen, cell culture techniques similar to those required for viral isolation are necessary. This may prove to be a logistic obstacle for proper identification.

Antigen Detection Methods

As a result of the inherent problems with cell culture, antigen detection methods have emerged as practical alternatives, albeit less specific and less sensitive. Both direct immunofluorescence and enzyme-linked immunoassay (ELISA) methods are available, and they are particularly useful for diagnosis of mucopurulent cervicitis, endometritis, pelvic inflammatory disease, acute urethritis, or acute proctitis.[19] Cross reactivity exists between various stains of *C. trachomatis*. Although there is some discrepancy about which method is most reliable, newer diagnostic tests, such as these and others being developed, hold promise for earlier recognition and more specific diagnosis of chlamydial genital infections.[19]

Vaginopancervical (Fast) Smears

Another convenient, but controversial, diagnostic method for detection of chlamydial infection is the Papanicolaou-stained vaginopancervical (fast) smear.[20–24] However, cytology has not been very successful for diagnosis of LGV. Criteria for evaluating such smears have been proposed and are being refined. Important features include an acute inflammatory background and chlamydial acidophilic intracytoplasmic, initial and intermediate morphologic forms within metaplastic cells.[20] If proven sensitive and specific, they will be of great value in detecting chlamydial infection[19–22,24] in women.

REFERENCES

1. Manire GP, Wyrick PB. The chlamydia. In: Brause AI, Davis CE, Fierer J, eds. *Infectious Diseases and Medical Microbiology*. 2nd ed. Philadelphia: WB Saunders Company; 1986:449.

2. Ward ME. Chlamydial classification, development and structure. *Br Med Bull.* 1983;39:109.

3. Schachter J. Chlamydial infections. *N Engl J Med.* 1978;298:428, 490.

4. Hammerschlat MR. Lymphogranuloma venereum. In: Felman YM, ed. *Sexually Transmitted Diseases.* New York: Churchill Livingstone; 1986:93.

5. Perine PL. Lymphogranuloma venereum. In: Strickland T, ed. *Hunter's Tropical Medicine.* 6th ed. Philadelphia: WB Saunders Co; 1984:238–242.

6. Schacter J, Osoba AO. Lymphogranuloma venereum. *Br Med Bull.* 1983;39:151.

7. Durand M, Nicolas J, Favre M. Lymphogranulomatose inguinale subaigue d'origine genital probable, peut-etre venerienee. *Bull Mem Soc Med Hops.* 1913;35:274–277.

8. Centers for Disease Control. Chlamydia trachomatis infections: Policy guidelines for prevention and control. *MMWR.* 1985;34(suppl):53S–73S.

9. Becker LE. Lymphogranuloma venereum. *Int J Dermatol.* 1976;15:26–33.

10. Quinn TC, Stamm WE, Goodell SE, et al. The polymicrobial origin of intestinal infections in homosexual men. *N Engl J Med.* 1983;309:576–582.

11. Sheldon WH, Heyman A. Lymphogranuloma venereum. *Am J Pathol.* 1947;23:653–664.

12. Stannus HS. *A Sixth Venereal Disease.* London: Bailliere, Tindall & Cox; 1933.

13. Kornblith BA. Observations on lymphogranuloma venereum. Clinical pathological study of sixty cases with observations on the histopathology of the Frei test. *Surg Gynecol Obstet.* 1936;63:99–102.

14. Smith EB, Custer RP. The histopathology of lymphogranuloma venereum. *J Urol.* 1950;63:546–548.

15. Von Lichtenberg F. Infectious diseases: viral, chlamydial, rickettsial, and bacterial diseases. In: Robbins SL, Cotran RS, Kumar V, eds. *Pathologic Basis of Disease.* 3rd ed. Philadelphia: WB Saunders Co; 1984;292–294.

16. Jorgensen L. Lymphgranuloma venereum: a study of the pathology and the pathogenic problems based on observation of eight cases examined post mortem. *Acta Pathol Microbiol Scand.* 1959;47:113–139.

17. Lever WF, Schaumburg-Lever G. Lymphogranuloma venereum. In: *Histopathology of the Skin.* 6th ed. Philadelphia: JB Lippincott Co; 1983:314–315.

18. Gamna C. Sur petiologie de la lymphogranulomatose inginale subaigue. *Presse Med.* 1924;32:404–405.

19. Stamm WE. Diagosis of *Chlamydia trachomatis* genitourinary infections. *Ann Intern Med.* 1988;108:710–717.

20. Gupta PK, Shurbaji MS, Mintor JL, et al. Cytopathologic detection of *Chlamydia trachomatis* in vaginopancervical (fast) smears. *Diag Cytopathol.* 1988.

21. Kiviat NB, Paavonnen JA, Brockway J, et al. Cytologic manifestations of cervical and vaginal infections: I: epithelial and inflammatory cellular changes. *JAMA.* 1985;253:989–996.

22. Kiviat NB, Peterson M, Kinney-Thomas E, et al. Cytologic manifestations of cervical and vaginal infections. II: confirmation of *Chlamydia trachomatis* infection by direct immunofluorescence using monoclonal antibodies. *JAMA.* 1985;253:997–1000.

23. Spence MR, Barbacci M, Kappus E, Quinn T. A correlative study of Papanicolaou smear, fluorescent antibody, and culture for the diagnosis of *Chlamydia trachomatis. Obstet Gynecol.* 1986;68:691–695.

24. Stamm WE, Harrison R, Alexander ER, et al. Diagnosis of *Chlamydia trachomatis* infections by direct immunofluorescence staining of genital secretions. *Ann Intern Med.* 1984;101:638–641.

CHAPTER 26

Mycobacterial Infections
James P. Fields and Wayne M. Meyers

TUBERCULOSIS

In the early 19th century, Laennec proposed the common etiology of the diverse lesions of tuberculosis and was the first to describe and recognize a cutaneous tubercle—the prosector's wart (tuberculosis verrucosa cutis). The genius of this observation is remarkable considering that Koch did not identify the etiologic agent *Mycobacterium tuberculosis* until 1882, more than half a century later. This early recognition of the etiology of tuberculosis and the high susceptibility of experimental animals made tuberculosis a paradigm for understanding granulomatous infections, and much of our knowledge of cell-mediated immunity and delayed-type hypersensitivity came from observations on tuberculosis.

Primary Tuberculosis

Primary Inoculation Tuberculosis

CLINICAL FEATURES. In individuals not sensitized to antigens of *M. tuberculosis,* the inoculation of tubercle bacilli into the skin produces a local lesion and inflammation of regional lymph nodes. The initial lesion appears as a small papule that becomes a painless ulcer with ragged undermined edges.

HISTOLOGIC FEATURES. Within 2 weeks, neutrophils infiltrate the inoculation site, and there is necrosis. After approximately 6 weeks, epithelioid cells and giant cells replace the suppuration. Tubercles may develop in the later stages, but caseation is not constant. Acid-fast bacilli are abundant in the early stages but become rare as granulomas develop. Prosector's paronychia in pathologists is a classic example of this lesion[1] (Fig. 26–1).

Generalized Miliary Tuberculosis

CLINICAL FEATURES. In anergic patients with fulminant tuberculosis, there may be hematogenous spread to the skin, especially in children. The lesions are present all over the body, but particularly on the trunk. They may be macules or papules, with or without purpura or central necrosis.

HISTOLOGIC FEATURES. In the dermis, there are perivascular infiltrations of neutrophils and lymphocytes with microabscesses. Acid-fast bacilli are numerous in severe forms but rare in milder cases.

Reinfection Tuberculosis

Patients sensitized to antigens of *M. tuberculosis*, either by healed or quiescent infections or coexisting tuberculosis, develop local delayed-type hypersensitivity reactions when reinfected in the skin by tubercle bacilli. Reinfection may be by hematogenous spread from reactivated foci or, less commonly, by local inoculation. Horwitz, in a study of 3902 patients with lupus vulgaris, found that one third eventually developed pulmonary tuberculosis, one third had pulmonary tuberculosis before lupus vulgaris, and one third had simultaneous onset of pulmonary tuberculosis and lupus vulgaris.[2]

Lupus Vulgaris

CLINICAL FEATURES. This is the most common form of cutaneous reinfection tuberculosis, with peak incidences at 20 years to 50 years of age. Lesions are usually solitary, brownish red, and soft and involve the head and neck. They are chronic and progressive, and if they remain untreated, scarring can cause marked disfigurement.

HISTOLOGIC FEATURES. There may be ulceration, but usually the epidermis shows hyperkeratosis, acanthosis, hyperplasia, or occasionally squamous cell carcinoma. Cellular infiltrations frequently involve only the upper dermis but may involve the entire dermis. There are admixtures of epithelioid cells, giant cells, and lymphocytes, and well-formed tuberculoid granulomas are common, with little or no necrosis (Fig. 26–2). Acid-fast bacilli are rare. With healing, there is extensive fibrosis leading to atrophic scars.

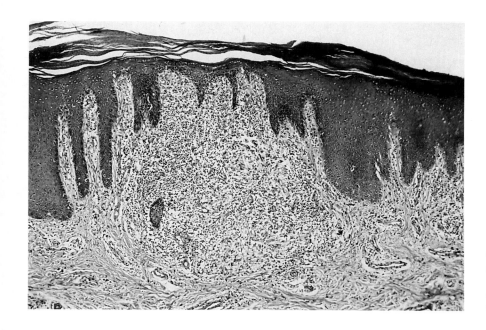

Figure 26–1. Inoculation tuberculosis in the finger of a pathologist. This lesion is in a granulomatous (late) phase. The granuloma is comprised of epithelioid cell nests, a few giant cells and large numbers of lymphocytes. (H&E ×80.) (*AFIP neg 87–5148.*)

Tuberculosis Verrucosa Cutis

CLINICAL FEATURES. Reinfection in exquisitely hypersensitive patients tends to provoke florid epidermal responses that produce an often solitary verrucous lesion usually seen on the hands in adults and the lower extremities in children.

HISTOLOGIC FEATURES. The epidermis shows hyperkeratosis, parakeratosis, acanthosis, or pseudoepitheliomatous hyperplasia. In the epidermis or upper dermis, there are neutrophils. Tuberculoid granulomas with slight to moderate necrosis infiltrate the upper or middermis (Fig. 26–3). Acid-fast bacilli are rare but usually can be demonstrated.

Scrofuloderma (Tuberculosis Cutis Colliquativa)

CLINICAL FEATURES. Scrofuloderma is extension of tuberculosis into skin from underlying mycobacterial infection. Cervical mycobacterial lymphadenitis is most common in children and is frequently nontuberculous, with scotochromogens (e.g., *Mycobacterium scrofulaceum*) being the most common, followed by *Mycobacterium avium-intracellulare*, Runyon group I (probably *Mycobacterium kansasii*) and rarely by rapid-growing mycobacteria.[3] *Mycobacterium bovis* is a well-known cause of scrofuloderma.

HISTOLOGIC FEATURES. A necrotic sinus tract extends through the dermis and ulcerates the epidermis. Chronic inflamma-

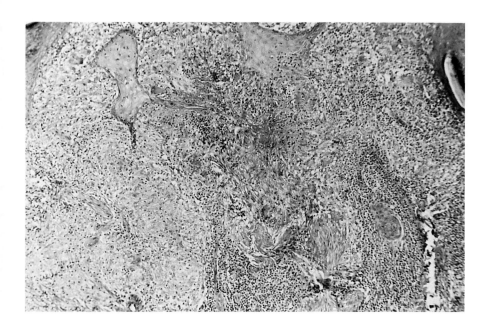

Figure 26–2. Lupus vulgaris. The epidermis is hyperplastic. In the dermis there are epithelioid cell granulomas with lymphocytes and occasional giant cells. There is a small focus of necrosis in the center of the photograph. (H&E ×50.) (*AFIP neg 57–9804.*)

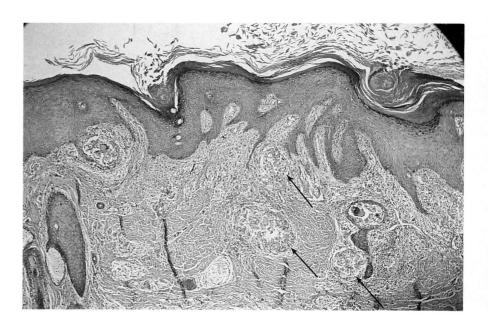

Figure 26–3. Tuberculosis verrucosa cutis. There are hyperkeratosis and acanthosis, with scattered tuberculoid granulomas in the dermis. (H&E ×50.) (*AFIP neg 58–4939.*)

tory cells and tuberculoid granulomas with caseation necrosis frequently surround the sinus. Acid-fact bacilli often are readily demonstrable.

Tuberculosis Cutis Orificialis

CLINICAL FEATURES. Tuberculosis cutis orificialis arises from autoinoculation of mucous membranes by *M. tuberculosis* from internal lesions and is rare where tuberculosis is well controlled. Frequent sites are the mouth, anus, and vulva.

HISTOLOGIC FEATURES. The mucous membrane is ulcerated, with acute inflammatory cells in the base underlaid by mixed acute and chronic inflammation. Chronic lesions may contain tuberculoid granulomas with caseation. Acid-fact bacilli are abundant.

Tuberculids

Some authorities argue that tuberculids are local hyperergic responses to mycobacteria or mycobacterial antigens disseminated hematogenously from foci of active tuberculosis.[4,5] Others consider tuberculids a misnomer and unrelated to tuberculosis. We believe that papulonecrotic tuberculids and lichen scrofulosorum are tuberculids and hypersensitivity responses to mycobacterial antigens. The pathogenesis of the tuberculid, erythema induratum of Bazin, may be less certain, but a relationship to tuberculosis is tenable.[6] Diagnosis of tuberculids depends not only on consistent histopathologic changes but also on the coexistence of tuberculosis, positive tuberculin reaction, and response to antituberculosis therapy.

Papulonecrotic Tuberculid. The lesions consist of multiple necrotizing papules occurring bilaterally on the extensor surfaces of the extremities. They tend to occur in crops and spontaneously involute, leaving residual scars.

HISTOLOGIC FEATURES. There is coagulation necrosis that usually is ovoid but becomes flask-shaped with ulceration. The necrotic area is surrounded by lymphocytes and histiocytes.

Vascular changes are prominent, can be at all levels of the dermis and subcutis, and range from mild lymphocytic vasculitis to fibrinoid necrosis and thrombosis. There may be occasional foci of epithelioid cells and giant cells at the periphery of the necrotic area but no tuberculoid granulomas. Acid-fast bacilli are not seen.

Lichen Scrofulosorum. Lesions are composed of small asymptomatic lichenoid papules usually confined to the trunks of children with tuberculosis.

HISTOLOGIC FEATURES. Tuberculoid granulomas develop in any area of the dermis, but especially around hair follicles and sweat glands. There is usually no necrosis. Acid-fast bacilli are not seen.

Erythema Induratum of Bazin. These chronic, recurrent, nodular, ulcerative lesions occur most commonly on the lower legs of women. The nodules often undergo central necrosis and ulceration. Resolution is accompanied by scarring.

HISTOLOGIC FEATURES. The initial changes are in the subcutis but may extend to the dermis and eventually ulcerate. Vasculitis and panniculitis are prominent. Vascular changes range from endothelial swelling to complete occlusion and necrosis. Fat lobules may be infiltrated with lymphocytes, plasma cells and neutrophils, or granulomatous inflammation. Acid-fast bacilli are not seen.

The histopathologic features of cutaneous tuberculosis are summarized in Table 26–1.

LEPROSY

Pathogenesis and Immunology

Mycobacterium leprae, initially observed by Hansen in 1873, was the first bacterium known to cause chronic disease in humans. It does so by its proclivity to survive and multiply

TABLE 26–1. HISTOPATHOLOGIC FEATURES OF CUTANEOUS TUBERCULOSIS

Type	Histologic Features	Acid-fast Bacilli
Primary		
Primary inoculation	Early: Neutrophils with necrosis Late: Tuberculoid granulomas Caseation variable	Early: many Late: rare
Miliary	Microabscesses	Rare to many
Reinfection		
Lupus vulgaris	Tuberculoid granulomas; little or no caseation	Rare
Tuberculosis verrucosa cutis	Acanthosis or pseudoepitheliomatous hyperplasia; abscesses in epidermis; tuberculoid granulomas with moderate caseation	Rare
Scrofuloderma (tuberculosis cutis colliquativa)	Sinus tract with ulceration, surrounded by chronic inflammation and tuberculoid granulomas with caseation	Few
Tuberculosis cutis orificialis	Ulcer with acute and chronic inflammation, or tuberculoid granulomas with caseation	Many
Tuberculids		
Papulonecrotic	Vasculitis prominent, ranging from mild lymphocytic infiltrates to necrosis and thrombosis; necrosis with surrounding epithelioid and giant cells but no well-formed granulomas	None
Lichen scrofulosorum	Tuberculoid granulomas, especially around adnexae; usually no caseation	None
Erythema induratum	Initial panniculitis with later extension to dermis; vasculitis ranging from endothelial swelling to occlusion and necrosis; acute and chronic inflammation, sometimes with tuberculoid granulomas	None

in macrophages. When infection occurs, if the host's cell-mediated immune response is optimal, macrophages will readily digest the organism and prevent the occurrence of clinical disease. On the other hand, with suboptimal immune response, *M. leprae* causes a clinical and histopathologic spectrum of disease that manifests in varying forms, generally reflecting the destructive rather than the protective aspects of the immune response. The two spectral poles are the high immune tuberculoid form and the low host resistant lepromatous form. The key feature of the latter seems to correlate with ineffective killing of *M. leprae* by macrophages.

Since no specific differences exist in vitro between lepromatous and normal macrophages, attention has been appropriately directed toward T lymphocytes, which activate macrophage function.[7] Qualitatively, there is a disturbance of the blood T:B lymphocyte ratio in lepromatous patients, characterized by a significant reduction in the total number of circulating T lymphocytes and a moderate increase in B lymphocytes.[8] Lepromatous patients demonstrate unresponsiveness in vivo by lepromin skin test and in vitro by lymphocyte transformation and macrophage migration inhibition tests to antigens of *M. leprae*.[9,10] Suppressor activity in the presence of lepromin is induced in normal mononuclear cells by T cell-enriched peripheral blood leukocytes from lepromatous patients but not from tuberculoid patients.[11] This antigen-specific suppression is mediated by activated lymphocytes of the T suppressor phenotype, with high correlation for Ia antigen positivity and Fc receptors for IgG.[12] Besides suppressor activity to account for the lack of proliferative T cell response and macrophage activation, insufficient production or availability of interleukin 2 (IL-2) appears to be an important immunologic defect in lepromatous leprosy. The peripheral blood mononuclear cells of lepromatous patients fail to produce the macrophage activator, gamma-interferon, but are capable of responding

to *M. leprae* antigens up to the point of IL-2-induced proliferation, and they will undergo clonal proliferation and produce gamma-interferon after the addition of IL-2 to the in vitro system.[13] Further, there are significantly fewer T helper and IL-2-producing cells in lepromatous as compared with tuberculoid infiltrates. IL-2 is known to be adsorbed to and consumed by T suppressor cells, which is the predominant subset in lepromatous lesions.[14–16]

Diagnosis and Bacteriologic Numerical Indices

M. leprae measures 0.3 to 0.5 μm wide by 4 to 7 μm long and morphologically resembles *M. tuberculosis*, although it possesses a weaker degree of acid-fastness. Bacilli that stain solidly are viable, whereas those that stain in a granular fashion are nonviable. The microscopic examination of skin slit smears obtained from the edge of leprosy lesions and ear lobes, stained by the Ziehl-Neelsen technique, is an important diagnostic screening and prognostic procedure. Incisional skin biopsies of approximately 1.5 cm in length taken from the active advancing border of a suspected lesion, extending deeply enough into the subcutis to include deep nerve bundles, are ideal specimens for diagnostic study. The tissue is fixed in 10% buffered neutral formalin and stained for acid-fast bacilli by the Fite-Faraco method or one of its modifications.[17]

The numerical index that measures the density of bacilli in a smear or biopsy is the Bacterial Index (BI).[18] It is determined by estimating the number of acid-fast bacilli using an oil immersion objective (100×) and is expressed on a logarithmic scale (Table 26–2). This index is important in classifying the various forms of leprosy and in measuring therapeutic response. Effective treatment is associated with an expected fall of 1 index point annually.

TABLE 26–2. THE BACTERIAL INDEX (BI)

BI	Average No. of Acid-fast Bacilli in Oil Immersion Field
6+	Over 1000/field (many clumps)
5+	100–1000/field
4+	10–100/field
3+	1–10/field
2+	1–10/10 fields
1+	1–10/100 fields
0	0/100 fields

The Morphologic Index (MI) is defined as the percentage of normal-appearing, solid-staining, acid-fast bacilli in smears or sections. It is broadly a measure of viability, although the time of biologic death and degenerate staining do not precisely coincide. The MI indicates the potential infectiousness of the patient, the therapeutic response, or development of relapse in treated patients.[19]

Histologic Criteria for Classification

Ridley and Jopling have devised a reproducible diagnostic classification of established leprosy based on immunopathologic data.[20,21] Five objective histopathologic criteria have been identified that correlate with the immunologic parameters in patients and form the microscopic basis for the Ridley–Jopling classification. These include the granuloma cell type, the bacterial load (BI), the number and distribution of lymphocytes, pathologic changes in nerves, and the presence or absence of encroachment of the subepidermal grenz zone and epidermis. The spectrum of established leprosy is continuous, extending from the high immune polar tuberculoid (TT) through borderline tuberculoid (BT), borderline (BB), borderline lepromatous (BL), and subpolar lepromatous (LLs) to the low immune polar lepromatous (LLp). The polar groups are immunologically stable, TT being incapable of downgrading and LL of upgrading. The borderline groups are unstable and are prone to shift toward either pole. Midborderline (BB) leprosy is so unstable that it is rarely observed and thus is not considered further.

Granuloma
Epithelioid cells are present in TT, BT, and occasionally in BL, but never in LL. Large, well-differentiated Langhans giant cells are a feature of TT that has upgraded from BT. Smaller Langhans giant cells may be fairly numerous in BT. No giant cells are present in BL. In LL, foreign body type giant cells containing fatty vacuoles may be seen. In any group, there may be no giant cells. Large numbers of undifferentiated giant cells may occur in the reversal (upgrading) reaction. Macrophages comprise the granuloma of BL and LL, and they contain more abundant foamy cytoplasm in LL than in BL.

Bacterial Load
The density of bacilli in granulomas delineates the position within the two halves of the spectrum, being low in tubercu-loid and high in lepromatous granulomas. Bacterial load is most useful in differentiating between BT and BL where classification is otherwise difficult. It also serves to authenticate the cell type. If the BI does not correlate with the identified cell type, it may indicate a misconception of the cell identity, that the patient has been treated, or that the staining technique has failed.

Lymphocytes
The number and distribution of lymphocytes are useful in subdividing both epithelioid and macrophage granulomas. In TT, lymphocytes are numerous and surround the periphery of well-developed epithelioid cell granulomas in the deep dermis. In BT, they vary in number and sometimes are numerous within the granuloma, forming clusters rather than being scattered diffusely throughout or peripheral to it. Numerous lymphocytes that diffusely infiltrate entire foci of macrophage granulomas or circumscribe a nerve signify BL. Lymphocytes are more sparse in LLs, where they form clusters that do not extend to the peripheral margin of the granuloma, and they are scant to absent in LLp.

Nerves
Marked swelling of nerves in the deep dermis or subcutis with or without central necrosis is indicative of TT. Cellular infiltration of nerves and lamination of perineurium also are useful criteria. In TT, there is minimal penetration of the perineurium, which seems to separate the epithelioid cell granuloma within the nerve from the lymphocytes without. There may be marked lymphocytic infiltration of the perineurium in both BT and BL, but perineural (onion skin) lamination is present in BL. Laminated perineurium without lymphocytes characterizes LLs, and dermal nerve changes are minimal in LLp.

Subepidermal Grenz Zone and Epidermis
The grenz zone is uninvolved in all forms of leprosy except TT and sometimes BT. Infiltration of the grenz zone with effacement of the epidermis usually is observed in TT unless the granuloma is situated deeply. The clinical and histopathologic features used to classify the various forms of leprosy are summarized in Table 26–3.

Classification and the Spectrum

Indeterminate Leprosy

CLINICAL FEATURES. Indeterminate leprosy is often the first manifestation, appearing as one or few hypopigmented or mildly erythematous macules or patches, with the capacity to heal spontaneously or progress to one of the more advanced stages.

HISTOLOGIC FEATURES. Microscopic changes reflect the absence of delayed hypersensitivity to mycobacterial antigens, manifested only by a mild lymphoid infiltrate surrounding neurovascular bundles and adnexae[22] (Fig. 26–4). Visualization of an acid-fast bacillus in a nerve structure is diagnostic (Fig. 26–5).

TABLE 26–3. CLASSIFICATION OF LEPROSY

	Indeterminate (I)	Polar Tuberculoid (TT)	Borderline Tuberculoid (BT)	Borderline Lepromatous (BL)	Subpolar Lepromatous (LLs)	Polar Lepromatous (LLp)
Clinical features						
Skin lesions	Ill-defined hypopigmented or mildly erythematous macule or patch	One or few anesthetic macules or plaques with well-defined borders	Lesions similar to TT but more numerous and with less distinct borders; satellite lesions may be present	Symmetrical circinate maculopapules, nodules, or plaques with vague borders	Residual BL Lesions with symmetrical macules, patches, papules, or plaques	Widespread symmetrical nodules, plaques, or diffuse infiltration
Peripheral nerves	Not clinically involved	Early involvement common	Early involvement common	Some nerve damage	Nerve damage late	Nerve damage late, with loss of sensation in acral regions
Lepromin reaction (Mitsuda)	Negative or weakly positive	Strongly positive	Positive	Negative	Negative	Negative
Histologic features						
Grenz zone	Present	Absent	Absent or present	Present	Present	Present
Granuloma	Absent	Large, well-developed epithelioid cell granuloma	Epithelioid cell granuloma	Macrophage granuloma with small foci of epithelioid cells	Compact macrophage granuloma; plasma cells may be present	Macrophage granuloma with foamy histiocytes
Giant cells	Absent	Numerous and often large Langhans type	Langhans and undifferentiated giant cells	Absent	Absent	Foreign body type containing fatty vacuoles
Lymphocytes	Mild lymphocytic infiltrate around neurovascular bundles and skin appendages	Large numbers surround granulomas	Moderate numbers invade granulomas	Numerous, diffusely infiltrate granulomas or surround nerves	Sparse, may form small clusters in granuloma	Scant to absent
Neural involvement	Perineural inflammation	Epithelioid granulomas in deep nerves with or without necrosis	Epithelioid granulomas in nerves; lymphocytic invasion of perineurium	Lymphocytic invasion of perineurium; laminated perineurium	Perineural lamination without lymphocytes	Minimal changes in dermal nerves
Density of acid-fast bacilli in biopsy specimen	Rare to none	Rare, usually seen in nerves or papillary dermis	Scanty, usually seen in nerves	Plentiful in nerves	Abundant	Numerous

343

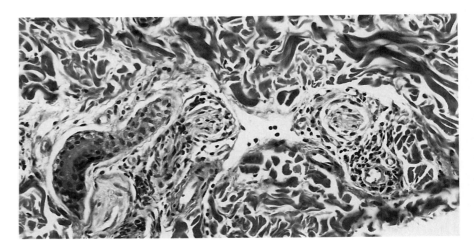

Figure 26–4. Indeterminate leprosy showing mild lymphocytic infiltrations along neurovascular bundles at lower limit of the dermis. (H&E ×325.) (*AFIP neg 84–7138.*)

Tuberculoid Leprosy (TT)

CLINICAL FEATURES. Tuberculoid lesions remain localized, are single or few in number, and are macular or annular plaques with sharply demarcated, sometimes fine papular borders. Centrally, they may be atrophic, hypopigmented, scaly, anesthetic, dry, and hairless. Painful peripheral nerves may be palpably enlarged.

HISTOLOGIC FEATURES. The epidermis is characteristically effaced by a dermal epithelioid cell granuloma associated

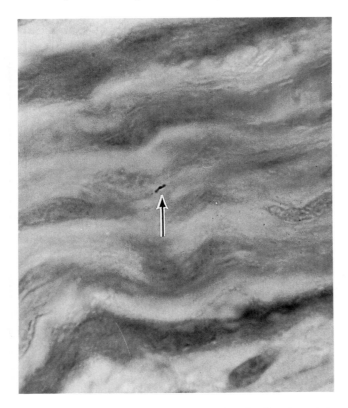

Figure 26–5. Indeterminate leprosy. Acid-fast bacillus (arrow) in nerve in lower dermis. (Fite-Faraco stain, ×1890.) (*AFIP neg 72–12469.*)

with Langhans giant cells and lymphocytes, which form a peripheral mantle around the deeply situated granulomas (Figs. 26–6, 26–7). A high proportion of T helper cells are distributed within the granuloma. Lesser numbers of suppressor cells are present, these being present in the peripheral mantle.[23] Large nerve structures are involved with epithelioid cell granulomas surrounded by lymphocytes (Fig. 26–8). Such nerves may undergo acute segmental necrosis and ultimate fibrosis. Rare acid-fast bacilli may be seen in nerves or in the superficial papillary dermis. BI is 0 to 1+.

Borderline Tuberculoid Leprosy (BT)

CLINICAL FEATURES. Clinically, BT lesions resemble TT lesions, but they are more numerous, somewhat less sharply delimited at their margins, and may exhibit smaller adjacent satellite lesions. Nerve damage occurs early and is associated initially with pain and later sensory and motor impairment in the involved nerve trunks.

HISTOLOGIC FEATURES. Beneath an epidermis that shows variably absent to slight effacement lies an epithelioid cell granuloma associated with moderate numbers of lymphocytes that spread into the granuloma (Fig. 26–9). Giant cells when present are undifferentiated. Nerve structures are more easily identifiable than in TT, although they, along with pilosebaceous units and sweat glands, may be involved by tuberculoid granulomas. BI is 0 to 2+.

Borderline Lepromatous Leprosy (BL)

CLINICAL FEATURES. Clinically, the skin lesions are bilaterally symmetrical, hypopigmented or erythematous circinate or irregularly shaped maculopapules, infiltrative nodules or plaques with smooth surfaces, not sharply delimited at their borders, and not associated with sensory impairment.

HISTOLOGIC FEATURES. Microscopically, there is an uneven mixture of macrophages, irregularly dispersed lymphocytes, and small foci of epithelioid cells. Nerve structures typically show perineural infiltration, thickening, and easily identifiable acid-fast bacilli (Fig. 26–10). BI is 4 to 5+.

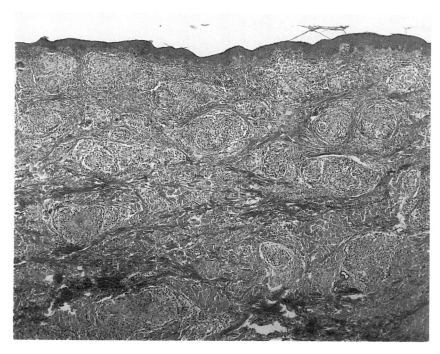

Figure 26–6. Tuberculoid leprosy (TT) showing dermal and subcutaneous granulomas. (H&E ×25.) (*AFIP neg 72–12492.*)

Subpolar Lepromatous Leprosy (LLs)

CLINICAL FEATURES. This form of leprosy may evolve from downgrading of BL, and one may see residual borderline skin lesions in association with widespread symmetrically distributed, hypopigmented or slightly erythematous discrete and coalescent macules, papules, patches, and thin plaques.

HISTOLOGIC FEATURES. Beneath a clear subepidermal grenz zone lies a compact macrophage granuloma containing few lymphocytes in small clumps or diffusely scattered, admixed with occasional plasma cells. Lymphocytes of both helper and suppressor phenotypes are diffusely distributed among the macrophages. T suppressor cells are about twice as numerous as T helper cells in untreated lepromatous leprosy, and treatment is followed by an increase in T helper cells.[24] As the macrophages age, they accumulate lipid and form a foamy cytoplasm. Regressing lesions may contain large foamy vacuoles within giant cells. Nerves with laminated perineurium are characteristic (Figs. 26–11, 26–12). BI is 5 to 6+.

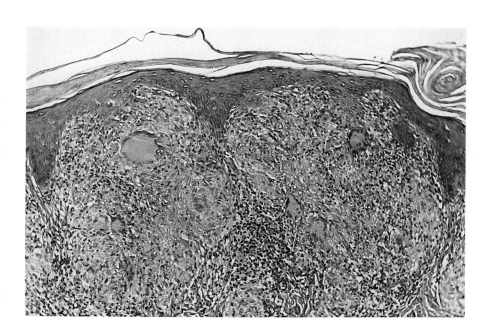

Figure 26–7. Tuberculoid leprosy (TT). Epithelioid and Langhans giant cell granuloma with lymphocytes, extending up to the lower epidermal margin. Focal parakeratosis is present. (H&E ×160.) (*AFIP neg 72–12465.*)

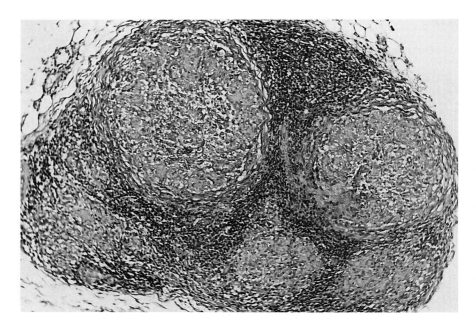

Figure 26–8. Tuberculoid leprosy (TT). Fascicles of nerves in subcutis, replaced by epithelioid cell granulomas, surrounded by lymphocytes. (H&E ×130.) (*AFIP neg 72–12463.*) *Note:* Figures 26–6, 26–7, and 26–8 are from the same specimen

Polar Lepromatous Leprosy (LLp)

CLINICAL FEATURES. In this form of leprosy are seen shiny, smooth nodules and infiltrative plaques and thickening of the skin of the ears and face, with loss of eyebrows and eyelashes. Nerve damage occurs late, with loss of sensation in the acral regions. A type of LLp called "diffuse lepromatous leprosy" occurs chiefly in persons from Mexico or Central America who are anergic and in whom the skin becomes diffusely infiltrated. These patients appear normal except for slight facial puffiness until facial hair is lost or the erythema nodosum leprosum reaction supervenes.

HISTOLOGIC FEATURES. Beneath a clear supepidermal grenz zone lies a macrophage granuloma composed of abundant, vacuolated, foamy cytoplasm (Virchow cells), initially surrounding cutaneous appendages and ultimately coalescing to form larger granulomas (Fig. 26–13). Lymphocytes and plasma cells are scant to absent. The active macropages are packed with globi of acid-fast bacilli (Fig. 26–14). BI is 5 to 6+. Large numbers of bacilli occupy dermal nerves, arrectores pilorum muscles, hair follicles, endothelial cells, and walls of blood vessels (Fig. 26–15). By immunofluorescence microscopy, IgM is deposited at the basement membrane zone region of about one third of lepromatous patients, including clinically uninvolved skin.[25]

Relapsing Lepromatous Leprosy. Leprosy in relapse has become increasingly important largely due to emergent

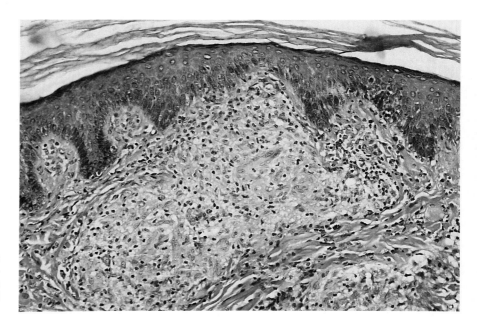

Figure 26–9. Borderline tuberculoid (BT) leprosy. Epithelioid cell granuloma not extending to the epidermis. Lymphocytes are scattered through the granuloma. (H&E ×200.) (*AFIP neg 87–5252.*)

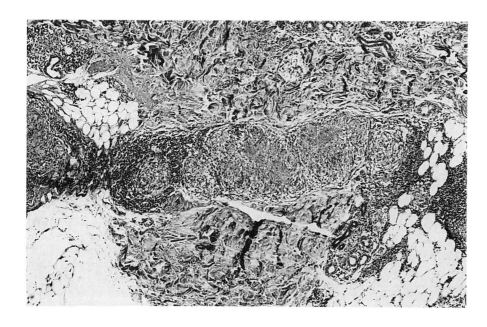

Figure 26–10. Borderline lepromatous (BL) leprosy. Nerve structure with granuloma, perineural thickening, and infiltration by lymphocytes. (H&E ×200.) (*AFIP neg 87–5261.*)

strains of *M. leprae* resistant to sulfone drug monotherapy. A characteristic histologic pattern of hyperreactivity is common in relapsing leprosy, although it does not occur in every example, and it may be occasionally observed in primary infection. Infiltrative or expansile granulomas are comprised of almost uniform young active macrophages, polyhedral, spindle-shaped, or flattened in appearance, with copious homogeneous cytoplasm, minimal vacuolization, and abundant solid-staining acid-fast bacilli. An extreme form of hyperreactivity is the histoid variety of lepromatous leprosy. Here, the skin lesions are multiple, nontender, hard nodules that both clinically and histopathologically resemble dermatofibromas except for the presence of nu-

merous solid-staining acid-fast bacilli in the cytoplasm of the spindle-shaped histiocytes[26] (Figs. 26–16, 26–17, 26–18).

Reactions

The course of leprosy irrespective of treatment may be marked by acute inflammatory reactions that are apparent both clinically and microscopically and that fall into two distinct immunologic types. Because they share clinical similarities, skin biopsies are useful in their differentiation and in separating reactional states from leprosy in relapse. In all such instances, a baseline prereaction biopsy specimen when available should be compared.

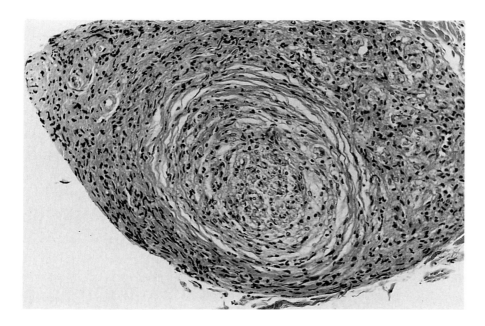

Figure 26–11. Subpolar lepromatous (LLs) leprosy. Nerve showing lamellar (onion skin) thickening of the perineurium surrounded by a compact macrophage granuloma. (H&E ×300.) (*AFIP neg 59–5469.*)

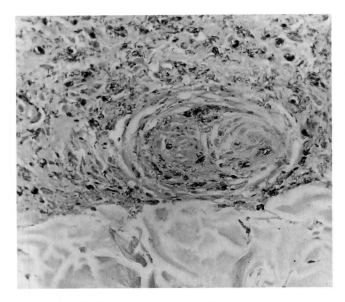

Figure 26–12. Subpolar lepromatous (LLs) leprosy. Laminated nerve and surrounding granuloma containing abundant acid-fast bacilli. (Fite-Faraco stain, ×504.) (*AFIP neg 73–7532.*)

Reversal Reaction

CLINICAL FEATURES. A delayed hypersensitivity phenomenon precipitated by the release of antigenic material from destroyed bacilli, the reversal reaction, is associated with an upgrading of the patient's cell-mediated immunity.[27] This response complicates mainly BT to BL leprosy but may occur in LLs patients after they have received antileprosy drug treatment and has been reported in LLp only after the use of transfer factor.[28] Existing lesions become more erythematous, and involved nerves become inflamed. Such patients must be closely monitored, with their reaction controlled by systemic corticosteroid administration if sensory loss and paralytic deformities are to be avoided.

HISTOLOGIC FEATURES. The enhanced T cell function is expressed microscopically by edema and increased numbers of lymphocytes, fibroblasts, and undifferentiated giant cells (Fig. 26–19). Severe reactions are marked by necrosis and dispersion of the granuloma, which later reforms into the new upgraded pattern.

Erythema Nodosum Leprosum (ENL)

CLINICAL FEATURES. This reactional episode occurs in approximately 50% of lepromatous patients, LLp, and LLs, and less often in BL, usually during regression within a year after institution of antileprosy drug therapy. It is manifested clinically by malaise, fever, and eruptive painful intracutaneous and subcutaneous nodules to plaques, which occur at the sites of small, frequently clinically inapparent regressing lepromatous granulomas. The eyes, nerves, lymph nodes, synovia, and testes may be involved as well.

HISTOLOGIC FEATURES. Erythema nodosum leprosum is characterized initially by endothelial swelling, vascular ectasia, influx of neutrophils within the dermal granuloma and between fat septae, and later by the accumulation of lymphocytes.[29] Leukocytoclastic vasculitis affecting venules and arterioles occurs in about half the cases (Fig. 26–20). Necrosis, abscess formation, and ulceration may occur in severe forms.[30] Immunoperoxidase studies have revealed that ENL lesions have a T helper phenotype excess in contrast to lepromatous lesions without ENL, which have a T suppressor excess.[31] Bacilli are usually scanty, fragmented, and beaded. Mycobacterial antigen has been demonstrated by immunoperoxidase staining at sites of the degenerate bacilli. That ENL is an immune complex disorder is supported by the presence of C3 in the vessel walls of ENL lesions,[25] by the presence of IgG and IgM in addition

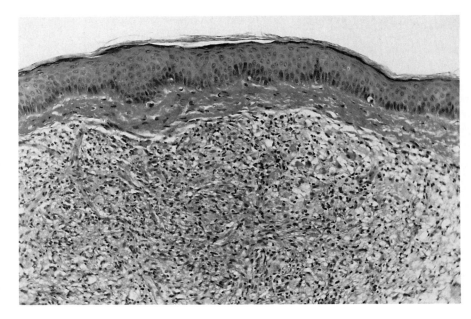

Figure 26–13. Polar lepromatous (LLp) leprosy. Underlying a clear grenz zone is a granuloma of undifferentiated and foamy macrophages. (H&E ×220.) (*AFIP neg 65–1653.*)

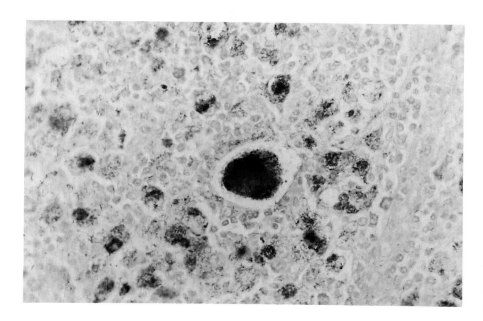

Figure 26–14. Polar lepromatous (LLp) leprosy. Macrophage packed with globi of acid-fast bacilli. (Fite-Faraco stain, ×645.) (*AFIP neg 72–2509.*)

to C3 in perivascular areas of neutrophilic infiltrates,[32] and by the detection of immune complexes in the sera of ENL patients.[33]

Lucio Phenomenon

In advanced forms of diffuse lepromatous leprosy in which there is heavy colonization of capillary endothelium by *M. leprae,* a severe obstructive vasculitis causes cutaneous infarcts, which are manifested clinically as irregular or stellate-shaped ulcerations. Components of immune complexes have been documented in the walls of blood vessels and perivascular areas of these lesions.[34]

Histologic Differential Diagnosis

Problems in differential diagnosis center mainly around indeterminate and tuberculoid forms of leprosy. Early leprosy in which granulomas have not fully developed must be differentiated from chronic nonspecific dermatitis. An infiltrate of lymphocytes and histiocytes may be all that is observed. The suspicion of leprosy relates in order of importance to the presence of acid-fast bacilli, a granuloma, or lymphoid infiltrate in nerve bundles, superficial papillary dermis, arrectores pilorum muscles, sweat glands, or neurovascular bundles. A mild infiltrate of lymphocytes and histi-

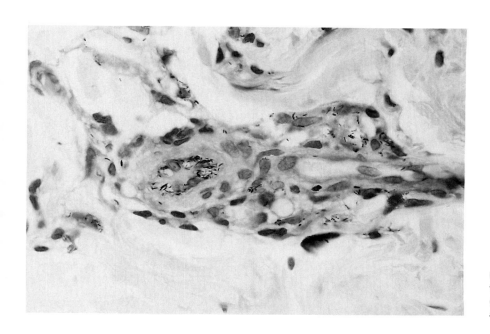

Figure 26–15. Lepromatous leprosy. Acid-fast bacilli in endothelium of blood vessels. (Fite-Faraco stain, ×775.) (*AFIP neg 87–5259.*)

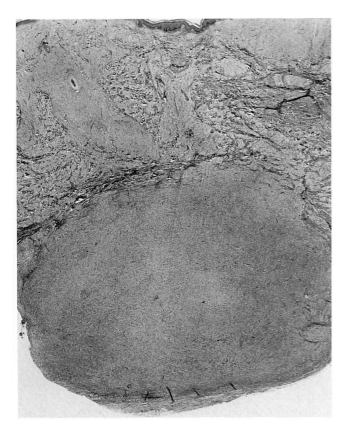

Figure 26–16. Lepromatous leprosy. Histoid nodule in lower dermis. (H&E ×20.) (*AFIP neg 87–5250.*)

nerve bundle is diagnostic. Disorientation of Schwann cell nuclei and disorganization of perineurium or nerve structure strongly favor leprosy. The finding of a small epithelioid cell granuloma without acid-fast bacilli at one of the sites of predilection for *M. leprae* carries great significance, since it may represent the site of their destruction.

Epithelioid cell granulomas may occur in sarcoid, foreign body granulomas of the silica, zirconium, or beryllium type, infection with other *Mycobacteria*, fungi, and some protozoa, and in granuloma multiforme. The differential diagnosis of lesions of tuberculoid leprosy is based on the same criteria employed in early leprosy. Acid-fast bacilli are indicative of leprosy if they are situated in nerve bundles, the subepidermal zone, or granulomatous masses that might represent the end-stage of nerve destruction. In the absence of bacilli, the finding of either an epithelioid cell granuloma in a nerve bundle, massive swelling of a nerve, or a patch of necrosis in the nerve parenchyma is almost conclusive for leprosy. Sarcoid is a compact epithelioid cell granuloma that often does not extend to the lower epidermal margin and, unlike lupus vulgaris, exhibits no caseation necrosis. Silica granulomas reveal birefringent foreign particles on polaroscopy. Granuloma multiforme, a tropical disease that histologically resembles granuloma annulare, unlike tuberculoid leprosy, maintains a clear subepidermal grenz zone and contains more plasma cells.[35] Histologic features that militate against leprosy include a perivascular lymphoid infiltrate sparing the adnexal structures, admixture of neutrophils, numerous plasma cells, spongiosis, pseudoepitheliomatous hyperplasia, and epithelioid or giant cell granuloma in conjunction with normal nerve bundles, caseation necrosis except when centered on nerves, or massive necrosis.

ocytes situated more around skin adnexae than blood vessels suggests leprosy and warrants the cutting of further sections in search of acid-fast bacilli, granuloma, or nerve involvement. A cuff of lymphocytes around a normal-appearing nerve twig is strong evidence in favor of leprosy, and the finding of one or more acid-fast bacilli within a

ATYPICAL MYCOBACTERIAL INFECTIONS

Following Koch's discovery of the typical *M. tuberculosis*, many pathogenic atypical mycobacteria were identified. Tiempe and Runyon in 1954 classified these diverse myco-

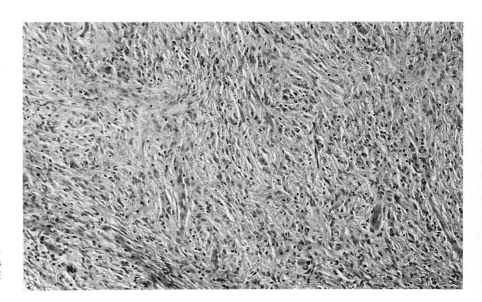

Figure 26–17. Histoid lepromatous leprosy. Abundant compressed active macrophages resembling pattern of dermatofibroma. (H&E ×200.) (*AFIP neg 87–5248.*)

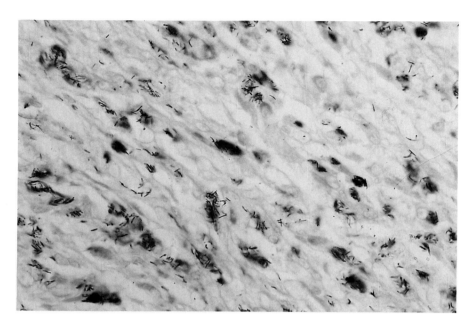

Figure 26–18. Histoid lepromatous leprosy. Abundant solid-staining acid-fast bacilli in histoid lesion. (Fite-Faraco stain, ×775.) (*AFIP neg 87–5258.*)

bacteria into four groups (I–IV) based on growth characteristics.[36] This classic effort was useful but has been largely abandoned in favor of identified species or species complexes of mycobacteria. The histopathologic changes produced by atypical mycobacteria are manifold, ranging from abscesses to tuberculoid granulomas to extensive coagulation necrosis.[37]

Mycobacterium ulcerans Infection (Buruli Ulcer)

CLINICAL FEATURES. *M. ulcerans* grows slowly, with optimal growth at 32° C, and causes extensive necrotic cutaneous ulcers that are frequently disfiguring and typically involve the extremities of children, especially over bony prominences. The disease prevails in swampy terrain of tropical and subtropical countries, notably East, Central and West Africa and Australia.[38] Koalas acquire infections in nature and may be reservoirs of *M. ulcerans*.[39] Infection begins by inoculation of *M. ulcerans* into the skin by trauma,[40] where the proliferating organisms elaborate a potent cytotoxin[41] that causes massive contiguous coagulation necrosis of the deep dermis and panniculus with destruction of fat, nerves, appendages, and vessels[42] (Fig. 26–21).

HISTOLOGIC FEATURES. Early lesions are closed, but necrosis eventually destroys the overlying dermis and epidermis in 2 to 3 months, leaving an ulcer with undermined borders and necrotic base. There is interstitial edema without conspicuous inflammatory cells. We have recently demonstrated marked in vitro immunosuppressive properties of the toxin, possibly explaining the absence of inflammatory

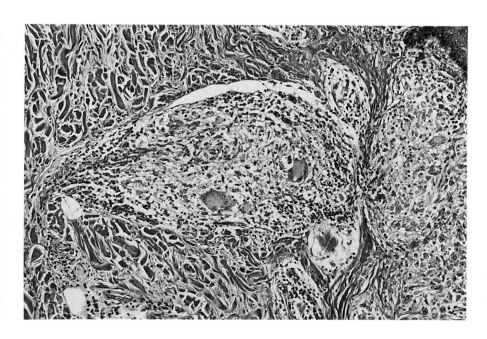

Figure 26–19. Reversal (upgrading) reaction in borderline tuberculoid (BT) leprosy. Edema, abundant lymphocytes, and scattered undifferentiated giant cells. (H&E ×160.) (*AFIP neg 87–5260.*)

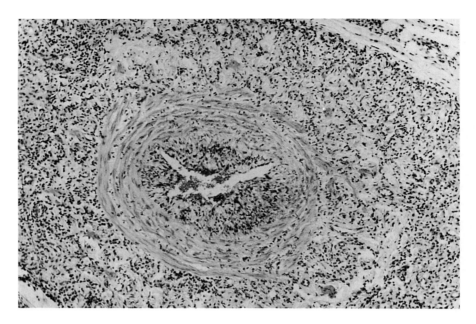

Figure 26–20. Erythema nodosum leprosum (ENL) in lepromatous leprosy. Large numbers of neutrophils are present throughout the granuloma and within wall of blood vessel. (H&E ×145.) (*AFIP neg 74–12821–3.*)

cells (unpublished data). Necrosis may spread to deep fascia and muscle and rarely to the bone. Acid-fast bacilli are numerous in the necrotic base of the ulcer but absent at the advancing margin of tissue necrosis (Fig. 26–22). In the healing phase, there is a granulomatous reaction and eventual scarring.

Mycobacterium marinum Infection (Swimming Pool Granuloma)

CLINICAL FEATURES.   Although this disease probably was first described in 1886, Linell and Norden first isolated the slow-growing *M. marinum* (*M. balnei*), with an optimal growth temperature of 32° C, from a group of patients who developed cutaneous lesions after swimming in the same pool in Sweden.[43,44] The organism is ubiquitous and enters the skin by trauma. The incubation period may be as short as 15 days,[45] and although spontaneous cure in several months is the rule, lesions may persist for many years. The low temperature growth requirement tends to limit infections to skin, usually to the site of inoculation. However, sporotrichoid spread[46] and disseminated cutaneous infections occa-

sionally are described in normal and immunosuppressed hosts.[47,48]

HISTOLOGIC FEATURES.   There is a spectrum of histopathologic responses.[49] In early lesions, in the dermis, there are focal infiltrates of lymphocytes, histiocytes, and often large numbers of neutrophils (Fig. 26–23). In older lesions, there are tuberculoid granulomas that may show caseation necrosis. There is usually some degree of epidermal hyperplasia with hyperkeratosis and parakeratosis. The epidermis is frequently ulcerated. Acid-fast bacilli usually are seen in early lesions but are rare in the granulomatous phase.

Mycobacterium scrofulaceum and *Mycobacterium avium-intracellulare* Infections

CLINICAL FEATURES.   *M. scrofulaceum* frequently is included with *M. avium-intracellulare* to form the MAIS-complex. However, *M. scrofulaceum* is not sufficiently close taxonomically to *M. avium-intracellulare* to warrant such association.[50] As has been noted previously, *M. scrofulaceum* is a common cause of scrofuloderma in children but has not been established as the cause of primary lesions in the skin of normal individuals. Dustin et al.[51] noted a fatal *M. scrofulaceum*

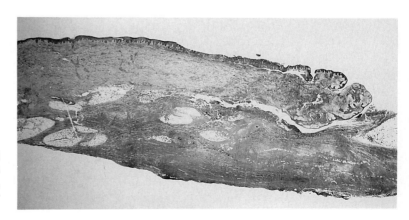

Figure 26–21. *Mycobacterium ulcerans* infection (Buruli ulcer). Margin of massive ulcer showing reepithelialization at the edge of the ulcer, wide undermining of the dermis, and contiguous coagulation necrosis of the subcutis. (Movat stain, ×4.5.) (*AFIP neg 74–803.*)

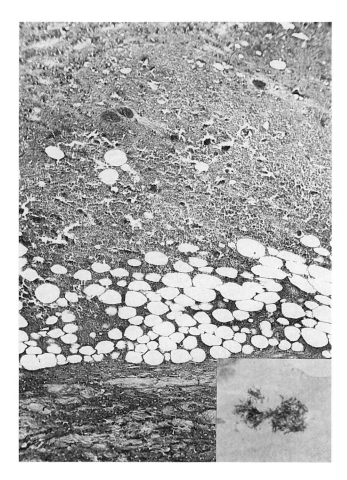

Figure 26–22. *Mycobacterium ulcerans* infection (Buruli ulcer). Massive necrosis of the subcutis with retention of ghosts of fat cells. Necrosis does not penetrate the underlying fascia. (Movat stain, ×120.) (*AFIP neg 74–800.*) *Inset.* Cluster of extracellular acid-fast bacilli in the necrotic subcutis. (Ziehl-Neelsen stain, ×750.) (*AFIP neg 74–802.*)

infection with extensive involvement of skin in an immunosuppressed boy and reviewed reports on six other patients.

Primary *M. avium-intracellulare* infections in the skin are rare in immunocompetent patients. An ulcer of the foot caused by a Runyon group III organism may be unique.[52] In the chronically ill, immunosuppressed patient, *M. avium-intracellulare* is being recognized with increased frequency.[53,54] Patients with acquired immunodeficiency syndrome (AIDS) are at high risk for disseminated *M. avium-intracellulare* infections, and the skin and subcutaneous tissue frequently are involved.[55]

HISTOLOGIC FEATURES. There is a histiocytic infiltration of the subcutis and adjacent dermis, sometimes with central abscesses. Histiocytes usually have swollen foamy cytoplasms but may assume a histoid pattern.[56] There are many acid-fast bacilli within histiocytes and in the necrotic debris.

Mycobacterium fortuitum Complex

CLINICAL FEATURES. Two species of rapid growers (i.e., growth on laboratory media within 5 days) are common human pathogens: *Mycobacterium fortuitum* and *Mycobacterium chelonei* (with subspecies *Mycobacterium abscessus*). These species and subspecies are often combined as the *M. fortuitum* complex. Identified first in 1938[57] as the cause of injection abscesses, the *M. fortuitum* complex is now recognized as a common pathogen where asepsis in surgery or hypodermic injections is lacking.[58] The organism may enter the skin by minor trauma, such as nail scratches.[59] *M. fortuitum* infections have been traced to hot tubs and hydrotherapy pools.[60,61]

HISTOLOGIC FEATURES. Early histopathologic changes have not been described. The first clinical manifestation usually is a fluctuant abscess that is frequently loculated. The abscess eventually ulcerates and discharges pus from one or more sinuses. In closed lesions, there is liquefactive necro-

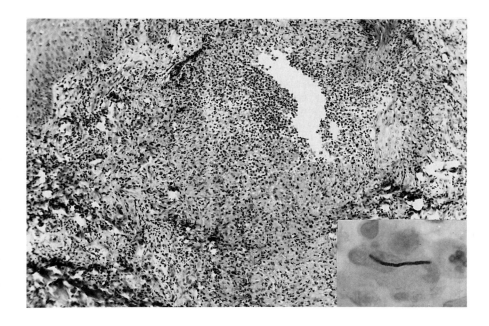

Figure 26–23. *Mycobacterium marinum* infection (swimming pool granuloma). An early lesion with a pyogranulomatous reaction in the upper dermis. (H&E ×130.) (*AFIP neg 73–3053.*) *Inset.* A single intracellular *M. marinum* in the area of inflammation. (Ziehl-Neelsen stain, ×1500.) (*AFIP neg 73–3054.*)

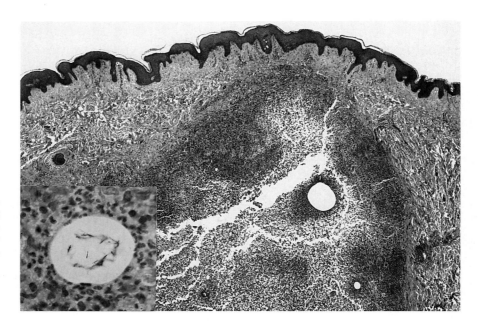

Figure 26–24. *Mycobacterium chelonei* infection. This lesion developed in the buttock after a hypodermic injection. An abscess with a granulomatous reaction at the periphery occupies much of the dermis. Vacuoles are dispersed in the abscess. (H&E ×35.) *Inset.* Acid-fast bacilli in a vacuole at the periphery of the lesion. (Ziehl-Neelsen stain, ×630.) *(AFIP neg 81–13871.)*

sis, with massive neutrophilic infiltrates in the dermis and subcutaneous tissue. There are often fibrosis and epithelioid cell granulomas. Scattered in the suppurative areas there are often spherical vacuoles. Acid-fast bacilli usually are found and are most consistently seen in the spherical vacuoles[62] (Fig. 26–24). In immunocompetent individuals, the lesions remain localized and heal readily after incision and draining. However, immunosuppression may cause multiple skin lesions and dissemination.[63]

Other Atypical Mycobacterial Infections

Of the more than 50 species of *Mycobacterium* known today, approximately half are recognized pathogens of humans or animals. In addition to those already discussed, some other species rarely may cause cutaneous disease. In fact, there is increasing belief that most of the mycobacteria may be pathogenic, given a large enough inoculum and a sufficiently immunosuppressed host.[50]

Mycobacterium kansasii Infection
M. kansasii is a common pulmonary pathogen, but only approximately 12 patients with cutaneous lesions are known. Types of lesions vary: verrucous nodules,[64] crusted ulceration,[65] papulopustules,[66] and cellulitis.[67] Some lesions are primary, but most of those in immunosuppressed patients disseminated from pulmonary disease.

HISTOLOGIC FEATURES. Histopathologic changes range from tuberculoid granulomas in the verrucous lesions to mixed acute and chronic inflammation in the pustular lesions. Acid-fast bacilli are scarce in most lesions.

Mycobacterium szulgai Infection
Of the two known and one presumed patients with primary cutaneous lesions caused by *M. szulgai*, two were immuno-

suppressed patients and one was a 6-month-old normal child.[68–70] The lesions were single or multiple and were ulcerated abscesses or cellulitis.

HISTOLOGIC FEATURES. The histologic changes seen in lesions range from mixed exudates of histiocytes, lymphocytes, and neutrophils to noncaseating tuberculoid granulomas and reactive fibrosis. Acid-fast bacilli are seen in some lesions.

Mycobacterium haemophilum Infection
Ten patients have been reported with multiple nodules, abscesses, and ulcers in the skin caused by *M. haemophilum* (so-called because iron-supplemented media are necessary for growth).[50,71] Although this infection is most common in immunosuppressed patients, normal individuals are susceptible to *M. haemophilum* infection.

HISTOLOGIC FEATURES. There is a granulomatous panniculitis without caseation necrosis. Acid-fast bacilli are present.

Mycobacterium gordonae Infection
A single patient has been described with cutaneous nodules on the dorsum of the hand in which *M. gordonae* was identified by culture.[72]

HISTOLOGIC FEATURES. There are reactive epidermal changes with acute and chronic inflammation in the dermis. No acid-fast bacilli are seen.

Bacillus of Calmette-Guerin (BCG) Infection
In young children and immunosuppressed patients, vaccination with BCG, an attenuated strain of *M. bovis*, produces ulcerative lesions with regional lymphadenopathy. Rarely, there is fatal systemic spread.[73] Local abscesses and lupus vulgaris-like lesions are sometimes seen at the vaccination site.

Anonymous Mycobacterial Infections

Noncultivable and nonidentifiable mycobacteria cause sporadic skin disease in humans. For example, Feldman and Hershfield described 29 patients in northern midwestern United States and Manitoba, usually with a single erythematous papule with regional lymphadenopathy.[74]

HISTOLOGIC FEATURES. The skin showed mixed lymphohistiocytic and neutrophilic infiltrations, sometimes with necrosis, and focal tuberculoid granulomas. Nerves were not involved. Most lesions contained large numbers of acid-fast bacilli in histiocytes and extracellular bacilli. Repeated attempts to cultivate the acid-fast bacillus were unsuccessful, but it was not *M. leprae*. At the AFIP, we have studied several lesions with similar features in immunosuppressed patients.[62]

We have conducted paired comparisons on serial sections stained with either the Fite-Faraco or the Ziehl-Neelsen stain and have observed that the former, although superior in the identification of *M. leprae* in paraffin-embedded tissue sections, offers no specific advantage over a proper Ziehl-Neelsen stain for identifying other mycobacterial species. The Auramine O immunofluorescent technique may be used as a companion stain to one of the conventional acid-fast stains.

REFERENCES

1. Goette DK, Jacobson KW, Doty RD. Primary inoculation tuberculosis of the skin. Prosector's paronychia. *Arch Dermatol.* 1978;114:567–569.
2. Horwitz O. Lupus vulgaris cutis in Denmark 1895–1954: its relation to the epidemiology of other forms of tuberculosis. Epidemiology and course of the tuberculosis infection based on 3902 cases from the Finsen Institute, Copenhagen. *Acta Tuberc Scand.* 1960;49(suppl):1–137.
3. Lincoln EM, Gilbert LA. Diseases in children due to mycobacteria other than *Mycobacterium tuberculosis. Am Rev Respir Dis.* 1972;105:683–714.
4. Wilson-Jones E, Winkelman RK. Papulonecrotic tuberculid: a neglected disease in Western countries. *J Am Acad Dermatol.* 1986;14:815–826.
5. Iden DL, Rogers RS, Schroeter AL. Papulonecrotic tuberculid secondary to *Mycobacterium bovis. Arch Dermatol.* 1978;114:564–566.
6. Lebel M, Lassonde M. Erythema induratum of Bazin. *J Am Acad Dermatol.* 1986;14:738–742.
7. Stoner GL, Touw J, Atlaw T, Bellehu A. Antigen specific suppressor cells in subclinical leprosy infection. *Lancet.* 1981;2:1372–1377.
8. Dwyer JM, Bullock WE, Fields JP. Disturbance of the blood T:B lymphocyte ratio in lepromatous leprosy. *N Engl J Med.* 1973;288:1036–1039.
9. Bullock WE. Studies of immune mechanisms in leprosy, I: depression of delayed allergic response to skin test antigens. *N Engl J Med.* 1968;278:298–304.
10. Myrvang B, Godal T, Ridley DS, et al. Immune responsiveness to *Mycobacterium leprae* and other mycobacterial antigens throughout the clinical and histopathological spectrum of leprosy. *Clin Exp Immunol.* 1973;14:541–553.
11. Mehra V, Mason LH, Fields JP, Bloom BR. Lepromin-induced suppressor cells in patients with leprosy. *J Immunol.* 1979;123:1813–1817.
12. Mehra V, Convit J, Rubinstein A, Bloom BR. Activated suppressor T cells in leprosy. *J Immunol.* 1982;129:1946–1951.
13. Nogueira N, Kaplan G, Levy E, et al. Defective interferon production in leprosy: reversal with antigen and interleukin 2. *J Exp Med.* 1983;158:2165–2170.
14. Modlin RL, Hofman FM, Horwitz DA, et al. In situ identification of cells in human leprosy granulomas with monoclonal antibodies to interleukin 2 and its receptor. *J Immunol.* 1984;132:3085–3090.
15. Longley J, Haregewoin A, Yemaneberhan T, et al. In vivo responses to *Mycobacterium leprae:* antigen presentation, interleukin 2 production, and immune cell phenotypes in naturally occurring leprosy lesions. *Int J Lepr.* 1985;53:385–394.
16. Harboe J. The immunology of leprosy. In: Hastings RC, ed. *Leprosy.* Edinburgh: Churchill Livingstone; 1985:53–87.
17. Job CK, Chacko CJG. A modification of Fite's stain for demonstration of *M. leprae* in tissue sections. *Indian J Lepr.* 1986;58:17–18.
18. Ridley DS, Hilson GRF. A logarithmic index of bacilli in biopsies. *Int J Lepr.* 1967;35:184–193.
19. Levy L, Fasal P, Murray LP. Morphology of *Mycobacterium leprae* in tissue sections. Correlation with results of mouse foot pad inoculation. *Arch Dermatol.* 1969;100:618–620.
20. Ridley DS, Jopling WH. Classification of leprosy according to immunity. A five-group system. *Int J Lepr.* 1966;34:255–273.
21. Ridley DS. *Skin Biopsy in Leprosy.* 2nd ed. Basel: Ciba-Geigy; 1985.
22. Liu T-C, Yen L-Z, Ye G-Y, Dung G-L. Histology of indeterminate leprosy. *Int J Lepr.* 1982;50:172–176.
23. Modlin RL, Hofman FM, Taylor CR, Rea TH. T lymphocyte subsets in the skin lesions of patients with leprosy. *J Am Acad Dermatol.* 1983;8:182–189.
24. Wallach D, Flageul B, Bach M, Cottenot F. The cellular content of dermal leprous granulomas: an immuno-histological approach. *Int J Lepr.* 1984;52:318–326.
25. Fields JP, Abel EA. Immunofluorescent abnormalities in leprosy patients. *Arch Dermatol.* 1975;111:1164–1165.
26. Desikan KV, Iyer CGS. Histoid variety of lepromatous leprosy. A histopathologic study. *Int J Lepr.* 1972;40:149–156.
27. Waters MFR, Turk JL, Wemambu SNC. Mechanisms of reactions in leprosy. *Int J Lepr.* 1971;39:417–428.
28. Bullock WE, Fields JP, Brandriss MW. An evaluation of transfer factor as immunotherapy for patients with lepromatous leprosy. *N Engl J Med.* 1972;287:1053–1059.
29. Mabalay MC, Helwig EB, Tolentino JF, Binford CH. The histopathology and histochemistry of erythema nodosum leprosum. *Int J Lepr.* 1965;33:28–49.
30. Job CK, Gude S, Macaden VP. Erythema nodosum leprosum. A clinico-pathologic study. *Int J Lepr.* 1964;32:177–184.
31. Modlin RL, Bakke AC, Vaccaro SA, et al. Tissue and blood T-lymphocyte subpopulations in erythema nodosum leprosum. *Arch Dermatol.* 1985;121:216–219.
32. Ridley MJ, Ridley DS. The immunopathology of erythema nodosum leprosum: the role of extravascular complexes. *Lepr Rev.* 1983;54:95–107.
33. Gelber RJ, Drutz DJ, Epstein WV. Clinical correlates of Clq-precipitating substances in the sera of patients with leprosy. *Am J Trop Med Hyg.* 1974;23:471–475.
34. Quismorio FP, Rea T, Chandor S, et al. Lucio's phenomenon: an immune complex deposition syndrome in leprosy. *Clin Immunol Immunopathol.* 1978;9:184–193.
35. Meyers WM, Connor DH, Shannon R. Histologic characteristics of granuloma multiforme (Mkar disease). *Int J Lepr.* 1970;38:241–249.
36. Timpe A, Runyon EH. Relationship of "atypical" acid-fast bacilli to human disease: preliminary report. *J Lab Clin Med.* 1954;44:202–209.

37. Santa Cruz DJ, Strayer DS. The histologic spectrum of the cutaneous mycobacteriosis. *Hum Pathol.* 1982;13:485–495.

38. Meyers WM, Connor DH, McCullough B, et al. Distribution of *Mycobacterium ulcerans* infections in Zaire, including the report of new foci. *Ann Soc Belg Med Trop.* 1974;54:147–157.

39. Mitchell PJ, Jerrett IV, Slee KJ. Skin ulcers caused by *Mycobacterium ulcerans* in koalas near Bairnsdale, Australia. *Pathology.* 1984;16:256–260.

40. Meyers WM, Shelly WM, Connor DH, Meyers EK. Human *Mycobacterium ulcerans* infection developing at sites of trauma to skin. *Am J Trop Med Hyg.* 1974;23:919–923.

41. Hockmeyer WT, Krieg RE, Reich M, Johnson RD. Further characterization of *Mycobacterium ulcerans* toxin. *Infect Immun.* 1978;21:124–128.

42. Connor DH, Lunn F. Buruli ulceration. A clinicopathologic study of 38 Ugandans with *Mycobacterium ulcerans* infection. *Arch Pathol.* 1966;81:183–189.

43. Collins CH, Grange JM, Noble WC, Yates MD. *Mycobacterium marinum* infections in man. *J Hyg (Lond).* 1985;94:135–149.

44. Linell F, Norden A. *Mycobacterium balnei.* A new acid-fast bacillus occurring in swimming pools and capable of producing skin lesions in humans. *Acta Tuberc Scand.* 1954;33(suppl): 1–84.

45. Chappler RR, Hoke AW, Borchardt KA. Primary inoculation with *Mycobacterium marinum. Arch Dermatol.* 1977;113:380.

46. Dickey RF. Sporotrichoid mycobacteriosis caused by *M. marinum (balnei). Arch Dermatol.* 1968;98:385–391.

47. King AJ, Fairly JA, Rasmussen JE. Disseminated cutaneous *Mycobacterium marinum* infection. *Arch Dermatol.* 1983;119:268–270.

48. Gombert ME, Goldstein EJC, Corrado ML. Disseminated *Mycobacterium marinum* infection after renal transplantation. *Ann Intern Med.* 1981;94:486–487.

49. Travis WD, Travis LB, Roberts GD, et al. The histopathologic spectrum in *Mycobacterium marinum* infection. *Arch Pathol Lab Med.* 1985;109:1109–1113.

50. Wayne LG. The "atypical" mycobacteria: recognition and disease association. *CRC Crit Rev Microbiol.* 1985;12:185–222.

51. Dustin P, Demol P, Derks-Jacobvitz D, et al. Generalized fatal chronic infection by *Mycobacterium scrofulaceum* with severe amyloidosis in a child. *Pathol Res Pract.* 1980;168:237–248.

52. Schmidt JD, Yeager H Jr, Smieth EB, Raleigh JW. Cutaneous infection due to a Runyon group III atypical mycobacterium. *Am Rev Respir Dis.* 1972;106:469–471.

53. Cox SK, Strausbaugh LJ. Chronic cutaneous infection caused by *Mycobacterium intracellulare. Arch Dermatol.* 1981;117:794–796.

54. Sanderson TL, Moskowitz L, Hensley GT, et al. Disseminated *Mycobacterium avium-intracellulare* infection appearing as a panniculitis. *Arch Pathol Lab Med.* 1982;106:112–114.

55. Reichert CM, O'Leary TJ, Levens DL, et al. Autopsy pathology in the acquired immune deficiency syndrome. *Am J Pathol.* 1983;112:357–382.

56. Wood C, Nickoloff BJ, Todes-Taylor NR. Pseudotumor resulting from atypical mycobacterial infection: a histoid variety of *Mycobacterium avium-intracellulare* complex infection. *Am J Clin Pathol.* 1985;83:524–527.

57. da Costa Cruz JP. *Mycobacterium fortuitum,* um novo bacilo acido-resistente patogenico para o homem. *Acta Med Rio de Janeiro.* 1938;1:297–301.

58. Wallace RJ Jr, Swenson JM, Silcox VA, et al. Spectrum of disease due to rapidly growing mycobacteria. *Rev Infect Dis.* 1983;5:657–679.

59. Hamrick HJ, Maddux DW, Lowry EK, et al. *Mycobacterium chelonei* facial abscess: case presentation and review of cutaneous infection due to Runyon group IV organisms. *Pediatr Infect Dis.* 1984;3:335–340.

60. Aubuchon C, Hill JJ Jr, Graham DR. Atypical mycobacterial infection of soft tissue associated with use of a hot tub. *J Bone Joint Surg.* 1986;68A:766–768.

61. Communicable Disease Surveillance Centre. *Mycobacterium chelonei* associated with a hydrotherapy pool. *Commun Dis Rep.* Oct 11, 1985:3–4.

62. Meyers WM. Mycobacterial infections of the skin. In: Braude AI, Davis CE, Fierer J, eds. *Infectious Diseases and Microbiology.* 2nd ed. Philadelphia: WB Saunders, 1986:1350–1361.

63. Graybill JR, Silva J, Fraser DW, et al. Disseminated mycobacteriosis due to *Mycobacterium abscessus* in two recipients of renal homografts. *Am Rev Respir Dis.* 1974;109:4–10.

64. Mayberry JD, Mullins JE, Stone OJ. Cutaneous infection due to *Mycobacterium kansasii. JAMA.* 1965;194:1135–1137.

65. Hirsch FS, Saffold OE. *Mycobacterium kansasii* infection with dermatologic manifestation. *Arch Dermatol.* 1976;112:706–708.

66. Bolivar R, Satterwaite TK, Floyd M. Cutaneous lesions due to *Mycobacterium kansasii. Arch Dermatol.* 1980;116:207–212.

67. Rosen T. Cutaneous *Mycobacterium kansasii* infection presenting as cellulitis. *Cutis.* 1983;31:87–89.

68. Sybert A, Tsou E, Garagusi VF. Cutaneous infection due to *Mycobacterium szulgai. Am Rev Respir Dis.* 1977;115:695–698.

69. Cross GM, Guill MA, Aton JK. Cutaneous *Mycobacterium szulgai* infection. *Arch Dermatol.* 1985;121:247–249.

70. Cookson BD, Dunger D. *Mycobacterium szulgai*—a case of cutaneous infection? *Tubercle.* 1985;66:65–67.

71. Davis BR, Brumbach J, Sanders WJ, Wolinsky E. Skin lesions caused by *Mycobacterium haemophilum. Ann Intern Med.* 1982; 97:723–724.

72. Shelly WB, Folkens AJ. *Mycobacterium gordonae*—infection of the hand. *Arch Dermatol.* 1984;120:1064–1065.

73. Aungst CW, Sokal JE, Jager BV. Complications of BCG vaccination in neoplastic diseases. *Ann Intern Med.* 1975;82:666–669.

74. Feldman RA, Hershfield E. Mycobacterial skin infection by unidentified species. *Ann Intern Med.* 1974;80:445–452.

CHAPTER 27
Spirochetal Infections

Edward Abell

The organisms producing spirochetal infections consist of four types of long, spiral, mobile organisms. They are responsible for a number of systemic diseases with worldwide distribution. Some have major dermatologic manifestations. The organisms and the diseases for which they are responsible are:

1. *Treponema:* syphilis, bejel, pinta, yaws
2. *Borrelia:* relapsing fevers and Lyme disease
3. *Leptospira:* Weil's disease and Canicola fever
4. *Spirillum:* rat-bite fever

The organisms of groups 3 and 4 may provoke cutaneous erythema, and the organisms of group 3 may produce petechiae during the course of febrile illness, but none, of themselves, produce primary dermatoses, and they are not considered here. Until the early 1970s, the same could have been said of the *Borrelia* spirochetes. During those years, however, unusual cases of arthritis with fever, clustered around the town of Lyme, Connecticut, were recognized.[1] Some cases were associated with large and often dramatic annular erythematous patches. Ultimately, the elucidation of Lyme disease and its causation by the *Borrelia* spirochete were established.[2] Infection is acquired by the bite of a vector tick.

THE TREPONEMAL DISEASES

A number of treponemes have been isolated from moist human skin, especially of the genital area and also from the oral cavity, but have not been shown to be pathogenic. *Treponema pallidum* is the cause of syphilis, and morphologically and immunologically identical organisms cause yaws and pinta. All three disorders are characterized clinically by evolution through three stages, but the expression and degree of systemic involvement are quite different in each. Only syphilis appears to be spread as a venereal disease.

SYPHILIS

The spirochete *T. pallidum* measures 6 to 15 μm in length and contains regularly spaced spiral coils at intervals of 1 μm. Motion is achieved by rotation around its longitudinal axis. The organism can be identified easily from exudate from primary chancres under darkfield microscopic illumination. Oral lesions may be very difficult to evaluate because of contamination by commensal spirochetes. In fixed tissue specimens, silver staining has been the traditional method of identification (Fig. 27–1) (Warthin Starry, Steiner, and Dieterle stains).[3–6] Identification of these organisms, in both smears and biopsy specimens, has been achieved more recently by immunofluorescence methods.[7] Using this technique, spirochetes have been identified often in considerable numbers even in gummas,[8] where previously silver stains had not proved a satisfactory method of identification.

Primary Syphilis

Clinical Features
Primary syphilis is heralded by the development of the chancre about 3 weeks (10 to 30 days) after infection is acquired. Untreated, the lesion usually resolves in 3 to 8 weeks, leaving an almost imperceptible superficial scar. The chancre, at first a papule, becomes a usually painless but hard indurated erosion or ulcer with sharply defined margins. Multiple lesions are not unusual. Genital, oral, and anal lesions are most common, but other sites occasionally are involved.

Histologic Features
The chancre is not primarily an ulcer. In its initial stages, the biopsy retains an edematous hyperplastic or attenuated epidermis, and this overlies an intense dermal infiltrate of lymphocytes and histocytes, with large numbers of plasma cells that extend deeply into the dermal connective tissue.[9] Infiltration occasionally can be so dense as to suggest

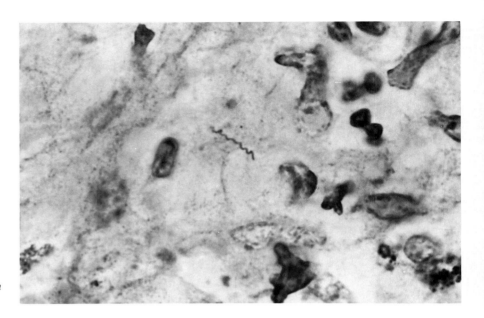

Figure 27–1. The spirochete, *Treponema Pallidum.* (Warthin-Starry stain, ×780.)

obliteration of the connective tissue. Ulceration ultimately may develop through complete erosion of the epidermal surface, which then becomes covered by a plasma fibrinous exudate, and neutrophils may be seen in and immediately beneath it. Dermal edema and dilated, sometimes thick-walled vessels usually are apparent, and this, combined with intense edema and cellular infiltrate, is responsible for the induration so characteristic of this lesion. Endothelial proliferation is said to occur in the primary lesion.

Secondary and Latent Syphilis

Clinical Features
The secondary syphilis follows primary disease by approximately 1 to 3 months. The onset is characterized by constitu-

tional symptoms, a diffuse lymphadenopathy, and skin rash. Mucous membrane involvement is common, and both the oral and anal cavity should be examined. The skin eruption, which may vary considerably in degree, extent, and distribution, is generally one of three major types: macular, papular, or papulosquamous lesions. Itching is rarely severe but does occur. Macular lesions may be evanescent and minimal and, occasionally, are not perceived by the patient. A rare ulcerative form—lues maligna—is described. Alopecia of the so-called moth-eaten pattern is sometimes seen and appears to represent the only significant inflammatory involvement of cutaneous appendages. Untreated, the eruptions may resolve and then relapse over several years. Sooner or later, a period of latency develops, during which the disorder appears to be entirely quiescent. In the majority

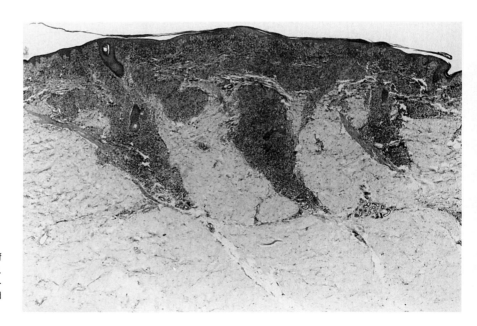

Figure 27–2. Papulosquamous lesion of secondary syphilis; biopsy of whole lesion. Diffuse superficial and deep perivascular infiltrate creates a triangular, or wedge-shaped outline. (H&E ×8).

of cases left without treatment, no tertiary disease of any type occurs. However, tertiary syphilis may develop within 3 or 4 years of the primary infection and may produce cardiovascular, neurologic, encephalitic, and cutaneous disorders.

Histologic Features

Although not entirely reproducible, there is a reasonably close histopathologic correlation in the clinical type of skin eruption seen in secondary disease.[10] When the biopsy is sufficiently large to encompass the entire lesion, the organization within the dermis shows a pattern of dermal and epidermal involvement in the shape of an inverted triangle (Fig. 27–2). A chronologic association of the inflammatory response occurs, and all lesions during the first weeks show a mixed infiltrate of lymphocytes and histiocytes and usually many plasma cells. Untreated cases occasionally demonstrate a granulomatous organization by 12 weeks, and all lesions become granulomatous by 4 months. It should be stressed that although plasma cells are characteristic of all stages of the histopathology of syphilis (Fig. 27–3), in secondary syphilis particularly, they may not be a constant finding.[10] In 10% of cases, plasma cells may be entirely absent, and in an additional 15% they may be quite sparse, so that in one quarter of all cases the presence of plasma cells may not provide the stimulus to consider syphilis. A pathologic feature sometimes overemphasized is vascular endothelial proliferation. Significant endothelial proliferation is uncommon (Fig. 27–4), and less than half of all biopsies show any vascular change. Some degree of epidermal involvement is nearly constant, and exceptions are seen only in macular lesions. It is appropriate to keep these considerations in mind when biopsy material is reviewed and syphilis is suspected (Table 27–1).

The macular eruption is characterized by a superficial and deep perivascular infiltrate of lymphocytes with plasma cells and occasional scattered histocytes (Fig. 27–5). Plasma cells may be absent, however, and only about half of the lesions are likely to show any significant epidermal involvement. This latter feature is usually mild and focal and consists of minor degrees of mononuclear cell exocytosis and spongiosis. Little alteration of the stratum corneum is to be expected. Vascular endothelial change, if present, is very mild.

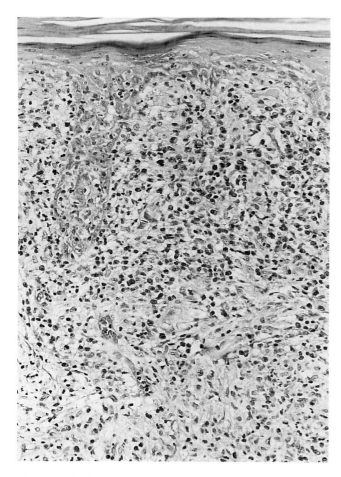

Figure 27–3. Papulosquamous lesion of secondary syphilis. Diffuse papillary dermal infiltrate of lymphocytes, histiocytes, and many plasma cells. Note exocytosis, epidermal edema, and developing scale (H&E ×40).

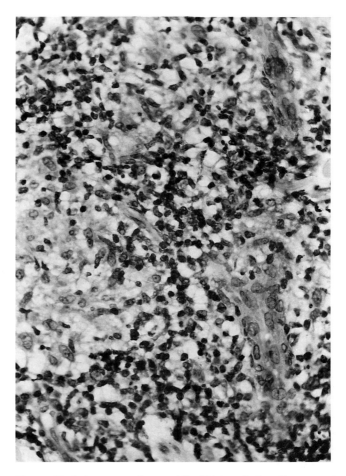

Figure 27–4. Late secondary syphilis. Thick-walled capillary vessel showing endothelial cell proliferation (*right*). The infiltrate shows granuloma formation with lymphocytes and plasma cells arranged around aggregated epithelioid histiocytes (H&E ×160).

TABLE 27–1. SKIN BIOPSY FINDINGS IN 62 CASES OF SECONDARY LUETIC DISEASE IN RELATIONSHIP TO THE CLINICAL APPEARANCE OF THE ERUPTION

Rash	Number	Exocytosis (All Types) % (No.)	Significant Plasma Cell Components of Dermal Infiltrate % (No.)	Proliferation of Vascular Endothelial Cells % (No.)
Macular	13	54 (7)	77 (10)	38 (5)
Papular	29	96 (28)[a]	69 (20)	34 (10)
Papulosquamous	20	90 (18)[a]	85 (17)	60 (12)

[a] 25% showing microabscess or spongiform pustule formation.
From ref. 10.

Alteration of the epidermis in the papular and papulosquamous lesions, however, is nearly obligatory, and exocytosis of mononuclear cells often is quite prominent (Fig. 27–6). Formation of microabscess-like lesions or, occasionally, spongiform pustular aggregates containing some neutrophils may occur in the stratum corneum. Papulosquamous lesions show scale crust (Fig. 27–7). The epidermal response to the inflammatory process may be a mild to moderate psoriasiform hyperplasia, or a somewhat edema-

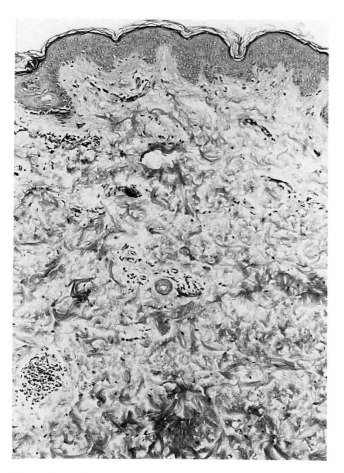

Figure 27–5. Macular lesion of secondary syphilis. A mild superficial and deep perivascular infiltrate without epidermal involvement (H&E ×16).

tous attenuated lichenoid appearance often is created.[10,11] (Fig. 27–8). Edema is often pronounced and diffuse. Solitary necrotic keratocytes are not uncommon. The dermal inflammatory process in papular and papulosquamous lesions is almost always moderate to dense and frequently may be accompanied by red blood cell extravasation from the superficial vessels. Plasma cells are usually prominent but may be sparse or absent, as stated previously. In a substantial series of biopsies of secondary luetic disease, there was the strong suggestion that significant vascular endothelial cell proliferation was seen only in the older lesions.[10] Eosinophils have been reported in the infiltrate, and dermal fibrosis has been described.[11] In older lesions, granulomas organize in a nodular perivascular and perifollicular pattern, with epithelioid histiocytes forming the central zone and lymphocytes and plasma cells arranged peripherally (Fig. 27–9).

Involvement of follicles can be seen in all lesions in addition to those from scalp biopsies of so-called motheaten alopecia. The pathologic features are essentially the same in all lesions. The follicles may be in either catagen or telogen phase, and the follicular epithelium may show pronounced spongiosis and mononuclear cell exocytosis (Fig. 27–10). The deep perivascular infiltrate is also accentuated around the vessels of the adventitial tissue of the involved follicular structures, and the usual mixture of lymphocytes, histiocytes, and plasma cells is found.

The ulceration of lues maligna is said in some cases to be associated with proliferative changes in small blood vessels and their occlusion by fibrin thrombi,[12,13] but not all patients are so affected, and other factors, perhaps nutritional or immunologic, must be associated with the tissue breakdown.[14,15]

Biopsy sections of condylomata lata lesions show somewhat modified papular or papulosquamous lesions. Epidermal hyperplasia is much more prominent and may become pseudoepitheliomatous.[11,16] Central erosion and ulceration can occur. Spirochetes are present as they are in all secondary lesions.

A differential diagnosis may be extensive in this stage of the disease. Macular lesions may easily mimic a deep type of gyrate or figurate erythema or a mild polymorphous light eruption. In papular and papulosquamous lesions, if the characteristic deep perivascular involvement is not apparent or if the deeper tissues are not included in the section, psoriasis and various lichenoid inflammatory reactions could be serious considerations. With adequate biopsy tissue, pityriasis lichenoides chronica and occasionally pityria-

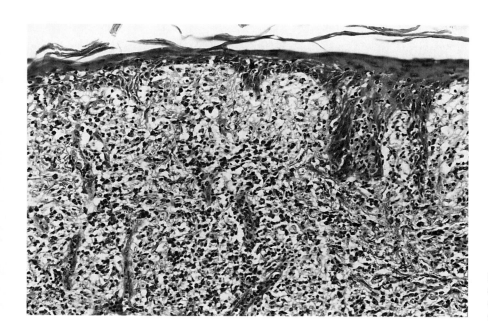

Figure 27–6. Papulosquamous lesion of secondary syphilis. Diffuse exocytosis into an attenuated epidermis and diffuse papillary dermal infiltrate (H&E ×80).

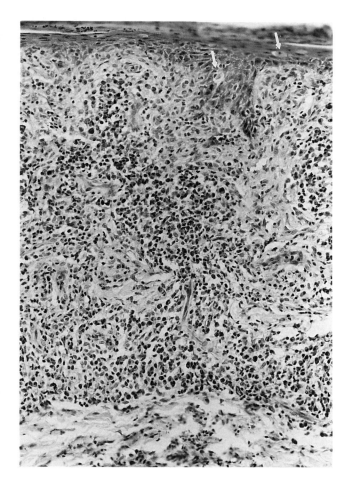

Figure 27–7. Papulosquamous lesion of secondary syphilis. The epidermis has a parakeratotic scale crust, intercellular edema and isolated necrotic keratinocytes (*arrows*). A mixed upper dermal infiltrate with many plasma cells is present (H&E ×80).

sis lichenoides varioliformis acuta can be easily confused, particularly where the plasma cell component of the infiltrate is not prominent or absent. Photocontact dermatitis and photolichenoid reactions also might be considered in some cases. Since atypical lymphoid cells are most unusual in the infiltrate in leutic disease, lymphomatoid papulosis would not normally be a diagnostic problem. However, the intensity of dermal infiltration and the extent of mononuclear cell exocytosis sometimes make actinic reticuloid and mycosis fungoides a difficult diagnostic problem, especially if clinical information is lacking.[17] When eosinophils are present in the infiltrate, the focal nature of the lesion may suggest an arthropod bite reaction.

In the granulomatous phase of secondary luetic disease, one may, on occasion, have to consider all forms of infectious granulomas and, rarely, sarcoidal granulomas.

Tertiary Syphilis

Clinical Features

Cutaneous lesions in this stage of the disease are either nodules or ulcerated nodules or plaques and may develop before, with, or after a wide variety of internal organ involvement. The nodular lesions may form scale and occasionally scale crust, and their organization and distribution often are irregular, focal, and asymmetrical. Gumma usually ulcerate eventually.

Histologic Features

NODULAR TERTIARY LESIONS. Small granulomas without gross tissue necrosis are seen throughout the dermis, set in a diffuse cellular infiltrate of lymphocytes, histocytes, and plasma cells in the nodular tertiary luetic lesion. Sparse multinucleate giant cells often are present either singly or in small clusters. Vascular swelling and endothelial proliferation are usually prominent features.[18] Caseous necrosis

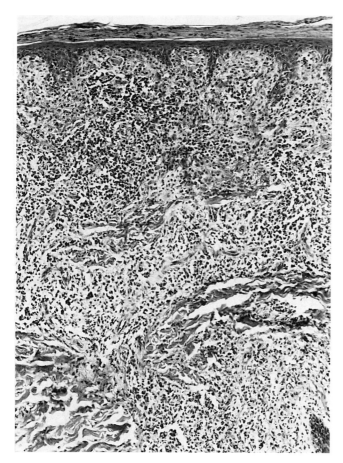

Figure 27–8. Papulosquamous lesion of secondary syphilis. An attenuated epidermis with scale crust and a mixed dermal infiltrate shows a lichenoid appearance, but with a deep perivascular extension (H&E ×16).

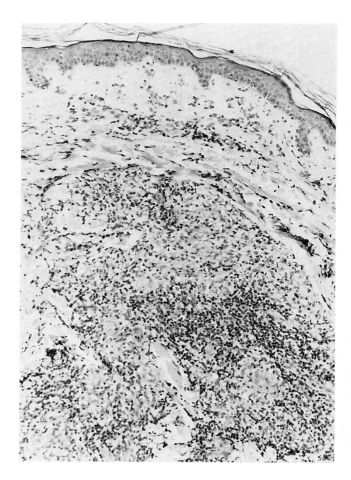

Figure 27–9. Late secondary syphilis, papular lesion. Extensive granulomatous infiltrate of reticular dermis (H&E ×16).

may develop within such nodular lesions, which gradually evolve into a gumma.

GUMMATOUS TERTIARY LESIONS. Gummatous lesions develop substantial central caseous necrosis around which extensive and often intense cellular infiltration and granuloma formation arise (Fig. 27–11).[19] Epithelioid cells and multinucleate giant cells may be numerous. Gumma may extend deeply into the subcutaneous tissue. As in granulomatous secondary syphilis, infectious granulomas may be a significant differential diagnosis in the nodular forms of tertiary luetic disease. Plentiful plasma cells and vascular change are useful pointers to the correct diagnosis. Scrofuloderma, especially, and erythema induratum may mimic gumma.

JUXTAARTICULAR NODES. Juxtaarticular nodes are nodular lesions, occasionally of considerable size, that may be found in late syphilis around the elbows and knees and that resemble rheumatoid nodules. As these lesions develop, the pathology is that of a diffuse dermal or subcutaneous infiltrate of mixed type, with histiocytes, epithelioid cells, occasional giant cells, and many plasma cells.[20,21] Later, fibrosis is seen developing in the central areas, with the granuloma-

tous infiltrate arranged around it so as to give a superficial resemblance to a palisading granuloma. Caseous necrosis in these lesions appears to be rare.[16]

YAWS

Clinical Features
Yaws is a nonvenereal treponematosis caused by *Treponema pertenue,* which is endemic in the humid tropics and spread by skin contact between children. This disease also evolves through three stages, although it is more practical to consider it as having an early and a late stage, with a latent period separating the two.

The primary yaw begins as a hyperkeratotic plaque, which eventually develops into a clean ulcer. This lesion usually is seen on an extremity but can be anywhere. It will eventually heal. The secondary lesions are smaller but similar and may be widely scattered over the body, although they favor the moist flexures and the mucocutaneous junctions. The tertiary lesions may evolve before the secondary lesions have healed, or there may be a period of latency. These late, or tertiary, lesions are gummas, which affect only the skin, subcutaneous tissue, and bone. Chronic hy-

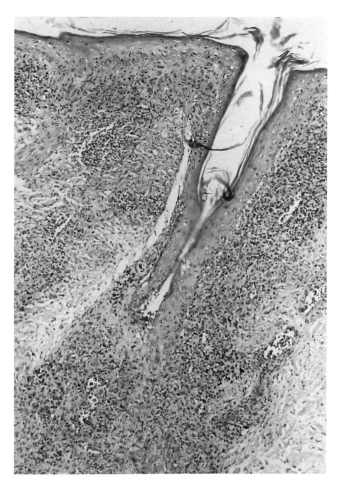

Figure 27–10. Follicular lesion of secondary syphilis. Extensive dermal infiltrate extending directly into follicular wall, with exocytosis and edema of upper infundibulum (H&E ×16).

pertrophic periostitis (saber tibia) is a common deformity. Juxtaarticular nodes may develop, as in late syphilis. These gummas produce deep draining ulcers.

Histologic Features

The histopathology of yaws differs little if at all from that of syphilis.[22-25] Treponemes are easily found in the early lesions; indeed they may be numerous. The principal variation in pathologic expression appears to be in the early lesion, in which pronounced epidermal hyperplasia is associated with spongiosis. This may be accompanied by heavy neutrophil exocytosis with the formation of intraepidermal microabscesses. Otherwise, the cellular infiltrate, tissue damage, and vessel involvement are not significantly different from that seen in luetic disease.

PINTA

Clinical Features

This disease, the mildest and least destructive of the treponematoses, is caused by *Treponema carateum* and appears only in the American tropics. The name is derived from Spanish and means "painted," referring to the characteristic cutaneous change: patches of altered skin color. It is a nonvenereal disease that tends to develop in the third decade. The primary lesions, as in yaws, usually begin on the extremities, which suggests skin to skin contact as the method of spread. Spirochetes are found consistently in the early lesions. Three stages of the disease occur, but, like yaws, it is simpler to consider the first two stages as a single early stage, since the lesions are very similar.

The primary lesion is a small, scaly papule that expands slowly to about 10 cm with irregular borders. The appearance of disseminated lesions (pentids) marks the onset of the secondary stage. These develop as the primary lesions but show various color changes—pink, red, purple, or black. The serologic tests may not become positive until this stage.

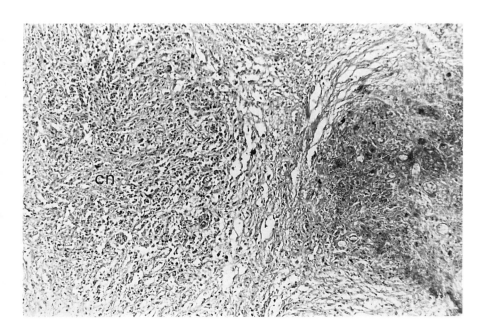

Figure 27–11. Tertiary syphilis, gumma. Dense inflammatory cell reaction (*right*) adjacent to gumma (*left*) with central caseous necrosis (CN) (H&E ×40).

In the tertiary stage, the secondary lesions become depigmented and resemble viteligo.

Histologic Features

Microscopically,[23,26] primary and secondary lesions are indistinguishable,[27] and the epidermis is spongiotic with hyperkeratosis and parakeratosis. Intraepidermal microabscess formation can occur. Dermal melanophages are seen, together with a superficial mononuclear infiltrate with plasma cells. Vessel changes may develop as in early syphilis. During the late, or tertiary, stage the inflammation subsides, and fibrosis develops in the upper dermis. Pigment is absent from epidermis and dermis, although an occasional melanophage may remain. Electron microscopy has shown an absence of melanocytes but persistant Langerhans cells.[28]

BORRELIAL DISEASES

LYME DISEASE

Clinical Features

This disorder derives its name from the small town in Connecticut around which were clustered a number of unusual cases of arthritis and a skin eruption usually consisting of a solitary patch or annulus of expanding erythema—erythema chronicum migrans. The skin eruption had been known for nearly 70 years when Lyme arthritis was described in 1976,[29] and involvement of spirochetes in the etiology of the rash had been postulated previously.[30] The disease starts in summertime with fever, myalgia, and arthralgia and frequently a spreading macular erythematous patch. Multiple lesions can occur. Neurologic and cardiac complications may sometimes develop. The evidence for a causative spirochete is now substantial, and in the United States, *Borrelia burgdorferi* is the etiologic agent, which is spread by the bite of the vector tick *Ixodes dammini* (in Europe *I. ricinus*).[31–34]

Histologic Features

Biopsy specimens are best taken from the edge of the active lesion. The most characteristic histopathologic findings are a superficial and deep perivascular lymphocytic infiltrate, with some plasma cells.[32] There may be a mild interstitial component to the dermal reaction and diffuse edema (Fig. 27–12). Eosinophils may replace the plasma cells in some lesions, when the reaction more closely resembles an arthropod bite. In a few cases, only lymphocytes are present. Warthin Starry silver stain may demonstrate *Borrelia* in about one quarter of the patients in either epidermis or dermis or both. *B. burgdorferi* is a spirochete 180 to 250 nm wide and about 3 µm long. The organism is found more easily in the periphery of the lesions.

ACRODERMATITIS CHRONICA ATROPHICANS

Clinical Features

This is an uncommon disease in the United States, which is seen particularly throughout northern, central, and east-

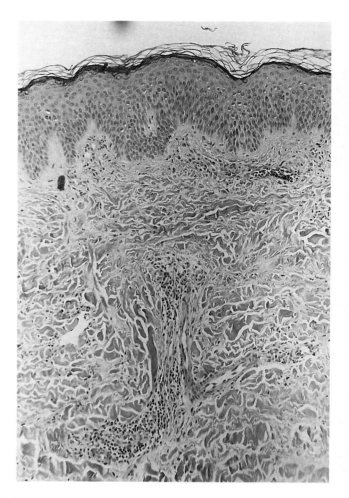

Figure 27–12. Erythema chronicum migrans (Lyme disease). Mild superficial and deep perivascular lymphocytic infiltrate with diffuse dermal edema (H&E ×32).

ern Europe. Erythematous plaques may arise on the dorsum of one hand or foot, on the elbow or knee, and persist for many years. Multiple lesions may develop, occasionally even on the trunk. Lesions closely resembling lichen sclerosus et atrophicus are also a feature of this odd condition, and lesions may suggest cutaneous scleroderma. Genital lesions are described. Skin atrophy may be very pronounced. The condition can be associated with a sensory peripheral neuropathy and distal joint deformity. Evidence suggests that acrodermatitis chronica atrophicans is associated with the same spirochetes that cause Lyme disease and erythema chronicum migrans and that the disorder represents a late manifestation of such infections.[35,36]

Histologic Features

Telangiectatic vessels in the upper dermis with a dense patchy or diffuse lymphocytic infiltrate with some plasma cells involving the whole dermis are seen.[37] The epidermis is atrophic and shows relative hyperkeratosis and basal cell hydropic degeneration. Scattered dermal vacuoles and diffuse dermal edema often are seen. In the lichen sclerosis et atrophicus and scleroderma-like lesions, the pathologic findings are not distinguishable from the real disease. Elastic fibers are lost or absent. Plasma cells, if present in significant numbers, may help to diagnose acrodermatitis chronica atrophicans.

REFERENCES

1. Steere AC, Malawista SE, Hardin JA, et al. Erythema chronicum migrans and Lyme arthritis. *Ann Intern Med.* 1977;86:685–698.
2. Steere AC, Grodzicki RL, Kornblatt AN, et al. The spirochetal etiology of Lyme disease. *N Engl J Med.* 1983;308:733–742.
3. Warthin AS, Starry AC. A more rapid and improved method of demonstrating spirochetes in tissues. *Am J Syph Gonor Vener Dis.* 1920;1:97.
4. Bridges CH, Luna L. Kerr's improved Warthin-Starry technic—study of permissible variations. *Lab Invest.* 1959;6:357–367.
5. Steiner G, Steiner G. Silver methods for spirochetes and Donovan bodies. *J Lab Clin Med.* 1944;29:868–871.
6. Van Orden AE, Greer PW. Modifications of the Dieterle spirochete stain. *J Histotechnol.* 1977;1:51–53.
7. Yobs AR, Brown L, Hunter EF. Fluorescent antibody technique in early syphilis. *Arch Pathol Lab Med.* 1967;77:220–225.
8. Handsfield HH, Lukehart SA, Sell S, et al. Demonstration of *Treponema pallidum* in a cutaneous gumma by indirect immunofluorescence. *Arch Dermatol.* 1983;119:677–680.
9. Unna PG. *The Histopathology of the Diseases of the Skin.* New York: Macmillan; 1896:517–570.
10. Abell E, Marks R, Wilson-Jones E. Secondary syphilis: a clinico-pathological review. *Br J Dermatol.* 1975;93:53–61.
11. Jeerapaet P, Ackerman AB. Histologic patterns of secondary syphilis. *Arch Dermatol.* 1973;107:373–377.
12. Fisher DA, Chang LW, Tuffanelli DL. Lues maligna. *Arch Dermatol.* 1969;99:70–73.
13. Degos R, Touraine R, Collart P, et al. Syphilis maligne précoce d'évolution mortelle (avec examen anatomique). *Bull Soc Fr Dermatol Syph.* 1970;77:10–15.
14. Adam W, Korting GW. Lues maligna. *Arch Klin Exp Dermatol.* 1960;210:14–26.
15. Petrozzi JW, Lockshin NA, Berger BJ. Malignant syphilis. *Arch Dermatol.* 1974;109:387–389.
16. Johnson WC. Venereal diseases and treponemal infections. In: Graham JH, Johnson WC, Helwig EB, eds. *Dermal Pathology.* New York: Harper & Row; 1972;371–373.
17. Cochran REI, Thomson JT, Fleming KA, et al. Histology simulating reticulosis in secondary syphilis. *Br J Dermatol.* 1976;95:251–254.
18. Pembroke AC, Michell PA, McKee PH. Nodulo-squamous tertiary syphilide. *Clin Exp Dermatol.* 1980;5:361–364.
19. Holtzmann H, Hassenpflug K. Tertiärsyphilitische Lymphknotenbeteilgung vom granulierenden Typ bei einem Kranken mit plattenargigen Gummen der Haut. *Arch Klin Exp Dermatol.* 1962;215:230–245.
20. Tuta JA, Coombs RA. Symmetric syphilitic granulomas of the elbow. *Arch Dermatol Syph.* 1942;46:375–378.
21. Kaltz F, Newton BL. Syphilitic juxtarticular nodules. *Arch Dermatol Syph.* 1943;48:626–634.
22. Dooley JR, Binford CH. Treponematoses. In: Binford CH, Connor DH, eds. *Pathology of Tropical and Extraordinary Diseases.* Washington, DC: Armed Forces Institute of Pathology; 1976; 1:116.
23. Hasselmann CM. Comparative studies on the histopathology of syphilis, yaws and pinta. *Br J Vener Dis.* 1957;33:5–23.
24. Williams HU. Pathology of yaws. *Arch Pathol.* 1935;20:596–630.
25. Ferris HW, Turner TB. Comparative histology of yaws and syphilis in Jamaica. *Arch Pathol.* 1937;24:703–737.
26. Pardo-Castello V, Ferrer I. Pinta. *Arch Dermatol Syph.* 1942; 45:843–864.
27. Dooley JR, Binford CH. Treponematoses. In: Binford CH, Conner DH, eds. *Pathology of Tropical and Extraordinary Diseases.* Washington, DC: Armed Forces Institute of Pathology; 1976;1:113.
28. Rodriguez HA, Albores-Saavedra J, Lozano MM, et al. Langerhans' cells in late pinta. *Arch Pathol.* 1971;91:302–306.
29. Steere AC, Malawista SE, Snyder DR, et al. A cluster of arthritis in children and adults in Lyme, Connecticut. *Arthritis Rheum.* 1976;20:824. Abstract.
30. Lennhoff C. Spirochaetes in aetiologically obscure diseases. *Acta Derm Venereol.* 1948;28:295–324.
31. Burgdorfer W, Barbour AG, Hayes SF, et al. Lyme disease—a tick-borne spirochetosis? *Science.* 1982;216:1317–1319.
32. Berger BW, Clemmensen OJ, Ackerman AB. Lyme disease is a spirochetosis. *Am J Dermatopathol.* 1983;5:111–124.
33. Waldo ED, Sidhu GS. The spirochete in erythema chronicum migrans. *Am J Dermatopathol.* 1983;5:125–127.
34. Mélotte P, Pierard GE. Spirochetosis in ticks. *Am J Dermatopathol.* 1984;6:414–415.
35. Frithz A, Lagerholm B. Acrodermatitis chronica atrophicans, erythema chronicum migrans and lymphadenosis benigna cutis—spirochetal diseases? *Acta Derm Venereol.* 1983;63:432–436.
36. Åsbrink E, Hovmark A, Hederstedt B. The spirochetal etiology of acrodermatitis chronica atrophicans Herxheimer. *Acta Derm Venereol.* 1984;64:506–512.
37. Åsbrink E, Brehmer-Andersson E, Hovmark A. Acrodermatitis chronica atrophicans—a spirochetosis. *Am J Dermatopathol.* 1986;8:209–219.

CHAPTER 28
Diseases Caused by Protozoa
Amal Kurban and Abdul-Ghani Kibbi

DEFINITION AND CLASSIFICATION

Protozoa are single-celled eukaryotic organisms that reproduce by binary fission. The various groups of protozoa share common fundamental structures but differ in size and form. Species of the two genera, *Leishmania* and *Entamoeba*, are discussed in this chapter.

CUTANEOUS LEISHMANIASIS

Pathogenesis
Human leishmaniasis, caused by members of the genus *Leishmania*, encompasses a heterogeneous spectrum of diseases.[1,2] Three major forms generally are distinguished: cutaneous, mucocutaneous, and visceral. Cutaneous leishmaniasis can be caused by species and subspecies of *Leishmania tropica*, *Leishmania braziliensis*, and *Leishmania mexicana*, and the mucocutaneous form is caused by subspecies of *L. braziliensis*.[3] The usual vectors are sandflies of the genera *Phlebotomus*, *Sergeutomyia*, and *Lutzomyia*, and the animal reservoirs are infected dogs, gerbils, rats, and other rodents.[2,4] The different species and strains of *Leishmania* cannot be differentiated morphologically. However, analysis of enzyme patterns, determination of the buoyant density of kinetoplastic DNA, and immunologic tests are useful methods for such differentiation.[2,5] Two distinct morphologic forms of leishmania exist: the flagellated promastigote in the insect vector and in culture media and the unflagellated amastigote (leishman bodies) in the mammalian host.[1,6] Following inoculation in human skin, the flagellated parasites are taken up by macrophages within which they transform into the unflagellated form. The parasites multiply rapidly, causing macrophage rupture and release of parasites.[7] These are than taken up by other macrophages or are ingested during a blood meal by female sandflies, which in turn transmit them into other hosts.[2]

Clinical Features
Two weeks to 8 months after inoculation, small erythematous papules appear at the sites of the insect bites, which are usually on exposed parts.[1,3] In acute cutaneous leishmaniasis (ACL), the papules progress to nodules that may ulcerate and then heal over a period of months, leaving depressed and disfiguring scars.[1] On rare occasions, satellite lesions[8] or sporotrichoid nodules develop.[9,10] Resolution imparts permanent immunity. Chronic cutaneous leishmaniasis (CCL) evolves from lesions that fail to heal and follows a protracted course over many years. The lesions are erythematous, scaly plaques,[1] and ulceration is very rare. An uncommon sequela of Old World ACL (5%) is recurrent cutaneous leishmaniasis (RCL) or leishmaniasis recidivans (LR).[6] Months to years after the partial or total resolution of the acute disease, yellowish brown translucent nodules develop in or around the healed scar.[1,11] The strongly positive response of the Montenegro skin test attests to the strong delayed hypersensitivity status of patients with RCL. In diffuse cutaneous leishmaniasis (DCL), there are disseminated macules, papules, nodules, and rarely ulcers rich in organisms.[12] Internal organs are not involved. The Montenegro skin test is negative, and the course is prolonged and progressive. Dissemination is by lymphatic and hematogenous routes.

In mucocutaneous leishmaniasis (MCL), cutaneous lesions are followed by mucosal involvement that is particularly destructive and does not heal spontaneously.[2] The nasopharynx is especially affected. In dermal post-kala-azar leishmaniasis, cutaneous lesions appear years after apparent recovery from visceral leishmaniasis (caused by *Leishmania donovani*). The lesions are polymorphic and range from hypopigmented or hyperpigmented macules to erythematous macules and nodules.[13]

Histologic Features
The varied histologic findings in cutaneous leishmaniasis relate to the duration of the lesions and the complex interre-

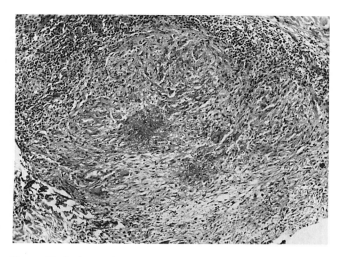

Figure 28–1. A granulomatous infiltrate composed of macrophages, lymphocytes, and plasma cells is seen. Note the focus of fibrinoid necrosis in the center of the granuloma (H&E ×125).

lationship between the parasite and its host.[14–17] Even though there is an overlap, the pathologic changes are somehow distinct for each of the aforementioned clinical forms.[15]

Acute Cutaneous Leishmaniasis. The epidermis shows nonspecific changes of hyperkeratosis, parakeratosis, epidermal atrophy or hyperplasia, and occasionally pseudoepitheliomatous hyperplasia.[15,16] Vacuolar degeneration of the basal cell layer may be seen, especially when the dermal inflammatory infiltrate abuts to the basement membrane zone. Intraepidermal abscesses composed of neutro-

phils and round cells occur infrequently, mainly in lesions of sporotrichoid leishmaniasis (SL).[15,18] Leishman bodies (LB) occasionally are seen within keratinocytes. It has been suggested that the epidermal hyperplasia is induced by γ-interferon released by the dermal T lymphocytes, leading to keratinocyte Ia expression and epidermal thickening.[19] Throughout the dermis, there is a diffuse infiltrate consisting predominantly of large macrophages, with interspersed lymphocytes and plasma cells (Fig. 28–1). Intracellular and extracellular parasites are numerous (Fig. 28–2). Eosinophils are usually absent.[15] Tubercle formation may be seen in the American-acquired[20] and sporotrichoid leishmaniasis.[18] Neutrophils are seen when there is ulceration or dermal necrosis.[21] Dermal necrosis may be diffuse, notably in lesions with an intermediate number of organisms, or focal in the centers of the granulomas, when the parasite load is low.

Chronic Cutaneous Leishmaniasis. The prominent histologic feature in CCL is the microtubercle, which consists of epithelioid cells and a few giant cells of the Langhans type.[6,15] The tubercles are surrounded by a mantle of lymphocytes, histiocytes, and sparse plasma cells (Fig. 28–3). Necrosis, although rare, may occur and is of the apoptotic type in which the necrotized cells undergo marked condensation of their nuclear chromatin and cytoplasm.[22] Eventually, this leads to disintegration into small fragments composed of nuclear debris and cytoplasmic remnants that might possibly represent hematoxyphilic bodies seen commonly by light microscopy in lesions of cutaneous leishmaniasis. Leishmania organisms are either absent or extremely difficult to see.[15] The epidermal alterations are variable, although ulceration is almost always absent. Immunohistochemically, S100-positive and lysosome-negative histiocytic cells are present in the inflammatory infiltrate, especially

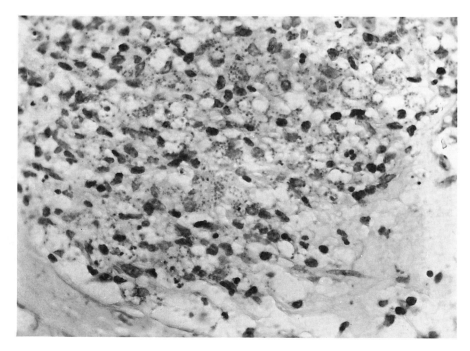

Figure 28–2. Numerous intracellular and extracellular leishman bodies are evident in this photomicrograph of ACL (H&E ×500).

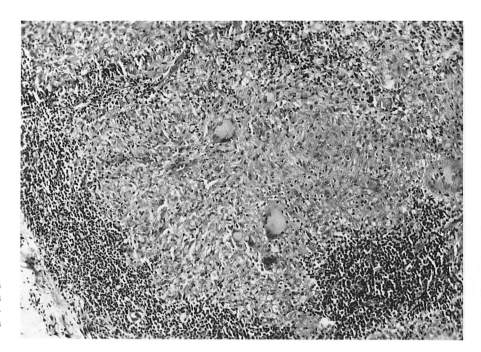

Figure 28–3. A cluster of epithelioid cells with interspersed giant cells of the Langhans type forms a microtubercle in CCL. An intense mononuclear cell infiltrate surrounds this tubercle (H&E ×125).

around the granulomas.[23] These cells with dendritelike projections presumably participate in antigen recognition and presentation and the release of mediators that in turn stimulate T cells. Ultrastructurally, an intimate contact between lymphocytes and macrophages has been noted, further substantiating the interaction between the two cell types.[22]

Recurrent Cutaneous Leishmaniasis. Features of both the acute and chronic forms of leishmaniasis occur.[6,15] The epidermis is variably hyperplastic, and the dermis is infiltrated by an admixture of histiocytes, lymphoid cells, and sparse plasma cells. There are tuberculoid granulomas with or without giant cells. Necrosis as well as necrobiosis in the centers of these granulomas may be observed. Organisms may be absent, scanty, or rarely numerous.

Diffuse Disseminated Leishmaniasis. This form is characterized by the presence of heavily parasitized macrophages throughout the dermis[12] (Fig. 28–4). On electron microscopy, the parasites are localized in either parasitophorous vacuoles or singly within the cytoplasm.[24]

Mucocutaneous Leishmaniasis. The changes are similar to those in ACL except for a lower parasite load.[25] In some cases, no parasites are demonstrable. There are, however, plasma cells containing Russell bodies, considered by some to be an adjunctive criterion for the histologic diagnosis.[26] The ulcerodestructive mucocutaneous lesions reveal a nonspecific inflammatory cell response with a few parasite-laden macrophages and few or no tuberculoid components.[2]

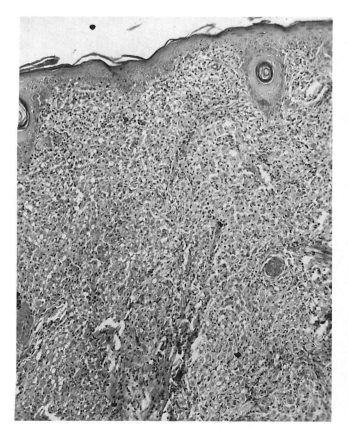

Figure 28–4. Throughout the dermis, a diffuse infiltrate of organism-rich macrophages is present. The infiltrate hugs the dermoepidermal junction, where there is basal cell vacuolization (H&E ×125). (*Courtesy of Dr. Sebastian Lucas, University College, London, UK.*)

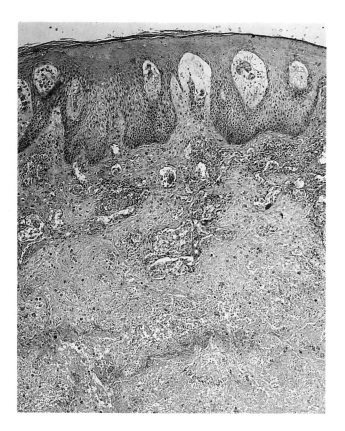

Figure 28–5. Cutaneous amebiasis with papillary dermal edema, dermal necrosis, and acute and chronic inflammation (H&E ×55).

Dermal Post-Kala-Azar Leishmaniasis. There is a dermal infiltrate of lymphocytes, plasma cells, and histiocytes.[13] The number of organisms is variable. The degree of the cellular infiltrate varies with the clinical presentation, being least in the macular lesions and most in the nodular. In the latter, epithelioid cells, a few giant cells, and numerous plasma cells are also seen.

Diagnosis and Differential Diagnosis

The diagnosis of cutaneous leishmaniasis depends on identification of the organism in tissue sections or in smears or culture.[1,26] Direct smear examination using Giemsa stain is positive in a high percentage (over 70%) in ACL and DCL but is usually negative in CCL and RCL.[6] In tissue sections, the organisms, if present, appear as round or oval bodies ranging in size from 2 μm to 4 μm.[27] The parasites usually are visible in routinely stained sections but are best seen when a Giemsa stain is employed. Each organism possesses a deeply basophilic round nucleus about 1 μm in diameter and a small rodlike paranucleus or kinetoplast. Both the nucleus and the kinetoplast stain bright red with the Giemsa stain.

Since the organisms are obligate intracellular parasites of macrophages, leishmaniasis must be distinguished from other cutaneous disorders characterized by parasite-filled macrophages.[27] These are rhinoscleroma, granuloma inguinale, and histoplasmosis. In rhinoscleroma, there are Mikulicz cells, Russell bodies, and a large number of plasma cells. In granuloma inguinale, encapsulated round to oval bodies are seen, as are neutrophil-containing small abscesses throughout the lesion. In histoplasmosis, round to oval bodies surrounded by a clear halo and foci of tissue necrosis are displayed. In the absence of organisms, especially in the chronic and recidivans forms, the differentiation

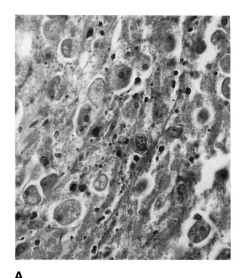

A

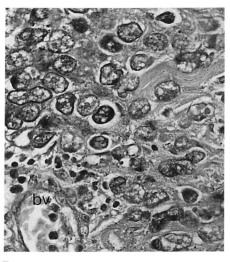

B

Figure 28–6. In biopsy specimens, organisms are more readily visualized with a PAS stain. Note size of organisms relative to erythrocytes in blood vessel (bv). (**A.** H&E ×575; **B.** Periodic acid-Schiff, ×575.)

of cutaneous leishmaniasis from lupus vulgaris is difficult. However, the lack of caseation necrosis and the sparsity of plasma cells are ancillary clues to establish a correct diagnosis.[15]

CUTANEOUS AMEBIASIS

Pathogenesis
Cutaneous amebiasis, a rare disorder chiefly encountered in endemic areas, is caused by *Entamoeba histolytica*.[28] Skin lesions arise from perianal extension of acute amebic colitis, rupture or open drainage of colonic, appendiceal, or hepatic lesions into the abdominal skin, or external skin contact with infectious material.

Clinical Features
The signs and symptoms are nonspecific. The lesion is usually a deeply invading ulcer with indistinct indurated borders and is rarely an exudative verrucous plaque.[28] Sites of predilection include the perianal region, buttocks, abdominal wall, face, legs, and genitalia.

Histologic Features
The histologic features are not diagnostic.[28] The ulcer has a base of necrotic debris and shows acute and chronic inflammation. The ulcer edges show pseudoepitheliomatous hyperplasia, especially in the verrucous lesions.[29] Organisms are not easily identified on routine hematoxylin and eosin staining (Figs. 28–5, 28–6). Hence, smear preparations become mandatory for a definitive diagnosis.[28]

Diagnosis and Differential Diagnosis
The diagnosis of cutaneous amebiasis rests on identification of the ameba organisms.[28] The trophozoites can be identified

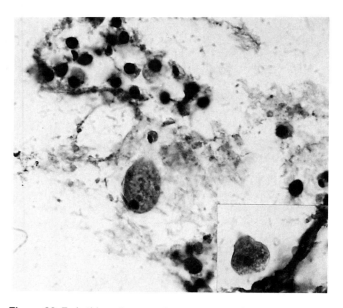

Figure 28–7. In this wet smear of cutaneous amebiasis, two trophozoites are shown. Note the difference in size between the organisms and the surrounding mononuclear cells (H&E ×788).

in saline mounts of skin scrapings or in smears that can be fixed and stained with Gomori's trichrome (Fig. 28–7). The trophozoites range in size from 10 to 60 μm in diameter and exhibit rather remarkable locomotion when examined in saline mounts.

REFERENCES

1. Farah FS, Malak JA. Cutaneous leishmaniasis. *Arch Dermatol.* 1971;103:467–474.
2. Kern P. Leishmaniasis. *Antibiot Chemother.* 1981;30:203–223.
3. Nelson DA, Gustafson TL, Spielvogel RL. Clinical aspects of cutaneous leishmaniasis acquired in Texas. *J Am Acad Dermatol.* 1985;12:985–992.
4. Gustafson TL, Reed CM, McGreevy PB, et al. Human cutaneous leishmaniasis acquired in Texas. *Am J Trop Med Hyg.* 1985;34:58–63.
5. Barbosa W, Moreira De Souza MdoC, De Souze JM, et al. Note on the classification of the *Leishmania* sp. responsible for cutaneous leishmaniasis in the east central region of Brazil. *Ann Trop Med Parasitol.* 1976;70:389–399.
6. Stratigos JD. New aspects on cutaneous leishmaniasis. *Derm Beruf Unwelt.* 1980;28:139–148.
7. Ridley MJ, Wells CW. Macrophage–parasite interaction in the lesions of cutaneous leishmaniasis: an ultrastructural study. *Am J Pathol.* 1986;123:79–85.
8. Bienzle U, Ebert F, Dietrich M. Cutaneous leishmaniasis in Eastern Saudi Arabia. Epidemiological and clinical features in a nonimmune population living in an endemic area. *Tropenmed Parasitol.* 1978;29:188–193.
9. Berger TG, Meltzer MS, Oster CN. Lymph node involvement in leishmaniasis. *J Am Acad Dermatol.* 1985;12:993–996.
10. Spier S, Medenica M, McMillan S, et al. Sporotrichoid leishmaniasis. *Arch Dermatol.* 1972;113:1104–1105.
11. Strick RA, Borok M, Gasiorowski HC, et al. Recurrent cutaneous leishmaniasis. *J Am Acad Dermatol.* 1983;9:437–443.
12. Convit J, Pinardi ME, Rondon AJ. Diffuse cutaneous leishmaniasis: a disease due to an immunological defect of the host. *Trans R Soc Trop Med Hyg.* 1972;66:603–610.
13. Girgla HS, Marsden RA, Singh GM, et al. Post-kala-azar dermal leishmaniasis. *Br J Dermatol.* 1977;97:307–311.
14. Azadeh B, Samad A, Ardehali S. Histological spectrum of cutaneous leishmaniasis due to *Leishmania tropica*. *Trans R Soc Trop Med Hyg.* 1985;79:631–636.
15. Kurban AK, Malak JA, Farah FS, et al. Histopathology of cutaneous leishmaniasis. *Arch Dermatol.* 1966;93:396–401.
16. Ridley DS. A histological classification of cutaneous leishmaniasis and its geographical expression. *Trans R Soc Trop Med Hyg.* 1980;74:515–521.
17. Ridley DS, Ridley MJ. The evolution of the lesion in cutaneous leishmaniasis. *J Pathol.* 1983;141:83–96.
18. Kibbi AG, Karam PG, Kurban AK. Sporotrichoid Leishmaniasis in patients from Saudi Arabia: clinical and histological features. *J Am Acad Dermatol.* 1987;17:759–764.
19. Kaplan G, Witmer MD, Nath I, et al. Influence of delayed immune reactions on human epidermal keratinocytes. *Proc Natl Acad Sci USA.* 1986;83:3469–3473.
20. Andrade-Narvaez F, Garcia-Miss MA.R, Cruz-Ruiz AL, et al. Preliminary study of clinical, histopathological and immunological correlation of mexican cutaneous leishmaniasis in man. *Arch Invest Med (Mex).* 1984;15:267–279.
21. Ridley DS. The pathogenesis of cutaneous leishmaniasis. *Trans R Soc Trop Med Hyg.* 1979;73:150–160.
22. El Hassan AM, Veress B, Kutty MK. The ultrastructural morphology of human cutaneous leishmaniasis of low parasite load. *Acta Derm Venereol.* 1984;64:501–505.

23. Veress B, El Hassan AM. Immunohistochemical demonstration of S100 protein antigen-containing cells in chronic cutaneous leishmaniasis. *Acta Pathol Microbiol Immunol Scand.* [*A*]. 1985; 93:331–334.

24. Zaar K, Wundelrich F. Electron microscopical studies on cutaneous leishmaniasis in Ethiopia. I: the diffuse form and its treatment with pentamidine. *Ann Trop Med Parasitol.* 1982; 76:595–605.

25. Price SM, Silvers DN. New World leishmaniasis. *Arch Dermatol.* 1977;113:1415–1416.

26. Babareschi M, Mariscotti C, Missoni E, et al. Russell bodies in New World cutaneous leishmaniasis. *Pathologica.* 1985; 77:87–90.

27. Lever WF, Schaumburg-Lever G. *Histopathology of the Skin.* Philadelphia: JB Lippincott Co; 1990:394–398.

28. Fujita WH, Barr RJ, Gottschalk HR. Cutaneous amebiasis. *Arch Dermatol.* 1981;117:309–310.

29. Majmudar B, Chaiken ML, Lee KW. Amebiasis of the clitoris mimicking carcinoma. *JAMA.* 1976;236:1145–1146.

CHAPTER 29
Diseases Caused by Fungi

Justin Roscoe and Evan R. Farmer

The purpose of this chapter is to provide a practical framework that will aid the histologic identification in the skin of fungal diseases and the fungi that cause them. It is not intended to be a compendium of all aspects of mycoses nor of all pathogenic fungi and their characteristics, since there are numerous excellent books on the subject. Furthermore, the classification of fungi is a matter of ongoing reformulation and discussion. For the sake of simplicity and to avoid controversy, we use the most widely accepted nomenclature and list synonymous names only when appropriate. Also, since this is predominantly a light microscopy text and distinguishing between hyphae and pseudohyphae requires electron microscopy, we use the terms "mycelia" or "hyphal elements," which are more general.

GENERAL PATHOGENESIS

Fungi are among the most ubiquitous microorganisms, but fortunately for both the human race and dermatopathologists, relatively few of them cause disease. Some, such as *Malassezia furfur* or *Candida albicans*, may be normal flora of the skin or mucous membranes. In order to be pathogenic, fungi must fulfill certain criteria: (1) have access, (2) invade, (3) establish and multiply, (4) produce an inappropriate host response, and (5) damage the host.

Access varies greatly depending on whether the fungus is a normal inhabitant of our skin, ubiquitous like *Aspergillus fumigatus,* or found only in certain environments like *Loboa loboi.* Once a fungus has access, it may or may not invade. The normal fungal flora of the skin is composed of yeastlike organisms that remain on the skin or mucosal surface. A change in environmental or host conditions is needed to provide an opportunity for the spores to form hyphal elements and invade the skin or mucosal surface. This ability of certain fungi to modify their morphology in response to environmental and host factors is known as "dimorphism." Several environmental factors are particularly important to fungi. For example, warmth and occlusion seem

to favor the growth of dermatophytes, antibiotic therapy favors the growth of *C. albicans,* temperature is critical to *Sporothrix schenkii,* and medium-length fatty acids are an absolute nutritional requirement for the growth of *M. furfur.*

The host immune response is of critical importance to permit the establishment and growth of the fungus and develop a particular histologic pattern. It is known that immunity to fungi largely depends on the cellular response, particularly the granulomatous reaction pattern. However, much work is still needed, since the majority of individuals with fungal disease apparently do not suffer from general immunosuppression of their cellular response but rather from specific defects that are as yet uncharacterized. Eosinophils or neutrophils may also figure prominently. In addition to the immune response, the epidermis is also capable of responding, ranging from desquamation to pseudoepitheliomatous hyperplasia.

Numerous mechanisms have been postulated to account for how fungi damage their host. Some fungi cause disease by the simple mass effect of their growth, such as *Cryptococcus neoformans* in the brain. Various toxins have been postulated as mediating pathogenic effects. It is likely that most pathogenic fungi exert multiple effects that damage the host. For example, *A. fumigatus* can induce fever presumably by liberating toxins, may induce pulmonary hypersensitivity, and can produce a space-occupying lesion or directly invade and destroy tissue, as well as embolize to blood vessels, producing infarction.[1] On the other hand, despite *A. fumigatus* being a ubiquitous fungus, it rarely is capable of producing any disease in a truly immunocompetent host.

CLASSIFICATION

There is no perfect way to classify the mycoses because one fungus may produce several disease entities or a single disease entity may be produced by more than one fungus. Nowhere is this more obvious than in the controversy surrounding the dematiaceous (endogenous pigment-producing) fungi, which cause several infections: tinea nigra, chromomycosis, phaeomycotic cyst, some phaeohyphomycosis, and eumycotic mycetoma. For example, *Phialophora* (Exophiala) *jeanselmei* has been identified as an etiologic agent of chromomycosis, phaeohyphomycosis, phaeomycotic cyst, and eumycotic mycetoma. On the other hand, chromomycosis is caused by multiple agents, of which *Fonsecaea pedrosoi*, *Phialophora verrucosa*, and *Cladosporium carrionii* are the three most common. For this reason, it is not possible to classify fungal disease merely on the basis of etiologic agent. In this chapter, we arbitrarily classify the mycoses as superficial, subcutaneous, or systemic, depending on where they most commonly produce lesions.

Superficial fungi are capable only of growth in dead corneocytes and the lipids that envelop them, although in special circumstances, they may invade. Subcutaneous fungal infections are caused by low virulence fungi found in water and soil that require direct inoculation for access. They are indolent growers but may be very difficult to eradicate. Systemic fungal infections are caused by either opportunistic or truly pathogenic fungi. The opportunistic fungi require a severely immunocompromised host and are either part of the normal human flora or are widespread soil organisms. There are few truly pathogenic fungi, and these, fortunately, are restricted to certain geographic areas, and most such infections resolve spontaneously. The portal of entry and initial site of infection are almost invariably pulmonary, followed by dissemination to multiple organs and the skin depending on the host immunity. All of the truly pathogenic fungi grow as hyphal elements at 25° C but become transformed and grow as yeasts in the body at 37° C, a characteristic known as "thermal dimorphism."

APPROACH TO DIAGNOSIS

The diagnosis of fungal disease in a skin biopsy stained by hematoxylin and eosin begins with suspecting that a fungus is involved. The stratum corneum should be surveyed for hyphae or pseudohyphae (Fig. 29–1). Budding yeasts are a sign of colonization but are not indicative of disease. An inflammatory infiltrate with eosinophils should increase the suspicion of a superficial fungal infection. This should also be the case in a folliculitis, with particular attention being given to the hair shaft.

Another pattern in which fungal infection becomes likely is that of pseudoepitheliomatous hyperplasia (Fig. 29–2), especially when accompanied by a granulomatous infiltrate with giant cells, neutrophilic abscesses, or eosinophils. It is particularly useful to look carefully at the cytoplasm of the giant cells or at the center of abscesses, although the fungi may be found standing free or be exceedingly difficult to find, as in sporotrichosis. Pattern becomes increasingly less important as the fungus grows deeper, particularly in the immunocompromised host (Fig. 29–3).

Several special stains can enhance detecting and properly identifying fungi in histologic sections. The two most commonly used are methenamine silver and periodic acid-Schiff (PAS). PAS stains all polysaccharides, which may

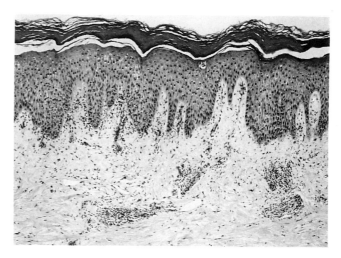

Figure 29–1. Dermatophytosis. The epidermis shows compact hyperkeratosis, acanthosis, mild spongiosis, exocytosis of lymphocytes, and a moderate perivascular lymphocytic infiltrate. (H&E, ×125).

result in glycogen granules being interpreted as fungi. It is, therefore, useful to predigest with diastase (amylase), which is incapable of digesting the chitin and cellulose found in fungus cell walls. Although immunologic stains may in the future afford greater specificity, the PAS-D stain is generally the most useful one on a routine basis in terms of diagnostic value, reproducibility, and cost. Mucicarmine is also useful for staining of cryptococcosis and rhinosporidiosis. All fungi in tissue produce either spores, pseudohyphae, or hyphae. The size and morphology of spores are compared in Table 29–1, and the mycelia are compared in Table 29–2.

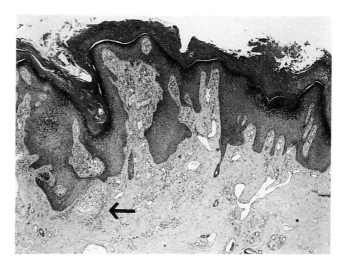

Figure 29–2. Chromomycosis. This specimen shows the typical pattern of pseudoepitheliomatous hyperplasia in association with granulomas (*arrow*) (H&E, ×45).

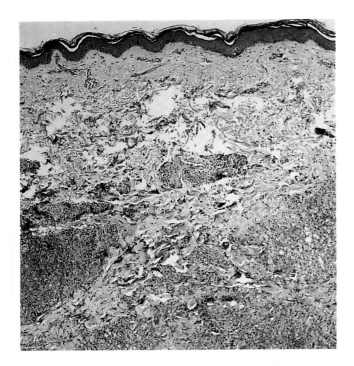

Figure 29–3. Cryptococcosis. This specimen from an immunocompromised patient shows a diffuse granulomatous infiltrate filling the lower two thirds of the reticular dermis with a normal overlying epidermis (H&E, ×60).

SPECIFIC DISEASES

SUPERFICIAL MYCOSES

Dermatophytoses

History

The first microorganism shown to cause a human disease was a dermatophyte. David Gruby published an article documenting the isolation of the fungus of favus on potato slices and the production of the disease by inoculation on human skin in 1841,[2] antedating Koch by 40 years. Unfortunately, because of the religious prejudices of the time, credit was given to Shoenlein when the fungus was named, although he was also not the first to describe it. The great dermatologist, Sabouraud, in his 1910 classic *Les Teignes*, classified dermatophytes into the genera *Microsporum, Trichophyton,* and *Epidermophyton.*[3] He developed the basic culture medium for fungi and a treatment regimen that was the standard until the advent of griseofulvin. The term "tinea" is properly reserved only for diseases caused by species of these genera, which are characterized not only on morphologic grounds but also by the production and tolerance of an alkaline pH, sensitivity to 20 μg/ml or less of griseofulvin, and resistance to 500 μg/ml of cycloheximide. In the United States, the term often is used to designate pityriasis (tinea) versicolor, which is not caused by a

TABLE 29–1. SPORES IN TISSUE

Name	Diameter	Shape (μm)	Differentiating Features
Pityriasis versicolor	2–8	Round	Variable number of thick (2–3μm), short mycelia may be seen
Candidiasis	3–6	Round/oval	Variable numbers of thin (1–2μm), long mycelia with blastoconidia
Sporotrichosis	4–6	Round/oval	Cigar bodies, mycelia very rare, asteroid bodies
Chromomycosis	6–12	Round/oval	Bronze-colored, thick walls (no budding), mycelia very rare
Phaeohyphomycosis	2–25	Round/oval	Brown, budding, chains of spores, mycelia predominate
Lobomycosis	9–10	Lemon-shaped	Single budding, narrow-base spores form chains that may branch; no mycelia, asteroid bodies
Rhinosporidiosis	6–10	Round	10–12μm spherule, 250–350μm sporangia also seen, mucicarmine positive
Coccidioidomycosis	2–5	Round	10–80μm spherule, asteroid bodies, mycelia very rare
Paracoccidioidomycosis	1–40	Round	Multiple narrow-neck budding
Blastomycosis	8–30	Round	Broad-based bud, thick wall
Histoplasmosis (var. capsulatum)	3	Round	Pseudocapsule (mucicarmine negative), narrow-neck budding. H & E stains cytoplasm dark blue, PAS and methenamine silver stain pseudocapsule
Histoplasmosis (var. duboisii)	10–15	Ovoid	4–5 cell chains may be seen
Cryptococcosis	3–20	Round	Narrow-neck budding; true capsule (mucicarmine positive), H & E negative, PAS & and methenamine silver stain spore but not capsule

TABLE 29–2. MYCOSES WITH PROMINENT MYCELIA

Regular mycelia
  Hyaline
    Dermatophytosis
    Pityriasis versicolor
    Candidiasis
  Dematiaceous
    Phaeohyphomycosis
    Phaeomycotic cyst
Irregular
  Septate
    Aspergillosis
  Coenocytic (nonseptate)
    Zygomycosis
Clumped
  Fungus ball
    Pseudoallescheria boydii
    Sporothrix schenkii
    Coccidioides immitis
    Aspergillus spp.
  Eumycetoma
  Scutula (favus)

TABLE 29–3. DERMATOPHYTES

Dermatophyte infections of hair
1. Caused only by *Microsporum* and *Trichophyton* spp., not by *Epidermophyton*
2. *Microsporum* produces ectothrix, and *Trichophyton* produces endothrix infections of the hair
3. *Microsporum* (*canis, adouinii, distortum, ferrugineum*) fluoresce yellow-green; of the *Trichophyton* spp., only *T. schoenleinii* fluoresces a dull blue-white
4. The fluorescent *Microsporum* exospores are much smaller (2–3μm) than *Trichophyton* endospores (8–10 μm); only nonfluorescent *M. gypseum* has 8μm exospores
5. *T. shoenleinii* does not produce spores in hair shafts, only hyphae that leave air spaces.
6. Nondermatophyte mycoses may also affect the hair: white piedra (*Trichosporum beigelii*) and black piedra (*Piedraia hortai*); trichomycosis axillaris (nodosum), despite the name, is caused by a corynebacterium

Dermatophyte infections of nail (tinea unguium)
1. Subungual involvement can be caused by any genus, but *Trichophyton rubrum* is by far the most common agent
2. Leukonychia mycotica (white spote disease) is caused exclusively by *Trichophyton mentagrophytes*
3. Other fungi affect the nail and produce onychomycosis, the most common being *Candida albicans, Candida parapsicosis,* and *Trichosporum beigelii*

dermatophyte, but by the yeast, *M. furfur.* Tinea nigra, caused by *Exophiala* (*Cladosporium*) *werneckii,* is also not a tinea.

Clinical Features

Dermatophyte infections have been known at least since Greek and Roman times. The Greeks used the adjective *herpes* to describe the tendency for the rash to move like a snake in a circular form. The Romans attributed its causation to insect larvae and called it *tinea.* The English term *ringworm* is a combination of both.

The clinical features of dermatophyte infections are determined by three factors: the particular species of fungus involved, the location of the infection, and the host response. Certain dermatophytes are known to infect hair and nails, whereas others do not (Table 29–3). Some fluoresce on Wood's light examination of hairs. Dermatophytes may be classified as zoophilic, geophilic, or anthropophilic depending on whether they are usually found on animals, soil, or humans. As a rule, zoophilic fungi produce more of a host response than do geophilic fungi, which produce more of a host response than do anthropophilic fungi. Dermatophyte infections are clinically described as tinea manum when occurring on the hands, tinea capitis when occurring on the scalp, and so on. For example, the zoophilic fungus *Microsporum canis,* which often produces inflammatory tinea capitis in children, may produce a generalized noninflammatory tinea corporis in an immunosuppressed individual.

Histologic Features

The histopathologic features of dermatophyte infections mirror the clinical appearance. Interestingly, the more inflammatory a lesion is, the more difficult it may become to demonstrate the fungus by either KOH, culture, or microscopy.

DERMATOPHYTE INFECTIONS OF THE HAIR. These most commonly occur on the scalp (tinea capitis) (Fig. 29–4) and on the beard area (tinea barbae), but actually any hair-bearing area may be involved. The involvement may be on the surface of the hair or may burrow into the hair.[4] Spore size and disposition in chains are other factors that aid in

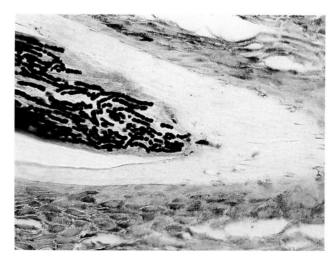

Figure 29–4. Tinea capitis. Hyphal elements are present, filling the follicular lumen and, in this field essentially replacing the hair shaft (PAS-D, ×480).

actually identifying the species involved, as shown in Table 29–1.

There is an entire spectrum of inflammatory response. A common finding is the follicular or perifollicular pustule or neutrophilic abscess, often with numerous eosinophils, and a variable number of lymphoid, histiocytic, and giant cells.[5] Plasma cells also may be seen. Hyphae may be seen in the dermis after follicular rupture. However, the response may range from practically none to the intense granulomatous reaction that characterizes Majocchi's granuloma,[6] a condition usually seen in women who shave their legs. Another special variant, tinea favosa or favus (L., honeycomb), is caused mainly by one species, Trichophyton schoenleinii, and is characterized by an intense inflammatory reaction,[7] leading to a cicatricial alopecia. It is histologically distinctive because of the air bubbles and hyphae seen, the absence of spores, and the clumps of hyphae known as scutula.

DERMATOPHYTE INFECTIONS OF NAILS. Tinea unguium can be of two major types: those that involve only the uppermost surface of the nail plate, also known as white spot disease or leukonychia mycotica, usually caused by Trichophyton mentagrophytes, and those that first involve the nailbed and only later involve the lowermost portion of the nail plate, usually caused by Trichophyton rubrum. The nail matrix is never involved, and a diagnostic biopsy should not be necessary in most cases. Although the nail plate is routinely examined by KOH and cultured for diagnosis, histologic sections are more likely to demonstrate the fungus than a KOH smear because of the difficulty in dissolving nail keratin (Fig. 29–5). The spores and hyphal elements may be seen clearly, but there usually is very little if any inflammatory response even if the nailbed and matrix are included.[8]

DERMATOPHYTE INFECTIONS OF GLABROUS SKIN. These comprise all remaining dermatophyte infections (Fig. 29–1). There may be very little inflammatory response and precious

few hyphal elements, perhaps visible only in transverse sections as small round spaces between corneocytes. There may only be psoriasiform hyperplasia with slight hyperkeratosis and a mild mononuclear perivascular infiltrate, yet abundant hyphae are seen. Very intense spongiosis with eosinophils may be present, which often may not have many hyphal elements. These features may be combined with those described for dermatophyte infections of hair. In summary, there is anywhere from minimal chronic dermatitis to acute spongiotic dermatitis, with variable degrees of hair involvement and amounts of hyphae.[9]

Differential Diagnosis

The differential diagnosis of dermatophyte infections of the hair includes alopecia, folliculitis, and parafolliculitis. The differential of nail involvement is psoriasis and pachyonychia secondary to circulatory changes. The reaction pattern on glabrous skin is identical to the spectrum from chronic dermatitis through acute spongiotic dermatitis.

The regular septate hyphae of dermatophytes in the stratum corneum must be distinguished from Candida sp. and M. furfur (spores should be seen, and the mycelia are less regular and usually pseudoseptate), as well as from Exophiala werneckii (dematiaceous). In the hair, piedra and trichomycosis nodularis (axillaris) must be considered. Fungi in the nails cover a very wide spectrum, with Candida sp. being common, followed by numerous occasionally encountered fungi that must be identified by culture. Dermatophytes may produce round arthrospores in nails, which may be difficult to distinguish from budding yeasts. The PAS-D stain is useful for enhancement.

Diseases Caused by *Malassezia furfur*

History

This fungus was first noted to cause the disease pityriasis versicolor by Eichstedt in 1846 and was classified as M. furfur in 1889 by Baillon. Other investigators have used the term "tinea versicolor" to designate the disease and the species Pityrosporum orbiculare and Pityrosporum ovale to designate the fungus, but they do not hold historical precedence, nor are they phylogenetically more accurate.

Clinical Features

M. furfur is a normal colonizer of the human skin, both on the surface and in hair follicles. It has an obligatory nutritional requirement, C12 to C24 fatty acids, which are found in nature only in human skin. The most common disorder it causes is pityriasis versicolor, so named for the branny scale (pityriasis) on patches that may be erythematous, hyperpigmented, or hypopigmented (versicolor). The variegation in color is most likely secondary to the mild inflammatory response. It is not known why certain people are affected and others are not, although its increased frequency in warm humid climates and in individuals with hyperthyroidism certainly implicates environmental factors. Two disorders apparently are caused by an excessive colonization by M. furfur resulting in obstruction of adnexal structures. These are pityrosporon folliculitis,[10] a disorder characterized by papules and pustules mainly on the trunk, and

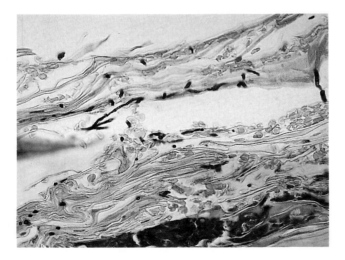

Figure 29–5. Tinea unguium. Branching hyphal elements are present in the hyponychium without any significant inflammatory response (PAS-D, ×480).

obstructive dacryocystitis, which inflames and interferes with the normal function of the lacrimal duct.[11] Very rarely, profoundly immunosuppressed individuals given intravenous lipid-containing medium-length fatty acids may develop *M. furfur* sepsis.[12]

Histologic Features

PITYRIASIS (TINEA) VERSICOLOR. The budding yeasts and hyphal elements usually are seen in the most superficial layers of the stratum corneum, perhaps more numerous at the hair follicle orifice. Sometimes, the round spores predominate over the hyphal elements, or vice versa. The hyphal elements are essential for diagnosis. A variable amount of hyperkeratosis, psoriasiform hyperplasia, and chronic inflammation with blood vessel dilatation may be seen, but these are characteristically very mild.[11]

The characteristic fungal morphology is a thick, short mycelium with variable numbers of round budding yeasts that have been described as "spaghetti and meatballs" on KOH examination (Fig. 29–6). The PAS-D stain is useful for enhancement in histologic sections.

PITYROSPORUM FOLLICULITIS. The basic process is a dilated follicle that is plugged by keratinaceous material in which numerous budding yeasts but no hyphal elements are seen[10] (Fig. 29–7). Varying degrees of follicular rupture and resultant inflammation may be seen, from none to a full-fledged follicular and perifollicular neutrophilic abscess with eosinophils and a giant cell foreign body reaction to keratin and spores in the dermis.

Differential Diagnosis

Pityriasis versicolor most commonly enters the differential diagnosis of "nothing" lesions but could also resemble a mild chronic dermatitis, such as pityriasis alba. Pityrosporum folliculitis must be differentiated from other causes

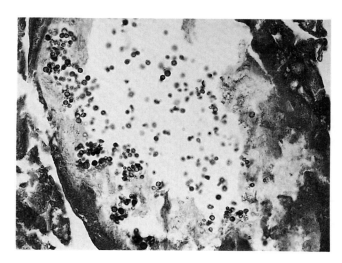

Figure 29–7. Pityrosporum folliculitis. The specimen shows a dilated follicle filled with keratinaceous material and numerous budding yeasts of varying sizes (PAS-D, ×480).

of folliculitis: bacteria, other fungi, acne, and acneiform drug eruptions.

Tinea Nigra

History
The disease was first described as keratomycosis nigricans palmaris by Alexandre Cerqueira of Brazil in 1891. The fungus was isolated and named *Cladosporium* (*Exophiala* or *Phaeoannellomyces*) *werneckii* in 1921 by another Brazilian, Parreiras Horta. The fungus produces its own pigment and is thus classified as dematiaceous. It is not a dermatophyte, but tinea nigra is the common usage.

Clinical Features
The initial presentation is an asymptomatic, minimally scaly, brown macule that slowly expands and becomes darker, almost always on the palm, but it may occur anywhere on the skin. It is far more common in tropical areas. The major clinical differential is melanoma, particularly acral lentiginous melanoma.[13]

Histologic Features
Large numbers of branching brown hyphal elements are easily visualized without PAS-D staining in the upper stratum corneum. Minimal parakeratosis and a minimal perivascular infiltrate are also noted. There is no increase in the number or activity of melanocytes.[11]

Differential Diagnosis
Other dematiaceous fungi that produce hyphal elements, that is, phaeohyphomycoses, fortunately are exceedingly rare and produce deeper lesions, which are not known to occur with the agent of tinea nigra. The agents of chromomycosis are dematiaceous but almost never produce mycelia.

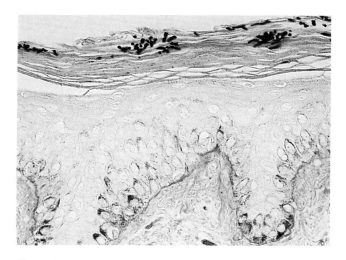

Figure 29–6. Pityriasis (tinea) versicolor. Short thick mycelia and yeasts are present in the outer layers of the stratum corneum (PAS-D, ×480).

Candidiasis

History

The fungus of thrush was first described by Lagenbeck in 1839, though the disease had been known since classical Greece. In 1875, Haussmann demonstrated that thrush in infants was related to vaginal candidiasis and proved that the fungus was pathogenic by inoculating a healthy gravid woman and inducing vaginitis.[14] Although we have placed it among the superficial fungal infections because that is where it is most commonly seen, it is easily capable of producing systemic disease in the compromised host.

Clinical Features

Numerous species of *Candida* are found colonizing normal human skin, mucosae, and gastrointestinal tract. *C. albicans* is the most common and most pathogenic, but their clinical manifestations are essentially interchangeable, so we refer to them all as *Candida*. The cutaneous involvement in individuals with normal immunity is almost always related to moisture or maceration. Classic examples are intertriginous candidiasis in the skinfolds of obese individuals, acute candidal paronychia from prolonged immersion of the hands in water, and candidal diaper dermatitis.[15] On mucosal surfaces, perleche, vulvovaginitis, and balanitis are common. On the other hand, thrush (other than in infants), esophagitis, or bronchitis caused by *Candida* should warrant a search for an underlying systemic cause, which may be as simple as broad-spectrum antibiotics or as complex as immunosuppression.[16] Systemic candidiasis, such as cellulitis with sepsis or endocarditis, should always lead to a full-scale investigation. Chronic mucocutaneous candidiasis is seen in several genetic disorders often associated with polyendocrinopathy or thymic dysfunction.[17]

The typical morphology of candidal lesions on the skin is a macerated, bright red, scaly or eroded plaque with satellite pustules. A rare variant, the candidal granuloma, may appear as a cutaneous horn.[18] Disseminated candidiasis most commonly appears as widespread erythematous papules and nodules that may be asymptomatic, but painful ecthyma gangrenosum-like lesions and cellulitis rarely may be seen.[19] On mucosal surfaces, a whitish, curdlike adherent plaque is the basic lesion, with erosions after removal of the plaque. Scrapings of the lesions usually reveal multiple budding oval spores and hyphal elements. Skin lesions of chronic mucocutaneous candidiasis are verrucous plaques.

Histologic Features

The scaly plaque will appear histologically as hyperkeratosis and acanthosis with variable amounts of spongiosis, whereas the pustules are subcorneal.[20] Hyphal elements and budding oval spores are seen in the stratum corneum and pustules. The pseudomembrane of thrush is a mat of food, bacteria, spores, hyphal elements, necrotic keratinocytes, and leukocytes. No fungus is seen beneath the stratum corneum, despite edema and abscesses in the corium. Vulvovaginitis and balanitis present a similar picture to thrush. In candidal granuloma, there is exuberant hyperkeratosis overlying an acanthotic epidermis under which is a granulomatous reaction with giant cells. Chronic mucocutaneous candidiasis presents a combination of all these

features.[18] The lesions of disseminated candidiasis often show very little inflammatory response despite vascular damage from clumps of hyphal elements that grow into the dermis. However, leukocytoclastic vasculitis or abscess formation may be seen.[21]

The 4 to 6 μm oval spores are often found budding in clumps around the mycelia, which are 2 to 4 μm in diameter and of variable length, usually longer than those of *M. furfur* and often shorter than dermatophytes. When spores are not seen, other features may sometimes be useful in identifying the mycelia of *Candida*: the branching occurs at a 90° rather than at a 45° angle, and the septations are not straight and complete but appear pinched off (pseudohyphae). However, these criteria are not absolute.

Differential Diagnosis

The differential diagnosis of a red, scaly, eroded plaque with subcorneal pustules includes pustular psoriasis, pemphigus foliaceus, impetigo, and impetiginized eczema. Candidal granuloma enters into the differential diagnosis of cutanous horn and verrucous lesion, which includes warts, actinic keratosis, squamous cell carcinoma, leishmaniasis, tuberculosis, and other fungal diseases. In the differential diagnosis of thrush is leukoplakia, but nuclear atypia is not seen in candidiasis. Disseminated candidiasis must be differentiated from other disseminated bacterial, mycobacterial, and fungal diseases. Finding oval spores with the hyphal elements suggests the diagnosis of *Candida*, but further mycologic confirmation may be needed.

SUBCUTANEOUS MYCOSES

Sporotrichosis

History

The disease was first described and the fungus isolated at the Johns Hopkins Hospital by Schenck in 1898.[22] The fungus was named *Sporothrix schenckii* by Hektoen and Perkins.

Clinical Features

The usual clinical presentation of sporotrichosis is produced by direct inoculation of the fungus into the dermis or subcutis. This produces an inoculation site from which the fungus may ascend via the lymphatics or grow only locally. In rare cases, the mucosae or bone may be the site of implantation; even more rarely, dissemination may occur from the initial site. The primary lesion is an erythematous nodule that suppurates and only later becomes a verrucous plaque.[23]

A second clinical presentation is produced by inhalation of conidia and is analogous to what is seen with the truly pathogenic fungi. One variant begins with an acute pneumonitis or bronchitis that is usually accompanied by malaise, fever, and cough and usually ends with a chronic cavity or may be entirely asymptomatic.[24] Another variant produces acute massive tracheobronchial lymphadenopathy but usually ends in resolution and recovery.[25]

Histologic Features

The nodules may show only a nonspecific inflammatory infiltrate with variable numbers of lymphoid cells, histio-

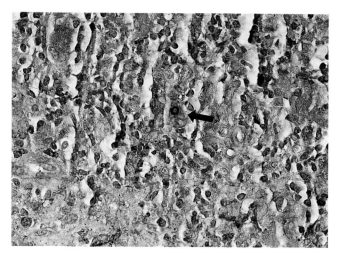

Figure 29–8. Sporotrichosis. This specimen shows a solitary yeast (*arrow*) within a dense inflammatory infiltrate (PAS-D, ×480).

cytes, neutrophils, and plasma cells (Fig. 29–8). As the lesion matures, microabscesses and granulomas with variable numbers of giant cells form. A characteristic arrangement into three zones may occur: a central neutrophilic suppurative zone surrounded by a tuberculoid zone, which is itself surrounded by a round cell zone with plasma and lymphoid cells. The epidermis may respond with pseudoepitheliomatous hyperplasia.[26]

Unless the lesion has injected with corticosteroids or there is significant immunosuppression, it may be exceedingly difficult to demonstrate the round to oval spores that measure 4 to 6 μm in diameter.[27] In order of frequency, single or multiple buds, cigar bodies, or nonseptate hyphal elements may be seen. Asteroid bodies, which represent an artifact produced by immune complexes deposited around the fungus, appear as an eosinophilic homogeneous asterisk with a diameter of about 20 μm, centered by the fungus.

Differential Diagnosis

Unfortunately, the clinical and histopathologic differentiation from infections by atypical mycobacteria may be impossible unless the microorganism can be identified. The dilemma is usually resolved only by culturing tissue for both fungi and atypical mycobacteria. On the bright side, *S. schenkii* is the fastest growing of the fungi that cause disease in humans and grows easily at 25° C within 5 days to be seen as a black to brown colony.

Chromomycosis (Chromoblastomycosis)

History

The first clinical case was observed by Pedroso in Brazil in 1911, although he did not publish until 1920,[28] when he had four cases. It was not until 1922 that Brumpt isolated the fungus from the index case and named it *Hormodendrum (Fonsecaea) pedrosoi*. Credit for the first published case that correctly identifies a mycotic etiology goes to Medlar, who described a New England patient with verrucous lesions in 1915.[29] The fungus isolated in this case was classified as *Phialophora verrucosa* by Thaxter.

Clinical Features

Chromomycosis is a clinicopathologic entity characterized by verrucous lesions whose etiologic agents are dematiaceous (pigmented) fungi that produce the sclerotic bodies (copper pennies, Medlar bodies) that reproduce by cissiparity (planate-dividing) in tissue. *F. pedrosoi*, *F. compacta*, *P. verrucosa* and *C. carrionii* are the most common etiologic agents of chromomycosis. The initial lesion is an erythematous papule that develops into one or multiple verrucous papules, nodules, and plaques. The presence of black dots in the verrucous plaques is a very characteristic finding, and KOH preparation of these hematic crusts will reveal the sclerotic bodies. The disease occurs commonly on an extremity secondary to traumatic implantation, and its clinical course is characterized by pruritus and extremely slow growth, leading to fibrosis, lymphedema, and elephantiasis.[30]

Histologic Features

As in all fungal diseases, a spectrum of histopathologic appearances may be seen, mirroring the clinical aspect.[31] A biopsy from the characteristic verrucous plaque will show hyperkeratosis and exuberant irregular acanthosis without significant atypia (pseudoepitheliomatous hyperplasia) (Fig. 29–2). A mixed infiltrate composed of varying numbers of lymphoid, epithelioid, giant, and plasma cells is seen in the dermis. There may be neutrophilic abscesses, granuloma formation without caseation, and a variable number of eosinophils. In long-standing lesions, fibrosis may be quite marked. A prominent and characteristic feature is transepidermal elimination of the fungus, resulting in the black dots that are observed clinically.[32]

The spores may be free-standing but often are found within giant cells, at the center of abscesses, or where transepidermal elimination is occurring. They are round to oval, bronze colored, measure 6 to 12 μm in diameter, and may be found singly or in clusters (Fig. 29–9). When septation is seen dividing such a spore, the diagnosis is made. Hyphal elements may rarely be seen.[33]

Differential Diagnosis

The overall pattern resembles other fungal and mycobacterial disorders that may be verrucous, such as blastomycosis, paracoccidioidomycosis, and tuberculosis verrucosa cutis. The pseudoepitheliomatous hyperplasia may suggest malignancy, but the lack of significant atypia and the presence of a mixed infiltrate help to differentiate. The distinction from phaeohyphomycosis is made on the basis of finding the sclerotic bodies, which are distinguished from the spores of phaeohyphomycosis only by the presence of septation and the absence of budding. Hyphal elements are much less abundant in chromomycosis.

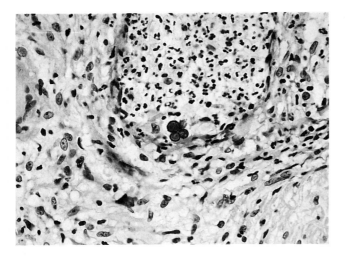

Figure 29–9. Chromomycosis. A cluster of yeasts is present in the center of the section at the edge of an abscess (H&E, eosin, ×480).

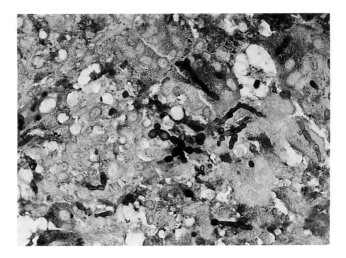

Figure 29–10. Phaeohyphomycosis. Budding spores and hyphal elements are present (PAS-D, ×480).

Phaeohyphomycosis

History

The term "phaeohyphomycosis" was arbitrarily created by Ajello et al.[34] in 1974 to encompass infections by dematiaceous fungi that grow in tissue by budding and have abundant hyphal elements. Numerous etiologic agents have been described, *E. jeanselmei* and *Wangiella dermatitidis* being the most common.

Clinical Features

Phaeohyphomycosis encompasses a variety of clinical presentations and is more common in hosts with at least mild degrees of immunocompromise. Phaeomycotic cysts are single or multiple deep-seated cysts in which abundant dematiaceous yeasts and hyphal elements are seen.[35] Subcutaneous phaeohyphomycosis encompasses two clinical presentations: either subcutaneous masses with little tendency to ulceration or verrucous lesions. *E. jeanselmei* is more common in the former, and *W. dermatitidis* is almost exclusively found in the latter.[36] Ocular, skeletal, and central nervous system involvement also have been reported. In the severely immunosuppressed host, dissemination without a marked response is the rule.

Histologic Features

The pattern in tissue reflects the clinical appearance and follows the general pattern seen in dermal fungal disease: a mixed infiltrate with lymphoid and epithelioid cells, along with variable numbers of neutrophils, eosinophils, and giant cells. Abscess or granuloma formation may be seen, and the epithelial response is pseudoepitheliomatous hyperplasia only if the lesion was clinically verrucous.[35,37]

The characteristically abundant fungi are varicus shades of brown and appear as budding spores that may be in chains or hyphal elements (Fig. 29–10). They usually range in size between 2 and 6 μm but have been seen up to 25 μm.

Differential Diagnosis

The diagnosis rests on finding the characteristic fungal forms. These fungal forms are distinguished from those seen in chromomycosis by the absence of true sclerotic bodies and by the presence of spores that bud in chains or produce abundant hyphal elements. It is not always easy to distinguish true sclerotic bodies from the spores in phaeohyphomycosis, which should have thinner walls and not have septae. Phaeohyphomycosis is separated from hyphomycosis by the ability to produce pigment; however, the pigment may not be readily apparent, and a culture may be needed for clarification. Phaeohyphomycosis can be differentiated from a dematiaceous eumycotic mycetoma because the fungal elements are not found clumped together to form a grain.

Eumycetoma

History

Mycetoma was first described as Madura foot in 1842 by Gill in the area of Madurai, India. Pinoy in 1913 was the first to suggest division into fungal and bacterial etiologies (eumycetoma and actinomycetoma).

Clinical Features

Mycetoma is a clinical entity characterized by indolent tumefaction involving all depths of tissue down to bone, sinus formation, and the presence of grains composed of the etiologic agent.[38] Mycetomas may be classified into one of three groups according to the micromorphology of the grains: botryomycosis (cocci or short rods), actinomycetoma (thin, branching, intertwined filaments), and eumycetoma (thick, branching, intertwined filaments). Eumycotic grains are black when produced by dematiaceous fungi and white otherwise. The most common agents of eumycetoma are *Pseudoallescheria boydii* (white grain) and *Madurella mycetomatis* (black grain). Table 29–4 compares the grains produced by the various etiologic agents of mycetomas.

TABLE 29–4. GRAINS IN TISSUE

Group	Micromorphology of Grains
Botryomycosis	Soft, yellow-white, lobulated, < 1mm Masses of cocci in 0.5–1μm unbranched filaments held together by PAS + cement Gram stain useful
Actinomycetoma	Soft or hard, white, yellow, pink, or red, variable size Masses of 0.5–μm branched filaments composed of cocci or bacilli Gram stain useful
Eumycetoma	Masses of mycelia of 2–5μm and larger swollen fungus cells might be hard or soft, dark or light, small or large, with or without cement Gram stain not useful

Note: Dark grains may be due to the fungus itself having pigment (i.e., dematiaceous) or the cement being pigmented; brown to black
Light grains indicate no pigment in either the mycelia or the cement

Histologic Features

The characteristic findings are a grain in a neutrophilic abscess surrounded by granulation tissue and fibrosis. Neutrophils are often seen attached to the edge of the granule, and a granulomatous reaction with giant cells is seen in the sinus tracts. The etiologic diagnosis can be narrowed significantly by examining the grain carefully. Eumycotic grains are a poorly organized collection of about 5 μm thick septate hyphal elements and distorted, cystlike cells. No cementing substance is noted. Dark brown or black pigment is noted if the fungus is dematiaceous[39,40] (Fig. 29–11).

Differential Diagnosis

Clumps of hyphal elements surrounded by a giant cell reaction are not sufficient for a diagnosis of eumycetoma, since they may be seen in many clinical settings with several fungi. Both eumycetoma and actinomycetoma stain by PAS-D and methenamine silver, so these are not helpful differentiating criteria. Actinomycetoma are distinguished by having branching filaments that are only 1 μm thick and by the grain being better organized, having a cementing substance, and not eliciting a giant cell reaction. Botryomycosis is differentiated by the absence of branching and the presence of cocci or short rods.

Lobomycosis

History

Jorge Lobo of Brazil described the first case[41] of keloidal blastomycosis in 1931, and it was distinguished histologically from paracoccidioidomycosis by Leite in 1954. *Loboa loboi* is the best name for the fungus at present, since it has not been cultured and its taxonomic position is a subject of controversy.

Clinical Features

The disease is seen almost exclusively in the Amazon region and occurs typically as a keloid on the ear or an extremity, but it may also appear verrucoid or atrophic and be on any part of the integument. Lesions begin as firm, often pruritic, flesh-colored to slightly hyperpigmented, smooth papules that are freely movable. Spread of lesions is believed to be due to autoinoculation. The course is characterized by slowly progressive growth that is not amenable to any form of antifungal treatment, and recurrence after surgical excision is common.[42]

Histologic Features

The epidermis is atrophic, and the process is predominantly dermal. There is a granulomatous infiltrate composed almost entirely of macrophages and massive fibrosis[43] (Fig. 29–12). An abundance of yeast cells is seen, either within giant cells or free in tissue. The characteristic shape is round with a tip, resembling a lemon. The size is uniformly around 10 μm, and they may be found in chains that occasionally branch. The wall is about 1 μm thick and stains deeply

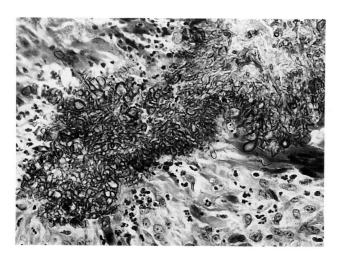

Figure 29–11. Mycetoma. This view of a grain shows a mass of pigmented hyphal elements (×480). (*Courtesy of Dr. William Merz.*)

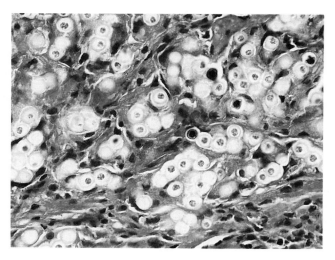

Figure 29–12. Lobomycosis. This section shows an abundance of uniform-sized yeasts tending to form chains, located in a fibrotic stroma (H&E, ×480).

with methenamine silver or PAS-D. Budding is almost invariably single. Eosinophilic amorphous spicules similar to those seen in the asteroid bodies of sporotrichosis may be seen.[43]

Differential Diagnosis

Keloids and other scars do not have as exuberant a granulomatous infiltrate nor the abundance of fungal elements. *Paracoccidioides brasiliensis* has a much greater variability in size (1 to 40 μm), and multiple sporulation is common. *Blastomyces dermatitidis* is about the same size but does not have the lemon shape, the buds are broader based, and it has no tendency to form long chains. *S. schenckii* is smaller (5 to 8 μm) and more oval. *Histoplasma capsulatum* is much smaller (3 μm).

Rhinosporidiosis

History

Rhinosporidiosis was first reported by Seeber of Argentina in 1900. Ashworth established that it was a fungus and named it *Rhinosporidium seeberi* in 1923. The fungus has yet to be cultured and classified.[44]

Clinical Features

The disease is most common in India, with South America a distant second.[45] The most frequent site involved is the nasal mucosa, but other mucosae may be involved. Patients first note what appears to be a foreign body, with pruritus and coryza. A papule forms and may enlarge, resulting in one or many papules, nodules, and polyps that can reach sizes capable of obstructing respiration and feeding. The skin itself is rarely affected unless it is immediately adjacent. Dissemination occurs very rarely.[46]

Histologic Features

The transitional epithelium responds to the fungus with hyperplasia and papillomatosis. A dense, mixed cellular infiltrate with lymphocytes, histiocytes, plasma cells, neutrophils, eosinophils, and some giant cells is seen in the chorium. The invaginated epithelium may form pseudocysts containing pus, mucus, and spores. Mature sporangia often are seen beneath areas of thinned epithelium. Asteroid bodies are not seen.[45] Mucicarmine stains the outer wall of the spores and inner wall of the sporangia.

Numerous life cycle forms of the fungus may be seen in tissue, ranging from a 6 to 10 μm spore, which grows into a 10 to 12 μm spherule that undergoes numerous cell divisions until it becomes a large sporangium with around 16,000 spores and a diameter of 250 to 350 μm. At this point, the sporangium ruptures, and spores can be seen spilling out from a pore in the cellulose-like wall[47] (Fig. 29–13).

Differential Diagnosis

The only other pathogenic fungus that produces sporangia is *Coccidioides immitis*, but these are much smaller (30 to 60 μm), asteroid bodies may be noted, and hyphae may be seen. Only the cell wall of *C. neoformans* also stains

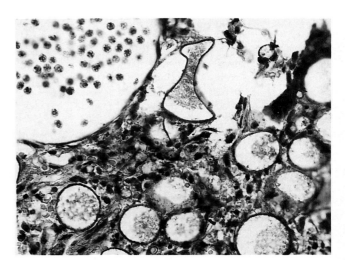

Figure 29–13. Rhinosporidiosis. Multiple cysts are present throughout the section, and a large sporangium containing numerous spores is present at the upper left corner. (H&E, ×480). (*Courtesy of Dr. William Merz.*)

with mucicarmine, but the morphology is so different that this is usually not a problem.

SYSTEMIC MYCOSES

Coccidioidomycosis

History

The first case was described in 1892 by Posadas[48] in Argentina, who also noted organisms in the tissue and reproduced the disease in animals by inoculation. The fungal nature of the disease was established in 1900 by Ophuls.

Clinical Features

This is the most virulent of the pathogenic fungi. Possibly the inhalation of only a single spore is sufficient to produce disease. Fortunately, 60% of affected individuals with primary infections are asymptomatic, and only 1 or 2 per 1000 of the remaining 40% progress beyond the initial acute pulmonary disease. The asymptomatic form is noted only by a positive skin test to coccidioidin and small areas of fibrosis and calcification on chest x-ray. Acute primary pulmonary disease is characterized by anorexia, cough, fever, chest pain, and respiratory distress.[49] Secondary coccidioidomycosis may remain confined to the lungs or may disseminate to multiple organ systems.

The existence of a pure cutaneous form secondary to traumatic implantation is controversial.[50] Erythema multiforme, erythema nodosum, or a morbilliform exanthem may be seen as a hypersensitivity reaction to the acute infection, even without clinically apparent disease. The chronic cutaneous disease is seen in secondary coccidioidomycosis and is characterized by infiltrated papules and plaques that develop a verrucous surface. Sinus tracts from subcutaneous and osseous lesions may be noted, especially over joints and bony prominences.

Histologic Features

There is no characteristic pattern beyond that seen in other deep fungal infections: a variable number of plasma cells, lymphocytes, histiocytes, eosinophils, neutrophils, and giant cells that may form abscesses or granulomas.[51] Depending on the state of the lesion, the epidermis may respond with pseudoepitheliomatous hyperplasia.

The diagnosis is established by finding the typical 10 to 80 μm spherule with multiple 2 to 5 μm endospores, either free or within giant cells (Fig. 29–14). A neutrophilic response frequently is seen when the endospores are released.[52] Asteroid bodies may be noted around spherules. Hyphal elements are rarely seen. Arthroconidia are typical at 25° C but not in tissue.

Differential Diagnosis

The pseudoepitheliomatous hyperplasia may be exuberant enough to be confused with squamous cell carcinoma, but the lack of true atypia and the presence of the mixed infiltrate are helpful. The same pattern is seen in other fungal and mycobacterial diseases. If spherules are found, the only possible confusion is with *R. seeberi*, which is larger. If only endospores are seen, they may be confused with those of other yeastlike fungi in tissue, such as *C. neoformans*, *P. brasiliensis*, *L. loboi*, *B. dermatitidis*, and *H. capsulatum*. These are differentiated in Table 29–1.

Paracoccidioidomycosis (South American Blastomycosis)

History

The first two cases were described, and a fungus similar in tissue to *C. immitis* was described and isolated in 1908 by Lutz[53] in Brazil. Splendore expanded on these descriptions, and the fungus was designated *Paracoccidioides brasiliensis* by Almeida in 1930.

Clinical Features

The overall clinical picture is similar to that of coccidioidomycosis, blastomycosis, and histoplasmosis with some variations. Although less common than with coccidioidomycosis, skin test positivity is prevalent in endemic areas, and there is a benign, primary, pulmonary form that resolves spontaneously with only calcification as sequela.[54] Reactivation in these cases may occur in immunosuppressed patients. Allergic manifestations, such as erythema multiforme or erythema nodosum, are uncommon. Progressive disease occurs only rarely, either acutely from the primary infection or chronically by dissemination from the pulmonary focus. The characteristic features are a tendency to develop mucocutaneous as opposed to purely cutaneous lesions, frequent involvement of lymphatics, with development of draining lesions, and a predisposition to affect the adrenal gland.[55]

Histologic Features

The pattern follows that of the other verrucous types of deep fungal infections: pseudoepitheliomatous hyperplasia with an underlying infiltrate composed of variable numbers of lymphocytes, histiocytes, plasma cells, neutrophils, and giant cells, with abscess and granuloma formation being common.[56]

The fungus may be seen free in tissue or within abscesses or giant cells (Fig. 29–15). The round yeast cells are characterized by their considerable variation in size from about 12 to 40 μm in diameter and the variation in the number of narrow-necked buds, which may range from one to over a dozen, giving the characteristic pilot's wheel appearance. They have no tendency to form chains.[57]

Differential Diagnosis

The overall pattern must be differentiated from other verrucous lesions to include leishmaniasis, pseudoepitheliomatous hyperplasia, mycobacteria, and verrucous lupus erythematosus. The spores of other fungi are compared in Table 29–1.

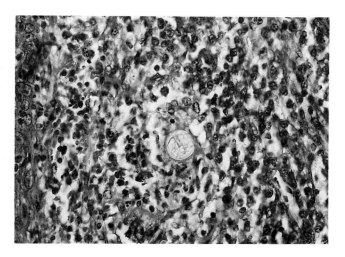

Figure 29–14. Coccidioidomycosis. This section from skin shows a solitary spherule and no hyphal elements. (PAS-D, ×480).

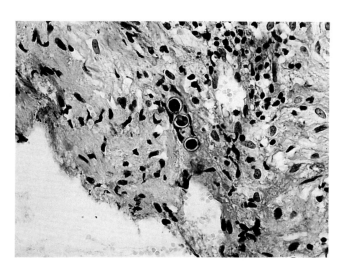

Figure 29–15. Paracoccidioidomycosis. Three yeasts are present in the center of the section, two of which are connected by a narrow neck. (PAS-D, ×480).

Blastomycosis (North American Blastomycosis)

History

The first case was described by Gilchrist in 1894,[58] and the fungus was named *Blastomyces dermatitidis* by Gilchrist and Stokes in 1898. Although the initial cases were all diagnosed in the United States, the disease is found worldwide.

Clinical Features

Unlike coccidioidomycosis and paracoccidioidomycosis, it is not known if subclinical infections can occur, although the usual portal of entry and infection is the lungs. Once established, the disease progresses primarily in one organ system and may eventually become systemic.[59] The organs most commonly involved are the lungs, bones, and skin. Inoculation blastomycosis is self-limited and only rarely the cause of the cutaneous lesions of blastomycosis. Approximately 70% of patients with systemic blastomycosis develop cutaneous lesions, which are either verrucous or ulcerated. Verrucous lesions are more common and consist of a plaque that is atrophic in the center and the verrucous border with a variable amount of pustules. The ulcerated lesions begin as pustules that break down to form an ulcer with well-defined borders and a granulation tissue base. The osseous lesions may extend into the subcutis and result in abscess formation. Mucosal lesions may occur but are less common than in paracoccidioidomycosis.

Histologic Features

This is the prototype disease for pseudoepitheliomatous hyperplasia. In biopsies taken from the verrucous border of a cutaneous lesion, there is hyperkeratosis overlying exuberant irregular acanthosis into a dermis infiltrated by a mix of inflammatory cells. Neutrophils often aggregate to form microabscesses, and giant cells may be seen within epithelioid granulomas or isolated among the rest of the infiltrate. In biopsies taken from the border of an ulcerated lesion, the dermal infiltrate is identical to that described previously, but the pseudoepitheliomatous hyperplasia is absent.[51]

The diagnostic feature of this yeast is its broad-based single bud (Fig. 29–16). Spores are round and measure about 10 μm but may be as small as 8 μm or as large as 30 μm in diameter.[59] The number of organisms is greater in lesions that are not verrucous. They may be free-standing but are more easily found at the center of neutrophilic abscesses or within giant cells. They are outlined as clear, round spaces within the cytoplasm of multinucleate giant cells when special stains have not been used. The fungus wall is thick and doubly refractile. The cytoplasm often collapses around the nucleus, forming a space between it and the cell wall, and multiple rather than single nuclei are often seen. Staining is variable with any method, although the number of organisms seen increases with PAS-D or methenamine silver.

Differential Diagnosis

The overall histologic reaction pattern must be differentiated from other verrucous lesions with pseudoepitheliomatous hyperplasia, such as leishmaniasis, mycobacterial infections, and verrucous lupus erythematosus. The yeast can

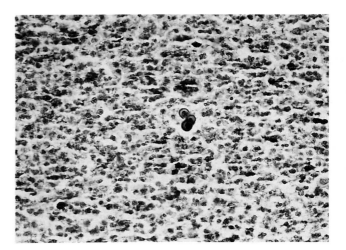

Figure 29–16. Blastomycosis. A cluster of three yeasts is present in the center of the specimen, two of which are joined by a broad-based connection. (PAS-D, ×480). (*Courtesy of Dr. Robert Taylor.*)

easily be confused with *H. capsulatum var. duboisii, C. immitis,* and *C. neoformans.* The most helpful differentiating features are shown in Table 29–1.

Histoplasmosis

History

The first cases were published in 1906 by Darling,[60] an American working in Panama. He named the organism *Histoplasma capsulatum* because it was found in histiocytes, resembled a plasmodium, and had a capsule. The fungal nature of the disease was established 7 years later by a Brazilian working in Germany, Rocha-Lima.

Clinical Features

The disease is found worldwide, especially in areas associated with bird and bat excrement, where it grows particularly well. As with the other pathogenic fungi, the vast majority of cases are acquired by inhalation, are asymptomatic, and are only diagnosed by the histoplasmin skin test and residual findings on chest films. The disease may occur in any of a bewildering array of patterns.[61] Unlike their occurrence with the other true pathogenic fungi, cutaneous lesions are uncommon and consist of papules or plaques that may undergo ulceration. In contrast, oral ulcerations are said to occur in half the patients.

Histologic Features

In patients with good immunity, yeasts are seen within histiocytes accompanied by a mixed infiltrate, with plasma cells, lymphocytes, histiocytes, neutrophils, and giant cells, often forming granulomas. When the immune system is more compromised, a very large number of organisms are seen within histiocytes, and there are relatively few of the other cells in the infiltrate.[62]

The organism is distinctive because of its very thick cell wall, which resembles a capsule surrounding a 3 μm

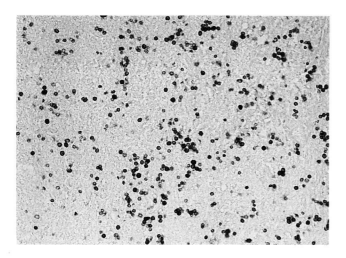

Figure 29–17. Histoplasmosis. Numerous small spores are scattered throughout the section, some connected by a narrow neck. (Methenamine silver, ×480). (*Courtesy Dr. William Merz.*)

spore that stains dark blue with either hematoxylin and eosin, Giemsa, Gram, or Wright's stain (Fig. 29–17). They can be shown by electron microscopy to be individually wrapped by a phagolysosome membrane when in histiocytes.[63] The size is quite uniform in active lesions, only one nucleus is seen, and the buds have a narrow neck.

Differential Diagnosis

The large number of small organisms within histiocytes may lead to confusion with *Leishmania donovani*, but the thick cell wall and the lack of a kinetoplast should allow differentiation. The thick cell wall may lead to confusion with *C. neoformans*, but a mucicarmine stain will not be positive in histoplasmosis. *B. dermatitidis* has a broad-based bud and is multinucleate. *Candida* in tissue tends to be predominantly hyphal.

African Histoplasmosis

History

The first case published that described a large cell type of histoplasmosis was by Catanei and Kervan in 1945.[64] It was not until 1957 that Drouet demonstrated that this was not a new species, and named it *Histoplasma capsulatum* var. *duboisii.*

Clinical Features

All reported cases, with one questionable exception, have been reported from equatorial Africa. The portal of entry has yet to be defined, but lesions may either involve a single organ system or be disseminated. The organs most frequently involved are the skin, bone, lymph nodes, and lungs.[65] Systemic symptoms vary in proportion to the degree of dissemination. The cutaneous lesions may be papules, nodules, or plaques. They may resemble molluscum contagiosum, eczema, figurate erythemas, or psoriasis. Ul-

ceration may occur in any of these lesions or from deeper subcutaneous lesions in which suppuration may develop. Mucosal involvement occasionally is seen.

Histologic Features

The epidermal reaction pattern mirrors the clinical appearance of the lesions. In the dermis, the presence of abundant giant cells is the distinctive feature of African histoplasmosis, particularly when compared to their relative rarity in other deep fungal infections. The giant cells are extremely large and are packed with the yeasts. A mixed infiltrate of histiocytes, lymphocytes, and plasma cells, as well as neutrophilic microabscesses, accompanies the giant cells.[66]

The yeast cells are thick-walled and ovoid and range from 8 to 15 μm in diameter.[67] They occasionally form short chains and may exhibit broad-based budding in rare instances. The methenamine silver and PAS-D stains are useful, though the fungus is visible on routine hematoxylin and eosin sections.

Differential Diagnosis

The differential diagnosis of yeasts is outlined in Table 29–1. The short chains and ovoid shape may be seen in lobomycosis, but the size is quite different. In the rare instances when broad-based budding is seen, it may be extremely difficult to distinguish from blastomycosis, and a fungal culture becomes imperative.

Cryptococcosis

History

The yeast was first isolated from cutaneous lesions by Busse, a German pathologist, in 1894. Its present name, *Cryptococcus neoformans*, only gained general acceptance in 1952.

Clinical Features

The etiologic agent is found ubiquitously in the environment, although it is not easily cultured from the soil. The urban pigeon is a common vector since *C. neoformans* is found abundantly in dry, alkaline bird excrement high in nitrogen and salt. The fungus also can be cultured from normal human skin or other areas open to the air.

Like the previous five mycoses discussed, the portal of entry is pulmonary, but the infection remains asymptomatic and heals without sequelae in almost all cases. As a rule, the host must be immunosuppressed in order to become affected, the degree of which determines how widespread it becomes. Primary inoculation cutaneous cryptococcosis is very rare. The most common site of infection is pulmonary, but the diagnosis is not usually made in the lungs.[68] Central nervous system disease is the most frequently diagnosed in the Americas, and in Europe, the presentation is more often cutaneous or mucocutaneous. The skin lesions consist of papules, pustules, nodules, plaques, abscesses, or ulcers.[69] The papules may be firm and resemble molluscum contagiosum. The plaques may resemble cellulitis or thrombophlebitis.

Histologic Features

The spectrum of tissue reaction ranges from essentially none to an intense infiltrate of lymphocytes, histiocytes, and giant

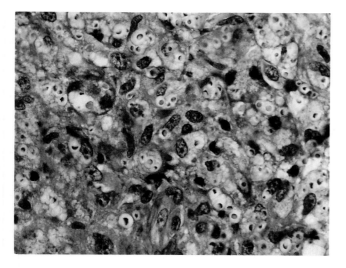

Figure 29–18. Cryptococcosis. This section is a high power view of the same biopsy as in Figure 29–3 and shows numerous spores within the granulomatous pattern. (H&E, ×480.)

cells. These two extremes are known as gelatinous and granulomatous (Fig. 29–3) and may both be seen in the same specimen.[70] The gelatinous pattern is composed almost entirely of masses of spores free in tissue and is due to the very small immunologic response elicited by the mucinous capsule. The capsule often is much diminished or absent in the granulomatous response (Fig. 29–18). It is not known whether it disappears because of the granulomatous response or if the granulomatous response appears because of the lack of a capsule.

The spore is round and varies in diameter from 3 to 20 μm, budding is narrow-based, and the diagnosis is established when the capsule does not stain well with hematoxylin and eosin but is red with the mucicarmine stain (Fig. 29–19A).[71] PAS-D (Fig. 29–19B) and methenamine silver stain the spore but not the capsule. Pertinent negative features include the absence of spherules and the extreme rarity of hyphal elements in tissue.

Differential Diagnosis

The tissue reaction pattern in very characteristic when gelatinous, but the granulomatous pattern may be seen with other granulomatous disorders. The yeasts are differentiated in Table 19–1. The lack of spherules rules out coccidioidomycosis, *Candida* does not vary as much in size and mycelia figure prominently, blastomycosis has wide budding, and histoplasmosis is not really "capsulatum" with mucicarmine.

Aspergillosis

History

The term aspergillosis was first used by Micheli in 1729 to describe the resemblance of the fungus to the aspergillum used in Roman Catholic ceremonies. The first case in humans was described by Sluyter in 1847.[72]

Clinical Features

Aspergillus sp. is an exceedingly common contaminant of dead organic masses and soil. Humans are constantly exposed to the fungus and inhale spores, but clinically significant disease fortunately is infrequent. The dermatopathologist or pathologist is usually involved only in the diagnosis

Figure 29–19. Cryptococcosis. **A.** This section from a case with the gelatinous pattern shows the spores outlined by a capsule. (Mucicarmine, ×480). **B.** The same section on PAS staining does not demonstrate capsules. (PAS-D, ×480).

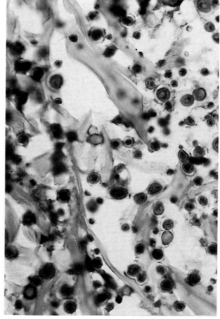

A

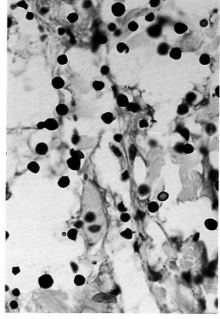

B

of cutaneous or disseminated disease in the immunocompromised host, but other manifestations occur: colonization of cavities by fungus balls, allergic reactions to spore inhalation, and poisoning by toxins released into foods.[73]

Primary cutaneous aspergillosis occurs as a result of direct inoculation into the skin. Intravenous boards are a common source.[74] The initial lesion is a red papule that develops a necrotic eschar and continues to expand if no diagnosis is made, with an obvious risk of dissemination. Chronic lesions have been reported but are unusual. Cutaneous aspergillosis secondary to dissemination from another primary focus almost always occurs in the setting of immunosuppression. The necrotic eschar also figures prominently in these lesions.

Histologic Features

In the severely immunosuppressed individual, there may be very little inflammatory response around the fungus, which is often found embolized in blood vessels and growing through them into the surrounding tissue[75] (Fig. 29–20). Necrosis secondary to the embolization is common, and the response, when it occurs, is characteristically neutrophilic, although it may be granulomatous on occasion.[76]

Aspergillus sp. stain with hematoxylin and eosin but may be enhanced by the methenamine silver stains. PAS-D stains variably. The classic morphology is a septate mycelium with dichotomous branching in the same direction at a 45-degree angle. The shape is irregular, and the diameter varies from 2.5 to 4.5 μm.

Differential Diagnosis

It must be emphasized that the histologic appearance of *Aspergillus* sp. cannot be differentiated from that of *Fusarium* sp. and *Pseudoallescheria boydii*, as well as several other much more rarely encountered organisms. Fortunately, it can readily be distinguished from *Candida* sp. by the absence of budding yeasts and from *Mucor* sp. by the presence of septations (Table 29–2).

Zygomycosis

History

The first case involving a *Mucor* organism in a human was described by Kurchenmeister in 1855. The classic article on rhinocerebral zygomycosis, which is the most common form, was published by Gregory in 1943.[77]

Clinical Features

There are four distinct clinical syndromes in addition to the metastatic lesions of disseminated disease. These are rhinocerebral, rhinofacial, cutaneous, and subcutaneous zygomycosis. Rhinocerebral zygomycosis is a fulminant disorder, usually caused by *Rhizopus* sp., that is commonly seen in the setting of immunosuppression or diabetic ketoacidosis. Lesions arise in the nose or mouth, and characteristically a black hematic eschar and discharge are noted, surrounded by a variable amount of swelling. The sinuses and eyes are involved early, and extension occurs via vessels and nerves into the brain. In cutaneous zygomycosis, a wide variety of lesions may be seen.[78] Chronic subcutaneous zygomycosis is most commonly an indurated well-defined plaque that is attached to the underlying fascia but not to the dermis above.[79] Rhinofacial zygomycosis is quite similar, a localized variant that manifests initially as a nasal swelling but may go on to produce airway obstruction. In these latter two forms, the patient usually has no other complaints, at least initially.

Histologic Features

The characteristic findings of acute rhinocerebral disease are direct neural invasion and necrosis secondary to direct invasion of blood vessel walls by the fungus, accompanied by either a granulomatous or a predominantly polymorphonuclear infiltrate. In contrast, neither neural nor blood vessel invasion is noted in the more chronic forms. Rather, multiple microabscesses composed of neutrophils and eosinophils surrounded by epithelioid and giant cells are seen

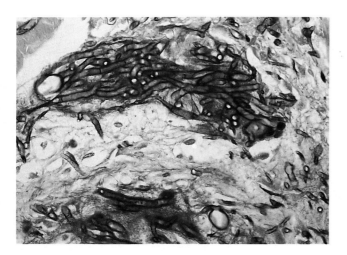

Figure 29–20. Aspergillosis. This section is from an immunocompromised patient and shows a blood vessel filled with hyphal elements and hyphal elements scattered throughout the dermis (PAS-D, ×480).

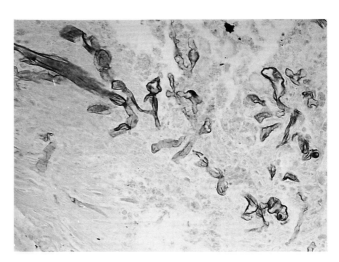

Figure 29–21. Zygomycosis. This section demonstrates the typical branching hyphal elements (PAS-D, ×480). (*Courtesy of Dr. William Merz.*)

reacting to the presence of the fungus.[80] The fungus often is encased by an eosinophilic material that results from immune complex deposition.

In either case, the hyphal form predominates (Fig. 29–21). The width varies from 10 to 25 μm, septation is rare, and branching occurs at odd intervals. Occasionally, rounded structures resembling yeast cells may be present. These are chlamydoconidia, and they range from 5 to 30 μm in diameter.[81] These fungi stain well with hematoxylin and eosin, but a PAS-D stain occasionally may be useful.

Differential Diagnosis

Zygomycosis must be differentiated from other nonpigmented fungi in which the hyphal form predominates in tissue (Table 29–2). The irregularity in width is helpful in differentiating from dermatophytes and *Candida* sp. The lack of septation and of dichotomous branching distinguishes it from *Aspergillus* sp., *Fusarium* sp., and *Pseudoallescheria boydii*.

REFERENCES

1. Henrici AT. An endotoxin from *Aspergillus fumigatus*. *J Immunol.* 1939;36:319–338.
2. Gruby D. Sur les mycodermes que constituent la teigne faveuse. *CR Acad Sci.* 1841;13:309–312.
3. Sabouraud R. *Les Teignes.* Paris: Masson et Cie; 1910.
4. Kligman AM. The pathogenesis of tinea capitis due to *Microsporum andouinii* and *Microsporum canis*. *J Invest Dermatol.* 1952; 18:231–246.
5. Graham JH, Johnson WC, Burgoon CF, et al. Tinea capitis. *Arch Dermatol.* 1964;89:528–543.
6. Majocchi D. Sopra una nuova tricofizia (granuloma tricofitico). *Studi clinici e micologi. Boll R Accad Med Roma.* 1883;9:220–223.
7. Dvoretzky I, Fisher BK, Movshovitz M, et al. Favus. *Int J Dermatol.* 1980;19:89–92.
8. Koskuakis CE, Scher RK, Ackerman AB. Biopsies of nails. What histologic findings distinguish onychomycosis from psoriasis? *Am J Dermatopathol.* 1983;5:501–503.
9. Negroni P. *Dermatomicosis, Diagnostico y Tratamiento.* Buenos Aires: Aniceto Lopez; 1942.
10. Potter BS, Burgoon CF Jr., Johnson WC. Pityrosporon folliculitis. *Arch Dermatol.* 1973;107:388–391.
11. Rippon JW. *Medical Mycology.* Philadelphia: WB Saunders; 1988.
12. Redline RW, Dahms BB. Malassezia pulmonary vasculitis in an infant on long-term intralipid therapy. *N Engl J Med.* 1981; 305:1395.
13. Vaffee AS. Tinea nigra palmaris resembling malignant melanoma. *N Engl J Med.* 1970;283:1112.
14. Haussmann D. Parasites des organes sexuals femeilles de l'homme et de quelques animaux avec une notice sur developpement *d'oidium albicans*. Robin Paris: JB Bailliere; 1875.
15. Rebora A, Marples RR, et al. Erosio interdigitalis blastomycetica. *Arch Dermatol.* 1973;108:66–68.
16. Bodey GP. Candidiasis in cancer patients. *Am J Med.* 1984; 77:13–19.
17. Jorizzo JL. Chronic mucocutaneous candidosis. *Arch Dermatol.* 1982;118:963–96.
18. Hauser FV, Rothman S. Monilial granuloma: report of a case and review of the literature. *Arch Dermatol Syph.* 1950;61:297–310.
19. File TM, Marina OA, Flowers FP. Necrotic lesions associated with disseminated candidiasis. *Arch Dermatol.* 1979;115:214–215.
20. Degos R, Garnier G, Civatte J. Pustulose par *Candida albicans* avec lesions psoriasiformes rappelant le psoriasis pustuleux. *Bull Soc Fr Dermatol Syph.* 1962;69:231–233.
21. Grossman ME, Silvers DN, Walther RR. Cutaneous manifestations of disseminated candidiasis. *J Am Acad Dermatol.* 1980; 2:111–116.
22. Schenck RB. On refractory subcutaneous abscesses caused by a fungus possibly related to sporotrichia. *Bull Johns Hopkins Hosp.* 1898;9:286–290.
23. Sampaio SAP, Lacaz CS, Almeida F. Aspectos clinicos da esporotricose em Sao Paulo. *Rev Hosp Clin Fac Med Univ S Paulo.* 1954;9:391–402.
24. Rippon JW. Pulmonary sporotrichosis mimicking tuberculosis. *Clin Microbiol Newsletter.* 1986;8:104–106.
25. Ridgeway NA, Whitcomb FC, Erickson EE, Law. Primary pulmonary sporotrichosis: report of two cases. *Am J Med.* 1962; 32:153–160.
26. Lurie HL. Histopathology of sporotrichosis. *Arch Pathol.* 1963; 75:121–137.
27. Bickley LK, Berman IJ, Hood AF. Fixed cutaneous sporotrichosis: unusual histopathology following intralesional corticosteroid administration. *J Am Acad Dermatol.* 1985;12:1007–1012.
28. Podroso A, Gomes JM. Sobre quatro casos de dermatite verrucosa produzida pela *Phialophora verrucosa*. *An Paul Med Cirurg.* 1920;11:53–61.
29. Medlar EM. A cutaneous infection caused by a new fungus *Phialophora verrucosa* with a study of the fungus. *J Med Res.* 1915;32:507–522.
30. McGinnis MR. Chromoblastomycosis and phaehyphomycosis: new concepts, diagnosis and mycology. *J Am Acad Dermatol.* 1983;8:1–16.
31. Tibirica PQT. *Anatomia Patologica da Dermatite Verrucosa Cromomicotica.* Sao Paulo, Brazil: Empresa Grafica da Revista dos Tribunais; 1939.
32. Batres E, Wolf JE Jr., Rudolph AH, et al. Transepithelial elimination of cutaneous chromomycosis. *Arch Dermatol.* 1978; 114:1231–1232.
33. Nodl F. Zur Histologie der Chromomydose. *Z Houtke.* 1963; 35:305–309.
34. Ajello L, Georg LK, Steigbigel RT, Wang CJK. A case of phaehyphomycosis caused by a new species of *Phialophora*. *Mycologia.* 1974;66:490–498.
35. Zeifer A, Connor DH. Phaeomycotic cyst. A clinicopathologic study of 25 patients. *Am J Trop Med.* 1980;29:901–911.
36. Kano K. A new pathogenic *Hormiscium* Kunze causing chromoblastomycosis (in Japanese). *Aichi Igakkai Zasshi.* 1934; 41:1657–1673.
37. Ravisse P, Vindos AJR. Lykystes mycosique etude histopathologique. *Bull Soc Pathol Exot.* 1981;74:46–54.
38. Mahgoub ES, Murray IG. *Mycetoma.* London: Heinemann Medical Books; 1973.
39. Hay RJ, Mackenzie DWRs. The histopathologic features of pale grain eumycetoma. *Trans R Soc Trop Med Hyg.* 1982;76:839–844.
40. Khandari KC, Mohapatra LN, Sehgal VN, et al. Black grain mycetoma of foot. *Arch Dermatol.* 1964;89:867–870.
41. Lobo J. Um caso de blastomicose produzida por uma especie nova, encontrada en Recife. *Rev Med Pernambuco.* 1931;1:763–765.
42. Dias LB, Sampaio MM, Silva D. Jorge Lobo's disease. Observations on its epidemiology and some unusual morphological forms of the fungus. *Rev Inst Med Trop S Paulo.* 1970;12:8–15.
43. Leite JM. Doenca de Jorge Lobo. Contribuicao a seu estudo anatomopatologico. Tese. *Oficinas Graficas da Revista Veterinaria.* Para, Brazil: Belem; 1954.

44. Seeber GR. *Un nuevo esporozoario parasito del hombre. Dos casos encontrados en polipos nasales.* Tesis, Universidad Nacional de Buenos Aires, Buenos Aires, 1900.

45. Karunaratne WAE. *Rhinosporidiosis in Man.* London: The Athlone Press; 1964.

46. Allen FRWK, Dave M. Treatment of rhinosporidionycosis in man based on sixty cases. *Indian Med Gaz.* 1936;71:376–395.

47. Ashworth JH. On *Rhinosporidium seeberi* (Wernicke 1903) with special reference to its sporulation and affinities. *Trans R Soc Edinb.* 1923;53:301–342.

48. Posadas A. Un nuevo caso de micosis fungoidea con psorospermias. *Circulo Med Argent.* 1892;5:587–597.

49. Dickson EC, Gifford MA. Coccidioides infection (coccidioidomycosis): the primary type of infection. *Arch Intern Med.* 1938; 62:853–871.

50. Carroll GF, Haley LD, Brown JM. Primary cutaneous coccidioidomycosis. *Arch Dermatol.* 1977;113:933–936.

51. Moore M. Mycotic granulomata and cutaneous tuberculosis: a comparison of the histopathologic response. *J Invest Dermatol.* 1945;6:149–181.

52. Trimble JR, Doucette J. Primary cutaneous coccidioidomycosis. *Arch Dermatol.* 1956;74:405–410.

53. Lutz A. Uma micose pseudococcidica localizada na boca e observada no Brasil. Contribuicao ao conhecimento das hifoblastomicoses americanas. *Brasil-Med* 1908;22:121–124, 141–144.

54. Lacaz CS, Passos-Filho MCR, Fava-Netto C, Macarron B. Contribuicao para o estudo da blastomicose-infeccao. Inquerito com a para coccidiodina. Estudo sorologico e clinico-radiologico dos paracoccidiodino-positivos. *Rev Inst Med Trop S Paulo.* 1959; 1:245–259.

55. Calle Velez G. *Dermatological Aspects of Paracoccidiodomycosis.* Scientific publication No. 254, pp. 118–121, Washington, DC: World Health Organization; 1971.

56. Motta LC, Pupo JA. Granulomatose paracoccidoidica (*Blastomycose brasileira*). *An Fac Med S Paulo.* 1936;12:407–426.

57. Almeida FP. Blastomyces e Paracoccidiodes. *An Fac Med S Paulo.* 1946;22:61–71.

58. Gilchrist TC. Protozoan dermatitis. J Cutan Dis. 1894; 12:496.

59. Schwarz J, Salfelder K. Blastomycosis: a review of 152 cases. *Curr Top Pathol.* 1977;65:165–200.

60. Darling STA. A protozoan general infection producing pseudotubercles in the lung and focal necrosis in the liver, spleen and lymph nodes. *JAMA.* 1906;46:1283–1285.

61. Goodwin RA, Des Prez RM. Histoplasmosis. *Am Rev Respir Dis.* 1978;117:929–956.

62. Studdard JW, Sneed F, et al. Cutaneous histoplasmosis. Am Rev Respir Dis. 1976;113:689–693.

63. Dumont A, Piche C. Electron microscopic study of human histoplasmosis. *Arch Pathol.* 1969;87:168–178.

64. Cantanei A, Kervan P. Nouvelle mycose humaine observee au Sondan francais. *Arch Inst Pasteur Alger.* 1945;23:169–172.

65. Cockshott WP, Lucas AO. Histoplasmosis duboisii, *Q J Med.* 1964;33:223–238,

66. Williams AO, Lawson EA, Lucas AO. African histoplasmosis due to *Histoplama duboisii.* Arch Pathol. 1971;92:306–318.

67. Nethercott JR, Schachter RK, Givan KF, et al. Histoplasmosis due to *H. capsulatum var. duboisii* in a Canadian immigrant. *Arch Dermatol.* 1978;114:595–598.

68. Kerkering TM, et al. The evolution of pulmonary cryptococcosis. Clinical implications from a study of 41 patients with and without compromising host factors. *Ann Intern Med.* 1981; 94:611.

69. Rook A, Woods B. Cutaneous cryptococcosis. *Br J Dermatol.* 1962;74:43–49.

70. Moore M. Cryptococcosis with cutaneous manifestations. *J Invest Dermatol.* 1957;28:159–182.

71. Baker RD, Hangen RK. Tissue changes and tissue diagnosis in cryptococcosis: a study of 26 cases. *Am J Clin Pathol.* 1955; 25:4–24.

72. Sluyter T. De vegetabilus organisimic animalis parasitis. *Diss Inaug Berolini.* 1847:14.

73. Seabury JH, Samuels M. The pathogenic spectrum of aspergillosis. *Am J Clin Pathol.* 1963;40:21–33.

74. McCarty JM, Flam MS, Pullen G, et al. Outbreak of primary cutaneous aspergillosis related to intravenous arm boards. *J Pediatr.* 1986;108:721–724.

75. Prystowski SD, Vogelstein B, Ettinger DS, et al. Invasive aspergillosis. *N Engl J Med.* 1976;295:655–658.

76. Canlile JR, Millet RE, Cho CT, et al. Primary cutaneous aspergillosis in a leukemic child. *Arch Dermatol.* 1978;114:78–80.

77. Gregory JE, Golden A, et al. Mucormycosis of the central nervous system. *Bull Johns Hopkins Hosp.* 1943;73:405–419.

78. Hammond DE, Winkelman NRD. Cutaneous phycomycosis. Report of three cases and identification of *Rhizopus. Arch Dermatol.* 1979;115:990–992.

79. Bittencourt AL, Londero AT, Arauso M, et al. Occurrence of subcutaneous zygomycosis caused by *Basidiobolus haptosporus* in Brazil. *Mycopathologia.* 1979;68:101–104.

80. Sands JM, Macher Am, Ley TJ, Neinhuis Z. Disseminated infection caused by *Cunninghamella bertholletiae* in a patient with B-thalassemia. Case report and review of literature. *Ann Intern Med* 1985;102:59–63.

81. Rabin ER, Lundberg GD, Mitchell ET. Mucormycosis in severely burned patients. *N Engl J Med.* 1961;264:1286–1289.

CHAPTER 30
Bites and Infestations

Thomas M. Chesney

Insects and related anthropods are ubiquitous in the world around us, and every human falls prey to them many times during life.[1] Most insect bites are trivial, however, and do not come to medical attention. Three major forms of reaction to anthropods are of importance to the dermatopathologist because each has a fairly characteristic histopathologic picture and because recognition of the lesion as an arthropod bite reaction may solve an enigmatic clinical problem or provide a foundation for further management. These forms of reaction are the acute insect bite reaction, the responses to scabies mite infestation, and the toxic–necrotic lesion of the brown recluse spider bite. An additional lesion of importance is the chronic tick bite granuloma or persistent insect bite reaction, which is important in the differential diagnosis of cutaneous lymphoma and pseudolymphoma.

ACUTE INSECT BITE REACTION

Clinical Features
Most insect bite reactions represent a host response to antigens present in the saliva of the insect that bites the human in search of a blood meal. The proboscis or sucker is inserted into the human skin, and the insect sucks in blood or interstitial fluid, at the same time injecting a minute volume of saliva. The first time a given type of insect bites a given individual, there is no response, but after multiple bites over time, there will develop a firm itchy papule as a manifestation of delayed hypersensitivity. Additional bites over time will then provoke an immediate wheal reaction, and further bites will provoke the papular response, the wheal response, or a combination of both. With further exposure, these responses may repeatedly recur, or there may be desensitization of the individual, with loss of response to the bites. This course of events obtains with mosquito, bedbug, flea, and sandfly bites, among others.[1]

Histologic Features
The cardinal feature of the acute insect bite reaction is the necrotizing nidus, or center of reaction, a small focus of tissue necrosis that may be centered at the dermal–epider-

mal interface or in the superficial dermis (Fig. 30–1). This nidus consists of homogenized necrotic tissue, including necrotic connective tissue, fibrin, and degenerating inflammatory cells. The background is usually eosinophilic but may be basophilic or may include basophilic strands that represent degenerated nuclear material. There may be proliferation of small blood vessels, and collagen bundles may stand out in and around the nidus, although they are not as pronounced as those in the flame figures of Well's syndrome. Inflammatory cells are characteristically present in and around the necrotizing nidus, especially polymorphonuclear leukocytes and eosinophils. The nidus is surrounded by mononuclear cells, which are mostly small lymphocytes in the immediate vicinity of the nidus in early bites. Larger lymphocytes and histiocytes become more prominent in the reaction as time passes.[2]

The low-power pattern of the acute insect bite reaction is typically triangular, with the epidermis at the base and with perivascular inflammation at the apex in the middermis. In earlier bites, this presents an inverted triangle shape, with the necrotizing nidus at the midbase area near the dermal–epidermal interface. With time, the low-power configuration of the infiltrate becomes more disciform and may extend deeper into the dermis while still occupying the upper dermis. The infiltrate away from the necrotizing nidus is a fairly well circumscribed perivascular cuff composed largely of lymphocytes but with scattered eosinophils, particularly around the periphery of the perivascular cuffs and also in the intervascular interstitium. In the interstitium, often single scattered eosinophils and single scattered lymphocytes are present in approximately equal numbers and in haphazard array. With time, eosinophils become less prominent, more histiocytes appear in the perivascular cuffs, and rare plasma cells may appear.

In the wheal form of reaction, the findings are as described, but, in addition, there is a localized focus of edema in the upper dermis immediately beneath the epidermis, constituting a subepidermal bulla (Fig. 30–2). This bulla may be traversed by thin fibrin strands and contain scattered lymphocytes and eosinophils (Fig. 30–3). The necrotic nidus

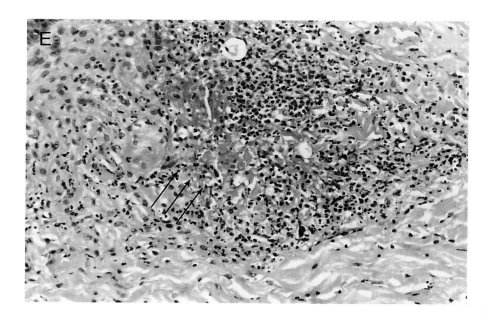

Figure 30–1. Acute insect bite reaction. The necrotizing nidus of the acute insect bite reaction contains a central focus of homogenized necrotic tissue (*arrow*) admixed with and surrounded by acute inflammatory cells (eosinophils and neutrophils). Note the relationship to the overlying epidermis (H&E, 100).

is usually located at or just beneath the floor of the subepidermal bulla. Whether or not the bulla is present, there may be changes in the overlying skin related to itching or excoriation, including early spongiosis, parakeratosis, and compaction of the stratum corneum, and later hyperkeratosis. An overtly eroded excoriation may be present with serous and inflammatory crust and with parakeratosis at the edges. Individually necrotic keratinocytes and degenerating inflammatory cells may be seen in the epidermis if the necrotic nidus involves the dermal–epidermal interface.

TICK BITE GRANULOMA

Tick bite granuloma (Fig. 30–4)[3,4] is a form of persistent allergic reaction that occurs when a portion of the tick remains embedded in the skin.

Histologic Features

The fragment of proboscis may be found in the upper dermis, with a dense, distinctly nodular infiltrate at all levels of the dermis, even extending into the subcutaneous tissue.

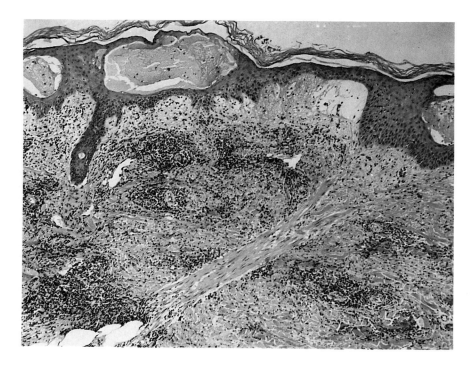

Figure 30–2. Acute insect bite reaction. Intraepidermal and subepidermal vesicle formation with a moderately intense superficial and deep perivascular infiltrate (H&E, ×65).

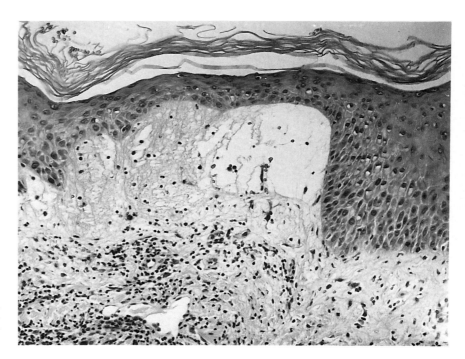

Figure 30–3. Acute insect bite reaction. Higher magnification of subepidermal bulla seen in Figure 30–2. Strands of fibrin and inflammatory cells are present within the blister cavity (H&E, ×135).

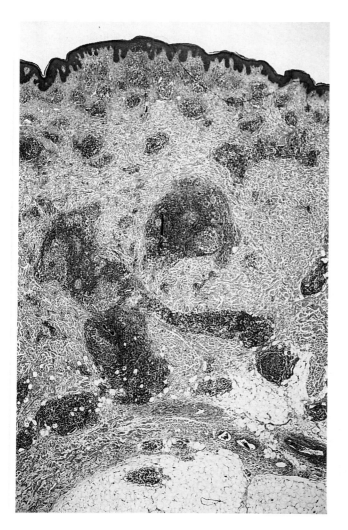

The nodules are characteristically polymorphous, with small and transformed lymphocytes, histiocytes, eosinophils, and plasma cells admixed in a dense perivascular infiltrate. Lymphoid follicular centers frequently are present, typically in the deeper component of the infiltrate.[3–6]

SCABIES INFESTATIONS

Clinical Features

There are several clinical presentations of scabies mite reactions. The scabies burrow is a clinically diagnostic lesion in which the gravid female scabies mite burrows through the skin at the level of the junction of the malpighian layer and the stratum corneum, depositing eggs and feces. Most of the symptomatology and most of the clinically observed papular lesions, are, however, related to the host inflammatory immune reaction. This inflammatory hypersensitivity response, an intensely pruritic, widespread papular eruption, is much more likely to be sampled in a small biopsy specimen.

In the rare variant known as Norweigian scabies, there is massive infestation of the skin, with marked hyperkeratosis and lichenification and with innumerable mite organisms embedded in the hyperkeratotic matrix. This form of scabies is typically seen in individuals with mental retardation or who are immunosuppressed by disease or therapy.

Histologic Features

Biopsy of the burrow will reveal a space between stratum corneum and the underlying keratinocytes within which

Figure 30–4. Chronic tick bite granuloma. There are perivascular nodules of chronic inflammation at all levels of the dermis, including the subcutis. Lymphoid follicular centers are present in the middermis (H&E, ×5).

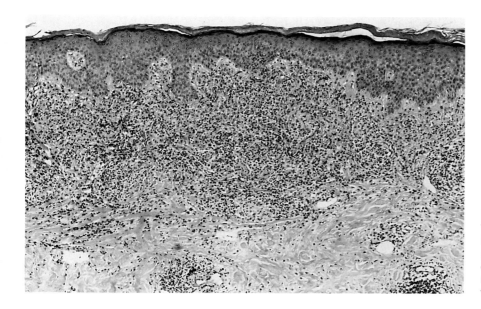

Figure 30–5. Chronic scabies reaction. There is a dense bandlike subepidermal polymorphous reaction in which eosinophils are prominent. Mites or mite products are typically not seen in the overlying stratum corneum. This appearance has been confused with cutaneous lymphoma (H&E, ×40).

one may find the female mite, her eggs, or her feces. The mite and the eggs are recognized by their chitin walls, which have strong homogeneous eosinophilia, are refractile, and are strongly PAS positive. This provides another good reason for routine performance of PAS stains on all cases of epidermal reactive dermatitis, in addition to the search for fungal spores and hyphae.

A biopsy specimen taken from a papular lesion will not display the mites or their products, but rather a dense bandlike inflammatory infiltrate in the upper dermis composed of lymphocytes, histiocytes, and variable but usually large numbers of eosinophils. This infiltrate fills the upper dermis but does not obscure the dermal–epidermal interface (Fig. 30–5). Epidermal changes are variable, as outlined previously,[7–10] and may include hyperplasia, spongiosis, or ulceration.

SPIDER BITE REACTION

Clinical Features

The brown recluse spider (*Loxosceles reclusa*) occupies a large portion of the southcentral United States in dry habitats, such as barns, garages, and homes. Its bite, frequently sustained while getting dressed or cleaning house, injects a complex venom containing many enzymes, principally hyaluronidase.[11,12] This results in an aggressively necrotizing skin lesion that ultimately manifests recalcitrant ulceration and scarring.[13]

Histologic Features

The early site displays extensive dermal and epidermal necrosis, often with bulla formation, with numerous perivascular and interstitial neutrophils (Fig. 30–6). A stage dominated by eosinophils then develops, during which fibrinoid

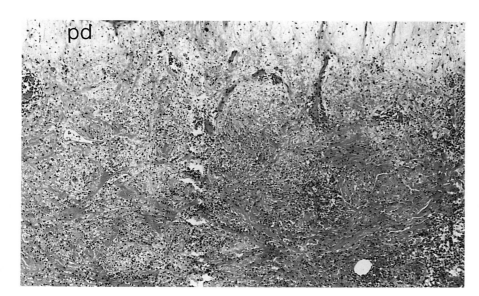

Figure 30–6. Acute brown recluse spider bite, toxic–necrotic lesion (at 48 hours). There is a marked edema of the papillary dermis (pd), with extensive necrosis throughout the subjacent dermis and an extensive acute and chronic inflammatory cell infiltrate both perivascular and interstitial. Neutrophils and eosinophils are present at this stage (H&E, ×10).

necrosis and the depth of involvement distinguish the recluse spider bite from the other arthropod reactions.

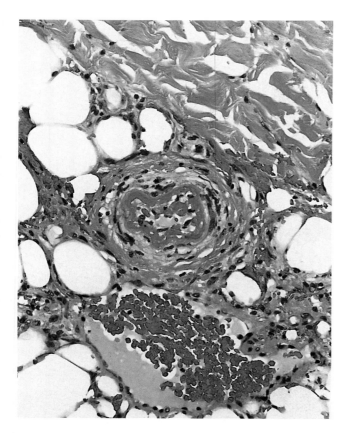

Figure 30–7. Brown recluse spider bite reaction. There is fibrinoid necrosis of the wall of an arteriole at the junction of the deep dermis and subcutaneous fat. The arteriole is surrounded by a few eosinophils and an early panniculitis (H&E, ×50).

necrosis of the walls of dermal and subcutaneous arterioles is characteristic (Fig. 30–7).[14] Finally, there is a stage of consolidating dermal change, panniculitis, and then dense scarring. The degree of phlebitis and arteriolar fibrinoid

REFERENCES

1. Rook A. Skin diseases caused by arthropods and other venemous or noxious animals. In: Rook A, Wilkinson DS, Ebling FJG, eds. *Textbook of Dermatology.* 3rd ed. Oxford: Blackwell Scientific Publications; 1979:911–950.
2. Bandman HJ, Boose K. Histologie des Muckenstiches (*Aedes aegypti*). *Arch Klin Exp Dermatol.* 1967;231:59–67.
3. Allen AC. Persistent "insect bites" (dermal eosinophilic granulomas) simulating lymphoblastomas, histiocytoses, and squamous cell carcinomas. *Am J Pathol.* 1948;24:367–387.
4. Tobias N. Tickbite granuloma. *J Invest Dermatol.* 1949;12:255–259.
5. Theis JH, Budwiser PD. *Rhipicephalus sanguineus:* sequential histopathology at the host–arthropod interface. *Exp Parasitol.* 1974;36:77–105.
6. Yesudian P, Thambiah AS. Persistent papules after tick bites. *Dermatologia.* 1974;147:214–218.
7. Thomson J, Cockrane T, Cochran R, McQueen A. Histology simulating reticulosis in persistent nodular scabies. *Br J Dermatol.* 1974;90:421–429.
8. Hejazi N, Mehregan AH. Scabies. Histological study of inflammatory lesions. *Arch Dermatol.* 1975;111:37–39.
9. Fernandez N, Torres A, Ackerman AB. Pathological findings in human scabies. *Arch Dermatol.* 1977;113:320–324.
10. Falk ES, Eide TJ. Histologic and clinical findings in human scabies. *Int J Dermatol.* 1981;20:600–605.
11. Wasserman GS, Anderson PC. Loxoscelism and necrotic arachnidism. *J Toxicol Clin Toxicol.* 1983–84;21:451–472.
12. Wong RC, Hughes SE, Vorhees JJ. Spider bites—review in depth. *Arch Dermatol.* 1987;123:98–104a.
13. Schenone H, Prats F. Arachnidism by *loxoscele laeta*—report of 40 cases of necrotic arachnidism. *Arch Dermatol.* 1961;83:139–142.
14. Pucevich MV, Chesney TM. Histopathologic analysis of human bites by the brown recluse spider. *Arch Dermatol.* 1983;119:851.

SECTION V
Non-Inflammatory Disorders

CHAPTER 31
Non-Inflammatory Disorders of the Skin

Thomas D. Horn

The following entities have in common disorders of the epidermis felt to be based primarily on noninflammatory etiologies. They constitute a heterogeneous group of diseases, some associated with known metabolic derangements (e.g., necrolytic migratory erythema) and others with heritable diatheses (e.g., Bloom's syndrome).

ICHTHYOSIS

The term *ichthyosis* is applied to a variety of entities, most having the feature of variably sized scaling patches occurring in characteristic patterns and often in association with predictable internal manifestations. The histopathology of these conditions, although often typical of ichthyosis, must usually be interpreted within the clinical setting to arrive at a specific diagnosis. For example, the histopathologic finding of epidermolytic hyperkeratosis may be incidental, may occur as a plamoplantar keratoderma, or may characterize the severe, generalized ichthyosis known as bullous congenital ichthyosiform erythroderma. The various entities featuring ichthyosis are described separately. Advances in the understanding of the biology of the stratum corneum merit further study for the interested reader.[1,2]

Ichthyosis Vulgaris

In this autosomal dominantly inherited condition, cutaneous changes are not present at birth; rather, they appear within the first few months of life and subsequently wax and wane, often seasonally. Some individuals experience a gradual improvement with age. The large, angular scales preferentially involve the extensor surfaces of the extremities in the typical patient. A plamoplantar keratoderma frequently accompanies the ichthyosis. Ichthyosis vulgaris is the most common of the ichthyoses.

The typical histologic changes (Fig. 31–1) are basket-weave or orthokeratotic hyperkeratosis overlying hypo-granulosis or an absent granular layer.

The observation of a diminished or absent granular layer is substantiated by electron microscopy, showing diminished or absent keratohyalin granules. Filaggrin, a protein of the keratohyalin granule responsible for keratin organization, and its precursor, profilaggrin, have been found to be absent from affected skin in ichthyosis vulgaris.[3] The rate of proliferation of the epidermis appears to be normal in ichthyosis vulgaris, favoring a retention of corneocytes as the cause of the hyperkeratosis.[4]

Recessive X-Linked Ichthyosis

Clinical Features
Recessive X-linked ichthyosis (RXLI) represents an inherited ichthyosis with normal epidermal proliferation. The cutaneous manifestations are variably present at birth and consist of ichthyotic scales similar to ichthyosis vulgaris, but with flexural involvement. Corneal opacities visible upon slit-lamp examination are a characteristic, albeit variably present manifestation.

Histologic Features
The histopathology of RXLI (Fig. 31–2) differs from that of ichthyosis vulgaris chiefly by the presence of a normal granular layer or hypergranulosis in association with basket-weave or othokeratotic hyperkeratosis.

Etiology
A wealth of information exists regarding the etiology of RXLI. These males are the product of pregnancies marked by low maternal urinary steroids resulting from a deficiency of fetal steroid sulfatase, an arylsulfatase. In the later stages of pregnancy, the maternal urinary estrogens are derived from the metabolism of fetal steroids which are deficient in affected individuals.[5] The gene encoding steroid sulfatase is located on the short arm of the X chromosome. The cutaneous expression of steroid sulfatase deficiency manifests as elevated levels of cholesterol sulfate, normally a substrate of this enzyme. Cholesterol sulfate is increased in the scale of RXLI; increased cholesterol sulfate from topical administration is associated with hyperkeratosis.[4]

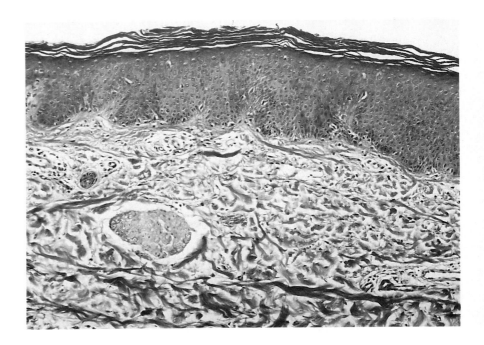

Figure 31–1. Acanthosis, hypogranulosis, and mild orthokeratotic hyperkeratosis typify ichthyosis vulgaris (H&E, ×145).

Bullous Congenital Ichthyosiform Erythroderma

Clinical Features

Bullous congenital ichthyosiform erythroderma (BCIE), also known as epidermolytic hyperkeratosis, is inherited as an autosomal dominant disorder. BCIE generally presents at birth with erythema, bullae, and, later, widespread, hyperkeratotic, muddy brown, verrucous plaques. Ichthyotic scale is not a feature of this entity. In particularly severe cases, routine personal hygiene is insufficient to eradicate the markedly unpleasant odor. The vesicobullous aspect of BCIE generally resolves in the first years of life.

Histologic Features

Epidermolytic hyperkeratosis is also used as a histopathologic term to describe a specific alteration in the epidermis. The epidermis is mildly acanthotic and notable for a process of reticular degeneration of keratinocytes, beginning immediately above the basal layer or at a higher level and resulting in perinuclear clear zones (Fig. 31–3). Confluence of this degeneration creates an intraepidermal cleavage characterizing bullous lesions. Associated with the reticular degeneration is a clumping of keratohyalin granules with deepened basophilia, scattered eosinophilic granules, and overall hypergranulosis. Marked overlying compact hyperkeratosis is present. Epidermolytic hyperkeratosis is the characteristic histopathologic change seen in BCIE.

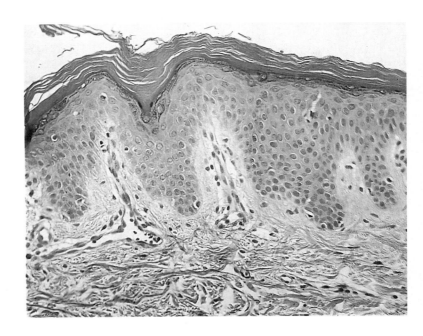

Figure 31–2. This biopsy of recessive X-linked ichthyosis displays slight acanthosis, a prominent granular layer, and orthokeratotic hyperkeratosis (H&E, ×225).

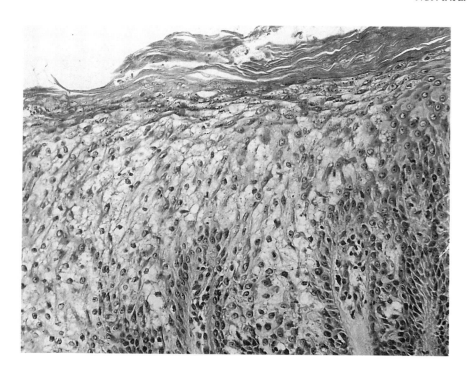

Figure 31–3. Hypergranulosis, keratinocytic reticular degeneration, and acanthosis characterize epidermolytic hyperkeratosis occurring in a patient with bullous congenital ichthyosiform erythroderma (H&E, ×230).

Etiology

Clues to the etiology of BCIE are less forthcoming than in other ichthyoses. Electron micrographic analysis has demonstrated clumping of tonofibrils and the appearance of keratohyalin granules at abnormally low levels of the epidermis. The rate of passage of keratinocytes through the epidermis is faster than normal; therefore, BCIE is classified as a hyperproliferative ichthyosis.[4] In a study of palmoplantar epidermolytic hyperkeratosis, the amount of 67-kDa high-molecular-weight keratin was found to be diminished and interpreted as abnormal terminal differentiation.[6]

Differential Diagnosis

As mentioned earlier, the histopathologic finding of epidermolytic hyperkeratosis is not specific for the ichthyosis clinically recognized as BCIE. Normal skin may contain foci of epidermolytic hyperkeratosis in addition to actinic keratoses, squamous cell carcinomas, seborrheic keratoses, verruca plana, epidermal nevus, palmoplantar epidermolytic hyperkeratosis, and solitary or disseminated epidermolytic acanthomas.[7]

Lamellar Ichthyosis

Lamellar ichthyosis, or congenital nonbullous ichthyosiform erythroderma, is inherited as an autosomal recessive trait. It presents at birth, often in the setting of a collodion baby, with persistent erythema and scaling.

The histopathology of lamellar ichthyosis resembles (Fig. 31–4) that of recessive X-linked ichthyosis with moderate hyperkeratosis and a normal to increased granular cell layer.

Some authors have further classified lamellar ichthyosis based on the amount of stratum corneum n-alkanes, a unique group of lipids of unknown origin. Patients with

normal levels of n-alkanes in the stratum corneum (normally n-alkanes constitute 5% to 7% of total lipid content) characteristically have larger, thicker scales, ectropion, and less erythroderma, whereas patients with elevated n-alkanes (25% of total stratum corneum lipid content) have finer scales, marked erythroderma, and no ectropion.[4]

Collodion Baby and Harlequin Fetus

The term *collodion* is derived from the Greek for "gluelike" and refers to the tightly adherent membrane surrounding certain newborns who usually later develop a currently classifiable type of ichthyosis. Approximately 60% have lamellar ichthyosis or bullous congenital ichthyosiform erythroderma, but a collodion may also herald the onset of ichthyosis vulgaris and trichothiodystrophy.[8] One study found that approximately 10% of cases lacked sequelae but noted an overall mortality of 11% from sepsis.[8] The harlequin fetus is encased in very thick, armourlike plates, which constrict chest wall motion and, therefore, respiration. These plates exhibit deep furrows running in irregular patterns. The condition is generally fatal.

Biopsy of the collodion membrane reveals an orthokeratotic hyperkeratosis, with the lower one third of the stratum corneum being markedly compact and the outer two thirds less dense.[8] The plates of the harlequin fetus consist of massive hyperkeratosis overlying a diminished granular cell layer.[9]

Acquired Ichthyosis

In general, acquired ichthyosis clinically resembles ichthyosis vulgaris. Numerous associated diseases have been described including sarcoidosis, hypothyroidism, leprosy, ac-

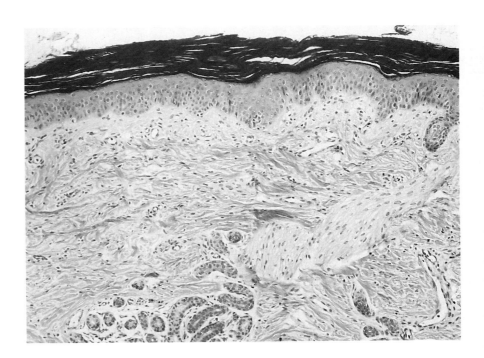

Figure 31–4. Marked hyperkeratosis overlies a normal granular layer in this biopsy of lamellar ichthyosis (H&E, ×125).

quired immunodeficiency syndrome, and lymphoma (particularly Hodgkin's disease) and other malignant neoplasms. Various medications, especially cholesterol-lowering agents such as triparanol, nicotinic acid, and dixyrazine, may induce ichthyosis.[10,11]

The histopathology of acquired ichthyosis resembles that of ichthyosis vulgaris. The notable exception to this similarity is ichthyosis associated with sarcoidosis or leprosy, which may show typical granulomas on biopsy.

Ichthyosis in Various Syndromes

Ichthyosis is a characteristic finding in numerous syndromes. Among these are CHILD syndrome (congenital hemidysplasia with ichthyosiform erythroderma, usually unilateral),[12] Dorfman-Chanarin syndrome (disordered neutral lipid metabolism affecting skin, liver, muscle, and central nervous system),[13] KID syndrome (keratitis, ichthyosis, and deafness),[14] Sjögren-Larsson syndrome (mental retardation and neurologic abnormalities), Conradi's syndrome (chondrodysplasia punctata and ocular deficits), Refsum's disease (see next section), Netherton's syndrome (ichthyosis linearis circumflexa; see later), and Rud's syndrome (mental retardation and hypogonadism).

Refsum's Disease

Refsum's disease (heredopathia atactica polyneuritiformis), an autosomal recessive disorder of phytanic acid degradation, consists of retinitis pigmentosa, deafness, polyneuropathy, and ichthyosis.[15] The cutaneous histopathology is striking in that lipid-containing vacuoles are present in the lower epidermal layers in addition to hyperkeratosis and hypergranulosis.[16] The vacuoles present in basilar and suprabasilar keratinocytes of Refsum's disease are not unique. The histopathology of the ichthyosis in Dorfman-Chanarin syndrome is characterized by lipid-containing vacuoles in keratinocytes of the basal and granular layers. Acanthosis, hypergranulosis, and hyperkeratosis accompany this change. Interestingly, elevated levels of n-alkanes have been reported, similar to one subset of patients with lamellar ichthyosis. Electron microscopy reveals structurally abnormal lamellar bodies and intercellular spaces within the stratum corneum.[17]

Ichthyosis Linearis Circumflexa

Ichthyosis linearis circumflexa (ILC), lamellar ichthyosis, trichorrhexis invaginata (bamboo hair), and atopic dermatitis are the chief dermatologic features of Netherton's syndrome. It is inherited as an autosomal recessive disorder. Aminoaciduria and mental retardation are reported associations.[18] ILC consists of erythematous patches with rapidly changing borders and a characteristic "double-edged scale." The eruption may generalize, resulting in erythroderma. The histopathology of ILC is rather nonspecific (Fig. 31–5), with acanthosis, parakeratosis, and occasionally spongiosis progressing to microvesiculation.[18,19] The scalp hair is short and brittle. Hair shafts with trichorrhexis invaginata have a nodose swelling and "ball and socket joint" abnormality microscopically. Similar but less well developed change is present in hair from other sites.[20] The hair tends to fracture at the site of the trichorrhexis invaginata defect.

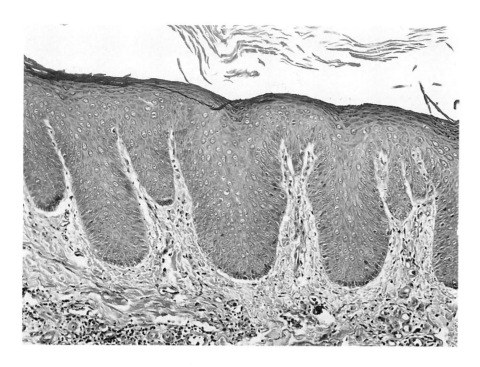

Figure 31–5. A biopsy of ichthyosis linearis circumflexa from a patient with Netherton's syndrome displays acanthosis and hypergranulosis (H&E, ×145).

KERATOSIS PALMARIS ET PLANTARIS

Clinical Features

Keratosis palmaris et plantaris is the term applied to hyperkeratotic thickening of the palms and soles occurring in diverse settings. The condition may be inherited in an autosomal dominant manner in Unna-Thost disease (with hyperhidrosis and bromhidrosis), epidermolytic hyperkeratosis localized to the palms and soles, Howel-Evans syndrome (with esophageal carcinoma in some family members), keratosis punctata, and pachyonychia congenita (with hyperkeratosis of the nail beds and benign white patches of the oral mucosa). Recessive forms of this disorder include Mal de Meleda, Papillon-Lefèvre syndrome (with periodontitis, loss of teeth, and calcification of the falx cerebri), and Richner-Hanhart syndrome (tyrosinemia II).

Histologic Features

Except as noted here, most forms of diffuse keratosis palmaris et plantaris possess a nonspecific histology, characterized by acanthosis with marked hyperkeratosis and accompanying hypergranulosis (Fig. 31–6). Parakeratosis and a mononuclear perivascular infiltrate are variably present.

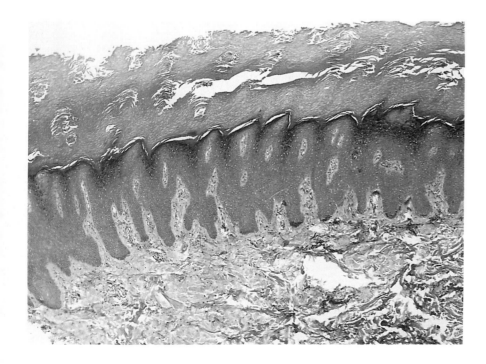

Figure 31–6. Acanthosis, hypergranulosis, papillomatosis, and marked orthokeratotic hyperkeratosis are seen in this palmar biopsy of keratosis palmaris et plantaris (H&E, ×140).

The stratum corneum and upper stratum malpighii in Richner-Hanhart syndrome may contain refractile eosinophilic deposits.[21]

Epidermolytic hyperkeratosis of the palms and soles displays histologic changes consistent with epidermolytic hyperkeratosis found elsewhere,[22,23] namely, compact hyperkeratosis, hypergranulosis, and distinct perinuclear vacuolation in the stratum spinosum and stratum corneum. In one patient studied, the rate of cellular proliferation was found to be increased, similar to the cellular kinetics of generalized epidermolytic hyperkeratosis.[22]

In kerotosis punctata, the hyperkeratosis and hypergranulosis occur in discrete foci indenting the epidermis, which is acanthotic but otherwise unremarkable. Underlying papillary dermal edema has been reported.[24]

In evaluation of a biopsy from the palm or sole, the presence of a cornoid lamella is indicative of porokeratosis punctata palmaris et plantaris.

Etiology

Evidence exists that there is abnormal maturation of fatty acids in the stratum corneum of patients with various forms of keratosis palmaris et plantaris. Affected patients, regardless of specific diagnosis, exhibited increased short-chain and monoene fatty acids compared with normal controls.[25] Inasmuch as intercellular lipids are believed to help regulate desquamation,[26] these alterations in fatty acid content may promote hyperkeratosis.

ACANTHOSIS NIGRICANS

Clinical Features

Hyperpigmented patches with a finely papillomatous quality, imparting a velvety sheen to the surface, characterize the lesions of acanthosis nigricans. These patches most commonly present in intertriginous areas, but may become widespread, thereby resembling systematized epidermal nevus. Involvement of the oral mucosa may occur. Acanthosis nigricans in the esophagus has been reported in a patient with a gastric carcinoma.[27] Acanthosis nigricans occurs idiopathically as well as in association with various systemic disorders and, therefore, may have important implications for the general health of the patient when diagnosed.

Most commonly, acanthosis nigricans appears as an isolated finding, frequently in an obese but otherwise healthy individual.

Acanthosis nigricans may accompany a wide variety of endocrine disorders, including diabetes mellitus, pituitary adenoma, acromegaly, Cushing's syndrome, Addison's disease, and Stein-Leventhal syndrome.[28] The association of acanthosis nigricans with insulin-resistant diabetes mellitus is particularly well recognized. This insulin resistance may result from deficient number of receptors in some patients or from a faulty postreceptor mechanism in others.[29,30]

Numerous medications have been reported to cause acanthosis nigricans. Among these are niacinamide,[31] oral contraceptives, and corticosteroids.[28] The eruption is reversible on discontinuation of therapy.

Individuals with Bloom's syndrome, Rud's syndrome,

Lawrence-Seip syndrome, and Crouzon's syndrome may exhibit acanthosis nigricans. Notably, Lawrence-Seip syndrome (congenital lipodystrophy) is associated with insulin-resistant diabetes.

Lastly, acanthosis nigricans may occur as a paraneoplastic manifestation, most commonly concomitant with the appearance of a malignant neoplasm, usually a gastrointestinal adenocarcinoma. The eruption may precede the appearance of the tumor and may reappear with the development of metastases.

Histologic Features

Regardless of the presence or absence of an underlying association, the histopathology of acanthosis nigricans remains the same.[32] Actual acanthosis is mild, instead; the major epidermal alteration is marked papillomatosis in thin upward projections, often with blunt rather than pointed tips (Fig. 31–7). The epidermis is thinned at the top and sides of these projections. Hyperkeratosis is also prominent with abundant accumulation of keratinaceous material in the valleys between epidermal peaks. The hyperpigmentation characteristic of acanthosis nigricans seems not to arise solely from increased melanin production as this feature is only variably present. Instead, the abundant hyperkeratosis may explain the dyschromia. There are no dermal changes except for an occasional mononuclear inflammatory infiltrate.

Differential Diagnosis

The differential diagnosis of acanthosis nigricans consists of those entities displaying primarily papillomatosis.

Hyperkeratotic seborrheic keratoses, some actinic keratoses, and epidermal nevi may closely simulate the epidermal changes of acanthosis nigricans. Clinicopathologic correlation may be required to distinguish between some epidermal nevi, hyperkeratotic seborrheic keratoses, and acanthosis nigricans. Confluent and reticulated papillomatosis of Gougerot and Carteaud typically displays similar features, making confident distinction between the two entities difficult. The role of *Pityrosporon* organisms in the etiology of confluent and reticulated papillomatosis is unclear.[33]

NECROLYTIC MIGRATORY ERYTHEMA

Clinical Features

Necrolytic migratory erythema (NME) represents one manifestation of the glucagonoma syndrome. The characteristic constellation of findings includes an alpha cell tumor of the pancreas that secretes glucagon, elevated circulating glucagon levels, a cutaneous eruption, mild diabetes or glucose intolerance, and hypoaminoacidemia. Not all elements must be present to make the diagnosis; up to 35% of patients may lack NME at the time of diagnosis.[34] Additional findings include normochromic, normocytic anemia; hypocholesterolemia; and an association with multiple endocrine neoplasia I and II in some cases. Renal failure, hepatic failure, stress, and prolonged hypoglycemia may be associated with elevated glucagon levels.[35] Glucagon is felt to promote the degradation of amino acids for glucose production and thereby to induce the hypoaminoacidemia.[36] The alpha cell tumor is located in the tail or body

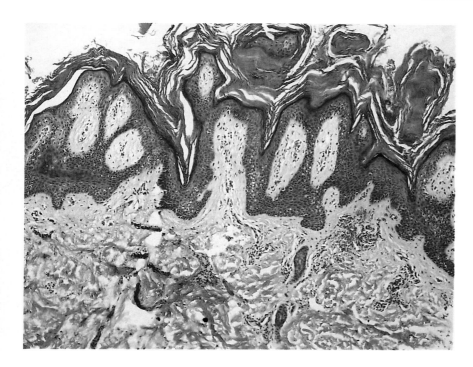

Figure 31–7. This biopsy of acanthosis nigricans shows mild acanthosis with papillomatosis and hyperkeratosis (H&E, ×45).

of the pancreas in more than 50% of cases and has metastasized in approximately 50% of patients at the time of diagnosis. Fully 80% of tumors are malignant as determined by the eventual occurrence at metastases.[34]

NME typically involves perioral and perineal skin as well as skin of the lower extremities, following a cyclic pattern of erythematous patches that become centrally edematous and vesicular with occasional bulla formation. Erosion and crusting ensue and resolve, leading to repetition of the process over 7 to 14 days.[37]

Administration of zinc or amino acids has been associated with clearing of the eruption, but complete surgical excision of the tumor remains the only definitive therapy and also results in resolution of the rash.[38] NME recurs in the presence of metastases.

Histologic Features
Biopsy of NME must be taken from a relatively fresh lesion to provide diagnostic information. The crusted stage of the eruption may show only nonspecific findings. A superficial perivascular mononuclear infiltrate is initially present which becomes mixed with an increasing number of neutrophils. Papillary dermal edema is often present. The most striking changes occur in the epidermis with the keratinocytes of the upper stratum malpighii undergoing intracellular edema, ballooning, and necrosis, resulting in pale eosinophilic cells, vesiculation, and occasionally bulla formation (Fig. 31–8). This process eventuates in crust formation with marked overlying parakeratosis. Moderate acanthosis occurs. The epidermis below the necrotic keratinocytes is uninvolved, and the cells appear relatively normal.[39]

Differential Diagnosis
Similar histologic features may be seen in acrodermatitis enteropathica, a syndrome related to zinc malabsorption;

pellagra, a disease related to nicotinic acid or tryptophan deficiency; and Hartnup disease, an inherited condition with an associated hypoaminoacidemia. The acquired or inherited nutrient deficiency common to these three diseases is an intriguing link. The precise mechanism by which inadequate quantities of zinc and/or amino acids causes NME remains unknown.

POROKERATOSIS

Clinical Features
Porokeratosis is a disorder of epidermal keratinization often inherited in an autosomal dominant fashion. Several distinct clinical patterns of porokeratosis exist, including porokeratosis of Mibelli, porokeratosis punctata, disseminated superficial actinic porokeratosis, linear porokeratosis, and disseminated superficial porokeratosis. The characteristic lesion is an erythematous annular patch displaying little or no abnormality centrally, but marked by a raised, thready keratotic ridge at the periphery.

The pathogenesis of the porokeratosis remains unclear. Cases have been reported in immunosuppressed individuals.[40] Squamous cell carcinoma arising in porokeratosis of Mibelli,[41] linear porokeratosis,[42] and disseminated superficial actinic porokeratosis[43] have been documented.

Histologic Features
The histologic hallmark of porokeratosis is the cornoid lamella (Fig. 31–9). A cornoid lamella is characterized by a column or wedge of parakeratosis extending through an otherwise orthokeratotic stratum corneum, often tangential to the epidermis. The epidermis immediately below this column may contain a few dyskeratotic cells in addition to a reduced or absent granular cell layer. As the annular

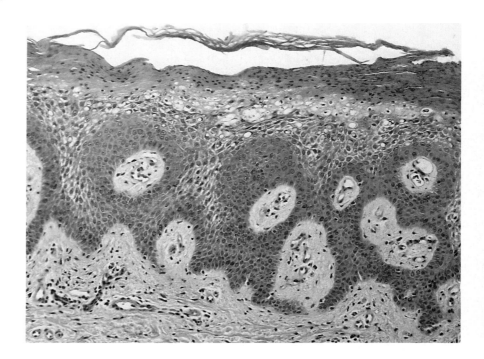

Figure 31–8. Edema and necrosis of the middle and upper epidermis are characteristic of necrolytic migratory erythema (H&E, ×145).

lesion of porokeratosis expands, the deepest point or tip of the wedge of the cornoid lamella moves outward and thus marks the lateral limit with the parakeratotic column or wedge pointing inward. The central epidermis may be normal or somewhat thin. Dermal changes are generally mild and consist of focal telangiectasia and mild perivascular mononuclear inflammatory cell infiltrate beneath the cornoid lamella.

Differential Diagnosis
Although characteristic of porokeratosis, the cornoid lamella is not specific. Other entitles in which a cornoid lamella has been found include seborrheic keratosis, scar, verruca vulgaris, milium, actinic keratosis, squamous cell carcinoma *in situ*, and basal cell carcinoma.[41] Additionally, a congenital anomaly of eccrine ducts exists in which cornoid lamellae arise within deep or superficial portions of adjacent

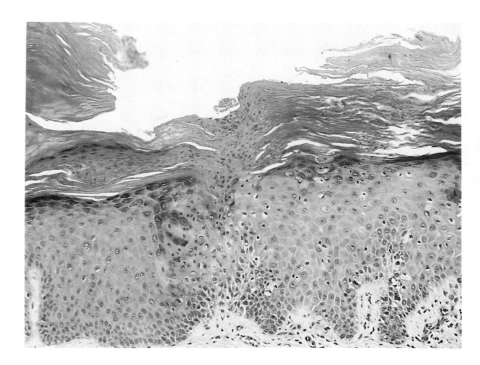

Figure 31–9. A well-formed cornoid lamella is present with underlying dyskeratotic keratinocytes in this biopsy of porokeratosis of Mibelli (H&E, ×140).

ducts. This entity has been termed porokeratotic eccrine ostial and dermal duct nevus.[45,46] Its clinical appearance is that of grouped keratotic papules, usually on the palm or sole.

POIKILODERMA

Clinical Features

Poikilo is derived from the Greek for "variegated" and refers to the typical clinical findings in poikilodermatous skin, namely, hyperpigmentation, hypopigmentation, telangiectasia, and atrophy. Therefore, the word *poikiloderma* describes a particular eruption, not a specific diagnosis. Poikiloderma occurs with mycosis fungoides where it is known as poikiloderma vasculare atrophicans. It may arise in the setting of a collagen vascular disease, most commonly dermatomyositis and lupus erythematosus. Injury to the skin may eventuate in poikiloderma as seen after radiation, prolonged sun exposure (poikiloderma of Civatte), and heat or cold exposure. Rothund-Thomson syndrome, dyskeratosis congenita, Werner's syndrome, Fanconi's anemia, and hereditary sclerosing poikiloderma[47] have all been described as having the characteristic cutaneous findings of poikiloderma. Most notably, Rothund-Thomson syndrome, or poikiloderma congenitale, displays the early onset of poikiloderma and sensitivity to sunlight in addition to short stature, juvenile cataracts, congenital skeletal defects, hypogonadism, nail abnormalities, and mental retardation.[48] Lastly, poikilodermatous change may arise in chronic graft-versus-host disease, acrodermatitis chronica atrophicans, and as a sequela to administration of various drugs (e.g., arsenicals, topical corticosteriods, and busulfan).[49]

Histologic Features

Used as a histopathologic term, *poikiloderma* defines a pattern of changes including flattening and thinning of the epidermis, some degree of basal layer vacuolization, pig-

ment incontinence with melanophages in the superficial dermis, telangiectasia, and variable epidermal hyper- and hypopigmentation (Fig. 31–10). The papillary dermis characteristically contains sclerotic collagen with loss of the papillae. This description is nonspecific, yet the changes described may often be accompanied by other findings that point to the true etiology underlying the poikiloderma. For example, a heavy bandlike infiltrate of mononuclear cells with hyperchromatic and convoluted nuclei, exocytosis, and possibly Pautrier's microabscesses suggests poikiloderma vasculare atrophicans. The infiltrating cells involved in this process have been shown to be T lymphocytes, predominantly of the T helper phenotype (OKT4/Leu-2A positive), with an admixture of T suppressor cells (OKT8/Leu-2A positive).[50] Poikilodermatomyositis is typically noninflammatory and accompanied by a thickened basement membrane zone.[51] Similarly, characteristic changes of lupus erythematosus may be noted in biopsies of poikilodermatous skin from affected individuals. Careful search for other histopathologic findings in the setting of poikiloderma is therefore of significant potential value.

BLOOM'S SYNDROME

Clinical Features

An autosomal recessive disorder, Bloom's syndrome consists of several characteristic features, including photodistributed, telangiectatic patches and plaques principally on the face; diminished growth; dolichocephaly; immunoglobulin deficiencies; increased spontaneous chromosome breakage (sister chromatid exchange) in metaphase lymphocytes in culture;[52,53] and an approximately 25% incidence of neoplasia by age 20. The malignancy most commonly is lymphoreticular, but may be a carcinoma. Ashkenazi Jews are particularly affected.

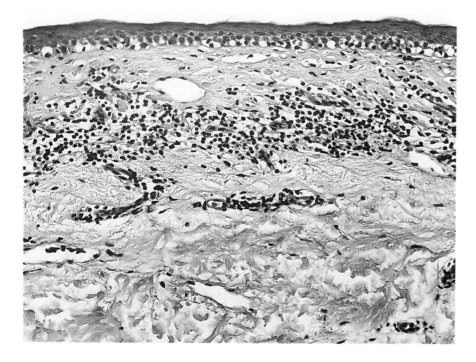

Figure 31–10. Epidermal atrophy, basal vacuolization, exocytosis, telangiectatic vessels, and a bandlike infiltrate of small mononuclear cells are present in this biopsy of poikiloderma (H&E, ×145).

The photosensitive eruption typically begins during the warmer months, usually by the second year of life. The rash may resemble lupus erythematosus and may eventuate in atrophy. Characteristically, the rash improves with time and may clear completely.[53]

Histologic Features

Biopsy specimens from the telangiectatic eruption show epidermal atrophy, basal layer vacuolar change, and dyskeratosis. Katzenellenbogen and Laron reported keratotic plugs in the epidermis.[54] Telangiectasia of superficial dermal vessels is present with or without a perivascular predominantly mononuclear inflammatory cell infiltrate.[54] Direct immunofluorescence has been reported to reveal cytoid bodies staining for IgG, IgM, C3, and fibrin.[55] Some fibrin was also found at the dermal–epidermal junction.

Differential Diagnosis

The presence of epidermal atrophy, basal layer vacuolar change, and dyskeratosis is suggestive of lupus erythematosus, which the eruption of Bloom's syndrome also resembles clinically. In the absence of significant atrophy, these epidermal changes may also resemble those of interface dermatitides in general; however, the inflammatory infiltrate in Bloom's syndrome is reported to be predominantly perivascular or entirely absent. A lichenoid pattern is not described, nor is periappendageal inflammation a prominent feature. The absence of linear basement membrane zone staining on direct immunofluorescence for immunoglobulins and complement further serves to distinguish the photosensitive rash of Bloom's syndrome from lupus erythematosus.

REFERENCES

1. Elias PM: Epidermal lipids, barrier function and desquamation. *J Invest Dermatol* 1983;8:44–49.
2. Williams ML: The dynamics of desquamation. Lessons to be learned from the ichthyoses. *Am J Dermatopathol* 1984;6:381–385.
3. Fleckman P, Holbrook KA, Dale BA, et al.: Keratinocytes cultured from subjects with ichthyosis vulgaris are phenotypically abnormal. *J Invest Dermatol* 1987;88:640–645.
4. Epstein EH, Williams ML, Elias PM: Biochemical abnormalities in the ichthyoses. *Curr Probl Derm* 1987;17:32–44.
5. France J, Liggins G: Placental sulfatase deficiency. *J Clin Endocrinol Metab* 1969;29:138–141.
6. Moriwaki S, Tanaka T, Horiguchi Y, et al.: Epidermolytic hereditary palmoplantar keratoderma. *Arch Dermatol* 1988;124:555–559.
7. Shapiro L, Baraf CS: Isolated epidermolytic acanthoma. *Arch Dermatol* 1970;101:220–223.
8. Larregue M, Ottavy N, Bressieux S-M, et al: Bébé collodion. Trente nouvelles observations. *Ann Dermatol Venereol* 1986;113:773–785.
9. Luderschmidt C, Dorn M, Basserman R, et al.: Kollodiumbaby und harlekinfetus. *Hautarzt* 1980;31:154–158.
10. Williams ML, Feingold KR, Grubauer G, et al.: Ichthyosis induced by cholesterol-lowering drugs. *Arch Dermatol* 1987;123:1535–1538.
11. Brenner S: Acquired ichthyosis in AIDS. *Cutis* 1987;39:421–423.
12. Hebert AA, Esterly NB, Holbrook KA, et al.: The CHILD syndrome. Histologic and ultrastructural studies. *Arch Dermatol* 1984;123:503–509.

13. Srebrnik A, Tur E, Perluk C, et al.: Dorfman-Chanarin syndrome. A case report and review. *J Am Acad Dermatol* 1987;17:801–808.
14. Harms M, Gilardi S, Levy PM, et al.: KID syndrome (keratinitis, ichthyosis, and deafness) and chronic mucocutaneous candidiasis: Case report and review of the literature. *Pediatr Dermatol* 1984;2:1–7.
15. Mize CE, Hernden Jr. JH, Tsai SC, et al.: Phytanic acid storage in Refsum's disease due to defective alpha-hydroxylation. *Clin Res* 1968;16:346.
16. Davies MG, Marks R, Dykes PJ, et al.: Epidermal abnormalities in Refsum's disease. *Br J Dermatol* 1977;97:401–406.
17. Elias PM, Williams ML: Neutral lipid-storage disease with ichthyosis. *Arch Dermatol* 1985;121:1000–1008.
18. Caputo R, Vanotti P, Bertani E: Netherton's syndrome in two adult brothers. *Arch Dermatol* 1984;120:220–222.
19. Hersle K: Netherton's disease and ichthyosis linearis circumflexa. *Acta Dermatol Venereol (Stockh)* 1972;52:298–302.
20. Netherton EW: A unique case of trichorrhexis nodosa—"bamboo hairs." *Arch Dermatol* 1958;78:483–487.
21. Goldsmith LA: Molecular biology and molecular pathology of a newly described molecular disease—Tyrosinemia II (the Richner-Hanhart syndrome). *Exp Cell Biol* 1978;46:96–113.
22. Klaus S, Weinstein GD: Localized epidermolytic hyperkeratosis. *Arch Dermatol* 1970;101:272–275.
23. Fritsch P, Honigsmann H, Jaschke E; Epidermolytic hereditary palmoplantar keratoderma. *Br J Dermatol* 1978;99:561–568.
24. Buchanan RN: Keratosis punctata palmaris et plantaris. *Arch Dermatol* 1963;88:644–650.
25. Nicollier M, Massengo T, Rémy-Martin J-P, et al.: Free fatty acids and fatty acids of triacylglycerols in normal and hyperkeratotic human stratum corneum. *J Invest Dermatol* 1986;87:68–71.
26. Elias PM: Epidermal lipids, barrier function and desquamation. *J Invest Dermatol* 1983;80(suppl):44s–49s.
27. Dyrszka H, Sanghavi B, Peddamatham K, et al.: Esophageal involvement in acanthosis nigricans. *NY State J Med* 1984;84:256–258.
28. Tasjian D, Jarratt M: Familial acanthois nigricans. *Arch Dermatol* 1984;120:1351–1354.
29. Stuart CA, Peters EJ, Prince MJ, et al.: Insulin resistance with acanthosis nigricans: The roles of obesity and androgen excess. *Metabolism* 1986;35:197–205.
30. Harrison LC, Dean B, Peloso I, et al.: Insulin resistance, acanthosis nigricans and polycystic ovaries associated with a circulating inhibitor of postbinding insulin action. *J Clin Endocrinol Metab* 1985;60:1047–1052.
31. Papa C: Niacinamide and acanthosis nigricans. *Arch Dermatol* 1984;120:1281.
32. Brown J, Winkelmann RK: Acanthosis nigricans: A study of 90 cases. *Medicine (Baltimore)* 1986;47:33–51.
33. Hamilton D, Tavafoghi V, Shafer JC Jr, et al.: Confluent and reticulated papillomatosis of Gougerot and Carteaud. *J Am Acad Dermatol* 1980;2:401–410.
34. Stacpoole PW: The glucagonoma syndrome: Clinical features, diagnosis, treatment. *Endocr Rev* 1981;2:347–361.
35. Bloom SR, Polak JM: Glucagonoma syndrome. *Am J Med 82* 1987;82(5B):25–35.
36. Skouge JW, Farmer ER: Papulosquamous eruption with weight loss. *Arch Dermatol* 1985;121:399–404.
37. Parker CM, Hanke CW, Madura JA, et al.: Glucagonoma syndrome: Case report and literature review. *J Dermatol Surg Oncol* 1984;10:884–889.
38. Vandersteen PR, Scheithauer BW: Glucagonoma syndrome. *J Am Acad Dermatol* 1985;12:1032–1039.
39. Wilkinson DS. L'érythème migrateur nécrolytique: Syndrome du glucagonome. *Ann Med Intern* 1984;135:654–657.

40. Lederman JS, Sober AJ, Lederman GS: Immunosuppression a cause of porokeratosis? *J Am Acad Dermatol* 1985;13:75–79.

41. Johnson ENM: Porokeratosis of Mibelli with squamous cell carcinoma. *Br J Dermatol* 1958;70:381.

42. Lozinski Az, Fisher BK, Walter JB, et al.: Metastatic squamous cell carcinoma in linear porokeratosis of Mibelli. *J Am Acad Dermatol* 1987;16:448–451.

43. Shrum JR, Cooper PH, Greer KE, et al.: Squamous cell carcinoma in disseminated superficial actinic porokeratosis. *J Am Acad Dermatol* 1982;6:58–62.

44. Wade TR, Ackerman AB: Cornoid lamellation: A histologic reaction pattern. *Am J Dermatopathol* 1980;2:5–15.

45. Abell E, Read SI: Porokeratotic eccrine ostial and dermal duct naevus. *Br J Dermatol* 1980;103:435–441.

46. Driban Ne Cavicchia JC: Porokeratotic eccrine ostial and dermal duct nevus. *J Cutan Pathol* 1987;14:118–121.

47. Weary PE, Hsu YT, Richardson DR, et al.: Hereditary sclerosing poikiloderma. *Arch Dermatol* 1969;100:413–422.

48. Berg E, Chuang T-Y, Cripps D: Rothmund-Thomson syndrome. *J Am Acad Dermatol* 1987;17:332–338.

49. Person JR, Bishop GF: Is poikiloderma a graft-versus-host–like reaction? *Am J Dermatopathol* 1984;6:71–72.

50. McMillan EM, Wasik R, Everett MA: In situ demonstration of T cell subsets in atrophic parapsoriasis. *J Am Acad Dermatol* 1982;6:32–39.

51. Janis JF, Winkelmann RK: Histopathology of the skin in dermatomyositis. *Arch Dermatol* 1968;97:640–650.

52. Vanderschueren-Lodeweyckx M, Fryn J-P, Van den Berghe H, et al.: Bloom's syndrome. *Am J Dis Child* 1984;138:812–816.

53. Gretzula JC, Hevia O, Weber PJ: Bloom's syndrome. *J Am Acad Dermatol* 1987;17:479–488.

54. Katzenellenbogen I, Laron Z: A contribution to Bloom's syndrome. *Arch Dermatol* 1960;82:609–616.

55. Dicken CH, Dewald G, Gordon H: Sister chromatid exchanges in Bloom's syndrome. *Arch Dermatol* 1978;114:755–760.

CHAPTER 32
Disorders of Collagen

Sharon R. Hymes

Collagen is the most abundant structural protein of connective tissue, accounting for greater than 70% of its dry weight.[1] The collagens of the dermis include types I,α1(I), III, IV, and V, as well as type I and III procollagen.[2,3] Type I collagen accounts for approximately 80% to 85% of mature dermal collagen and is the principal constituent of the large-diameter fibrils in the reticular dermis.[3,4] Type III collagen constitutes about 10% to 15% of the remaining collagen and tends to form the small-diameter fibrils of the smaller fiber bundles.[3,4] Together with the dermal elastic fibers, collagen fibrils are largely responsible for the structural integrity, as well as the physiologic and functional properties, of normal dermis. Not surprisingly, alterations in collagen directly modify these properties, although not necessarily in a disease-specific manner.

Exogenous factors, altered gene products, and metabolic abnormalities interfere with the complex interactions between collagen and its matrix. The relationship of collagen to the surrounding epithelium, adnexae, and vascular system affects dermal histology. These dermal changes provide an easily accessible window through which collagen pathophysiology may be viewed.

The collagen of the dermis is structurally divided by light microscopy into two relatively distinct regions: the papillary dermis and the reticular dermis. The fine-diameter, loosely woven collagen fibrils of the papillary dermis are distinct from the broader collagen bundles of the reticular dermis. The latter densely interwoven bundles form a "wickerwork" pattern that may become disturbed by a variety of exogenous and endogenous factors.[5] Structural collagen changes resulting in recognizable dermal pathology are the major focus of this chapter.

EHLERS-DANLOS SYNDROME (CUTIS HYPERELASTICA)

Clinical Features
Ehlers-Danlos syndrome is a genetically determined disorder of connective tissue characterized by clinical and histologic heterogenity. At least 11 subtypes, linked loosely together by similarity of clinical findings, manifest a variety of genetic, ultrastructural, and biochemical abnormalities. Precise classification is difficult because of the relatively small number of patients with identifiable biochemical or ultrastructural defects, as well as the marked clinical diversity of the disease. The skin, the gastrointestinal tract, and the cardiovascular and musculoskeletal systems are the principal sites of involvement.

Clinical and histologic skin alterations may be useful in determining the subtype and the prognosis of the disease. Classically, the skin is characterized by redundancy, velvety soft texture, and excessive fragility. Lacerations tend to heal slowly and form "cigarette paper–like" scars. Firm round nodules and blue-gray spongy tumors (molluscoid pseudotumors) may appear at body sites that are subject to traumatic injury. Hernias, varicose veins, distinctive facies, and easy bruisability are notable in some patients.

Histologic Features
The histologic changes of Ehlers-Danlos syndrome are often nonspecific and inconsistent. In most cases, light microscopy cannot be used to distinguish between the biopsies of affected and nonaffected individuals.[6] Alterations, if present, are usually confined to the mid- and deep dermis with papillary dermal sparing. Dermal thinning, decreased density and number of collagen fibrils, disturbances of the "wickerwork" pattern, and a disproportional increase in the number of elastic fibers have been noted[6,7] (Fig. 32–1). Pseudotumors, when present, consist of fat and mucoid material in fibrous capsules, along with variable areas of calcification.[8]

Electron Microscopy
Electron microscopy is a sensitive, but relatively nonspecific, tool used to detect collagen abnormalities. Although it is intriguing to postulate a causal relationship between ultramicroscopic collagen alterations in packing, size, and organization and a specific biochemical defect or genetic disorder, no direct correlation exists. Table 32–1 summarizes the pathogenesis and the clinical and the histologic features of Ehlers-Danlos syndrome. Changes

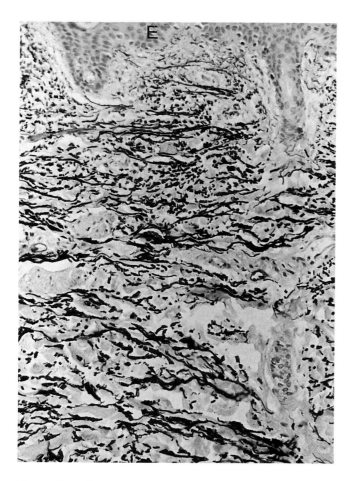

Figure 32–1. Ehlers-Danlos syndrome. Note the disproportional increase in elastic tissue. This is an inconsistent finding in biopsies from affected patients. E = epidermis. (Acid orcein, ×175.)

in the size, orientation, morphology, and integration of the collagen fibers are frequently seen.[9–13] So-called "collagen flowers" are large-diameter, loosely associated fibrils named for their cross-sectional appearance. These are present in a large variety of connective tissue disorders[3] (Fig. 32–2). Dilatation of regions of the rough endoplasmic reticulum appears to be helpful in distinguishing Ehlers-Danlos syndrome type IV from the other subtypes.[14]

ATROPHODERMA

Clinical Features

Based largely on the observations of Pasini, Pierini, and Vivoli, Canizares described an insidious and usually asymptomatic form of cutaneous atrophy named the idiopathic atrophoderma of Pasini and Pierini.[15–17] This distinctive clinical syndrome is characterized by sharply but irregularly demarcated areas of dermal atrophy that create solitary or confluent areas reminiscent of "inverted plateaus" or "cliff drops." Fully developed lesions tend to be a bluish violet to slate gray or brown. Idiopathic atrophoderma of Pasini and Pierini is most commonly present on the trunk and proximal extremities in a symmetric or occasionally a zosteri-

form pattern, with the long axis parallel to cleavage lines. Although the presence of telangectasia is not characteristic, large blood vessels may be seen through the atrophic dermis. Dermal herniation, as seen in macular atrophy (anetoderma), is not characteristic of atrophoderma. Sclerodermatous changes may occur within the atrophic plaques, suggesting a clinical and morphologic relation to morphea in some cases.[18] Dermal atrophy, when present primarily around hair follicles, suggests the diagnosis of follicular atrophoderma. The constellation of this finding in association with basal cell carcinomas, hypotrichosis, and hypohidrosis is characteristic of the Bazex syndrome.[19]

Histologic Features

Comparisons between normal and affected skin are imperative when diagnosing atrophoderma. Ideally, a full-thickness, elliptical excisional biopsy that passes through both normal and atrophic skin should be obtained. Alternately, symmetric biopsies of affected and nonaffected skin from comparable body sites are helpful. The affected dermis may be 25% to 75% thinner than nonaffected skin[17,18,20] (Fig. 32–3). Apart from the occasional finding of atrophy, the epidermis appears normal with little or no inflammatory or pigmentary change.[21] Early in the disease course, the collagen may exhibit some thickening and mild mononuclear perivascular infiltration.[22] Morphea-like changes characterized by edema, homogenization, and sclerosis may be present, but collagen degradation is not a feature.[17] Because morphea and atrophoderma may share common histologic features, their classification as independent entities has been challenged.[23]

The elastic tissue is usually normal, although some cases showing fragmented, shortened, rarefied, or decreased fibers have been reported.[21–23] When present, these changes are located in the deep dermis and seem to be influenced by the degree of dermal edema. The elastic changes return to normal when the edema subsides.[21–23]

The histologic changes of follicular atrophoderma are variable. Disfigured or underdeveloped follicular units have been noted,[24] as has an absence of follicular units below the level of the sebaceous glands.[25] The pilosebaceous units may appear normal, or there may be flattening of the epidermis at the base of the pit.[26] Epidermal thinning, absence of rete ridges, diminution of skin appendages, and epidermal proliferation of the follicular lining have also been reported. An inflammatory infiltrate is inconstantly present.[27] Ultrastructurally, abnormal melanosome aggregates in epithelial cells and a paucity of half-desmosomes in some areas has been reported.[24]

FOCAL DERMAL HYPOPLASIA (GOLTZ SYNDROME)

Clinical Features

Focal dermal hypoplasia is a multisystem disease characterized by both ectodermal and mesodermal defects. The cutaneous changes may include the presence of widespread areas of linear or cribriform hypoplasia of the dermis through which fat herniation produces yellowish nodules in a reticular pattern. Ulcers which heal secondarily, are

TABLE 32–1. EHLER-DANLOS SYNDROME

Type	References	Inheritance	Clinical Characteristics	Pathology	Biochemical and Structural Defect
I (gravis)	3,11,12	AD[a] AR	Joint laxity Fragile velvety skin "Cigarette paper-like scars" Aortic dilatation Visceral diverticulosis Premature rupture of fetal membranes	*Light Microscopy* Normal Disorganized collagen with decrease in birefringence and decrease in number of collagen bundles *Electron Microscopy* Collagen flowers Large-diameter fibrils Unraveled collagen fibrils Variability of width and shape of fibrils Unaltered or fragmented elastic	Unknown
II (mitis)	3,12,13	AD	Milder skin and joint changes Aortic dilatation or dissection Varicose veins	*Light Microscopy* Normal Disorganized pattern with decreased birefringence *Electron Microscopy* Collagen flowers Large-diameter fibrils Variable-diameter fibrils Bent, curled, or twisted collagen fibrils Unaltered or fragmented elastic	Unknown
III (benign hypermobility)	3,11–13	AD	Minimal skin changes Marked joint hypermobility Aortic dilatation or dissection	*Light Microscopy* Normal *Electron Microscopy* Collagen flowers Large-diameter fibrils Variable-diameter fibrils Unaltered elastic	Unknown
IV (ecchymotic, arterial, Sack-Barabas)	3,7,9,11,12,14	Four subtypes: AD, AR, ?	Minimal hyperextensibility Normal scar formation, healing Gut perforation Arterial rupture Aortic dilatation or dissection Prominent vascular markings Skin tightness over fingers, face, and ears Easy bruisability	*Light Microscopy* Normal or dermal thinning or disorganized collagen bundles *Electron Microscopy* Small-, variable-, or large-diameter fibrils Unaltered or fragmented elastic Elastic possibly increased in proportion to collagen RER possibly dilated in dermal fibroblasts Lack of cohesion of collagen fibers within bundles	Decreased type III collagen synthesis Abnormal type III collagen metabolism Unstable triple helix
V	3,11–14	X-linked	Similar to type I Easy bruisability Floppy mitral valve	*Light Microscopy* Normal *Electron Microscopy* Collagen flowers Large-diameter fibrils Small-diameter collagen fibrils Bent, curled, or twisted collagen fibrils Unaltered or fragmented elastic	Lysyl oxidase deficiency Unknown

Type		Inheritance	Clinical features	Microscopy	Biochemical defect
VI (ocular–scoliotic)	3,11–14	AR	Ocular rupture Kyphoscoliosis Joint laxity Hyperelastotic skin Premature rupture of fetal membranes	*Light Microscopy* Normal or dermal thinning *Electron Microscopy* Collagen flowers Large- or small-diameter fibrils Bent, curled, or twisted collagen fibrils Unaltered or electron-dense elastic	Lysyl hydroxylase deficiency or other
VII (arthrochalasis multiplex congenita)	3,11,12,14	AR AD ?	Joint laxity, stretchable, velvety skin Congenital hip dislocation	*Light Microscopy* Normal or dermal thinning *Electron Microscopy* Collagen flowers Variable-diameter fibrils Unaltered or small, irregularly stained elastic	Procollagen N peptidase deficiency Structural collagen mutation
VIII (peridontosis type)	3,11–13	AD	Peridontal disease Pretibial scarring No hypermobility	*Light Microscopy* Normal *Electron Microscopy* Variable-diameter fibrils Lack of cohesion of collagen fibers within bundles Bent, curled, or twisted collagen fibrils Unaltered elastic	Unknown
IX	3,11,12,14	X-linked	Joint laxity Moderate skin distensibility Visceral diverticulosis Striae Platelet aggregation defect	*Light Microscopy* Normal *Electron Microscopy* Collagen flowers Large-diameter fibrils Lack of cohesion of collagen fibers within bundles Unaltered elastic	Defective crosslinking Defective copper metabolism Unknown
X (dysfibronemic)	3,11,12	AR	Mild cutaneous changes Defective platelet aggregation in response to collagen	*Light Microscopy* Normal *Electron Microscopy* Collagen flowers	Fibronectin deficiency Functionally abnormal fibronectin
XI	?	?	Familial joint instability syndrome	?	Unknown

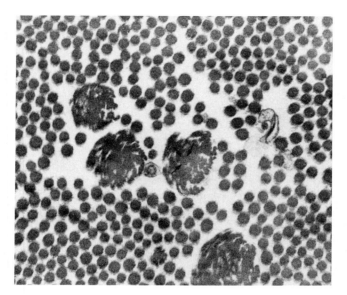

Figure 32–2. Ehlers-Danlos syndrome. Large, lobulated composite collagen fibrils (collagen flowers) are nonspecific electron microscopic findings in some types of Ehlers-Danlos syndrome, as well as in other disorders of connective tissue. A fibril with a normal-appearing diameter is indicated by the arrows. (×27,150). *(From Ref. 3.)*

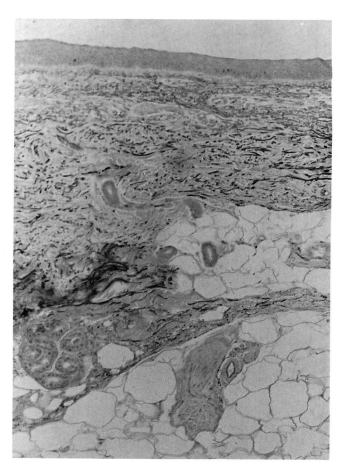

Figure 32–3. Atrophoderma. Dermal thinning may be the only manifestation. Elastic tissue is usually unaltered. (H&E, ×157.)

sometimes present at birth. Periorificial papillomatous lesions, linear or reticular areas of pigment changes, and hypoplasia or aplasia of the nails are prominent features in some affected individuals. Hair, teeth, and ocular and soft tissues may be abnormal, and bone may show the characteristic radiographic changes of osteopathia striata.[28,29] Because more than 90% of affected individuals are female, focal dermal hypoplasia is thought to be genetically transmitted as an X-linked dominant trait and to result in high intrauterine mortality of hemizygous males.[29]

Histologic Features

The predominant pathology is dermal with epidermal sparing. Affected areas show marked dermal thinning and morphologically abnormal collagen that appears to be arranged in thin nonbundled fibers.[28–30] Subcutaneous fat may extend upward through the dermis and encroach on the epidermis, which is separated from fat only by a thin layer of reticular fibers.[28] Figure 32–4 demonstrates the extreme dermal attenuation that may be characteristic.

The remaining collagen contains small but morphologically normal ultrastructural fibers. The fibroblasts may be normal in appearance or may show a decrease in number of intracellular organelles.[28] Phase contrast microscopy of affected skin has demonstrated the presence of abnormal vacuoles within the granular cytoplasm of fibroblasts.[31] Incomplete collagen fibers may also be predominant. Herniated fat contains multilocular fat cells consisting of young adipocytes, suggesting that active adipose proliferation rather than connective tissue involution is important in pathogenesis.[32] Clinical correlation is helpful in distinguishing focal dermal hypoplasia from nevus lipomatosus superficialis.[2]

The molecular basis of the connective tissue abnormality is unknown. Skin fibroblasts from affected areas do show

abnormal growth patterns characterized by long mean doubling time. This is suggestive of an abnormality in growth kinetics rather than an abnormality in the synthetic capacity of the fibroblasts.[31] The same abnormal growth is not demonstrable in the normal skin of affected individuals.

ACTINIC ELASTOSIS

Clinical Features

Chronic exposure to sunlight over many years produces a well-recognized clinical spectrum of cutaneous change in susceptible individuals. Yellowish, leathery, dry, atrophic, and telangiectatic skin is especially prominent in the exposed skin of the head, neck, and extremities. Pigmentary changes and loss of elasticity resulting in skin laxity are common. Although aging skin produces some overlapping clinical features, the pathogenesis of actinic changes and the pathogenesis of aging changes are clinically, histologically, and pathophysiologically quite distinct.[33]

Histologic Features

Epidermal atrophy is variably present but the predominant changes are dermal. In the papillary dermis, a thin band of normal-appearing collagen usually remains. Early on, there is proliferation of normal or slightly thickened

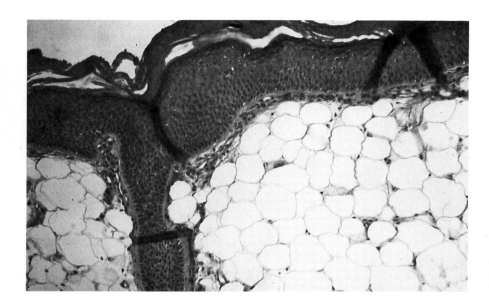

Figure 32–4. Focal dermal hypoplasia. Marked dermal thinning is present. The subcutaneous fat is encroaching upon the epidermis, separated only by a few fibrous strands. (*Courtesy of Dr. Robert Goltz.*)

elastic fibers in the papillary and superficial reticular dermis. Later, a basophilic and amorphous or granular material appears in the upper one third of the dermis under the few remaining normal collagen strands. This is referred to as elastotic material or solar elastosis. The elastic fibers in the papillary and superficial reticular dermis are increased and have a thick and tangled appearance in cases of severe actinic damage.[33] In contrast, aged and actinically protected skin demonstrates a slow spontaneous degradative process with elastic fragmentation and loss.[34,35] The compact appearance of both the collagen and elastic may result from the loss of ground substance (Fig. 32–5).

The derivation of the actinic, elastotic material remains controversial. Its staining characteristics are very similar to those of elastic tissue, hence its name. Biochemical analysis has shown that the elastotic material has an amino acid composition similar to that of elastin, with a hydroxyproline and proline content lower than that of collagen.[36] Recently, indirect immunofluorescence has demonstrated the material to consist primarily of elastin, microfibrillar proteins, fribronectin, and a lesser degree of interstitial collagens.[37]

The role of collagen degradation in the formation of elastotic material continues to be debated.[38–40] Fibroblasts have been shown to produce elastin after chronic ultraviolet exposure. This abnormal material is incorporated into microfibril dense zones after fiber assembly.[33] Close spatial contact between elastotic material and active fibroblasts supports the notion that this material is a newly sythesized

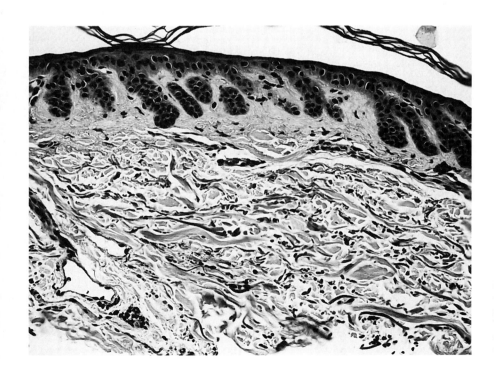

Figure 32–5. Solar elastosis. Thickened and tangled elastic fibers, as well as amorphous granular material, are present in the dermis. The overlying epidermis shows elongation of the rete and hyperpigmentation of a lentigo. (H&E, ×210.)

product rather than the result of collagen or elastic tissue breakdown.[39]

SCAR: HYPERTROPHIC AND KELOIDAL

Clinical Features

Keloidal and hypertrophic scars generally appear within a year at sites of local surgery or trauma. Although some patients remain asymptomatic, others complain of pruritis, tenderness, or pain. Keloids tend to persist or even grow and ultimately may extend far beyond the site of the original injury. Hypertrophic scars remain circumscribed and tend to flatten with time. The tendency to form keloids may be related to genetic and endocrinologic factors, as well as to skin tension lines and to body site of injury.[41,42]

Histologic Features

The epidermis is either normal or slightly flattened with adnexal displacement secondary to the fibrous proliferation. The wound healing sequences followed by normal, hypertrophic, and keloidal scars are largely identical, and the morphologic differences are the result of differences in fibroplasia, amount of tissue present, and time frame.[43]

Early on, all scars show prominent vasculature, inflammation, myxoid stroma, and fibroblasts. Normal mature scars are characterized by an ultimate decrease in the number of fibroblasts and an increase in orderly arranged, mature collagen.[42–44] Both keloidal and hypertrophic scars histologically and biochemically demonstrate an abnormally persistent accumulation of extracellular connective tissue matrix consisting predominantly of collagen.[42] As opposed to the profile of normal dermal collagen, an increase is noted in type III collagen, soluble collagen, and immature collagen, particularly in early lesions. Proteoglycan content, mostly chondroitin 4-sulfate, and water are increased.[42,45] Collagen degradation may be abnormal, and increases in collagenase, α_1-antitrypsins, and β_2-macroglobulin are detectable. Collagenase is usually inhibited by these substances.[42,46]

The end result of these changes is the characteristic morphologic picture of dermal nodules oriented in random whorls and bundles of hyalinized collagen fibers. Both keloids and hypertrophic scars are vascular and cellular. Fibroblasts, mast cells, and plasma cells are present in increased numbers. In the case of hypertrophic scars and mature normal scars, the number of fibroblasts and capillaries slowly decreases by the fifth week and the collagen bundles eventually are oriented parallel to the surface of the skin.[42,44] This arrangement is less commonly seen in the well-developed keloid, which exhibits persistent randomly oriented nodules. Figures 32–6 to 32–8 compare keloidal, hypertrophic, and normal scars with respect to histology.

Electron Microscopy

Electron microscopy confirms the randomly oriented arrangement of collagen bundles in keloid scars and the tendency of the collagen bundles to lie parallel to the surface in hypertrophic scars.[47] The keloidal ground substance is increased and has a fibrillar appearance. Early keloids and hypertrophic scars contain many myofibroblasts.[48] These are stimulated fibroblastic cells that demonstrate functional and structural properties of smooth muscle. Although these may be seen in any immature scar, few, if any are present in mature normal scars.[49]

CHRONIC RADIATION DERMATITIS

Clinical Features

Chronic tissue damage following the use of x-ray was noted as early as 1909.[50] Enthusiasm for the use of therapeutic radiation in the treatment of benign disorders has subsequently waned considerably. Acute cutaneous radiation injury produces erythema, pain, and ulceration. Radiation-induced connective tissue injury manifests months to years after the initial insult, perhaps because of its slower rate of proliferation.[51] The insidious clinical onset of hair loss, pigmentary changes, atrophy, and telangiectasia heralds chronic radiation damage. Thickened and fibrotic skin, as well as the changes of endarteritis obliterans, is characteristic. Hyperkeratosis and ulceration may be complicated by the malignant transformation of epidermal, dermal, and subcutaneous structures.

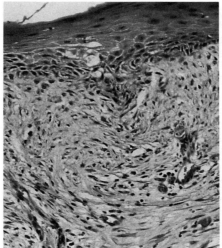
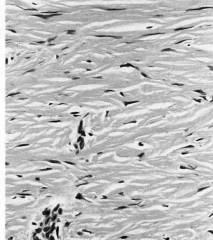

Figure 32–6. Scar. The orderly parallel orientation of the collagen bundles is demonstrated. Hyalinized fibers are not apparent. **A, B,** (H&E, ×160.)

A   **B**

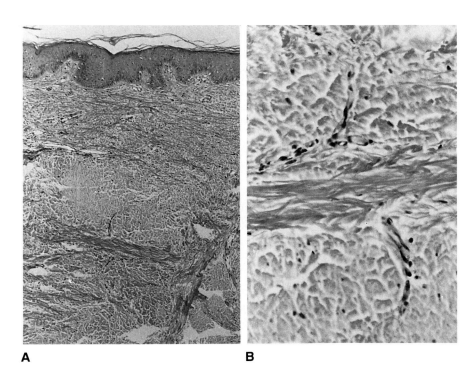

A   **B**

Figure 32–7. Hypertrophic scar. Areas of nodule formation, as well as normally oriented collagen, characterize an evolving hypertrophic scar. (H&E, **A,** ×40; **B,** ×160.)

Histologic Features

Depending on the severity and the depth of the ionizing radiation, both superficial and deep structures are the focus of chronic radiation damage. The epidermis tends to become atrophic with patchy hyperkeratosis. The rete ridges may appear hyperplastic with an elongated downward growth pattern. Atypical and dyskeratotic keratinocytes are easily observed in some cases.[52] Damage to the dermal–epidermal junction produces prominent vacuolar changes as well as pigmentary incontinence. Dermal damage is characterized by dense sclerosis and obliteration of adnexal structures.[52,53] Collagen bundles exhibit variable degrees of hyalinization, edema, and fragmentation, as well as marked thinning and

basophilic degeneration. So-called "radiation fibroblasts" are stellate cells with large hypochromatic, actively dividing nuclei (Fig. 32–9).

Injury to vascular structures results in the dilatation of lymphatic vessels as well as telangiectasia. Subendothelial connective tissue proliferation obliterates the lumen of superficial and deep structures. Subendothelial foam cells may be seen in association with these fibrinoid and thrombotic changes.[52] Megavolt radiation can produce a deep band of fibrosis overlying degenerated skeletal muscle.[52]

Superficial tumors arising in areas of chronic radiation dermatitis are similar to those arising in actinically damaged skin. Basal cell and squamous cell carcinomas predominate,

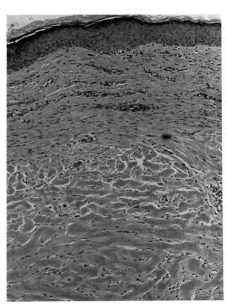

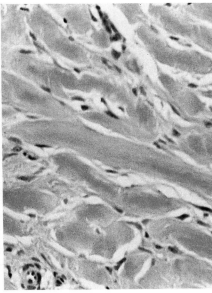

A   **B**

Figure 32–8. Keloidal scar. The collagen is hyalinized, nodular, and disordered. (H&E, **A,** ×40; **B,** ×160.)

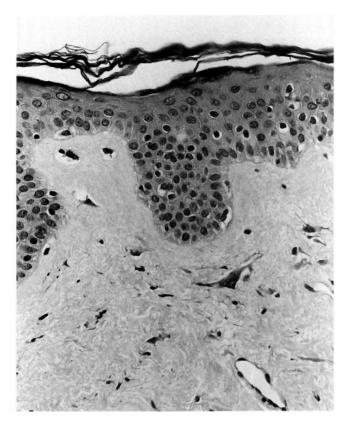

Figure 32–9. Chronic radiation dermatitis. Dermal sclerosis, vascular ectasia, and stellate fibroblasts are evident in this biopsy specimen. (H&E, ×175.)

but mesenchymal, adnexal, and melanocytic tumors also occur with increased frequency.

Electron Microscopy

Ultrastructural changes are comparable to those found in actinic elastosis.[54] Normal elastic fibers are replaced entirely, but not necessarily homogeneously, by elastotic fibers. The microfibrillar fringes disappear from the extremities of the elastic fibers, and matrix changes may be prominent. The collagen fibers are decreased in number but not necessarily ultrastructurally altered.

ANGIOFIBROMA

Clinical Features

An angiofibroma is a specific histologic entity that describes a number of distinct clinical lesions. To some authors, the fibrous papule of the nose and face, adenoma sebaceum, pearly penile papules, oral fibromas, and some perifollicular fibromas are all examples of angiofibromas.[55] Others believe that some of these entities have distinguishing histologic features.[56–59] Further study using sophisticated equipment will likely settle this controversy in the future. At present, the clinical history is often helpful in distinguishing these fibrovascular lesions.

Histologic Features

Epidermal alterations of acanthosis, hypergranulosis, hyperkeratosis, and thinning are variably present. The rete ridges may be normal or flattened.[55] When melanocytic hyperplasia is prominent in a clinical fibrous papule of the nose, the name *melanocytic angiofibroma* is sometimes used.[57] The proliferation of dermal fibrovascular tissue is the hallmark of all angiofibromas (Fig. 32–10). Delicate fibrosis and vascular or lymphatic ectasis are prominent. Young fibrous

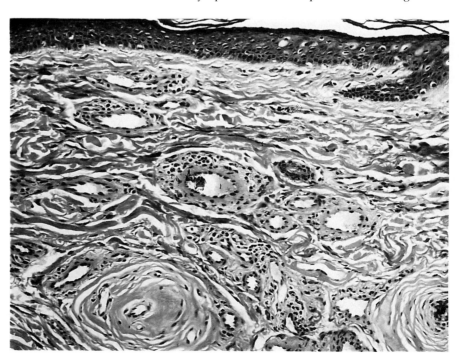

Figure 32–10. Angiofibroma. The hallmark of this tumor is the proliferation of dermal fibrovascular tissue. (H&E, ×180.)

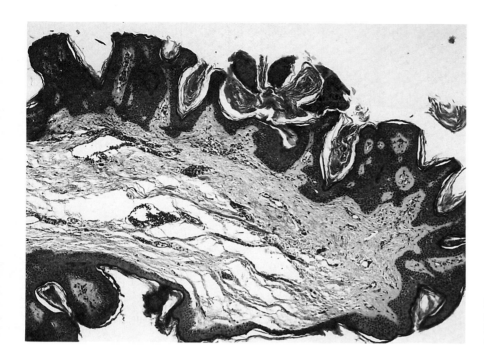

Figure 32–11. Fibroepithelial polyp. Papillomatosis, loose arrangement of collagen fibers, and scarcity of adnexal structures are evident. (H&E, ×40.)

papules exhibit a subepidermal pale staining zone and coarse upper dermal collagen bundles.[55] Concentric perivascular fibrosis is seen in some facial lesions, but not in acral angiofibromas, pearly penile papules, or oral fibromas. Perifollicular fibromas particularly manifest this finding, and are thought to be a distinct histologic entity by some authors.[56]

Angiofibromas demonstrate little or no elastic tissue.[55] There is an increase in the number of histiocytic and mast cells. The presence of large, occasionally multinucleate stellate-appearing cells is quite characteristic. They may demonstrate prominent cytoplasm and granular inclusions. Because of their similarity to nevus cells, fibrous papules have long been thought to represent involuting nevi.[58] Recent electron microscopic data points to their origin as probably fibrohistiocytic instead.[59,60]

FIBROEPITHELIAL POLYP

Clinical Features
Also termed acrochordons, skin tags, and fibromas, fibroepithelial polyps are flesh-colored benign growths, often multiple and occasionally pedunculated. One of the most common skin lesions in adults, often found around the neck, chest, and intertriginous folds.

Histologic Features
The epidermis shows a variable degree of papillomatosis, hyperplasia, and hyperkeratosis. Loose collagen fibers and prominent capillaries are common. Adnexal structures are either absent or reduced in number. Horn cysts are occasionally seen. Figure 32–11 illustrates a typical fibroepithelial polyp.

When fat cells are superficially present in the dermis,

the diagnosis of nevus lipomatosus superficialis should be considered. The presence of nevus cells suggests a preexisting nevoid lesion, perhaps in a stage of regression.

Acknowledgments

My thanks to Dr. Carmen Espinoza, Dr. Evan Farmer, and Dr. Antoinette Hood for their photographic assistance, and to Dr. Karen Holbrook for her valuable input into the Ehlers-Danlos syndrome.

REFERENCES

1. Grant ME, Prockop DJ: The biosynthesis of collagen. *N Engl J Med* 1972;286:194–199, 242–249, 291–300.
2. Uitto J, Santa Cruz DJ, Eisen AZ: Connective tissue nevi of the skin. *J Am Acad Dermatol* 1980;3:441–461.
3. Holbrook KA, Byers PH: Diseases of the extracellular matrix. Structural alterations of the collagen fibrils in skin, in *Connective Tissue Disease: Molecular Pathology of the Extracellular Matrix.* New York/Basel, Marcel Dekker, 1987, p 104.
4. Epstein EH Jr: α_1, (III)1$_3$ Human skin collagen. *J Biol Chem* 1974;249:3225–3231.
5. Jansen LH: The structure of the connective tissue, an explanation of the symptoms of the Ehlers-Danlos syndrome. *Dermatologica* 1955;110:108–120.
6. Sulica VI, Cooper PH, Pope FM, et al.: Cutaneous histologic features in Ehlers-Danlos Syndrome. *Arch Dermatol* 1979; 115:40–42.
7. Byers PH, Holbrook KA, McGillivray B, et al.: Clinical and ultrastructural heterogeneity of type IV Ehlers-Danlos syndrome. *Hum Genet* 1979;47:141–150.
8. Wechsler HL, Fisher ER: Ehlers-Danlos syndrome. Pathologic, histochemical and electron microscopic observations. *Arch Pathol* 1964;77:613–619.

9. Holbrook KA, Byers PH, Pinnell SR: The structure and function of dermal connective tissue in normal individuals and patients with inherited connective tissue disorders. *Scanning Electron Microsc IV* 1982:1731–1744.

10. Holbrook KA, Byers PH: Structural abnormalities in the dermal collagen and elastic matrix from the skin of patients with inherited connective tissue disorders. *J Invest Dermatol* 1982;9:7s–16s.

11. McKusick VA: *Heritable Disorders of Connective Tissues.* St Louis, Mo, CV Mosby, 1986.

12. Kobayasi T, Oguchi M, Asboe-Hansen G: Dermal changes in Ehlers-Danlos syndrome. *Clin Genet* 1984;25:477–484.

13. Prockop DJ, Kivirikko KI: Heritable diseases of collagen. *N Engl J Med* 1984;376–386.

14. Holbrook KA, Byers PH: Ultrastructural characteristics of the skin in a form of the Ehlers-Danlos syndrome type IV. Storage in rough endoplasmic reticulum. *Lab Invest* 1981;44:342–350.

15. Pasini A: Atrofodermia idiopatica progressiva. *G Ital Dermatol Sifol* 1923;58:785.

16. Pierini LE, Vivoli D: Atrofodermia idiopatica progressiva (Pasini). *G Ital Dermatol Sifol* 1936;77:403.

17. Canizares O, Sachs PM, Jaimovich L, et al.: Idiopathic atrophoderma of Pasini and Pierini. *Arch Dermatol* 1948;77:142–160.

18. Pullara TJ, Lober CW, Fenske NA: Idiopathic atrophoderma of Pasini and Pierini. *Int J Dermatol* 1984;23:643–645.

19. Bazex A, Dupre A, Christol B: Atrophodermie folliculaire proliferations basocellaires et hypotrichose. *Ann Dermatol Syphilol* 1966;93:211–254.

20. Brownstein MH, Rabinowitz AD: The invisible dermatoses. *J Am Acad Dermatol* 1983;8:579–588.

21. Miller RF: Idiopathic atrophoderma. *Arch Dermatol* 1965;92:653–660.

22. Quieroga I, Woscoff A: L'atrophodermie idiopathique progressive (Pasini–Pierini) et le sclerodermie atypique liliacee non induree (Gougerot). *Ann Dermatol Syphilol* 1961;88:507–520.

23. Jablonska S, Szczepanski A: Atrophoderma Pasini–Pierini: Is it an entity? *Dermatologica* 1962;125:226–242.

24. Plosila M, Kilstala, Niemi K-M: The Bazex syndrome: Follicular atrophoderma with multiple basal cell carcinomas, hypotrichosis and hypohidrosis. *Clin Exp Dermatol* 1981;6:31–41.

25. Curth HO: Follicular atrophoderma and pseudopelade associated with chondrodystrophia calcificans congenita. *J Invest Dermatol* 1949;13:233–247.

26. Tasker WG, Mastri AR, Gold AP: Chondrodysplasia calcificans congenita (dysplasia epiphysalis punctata). *Am J Dis Child* 1970;119:122–127.

27. Curth HO: The genetics of follicular atrophoderma. *Arch Dermatol* 1978;114:1479–1483.

28. Goltz RW, Henderson RR, Hitch JM, et al.: Focal dermal hypoplasia syndrome. A review of the literature and report of two cases. *Arch Dermatol* 1970;101:1–11.

29. Hall EH, Terezhalmy GT: Focal dermal hypoplasia syndrome. *J Am Acad Dermatol* 1983;9:443–451.

30. Howell JB: Nevus angiolipomatosus vs focal dermal hypoplasia. *Arch Dermatol* 1965;92:238–248.

31. Uitto J, Bauer EA, Santa Cruz PJ, et al.: Focal dermal hypoplasia. Abnormal growth characteristics of skin fibroblasts in culture. *J Invest Dermatol* 1982;75:170–175.

32. Tsuji T: Focal dermal hypoplasia syndrome. An electron microscopic study of the skin lesions. *J Cutan Pathol* 1982;9:271–281.

33. Braverman IM: Elastic fiber and microvascular abnormalities in aging skin. *Dermatol Clin* 1986;4:391–405.

34. Braverman IM, Fonferko E: Studies in cutaneous aging. 1. The elastic fiber network. *J Invest Dermatol* 1982;78:434–448.

35. Uitto J: Connective tissue biochemistry of the aging dermis. Age-related alteration of collagen and elastin. *Dermatol Clin* 1986;4:433–446.

36. Smith JG, Davidson EA, Clark RD: Dermal elastin in actinic elastosis and pseudoxanthoma elasticum. *Nature* 1962;195:716–717.

37. Chen VL, Fleischmajer R, Schwartz E, et al.: Immunochemistry of elastotic material in sun-damaged skin. *J Invest Dermatol* 1986;87:334–337.

38. Mitchell RE: Chronic solar elastosis. A light and electron microscopic study of the dermis. *J Invest Dermatol* 1967;48:203–220.

39. Nurenberger F, Schober E, Marsch W Ch, et al.: Actinic elastosis in black skin. *Arch Dermatol Res* 1978;262:7–14.

40. Danielson L, Kobayesi T: Degradation of dermal elastic fibers in relation to age and light exposure. *Acta Derm Venereol* 1972;52:1–10.

41. Cosman B, Crikelair GF, Gauler JC, et al.: The surgical treatment of keloids. *Plast Reconstr Surg* 1961;27:33–57.

42. Murray JC, Pollack SV, Pinnell SR: Keloids: a review. *J Am Acad Dermatol* 1981;4:461–470.

43. Mancini RE, Quaife JV: Histogenesis of experimentally produced keloids. *J Invest Dermatol* 1962;38:143–181.

44. Linares HA, Kischer CW, Dobrkovsky M, et al.: The histiotypic organization of the hypertrophic scar in humans. *J Invest Dermatol* 1972;59:323–331.

45. Kischer CW, Shetlar MR: Collagen and mucopolysaccharides in the hypertrophic scar. *Connect Tissue Res* 1974;2:205–213.

46. Milsom JP, Craig RDP: Collagen degradation in cultured keloid and hypertrophic scar tissue. *Br J Dermatol* 89:635–643.

47. Knapp TR, Daniels JR, Kaplan EN: Pathological scar formation. *Am J Pathol* 1977;86:47–63.

48. James WD, Besanceney CD, Odom RB: The ultrastructure of a keloid. *J Am Acad Dermatol* 1980;3:50–57.

49. Baur PS, Larson DL, Stacey TR: The observation of myofibroblasts in hypertrophic scars. *Surg Gynecol Obstet* 1975;141:22–26.

50. Wolbach SB: Pathological histology of chronic X-ray dermatitis and early X-ray carcinoma. *J Med Res* 1909;21:415–449.

51. Rudolph R, Aragahese T, Woodward M: The ultrastructure and etiology of chronic radiotherapy damage in human skin. *Ann Plast Surg* 1982;9:282–292.

52. Hood IC, Young JEM: Late sequelae of superficial irradiation. *Head Neck Surg* 1984;7:65–72.

53. Teloh HA, Masch MC, Wheelock MC: A histopathologic study of radiation injuries of the skin. *Surg Gynecol Obstet* 1950;90:335–348.

54. Ledoux-Corbousier M, Achten G: Elastosis in chronic radiodermatitis: An ultrastructural study. *Br J Dermatol* 1974;91:287–294.

55. Meigel WN, Ackerman AB: Fibrous papule of the face. *Am J Dermatopathol* 1979;1:329–340.

56. Pinkus H: Perifollicular fibromas. Pure periadnexal adventitial tumors. *Am J Dermatopathol* 1979;1:341–342.

57. Reed R: Fibrous papule of the face. Melanocytic angiofibroma. *Am J Dermatopathol* 1979;1:343–344.

58. McGibbon DH, Wilson Jones E: Fibrous papule of the face (nose). Fibrosing nevocytic nevus. *Am J Dermatopathol* 1979;1:345–348.

59. Santa Cruz DJ, Prioleau PG: Fibrous papule of the face. An electron microscopic study of two cases. *Am J Dermatopathol* 1979;1:349–352.

60. Ragaz A, Berezowsky V: Fibrous papule of the face. A study of five cases by electron microscopy. *Am J Dermatopathol* 1979;1:353–355.

CHAPTER 33
Alterations in Elastic Fibers

Ken Hashimoto

One of the three major components of the dermis is elastic fiber. Together with collagen and ground substance, elastic fibers are crucial to maintenance of the integrity and, particularly, the elasticity of the skin. The importance of this element is best seen when its deficiency occurs in such diseases as cutis laxa, macular atrophy, and actinic elastosis. In this chapter, several disorders that involve either loss or structural alteration of elastic fiber are discussed.

CUTIS LAXA

Also called dermatochalasis, generalized elastolysis, and dermatomegaly, cutis laxa may be congenital or acquired and affects both sexes. Autosomal dominant, recessive, and X-linked forms have been observed.

Clinical Features

In congenital cases, growth retardation, multiple dislocations of joints, particularly hip joints, and laxity of joint ligaments may be observed[1-5] in addition to the typical skin appearance. Skin is markedly redundant, forming large folds that droop down; the appearance is that of a baby wearing an oversized cape. The patient often develops an elderly facies. The acquired type may be induced by various drugs[6,7] or associated with multiple myeloma.[8-9] It shows similar skin changes. In both types of cutis laxa, inguinal and hiatus hernia, diverticula of the gastrointestinal tract and bladder, rectal prolapse, pulmonary emphysema, cardiovascular abnormalities, and other symptoms related to elastic and collagen fiber abnormalities are often encountered. Localized acquired lesions affecting axillary skin have been reported under the name of *progressive, atrophying, chronic granulomatous dermohypodermitis*.[10] Recently, Fisher et al[11] reported a case of acral localized acquired cutis laxa in which ventral skin of fingers and toes became edematous and then redundant. Neutrofils are attached to elastic fibers which eventually destroyed them.

Histologic Features

The elastic fiber abnormalities vary from marked diminution, fragmentation, and dustlike granulation to complete absence, and also vary from one lesion to another. Severely affected, folded, or wrinkled skin will give the diagnostic findings when stained with Verhoeff or orcein and Giemsa. Fragmented, short, curled elastic fibers are seen in early or mildly affected lesions (Fig. 33–1A). These may show tapered ends, an irregular contour, aggregation, and nodular and thin portions. Others are simply dotlike or dustlike specks. In some lesions, normal-sized and normal-shaped elastic fibers are found but they tend to aggregate or entangle. In severely affected areas, there are no normal elastic fibers (Fig. 33–1B). Inflammatory infiltrate may be present and increased acid mucopolysaccharides could be stained; these may be secondary phenomena.

Electron Microscopy

A longitudinal section of the normal elastic fiber reveals medium electron-dense layers or fascicles (skeleton fibrils) separated by very electron-dense septae, giving rise to zebra skin pattern[7] (Fig. 33–2). In cross section, electron-dense layers are seen (embedded in a medium electron-dense background, giving a leopard skin pattern[7] (Fig. 33–2). The typical zebra skin or leopard skin pattern of normal dermal elastic fiber is not observed in cutis laxa because skeleton fibrils are not tightly bound and elastin deposition is deficient in many fibers; on the other hand, microfibrils are normal[7] (Fig. 33–3A). In some cases, however, the opposite is true.[13] In the vicinity of these abnormal fibers are found electron-dense amorphous or granular aggregations that may represent abnormal elastin (Fig. 33–3B). Elastin is often dissociated from microfibrils. Pure aggregation of microfibrils is also observed in some cases.[12] The histogenesis of cutis laxa is not clear but more synthetic than degenerative abnormalities seem to be involved.[12]

Collagen abnormalities[12] are ultrastructually nonspecific and include broad, curved, or bent fibers which may show frayed ends (Fig. 33–3B).

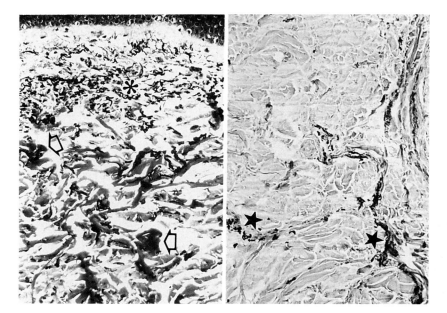

Figure 33–1. Cutis laxa. **A.** Fibers are fragmented but not diminished in the upper dermis (∗). They are irregularly shaped, aggregated, granular, or dustlike in the middermis (arrows). **B.** There are almost no elastic fibers except those that are aggregated or clumped irregularly (∗); these may be mistaken as dirt or staining artifacts. (**A, B,** Verhoeff stain; ×65.)

PSEUDOXANTHOMA ELASTICUM

The mode of inheritance of pseudoxanthoma elasticum is autosomal recessive or dominant. The pattern of inheritance and the severity of the disease vary widely.

Clinical Features

In the second or third decade of life, patients with pseudoxanthoma elasticum develop yellowish plaques with pebbly surfaces in flexural areas of the body, such as antecubital fossa, groin, axillae, and particularly the lateral sides of the neck. The lower abdomen may be diffusely affected in severe cases. Those areas of the skin subject to flexion and extension are where elastic fibers seem to be damaged most severely. In white skin, the lesions are sometimes confused with actinic elastosis or xanthoma.

Tissues in which elastic fibers constitute a significant component are similarly affected; for example, rupture of Bruch's membrane causes angioid streaks of the ocular fundus. Calcification and degeneration of perivascular elastic fibers causes gastrointestinal bleeding, renal hypertension, anomalies of pulsation, angina pectoris, and intermittent claudication of extremities.

Histologic Features

Hematoxylin and eosin stain reveals numerous short, wavy, or granular substances in the middermis (Fig. 33–4A) which may stain deeply basophilic because of their calcium con-

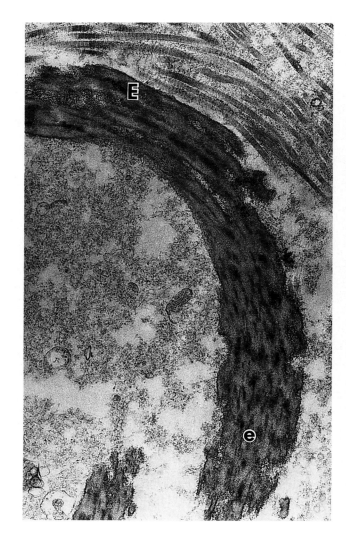

Figure 33–2. Normal elastic fibers are cut longitudinally (E) as well as in cross section (e). In the former, dense septae divide medium-dense skeleton fibrils to produce a zebra skin pattern. In the latter, the dense layers are seen as dots and speckles and produce a leopard skin pattern. (×30,000.)

tent. Papillary dermis shows normal elastic fibers with elastic fiber stain (Fig. 33–4B), probably because the vertically directed fibers in this area are under less mechanical tension when the skin is stretched and, thus, escaped severe damage. The abnormal elastic fibers have been variously described as fragmented, frayed, curled, lumpy, or raveled wool–like. These changes can best be demonstrated with elastic fiber stains (Fig. 33–4B) or calcium stains (Fig. 33–4C).

Electron Microscopy

Some small, young elastic fibers may be spared from degeneration and calcification, albeit they are abnormal (Fig. 33–5). Most of the large fibers show dense calcium deposition or an empty center; only the periphery of these fibers may have elastic fiberlike structures[15] (Fig. 33–5). Several

dense lines may crisscross and calcium apatites that exhibit snow crystal shapes are scattered within the degenerated center (Fig. 33–5). Medium electron-dense materials (ground substance), either amorphous or finely filamentous, are increased in some areas and are embedded in abnormal elastic fibers and collagen fibers in the vicinity.[15] They may represent abnormal elastic fiber microfibrils (elastofibrils) and elastin. Collagen fibers are essentially normal, although broad, curved, or irregularly shaped fibers may be found.

ELASTOSIS PERFORANS SERPIGINOSA

The idiopathic form of elastosis perforans, serpiginosa, typically affects young individuals without any hereditary back-

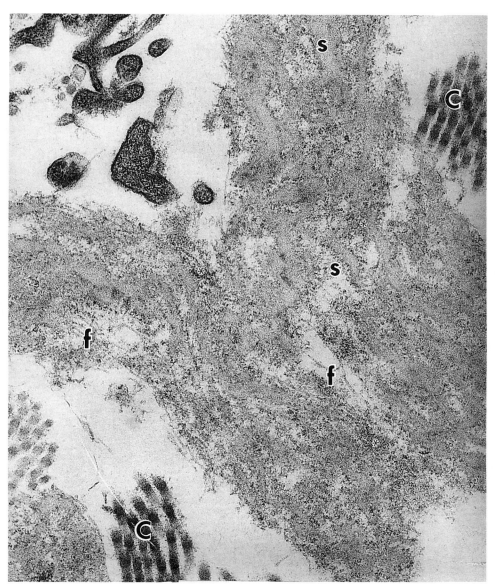

Figure 33–3. A. Cutis laxa, acquired type. Individual skeleton fibrils (s) are only loosely bound and the dense septae (∗) are not longitudinally organized between these skeleton fibrils. Microfibrils (elastofibrils) (f) are apparently normal. Collagen fibers (C) are normal in this field.
(*Continued*)

A

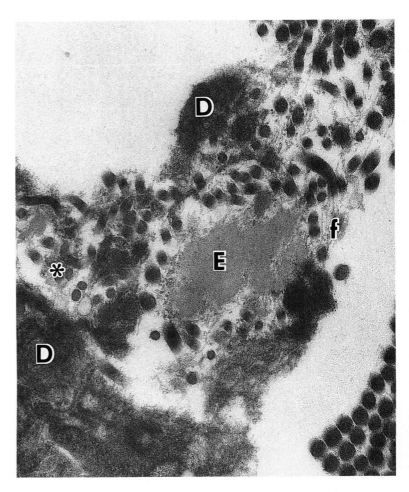

Figure 33–3 (*Continued*) **B.** Cutis laxa, congenital type. A fragment of normal elastic fiber (E) is surrounded by amorphous dense materials (D) in which microfibrils (f) are visible. Some collagen fibers are thick and bent (∗). (**A,** ×50,000; **B,** ×45,900.)

B

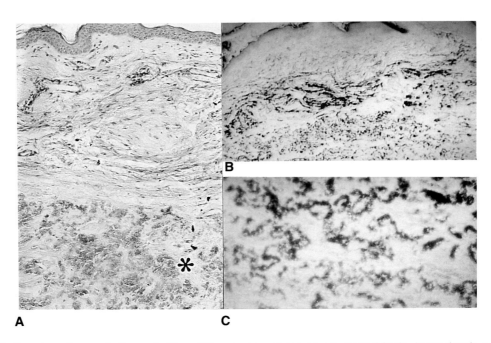

A   **C**

Figure 33–4. Pseudoxanthoma elasticum. **A.** Basophilic granular masses (∗) are located in the lower dermis and represent degenerated and calcified elastic fibers. **B.** Verhoeff stain demonstrates short, broken elastic fibers in the lower dermis as crumbled dark masses and normal elastic fibers in the upper dermis. **C.** Calcium stain (von Kossa stain) delineates abnormal fibers. (**A, B,** ×40; **C,** ×500.)

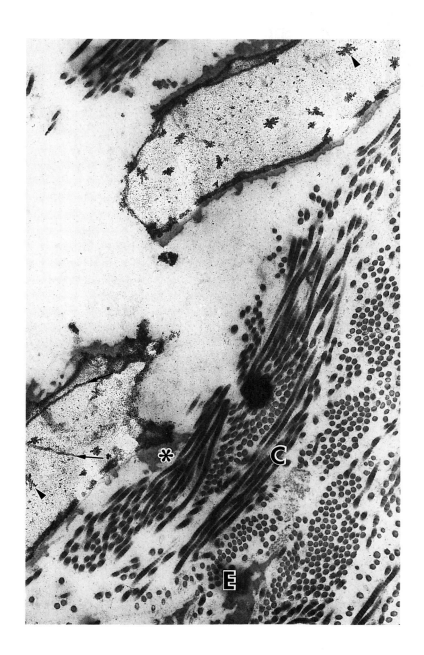

Figure 33–5. Pseudoxanthoma elasticum. Large elastic fibers show an empty center through which electron-dense lines (arrows) crisscross and to which medium electron-dense material (∗), which could be the remnant of a normal elastic fiber, attaches along the periphery. Star-shaped or snow crystal–like calcium apatite (arrowheads) depositions are seen. Small elastic fibers (E) and collagen fibers (C) seem to be normal (×5,000).

ground for the disorder.[16,17] A second type is associated with various connective tissue disorders, such as pseudoxanthoma elasticum, Ehlers-Danlos syndrome, osteogenesis imperfecta, Marfan's syndrome, and Down's syndrome.[17,18] A third variety is related to long-term penicillamine therapy for Wilson's disease or cystinuria.[19–23]

Clinical Features

In the idiopathic type, multiple keratotic papules (3–5 mm) surrounded by slight erythema are arranged in ring or arciform fashion, typically on the nape of the neck of teenage patients.[16,17] Elastosis perforans serpiginosa associated with connective tissue diseases shows similar eruptions, but the preferred sites are near the joints or extremities and the eruptions may be disseminated.[17,18] The penicillamine-induced type also presents annular or circinate papular eruptions.[19,20] It may be accompanied by penicillamine dermopathy[21–23] such as hemorrhage or hemorrhagic blister with subsequent formation of milia, cutis laxa–like lesions, or anetoderma. From these observations, it is seen that elastic fiber degeneration, no matter what the etiology, produces similar skin manifestations.

Histologic Features

In both the idiopathic type and the type associated with connective tissue diseases, an increased number of elastic fibers are observed in the papillary dermis, often aggregated focally[16,17] (Fig. 33–6A). These fibers are thick and stain brightly eosinophilic. The epidermis above these aggregations is often perforated with a canal into which debris of these fibers, keratin, and inflammatory cells are expelled (Fig. 33–6B). These changes are best observed with elastic

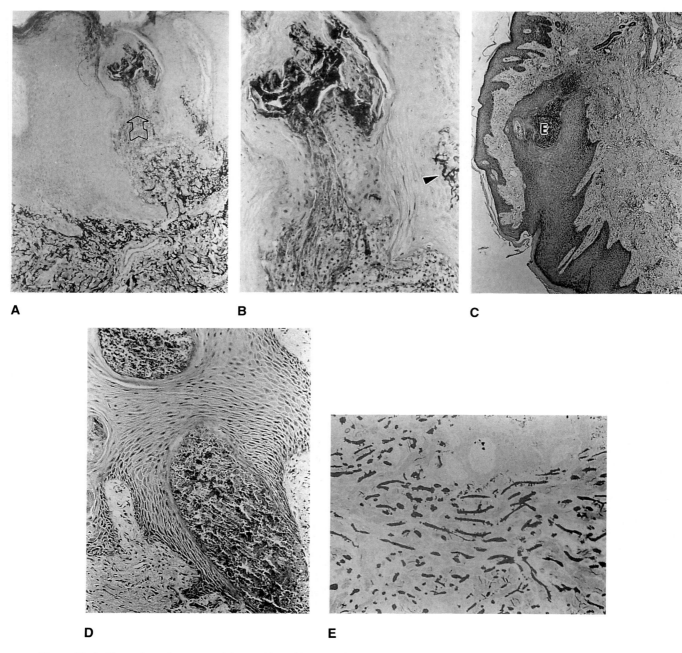

Figure 33–6. Elastosis perforans serpiginosa, idiopathic type. **A.** Verhoeff stain demonstrates an increased number of elastic fibers in the upper dermis and a transepidermal elimination canal (*arrow*) filled with degenerated elastic fiber. **B.** This canal is enlarged to show degenerated elastic fibers, keratin, and debris of inflammatory infiltrates (Verhoeff stain). Elastic fibers, which are abnormally thick for dermal papilla, invade the basal layer of the epidermis (arrowhead). **C.** Penicillamine-induced type of elastosis perforans serpiginosa. An acanthotic rete ridge picks up an aggregate of abnormal elastic fibers (**E**) with its tonglike tips (H&E stain). **D.** The penicillamine-induced lesion shows a perforation canal formed from the debris through the acanthotic rete ridge. Brightly eosinophilic thick elastic fibers and cellular debris are contained in this canal (hematoxylin and eosin stain). **E.** In the penicillamine-induced lesion elastic fibers have laterally projected thorns or dentils and thus resemble a bramble bush (orcein–Giemsa stain) (**A,** ×16; **B, D, E,** ×520; **C,** ×65).

fiber stains (Figs. 33–6A, B). Fine elastic fibers encroach on the basal layer of the epidermis (Fig. 33–6B) and hair follicle; this may represent an active invasive activity of abnormal elastic fibers which may lead to perforation of the epidermis and transepidermal elimination of these ab-

normal fibers.[17] The epidermis becomes acanthotic and hyperkeratotic in response to these activities. In the upper dermis, degenerated elastic fibers are admixed with lymphocytic or occasionally granulomatous infiltrations.

In penicillamine-induced elastosis perforans serpigi-

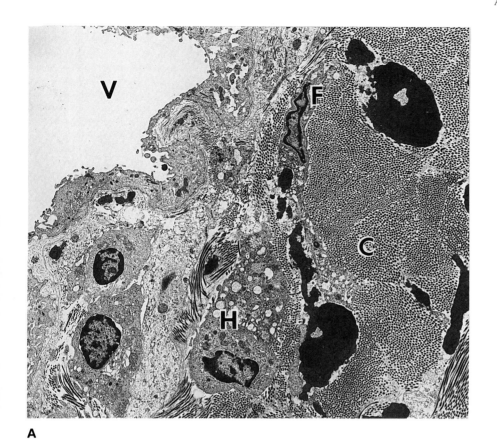

A

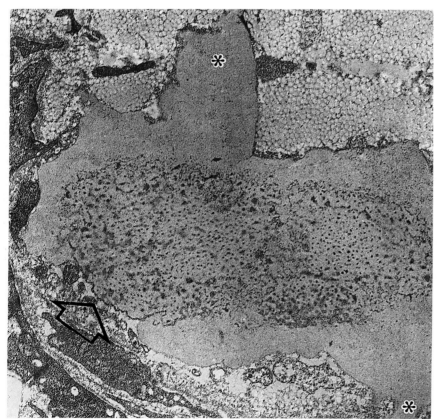

B

Figure 33–7. A. Elastosis perforans serpiginosa, idiopathic type. The increased density of these abnormal elastic fibers masks the internal structures. These fibers are fragmented, irregularly fused, or bizarre-shaped. Collagen fibers (C) are essentially normal. F = fibroblast, H = histiocyte, V = blood vessel. **B.** Elastosis perforans serpiginosa, penicillamine-induced type. The center of this fiber displays the leopard skin pattern (cf. Fig. 33–2), whereas the outer coat is abnormal and projects thornlike process (∗). This coat is incomplete in one area (arrowhead). E = epidermis.
(*Continued*)

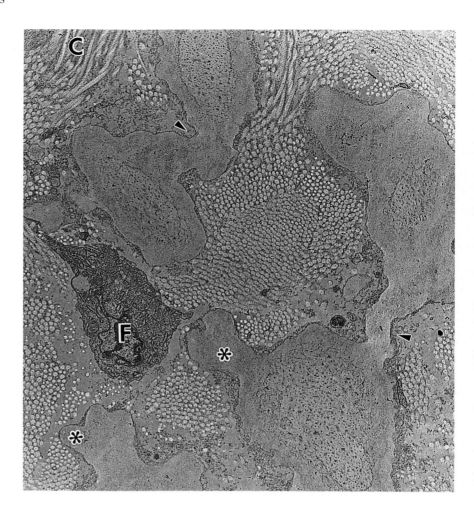

Figure 33–7 (*Continued*) **C.** Elastosis perforans serpiginosa. Lumpy-bumpy fibers of the penicillamine-induced type. The center or core of each cross-sectioned elastic fiber is normal and exhibits a leopard skin pattern (cf. Fig. 33–2). The medium electron-dense outer coat is amorphous and sticks to form projections (∗) or to connect two neighboring fibers like glue (arrowheads). Collagen Fibers (C) are greatly variable in diameter but otherwise essentially normal (**A**, ×2,500; **B**, ×7,700; **C**, ×2,750).

nosa, all of the features just described are seen (Figs. 33–6C, D). Degenerated elastic fibers are characteristically serrated or dentated[19,20] (Fig. 33–6E). The overall configuration of these fibers in aggregation is suggestive of a bramble bush.[20] Elastic fiber stains delineate these changes nicely (Fig. 33–6E). In some areas, the epidermal ridges surround a ball of degenerated elastic fibers as would a pair of tongs around a meatball (Fig. 33–6C); transepidermal canals appear to be formed within these ridges (Fig. 33–6D).

Electron Microscopy
In the idiopathic type, elastic fibers are irregularly shaped, fragmented, and often much more electron dense (Fig. 33–7A) than normal dermal elastic fibers. Disarray of internal structure is also observed. These changes in the abnormal elastic fibers indicate that they have been abnormal from the beginning. Penicillamine-induced elastosis perforans serpiginosa is characterized by peculiar elastic fibers; essentially normal in the center but enveloped by a mantle or coat of medium electron-dense, amorphous substance that may project out like thorns or dentils[19,20] (Fig. 33–7B). This substance may extend to connect with the similar mantle of neighboring abnormal fibers (Fig. 33–7C). These irregularly shaped, sticky elastic fibers are called lumpy-bumpy

elastic fibers.[19] In the penicillamine-induced type, it is therefore assumed that the core part, which may have been produced before the therapy, is normal, and the coat, which may be added after the therapy, is abnormal. The body seems to recognize these fibers as abnormal and reacts to eliminate them through the formation of transepidermal canals.

MACULAR ATROPHY (ANETODERMA)

It is customary to classify macular atrophy into three types: (1) preceded by inflammation (Jadassohn-Pellizzari type), (2) non-inflammatory type (Schweninger-Buzzi type), and (3) penicillamine-induced disease. A hereditary background has not been associated with any of these three types.

Clinical Features
In all three varieties, round or oval, slightly puffed macules are distributed mainly on the trunk. These macules are sharply defined, soft skin that may appear almost like a flaccid bulla. A well-demarcated herniation can be palpated over the macule. The color of the lesion ranges from a bluish gray to yellow.

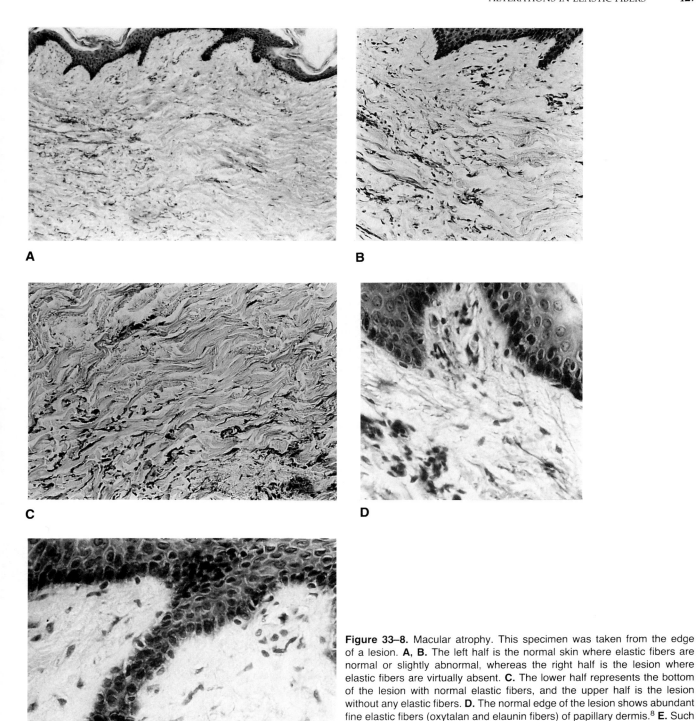

A

B

C

D

E

Figure 33–8. Macular atrophy. This specimen was taken from the edge of a lesion. **A, B.** The left half is the normal skin where elastic fibers are normal or slightly abnormal, whereas the right half is the lesion where elastic fibers are virtually absent. **C.** The lower half represents the bottom of the lesion with normal elastic fibers, and the upper half is the lesion without any elastic fibers. **D.** The normal edge of the lesion shows abundant fine elastic fibers (oxytalan and elaunin fibers) of papillary dermis.[8] **E.** Such fine fibers are absent from the lesion. Verhoeff stain. (**A,** ×33; **B, C,** ×130; **D, E,** ×160.)

Histologic Features

In the early stages of the disease, elastic fibers may be still normal, but in well-developed lesions they are totally absent (Figs. 33–8A, B, C), including the fine fibers in the papillary dermis (Figs. 33–8D, E). These changes are limited to the focal macular lesion; the elastic fibers in the surrounding dermal connective tissue are normal (Figs. 33–8A, B, C, D). Inflammatory cells may surround degenerated elastic fibers.[24] Deposition of C_3 and IgM has been described in the inflammatory type of macular atrophy.[24]

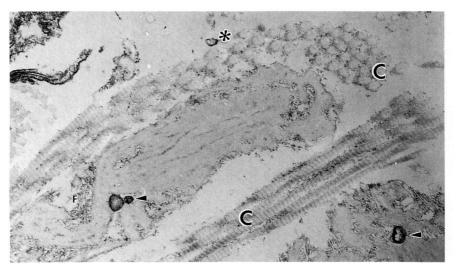

A

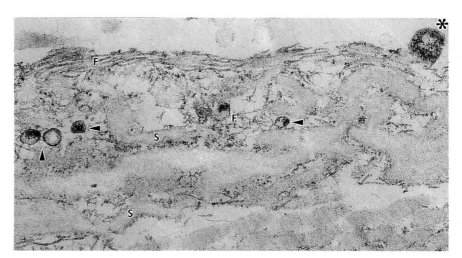

B

Figure 33–9. Macular atrophy. **A.** Two small fragments of elastic fibers are surrounded by collagen bundles (**C**). These fibers contain cellular debris (arrowheads) identical to that found in the vicinity (∗). Elastofibrils (**F**) are increased at the periphery as well as inside these fibers. **B.** The thinning of individual skeleton fibrils (**S**) loosens this elastic fiber and reveals the underlying elastofibrils (**F**). Cellular debris similar to that found outside this fiber (∗) is incorporated into this fiber (arrowheads). (**A,** ×30,000; **B,** ×60,000.)

Electron Microscopy

The affected elastic fibers are mostly small and round rather than stretched fibers (Fig. 33–9A, B). They are often surrounded by macrophages. The ultrastructure of these fibers, including small fragments, is essentially normal, suggesting that on their initial formation, these fibers are normal, and the changes are secondary. Abnormal changes include an increased number of elastofibrils, loosening of skeleton fibrils, incorporation of cellular debris between skeleton fibrils, and admixture of collagen bundles (Figs. 33–9A, B). Dissolution of the elastin might cause thinning of the skeleton fibrils and reveal underlying elastofibrils. Inflammation, immune reactions, and autophagocytosis of elastic fibers may play a role in pathogenesis.

ACTINIC ELASTOSIS

Individuals with a fair complexion develop actinic elastosis on sun-exposed body parts, particularly the face, neck, ex-

tensor surface of forearm, and dorsum of hands. Age may not be directly related as much as complexion and intensity of sun exposure. Blacks and orientals, except outdoor workers, are less prone to sustain actinic damage.

Clinical Features

The lesion is yellowish gray, thin, and finely wrinkled. The uneven elevations and deep furrows observed may be exaggerated to form cutis rhomboidalis nuchae or elastomas. Dilated hair follicles in lesions on the cheeks or periorbital or neck regions may be plugged with comedones (Favre-Racouchot's disease). The yellowish area on the neck may be mistaken for pseudoxanthoma elasticum.

Histologic Features

Elastic fibers in this condition stain grayish blue with hematoxylin and eosin (Fig. 33–10A); in contrast, the normal elastic fiber does not stain with the same method. The amorphous substance and fibrous components are positively stained with elastic fiber stain (Fig. 33–10B) and to-

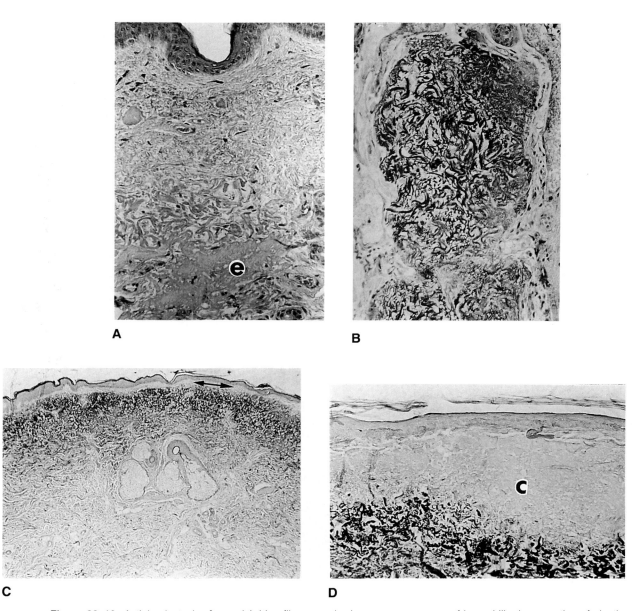

Figure 33–10. Actinic elastosis. **A.** grayish-blue fibrous and a homogeneous mass of basophilic degeneration of elastic fibers (elastoid material) (**E**) are seen. **B.** Fibrous and amorphous components of the elastoid materials are stained by Verhoeff stain. **C.** A band of normal collagen (grenz zone) (arrows) interposes between the epidermis and the Verhoeff stain–positive elastoid materials. **D.** Amorphous component in the upper dermis became unstainable with Verhoeff stain; this type of degeneration represents colloid substance. **(C).** (**A, B,** ×160; **C, D,** ×40.)

gether are referred to as elastotic materials. The collagen in the lesion decreases in proportion to the increase in elastotic material. Eosinophilic collagen fibers are virtually absent in the well-developed lesion, except for a thin layer below the epidermis (grenz zone) (Fig. 33–10C). Elastic fiber stains reveal entangled, thick, wirelike elastic fibers within amorphous ground substance; these are increased in the upper dermis (Fig. 33–10C). In old lesions, fibrous components are diminished and amorphous materials increased. Finally, elastic fiber stains become negative in some areas (Fig. 33–10D). Immunohistochemical methods using antibodies against amyloid P-component[25] and monoclonal anti-

body NKH-1,[26] both of which recognize the microfibril component of elastic fibers (elastofibrils), demonstrate that elastotic materials indeed contain elastofibril or proteins related to it.

Electron Microscopy
In early lesions of actinic elastosis, the electron-dense septal components of elastic fibers are increased in amount and size[23,24] (Fig. 33–11A). In more advanced stages, the electron-dense materials are irregularly aggregated (Fig. 33–11A) rather than arranged in septae between skeleton fibrils; the skeleton fibrils are thus loosened and individually

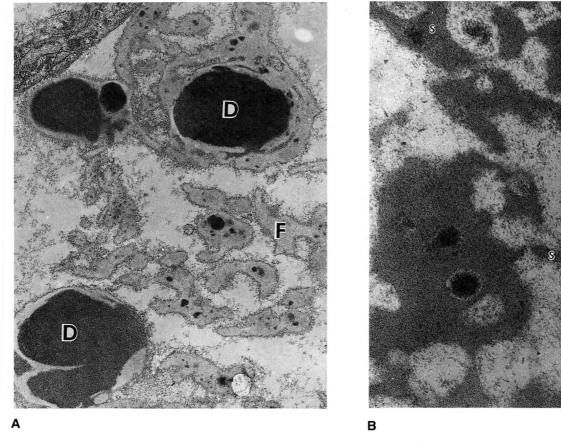

A

B

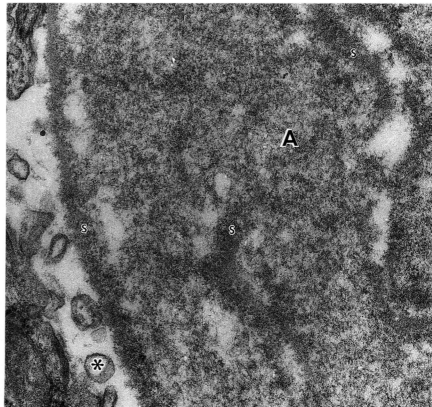

Figure 33–11 Actinic elastosis. **A.** severe disruption of skeleton fibrils (F) and aggregation of dense materials (D) are observed. **B.** An increase in the density of degenerated skeleton fibrils (S) is noted. **C.** The final stage of degeneration consists of an amorphous substance of low electron density (A), cellular debris (∗), and barely recognizable skeleton fibrils (S). F = fibroblast. (**A,** ×15,000; **B,** ×10,000; **C,** ×60,000.)

C

scattered. Such dense materials may occupy the major part of the elastotic fibers.[27,28] Degenerated skeleton fibrils may increase their electron density (Fig. 33–11B). In the final stage of degeneration, elastoid materials completely lose their electron density and transform into amorphous material; this final stage of degeneration corresponds to colloid as it is seen in colloid milium.[25,27,28] Amorphous material may contain numerous cellular debris (Fig. 33–11C) and/ or barely recognizable skeleton fibrils scattered in the amorphous substance.[28]

REFERENCES

1. Reisner SH, Seelenfreund M, Ben-Bassat M: Cutis laxa associated with severe congenital growth retardation and congenital dislocation of the hip. *Acta Paediatr Scand* 1971;60:357–360.
2. Philip AGS: Cutis laxa with intrauterine growth retardation and hip dislocation in a male. *J Pediatr* 1978;93:150–151.
3. Karrar ZA, Elidrissy ATH, Adam KA: Cutis laxa, intrauterine growth retardation and bilateral dislocation of the hips: A report of five cases, in Adam KA (ed): *Skeletal Dysplasias: Progress in Chemical and Biological Research.* New York, Alan R. Liss, 1982, vol 7, pp 215–221.
4. Sakati NO, Nyhan WL, Shear CS, et al.: Syndrome of cutis laxa, ligamentous laxity and delayed development. *Pediatrics* 1983;72:850–856.
5. Gardner LI, Sanders-Fay K, Bifano EM: Congenital cutis laxa syndrome: Relation to joint dislocations to oligohydramnios. *Arch Dermatol* 1986;122:1241–1243.
6. Kerl H, Burg G, Hashimoto K: Fatal, penicillin-induced, generalized, postinflammatory elastolysis (cutis laxa). *Am J Dermatopathol* 1983;5:267–276.
7. Hashimoto K, Kanzaki T: Cutis laxa. *Arch Dermatol* 1975; 111:861–873.
8. Scott MA, Kauh YC, Luscombe HA: Acquired cutis laxa associated with multiple myeloma. *Arch Dermatol.* 1976;112:853–855.
9. Ting HC, Foo MH, Wang F: Acquired cutis laxa and multiple myeloma. *Br J Dermatol* 1984;110:363–367.
10. Convit J, Kerdel F, Goihman M, et al: Progressive, atrophying, chronic granulomatous dermohypodermitis. Autoimmune disease. *Arch Dermatol* 1973;107:271–274.
11. Fisher BK, Page E, Hanna W: Acral localized acquired cutis laxa. *J Am Acad Dermatol* 1989;21:33–40.
12. Sephel GC, Byers PH, Holbrook KA, Davidson JM: Heterogeneity of elastin expression in cutis laxa fibroblast strains. *J Invest Dermatol* 1989;93:147–153.
13. Sayers CP, Goltz RW, Mottaz J: Pulmonary elastic tissue in generalized elastolysis (cutis laxa) and Marfan's syndrome. *J Invest Dermatol* 1975;65:451–457.
14. Marchase P, Holbrook K, Pinnell S: A familial cutis laxa syndrome with ultrastructural abnormalities of collagen and elastin. *J Invest Dermatol* 1980;75:399–403.
15. Hashimoto K, DiBella RJ: Electron microscopic studies of normal and abnormal elastic fibers in the skin. *J Invest Dermatol* 1967;48:405–423.
16. Hashimoto K, Hill WR: Elastosis perforans serpiginosa: A case report with histochemical and enzyme digestion studies. *J Invest Dermatol* 1960;35:7–14.
17. Mehregan AH: Elastosis perforans serpiginosa. A review of the literature and report of 11 cases. *Arch Dermatol* 1968;97:381–393.
18. Rasmussen JE: Disseminated elastosis perforans serpiginosa in four mongoloids. *Br J Dermatol* 1972;86:9–13.
19. Bardach A, Gebhart W, Niebauer G: "Lumpy-bumpy" elastic fibers in the skin and lungs of a patient with penicillamine-induced elastosis perforans serpiginosa. *J Cutan Pathol* 1979; 6:243–252.
20. Hashimoto K, McEvoy B, Belcher R: Ultrastructure of penicillamine-induced skin lesions. *J Am Acad Dermatol* 1981;4:300–315.
21. Sternlieb I, Fisher M, Scheinberg IG: Penicillamine-induced skin lesions. *J Rheumatol Suppl* 1981;7:149–154.
22. Thomas RHM, Light N, Stephens AD, et al.: Pseudoxanthoma elasticum–like skin changes induced by penicillamine. *J Roy Soc Med* 1984;77:794–798.
23. Light N, Meyrick T, Stephens A: Collagen and elastin changes in D-penicillamine-induced pseudoxanthoma elasticum-like skin. *Br J Dermatol* 1986;114:381–388.
24. Kossard S, Kronman KR, Dicken CH, et al.: Inflammatory macular atrophy: Immunofluorescent and ultrastructural findings. *J Am Acad Dermatol* 1979;1:325–334.
25. Hashimoto K, Black M: Colloid milium: A final degeneration product of actinic elastoid. *J Cutan Pathol* 1985;12:147–156.
26. Kambe N, Hashimoto K: Anti-elastofibril monoclonal antibody NKH-1: Production and application. *J Invest Dermatol,* in press.
27. Kobayashi H, Hashimoto K: Colloid and elastic fibre: Ultrastructural study on the histogenesis of colloid milium. *J Cutan Pathol* 1983;10:111–122.
28. Hashimoto K, Niizuma K: *Skin pathology by Light and Electron Microscopy.* New York, Igaku-Shoin Medical Publishers, 1983.

CHAPTER 34
Cutaneous Deposition Disorders

W. Clark Lambert

Cutaneous deposits may be either endogenous or exogenous. Endogenous deposits may occur spontaneously, may be secondary to systemic disease, as in myxedema, or may be caused by an external stimulus, as in mucinous pseudocyst. Exogenous deposits may be due to more or less site-specific metabolic processing, as in argyria, or to direct deposition in tissues, as in tattoos, often followed by limited local alteration and processing, primarily by macrophages. Cutaneous deposition disorders thus comprise a diverse group, including some of the most interesting and sometimes confusing entities in medicine. Because many of these disorders may cause only subtle changes in skin biopsy specimens, they must be considered when evaluating a slide showing apparently normal skin.

Many of the exogenous deposition disorders have been described in other chapters. In this chapter, endogenous disorders are primarily discussed.

THE AMYLOIDOSES

The term *amyloidosis* denotes any condition characterized by deposition in tissues of any of a group of chemically unrelated proteins that share certain properties.[1,2] Recent overall reviews have been provided by Breathnach[1] and by Hashimoto.[3] Ideally, the deposited protein, known as amyloid, has definitive characteristics that are readily detectable by light microscopy, both on routine hematoxylin and eosin (H&E) stained sections and using a number of special stains, as well as by electron microscopy and x-ray diffraction. In practice, however, amyloid deposited in tissues, particularly skin, often fails to demonstrate some of these properties, particularly when using light microscopy combined with special stains for amyloid.

Chemical Nature of Amyloid: X-Ray Diffraction, Infrared Spectroscopic, and Ultrastructural Demonstration of Amyloid

Protein molecules of permissive amino acid sequences can exist as either of two ordered tertiary molecular structures,

the alpha, or helical, form and the beta, or pleated sheet, form.[1,2] The former is physiological, occurring in a number of normal proteins; the latter is abnormal in human tissue. In the beta form, the amino acid chains lie flat, one beside the other, like ties in a railroad bed. Each lies just below or above the level of the one just before or after it in the plane described by the sheet, thus forming the pleated sheet. In amyloid, adjacent amino acid chains in the pleated sheet lie in opposite directions, so that at one edge of this sheet the polarity of the amino acid chains alternates, the carboxyl end of one chain adjacent to the amino end of the next chain lying beside it, and so on. This arrangement is called antiparallel. This railroad bed thus forms a ribbon, with the amino acid chains lying side by side perpendicular to the long axis of the ribbon in their antiparallel, beta, pleated sheet configuration.[2–5]

In addition to the tertiary protein structure detected in concentrations of extracted amyloid fibrils by x-ray diffraction crystallography and by infrared spectroscopy, amyloid also has a higher, much less well-characterized, quaternary structure, thought to be formed as follows[3–5]: The pleated sheet railroad bed does not lie completely flat, but is twisted to form a spirallike structure. The amino acid chains—the ties in our figurative railroad bed—thus are rotated around the axis of the spiral, so that in truncated cross section they would look like the spokes of a wheel, except that the spokes all pass to one side of the center of the wheel, which is left open. This is known as meridional array. The final result is identified on electron microscopy as a hollow, nonbranching, rigid fibril with a hollow core. The fibrils may show periodic cross-banding, apparently related to how tightly the underlying spiral is wound. These fibrils measure approximately 7.5 to 10 nm in diameter, are of indefinite length, and tend to occur in pairs; all of this is found in aggregates within a loose meshwork.[2,6] Wavy, thicker filaments may also be seen in apoptotic cells in macular and lichenoid amyloidosis, a process known as filamentous degeneration.[3]

It has been hypothesized that the meridional, antiparallel, pleated sheet (beta) configuration is the underlying common feature of all amyloid proteins, that any protein capable of forming this structure is a potential amyloid protein, and that once it has formed this structure it has, in fact, become amyloid. Although this hypothesis, proposed by Glenner,[2] is attractive and is supported by elegant experimental evidence, it is important to understand that it has not been verified in all amyloids, particularly many cutaneous amyloids, and that the quaternary structure remains largely hypothetical for all amyloids. It is likely that many amyloids show at least some degree of variation of this general structure. Based on his hypothesis, Glenner has proposed the term *beta-fibrilloses* to denote the amyloidoses.[2]

Amyloid deposits also contain a nonfibrillar tissue protein, called amyloid substance P, which constitutes as much as 14% of the dry weight of amyloid.[7,8] In vitro, amyloid P shows calcium-dependent binding to isolated amyloid fibrils.[9] Amyloid P is also an integral constituent of the microfibrillar sheath of normal elastic fibers, both in the skin and elsewhere. Amyloid P is identical antigenically to a circulating plasma alpha globulin that is present in all persons and is known as *serum amyloid P*. It has been speculated that amyloid P may play a part in the deposition and persistence of amyloid deposits of all types[9,10]; however, it has recently been found that amyloid binds to keratin whether or not it is in the form of amyloid.[11] It is thus not clear what, if any, role amyloid P has in the pathogenesis of amyloidosis.

The Committee on Nomenclature of the Third International Symposium on Amyloidosis recommended a classification of amyloidosis based on the chemical composition of the amyloid fibrillar proteins for those amyloidoses for which information regarding these proteins is available.[3] Table 34-1 is based on this scheme.

Histologic Demonstration of Amyloid: Special Stains for Amyloid

Regardless of the protein composition of their fibrils, all amyloids ideally share certain histochemical characteristics on light microscopy. These histochemical characteristics ap-

TABLE 34-1. CLASSIFICATION OF CUTANEOUS AMYLOIDOSIS BY FIBRIL BIOCHEMISTRY

Clinical Type of Amyloidosis	Precursor Substance	Amyloid Fibril Protein
Systemic		
Primary	Immunoglobulin light chains	AL
Myeloma associated	Immunoglobulin light chains	AL
Secondary	SAA	AA
Hemodialysis associated		β_2-microglobulin
Heredofamilial		
Familial Mediterranean	SAA	AA
Muckle-Wells syndrome	SAA	AA
Familial amyloid neuropathy	?	Prealbumin
Limited to Skin and Soft Tissues		
Nodular	Immunoglobulin light chain	AL
Macular and lichenoid	Keratin filaments	Keratin filaments

AA, amyloid A; AL, amyloid L; SAA, serum amyloid.

pear to be related to the meridional, antiparallel, pleated sheet (beta) tertiary and perhaps also the quaternary structure of the amyloid fibers, rather than to their primary (i.e., amino acid sequence) or secondary structure.[2] In practice, many amyloids in tissue, particularly skin, fail to stain with one or more of these special stains, so that if necessary several should be used to establish a diagnosis. In general, amyloid in frozen sections is more likely to stain with these reagents, but formalin-fixed tissue is usually adequate. It is important to note that amyloid itself does not become visible on a special stain. Rather, an amorphous material often showing fissures and sometimes hemosiderin or even hemorrhage is identified by the special stain. One should be able to note the amorphous material before obtaining the special stain. This is made *much* easier by constricting the aperture diaphragm. (The aperture diaphragm is the one that when constricted does not become visible at the edge of the microscopic field as one peers through the ocular; instead it becomes visible at the edge if one constricts it with the ocular removed while peering down the tube of the microscope.) Alternatively, the condenser may be defocused downward to obtain a partial "phase" effect (Huygens' effect). Manipulating the microscopic illumination in this manner often reveals a sharp outline of the amyloid deposits, causing the fissures within these deposits to become more easily visible. This technique often establishes the diagnosis of amyloidosis better than a battery of special stains. It is particularly helpful in establishing a diagnosis of macular or lichenoid amyloidosis. It should be done on all biopsy specimens that appear to show normal skin. In the author's practice, special stains for cutaneous amyloid are used almost exclusively for teaching purposes; the manipulation described is usually all that is needed to establish a diagnosis of amyloidosis. The special stains are, however, extremely important in establishing a diagnosis of amyloidosis in deeper tissues.

Special stains for amyloid that are routinely employed in various laboratories, and the feature that is indicative of amyloid using each, are summarized as follows:[1,12]

1. *Periodic acid-Schiff (PAS)*: The indicative feature is a *well-circumscribed red mass in the dermis.*[12] This stain lacks specificity; many things stain with it.
2. *Methyl violet* and *crystal violet*, both triphenylmethane dyes: The indicative feature is *metachromasia.*[13] These stains may give equivocal results and may fail to stain small deposits, such as in macular amyloidosis. False-positive staining of the deposits in colloid milium and of lipoid proteinosis may occur.
3. *Congo red, sirius red, pagoda red, RIT scarlet number 5, RIT cardinal red number 9,* and *dylon stain:* All are cotton dyes used in the clothing industry in the past or at present. The indicative feature is a *change in color, usually green, on fluorescence microscopy* and/or *circular dichroism,* measuring the color changes on rotation of one of the polarizing lenses, on polarization microscopy.[3,13–18] These stains may give equivocal results and especially may fail to stain small deposits of amyloid, such as those seen in macular amyloidosis. False-positive staining of the deposits of colloid pseudomilium (colloid milium) and of lipoid proteinosis may occur with these stains.

4. *Thioflavin T,* a thiazide dye, and possibly other thiazide dyes: The indicative feature is *fluorescence* on fluorescence microscopy.[19–22] This method is very sensitive, but false-positive staining of collagen fibers, of stromal hyaline deposits, and, in lichen planus and in some other interface dermatitides, of colloid bodies may occur.

5. *Phorwhite BBU,* a brightener for cellulose: The indicative feature is *fluorescence* on fluorescence microscopy.[23] Experience using this method is limited.

It is often possible to distinguish amyloid deposits composed of amyloid A, the precursor of which is serum amyloid A protein, from amyloid composed of amyloid L, the precursor of which is immunoglobulin light chain, based on the fact that amyloid A in tissue is sensitive to exposure to potassium permanganate, losing its affinity for Congo red and its amyloid characteristic polarization properties after exposure to this chemical.[24] Amyloid L is not affected by this treatment.

Special stains that distinguish between amyloidosis and colloid pseudomilium (colloid milium) are discussed later under that entity.

Immunohistochemical Identification of Amyloid
As a universal immunohistochemical stain for amyloid, antiserum amyloid P has been used. Although this substance is present in all amyloids, it is also present in low levels in elastic tissue normally present in the skin as well as in high levels in solar elastosis.[7] Thus its specificity is limited. Antisera specific for different types of amyloid fibrillar protein are becoming popular for immunohistochemical identification of amyloid.[25]

Electron Microscopic Identification of Amyloid
Electron microscopy may become necessary if the other methods for identification fail.[17] The characteristic picture seen was described earlier. Colloid pseudomilium (colloid milium) also shows fibrillar protein, but the fibers are wavy, with only short straight filaments seen, and then only occasionally.[3] Lipoid proteinosis shows a stringy network of irregular filaments, a few straight filaments, and collagen fibers.[3] An advantage of using electron microscopy for identification of amyloid is that formalin-fixed, paraffin-embedded tissue may be used.

X-Ray Diffraction Crystallography and Infrared Spectroscopy
X-ray diffraction crystallography and infrared spectroscopy are currently used only for research purposes, to determine the molecular structure of amyloids, particularly the tertiary structure. These methods are not diagnostic modalities at present.[1,2]

CLINICAL AND HISTOLOGIC TYPES OF AMYLOIDOSIS

SYSTEMIC, WITH CUTANEOUS INVOLVEMENT

Systemic amyloidosis is commonly classified into several major categories: primary, myeloma associated, herdofamilial (associated with familial Mediterranean fever,

the Muckle-Wells syndrome, or familial amyloid neuropathy), and that associated with hemodialysis.

Primary and Myeloma-Associated Amyloidosis

Primary and myeloma-associated amyloidosis differ only in the presence or absence of known myeloma and may represent variants of the same disease. Amyloidosis occurs in about 15% of patients with myelomatosis. In both conditions, material deposited as amyloid is derived from immunocytes, apparently as a result of a plasma cell dyscrasia, and, in both, monoclonal (i.e., of identical amino acid sequence) light chains are virtually always found in serum, urine, or both.[26,27] The amyloid protein in these disorders is largely composed of immunoglobulin light chain and is known as AL protein. Most amyloid fibril AL proteins are of lambda type, as are the serum monoclonal proteins from which they are thought to be derived. Bence Jones proteins in the urine of patients with myeloma may also contain fibrils with physiochemical properties of amyloid, which may be obtained by proteolytic digestion.[28]

Clinical Features, Systemic
Primary and myeloma-associated amyloidosis tend to occur in the elderly, with a slight male predominance; this tendency has remained unchanged in extensive studies obtained over several decades.[1,29–40] Presenting signs and symptoms are relatively nonspecific, often leading to a delay in diagnosis. Fatigue, weight loss, paresthesias, peripheral edema, dyspnea, hoarseness, and signs of orthostatic hypotension are common. When the condition is first seen by the physician, macroglossia, carpal tunnel syndrome, hepatomegaly, and edema are characteristically present, but usually not all in the same individual. Clinically evident cutaneous lesions and/or lesions on mucous membranes are present in approximately 29 to 40% of cases.[31,38,41] Cutaneous lesions may be an early sign of an occult plasma cell dyscrasia.[29,30,32,33,38,39] Less common manifestations include lymphadenopathy, which occurs in approximately 10% of patients and may be the presenting sign of the disease[35,42]; amyloid infiltration of the lacrimal and parotid glands, leading to the sicca syndrome (i.e., xerophthalmia and xerostomia)[43]; amyloid infiltration of soft tissues around the shoulders, producing extensive enlargement of these tissues (the "shoulder pad sign")[44]; and amyloid deposition in joints, mimicking rheumatoid arthritis.[44] Gastrointestinal bleeding or malabsorption is often encountered, as well as a bleeding diathesis and/or disseminated intravascular coagulation.[1] Cardiac changes are common, accounting for 40% of fatalities. Peripheral neuropathies, including sympathetic neuropathies, are also often noted in addition to the carpal tunnel syndrome; together they occur in about 17% of patients with primary systemic amyloidosis.[35,36]

Clinical Features, Mucocutaneous
Cutaneous and mucous membrane lesions of primary and myeloma-derived amyloidosis are extremely varied. The most common sign is purpura, either petechiae, ecchymoses, or both, occuring either spontaneously or after minor trauma. This sign is seen in 15 to 17% of cases[35] and occurs as a result of infiltration of amyloid into blood vessel walls and tissue immediately surrounding blood vessels. Purpura

is most frequently seen in the following sites: eyelids, naso-labial folds, neck, umbilicus, axillae, anogenital region, mouth, and flexural creases. Purpura following mild com-pression (so-called pinch purpura) is especially characteris-tic and may be deliberately elicited as a clinical sign. Facial purpura, especially perioral purpura, may occur after a Val-salva's maneuver, coughing, vomiting, forced expiration (during spirometry), or proctoscopy (so called postprocto-scopic purpura), and constitutes a highly diagnostic sign of systemic amyloidosis.[1] Pigmentary changes may occur secondarily in areas of hemorrhage.

More characteristic but less common cutaneous lesions of primary and myeloma-associated systemic amyloidosis are papules, nodules, and plaques containing deposited amyloid. These are smooth, nontender, and nonpruritic and have a waxy to translucent appearance. Hemorrhage is often present. Color varies from skin color to amber or yellow. These masses tend to occur in the same sites as listed earlier for purpuric lesions, as well as in the retroau-ricular areas, central face, lips, tongue, and buccal mucosa.[45] Widespread nodules may resemble xanthomas[46]; more lo-calized lesions may be confused with other nodular or papil-lary processes. Perineal lesions may be mistaken for condy-lomata lata.[33] Plaques may coalesce to form tumefactive lesions or may resemble scleroderma,[47] myxedema, or cutis verticis gyrata.[30,33,34] Bullous lesions, dystrophic nail changes, occlusion of the external auditory meatus, and loss of viability of fingers and hands due to amyloid deposi-tion all have been reported.[30,33,47–50] Nail changes may be the only sign of systemic amyloidosis. Lesions with bullae may resemble porphyria cutanea tarda.[51] Rare variants in-clude amyloid elastosis, characterized by papulonodular lesions and diffuse infiltration of cutaneous and visceral blood vessels by amyloid, with a tendency to involve elastic fibers,[52] and more extensive infiltration of cutaneous vessels by amyloid, leading to a ropelike or cordlike thickening of these vessels.[53] Cutis laxa associated with a plasma cell dyscrasia and amyloidosis has also been reported.

Secondary Systemic, Heredofamilial, and Hemodialysis-Associated Amyloidosis

Secondary systemic amyloidosis characteristically occurs in association with a chronic systemic disease, such as tubercu-losis, and only occasionally shows cutaneous involvement. This usually consists of purpura, similar to that described earlier, but nodular lesions may also occur. The distribution is the same as for primary amyloidosis. In contrast to that disorder, however, the amyloid fibers in secondary systemic amyloidosis have been found to consist of a nonimmunoglo-bulin protein known as protein amyloid A.[54] It has a precur-sor in serum designated serum amyloid A protein, which is an apolipoprotein of high-density lipoprotein that is pres-ent in the serum of normal individuals but that also func-tions as an acute phase reactant. It is synthesized in the liver.[54]

Familial Mediterranean fever and the Muckle-Wells syndrome also are characterized by amyloid fibers com-posed of protein amyloid A. Both produce amyloid deposits primarily in the kidneys; cutaneous changes in these dis-eases are usually not due to cutaneous amyloidosis.[55,56] Familial amyloid polyneuropathy is characterized by amy-

loid fibers composed of prealbumin involving peripheral nerves.[55,57] Cutaneous lesions are due mainly to trophic skin changes related to involved nerves.[58] Deposition of amyloid material in internal organs is a known complication of hemodialysis. The deposited material has been identified as beta$_2$ microglobulin. This substance is also known as a prealbumin, a confusing name that refers to its motility on an electrophoretic gel compared with that of albumin; it is not a precursor of albumin.

Histopathology of Systemic Amyloidosis

Biopsy of clinically apparent cutaneous lesions in systemic amyloidosis provides a safe, relatively noninvasive method of establishing a diagnosis. Even in the absence of clinically evident cutaneous involvement, biopsy of forearm skin is positive in up to 50% of primary and myeloma-associated amyloidosis.[33,38] Moreover, fine-needle biopsy of abdomi-nal subcutaneous fat underlying clinically normal skin has been reported to be positive in as many as 95, 60, and 86% of cases of primary and secondary systemic and heredo-familial amyloidosis, respectively.[59,60] In contrast, rectal biopsy, the traditional diagnostic method of diagnosis, is positive in 80% of cases of primary systemic amyloidosis if submucosa is included, but none if it is not, whereas peroral jejunal and gingival biopsies are positive in about 67 and 19% of cases, respectively.[36,41]

Biopsy specimens of skin and/or subcutaneous tissue in cases of systemic amyloidosis show three distinctive pat-terns of amyloid deposition, all, some, or uncommonly none of which may be present in an individual patient or specimen. The first of these is deposition of amyloid around adnexal structures, particularly eccrine and apocrine sweat glands (Figs. 34–1 and 34–2). The appearance of the amyloid may be very variable; one may see broad areas of hyalinized material (Fig. 34–1) or a much narrower band of darker staining material (Fig. 34–2). A common error in evaluating skin biopsy specimens of systemic amyloidosis is failure to appreciate the variability in intensity of staining of amy-loid, on all stains including H&E, and the amount deposited. The second pattern of deposition is within mesenchymal-derived structures such as nerves and blood vessels (Fig. 34–3). Both of these types of amyloid deposition are much more frequently found on skin biopsy than on subcutaneous fat aspiration, but may be seen on both in individual cases. The third pattern is deposition of amyloid between lipocytes in subcutaneous fat. This can be the most easily recognized and most diagnostic sign of systemic amyloidosis, but sev-eral cautions must be observed. First, not all adipose tissue shows this sign, and it may be necessary to examine step sections to see it. Alternatively, fat close to a large lesion of nodular amyloidosis may show this sign, even though systemic disease is not present. Second, the amount and intensity of staining of deposited amyloid may be quite variable, as noted earlier for periadnexal deposits. Third, the adipose tissue is likely to be disrupted by the biopsy procedure, especially in needle aspiration biopsies, because the deposited amyloid may cause the tissue to be brittle. Ideally, the individual lipocytes are surrounded by amyloid to form a very distinctive lattice (Fig. 34–4), but this is often disrupted on needle biopsy (Fig. 34–5), or may be very pale staining (Fig. 34–6). The amyloid may stain inten-

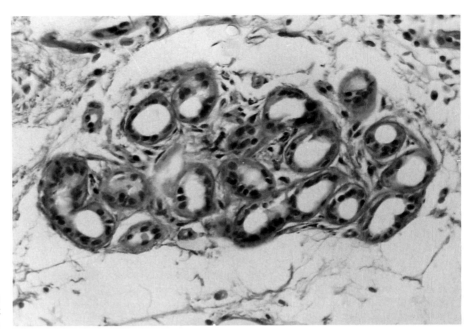

Figure 34–1. Systemic amyloidosis showing deposition of amyloid around basement membrane of sweat gland acini (H&E, ×100).

sively with all stains but may be so disrupted as to be mistaken for debris (see Fig. 34–5). An important diagnostic sign in such cases, and sometimes the only recognizable sign present on a needle aspiration biopsy of subcutaneous fat, is the *amyloid ring* (see Figs. 34–4 and 34–5). An amyloid ring consists of an individual lipocyte, encased in amyloid, that has remained intact during the biopsy. It is often found amid a mass of debris. Finally, in addition to the types of amyloid deposition that occur only in systemic amyloidosis, any of the patterns described later for localized amyloidosis may also be seen in biopsy specimens of systemic amyloidosis, with the possible exception of macular amyloidosis, which is almost always a localized process.

LOCALIZED CUTANEOUS AMYLOIDOSIS

There are a large number of reports of localized amyloidosis occurring in various tissues, particularly skin, lung, and respiratory tract. Localized cutaneous amyloidosis occurs in two major distributions, nodular and macular/lichenoid.

Nodular Amyloidosis

Clinical Features
Nodular localized cutaneous amyloidosis occurs as intracutaneous or subcutaneous nodules that are firm to rock hard on palpation and may vary from barely palpable to several

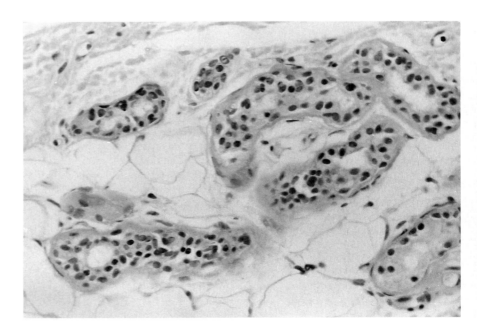

Figure 34–2. Systemic amyloidosis showing deposition of amyloid around basement membrane of sweat gland acini. Note lighter stain of amyloid than in Figure 34–1 (H&E, ×118).

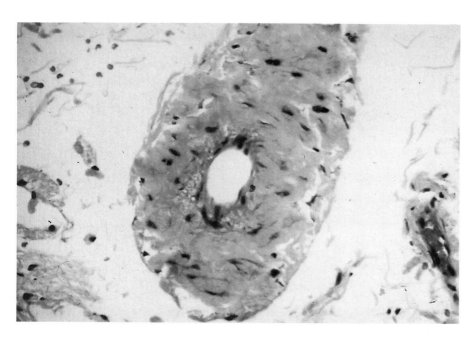

Figure 34–3. Cutaneous blood vessel in systemic amyloidosis showing accumulation of amyloid in wall (H&E, ×204).

centimeters in diameter. These deposits are often knobby and may be mistaken clinically for carcinoma. One or more lesions may occur on the face, trunk, or perineum, but they may occur anywhere.

Nodular cutaneous amyloidosis is often associated with a plasma cell dyscrasia.[1,2] This is often localized, in the same area as an isolated cutaneous plasmacytoma, and numerous plasma cells are usually seen in or near an isolated lesion. Nodular cutaneous amyloidosis may run a totally benign and innocuous course, or full-blown systemic amyloidosis with an associated paraproteinemia may develop.[13,61,62]

Histologic Features

Histologically, a large nodular lesion is seen in the dermis and/or subcutis. It may be either well or poorly demarcated. The amyloid may be for the most part relatively amorphous, with only certain areas showing frankly hyalinized material (Fig. 34–7), or a large area may be easily recognized as amyloid (Fig. 34–8). Special stains for amyloid are usually unequivocally positive. Numerous plasma cells are often seen.[13,23] In contrast, in nodular lesions of systemic primary or myeloma-associated amyloidosis, plasma cells are usually sparse or absent. The presence of numerous plasma cells therefore suggests that the lesion is localized.

Diagnosis of primary cutaneous nodular amyloidosis should be followed by an attempt to rule out systemic myeloma. Radiological evidence of bone involvement by plasmacytoma is present in 50% of patients with systemic myeloma, however 6% of cases with primary cutaneous nodular

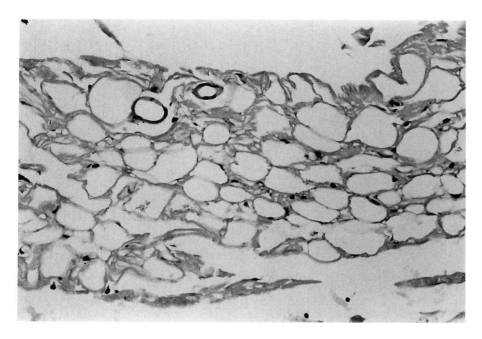

Figure 34–4. Subcutaneous fat needle biopsy in systemic amyloidosis showing deposition of amyloid between lipocytes. Note two amyloid rings in upper left center (H&E, ×200).

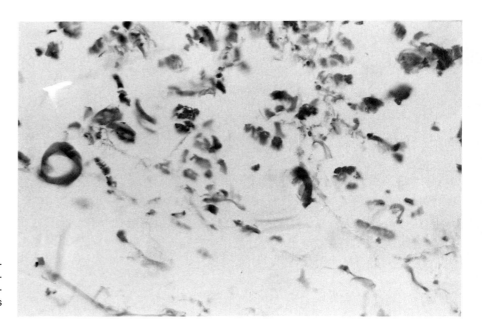

Figure 34–5. Subcutaneous fat biopsy specimen in systemic amyloidosis showing fragments of amyloid. Note dense stain and brittleness of structures. An amyloid ring is present on the left (H&E, ×120).

amyloidosis show such evidence as well without having systemic disease.[1] On the other hand, it has been reported that more than half of myeloma patients have in excess of 15% plasma cells on bone marrow biopsy (mean, 23%), versus none in cases of primary cutaneous nodular amyloidosis (mean, 4% plasma cells).[33]

Macular and Lichenoid Amyloidosis

Clinical Features

Macular amyloidosis classically presents as a pruritic process symmetrically distributed on the superior aspect of the back and upper and/or lower extremities. Less commonly, lesions may appear on the chest and/or buttocks.

Individual lesions are 1- to 3-mm brown to gray papules; together they may have a wavelike or rippled appearance. Lesions persist for years without changing.[1,13,61,63–65] Lichenoid amyloidosis tends to occur first on the shins and subsequently to spread to the dorsa of the feet, ankles, calves, and thighs. Less commonly it may involve the extensor aspects of the arms and abdominal or chest wall.[5,66] The two variants may occur together as "biphasic" amyloidosis.[67–69] There are marked racial preferences, with nodular amyloidosis occurring more frequently among Chinese,[5,66] and macular amyloidosis occurring more commonly among Central and South Americans,[64,70] Middle Eastern races,[65,71] and all Asians.[63] Familial cases of both types have also been reported.[40,66,72,73]

Numerous rarer forms of cutaneous amyloidosis have also been reported. A form occurring on the auricular concha

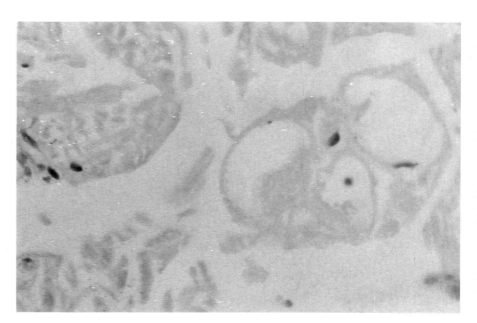

Figure 34–6. Subcutaneous fat biopsy specimen in systemic amyloidosis showing pale-staining amyloid material (H&E, ×122).

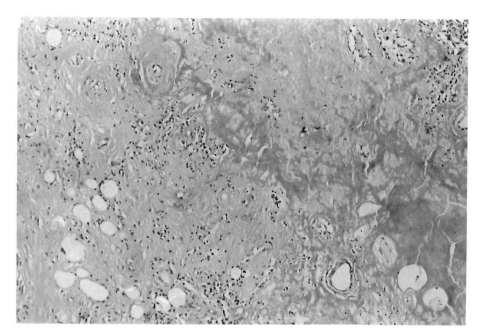

Figure 34–7. Nodular cutaneous amyloidosis showing masses of amorphous material replacing normal structures (H&E, ×148).

has been described,[74] as has a macular form occurring on the back of Orientals who habitually bathe using a nylon brush to scrub their bodies ("nylon brush macular amyloidosis").[75] Macular amyloidosis has been described as a cause of periocular hyperpigmentation,[76] as a simulant of nevoid hyperpigmentation,[77] and as a cause of or in association with poikiloderma.[71] Elderly Japanese men have been reported to develop macular and sometimes hyperkeratotic lesions radiating out from the anus.[78]

Primary localized macular/lichenoid amyloidosis has been found to occur in association with other diseases, including connective tissue disorders,[61] eczema occurring in association with celiac disease,[79] radiodermatitis,[3] and Riehl's melanosis.[3]

Histologic Features

Histologically, changes are limited to the papillary dermis in both macular and lichenoid amyloidosis. Particularly in macular amyloidosis, it is possible to overlook the amyloid deposits altogether and to mistake the lesion for normal skin. One sees small, well-demarcated deposits, often containing clefts and sometimes showing hemosiderin or hemorrhage, mainly in dermal papillae, which may be expanded, especially in lichenoid lesions (Figs. 34–9 through 34–11). One should constrict the aperture condenser of the microscope when searching for these deposits, as noted earlier. Special stains for amyloid are quite variable but may be positive (Figs. 34–12 through 34–15). Monoclonal antikeratin antibodies, such as EKH4, are often reactive

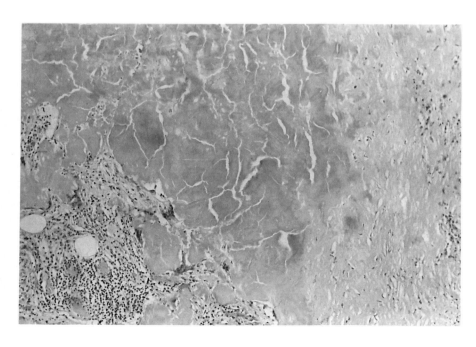

Figure 34–8. Nodular cutaneous amyloidosis showing masses of amorphous material, replacing normal structures. Note clefting of amyloid deposit (H&E, ×190).

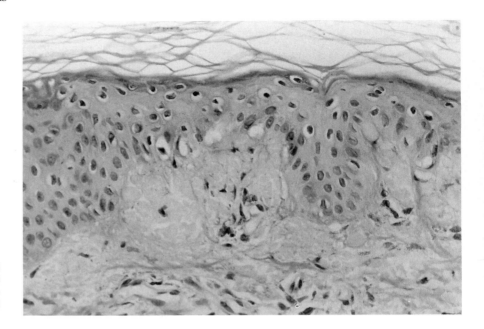

Figure 34–9. Macular amyloidosis showing amyloid deposits in papillary dermis. This photograph was taken with the aperture condenser constricted to show the amyloid (H&E, ×40).

with (i.e., positive for) these deposits.[74,80,81]

Amyloid also is frequently found deposited in the stroma of certain tumors and tumorlike conditions, including basal cell carcinoma, Bowen's disease, seborrheic keratosis, porokeratosis, and melanocytic nevus, as well as mycosis fungoides.[1,3,74] It has no special significance in this setting.

COLLOID PSEUDOMILIUM (COLLOID MILIUM)

Clinical Features

Although widely known as colloid milium, this disease shows no involvement of sweat ducts and thus is more accurately called colloid pseudomilium.[82] An excellent general review has been provided by Hashimoto.[83] This disorder is fairly common among light-complexioned individuals who are exposed to extensive sunlight, and it occurs in sun-exposed areas of the body.[84] Lesions typically occur as amber papules over the buccal regions (i.e., cheeks), nose, brow, pinnae of the ears, and dorsal surfaces of the hands.[83] These lesions, especially when mild, are often ignored by both patients and physicians. Through a slit incision, pure colloid material can be squeezed out of larger lesions. This technique may actually be used as a form of treatment.

There also exists a rare juvenile type of colloid pseudomilium that is not related to sunlight exposure.[83] Moreover,

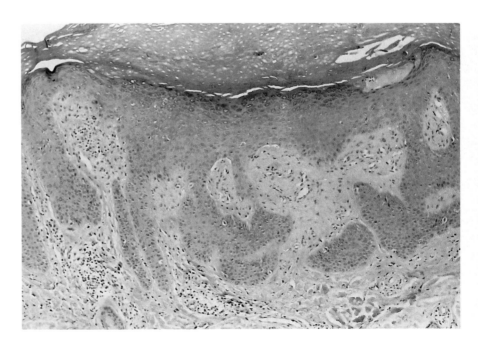

Figure 34–10. Lichenoid amyloidosis, showing amorphous deposits in papillary dermis (H&E, ×40.)

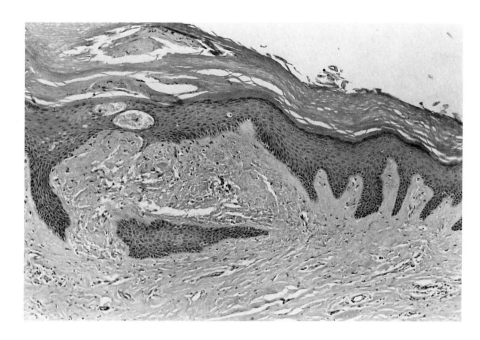

Figure 34–11. Lichenoid amyloidosis, showing amorphous deposits in papillary dermis. Partly lichenoid (left) and partly macular (right) lesion (H&E, ×26).

in South Africa, colloid may accumulate on the face of blacks who use hydroquinoine bleaching creams, a disorder that has been called cosmetic ochronosis.[84]

Histologic Features

Histologically, a large, solid-appearing accumulation of colloid is usually seen in the upper dermis (Figs. 34–16 and 34–17). After routine tissue processing, it usually appears fissured.[85,86] A few fibroblasts are seen in this mass along the cleavage lines. Inflammation is completely lacking. Overlying the lesion is a rim of collagen; the epidermis often shows pressure atrophy. Actinic elastosis is a regular feature but occurs around, rather than in, the colloid mass.

Histochemically, amyloid stains are positive, except that the dylon stain is said to be negative in paraffin-embedded sections.[87] The van Geison's stain shows amyloid as pink to red and colloid as yellow. Amyloid P component is present in abundance, as it is in actinic elastosis.[88] Because intermediate forms exist ultrastructurally, it has been proposed that actinic colloid pseudomilium is an end product of actinic degeneration of dermal elastic fibers.[88,89] Ultrastructurally, one sees a medium electron-dense amorphic material. A small number of filamentous structures are seen; these are of smaller diameter (1.5 to 2.0 nm) than amyloid filaments and, unlike amyloid, are short, curved, and anastomosed.[83]

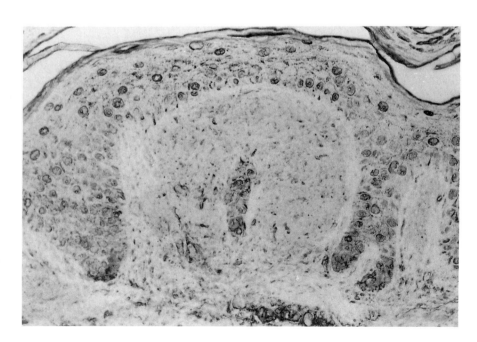

Figure 34–12. Macular amyloidosis (PAS, ×180).

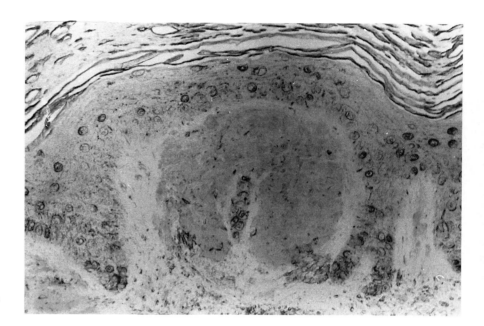

Figure 34–13. Macular amyloidosis (methylene blue, ×180).

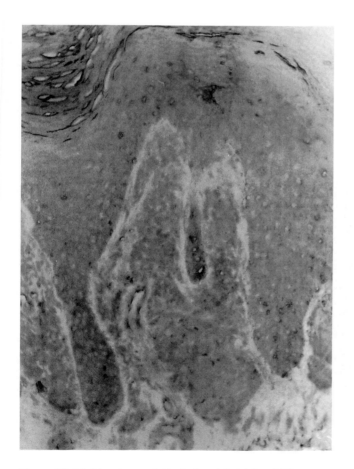

Figure 34–14. Macular amyloidosis (crystal violet, ×140).

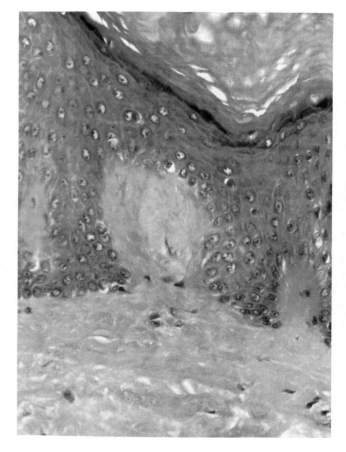

Figure 34–15. Macular amyloidosis, congo red stain with polarized light. Dichroic effect is manifest as bright (green) area in center of deposit. This is often difficult to demonstrate in small cutaneous deposits (×120).

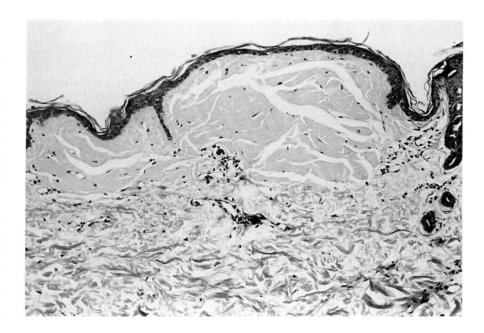

Figure 34–16. Colloid pseudomilium, large nodular lesion on face. Note well-circumscribed deposit within which large clefts are present (H&E, ×80).

LIPOID PROTEINOSIS (LIPODOSIS CUTIS ET MUCOSAE; HYALINOSIS CUTIS ET MUCOSAE)

Clinical Features

Lipoid proteinosis is a rare autosomal recessive disorder affecting skin, mucous membranes, and a number of internal organs.[90] Affected individuals have flesh-colored papules, verrucous nodules and plaques, and diffuse involvement of the skin.[91–93] Verrucous lesions are found on extensor surfaces, apparently related to minor trauma. Tissue infiltration of the tongue, larynx, and eyelids is present. The typical presenting sign, occurring in infancy, is a hoarse cry due to laryngeal involvement; this precedes clinically apparent organ involvement elsewhere.[94]

Histologic Features

Histologically, one sees a pink hyalin-like material deposited in the dermis (Fig. 34–18). This material is also deposited within and around basement membranes, often densely (Fig. 34–19). Capillaries may thus appear to be very thick walled. This material stains positive with PAS reagent and is largely diastase resistant, implying the presence of glycoprotein and/or proteoglycan complexes.[95] A large number of hypotheses have been put forward regarding the nature and origin of this material.[93]

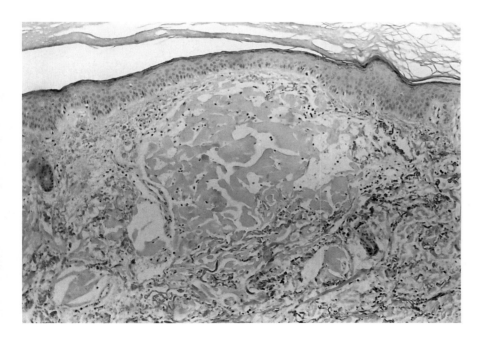

Figure 34–17. Colloid pseudomilium, small macular lesion on face. This lesion is less well demarcated than that in Figure 34–16 (H&E, ×75).

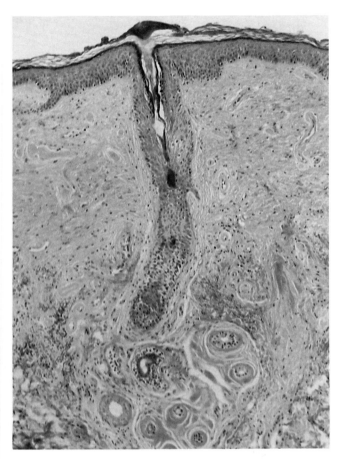

Figure 34–18. Lipoid proteinosis, chest lesion. Hyalinized material is abundant both in the dermis and around sweat gland acini (H&E, ×70).

THE PORPHYRIAS

The porphyrias comprise a heterogeneous group of diseases, each of which is associated with a metabolic defect in the synthesis of the tetrapyrrole heme, an essential structural component of several important, metabolically active proteins. Excellent general reviews have been provided by Bickers[96] and by Poh-Fitzpatrick.[97]

The Normal Heme Synthesis Pathway

Briefly, heme synthesis proceeds as follows:

1. It begins in the mitochondria, where δ-aminolevulinic acid synthetase (ALA-S) catalyzes condensation of the amino acids succinate (as succinyl coenzyme A) and glycine to form the water-soluble aminoketone δ-aminolevulinic acid (ALA), eight molecules of which are eventually condensed to form a single heme moiety.
2. The ALA then diffuses into the cytoplasm, where two molecules of ALA are condensed by the water-soluble cytosol enzyme ALA dehydrase (ALA-D) to form the water-soluble monopyrrole (one-ring structure) prophobilinogen (PBG).
3. Four molecules of PBG are then condensed by the water-soluble cytosol enzyme porphobilinogen deaminase (PBG-D) to form the water-soluble compound hydroxymethylibilane (HMB), which consists of four pyrrole ring structures linked in a chain.
4. The molecule of HMB then spontaneously cyclizes into a large ring structure composed of the four smaller rings (i.e., a tetrapyrrole), known as uroporphyrinogen I (UROGEN I). The designation "I" means that all of the pyrrole rings have their two side chains oriented the same way, so that as we proceed around this ring, we

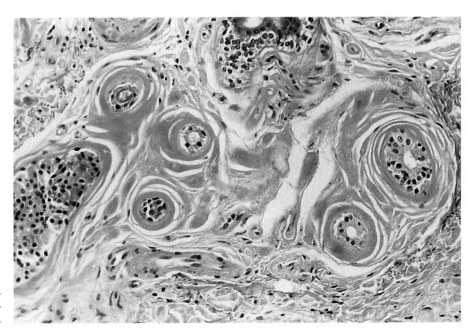

Figure 34–19. Lipoid proteinosis, chest lesion. Abundant hyalinized material is deposited around sweat gland acini (H&E, ×160).

encounter first the acetyl ($-CH_2COOH$) and then the propionyl ($-CH_2CH_2COOH$) side chain of each, never the reverse. Alternatively, one or more of the rings may be "flipped" so that their side chains are present in reverse order (i.e., first propionyl and then acetyl), producing other isomers with different roman numerical designations. The isomer family in which a single one (i.e., one and only one) of the four pyrrole rings is flipped in this manner is called III. This is important because only the III isomers of the porphyrinogens can form heme.

5. UROGEN I is converted into UROGEN III by the water-soluble enzyme uroporphyrinogen cosynthetase (URO-COS). All of the UROGENs are extremely water soluble and are readily excreted in the urine. This is also true of the oxidized forms of the UROGENs, the uroporphyrins (UROs).

6. Each of the four acetyl side chains of UROGEN III (and UROGEN I) is then sequentially decarboxylated by the enzyme UROGEN decarboxylase (UROGEN-D) to form a methyl group, producing coproporphyrinogen III (and I) (COPROGEN III and I). COPROGENs III and I are less water soluble than UROGENs III and I and are excreted partially in urine and partially in feces. This is also true of the oxidized forms of the COPROGENs, the coproporphyrins (COPROs).

7. First one and then the other of the two propionyl side chains that are not adjacent (the flipping of one pyrrole ring by URO-COS rendered the other two propionyl side chains on adjacent pyrrole rings adjacent to each other) on COPROGEN III are then oxidatively decarboxylated to form unsaturated vinyl groups by the mitochondrial enzyme COPROGEN oxygenase (COPROGEN-O), forming, successively, harderoporphyrinogen (HARDEROGEN) and then protoporphyrinogen (PROTOGEN). COPROGEN-O acts exclusively on the III isomer, so that COPROGEN I proceeds no further in the heme pathway.

All of the described tetrapyrrole compounds are porphyrinogens, not porphyrins. This distinction is important, because the porphyrinogens consist of reduced, hexahydro-, nonresonating, nonphotosensitizing compounds. By contrast, porphyrins are *oxidized* porphyrinogens that are both resonating and photosynthesizing and are therefore vastly different in chemical properties and pathogenic potential. Porphyrins as a group are highly photoreactive, absorbing light in the visible range with maximum absorption in the Soret band, 400 to 410 nm,[98] and a lesser but significant absorption in the range of 580 to 650 nm.[96] In all of these reactions, porphyrinogens, not porphyrins, are substrates for the respective enzymes in the pathway.

The final two steps in the pathway are as follows:

8. Protoporphyrinogen (PROTOGEN) is oxidized by the mitochondrial enzyme PROTOGEN oxidase (PROTOGEN-O) (this oxidation occurs in two of the four pyrrole rings) to form the first porphyrin in the pathway, protoporphyrin IX (PROTO). Then,

9. A ferrous iron (Fe^{2+}) ion is inserted by the mitochondrial enzyme ferrochelatase (FCHASE), also known as heme synthetase, to form the final product, heme. This enzyme

may also, in pathological states, insert other divalent cations without itself being abnormal and is responsible for the Zn-protoporphyrins in erythrocytes in hepatoerythrocytic porphyria.

Definitions and Biochemical Abnormalities of the Porphyrias

The porphyrias are a group of diseases associated with a series of partial enzyme deficiencies in heme biosynethesis (Table 34–2) that are expressed mainly in heme-synthesizing cells of the liver or bone marrow.[93,97] They are classified as *hepatic*[99] or *erythropoietic*,[100] depending on which organ system is more severely affected. The clinical features characteristic of each of these disorders are due to accumulation of either precursors of porphyrins, porphyrin by-products of the heme pathway, or both, in characteristic locations. Both the site of deposition and the type of porphyrin deposited are ultimately determined by the enzyme deficiency responsible for each disease.

Hepatic Porphyrias

Acute Intermittent Porphyria. Acute intermittent porphyria (AIP) is an uncommon autosomal dominant disease characterized by intermittent attacks of acute abdominal pain and/or other symptoms that appear to represent a central and peripheral neuropathy. It is precipitated by a number of factors, particularly administration of drugs, especially barbiturates. The disease is characterized by a deficiency of porphobilinogen deaminase (PBG-D). Patients with AIP excrete large amounts of both PBG and ALA in the urine, both during and between attacks. There are no skin manifestations except for the occasional finding of numerous abdominal surgical scars secondary to surgery during acute attacks due to erroneous diagnoses of appendicitis or an "acute abdomen." The Watson-Schwartz test detects ALA, which is otherwise colorless and undetected, in the urine of these patients.

Porphyria Cutanea Tarda. Porphyria cutanea tarda (PCT) is a very common disease occurring either sporadically or as an autosomal dominant condition. It is associated with a deficiency in UROGEN-D in the liver in the sporadic form and in both liver and bone marrow in the inherited form.[101] The sporadic form of the disease occurs primarily in individuals who are exposed to certain environmental or metabolic factors, particularly ethanol, estrogens, and chemicals such as chlorinated hydrocarbons. Inhibition of UROGEN-D by accumulated divalent cations, particularly ferrous iron, in the liver may be an important etiologic factor. Clinically, one sees chronic photosensitivity with increased cutaneous fragility, blistering, milia, hypertrichosis, and induration and scarring resembling scleroderma on chronically sun-exposed skin. The disease may be exacerbated by pregnancy or birth control pills (estrogens).

The biochemical changes in urine and feces that characterize PCT are complex. There is increased urinary URO (the oxidized form of UROGEN), with the I isomer greater than the III isomer. The urine also contains (elevated) 7-carboxylporphyrin (the III isomer greater than the I isomer),

TABLE 34-2. PORPHYRIAS WITH KNOWN BIOCHEMICAL DEFICIENCIES

Heme Pathway[a]	Disease	Porphyria Type	Frequency	Clinical Manifestations	Onset	Laboratory[b] Manifestations
Glycine + Scucinyl CoA (1) ↓ ALA-S[c] ALA (2) ↓ ALA-D PBG						
(3) ↓ PBG-D → → → → → HMB	Acute intermittent porphyria (AIP) (Autosomal dominant)	Hepatic	Uncommon	No skin disease. Surgical scars over abdomen may be present. Neurological disease: episodic abdominal pain, psychoses, neuropathy	Young adulthood	*Urine:* Increased PBG and ALA *Feces:* Negative *Erythrocytes:* Negative *Other:* Usually none
(4) ↓ (spontaneous) UROGEN I						
(5) ↓ URO(III)-COS → → → → → → → UROGEN III	Congenital erythropoietic prophyria (CEP) (Günther's disease) (Autosomal recessive)	Erythropoietic	Rare	Marked photosensitivity. Severe blistering, destructive mutilating skin lesions. Red teeth. Hemolytic anemia.	Infancy	*Urine:* URO I (marked increase resulting in red color) *Feces:* COPRO I *Erythrocytes:* URO I; stable fluorescence *Other:* Hemolytic anemia skeleton shows red fluorescence
(6) ↓ UROGEN-D → → → → → → → → → → → →	Porphyria cutanea tarda (PCT) (heterozygous deficiency of UROGEN-D) (Autosomal dominant or sporadic)	Hepatic	Common	Chronic sun-sensitive skin disease with fragility, bullae, milia, induration and scarring, especially on the head and overlying bony prominences. Lesions may resemble scleroderma. Photophobia and altered liver function may not be clinically apparent. Hypertrichosis on face.	Adulthood, usually in middle age	*Urine:* URO (I > III), 7-carboxylporphyrin (III > I), 6-carboxylporphyrin, 5-carboxylporphyrin, and COPRO (I > III); continuous fluorescence *Feces:* ISOCOPRO *Erythrocytes:* Negative *Other:* Altered serum liver function enzymes; Siderosin (iron deposition in hepatocytes) on liver biopsy

Pathway	Disorder	Type	Frequency	Clinical manifestations	Age of onset	Laboratory findings
→ → → → → → COPROGEN III	Hepatoerythrocytic porphyria (homozygous deficiency of URO-GEN-D) (HEP) (Autosomal recessive)	Hepatic	Rare	Marked photosensitivity. Severe blistering, scarring skin disease with thickening of skin. Altered liver function which may or may not be clinically apparent.	Infancy to childhood	*Urine:* Same as PCT, alterations may be more marked *Feces:* ISOCOPRO *Erythrocytes:* ZnPROTO *Other:* Same as PCT, alterations may be more marked
(7) ↓ → → → → → → HARDEROGEN	Hereditary coproporphyria (HCP) (Autosomal dominant)	Hepatic	Rare	Cutaneous features may show changes similar to PCT. Extracutaneous features are similar to AIP.	Childhood or young adulthood	*Urine:* COPROGEN III, COPRO III, ALA, and PBG during exacerbations *Feces:* COPROGEN III and COPRO III continuously *Erythrocytes:* Negative *Other:* May see altered serum liver function enzymes
(7) ↓ COPROGEN-O PROTOGEN	Variegate porphyria (VP) (Autosomal dominant)	Hepatic	Uncommon (common in South Africa)	Cutaneous features may show changes similar to PCT. Extracutaneous features are similar to AIP.	Adulthood; usually young adulthood	*Urine:* PBG and ALA, may be elevated only during exacerbations *Feces:* PROTO, COPRO III (and I) continuously *Erythrocytes:* Negative *Other:* May see altered liver function
(8) ↓ → → → → → PROTO						
(9) ↓ FCHASE HEME	Erythropoietic protoporphyria (EPP) (? Autosomal dominant)	Erythropoietic	Common	Acute burning sensation on sun exposure with edema and fine scarring. Rarely, blisters and/or fatal hepatic disease.	Childhood; cases often undiagnosed until many years after onset	*Urine:* Negative *Feces:* PROTO, continuously *Erythrocytes:* PROTO (may be transient); transient fluorescence *Other:* Plasma may contain PROTO transiently

---

[a] Numbers refer to numbered reactions in the home pathway given in the text.

[b] All biochemical manifestations variably continuous unless otherwise specified. Other, nonindicated, manifestations may be present in individual cases.

[c] Abbreviations defined in the text.

6-carboxylporphyrin, 5-carboxylporphyrin, and COPRO (the oxidized form of COPROGEN) (again the I isomer exceeding the III isomer). There is also increased fecal excretion of isocoproporphyrin (ISOCOPRO). The 5-, 6-, and 7-carboxylporphyrins are porphyrins partially digested by UROGEN-D with some but not all of the acetyl side chains decarboxylated to form methyl side chains. ISOCOPRO is a product formed by the next enzyme in the normal sequence, COPROGEN-D, acting prematurely on 5-carboxylporphyrinogen. ISOCOPRO is normally not present or is present only in trace amounts.

Hepatoerythrocytic Porphyria. Hepatoerythrocytic porphyria (HEP) is an extremely rare autosomal recessive disease that is thought to result from a homozygous deficiency of the gene for UROGEN-D.[102] (Hereditary PCT is presumably due to the heterozygous condition.) It is associated with very severe skin photosensitivity occurring early in life.

Hereditary Coproporphyria. Hereditary coproporphyria (HCP) is a rare autosomal dominant condition that is associated with a deficiency in COPROGEN-O. It is characterized by attacks resembling those of acute intermittent porphyria, as well as variable cutaneous photosensitivity somewhat resembling porphyria cutanea tarda.[103] Biochemically there is a major increase in fecal excretion, and a lesser increase in urinary excretion, of both COPROGEN III and COPRO III.

Variegate Porphyria. Variegate porphyria (VP) is an uncommon autosomal dominant disease characterized by intermittent attacks similar to those of AIP and HCP.[104] Affected individuals may show skin changes typical of porphyria cutanea tarda or may show no cutaneous manifestation at all. A large affected kindred in South Africa has been traced to a probable single mutation in Holland in the 17th century.[105] The characteristic biochemical changes are increased fecal excretion of PROTO and COPRO and increased urinary excretion of ALA and PBG. The latter are often increased in the urine only during attacks, in contrast to AIP, in which they are also increased between attacks.

Erythropoietic Porphyrias

Congenital Erythropoietic Porphyria (Günther's Disease). Congenital erythropoietic porphyria (CEP) is a rare autosomal recessive disease characterized by onset in infancy of severe, mutilating cutaneous photosensitivity. Patients may die prematurely because of anemia and recurrent infections. Hemolytic anemia is characteristically present. Current evidence suggests that these patients have a deficiency of URO-COS in their bone marrow cells.[106] They excrete large amounts of URO I in their urine, so much as to impart to their urine a characteristic reddish-pink to mahogany color. COPROGEN I is synthesized from UROGEN I by UROGEN-D, giving rise to large amounts of COPRO-I in feces.

Erythropoietic Protoporphyria. Erythropoietic protoporphyria (EPP) is a common disease characterized by an acute, intense burning and stinging of the skin on sun-exposed sites during or immediately after exposure to sunlight.[107] Careful examination of the skin shows fine to coarse scarring over sun-exposed sites. The disorder has been thought to be autosomal dominant, but the genetics may be complex and remain incompletely worked out.[98] A deficiency in ferrochelatase has been found in afflicted individuals.[108] The characteristic biochemical abnormality in these patients is increased PROTO in erythrocytes, plasma, and feces. The PROTO in erythrocytes may be detected by fluorescence microscopy of peripheral blood. Rarely, patients with EPP may develop hepatic insufficiency as a result of diminished clearance of PROTO by the liver; this is a serious complication and is potentially fatal.[109]

Ferrochelatase is a sulfhydryl-rich enzyme that is especially susceptible to inhibition by heavy metals such as lead. Excessive accumulation of PROTO in erythrocytes is a sensitive marker of lead poisoning. Because the PROTO in lead poisoning is chelated to the heavy metal, it does not diffuse out to cause photosensitivity, however. ALA-D, also a sulfhydryl-rich enzyme, is also sensitive to lead, so that urinary accumulation of ALA is an additional sign of lead poisoning that is diagnostically useful.[110]

Other Porphyrias

The heme synthesis pathway is complex and subject to many feedback and other mechanisms that may be defective in various conditions. Several rare porphyrias in which the biochemical mechanisms are unknown have been identified. An example is the rare childhood disorder known as erythropoietic coproporphyria.[96,97]

Cutaneous Lesions

Clinical Features

Photosensitive skin disease in porphyria is of two principal types, acute and chronic. Acute photosensitivity is most severe in the erythropoietic porphyrias. It is characterized by acute burning, sometimes pruritic, and stinging sensations, often associated also with edema, during or immediately after sun exposure. After repeated exposure, fine scarring progresses to waxlike linear bands prominent on acral areas, such as the nose, ears, and dorsa of the hands. In EPP these physical changes are relatively mild, whereas in erythropoietic porphyria they are severe and become mutilating.

Chronic photosensitivity is characterized by gradual onset and slow progression of fragility of the dermis in chronically light-exposed areas. Both chronic trauma and light have a role, so that skin stretched over bony projections such as the clavicles or interphalangeal joints is more affected than other light-exposed areas. The disease is characterized by vesicles; bullae, sometimes with a hemorrhagic base and crusting; milia; and hypertrichosis with induration and sometimes scarring, resembling scleroderma. Some patients also have edema. The photosensitivity itself is asymptomatic, and patients are often unaware of the role of sunlight in the pathogenesis of the disease. Hepatic porphyrias tend to manifest chronic photosensitization. The most typi-

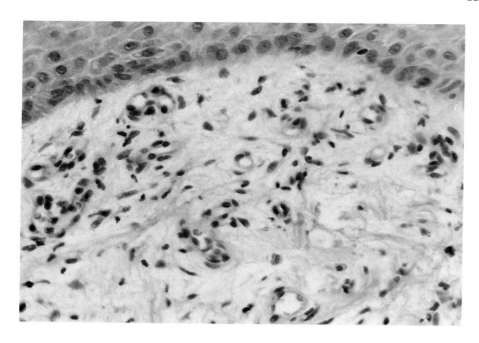

Figure 34–20. Erythropoietic protoporphyria. Moderate hyalin change limited to area around blood vessels. It is important not to mistake this process for normal skin (H&E, ×103).

cal example of this type of photosensitivity is that observed in PCT.

Histologic Features

The histopathologic findings correspond to the type and degree of changes in the skin specimen. In both bullous and nonbullous lesions are found markedly thickened walls around papillary dermal capillaries, as well as deposition of an amorphous, hyalin-like material both around the capillaries and scattered throughout the dermis.[111,112] The PAS stain readily reveals these deposits, which are diastase-resistant mucopolysaccharides (Figs. 34–20 and 34–21).[111,112] Indirect immunofluorescence reveals, in addition, immunoglobulin and complement in these deposits.[111] On light microscopy, these deposits may be readily apparent or their routine H&E staining and optical qualities may resemble normal dermis. Thus, they may not be appreciated without the PAS stain. Ultrastructurally, examination of the capillary walls shows replicated, redundant basal lamina, suggesting that the deposits seen may in part represent repetitive cycles of damage and repair with a new basal lamina laid down after each episode.[111,113,114] These changes around blood vessel walls are especially marked in EPP, and when especially severe in the absence of other changes are suggestive although not diagnostic of that form of porphyria.

Bullous lesions show the described changes plus noninflammatory subepidermal bullae. The changes within the papillae impart to them a rigidity, so that they remain at the base of the bullae as abnormally prominent, rigid structures, a change known as *festooning* (Figs. 34–22 through 34–25). Especially in bullous and scarred lesions, a PAS-positive linear deposit may also be seen at the dermal-epidermal interface, but this has not been found by electron microscopy to be due to redundant epidermal basal lamina, as has the PAS-positive linear deposit seen in lupus erythematosus, which it resembles histologically.

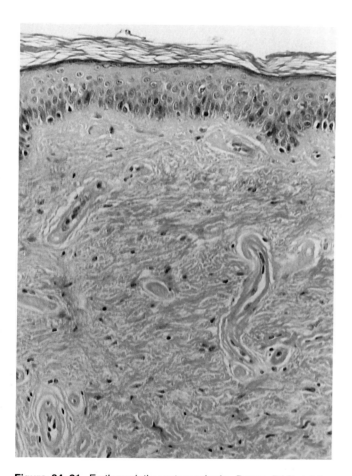

Figure 34–21. Erythropoietic protoporphyria. Dense PAS-staining hyalin change limited to area immediately around blood vessels (PAS, ×87).

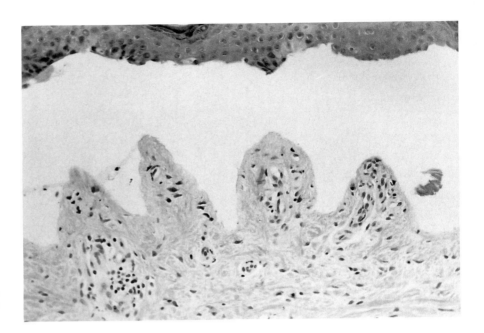

Figure 34–22. Porphyria (PCT), subcutaneous bulla with festooning of dermal papillae but no inflammation (H&E, ×35).

Pathogenesis

Two major hypotheses have been proposed to account for the cutaneous photosensitivity evoked by porphyrins—lipid peroxidation and complement activation. In the former, molecular oxygen is converted by energy from photoexcited porphyrin molecules to excited molecular species that react with unsaturated lipids in membranes.[115] Lysosomes and/or other cellular organelles may play a part in this process, probably via their membranes.[116] In the second hypothesis, porphyrin photoactivation leads to direct activation of complement components, leading to tissue injury, probably through direct release of the chemotactant complement component, C5a.[117–119] These mechanisms are not mutually exclusive, and it is possible that either or both may apply in different settings.

GOUT

Clinical Features

Gout is a metabolic disease in which a severe, recurrent monoarticular arthritis is the typical presentation. It occurs predominantly in males in middle adulthood and older. A family history of gout is often present. The first acute attack is preceded by hyperuricemia for many years, leading to the deposition of monosodium urate crystals in affected tissues.[120–122] Alternatively, the disease may occur

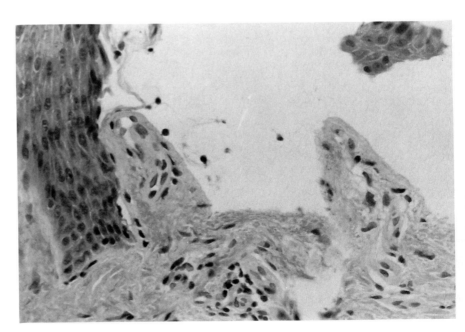

Figure 34–23. Porphyria (PCT), subcutaneous bulla with festooning but no inflammation. Note also apparent thickening of blood vessel walls in papilla on left (H&E, ×120).

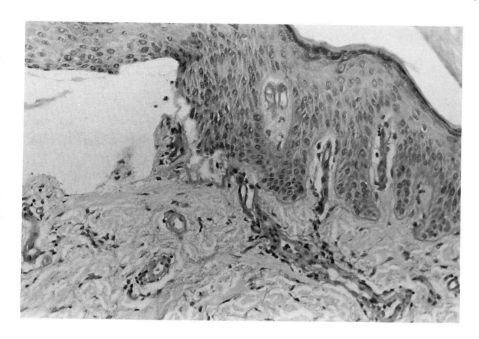

Figure 34–24. Porphyria (PCT), PAS-stained section showing festooning and hyalinized change around blood vessels (×180).

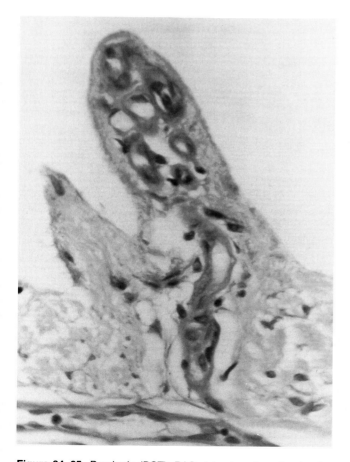

Figure 34–25. Porphyria (PCT), PAS-stained section showing festooning and hyalinized change around blood vessels (×285).

in a number of other settings in which purine metabolism is abnormal, such as in psoriasis (when in poor control), in certain leukemias treated with chemotherapy, and in von Gierke's disease.

In the skin, acute inflammatory changes are seen overlying inflamed joints. The more characteristic cutaneous sign, however, is the subcutaneous or intracutaneous tophus. This lesion occurs most commonly on the helix of the ear, dorsa of the elbow, and on the digits of the hands and feet, but it may occur anywhere. It first appears as a salmon-pink nodule but when large appears whiter. When it is very large it may drain a chalky white material composed of crystals of monosodium urate.

Histologic Features

Histopathologic findings include large, amorphous deposits that may contain needle-shaped to stellate impressions made by urate deposits. The deposits correspond to monosodium urate crystals, which are dissolved away during routine processing because they are water soluble. Processing (including fixation) of tissue in absolute alcohol or by freezing is required if one wishes to preserve this material in the tissue. Crystals of monosodium urate are brilliantly anisotropic on polarized light examination and in the De Galantha stain appear brownish black. The histiocytic response to these deposits has a characteristic appearance, with the nuclei of the macrophages distorted by the shapes of the crystals (Figs. 34–26 and 34–27). It is important that inexperienced pathologists not mistake these for malignant cells. Sometimes only these cells, and little deposited material, are recognizable.

THE CUTANEOUS MUCINOSES

The cutaneous mucinoses consist of a set of disorders involving connective tissue in which mucin accumulates in

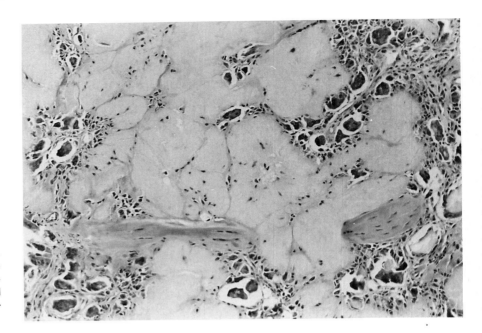

Figure 34–26. Gouty tophus, showing light-staining amorphous areas with spindle-shaped to stellate empty spaces, corresponding to monosodium urate crystals, and a marked histiocytic response. Note prominent macrophage nuclei (H&E, ×41).

the dermis as a prominent feature. In all cases, the mucin itself is a jellylike acid mucopolysaccharide (i.e., glycosaminoglycan) that consists of hyaluronic acid bound to small quantities of condroitin sulfate and heparin. This substance is produced normally, but in small quantities, by fibroblasts. These same cells produce and excrete precursors of collagen fibers, but under pathological conditions may produce mucin instead.[123–126] This group of disorders has been reviewed by Truban and Roenick.[127]

Certain rare genetic diseases, such as Hurler and Hunter's syndromes, are characterized by diffuse accumulation of a mucin that is biochemically different from hyaluronic acid. In these two examples, the principal accumulated substance is chondroitin sulfate. These diseases, all rare, are known as mucopolysaccharidoses. They should be considered when evaluating a child who has an undiagnosed generalized disease and who shows extensive mucin deposition on skin biopsy.

Histologically, mucin stains poorly with H&E but may be readily stained with special stains as follows[123,126]:

1. Colloidal iron, which stains acid mucopolysaccharides bluish-green.

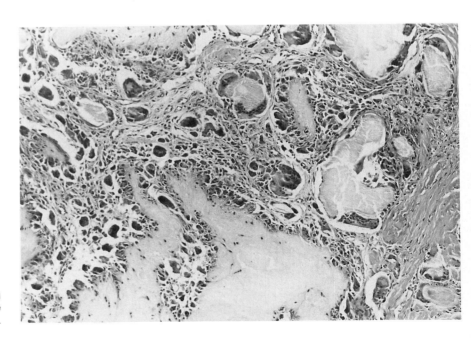

Figure 34–27. Gouty tophus, showing changes as in Figure 34–26 and connective tissue changes at edge of lesion (H&E, ×41).

2. Alcian blue, pH 2.5, which stains acid mucopolysaccharides blue. (At pH 0.5, this stain does *not* stain acid mucopolysaccharides, but rather neutral mucopolysaccharides.)
3. Mucicarmine, which stains acid mucopolysaccharides red.
4. Toluidine blue, methylene blue, and thionine, which stain acid mucopolsaccharides metachromatically.

Mucin consists of hyaluronic acid and can be almost completely removed by application of hyaluronidase.

Sulfated mucopolysaccharides, which include chondroitin sulfate and heparin, stain faintly violet with aldehyde-fuchsin.[126] Neutral mucopolysaccharides stain with the PAS reagent and, as noted earlier, with alcian blue, pH 0.5, which do not stain mucin.

CUTANEOUS FOCAL MUCINOSIS

Clinical Features

Cutaneous focal mucinosis is characterized by accumulation of mucin in the superficial dermis.[123,128] Lesions usually occur in adults, are usually solitary, and are found on the face, neck, trunk, or extremities, but not over the joints of the hands, wrists, or feet. Lesions are flesh colored to white, smooth surfaced, and approximately 1 cm in diameter.

Histological findings include an area of replacement of collagen by mucin with variable numbers of large, spindle-shaped fibroblasts in the upper dermis (Fig. 34–28). In early lesions, fibroblasts are numerous at the center of the lesion; in older lesions, the center contains only a few fibroblasts, but they may accumulate at the periphery. These lesions resemble the early stages of development of a myxoid pseudocyst; however, in contrast to a myxoid pseudocyst, no pseudocyst is formed, although cleftlike spaces containing mucin may be seen between fibroblasts.

MYXOID PSEUDOCYST (MYXOID CYST; MUCINOUS CYST; SYNOVIAL CYST; GANGLION; MUCOCELE)

Clinical Features

A confusing battery of names applies to various stages of the same process. Because it does not have an epithelial lining, the lesion should be called a pseudocyst rather than a cyst. It typically occurs as a translucent dome-shaped nodular process over the dorsal aspect of the interphalangeal joints of the fingers (especially the distal interphalanged joints) and, less commonly, on the toes and sometimes feet.[129] It occurs at any age and is slightly more common in women. The lesion may be covered by wartlike epidermal hyperplasia and/or may be associated with longitudinal grooving of the nail. If it is incised, clear to yellow mucinous fluid may be expressed. Osteoarthritis may afflict the associated joint.

Histologic Features

Histologically, in early lesions one sees the same changes noted earlier for cutaneous focal mucinosis. With time, however, there develops a small pseudocyst without a lining. It later enlarges. The overlying epidermis may be atrophic. The lesion often forms an exophytic nodule surrounded by a collarette of epidermis (Fig. 34–29).[123,129] The connective tissue around the pseudocyst may later become dense and collagenous and may form projections into the pseudocyst. This change is apparently the result of further trauma or chronic pressure. This latter lesion is known as a ganglion (Figs. 34–30 and 34–31).

The term *mucocele* is also used to describe an entirely different process caused by obstruction and subsequent distension of the ducts of the salivary glands.

GENERALIZED MYXEDEMA

Clinical Features

Generalized myxedema occurs as a result of a quantitative

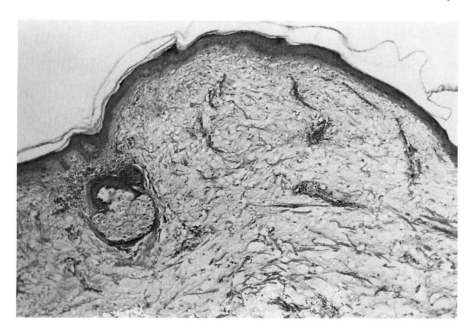

Figure 34–28. Focal mucinosis. Lesion showing mucin and large stellate to spindle-shaped fibroblasts in the papillary dermis (H&E, ×31).

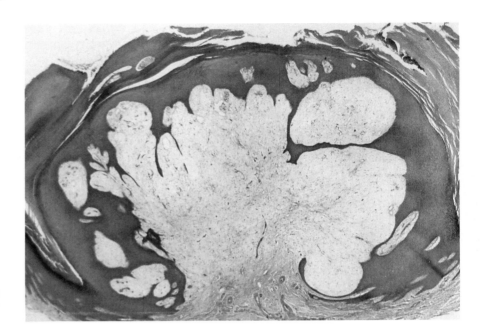

Figure 34–29. Mucous pseudocyst. A mass of mucin and large fibroblasts fills an exophytic nodule (H&E, ×8.1).

or functional deficit of thyroid hormone. Congenital hypothyroidism, or cretinism, is an extremely severe form occurring in infancy, usually as a result of agenesis of the thyroid. In adults, ablative surgery, primary idiopathic hypothyroidism, or any of several other thyroid or pituitary diseases may produce the hypothyroid state.[126] Clinically, lesions usually develop during the course of several months. The noncutaneous findings, such as mental and physical sluggishness and weight gain, are accompanied by accumulation of dermal mucin. The skin around the eyes is involved, the lips are thick, and the nose broad. The tongue is enlarged; the speech may be hoarse. The hands and feet may show a nonpitting edema. Carotenemia may develop be-

cause of an inability of the liver to form vitamin A. The skin is cool, waxy, and dry, with reduced sweat gland function. Ichthiotic changes, pruritus, or eczema craquelé may be noted. Keratotic lesions may occur on the elbows, knees, and buttocks, resembling hypovitaminosis A. The hair is dry and the nails brittle.

Histologic Features

Histological findings include extensive deposition of mucin in the dermis and sometimes in the subcutis, resembling changes encountered in pretibial myxedema (see below). Mild hyperkeratosis with follicular plugging may also be noted.

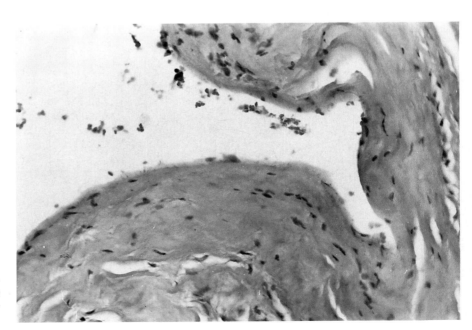

Figure 34–30. Mucous pseudocyst (ganglion, or well-developed, stage) showing the well-developed fibrous wall with no lining epithelium (H&E, ×244).

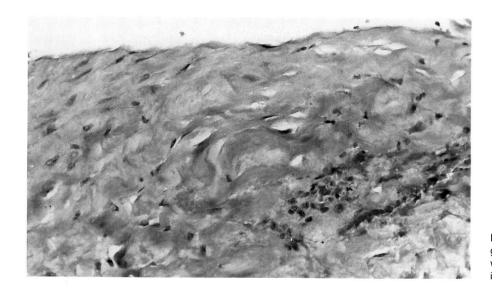

Figure 34–31. Mucous pseudocyst (ganglion, or well-developed, stage) showing the well-developed fibrous wall with no lining epithelium (H&E, ×291).

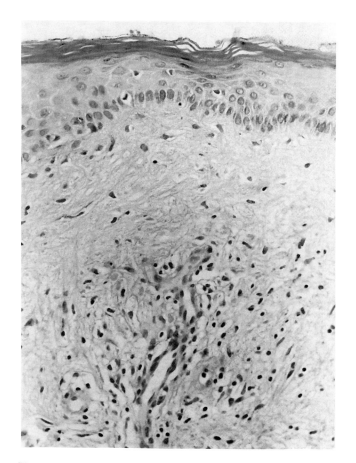

Figure 34–32. Pretibial myxedema, showing deposition of mucinous material in the dermis (H&E, ×35).

PRETIBIAL MYXEDEMA (LOCALIZED MYXEDEMA)

Clinical Features

Pretibial myxedema is produced by excessive amounts of thyroid hormone. The most common association is with Graves' disease. Patients may be euthyroid, however. Skin lesions may occur just after therapy for Graves' disease. Skin signs include elevated temperature and a soft, moist, smooth texture.

Nodules or plaques of dermal mucin appear focally, most commonly on the lower extremities. They are usually bilateral and are flesh colored to yellow or red. Follicular orifices may be very prominent. The overlying skin may become coarse and hyperkeratotic, resembling elephantiasis. Large lesions may be painful.

Histologic Features

Histological findings include accumulation of hyaluramic acid in the dermis and sometimes in the subcutis (Figs. 34–32 through 34–35). Marked hyperkeratosis may be present as well. Those lesions clinically appear verrucous (Fig. 34–36).

SCLEREDEMA (SCLEREDEMA ADULTORUM OF BUSCHKE)

Scleredema occurs in two forms, as a complication of diabetes mellitus and as a sequela of an upper respiratory tract infection.[130] Massive induration of the skin of the dorsal aspect of the upper body and upper extremities occurs in both forms. Histological findings include accumulation of mucin and collagenous material at the interface between subcutaneous fat and dermis, so that the dermis is markedly

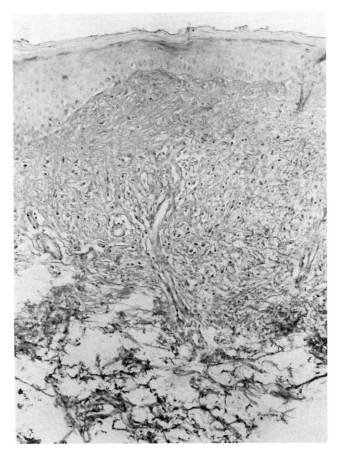

Figure 34–33. Pretibial myxedema, showing deposition of mucinous material in the dermis and extending into the subcutis (colloidal iron, ×8.3).

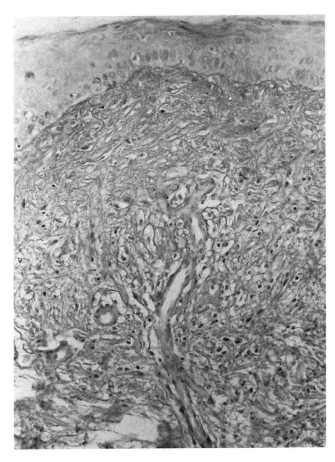

Figure 34–34. Pretibial myxedema, showing deposition of mucinous material in the dermis (colloidal iron, ×32).

thickened. The appendages retain their mantle of fat but are seen to lie much higher than normal in the thickened dermis. The collagen bundles may show "fenestrations," with mucin lying between them.

LICHEN MYXEDEMATOSUS (PAPULAR MUCINOSIS; SCLEROMYXEDEMA)

Lichen myxedematosus is a rare disease consisting of numerous small papules that tend to occur on the upper body. The papules can evolve into a lichenoid form, and several variants of the disease exist. The disease affects adults 30 to 50 years of age. A monoclonal gammopathy is often present, but it does not appear to progress to multiple myeloma. The paraprotein appears to be an IgG in most cases, but IgA and IgM have been found in others.[127,131]

Histological findings include collagen fibers fragmented into a fine fiber meshwork in the dermis and around appendages. These are associated with stellate fibroblasts in places (Fig. 34–37). In generalized disease, known as scleromyxedema, more and larger fibroblasts and more mucin are seen.

RETICULAR ERYTHEMATOUS MUCINOSIS (PLAQUELIKE MUCINOSIS; REM SYNDROME)

Reticular erythematous mucinosis is characterized by widespread, persistent, sharply marginated blue-red macules to plaques on the upper body of adults.[127,132] Women are twice as often affected as men. Plaquelike cutaneous mucinosis is either a very similar condition or a variant of the same condition (the author believes the latter), in which the lesions occur in the same population in the same areas but as papules and/or annular or arciform lesions with palpable borders. Lesions are asymptomatic and may be aggravated by sunlight. No one associated systemic disease occurs, but numerous associations of individual cases with a number of other disorders have been reported. These include thrombocytopenic purpura, hypothyroidism, hyperthyroidism, diabetes mellitus, and cancers of the colon or breast. Both menses and anovulatory agents have also been implicated.

Histological findings include a mild lymphocytic infiltrate, which is more marked at the edge of the lesion, and

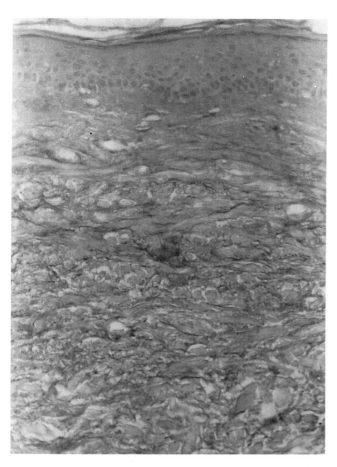

Figure 34–35. Pretibial myxedema, showing deposition of mucinous material in the dermis (alcian blue, ×36).

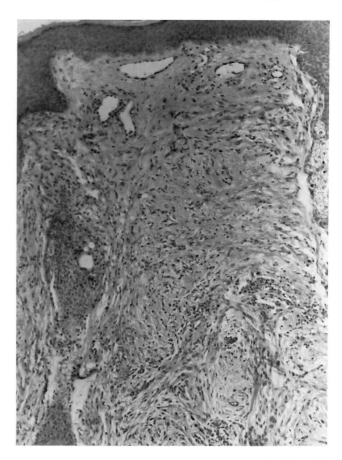

Figure 34–37. Scleromyxedema. Mucinous material and swollen fibroblasts are seen in the dermis (H&E, ×44).

deposition of mucinous material between collagen bundles in the upper dermis. The material is probably hyaluronic acid. These changes are relatively nonspecific (Fig. 34–38).

CUTANEOUS CALCIFICATIONS; OSTEOMA CUTIS

Cutaneous calcifications may occur as part of dystrophic or metastatic calcification (Figs. 34–39 through 34–43), secondary to local trauma or another pathological change in the former case and to metabolic calcium imbalance in the latter, as is true for any other tissue.[133,134] In particular, in late lesions of scleroderma, or in the CREST variant of scleroderma, or in dermatomyositis, calcinosis cutis may occur over extensor surfaces, such as elbows.[135]

In addition, there are several distant variants of calcinosis cutis, as follows:

1. Calcinosis secondary to deposition of calcium in tissues, as from an intravenous line or sometimes percutane-

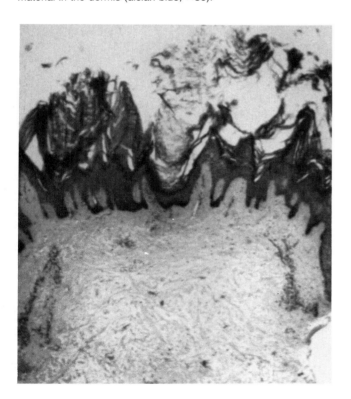

Figure 34–36. Pretibial myxedema, with overlying papillary and hyperkeratotic changes (H&E, ×9.4).

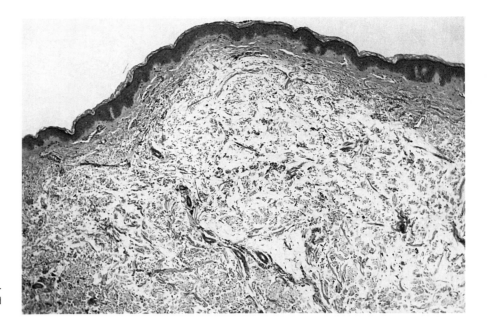

Figure 34–38. Reticular erythematous mucinosis. The dermal structures are separated by mucin (H&E, ×18).

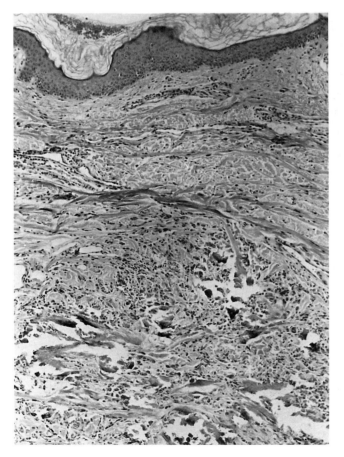

Figure 34–39. Metastatic calcification. Note the diffuse deposits of calcium (H&E, ×28).

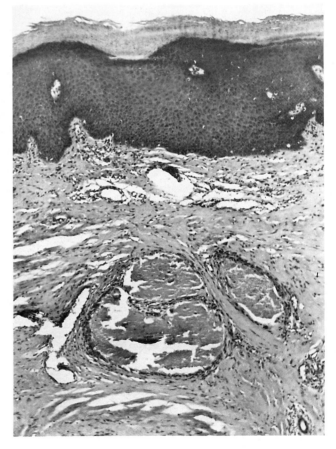

Figure 34–40. Dystrophic calcinosis. Note the well-demarcated areas of calcificaiton (H&E, ×46).

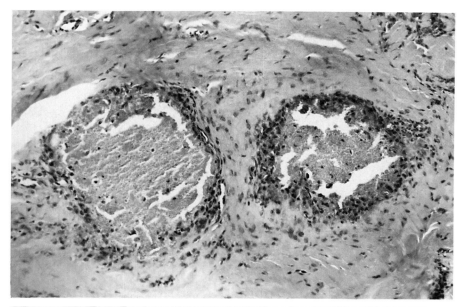

Figure 34–41. Dystrophic calcinosis. Note the well-demarcated areas of calcification and the histiocytic response (H&E, ×94).

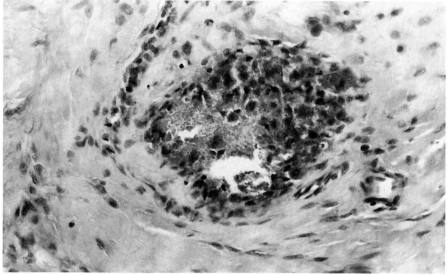

Figure 34–42. Dystrophic calcinosis. Note the histiocytic response with very little calcium present in this early lesion. Early lesions should not be mistaken for a different process (H&E, ×101).

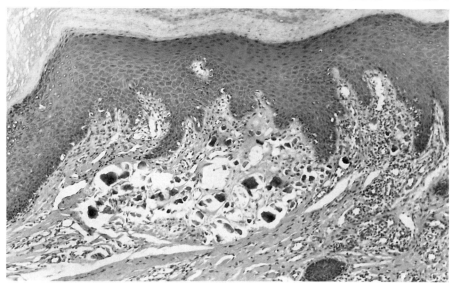

Figure 34–43. Dystrophic calcification. The process is more diffuse than in Figures 34–39 through 34–41 (H&E, ×38).

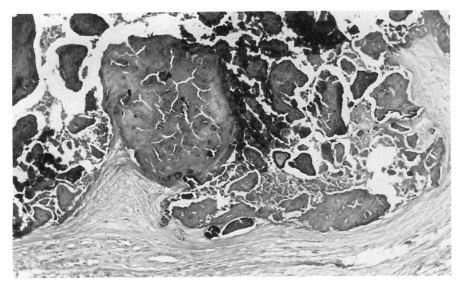

Figure 34–44. Tumoral calcinosis. A large mass of calcified material is seen in the dermis (H&E, ×27).

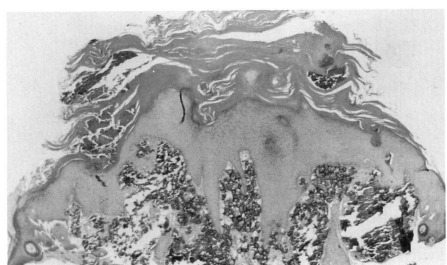

Figure 34–45. Subepidermal calcified nodule, showing exophytic papillated process containing calcified bodies (H&E, ×3.8).

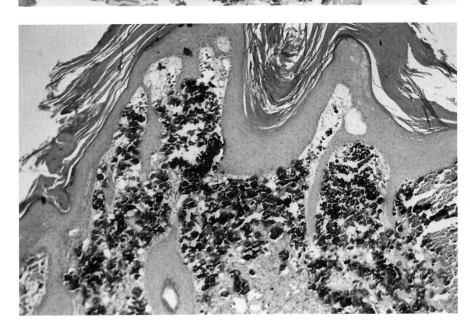

Figure 34–46. Subepidermal calcified nodule. Von Kossa's stain shows calcified bodies in an exophytic papillated process (×24).

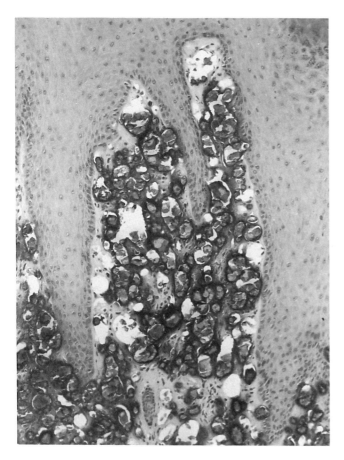

Figure 34–47. Subepidermal calcified nodule. Von Kossa's stain shows calcified bodies in expanded dermal papilla (×103).

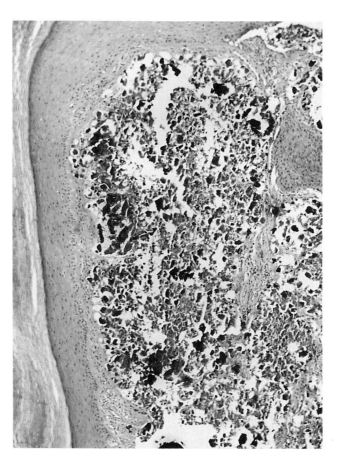

Figure 34–48. Subepidermal calcified nodule. The exophytic process is less well structured than in the classic presentation of this entity. This variant is fairly common (H&E, ×54).

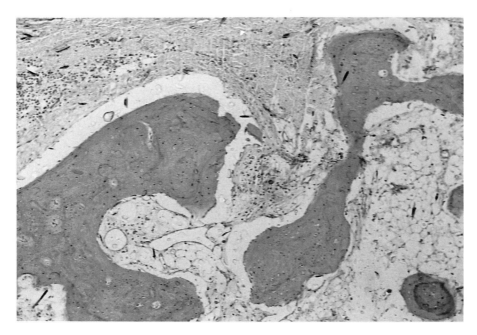

Figure 34–49. Osteoma cutis. Laminated bony trabeculae and fat cells suggestive of attempts at erythropoiesis are seen (H&E, ×88).

ously, as in electroencephalograhic studies. This occurs particularly in children.[136,137]

2. *Nodular (tumoral) calcinosis cutis.* Idiopathically, large tumorous nodules of calcinosis may occur, especially near large joints (Fig. 34–44). This rare process, which is sometimes inherited as an autosomal recessive or dominant condition, is thought to be associated with an abnormality of calcium and phosphate metabolism.

3. *Scrotal calcinosis.*[138,139] Nodular calcified lesions, usually numerous, occur on the scrotum. This pattern may represent dystrophic calcification of cysts.

4. *Subepidermal calcified nodule.*[140] This occurs as a verrucous, hard process in children and young adults. Histological findings include numerous calcified bodies within a verrucous structure (Fig. 34–45 through 34–48). It is thought to arise from a calcification of a previous lesion such as a verruca vulgaris or a nevocellular nevus.

Osteoma cutis is rare. It may occur at any site where a large mass of calcification has accumulated. Bony traebculae, sometimes with fat between them and even primitive attempts at hematopoiesis, may be noted (Fig. 34–49). Where blood dyscrasias are present, these may be reflected in this hematopoietic element.

REFERENCES

1. Breathnach SM. Amyloid and amyloidosis. *J Am Acad Dermatol. 1988; 18:1.*

2. Glenner GG. Amyloid deposits and amyloidosis: the β-fibrilloses. *N Engl J Med.* 1980; 302:1283.

3. Hashimoto K. Diseases of amyloid, colloid, and hyalin. *J Cutan Pathol.* 1985; 12:322.

4. Eanes ED, Glenner GG. X-ray diffraction studies on amyloid filaments. *J Histochem Cytochem.* 1968; 16:673.

5. Termine JD, Eanes ED, Ein D, et al. Infrared globulin proteins. *Biopolymers.* 1972; 11:3.

6. Shirahama T, Cohen AS. High-resolution electron microscopic analysis of the amyloid fibril. *J Cell Biol.* 1967; 33:679.

7. Breathnach SM, Bhogal B, Dyck RF, et al. Immunohistochemical demonstration of amyloid P component in skin of normal subjects and patients with cutaneous amyloidosis. *Br J Dermatol* 1981; 105:115.

8. Skinner M, Pepys MB, Cohen AS, et al. Studies on amyloid protein AP. In: Glenner GG, Pinho e Costa P, Falcao de Freitas A, eds. *Amyloid and Amyloidosis.* Amsterdam, Netherlands: Excerpta Medica: 1980:384.

9. Pepys MB, Baltz ML, de Beer FC, et al. Biology of serum amyloid P component. *Ann NY Acad Sci.* 1982; 389:286.

10. Breathnach SM. The cutaneous amyloidoses: pathogenesis and therapy. *Arch Dermatol* 1985;121:470.

11. Hintner H, Booker J, Ashworth J, et al. Amyloid P component binds to keratin bodies in human skin and to isolated keratin filament aggregates in vitro. *J Invest Dermatol.* 1988; 91:22.

12. Black MM. The nature, pathogenesis and staining properties of amyloid. *Br J Dermatol.* 1972; 87:280.

13. Brownstein MH, Helwig EB. The cutaneous amyloidoses. I: localized forms. *Arch Dermatol.* 1970; 102:8.

14. Cooper JH. An evaluation of current methods for the diagnostic histochemistry of amyloid. *J Clin Pathol.* 1969; 22:410.

15. Puchtler H, Sweat F. Congo red as a stain for fluorescence microscopy of amyloid. *J Histochem Cytochem.* 1965; 13:693.

16. Puchtler H, Sweat F, Levine M. On the binding of Congo red by amyloid. *J Histochem Cytochem.* 1962; 10:355.

17. Shapiro L, Kurban AK, Azar HA. Lichen amyloidosus: a histochemical and electron microscopic study. *Arch Pathol.* 1970; 90:499.

18. Yanagihara M, Mehregan AH, Mehregan DR. Staining of amyloid with cotton dyes. *Arch Dermatol.* 1984; 120:1184.

19. Heyl T: Amyloid staining with thioflavine T in dermatopathology. *Trans St Johns Hosp Dermatol Soc.* 1966; 52:84.

20. Hobbs JR, Morgan AD. Fluorescence microscopy with thioflavine-T in the diagnosis of amyloid. *J Pathol Bacteriol.* 1963; 86:437.

21. Kurban AK. Fluorescent stain for amyloid: an easy histological differentiation between cutaneous amyloidosis, colloid milium and senile elastosis. *Bull Johns Hopkins Hosp.* 1960; 107:320.

22. Vassar PS, Culling CFA. Fluorescent stains, with special reference to amyloid and connective tissues. *Arch Pathol.* 1959; 68:487.

23. Westermark P. Amyloidosis of the skin: a comparison between localized and systemic amyloidosis. *Acta Derm Venereol (Stockh).* 1979; 59:341–345.

24. Wright JR, Calkins E, Humphrey RL. Potassium permanganate reaction in amyloidosis: a histologic method to assist in differentiating forms of this disease. *Lab Invest.* 1977; 36:274.

25. Fujihara S, Balow JE, Costa JC, et al. Identification and classification of amyloid in formalin-fixed, paraffin-embedded tissue sections by the unlabelled immunoperoxidase method. *Lab Invest.* 1980; 43:358.

26. Isobe T, Ossermann EF. Patterns of amyloidosis and their association with plasma cell dyscrasia, monoclonal immunoglobulina and Bence Jones proteins. *N Engl J Med.* 1974; 290:473.

27. Terry WD, Page DL, Kimura S, et al. Structural identity of Bence-Jones and amyloid fibril proteins in a patient with plasma cell dyscrasia and amyloidosis. *J Clin Invest.* 1973; 52:1276.

28. Glenner GG, Ein D, Eanes ED, et al. Creation of "amyloid" fibrils from Bence-Jones proteins in vitro. *Science.* 1971; 174:712.

29. Breathnach SM, Black MM. Systemic amyloidosis and the skin: a review with special emphasis on clinical features and therapy. *Clin Exp Dermatol.* 1979; 4:517.

30. Brownstein MH, Helwig EB. The cutaneous amyloidoses. II: systemic forms. *Arch Dermatol.* 1970; 102:20.

31. Eisen HN. Primary systemic amyloidosis. *Am J Med.* 1946; 1:144.

32. Franklin EC. Amyloid and amyloidosis of the skin. *J Invest Dermatol.* 1976; 67:451.

33. Goltz RW. Systematized amyloidosis: a review of the skin and mucous membrane lesions and a report of two cases. *Medicine.* 1952; 31:381.

34. Higgins WH, Higgins WH Jr. Primary amyloidosis: a clinical and pathological study. *Am J Med Sci.* 1950; 220:610.

35. Kyle RA, Bayrd ED. Amyloidosis: review of 236 cases. *Medicine* 1975; 54:271.

36. Kyle RA, Greipp PR. Amyloidosis (AL): clinical and laboratory features in 229 cases. *Mayo Clin Proc.* 1983; 58:665.

37. Mathews WH. Primary systemic amyloidosis. *Am J Med Sci.* 1954; 228:317.

38. Rubinow A, Cohen AS. Skin involvement in generalized amy-

loidosis: a study of clinically involved and uninvolved skin in 50 patients with primary and secondary amyloidosis. *Ann Intern Med*. 1978; 88:781.

39. Rukavina JG, Block WD, Jackson CE, et al. Primary systemic amyloidosis: a review and an experimental, genetic and clinical study of 29 cases with particular emphasis on the familial form. *Medicine*. 1956; 5:239.

40. Symmers WStC. Primary amyloidosis: a review. *J Clin Pathol*. 1956; 9:187.

41. Barth WF, Willerson JT, Waldmann TA, et al. Primary amyloidosis: clinical, immunochemical and immunoglobulin metabolism studies in fifteen patients. *Am J Med*. 1969; 47:259.

42. Ko HS, Davidson JW, Pruzanski W. Amyloid lymphadenopathy. *Ann Intern Med*. 1976; 85:763.

43. Kuczynski A, Courtenay Evans RJ, Mitchinson MJ. Sicca syndrome due to primary amyloidosis. *Br Med J*. 1971; 2:506.

44. Katz GA, Peter JB, Pearson CM, et al. The shoulder-pad sign: a diagnostic feature of amyloid arthropathy. *N Engl J Med*. 1973; 288:354.

45. Natelson EA, Duncan WC, Macossay CR, et al. Amyloidosis palpebrarum. *Arch Intern Med*. 1970; 125:304.

46. Chapman RS, Neville EA, Lawson JW. Xanthoma-like skin lesions as a presenting feature in primary systemic amyloidosis. *Br J Clin Pract*. 1973; 27:271.

47. Leach WB, Vassar PS, Culling CFA. Primary systemic amyloidosis presenting as scleroderma. *Can Med Assoc J*. 1960; 83:263.

48. Chow C, Burns RE. Bullous amyloidosis: a case report. *Arch Dermatol*. 1967; 95:622.

49. Northover JMA, Pickard JD, Murray-Lyon IM, et al. Bullous lesions of the skin and mucous membranes in primary amyloidosis. *Postgrad Med J*. 1972; 48:351.

50. Wheeler GE, Barrows GH. Alopecia universalis: a manifestation of occult amyloidosis and multiple myeloma. *Arch Dermatol*. 1981; 117:815.

51. Hunter JAA. Primary systemic amyloidosis imitating porphyria cutanea tarda. *Proc R Soc Med*. 1976; 69:235.

52. Winkelmann RK, Peters MS, Venencie PY. Amyloid elastosis: A new cutaneous and systemic pattern of amyloidosis. *Arch Dermatol*. 1985; 121:498.

53. Breathnach SM, Wells GC. Amyloid vascular disease: cord-like thickening of mucocutaneous arteries, intermittent claudication and angina in a case with underlying myelomatosis. *Br J Dermatol*. 1980; 102:591.

54. Benditt EP, Eriksen N. Amyloid protein SAA is associated with high density lipoprotein from normal serum. *Proc Natl Acad Sci USA*. 1977; 74:4025.

55. Glenner GG, Ignaczak TF, Page DL. The inherited systemic amyloidoses and localized amyloid deposits. In: Stansbury JB, Wyngaarden JB, Fredrickson DF, eds. *Metabolic Basis of Inherited Disease*, 4th ed. New York, NY: McGraw-Hill International Book Co., 1978:1308.

56. Sohar E, Gafni J, Pras M, et al. Familial Mediterranean fever: a survey of 470 cases and a review of the literature. *Am J Med*. 1967; 43:227.

57. Muckle TJ. The Muckle-Wells' syndrome. *Br J Dermatol*. 1979; 100:87.

58. Rubinow A, Cohen AS. Skin involvement in familial amyloidotic polyneuropathy. *Neurology*. 1981; 31:1341.

59. Libbey CA, Skinner M, Cohen AS. Use of abdominal fat tissue asirate in the diagnosis of systemic amyloidosis. *Arch Intern Med*. 1983; 143:1549.

60. Westermark P, Stenkvist B. A new method for the diagnosis of systemic amyloidosis. *Arch Intern Med*. 1973; 132:522–523.

61. Black MM. Primary localized amyloidosis of the skin: clinical

variants, histochemistry and ultrastructure. In: Wegelius O, Pasternak A, eds. *Amyloidosis*. London, England: Academic Press, 1976:479–513.

62. Northcutt AD, Vanover MJ. Nodular cutaneous amyloidosis involving the vulva: Case report and literature review. *Arch Dermatol*. 1985; 121:518.

63. Black MM, Wilson Jones E. Macular amyloidosis: a study of 21 cases with special reference to the role of the epidermis in its histogenesis. *Br J Dermatol*. 1971; 84:199.

64. Brownstein MH, Hashimoto K, Greenwald G. Biphasic amyloidosis. *Dermatologica*. 1979; 153:243.

65. Shanon J, Sagher F. Interscapular cutaneous amyloidosis. *Arch Dermatol*. 1970; 102:195.

66. Tay Ch, Dacosta JL. Lichen amyloidosis: clinical study of 40 cases. *Br J Dermatol*. 1970; 82:129.

67. Bedi TR, Datta BN. Diffuse biphasic cutaneous amyloidosis. *Dermatologica*. 1976; 158:433.

68. Brownstein MH, Hashimoto K. Macular amyloidosis. *Arch Dermatol*. 1972; 106:50.

69. Piamphongsant T, Kullavanijaya P. Diffuse biphasic amyloidosis. *Dermatologica*. 1979; 153:243.

70. Wolf M, Tolmach JA. Macular amyloidosis. *Arch Dermatol*. 1969; 99:373.

71. Ogino A, Tanaka S. Poikiloderma-like cutaneous amyloidosis: report of a case and review of the literature. *Dermatologica*. 1977; 155:301.

72. Isaak L. Localized amyloidosis cutis associated with psoriasis in siblings. *Arch Dermatol Syphilol*. 1950; 61:859.

73. Sagher F, Shanon J. Amyloidosis cutis: familial occurrence in three generations. *Arch Dermatol*. 1963; 87:171.

74. Hicks BC, Weber PJ, Hashimoto K. Primary cutaneous amyloidosis of the auricular concha. *J Am Acad Dermatol*. 1988; 18:19.

75. Hashimoto K. Nylon brush macular amyloidosis. *Arch Dermatol*. 1987; 123:633.

76. Van den Bergh WHHW, Starink TM. Macular amyloidosis, presenting as periocular hyperpigmentation. *Clin Exp Dermatol*. 1983; 8:195–197.

77. Black MM, Maibach HI. Macular amyloidosis simulating naevoid hyperpigmentation. *Br J Dermatol*. 1974; 90:461.

78. Ive FA, Wilkinson DS. Diseases of the umbilical, perianal and genital regions: anosacral cutaneous amyloidosis. In: Rook A, Wilkinson DS, Ebling FJG, Champion RH, Burton J, eds. *Textbook of Dermatology*. 4th ed. Oxford, England, Blackwell Scientific Publishers, 1986:2173.

79. Presbury DGC, Griffiths WAD. Coeliac disease with primary cutaneous amyloidosis. *Br J Dermatol*. 1975; 92:109.

80. Kobayashi H, Hashimoto K. Amyloidogenesis in organ-limited cutaneous amyloidosis: an antigenic identity between epidermal keratin and skin amyloid. *J Invest Dermatol*. 1983; 80:66.

81. Masu SI, Hosokawa M, Seiji M. Immunofluorescence studies on cutaneous amyloidosis with anti-keratin antibody. *Tohoku J Exp Med*. 1980; 132:121.

82. Arnold HLJ. Colloid pseudomilium. *Arch Dermatol Syplilol*. 1943; 48:262.

83. Hashimoto K. Diseases of amyloid, colloid and hyaline. *J Cutan Pathol*. 1985; 12:322.

84. Findlay GH, De Beer HA. Chronic hydroquinone poisoning of the skin from skin lightening cosmetics. *S Afr Med J*. 1980; 57:187.

85. Hashimoto K, Kalzman RL, Kang AA, et al. Electron microscopical and biochemical analysis of colloid milium. *Arch Dermatol*. 1975; 111:49.

86. Hashimoto K, Miller F, Bereston EF. Colloid milium: histo-

chemical and electron microscopical studies. *Arch Dermatol.* 1972; 105:684.

87. Yanagihara M, Mehregan AH, Mehregan DR. Staining of amyloid with cotton dyes. *Arch Dermatol.* 1984; 120:1184.

88. Hashimoto K, Black MM. Colloid milium: a final degeneration product of actinic elastoid. *J Cutan Pathol.* 1985; 12:147.

89. Kobayoshi H, Hashimoto K. Colloid and elastic fibre: ultrastructural study on the histogenesis of colloid milium. *J Cutan Pathol.* 1983; 10:111.

90. Caplan RM. Visieral involvement in lipoid proteinosis. *Arch Dermatol.* 1967; 95:149.

91. Caro I. Lipoid proteinosis. *Int J Dermatol.* 1978; 17:388.

92. Hofer P-A. Urbach-Weithe disease (lipoglycoproteinosis; lipoid proteinosis; hyalinosis cutis et mucosae): a review. *Acta Dermatol Venerol (Stockh).* 1973; 53(suppl 71):1.

93. Moy LS, Moy RL, Matscroka LY. Lipoid proteinosis. ultrastructural and biochemical studies. *J Am Acad Dermatol.* 1987; 16:1193.

94. Harper JI, Duguid KP, Stanghton RCD, et al. Oropharangeal and laryngeal lesions in lipoid proteinosis. *J Laryngol Otol.* 1983; 97:77.

95. Fleishmajer R, Nedwick A, Ramos E, et al. Hyalinosis cutis et mucosae: a histochemical staining and analytical biochemical study. *J Invest Dermatol.* 1969; 52:495.

96. Bickers DR. Porphyria: basic science aspects. *Dermatol Clin.* 1986; 4:277.

97. Poh-Fitzpatrick MB. The porphyrias. *Dermatol Clin.* 1987; 5:55–61.

98. Went LN, Klasen EC. Genetic aspects of erythropoietic protoporphyria. *Ann Hum Genet.* 1984; 48:105–117.

99. Grossman ME, Poh-Fitzpatrick MB. Porphyria cutanea tarda: diagnosis, management, and differentiation from other hepatic porphyrias. *Dermatol Clin.* 1986; 4:297.

100. Poh-Fitzpatrick MB. The erythropoietic porphyrias. *Dermatol Clin.* 1986; 4:291.

101. de Verneuil H, Aitken G, Nordmann Y. Familial and sporadic porphyria cutanea: two different diseases. *Hum Genet.* 1978; 44:145–151.

102. de Verneuil H, Beaumont C, Deybach JR, et al. Enzymatic and immunological studies of uroporphyrinogen decarboxylase in familial porphyria cutanea tarda and hepatoerythropoietic porphyria. *Am J Hum Genet.* 1984; 36:613–622.

103. Brodie NJ, Thompson GG, Moore MR, et al. Hereditary coproporphyria. *Q J Med.* 1977; 46:229–241.

104. Brenner DA, Bloomer JR. The enzymatic defect in variegate porphyria studies with human cultured skin fibroblasts. *N Engl J Med.* 1980; 302:765–769.

105. Dean G. *The Porphyrias.* Philadelphia, Pa: JB Lippincott, 1963.

106. Romero G, Glenn BL, Levin EY. Uroporphyrinogen III cosynthetase activity in an asymptomatic carrier of congenital erythropoietic porphyria. *Biochem Genet.* 1970; 4:719–726.

107. DeLeo VA, Poh-Fitzpatrick MB, Matthews-Roth MM, et al. Erythropoietic protoporphyria. *Am J Med.* 1976; 60:8–22.

108. Bloomer JR. Characterization of deficient heme synthase activity in protoporphyria with cultured skin fibroblasts. *J Clin Invest.* 1980; 65:321–328.

109. Bloomer JR, Phillips MJ, Davidson DL, et al. Hepatic disease in erythropoietic protoporphyria. *Am J Med.* 1975; 58:869–882.

110. Granick S, Sassa S, Granick JL, et al. Assays for porphyrins, δ-aminolevulinic acid dehydratase and porphyrinogen synthetase in microliter samples of whole blood: applications to metabolic defects involving the heme pathway. *Proc Natl Acad Sci USA.* 1972; 69:2381–2385.

111. Epstein JH, Tuffanelli DL, Epstein WL. Cutaneous changes in the porphyrias: A microscopic study. *Arch Dermatol.* 1973; 107:689.

112. Ryan EA. Histochemistry of the skin in erythropoietic porphyria. *Br J Dermatol.* 1971; 78:501.

113. Anton-Lamprecht I, Berach A. Histopathology of the skin in erythropoietic porphyria. *Virchows Arch.* 1981; 352:75.

114. Ryan EA, Madill GT. Electron microscopy of the skin in erythropoietic porphyria. *Br J Dermatol.* 1968; 80:561.

115. Lamola A, Doleiden FH. Cross-linking of membrane proteins and protoporphyria-sensitized photohemolysis. *Photochem Photobiol.* 1980; 31:597.

116. Magnus IA. Action spectrum of the skin in porphyria. *Acta Dermatol Venereol (Stockh).* 1982; 100(suppl):47.

117. Gigli I, Schothorst AA, Soter NA, et al. Erythropoietic protoporphyria: photoactivation of the complement system. *J Clin Invest.* 1980; 66:517.

118. Lim HW, Perez HO, Poh-Fitzpatrick MB, et al. Generation of chemotactant activity in serum from patients with erythropoietic protoporphyria and porphyria cutanea tarda. *N Engl J Med.* 1981; 304:212.

119. Lim HW, Poh-Fitzpatrick MB, Gigli I. Activation of the complement system in patients with porphyrias often irradiation in vivo. *J Clin Invest.* 1984; 74:1961.

120. Eisen AZ, Seegmiller JE. Uric acid metabolism in psoriasis. *J Clin Invest.* 1961; 40:1486.

121. Seegmiller JE. Diseases of pruine and pyrimidine metabolism. In: Bandy PK, Rosenberg LE, eds. *Metabolic Control and Disease,* 8th ed. Philadelphia, Pa: WB Saunders Co., 1980:777.

122. Wyngaarden JB, Kelly WN. *Gout and Hyperuricania.* New York, NY: Grune & Stratton; 1976.

123. Johnson WC, Helwig HB. Cutaneous focal mucinosis: a clinicopathologic and histochemical study. *Arch Dermatol.* 1966; 93:13.

124. Johnson WC, Helwig EB. Histochemistry of the acid mucopolysaccharides of skin in normal and certain pathologic conditions. *Am J Clin Pathol.* 1963; 40:123.

125. Montgomery H, Underwood LJ. Lichen myxedematosus: differentiation from cutaneous myxedemas or mucoid states. *J Invest Dermatol.* 1953; 20:213.

126. Schermer DR. Cutaneous myxedematous (mucoid) states. *Cutis.* 1968; 4:939.

127. Truban AP, Roenizk HH. The cutaneous mucinosis. *J Am Acad Dermatol.* 1986; 14:1.

128. Hazelrigg DE. Cutaneous focal mucinosis. *Cutis.* 1974; 14:241.

129. Johnson WC, Graham JH, Helwig EB. Cutaneous myxoid cyst: A clinico-pathologic and histochemical study. *JAMA.* 1965; 191:15.

130. Venensis PY, Powell FC, Su WPD, et al. Scleredema: a review of 33 cases. *J Am Acad Dermatol.*1984; 11:128.

131. Rudner EJ, Mehregan A, Pinkus H. Scleromyxedema: a variant of lichen myxedematosus. *Arch Dermatol.* 1966; 93:3.

132. Braddock SW, Davis CS, Doris RB. Reticular erythematous mucinosis and thrombocytopemic purpura: report of a case review of the world literature, including plaquelike cutaneous mucinosis. *J Am Acad Dermatol.* 1988; 19:859.

133. Anderson HC. Calcific disease. *Arch Pathol Lab Med.* 1983; 107:341.

134. Steward VL, Herling P, Dalinka M. Calcification in soft tissue. *JAMA.* 1983; 250:78.

135. Bowyer SL, Blane CE, Sullivan DB, et al. Childhood dermatomyositis: factors predicting functional outcome and developmental of dystrophic calcification. *J Pediatr.* 1983; 103:882.

136. Goldminz D, Barnhill R, McGuire J, et al. Calcinosis cutis following extravasation of calcium chloride. *Arch Dermatol.* 1988; 124:922.

137. Weeland RG, Roundtree JM. Calcinosis cutis resulting from percutaneous penetration and deposition of calcium. *J Am Acad Dermatol.* 1985; 12:172.

138. Dare AJ, Oxelson RA. Scrotal calcinosis: origin from dystrophic calcification of exocrine duct milia. *J Cutan Pathol.* 1988; 15:142.

139. Harris MD. Idiopathic scrotal calcinosis. *J Pathol.* 1987; 152:238.

140. Shmunes E, Wood MG. Subepidermal calcified nodules. *Arch Dermatol.* 1972; 105:593.

CHAPTER 35
Developmental Defects of the Skin

Thomas D. Horn

Most developmental defects of the skin represent underdevelopment of one or many components of normal cutaneous anatomy or arise from ectopically placed tissue. The following entities exemplify the spectrum of these disorders.

APLASIA CUTIS CONGENITA

Aplasia cutis congenita (ACC) represents a localized or widespread congenital absence of the skin that may be associated with other congenital anomalies or may occur as an isolated finding. The depth of the defect within the skin is variable. ACC is not a homogeneous disorder; rather nine groups have been categorized by Frieden depending upon the constellation of clinical findings.[1] A unifying pathogenesis does not exist.

Clinical Features
The vertex of the scalp is the most common location of ACC and approximately three fourths of lesions are solitary in this location.[2] The defect may have arisen and subsequently healed in utero, resulting in a depressed alopecic patch. Alternatively, ulcers penetrating the dermis, subcutis, and even dura and meninges have been reported.[3] Similarly variable is the surface area of the defect with a range of 0.5 to 100 cm^2 reported.[1]

ACC of the scalp as an isolated finding constitutes Frieden's group 1. Group 2 combines midline scalp lesions with limb abnormalities. The occasional association of ACC with an epidermal nevus or nevus sebaceus and a more serious congenital malformation such as meningomyeloceles defines groups 3 and 4, respectively.[4] In group 5, ACC occurs in a fetus papyraceus or with placental infarcts. Group 6 is associated with epidermolysis bullosa, group 7 with localization to the extremities, group 8 with specific teratogens (e.g., herpes group virus infection[5]), and group 9 with specific syndromes.

Histologic Features
Unfortunately, most reported cases of ACC lack pathological findings. It is, however, clear that the histopathology of ACC depends upon which anatomic layers of the skin are lacking. Absence of the dermis reveals subcutaneous fat[6] as the uppermost tissue, whereas complete absence of skin may expose bone or deeper structures.[3] Changes noted in healed lesions are characteristic of a scar, with dermal fibrosis underlying a flattened epidermis. Adnexal structures are lacking.

ECTODERMAL DYSPLASIA

The term *ectodermal dysplasia* encompasses a wide range of clinical disease of great diversity. Solomon and Keuer suggest three criteria in defining an ectodermal dysplasia.[7] The entity must be (1) congenital, (2) diffusely involving the epidermis and at least one adnexal structure, and (3) not progressive. Overviews of the ectodermal dysplasias are recommended,[7,8] as in this section, only the two most commonly encountered forms, hidrotic and anhidrotic ectodermal dysplasia, are considered.

Clinical Features
Hidrotic ectodermal dysplasia (Clouston syndrome) exhibits autosomal dominant inheritance and consists of hypotrichosis, dysplastic nails, and palmoplantar dyskeratosis.[9] Extreme cases lack hair and nails entirely. Clouston noted additional anomalies including hyperpigmentation, mental retardation, and ocular abnormalities (conjunctivitis, pterygium, strabismus).[9]

Anhidrotic ectodermal dysplasia (Christ-Siemens-Touraine syndrome) occurs predominantly in males and is considered a sexlinked disorder. Patients display anhidrosis or hypohidrosis, hypotrichosis, hypodontia, and possibly onychodysplasia.[10] Difficulty with temperature regulation may result from defective sweating. Atopic dermatitis and hypopigmentation are found frequently. Asthma and upper respiratory tract infections have been noted to occur commonly in anhidrotic ectodermal dysplasia and may result from the lack of glandular structures responsible for producing upper airway secretions.[9,10]

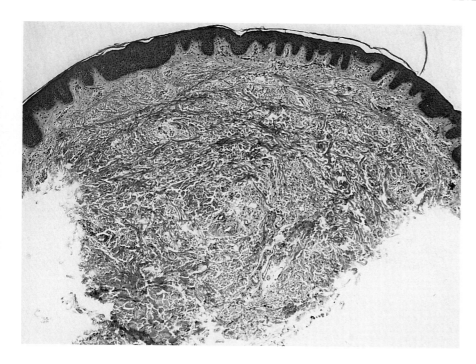

Figure 35–1. This punch biopsy from the buttock of a patient with anhidrotic ectodermal dyplasia shows the absence of any eccrine or pilosebaceous structures. (H&E, ×10.)

Histologic Features

The epidermis and dermal collagen and elastic fiber matrices are generally normal; however, eccrine glands and ducts are either completely absent,[9,11] poorly developed,[11] or present only in localized areas[12] in the anhidrotic form (Fig. 35–1). Hypoplasia and a diminished number of pilosebaceous units characterize the hidrotic and anhidrotic ectodermal dysplasias to varying degrees.[11] Scanning electron microscopy of the hair shafts in anhidrotic ectodermal dysplasia revealed abnormal longitudinal clefting present approximately 1 cm distal to the base of the follicle.[7,13] Chemical analysis of the hair shafts in ectodermal dysplasias has revealed altered sulfur content[13] and abnormally low-molecular-weight proteins.[14]

SUPERNUMERARY NIPPLES (POLYTHELIA)

Most supernumerary nipples reside along a curved line from the anterior axillary fold to the inner thigh known as the embryologic milk line. Underlying breast tissue may be present (polymastia) and may enlarge during puberty or pregnancy. Occasionally, supernumerary nipples and breasts are found near the vulva.[15] The histology of the supernumerary nipple (Fig. 35–2) is that of a normal nipple with abundant dermal smooth muscle bundles. Breast tissue, if present, resembles normally situated breast tissue and varies in size with varying hormonal influence.

ACCESSORY TRAGUS

Accessory tragi arise as a developmental defect of the first pharyngeal arch as it expands to form the mandible and the normal tragus. The second arch accounts for the majority of the external ear. Accessory tragi are present at birth and located in the immediate preauricular area or, less commonly, on the neck, anterior to the sternocleidomastoid muscle.[16] They are flesh-colored papules with variable consistency on palpation and rarely with erosion or inflammation. The majority of accessory tragi occur sporadically, however; rarely do they exist as part of a syndrome.[16,17]

Histologic Features

The accessory tragus occurs as a polypoidal lesion potentially exhibiting all adnexal structures (Fig. 35–3). As noted by Brownstein et al., hair follicles usually contain vellus hair shafts, but a few terminal hairs may be noted.[16] Mature sebaceous glands may be associated with these follicles depending on androgen stimulation. Additionally, eccrine and apocrine glands have been noted. Characteristically, cartilage occupies the center of the polyp, enveloped by often abundant adipose tissue. Occasional accessory tragi lack cartilage. The epidermis and dermis are generally not significantly abnormal.

Differential Diagnosis

Mature cutaneous and connective tissue elements comprise the accessory tragus. The particular combination of fully developed adnexae and a central cartilaginous plate serves to distinguish this lesion from the skin tag, which lacks cutaneous appendages entirely. Branchial cleft cysts, thyroglossal cysts and bronchial cysts are lined by their typical epithelia. Furthermore, a cystic structure is not a feature of an accessory tragus.

SUPERNUMERARY DIGIT

The supernumerary digit typically resides on the ulnar aspect of the base of the fifth finger, and may be completely

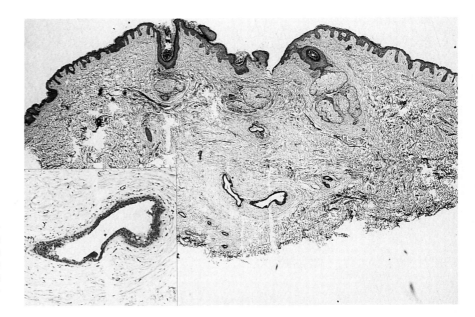

Figure 35–2. An elliptical excision of a supernumerary nipple reveals a ductal structure in the deep dermis surrounded by fibrous tissue and smooth muscle cells. *Inset:* Higher-power view of the duct with evidence of apocrine-type epithelium. (H&E, ×17; inset, ×60.)

formed or, more often, partially developed. Bone, cartilage, and nail structures are variably present. The pathogenesis of supernumerary digits is not known. Familial cases exist.[18] Autoamputation of a sixth finger in utero has been proposed to explain the small papule often present.[19] Some authors, however, suggest that the lesions represent amputation neuromas.[20]

Histologic Features

A variably sized papule exhibiting relatively normal epidermis and dermis is present. Bone and cartilage may be found in the center of the lesion. Adnexal structures are present. A proliferation of nerve trunks at the base of the papule characterizes the supernumerary digit.

Differential Diagnosis

The supernumerary digit must be chiefly differentiated from the acquired fibrokeratoma, which may be located at the base of the fifth finger but which lacks significant neural proliferation at its base. Amputation neuromas can be differentiated only by the history of trauma.

ACQUIRED FIBROKERATOMA

The acquired fibrokeratoma is a conical, hyperkeratotic growth of adults, often with a collarette at its base and usually solitary. Although characteristically situated on a

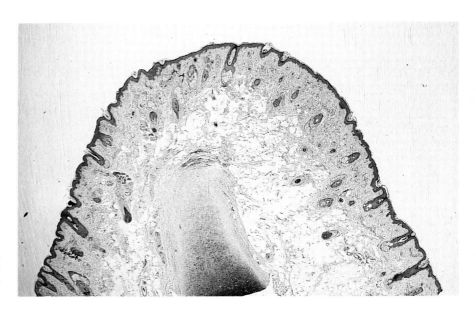

Figure 35–3. Cartilage and abundant adipose tissue constitute the core of this accessory tragus. Numerous vellus hairs are evident. (H&E, ×4.)

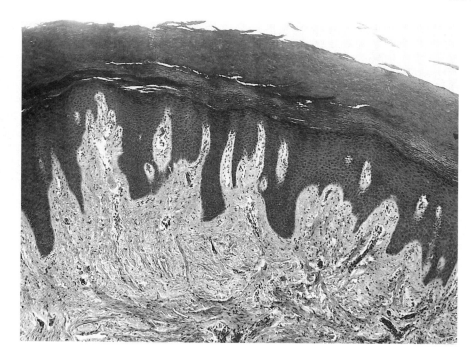

Figure 35–4. The epidermis in this acquired digital fibrokeratoma is irregularly acanthotic with orthohyperkeratosis. The papillary dermis is widened and fibrotic with vertically oriented collagen bundles. (H&E, ×20.)

digit, frequently near a joint, it may occur in other locations, notably the palm and sole.[21]

Histologic Features

Coarse bundles of collagen constitute the center of the tumor, merging smoothly with the underlying dermis. These collagen bundles as well as dilated capillaries are oriented parallel to the long axis of the fibrokeratoma. Generally, the epidermis exhibits acanthosis, hyperkeratosis, and hypergranulosis with prominent rete ridges (Fig. 35–4). The occasional acquired fibrokeratoma may have a thinned epidermis.[22] Elastic fibers are usually sparse or absent and adnexal structures are lacking. Nerve bundles may be located near the base of the lesion, but are not conspicuous.[22] Dermal hyaluronic acid deposition may be increased.[23]

Differential Diagnosis

Acquired fibrokeratomas are histologically distinct from supernumerary digits by the presence in the latter of prominent nerve bundles at the base of the lesion. Additionally, supernumerary digits are congenital and frequently bilateral. Verallo noted that the periungual fibroma associated with tuberous sclerosis may closely resemble histologically the acquired fibrokeratomas that have been reported to occur near the nail plate.[23] Kint and Baran classify the periungual fibroma as a fibrokeratoma and distinguish between lesions arising from dermal connective tissue (acquired digital fibrokeratoma) and those arising from or near the proximal nail fold (tuberous sclerosis and garlic-clove fibroma).[24] A cutaneous horn consists mainly of hyperkeratosis and is associated with an underlying epidermal disorder and thus should not be confused with the acquired fibrokeratoma.

UMBILICAL OMPHALOMESENTERIC DUCT POLYP

The omphalomesenteric (vitelline) duct is the embryologic structure connecting the yolk sac to the midgut, and normally regresses by the sixth to seventh week of development. Persistence of tissue forming this duct may result in an umbilic-enteric fistula, Meckel's diverticulum (most common), sinuses, cysts, or an umbilical polyp.[25] The polyp may present at birth as a brightly erythematous papule, often eroded, which may exhibit a serous, mucoid, serosanguineous, or bloody discharge.[26] Omphalomesenteric duct remnants in deeper soft tissue may coexist with the umbilical polyp and may become symptomatic.

Histologic Features

The hallmark of the umbilical omphalomesenteric duct polyp is ectopic gastrointestinal epithelium of either gastric, small intestine, large intestine, or mixed origin (Fig. 35–5). This epithelium may cover the polyp or line a sinus or cyst within a polyp covered by skin. The junction between skin and gastrointestinal epithelium is abrupt. Secondary changes of erosion in association with acute and chronic inflammation occur in most polyps.[26]

Differential Diagnosis

A finding of mature gastrointestinal epithelium in an umbilical polyp in an infant, child, or young adult should not be readily confused with other entities arising in the umbilical region, such as pyogenic granulomas, urachal remnants, and metastatic lesions. The diagnosis of an umbilical omphalomesenteric duct polyp may signal the presence

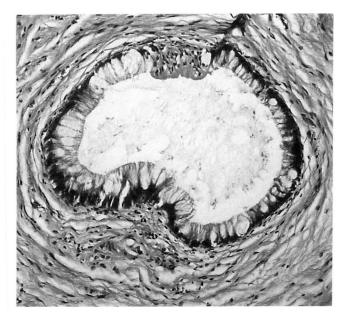

Figure 35–5. Gastrointestinal epithelium with numerous goblet cells in the center of an umbilical polyp characterizes this omphalomesenteric duct remnant. (H&E, ×252.)

of deeper remnants of potential clinical significance later in life, although the frequency of this association remains unknown.[26]

POROKERATOTIC ECCRINE OSTIAL AND DERMAL DUCT NEVUS

Porokeratotic eccrine ostial and dermal duct nevus presents at birth usually on the palm or sole as grouped comedonal papules in a linear array.[27] The involved cutaneous surface is anhidrotic.[27,28] The lesion persists into adult life and is usually unassociated with other congenital cases.[27–30]

The histopathology is distinctive: Columns of parakeratosis characteristic of cornoid lamellae plug dilated eccrine ducts at a middermal level or more superficially. The glandular portion of the eccrine unit is normal.[27] As in porokeratosis elsewhere, hypogranulosis and dyskeratotic epithelial cells are present below the cornoid lamella.[29]

The combination of the characteristic clinical morphology and the presence of cornoid lamellae in dilated eccrine ducts serves to distinguish this lesion from nevus comedonicus, which has been reported to occur on the palms and soles[29] but which lacks a clear association with eccrine structures and the cornoid lamella. Porokeratosis punctata on the palms and soles lacks the typical clinical presentation and eccrine duct involvement of porokeratotic eccrine ostial and dermal duct nevus.

REFERENCES

1. Frieden IJ: Aplasia cutis congenita: A clinical review and proposal for classification. *J Am Acad Dermatol* 1986;14:646–660.
2. Ingalls NW: Congenital defects of the scalp. III. Studies in the pathology of development. *Am J Obstet Gynecol* 1933;25:861–873.
3. Demmel J: Clinical aspects of congenital skin defects. *Eur J Pediatr* 1975;121:21–50.
4. Anderson NP, Novy FG Jr: Congenital defect of the scalp. *Arch Dermatol Syphilol* 1942;46:257–263.
5. Bailie FB: Aplasia cutis congenita of neck and shoulder requiring a skin graft: A case report. *Br J Plast Surg* 1983;36:72–74.
6. Deeken JH, Caplan RM: Aplasia cutis congenita. *Arch Dermatol* 1970;102:386–389.
7. Solomon LM, Keuer EJ: The ectodermal dysplasias. *Arch Dermatol* 1980;116:1295–1299.
8. Freire-Maia N: Ectodermal dysplasias. *Hum Hered* 1971;21:309–312.
9. Clouston HR: The major forms of hereditary ectodermal dysplasia. *Can Med Assoc J* 1939;40:1–7.
10. Reed WB, Lopez A, Lauding B: Clinical spectrum of anhidrotic ectodermal dysplasia. *Arch Dermatol* 1970;102:134–143.
11. Upshaw BY, Montgomery H: Hereditary anhidrotic ectodermal dysplasia. *Arch Dermatol Syphilol* 1949;60:1170–1183.
12. Malagon V, Traveras JE: Congenital anhidrotic ectodermal and mesodermal dysplasia. *Arch Dermatol* 1956;74:253–258.
13. Aoyagi T, Porter PS: Genetic disorders of hair growth: pathogenesis of human hair defects, in Kotori T, Montagna W, Kiyoshi T, et al. (eds): *Biology and Diseases of the Hair.* Baltimore, University Press, 1975, pp 473–488.
14. Hordinsky M, Berry S, Sundby S, et al.: Hair protein patterns in a new autosomal dominant form of ectodermal dysplasia. *J Invest Dermatol* 1987;88:495A.
15. Tow SH, Shanmugaratnam K: Supernumerary mammary gland in the vulva. *Br Med J* 1962;2:1234–1236.
16. Brownstein MH, Wanger N, Helwig EB: Accessory tragi. *Arch Dermatol* 1971;104:625–631.
17. Wildervanck LS: Hereditary malformations of the ear in three generations. *Acta Otolaryngol* 1961;54:553–560.
18. Hare PJ: Rudimentary polydactyly. *Br J Dermatol* 1954;66:402–408.
19. Cummins H: Spontaneous amputation of human supernumerary digits: Pedunculated postminimi. *Am J Anat* 1932;51:381–416.
20. Shapiro L, Juhlin EA, Brownstein MH: Rudimentary polydactyly: An amputation neuroma. *Arch Dermatol* 1973;108:223–225.
21. Hare PJ, Smith PAJ: Acquired (digital) fibrokeratoma. *Br J Dermatol* 1969;81:667–670.
22. Bart RS, Andrade R, Kopf AW, et al.: Acquired digital fibrokeratomas. *Arch Dermatol* 1968;97:120–129.
23. Verallo VVM: Acquired digital fibrokeratomas. *Br J Dermatol* 1968;80:730–736.
24. Kint A, Baran R: Histopathologic study of Koenen tumors. *J Am Acad Dermatol* 1988;18:369–372.
25. Hejazi N: Umbilical polyp: A report of two cases. *Dermatologica* 1975;150:111–115.
26. Steck WD, Helwig EB: Cutaneous remnants of the omphalomesenteric duct. *Arch Dermatol* 1964;90:463–470.
27. Abell E, Read SI: Porokeratotic eccrine ostial and dermal duct nevus. *Br J Dermatol* 1980;103:435–441.
28. Aloi FG, Pippione M: Porokeratotic eccrine ostial and dermal duct nevus. *Arch Dermatol* 1986;122:892–899.
29. Moreno A, Pujol RM, Salvatella N, et al.: Porokeratotic eccrine ostial and dermal duct nevus. *J Cutan Pathol* 1988;15:43–48.
30. Driban NE, Cavicchia JC: Porokeratotic eccrine ostial and dermal duct nevus. *J Cutan Pathol* 1987;14:118–121.

CHAPTER 36
The Perforating Dermatoses

Philip G. Prioleau and Mathew C. Varghese

The term *perforating disorder of skin* has been used to describe a variety of conditions characterized by transepithelial passage of either an altered component of normal body tissue, a product derived from body tissue, or possibly a foreign body. This broad, cumbersome definition has been applied to a variety of unrelated disorders, for many of which transepithelial elimination is only a minor feature of the disease.

Four diseases have commonly been called the major perforating diseases because their most prominent microscopic feature is transepidermal elimination of a substance (Table 36–1): elastosis perforans serpiginosa, perforating folliculitis, reactive perforating collagenosis, and hyperkeratosis follicularis et parafollicularis in cutem penetrans (*Kyrle's disease*).

To these four we have added a fifth condition, which we term *perforating disorder of renal disease*. All patients with this disorder have renal disease and most, but not all, have severe diabetic nephropathy and are on dialysis. This disorder has been variously called reactive perforating collagenosis, hyperkeratosis follicularis et parafollicularis in cutem penetrans (*Kyrle's disease*), and perforating folliculitis; however, the perforating disorder of renal disease differs significantly either clinically or microscopically from the original descriptions of these other diseases, and we believe that it is a distinct entity.

Hyperkeratosis follicularis et parafollicularis in cutem penetrans (*Kyrle's disease*) may not exist. Kyrle's original description is quite detailed, and differs considerably from the perforating disorder of renal disease, although it is conceivable that Kyrle's patient, a diabetic, represents one end of the spectrum of the disorder we have observed in renal disease. Until this can be convincingly demonstrated, however, we prefer to consider Kyrle's disease a separate but extremely rare entity.

PERFORATING DISORDER OF RENAL DISEASE

History

In Kyrle's original description as well as in many subsequent reports, the perforating disorder known as hyperkeratosis follicularis et parafollicularis in cutem penetrans (*Kyrle's disease*) was associated with diabetes mellitus. This disorder has been considered extremely rare, however.

A relatively common association of renal failure with a perforating disease has been observed. In 1982, three groups published cases of a perforating disorder associated with diabetes mellitus and/or renal failure. Although similar clinically and histologically, this disorder was variously termed reactive perforating collagenosis, Kyrle's disease, and perforating folliculitis.[1-4]

Despite the differing names ascribed to these lesions, we believe that each group was describing the same condition. In retrospect, this disorder might better have been termed "perforating disorder of renal disease," as it differs either clinically or histologically from the other known types of perforating disease.

Kyrle's report described a patient with an extremely dense papular eruption with coalescence of papules. This clinical presentation has not been seen in the chronic dialysis/diabetic population. It is conceivable, however, that Kyrle's patient, a severe diabetic, did have the same disorder found in chronic renal disease and represented the far end of a spectrum that we have not observed.

A form of perforating folliculitis is another possibility for its pathogenesis. Clinically, the lesions are in a follicular distribution, but, microscopically, hair follicles are observed only very rarely. Perhaps the two conditions coexist in some cases.

471

TABLE 36–1. PERFORATING DERMATOSES

Disorders	Microscopic Findings	Type of Perforation	Eliminated Material	Pathogenesis
Perforating disorder of renal disease	Dome-shaped papule with crater containing parakeratotic and neutrophilic debris; focal epithelial perforation by collagen	Transepithelial (transfollicular in some cases)	Collagen	Unknown (possibly follicular in some cases)
Reactive perforating collagenosis	Same as above	Transepithelial	Collagen	Necrobiosis of collagen following superficial trauma; probable genetic predisposition
Perforating folliculitis	Follicular and perifollicular inflammation with focal perforation of infundibular epithelial lining	Transfollicular	Basophilic, keratinous debris and degenerated inflammatory cells, collagen, and elastic fibers	Perforation of follicular epithelium caused by hair or friction
Kyrle's disease	Parakeratotic keratinization of all epithelial cells resulting in disruption of epidermis; dyskeratotic cells penetrate dermis, inciting granulomatous reaction	Transfollicular or parafollicular	Basophilic cellular debris	Abnormally rapid keratinization causing disruption of epithelial lining
Elastosis perforans serpiginosa	Accumulation of coarse, thick and clumped elastic tissue in dermal papillae with formation of narrow epidermal channels	Transepidermal, transfollicular, and parafollicular	Elastic fibers with basophilic cellular debris	Primary defect of elastin with structural alteration
Perforating granuloma annulare	Necrobiosis in papillary dermis	Transepidermal	Cellular debris and mucinous material	Unknown
Perforating pseudoxanthoma elasticum	Alteration of elastic fibers in reticular dermis	Transepidermal	Altered basophilic elastic fibers	Unknown; probably an acquired focus of pseudoxanthoma elasticum with only localized cutaneous manifestation

A variant of reactive perforating collagenosis was thought to be another possibility because it was similar microscopically to the disorder described by Mehregan et al.[1,5] On close examination, strands of collagen can usually be seen perforating the epidermis. Although the perforating disorder of renal disease appears grossly and microscopically similar to the reactive perforating collagenosis of Mehregan et al., the latter is an extremely rare disease that arises in infancy or early childhood. In some cases, the entity described by Mehregan et al. appears to be hereditary. This clinical presentation, therefore, does not resemble the disorder seen in chronic renal disease.

Clinical Features

All patients with this disorder have chronic renal disease and most have diabetic nephropathy and retinopathy. The disease appears to be relatively common in the dialysis populus and has been found in 4.5% to 10% of the patients undergoing dialysis. Most of the patients are black, and have advanced diabetes mellitus as evidenced by the presence of diabetic retinopathy. The ages have ranged from the third to the ninth decades with a median age of 55. The skin lesions consist of numerous umbilicated, hyperpigmented papules, which range in diameter from 2 to 10 mm, each containing a central plug. They occur mainly on the extensor surfaces of the extremities, particularly around knees and elbows. They may also be present on the trunk and, rarely, the face.

Almost all have associated pruritus which is often intense. The Koebner phenomenon is also common.

Without treatment, the lesions tend to persist. Spontaneous resolution does occur, however, and results in atrophic scars.

Although all cases have been associated with renal

disease, and almost all of these have had diabetic nephropathy, this perforating disorder has been seen in nondiabetic patients with obstructive uropathy and hypertensive nephrosclerosis, anuria, and chronic nephritis.[2] Usually this disorder is associated with dialysis; however, it has also been observed in patients who have never received dialysis.

Pathogenesis

The pathogenesis of this disorder is unknown. Although these papules are usually pruritic and show clinical and microscopic evidence of rubbing, the microscopic picture differs significantly from that of prurigo nodularis.

It is possible that the perforating disorder of renal disease represents an old folliculitis, as these patients usually have lost much of the hair on their extremities. Hurwitz et al. described hair shafts in the infundibular wall or site of infundibular perforation of nondiabetic patients on dialysis, and they hypothesized that the disorder is a form of perforating folliculitis and that the hair shaft is often removed by rubbing and scratching[4]; however, the rarity with which follicular remnants are seen does not support this pathogenesis in all cases.

Another possibility may be that the extruded collagen is altered and is therefore rejected from the dermis; however, microscopically altered collagen has not been demonstrated.

Histologic Features

There is a dome-shaped papule with a central crater filled with parakeratotic debris and neutophils. The diameter of the crater may vary considerably from the size of the infundibulum of a terminal hair follicle to one many times larger. The base is usually only at the papillary dermal or upper reticular dermal level (Fig. 36–1A).

The base of the crater may or may not have an epithelial lining. Bundles of collagen can be seen penetrating through this epidermis, or occasionally directly into the crater if no lining is present. Multiple step-sections may be required to demonstrate this finding (Figs. 36–1B,C).

Large collections of neutrophils may be present within the crater, within the epithelial lining, or in the adjacent upper dermis (Fig. 36–2). Within the upper and middermis, there is a moderately dense predominantly perivascular infiltrate which consists of lymphocytes and histiocytes as well as neutrophils. Rarely, the inflammation extends to the subcutaneous fat.

The epithelium adjacent to the crater is quite hyperplastic with a prominent granular layer and a thickened compact orthokeratotic layer, which suggest chronic rubbing. The cornified material within the crater is usually parakeratotic. The epithelial lining of the crater wall may comprise cells with abundant, pale cytoplasm with more intracytoplasmic glycogen than the adjacent epithelium. There is a reactive vascular hyperplasia below the crater, and the vessels at the tips of adjacent dermal papillae are frequently dilated with prominent endothelial cells.

Rarely, a fragmented hair shaft is present within the crater. In our experience, these are found in the smaller-diameter, deeper craters which resemble a follicular infundibulum (Fig. 36–3).

Differential Diagnosis

In a patient with severe renal disease, the lesions are quite characteristic, but could possibly be confused with perforating folliculitis, Majocchi's granuloma, or prurigo nodularis. Lack of a demonstrable hair shaft, or presence of a fungus or presence of a crater with collagen perforating through the epidermis helps to exclude these disorders.

REACTIVE PERFORATING COLLAGENOSIS

History

Mehregan et al. first recorded the classic form of reactive perforating collagenosis in 1967.[5] They described a 6½-year-old girl who developed an eruption of her upper and lower extremities at age 9 months, and, noting a Koebner phenomenon, they postulated that superficial trauma altered the collagenous tissue and precipitated these lesions.

Clinical Features

The classic form of reactive perforating collagenosis is a rare disorder beginning in early childhood in which traumatically altered collagen is extruded by the process of transepidermal elimination.

Characteristically, this disorder arises in early childhood as tiny papules on exposed surfaces, but it may also occur on the trunk. Over a several-week period, the papules progress to 5 to 10 mm centrally umbilicated papules with erosions, and in 6 to 8 weeks, they regress, leaving a small scar with altered pigmentation.[6] The lesions are precipitated by superficial trauma; deep trauma such as surgical incision may fail to cause them. At any one time, these papules are in varying stages of development. The Koebner phenomenon is characteristic and has been demonstrated experimentally.[7] Lesions have arisen in sites of acne vulgaris.

Males and females are equally affected. Although sporadic cases have been reported, Nair et al. reported a father and three children with reactive perforating collagenosis, which suggests an autosomal dominant mode of inheritance in at least some cases.[8]

The disorder lasts many years and is less active during the summer months. It appears to be primarily a disease of childhood, although it has been reported in adulthood. The classic form has no associated diseases.

Pathogenesis

The pathogenesis is unknown. A possible cause is an abnormality of collagen precipitated by superficial trauma.

Histologic Features

In their original description, Mehregan et al. studied lesions at different stages of development.[5] Early, nonumbilicated papules were characterized by moderately acanthotic epidermis. The central widened dermal papillae contained connective tissue, which stained a bluish color with hematoxylin and eosin. No inflammatory infiltrate was present, and the suprapapillary epidermis was atrophic and contained a thin layer of parakeratotic cells.

A well-developed lesion shows a dome-shaped papule with a central crater filled with basophilic keratinous and

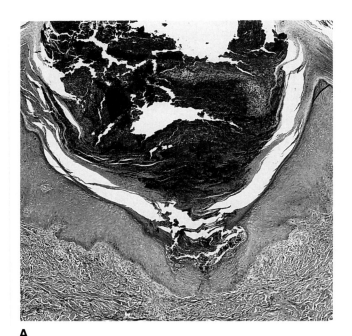

A

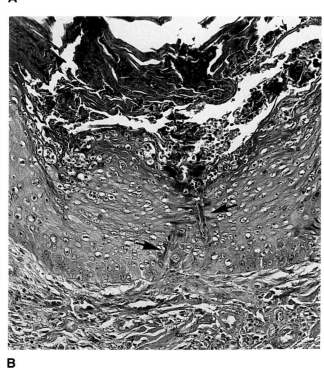

B

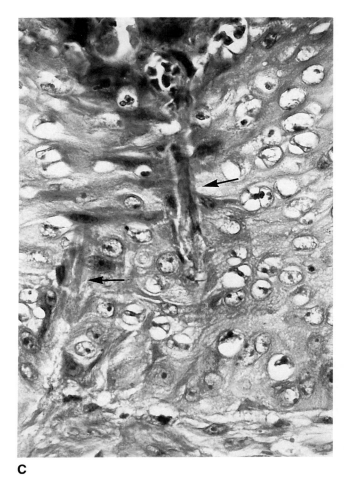

C

Figure 36–1. Perforating disorder of renal disease. **A.** Central crater contains keratinous debris. Adjacent hyperkeratosis with epidermal hyperplasia is characteristic. **B.** Base of crater containing parakeratotic and neutrophilic material. Collagen bundles perforate epithelium (arrows). **C.** Epithelial perforation by collagen bundles (arrows). (H&E, **A,** ×100; **B,** ×250; **C,** ×400.)

neutrophilic cellular debris as well as neutrophils. Epithelial cells line much of the crater, but are often absent at the base. Collagen bundles pass through this epithelium, and are easily demonstrable with a Fontana-Mason stain. Collagen bundles also extend from the dermis through the non-epithelialized portion into the base of the crater. Elastic tissue is not seen. By light microscopy, no abnormalities of collagen can be detected. The epidermis adjacent to the crater is moderately hyperplastic, and there is a thickened

orthokeratotic layer. These adjacent findings are similar to those of lichen simplex chronicus or prurigo nodularis, and indicate that the lesion was probably rubbed. Electron microscopic studies have confirmed the light microscopic findings; however, it is interesting that the collagen fibers being eliminated have a relatively normal configuration and periodicity and do not show substantial alteration.[9] Elastin is not concentrated at the site and usually does not perforate with the collagen.

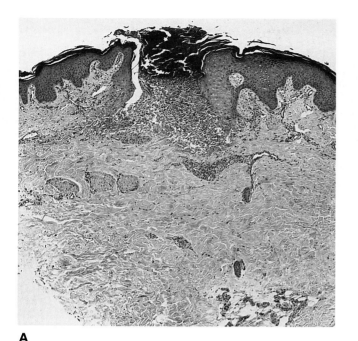

A

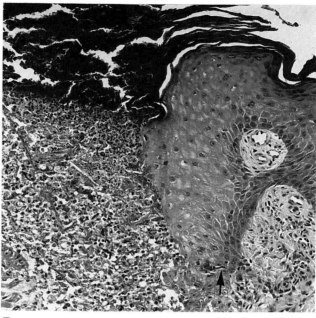

B

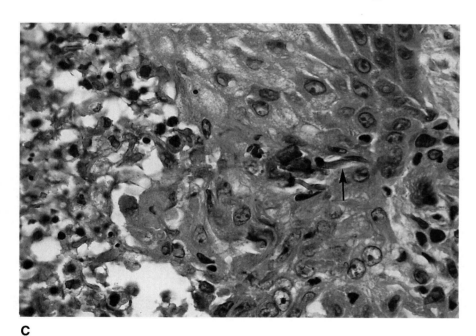

C

Figure 36–2. Perforating disorder of renal disease. **A.** Dome-shaped papule with central crater. **B.** Epithelial lining of base of crater is disrupted. Note the vascular dilatation with prominent endothelial cells and abundant neutrophilic debris. Collagen perforates epithelium (arrow). **C.** Bundles of collagen perforate epithelial lining (arrow). (H&E, **A,** ×25; **B,** ×250; **C,** ×400.)

Differential Diagnosis

Reactive perforating collagenosis must be differentiated from perforating folliculitis, Majocchi's granuloma, Kyrle's disease, elastosis perforans serpiginosa, and the perforating disorder of renal disease.

PERFORATING FOLLICULITIS

History

In 1968, Mehregan and Coskey described 25 patients with a discrete, keratotic, follicular eruption that involved mainly the extremities. They termed this disorder *perforating folliculitis.*[10]

Clinical Features

Perforating folliculitis is a not-uncommon disorder characterized by disruption of the follicular infundibulum with perforation. It appears as slightly elevated erythematous, follicular papules 2 to 8 mm in diameter. A central keratin-filled crater is present.

The papules usually occur on the extremities, especially the hair-bearing areas of the arms, forearms, thighs, and buttocks, and are usually asymptomatic or, less commonly

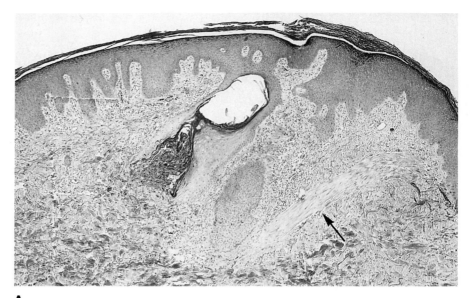

A

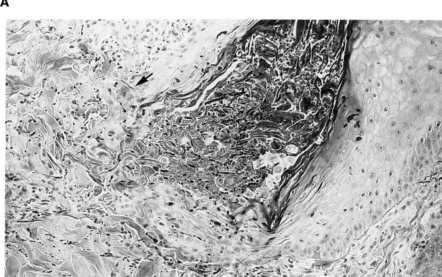

Figure 36–3. Perforating folliculitis in patient with renal disease. **A.** Note arrector pili muscle (arrow). Hair shaft was noted in other sections. **B.** Keratinous and neutrophilic debris are within follicle which shows focal perforation (left). Perforating bundle of collagen is present (arrow). (H&E, ×250) (*continued.*)

B

are associated with mild pruritus. The papules may be widely scattered.

Mehregan's original report included 17 women and 8 men who ranged from 10 to 64 in age, the average being 29.[10]

This disorder may last several months to several years and may show periods of remission and exacerbation.

Perforating folliculitis has been associated with psoriasis, juvenile acanthosis nigricans, and arteriosclerotic cardiovascular disease with hypertension. Reports have also linked this disorder with diabetes mellitus and renal failure, but in our opinion this represents a disorder best placed in a separate category.

Pathogenesis

The pathogenesis of perforating folliculitis is not known. Mehregan, in 1977, noted a great reduction in the prevalence

and speculated that the causative factor had been at least partially eliminated.[6] He suspected formaldehyde in clothing and demonstrated its presence in cloth material, but could not elicit an allergic reaction in skin tests.

Burkhart believed that the most significant factor is perforation of the follicular epithelium and not the elimination of connective tissue.[11] As perforating folliculitis usually occurs on the extensor surfaces, it is quite possible that friction may be an important causative factor.

Histologic Features

By light microscopy, the follicular infundibulum is dilated and contains an admixture of keratinous debris and degenerated inflammatory cells (Fig. 36–4). With step-sectioning, focal perforations of the infundibular lining can be found through which necrotic tissue, collagen, and elastic fibers can gain access to the follicular cavity. Curled-up hair is

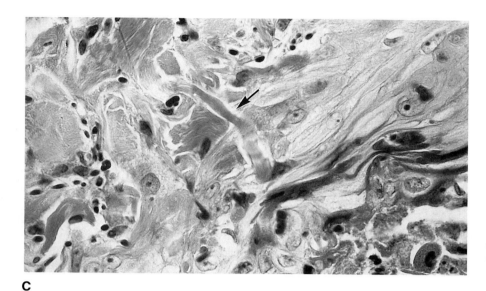

Figure 36–3.C. (*continued*) Collagen bundle perforates epithelium (*arrow*). (H&E, ×400)

C

often present within the keratinous plug, but cannot always be demonstrated. Sometimes the hair is within the dermis where it incites a foreign body reaction.

The dermis shows a mild, perifollicular, inflammatory infiltrate with degenerative changes of elastic fibers at the perforation site. The adjacent epidermis exhibits slight reactive hyperplasia.

Differential Diagnosis

Majocchi's granuloma and bacterial folliculitis are most readily confused with perforating folliculitis. Acne vulgaris, oil folliculitis, and other perforating diseases such as reactive perforating collagenosis, perforating disorder of renal disease, and elastosis perforans serpiginosa must also be considered.

HYPERKERATOSIS FOLLICULARIS ET PARAFOLLICULARIS IN CUTEM PENETRANS (KYRLE'S DISEASE)

History

In 1916, Kyrle described a 22-year-old diabetic woman with numerous papules with central hyperkeratotic plugs, and termed this condition *hyperkeratosis follicularis et parafollicularis in cutem penetrans.*[12] Kyrle's illustrations show hundreds of keratotic papules; some are discrete and others coalesce into plaques (Fig. 36–5A). The number of papules is far greater than we have observed in the perforating disorder of renal disease; however, Kyrle's microscopic illustrations show changes quite similar to those we observed in patients with renal disease.

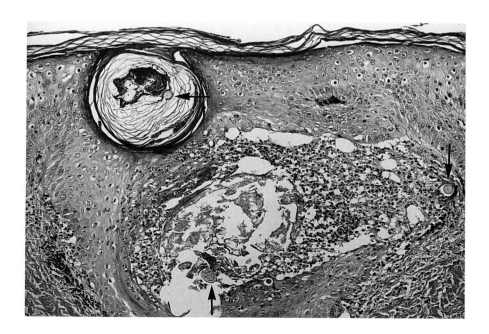

Figure 36–4. Perforating folliculitis. Dilated infundibulum contains keratinous debris with neutrophils and fragmented hair shafts (arrows). Epithelial lining is disrupted (far right). (H&E, ×100.)

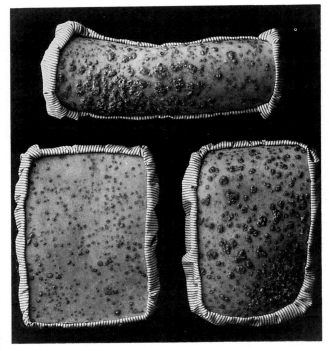

A

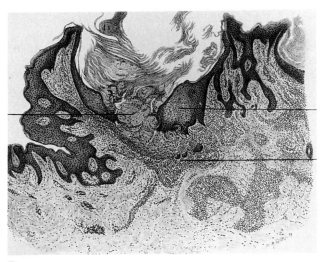

B

Figure 36–5. Hyperkeratosis follicularis et parafollicularis in cutem penetrans (Kyrle's disease). **A.** Numerous, sometimes coalesced papules as illustrated in Kyrle's original paper. **B.** Illustration from Kyrle's original paper showing centrally umbilicated papule filled with keratinous material. (*From Ref. 12.*)

Whether hyperkeratosis follicularis et parafollicularis in cutem penetrans is a distinct entity has been a source of debate. Mehregan, in 1977, stated that he believed that Kyrle's disease was not a distinctive clinicopathologic entity, but represented a histologic pattern of tissue reaction produced by a variety of conditions, including perforating folliculitis, hypertrophic Darier's disease, and keratosis pilaris.[6]

The presence of diabetes mellitus in Kyrle's original patient suggests that Kyrle might have been describing the same clinicopathologic condition that has subsequently been observed in patients with renal disease. Abele and Dobson described the first case of Kyrle's disease in the American literature. Their patient, a 36-year-old black man, also had diabetes mellitus, which they described as poorly controlled, and numerous related complications.[13]

Clinical Features

The eruption can occur everywhere on the body except the palms, soles, and mucosae. The primary lesion is a pinhead-shaped papule, which is skin-colored or grayish. Most but not all lesions are follicular.

The lesions subsequently develop into dome-shaped papules with central keratotic plugs. Usually, they are discrete and scattered, especially over the proximal thighs and around the elbows, but sometimes they are extremely prevalent and have coalesced into plaques. This coalescence is especially well illustrated by Kyrle[12] and Aram et al.[14]

The average age of onset is 30 years, and there is no sexual predilection. The eruption may be asymptomatic or pruritic. Most patients have a disturbance of carbohydrate metabolism; many patients are diabetic.

A major problem in reviewing reported cases of hyperkeratosis follicularis et parafollicularis in cutem penetrans is determining which patients should have been classified as having this disease. In 1968, Carter and Constantine carefully reviewed the previously reported cases and accepted only 12 of the 45 so designated in the literature.[15,16]

The patient that Kyrle reported had diabetes mellitus. Carter and Constantine hypothesized that hyperkeratosis follicularis et parafollicularis in cutem penetrans might be an unusual manifestation of the diabetic syndrome.[15] Hepatic insufficiency and congestive heart failure have also been associated with Kyrle's disease.

The disease tends to be persistent. No patients have been recorded as "cured," but correction of the associated systemic disease has resulted in clearing of the cutaneous lesions of Kyrle's disease.[15]

Pathogenesis

The pathogenesis of Kyrle's disease has been ascribed to an abnormal keratinization process that forms a keratotic plug. The keratinization proceeds faster than the adjacent normal epithelial proliferation, with resulting abnormal keratinization of the epidermis in all layers of that focus. This causes disruption of the epidermis, release of horny material, and a resulting foreign body reaction.[16]

Because of the improved results with tretinoin, Petrozzi and Warthan hypothesized that the keratinization is excessive in comparison with epidermal perforation, and that this may be important in the pathogenesis of this disorder.[17]

Histologic Features

The lesions, which may be either follicular or parafollicular, have an epithelial invagination filled with a keratotic plug that is partly parakeratotic. In addition, there is basophilic cellular debris, which does not stain with elastic tissue stains. There is abnormal parakeratotic keratinization of all the epithelial cells, including the basal cells in at least one region of the plug. Here, there are keratinized cells within the dermis accompanied by a granulomatous reaction and disruption of the epidermis (Fig. 36–5B).[16]

Constantine and Carter also noted that the epidermis surrounding the keratotic plug was acanthotic. Frequently, there was thinning of the epidermis with a parakeratotic horny layer. Neutrophils were sometimes observed and a lymphocytic infiltrate was present.[16]

Differential Diagnosis
Kyrle's disease must be differentiated from prurigo nodularis, perforating folliculitis, elastosis perforans serpiginosa, reactive perforating collagenosis, and the perforating disorder of renal disease.

ELASTOSIS PERFORANS SERPIGINOSA

History
Elastosis perforans serpiginosa was first clearly described by Lutz as keratosis follicularis serpiginosa.[18] Beening and Ruiter reported an association with Down's syndrome.[19]

Elastosis perforans serpiginosa is a not-too-rare disorder in which abnormal elastic fibers are extruded through the epidermis. It affects males four times more frequently than females, can be familial, and usually presents in the third decade, with 90% of patients being under age 30.

The lesions of elastosis perforans serpiginosa are usually confined to one anatomic site with areas of predilection in the following order: (1) nape and sides of neck, (2) upper extremities, (3) face, (4) lower extremities, and (5) trunk.[20] Disseminated elastosis perforans serpiginosa has been reported.

Characteristically, the lesions start as keratotic papules which may be skin-colored or erythematous. They measure 2 to 5 mm in diameter, and may be in either an annular or a serpiginous distribution. Sometimes, no arrangement is observed initially. Frequently, there is symmetry of these papules with contralateral involvement such as on both sides of the neck. Satellite lesions may occur. Usually, they are asymptomatic, although mild pruritus may be present. The Koebner phenomenon has been observed.

Individual lesions last from about 6 months to 5 years, and then involute spontaneously, leaving a superficial scar. New lesions often form as older ones resolve and the condition may be quite persistent.

Elastosis perforans serpiginosa has been associated with numerous diseases, Mehregan having noted an association in 26% of his cases.[20] The most common associations are Down's syndrome, Ehlers-Danlos syndrome, osteogenesis imperfecta, pseudoxanthoma elasticum, and Marfan's syndrome. Less commonly associated conditions are argyria, Rothmund-Thomson syndrome, systemic sclerosis, and morphea.

Pathogenesis
The exact cause of elastosis perforans serpiginosa is not known; however, there appears to be a primary defect of elastin with alteration of both the chemical composition and the morphologic configuration.

Patterson has reviewed the possible pathogenic mechanisms in detail.[23] He theorizes that elastosis perforans serpiginosa may be the final common pathway for more than one abnormality of elastic fibers, as both genetic and environmental factors have been implicated in some, but not all, cases.

It is well documented that copper is essential to the formation of elastin. Penicillamine chelates copper, a necessary cofactor of lysyl oxidase, and copper deficiency results in a decrease in the elastin covalently incorporated into fibers. Patients with Wilson's disease treated with penicillamine occasionally develop an elastosis perforans serpiginosa–like disorder, but ultrastructural studies show morphologic changes that differ from idiopathic elastosis perforans serpiginosa.[24] Not all patients with penicillamine-treated Wilson's disease developed this disorder. Furthermore, those with Menkes' kinky-hair syndrome, a disorder of copper deficiency, do not develop elastosis perforans serpiginosa. Therefore, copper is likely important but only in combination with other not-yet-identified factors.

Histologic Features
Mehregan performed step-sections and found areas of perforation in the form of narrow channels.[20] These occur in completely transepidermal, parafollicular, or transfollicular positions, and may have a straight vertical or corkscrew configuration. When transected, they can resemble asbestosis.

Peripherally, within these channels, there is loose parakeratotic, keratinous material; centrally, there is a basophilic, staining, necrobiotic mass consisting of a mixture of degenerating epithelial cells, nuclei of inflammatory cells, and fibers. Slight adjacent epithelial hyperplasia is present.

Elastic tissue stains show abundant, clumped elastic tissue within the upper papillary dermis (Fig. 36–6A). These fibers appear thicker than normal and extend across the basement membrane. The fibers within the dermis stain as elastic tissue, but as they enter the perforating channel, they lose their characteristic staining quality. Focal granulomatous inflammation may be present. In some areas, there may be strikingly widened dermal papillae containing collections of this abnormal elastic tissue (Fig. 36–6B).

By electron microscopy, the papillary dermis is filled with coarse, thick elastic fibers. These large-caliber fibers have an amorphous quality with low electron density, with fine, dense feltwork at the edges.[21] The fibers have a branching configuration, and there are numerous fine, surface filaments that resemble normal embryonic elastic fibers.[22]

Differential Diagnosis
The differential diagnosis includes perforating granuloma annulare, porokeratosis, and perforating pseudoxanthoma elasticum.

DISORDERS ASSOCIATED WITH OCCASIONAL EPIDERMAL PERFORATION

Epithelial perforation with transepidermal elimination has been reported in several other unrelated diseases; however, transepidermal elimination appears as only a minor compo-

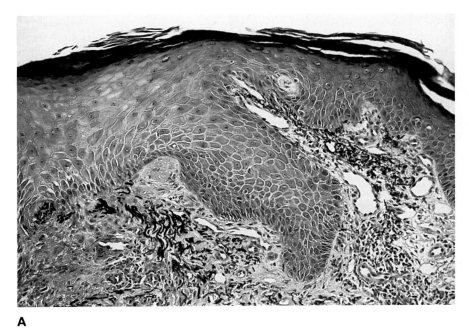

A

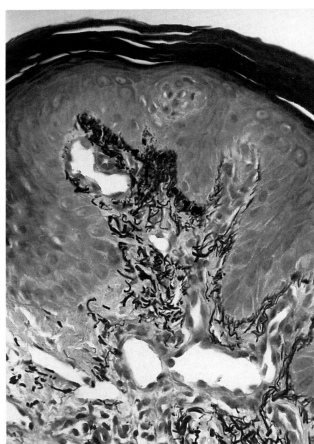

Figure 36–6. Elastosis perforans serpiginosa. **A.** Dome-shaped papule showing collections of black-staining elastic tissue in dermal papillae. Verhoeff–van Gieson elastic tissue stain. **B.** Different microscopic field shows collections of elastic tissue in dermal papilla with dilated blood vessels and prominent endothelial lining. (**A,** ×100; **B,** ×250.)

B

nent of the pathologic process in these. The important disorders with this occasional finding are granuloma annulare and perforating pseudoxanthoma elasticum, although various other disorders also show occasional epidermal perforation with transepidermal elimination.

Perforating Granuloma Annulare

History
Civette (1952)[25] and Calvan (1953)[26] observed epidermal perforation in granuloma annulare. Civette described ulcerative forms of granuloma annulare which he called tuberculo-ulcerous granuloma annulare. Owen and Freeman and others[27–30] have confirmed these observations.

Clinical Features
Most of the occurrences reported have been on the extremities of children and have been associated with generalized granuloma annulare. The skin lesions begin as flesh-colored papules; these enlarge and then develop an umbilication with a crust. Often there is a collarette of scale around the crust. The Koebner phenomenon is not present.[29,30]

Diabetes has been reported rarely in association with generalized perforating granuloma annulare.[28]

Pathogenesis
The pathogenesis of granuloma annulare and its perforating variant is unknown.[29]

Histologic Features
Histological findings vary with the clinical stage of development of these lesions.[27,30] In well-developed nonumbilicated papules, accumulations of necrobiotic tissue surrounded by palisading histiocytes and a lymphocytic inflammatory infiltrate are present in the papillary dermis. Multinucleated giant cells may also be seen. The inflammatory cells extend into epidermis in foci through which transepidermal elimination occurs later.

In well-developed umbilicated papules, there are epidermal perforations that communicate with areas of necrobiosis in the papillary dermis. The perforating channel contains a column of cellular debris, necrotic tissue, and mucinous material. Adjacent to the site of perforation, there are mild acanthosis and hyperkeratosis. These necrobiotic areas perforating through the epidermis are located in the superficial dermis and are surrounded by palisading histiocytes. Similar areas of necrobiosis, characteristic of granuloma annulare, are present in the deeper dermis. Follicular perforation with elimination of necrobiotic material in the dermis through a hair follicle has also been noted.[31] The necrobiotic plug contains no elastic or collagen fibers.[27,30]

Differential Diagnosis
The differential diagnosis includes other disorders with epithelial perforation such as elastosis perforans serpiginosa, perforating pseudoxanthoma elasticum, and perforating rheumatoid nodule.

Perforating Pseudoxanthoma Elasticum

History
In 1976, Lund and Gilbert[32] reported a case of pseudoxanthoma elasticum with focal epidermal perforation by calcified elastic tissue.

Clinical Features
All reported cases have occurred in middle-aged multiparous women, who developed solitary hyperpigmented reticulated atrophic patches or plaques.[32–35] Characteristically, these occur in the periumbilical region.

Obesity and hypertension are common associations.[35] Angioid streaks of the eye are rarely present. No other clinical manifestation of pseudoxanthomas elasticum has been noted. There is no family history of pseudoxanthoma elasticum in any of the reported cases.

Skin lesions remain solitary and persist for years without apparent resolution.

Pathogenesis
The etiology of this localized disorder is unknown. It appears to be a nonheritable form of pseudoxanthoma elasticum and has only a localized cutaneous manifestation.[35] Cutaneous as well as histopathological changes similar to those of pseudoxanthoma elasticum are seen in individuals exposed to saltpeter.[37]

Histologic Features
The epidermis shows slight acanthosis with a focal area of perforation, with extrusion of altered elastic fibers through the channel.[32–36] The altered elastic fibers are confined to the middermis; are short, granular, fragmented, curled and frayed, and basophilic; and exhibit all the changes characteristic of pseudoxanthoma elasticum.

MISCELLANEOUS DISORDERS

Goette, in 1980, reviewed 17 cases of chondrodermatitis nodularis helicis, and in 13 of these cases, he found elimination of necrobiotic material from the dermis through transepidermal channels, slits, or erosions overlying the necrobiotic granuloma.[38] Transepidermal elimination was also found in necrobiosis lipoidica, and Parra observed elimination of necrotic material and collagen through the follicular opening in three diabetic women.[39] A similar association of epidermal perforation has been observed in rheumatoid arthritis, as superficial ulcerating necrobiosis and perforating rheumatoid nodules,[40,41] and in lichen nitidis.[42] Elimination of calcium-impregnated connective tissue through an epidermal channel has been noted in calcinosis cutis after application of electrode paste containing calcium chloride to the skin. The epidermal necrosis observed in foreign body reactions to silica, beryllium, or contents of follicular cysts was thought to represent transepidermal elimination. Several other disease processes can be theoretically included as causes of transepidermal elimination.[43–45] Among these are amyloid; subepidermal hemorrhage of black heel; thrombosis of capillary hemangioma; infectious processes such as leprosy, tuberculosis, chroblastomycosis, histoplasmosis, North American blastomycosis, leishmaniasis, cryptococcosis, and epidermotropism of mycosis fungoides; malignant melanoma; and Spitz nevus.

REFERENCES

1. Poliak SC, Lebwohl MG, Parris A, et al.: Reactive perforating collagenosis associated with diabetes mellitus. *N Engl J Med* 1982;306:81–84.
2. Hood AF, Hardegen GL, Zarate AR, et al.: Kyrle's disease in patients with chronic renal failure. *Arch Dermatol* 1982;118:85–88.
3. White CR Jr, Heskel NS, Pokorny DJ: Perforating folliculitis of hemodialysis. *Am J Dermatopathol* 1982;4:109–116.
4. Hurwitz RM, Weiss J, Melton ME, et al.: Perforating folliculitis in association with hemodialysis. *Am J Dermatopathol* 1982; 4:101–108.
5. Mehregan AH, Schwartz OD, Livingood CS: Reactive perforating collagenosis. *Arch Dermatol* 1967;96:277–282.
6. Mehregan AH: Perforating dermatoses: A clinicopathologic review. *Int J Dermatol* 1977;16:19–27.
7. Bovenmyer DA: Reactive perforating collagenosis. *Arch Dermatol* 1970;102:313–317.
8. Nair BKH, Sarojini PA, Basheer AM, et al.: Reactive perforating collagenosis. *Br J Dermatol* 1974;91:399–403.
9. Fretzin DF, Beal DW, Jao W: Light and ultrastructural study of reactive perforating collagenosis. *Arch Dermatol* 1980; 116:1054–1058.
10. Mehregan AH, Coskey RJ: Perforating folliculitis. *Arch Dermatol* 1968;97:394–399.
11. Burkhart CG: Perforating folliculitis. *Int J Dermatol* 1981;20:597–599.
12. Kyrle J: Hyperkeratosis follicularis et parafollicularis in cutem penetrans. *Arch Dermatol Syphilol* 1916;123:466–493.
13. Abele DC, Dobson RL: Hyperkeratosis penetrans (*Kyrle's disease*). *Arch Dermatol* 1961;83:277–283.
14. Aram H, Szymanski FJ, Bailey W: Kyrle's disease. *Arch Dermatol* 1969;100:453–456.
15. Carter VH, Constantin VS: Kyrle's disease. *Arch Dermatol* 1968;97:624–632.
16. Carter VH, Constantine VS: Kyrle's disease. *Arch Dermatol* 1968;97:633–639.
17. Petrozzi JW, Warthan TL: Kyrle's disease. *Arch Dermatol* 1974;110:762–765.
18. Lutz W: Keratosis follicularis serpiginosa. *Dermatologica* 1953;106:318–320.
19. Beening GW, Ruiter M: Keratosis follicularis serpiginosa (Lutz). *Dermatologica* 1955;110:175.
20. Mehregan AH: Elastosis perforans serpiginosa. *Arch Dermatol* 1968;97:381–393.
21. Cohen AS, Hashimoto K: Electron microscopic observations on the lesions of elastosis perforans serpiginosa. *J Invest Dermatol* 1960;35:15–19.
22. Meves C, Vogel A: Elektronenmikroskopische untersuchungen in einen fall von elastosis perforans serpiginosa. *Dermatologica* 1973;145:210–221.
23. Patterson JW: The perforating disorders. *J Am Acad Dermatol* 1984;10:561–581.
24. Kirsch N, Hukill PB: Elastosis perforans serpiginosa induced by penicillamine. *Arch Dermatol* 1977;113:630–635.
25. Civette PA: Les formes tuberculo-ulcereuses et tuberculogommeuses du granuloma annulaire. *Ann Dermatol Syphol* 1952;79:387.
26. Calnan CD: Granuloma annulare. *Br J Dermatol* 1954;66:254.
27. Owens DW, Freeman EG: Perforating granuloma annulare. *Arch Dermatol* 1971;103:64–67.
28. Delaney TJ, Gold SC, Leppard G: Disseminated perforating granuloma annulare. *Br J Dermatol* 1973;89:523.
29. Izumi AK: Generalized perforating granuloma annulare. *Arch Dermatol* 1973;108:708–709.
30. Duncan WC, Smith JD, Knox JM: Generalized perforating granuloma annulare. *Arch Dermatol* 1973;108:570–572.
31. Bardach HG: Granuloma annulare with follicular perforation. *Dermatologica* 1982;165:47–53.
32. Lund HZ, Gilberg CF: Perforating pseudoxanthoma elasticum. *Arch Pathol Lab Med* 1976;100:544–546.
33. Hicks J, Carpenter CL, Reed RJ: Periumbilical perforating pseudoxanthoma elasticum. *Arch Dermatol* 1979;115:300–303.
34. Schwartz RA, Richfield DF: Pseudoxanthoma elasticum with transepidermal elimination. *Arch Dermatol* 1978;114:279–280.
35. Neldner KH, Martinez-Hernandez A: Localized acquired pseudoxanthoma elasticum. *J Am Acad Dermatol* 1979;1:523–530.
36. Reed RJ, Clark WH, Mihm MD: The cutaneous elastoses. *Hum Pathol* 1973;4:187–199.
37. Neilson AW, Christensen OB, Hentzer B, et al.: Saltpeter-induced dermal changes electron-microscopically indistinguishable from pseudoxanthoma elasticum. *Acta Dermatol Venereol* 1978;58:323–327.
38. Goette DK: Chondrodermatitis nodularis chronica helicis: A perforating necrobiotic granuloma. *J Am Acad Dermatol* 1980; 2:148–154.
39. Parra LA: Transepithelial elimination in necrobiosis lipoidica. *Br J Dermatol* 1977;96:83–86.
40. Jorizzo JL, Olansky AJ, Stanley RJ: Superficial ulcerating necrobiosis in rheumatoid arthritis. *Arch Dermatol* 1982;118:255–259.
41. Patterson JW, Demos PT: Superficial ulcerating rheumatoid necrobiosis: A perforating rheumatoid nodule. *Cutis* 1985; 36:323–325, 328.
42. Bardach H: Perforating lichen nitidus. *J Cutan Pathol* 1981;8:111–116.
43. Mehregan AH: Transepithelial elimination. *Curr Probl Dermatol* 1970;3:124–127.
44. Malak JA, Kurban AK: "Catharsis" an excretory function of epidermis. *Br J Dermatol* 1971;84:516–522.
45. Batres E, Wolfe JE, Rudolph AH, et al.: Transepithelial eliminations of cutaneous chromomycosis. *Arch Dermatol* 1978; 114:1231–1232.

CHAPTER 37
Non-inflammatory Subepidermal Blisters

Robert A. Briggaman

When faced with a skin biopsy that demonstrates a subepidermal blister with little or no inflammatory cell infiltrate, a limited list of diagnostic possibilities is suggested (Table 37–1). Examination of the presenting specimen may give some clue as to the correct diagnosis. For example, in porphyria cutanea tarda or pseudoporphyria, the presence of solar-induced changes suggests a light exposure distribution, or a few eosinophils along the basement membrane zone support cell-poor bullous pemphigoid. For the most part, however, further help must be sought. Careful correlation of clinical and pathologic features and further investigative studies, such as porphyrin determinations, electron microscopy, and immunohistochemical studies, are required to establish the correct diagnosis. The purpose of this chapter is to aid the dermatopathologist in sorting out the varied entities that present with a noninflammatory subepidermal blister.

EPIDERMOLYSIS BULLOSA HEREDITIA

Epidermolysis bullosa (EB) constitutes a heterogeneous group of inherited disorders that produce blister formation in response to minimal skin trauma. Classification of the various types of EB is based on the mode of inheritance, the level of separation within the skin, and special clinical features including disease severity and the presence or absence of scarring.[1–6] No classification is universally accepted at this time. A useful current classification is presented in Table 37–2.[7]

Determination of the level of separation within the skin is one of the most helpful aids to diagnosis of epidermolysis bullosa because it defines the major subdivisions.[7,8] These major subdivisions are a group of genetic diseases that produce separation in the epidermis (EB simplex group); a group that produce separation at the level of the plasma membrane of basal keratinocytes, hemidesmosomes, and lamina lucida (junctional EB group); and a group that produces separation at the level below the lamina densa

in the subbasal reticular zone (dermolytic or dystrophic EB group).

Routine histopathology is of limited value in the diagnosis of EB except in EB simplex. Epidermolytic changes are usually evident within the epidermis in EB simplex. Early cytoplasmic vesiculation leads to disruption of the cells within the basal and spinous layers and subsequent blister formation. In many cases of generalized EB simplex, however, these changes may be limited to the basal cells, in which case blisters appear to be subepidermal and mislead the observer into a diagnosis of junctional or dystrophic disease. In the junctional or dystrophic form of EB, a subepidermal blister with little or no inflammatory cell infiltration is seen. Routine light microscopic examination, even with the use of special basement membrane stains, is of no benefit in distinguishing between the junctional and dystrophic forms of EB. The reaction product produced by these stains (PAS, silver) is located in a broad area in the sub–lamina densa reticular zone[9] so that discrimination between lamina lucida and sub–lamina densa separation cannot be made.

Electron microscopy performed on appropriately selected and biopsied specimens remains the standard for defining a level of separation by which the main categories of EB are distinguished. In addition, specific alterations of morphologic components of the junction, such as hemidesmosomes and anchoring fibrils, characterize some forms of EB and these defects can only be recognized ultrastructurally.

Proper selection and performance of skin biopsies are of paramount importance in the diagnosis of EB.[8] The best biopsy specimen is a freshly induced blister that can be produced with ease in almost all forms of junctional epidermolysis bullosa and the severe generalized form of dystrophic recessive EB. On the other hand, blisters are difficult to produce in localized recessive dystrophic EB and dominant dystrophic EB, in which case a fresh (less than 12 hours old) spontaneous blister biopsied at the margin is satisfactory. Older spontaneous blisters contain many sec-

TABLE 37–1. NONINFLAMMATORY SUBEPIDERMAL BLISTERS

Epidermolysis bullosa, hereditary
Epidermolysis bullosa, acquired
Porphyrias
    Porphyria cutanea tarda
    Mixed porphyria
Pseudoporphyrias
    Drug-induced
    Hemodialysis/chronic renal failure
Penicillamine dermopathy
Bullous pemphigoid (noninflammatory)
Bullous amyloidosis
Traumatic blisters
    Suction
    Thermal
Blisters overlying recently healed wounds and scars

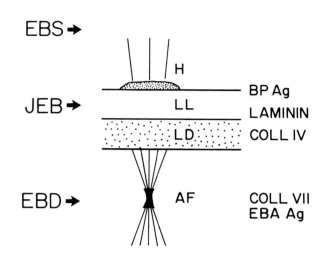

Figure 37–1. Diagrammatic scheme of epidermal–dermal junction in the area of a hemidesmosome (H). Anatomic structures, biochemical components, and levels of separation (arrows) for the major subdivisions of epidermolysis bullosa are shown. AF = anchoring fibril, LL = lamina lucida, LD = lamina densa, BP Ag = bullous pemphigoid, antigen, COL IV = type IV collagen, COL VII = type VII collagen, EBA Ag = epidermolysis bullosa antigen.

ondary changes that make interpretation difficult and occasionally lead to misinterpretation. It is desirable to supply specimens of both blistered and nonblistered, normal-appearing skin, as the specific morphologic alterations of anchoring fibrils and hemidesmosomes are best demonstrated in the unblistered skin.

TABLE 37–2. CLASSIFICATION OF INHERITED EPIDERMOLYSIS BULLOSA

Nonscarring Epidermolysis Bullosa With Intraepidermal Blisters and Dominant Inheritance

Epidermolysis bullosa simplex, generalized (Koebner) type
Epidermolysis bullosa simplex, localized (Weber-Cockayne) type
Epidermolysis bullosa simplex, with mottled pigmentation
Epidermolysis bullosa simplex, Ogna type
Epidermolysis bullosa herpetiformis (Dowling-Meara)

Nonscarring Epidermolysis Bullosa With Junctional Separation, Atrophy, and Recessive Inheritance

Epidermolysis bullosa atrophicans generalisata gravis (Herlitz-Pearson type epidermolysis bullosa letalis)
Epidermolysis bullosa atrophicans generalisata mitis
Epidermolysis bullosa atrophicans localisata
Epidermolysis bullosa atrophicans inversa

Scarring Epidermolysis Bullosa With Dermolytic Separation and Recessive Inheritance

Epidermolysis bullosa dystrophica recessive (Hallopeau-Siemens)
    Generalized sublethal, mutilans type
    Generalized mitis type
    Localized type
Epidermolysis bullosa dystrophica inversa

Scarring Epidermolysis Bullosa With Dermolytic Separation and Dominant Inheritance

Epidermolysis bullosa dystrophica, Cockayne-Touraine type
Epidermolysis bullosa dystrophica, albopapuloid Pasini type

Recently, immunofluorescence antigen mapping has proven useful in determining the level of blister separation using antibodies to specific basement membrane components whose localization is known within the skin.[10–12] The commonly employed antibodies are bullous pemphigoid, antilaminin, and anti–type IV antibodies. The localization of these antibodies is depicted in Figure 37–1. By applying these antibodies to biopsies of patients with EB, the level of cleavage within the skin can be defined. For example, referring to Fig. 37–1, junctional EB produces a separation in which bullous pemphigoid antigen is found on the roof of the blister and laminin and type IV collagen at the base. Dystrophic EB, on the other hand, produces a blister separation in which all antibodies are at the roof of the blister. The reagents for these studies either are available commercially or can be obtained from patients with bullous pemphigoid so that these studies are within the capability of many immunofluorescence laboratories.

In addition to immunofluorescence mapping, recent studies indicate that several monoclonal antibodies may prove useful in the diagnosis of specific types of epidermolysis bullosa.[8,12] These are discussed in more detail when specific types of EB are considered later.

JUNCTIONAL EPIDERMOLYSIS BULLOSA

Clinical Features

The junctional EB group comprises several distinct genetic disorders all of which have autosomal recessive inheritance and produce separation in the lamina lucida (junctional separation). Within the group, variants are distinguished by their clinical characteristics.[1–7]

The most severe subtype, Herlitz syndrome or EB letalis, appears at birth or soon thereafter as extensive blisters and erosions.[13,14] Skin is very fragile and separates easily with insignificant mechanical trauma. Both skin and mucous membranes are involved, especially the mucous membranes of the mouth, larynx, genitalia, and esophagus. Perioral cutaneous involvement is characteristic of this entity. Teeth exhibit a highly specific dysplastic enamel defect that gives the tooth surface a pitted or cobblestone appearance.[15] Infants with this variant usually do not survive beyond 2 years of age and many die in the first 3 months of life.

Another group of patients with junctional separation are long survivors, many of whom survive into adulthood.[16,17] In infancy, these patients are difficult to distinguish from the former letalis group but, in general, exhibit a more mild disease with less severe cutaneous and mucosal involvement. Blisters heal without the severe scarring characteristic of dystrophic types of EB, although atrophic changes may be seen. Enamel dysplasia is a characteristic feature of these patients also. Some of these patients have persistent areas of markedly exaggerated granulation tissue, especially in the perioral, neck, and buttock areas.

It is presently unknown whether these clinical subtypes are the result of different genes or different alleles at the same gene locus.

Histologic Features

Patients with junctional EB produce subepidermal blisters with little or no inflammatory reaction indistinguishable from other types of EB. A definitive diagnosis requires further studies such as electron microscopy and/or antigen mapping. A blister cleavage plane in the lamina lucida is a cardinal feature of this group and is evident in spontaneous or induced blisters and frequently even in intact skin as a result of the trauma induced by a biopsy or tissue processing (Figs. 37–1, 37–2). Both qualitative and quantitative alterations of hemidesmosomes have been reported.[18–21] Reduction in the number of hemidesmosomes may be seen as well as morphologic alterations of the hemidesmo-

somes including rudimentary attachment plaques and a lack of the normal subbasal dense plate of the hemidesmosome. Recent evidence indicates that not all patients with junctional EB exhibit abnormalities of the hemidesmosomes. Tidman and Eady[21] have recently reported normal numbers and appearance of hemidesmosomes in some patients with junctional EB, especially the nonlethal long-survivor forms. These studies suggest that heterogeneity may exist within the junctional group with regard to both clinical features and ultrastructural abnormalities.[19] Further study is needed to clarify the relationship of clinical features and specific ultrastructural abnormalities in varous subvariants of junctional EB.

As indicated previously, immunofluorescence mapping with specific basement membrane antigens is useful in determining the level of separation within the skin.

Although both electron microscopy and antigen mapping are useful in establishing the diagnosis of junctional EB, these procedures do not allow separation of different subtypes of junctional EB nor do they allow predictions of prognosis.

Recently, a murine monoclonal antibody (GB3) has been identified that recognizes an antigen localized to the lamina lucida, possibly related to hemidesmosomes. Localization by the antibody is absent in the skin of patients with various types of junctional epidermolysis bullosa.[22,23] Although presently an investigational tool, this antibody may prove useful in the diagnosis of junctional epidermolysis bullosa in the future.

DYSTROPHIC EPIDERMOLYSIS BULLOSA

Clinical Features

Diseases that produce separation beneath the lamina densa result in dystrophic scarring and are referred to as EB dystrophica or dermolytic EB.[1–8] Traditionally, these are subdi-

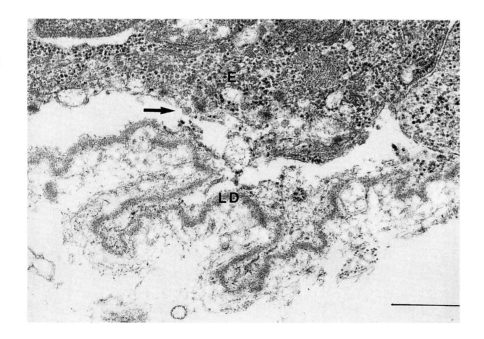

Figure 37–2. Junctional epidermolysis bullosa. Electron micrograph of incipient epidermal–dermal separation in lamina lucida (arrow) between epidermal cell (E) and lamina densa (LD). Calibration bar = 0.5 μm.

vided according to their mode of inheritance into autosomal dominant and recessive types. Further subtypes are distinguished within these larger groups on the basis of specific clinical characteristics. Four clinical subtypes of recessive dystrophic EB are recognized by Gedde-Dahl: generalized gravis, generalized mitis, localized, and inverse.[8] Generalized severe recessive dystrophic EB, the most clinically distinctive form, begins in infancy and affects the entire skin surface and stratified squamous mucous membranes of the mouth, pharynx, esophagus, and anal canal. The disease is accentuated in trauma-prone areas. Dystrophic scarring results from repeated cycles of blistering and frequently leads to a variety of complications including characteristic hand and foot deformities with pseudosyndactyly, nail loss, joint contractures, and esophageal and anal strictures. Growth retardation, anemia, and malnutrition from cutaneous protein loss and limited nutritional intake further complicate this picture.

Localized recessive dystrophic epidermolysis bullosa shows a predilection for trauma-prone regions such as the hands, feet, elbows, and knees. Blisters eventuate in dystrophic scarring and milia. Nails are dystrophic. Early on, the involvement may be more extensive, but usually becomes limited to the above trauma-prone sites in later life. Mucosal involvement is less frequent and severe than in the generalized forms although esophageal strictures may be seen occasionally. The inverse form of dystrophic recessive EB is rare and takes it name from its predilection for intertriginous sites of the central trunk while relatively sparing the extremities. Mucosal involvement with corneal, esophageal, oral, and anal erosion and scarring is comparatively common and may be severe.

Autosomal dominant forms of dystrophic epidermolysis bullosa are traditionally divided into two subtypes: albopapuloid (Pasini) and hypertrophic (Cockayne-Touraine). Common features of these are autosomal dominant inheritance pattern, dystrophic skin lesions with milia, nail dys-

trophy, and blisters that produce separation below the lamina densa. The albopapuloid variety tends to form atrophic scars, commonly involves the mucosa, and produces characteristic albopapuloid lesions, which are hypopigmented, scarlike, lichenoid papules on the trunk and, less commonly, the extremities. Albopapuloid lesions are variably expressed and may be present in some members and absent in others of the same kindred. In the hyperplastic subtype, scarring tends to be hypertrophic, mucosal involvement is rare, and albopapuloid lesions are absent.

Squamous cell carcinomas rise in the chronically scarred skin of all dystrophic EB types, more commonly in the severe forms.[24-25] The carcinomas may be aggressive and tend to metastasize frequently.

Histologic Features

Ultrastructural studies of the skin of patients with dystrophic EB show that the skin is separated in the area beneath the lamina densa. This cleavage plane can be demonstrated with ease in severe generalized recessive dystrophic EB by mechanically separating epidermis and dermis. The lamina densa, lamina lucida, and basal cell plasma membrane with its hemidesmosomes are intact on the blister roof (Figs. 37–1, 37–3). The dermal side of the blister separation may show collagen degeneration, especially in older blisters.

Abnormalities of anchoring fibrils are seen in all forms of dystrophic EB. In the recessive dystrophic forms, particularly of the severe generalized type, anchoring fibrils are completely absent in the clinically nonblistered skin.[26-29] There has been some confusion about this point,[30] although recent quantitative electron microscopic studies substantiate the absence of anchoring fibrils in this form.[28] In the localized, milder forms of dystrophic recessive disease, anchoring fibrils are diminished in number.[28]

Previous studies have indicated that the two forms of dystrophic dominant disease can be distinguished ultra-

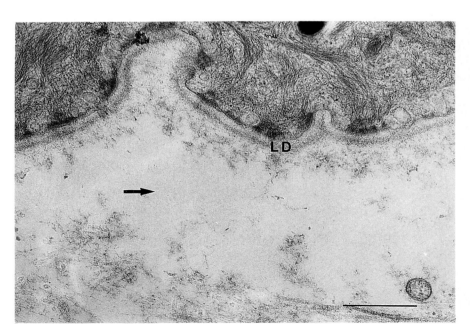

Figure 37–3. Epidermolysis bullosa dystrophica recessive. Electron micrograph showing incipient epidermal–dermal separation (arrow) beneath lamina densa. Anchoring fibrils are absent in the area. Calibration bar = 0.5 μm.

structurally.[31–33] In the albopapuloid subtype, anchoring fibrils are abnormal and reduced in number in both blister-prone and non–blister-prone areas.[31,32] In the hyperplastic subtype, anchoring fibrils are diminished in number and are abnormal only in the blister-prone skin, whereas the epidermal–dermal junction is completely normal in uninvolved areas.[33] These studies suggested that an anchoring fibril defect was the primary abnormality in these diseases. Recent studies using quantitative morphometric analysis have indicated that anchoring fibrils are diminished in number in all forms of dominant dystrophic EB and further show that the two subtypes cannot be clearly distinguished ultrastructurally.[28] Indeed, ultrastructural distinction cannot be made between localized recessive dystrophic and dominant dystrophic EB.

Immunofluorescence mapping is useful in distinguishing the level of separation in dystrophic EB. Here all basement membrane components, bullous pemphigoid antigen, laminin, and type IV collagen are found on the epidermal blister roof and none of the components are at the dermal floor of the blister (Fig. 37–1). Antibody mapping is of little use, however, in separating different forms of EB dystrophica. Monoclonal antibodies to specific antigens within the epidermal–dermal junction may prove useful in this regard.[12,34–36] Recent studies indicate that a monoclonal antibody, LH7:2, distinguishes localized dystrophic disease from the dominant forms of dystrophic EB.[36] This would be helpful, as this distinction is not possible ultrastructurally.

EPIDERMOLYSIS BULLOSA ACQUISITA

Epidermolysis bullosa acquisita (EBA) is a term that requires some discussion as concepts regarding its definition have evolved over the years. Early on, EBA was used operationally for a category of patients with the following features: (1) trauma-induced bullae over the hands, feet, elbows, and knees, atrophic scars, milia, and nail dystrophy; (2) adult onset; (3) absence of a family history of epidermolysis bullosa; and (4) exclusion of all other bullous diseases at least as then defined.[37] Through the years, specific diseases that might have been included under the term *EBA* have been recognized as specific entities. These include bullous amyloidosis; various types of porphyria; porphyria cutanea–like or EBA-like drug reactions to penicillamine, furosamide, tetracycline, and nalidixic acid; and the bullous eruption of chronic dialysis and/or renal failure (pseudoporphyria).

A group of patients with a clinical picture consistent with that described above was identified with immunoreactants at the epidermal–dermal junction.[38–40] These patients have been designated EBA of the immunopathologic type (EBA-IP). On extensive evaluation, this disease has the following characteristics: a chronic bullous disease, subepidermal blisters, linear deposits of IgG at the basement membrane zone, and IgG deposits in the upper dermis beneath the lamina densa. Some confusion has arisen regarding the term *epidermolysis bullosa acquisita* because it has been applied both to the generic category of patients fitting the former definition and the specific immunopathologic form (EBA-IP). One way out of this confusion might be to rename the latter disease *dermolytic pemphigoid,* which we have suggested.[41] There is some reason to retain the generic designation EBA, as patients with blistering, dystrophic scarring, adult onset, and absence of another defined bullous disease continue to be seen on rare occasions.

EBA of the immunopathologic type exhibits varied clinical features with inflammatory and/or noninflammatory bullous involvement.[41] The inflammatory phase may mimic other vesiculobullous diseases, especially bullous pemphigoid, cicatricial pemphigoid, and even dermatitis herpetiformis. The noninflammatory phase may mimic generalized or localized dystrophic epidermolysis bullosa. Some patients present a mixed picture of inflammatory and noninflammatory features. Mucous membrane involvement may be severe in EBA-IP and may even lead to scarring sequelae such as laryngeal or esophageal stricture. EBA of the immunopathologic form usually responds poorly to corticosteroids and other immunosuppressive agents.

Histopathology of the inflammatory phase lesion shows a subepidermal blister, usually with a predominance of neutrophils along the epidermal–dermal junction. The noninflammatory lesion presents as a subepidermal blister with little or no inflammatory cell infiltrate. In those patients who exhibit marked skin fragility, incipient epidermal–dermal separation can be seen, even in biopsies of unblistered skin.

On immunofluorescence studies, linear deposits of IgG are present at the epidermal–dermal junction. The ultrastructural localization of these deposits is beneath the lamina densa or both in the lamina densa and beneath. The "EBA antigen" has been identified as a normal component of human skin basement membrane (290- and 145-kDa proteins) and recently was shown to be identical to type VII collagen, the structural component of anchoring fibrils.[42–44]

PORPHYRIA AND PSEUDOPORPHYRIA

Porphyria and pseudoporphyria are difficult to distinguish clinically and histologically. Both feature increased skin fragility that leads to trauma-induced erosions and blister formation on light-exposed areas.[45,46] The backs of the hands and arms are particularly vulnerable sites. Histopathologic examination of the involved skin shows a subepidermal blister separation. Usually the dermal papilllae are preserved along the previous epidermal–dermal interface. Few, if any, inflammatory cells are present although the blisters are occasionally hemorrhagic. Evidence of solar damage within the dermis suggests the involvement of a light-exposed area. Another clue is the thickened walls of superficial dermal blood vessels. If immunofluorescent studies are performed, IgG and occasionally other immunoglobulins, but not complement, may be seen in some of the patients in a vascular distribution in the superficial dermis. Distinction between porphyria and the pseudoporphyrias requires further studies. The porphyrias are distinguished by the presence of porphyrin abnormalities in the plasma and/or urine. In pseudoporphyria, no detectable porphyrin abnormality can be demonstrated. Patients with pseudoporphyria fall into two categories: a drug-induced group and a hemodialysis/chronic renal failure group. Nalidixic acid, tetracycline, furosamide, and naproxen have been incriminated as etiologic agents in the former group.[47–49] Exposure to sunlight appears to be an important contributing factor in addition to the drug. Discontinuation of the drug results in clearing of the disorder, usually over a several-month period.

Increased skin fragility and blister formation with production of subepidermal blisters may be seen in patients with chronic renal failure and in patients undergoing hemodialysis.[50] The etiology and pathologic mechanisms in these patients are presently uncertain. It may well be that this represents a heterogeneous group. Some patients have elevated plasma porphyrins and may actually have porphyria cutanea tarda.[51] Patients with renal failure, with or without hemodialysis, may also have other vesiculobullous diseases and this should be borne in mind in the evaluation of such patients.

PENICILLAMINE DERMATOPATHY

Prolonged administration of penicillamine, especially of the high doses used in Wilson's disease or cystinuria, leads to a characteristic cutaneous lesion, penicillamine dermatopathy.[52–55] Wrinkled, atrophic plaques, frequently associated with purpura, are present in trauma-prone areas such as the knees, elbows, shoulder, buttocks, and feet. Milia commonly stud the plaques. In some patients, increased skin fragility leads to blister formation usually within the plaques.

Histologically, the reticular dermis is markedly thinned as a result of dimunition of collagen and elastic fibers. Moreover, both collagen and elastic fibers are qualitatively deranged. In those cases with blister formation, the blister cleft occurs within the abnormal reticular dermis. The epidermis and a grenz zone of more normal-appearing papillary dermis form the roof of the blister.[55]

This disorder results from decreased activity of the copper-requiring enzyme, lysyl oxidase, which is needed for essential crosslinkages in both collagen and elastic fibers.[54,55]

BULLOUS AMYLOIDOSIS

Bullae are a rare manifestation of primary cutaneous amyloidosis or myeloma-associated amyloidosis. Bullae and erosions are frequently induced by mild trauma and usually are accompanied by purpura. The changes may be localized or extensive, in which case they resemble epidermolysis bullosa acquisita.[56–59] Histologically, a subepidermal blister without significant inflammation is seen. The plane of separation appears in the dermis, usually with fragments of dermis attached at the blister roof. Amyloid deposits can usually be seen within the dermis but may be present in minimal amounts detectable only with special stains or electron microscopy. Extravasation of red blood cells within the dermis is common.

PHYSICAL AGENTS

Noninflammatory subepidermal bullae may be produced by various forms of physical injury including cold, heat, and pressure. The actual form and degree of the injury induced is dependent on the physical agent and its intensity and duration of application. Cold injury (frostbite) produces extensive cutaneous necrosis involving both epidermis and dermis. A subepidermal blister commonly accompanies frostbite. Experimental or therapeutic application of liquid nitrogen to the skin for brief periods induces a subepidermal blister with a cleavage plane in the lamina lucida.[60] In this type of blister, the basement membrane per se is intact and scarring seldom results. More prolonged liquid nitrogen application, as in cryosurgery, produces extensive skin damage.

Second-degree thermal burns result in skin necrosis involving both epidermis and upper dermis. Again, subepidermal bullae may result from these necrotic changes.[60]

Pressure applied to an area of skin for prolonged periods, as in drug-induced or carbon monoxide coma, results in a variety of changes including epidermal necrosis and sweat gland necrosis. Blister formation, as well as intraepidermal blister formation, may be present.[61]

Other conditions associated with extensive epidermal and dermal necrosis may also result in subepidermal blister formation. Some of these include gas gangrene and postmortem autolysis.

BLISTERS IN RECENTLY HEALED SPLIT-THICKNESS SITES AND SCARS

Newly healed split-thickness graft donor sites may show increased skin fragility and bullae or erosions induced by minimal trauma.[62,63] Similar changes may be seen overlying scars. This is an interesting situation in which subepidermal blisters may result from the failure to re-form structural components of the junction essential for adherence.

REFERENCES

1. Bauer EA, Briggaman RA: The mechanobullous diseases (epidermolysis bullosa), in Fitzpatrick TB, Eisen AZ, Wolff K, et al (eds): *Dermatology in General Medicine*, ed 2. New York, McGraw-Hill, 1979, pp 334–347.
2. Cooper TW, Bauer EA: Epidermolysis bullosa: A review. *Pediatr Dermatol* 1984;1:181–188.
3. Briggaman RA: Hereditary epidermolysis bullosa with special emphasis on newly recognized syndromes and complications. *Dermatol Clin* 1983;1:263–280.
4. Haber RM, Hanna W, Ramsey CA, et al.: Hereditary epidermolysis bullosa. *J Am Acad Dermatol* 1985;13:252–278.
5. Fine JD: Epidermolysis bullosa: Clinical aspects, pathology, and recent advances in research. *Int J Dermatol* 1986;25:143–157.
6. Tabas M, Gibbons S, Bauer EA: The mechanobullous diseases. *Dermatol Clin* 1987;5:123–136.
7. Gedde-Dahl T Jr: Sixteen types of epidermolysis bullosa. *Acta Dermatol Venereol* [*Suppl*] (*Stockh*) 1981;95:74–87.

8. Eady RAJ, Tidman MJ: Diagnosing epidermolysis bullosa. *Br J Dermatol* 1983;108:621–626.

9. Briggaman RA, Wheeler CE Jr: The epidermal–dermal junction. *J Invest Dermatol* 1975;65:71–84.

10. Briggaman RA: Biochemical composition of the epidermal–dermal junction and other basement membranes. *J Invest Dermatol* 1982;78:1–6.

11. Katz SI: The epidermal basement membrane zone—Structure, ontogeny, and role in disease. *J Am Acad Dermatol* 1984;11:1025–1037.

12. Fine JD: The skin basement membrane. *Adv Dermatol* 1986; 2:283–303.

13. Pearson RW, Potter B, Strauss F: Epidermolysis bullosa hereditaria letalis. *Arch Dermatol* 1974;109:349–355.

14. Schachner L, Lazarus GS, Dembitzer H: Epidermolysis bullosa hereditaria letalis: Pathology, natural history, and therapy. *Br J Dermatol* 1977;96:51–58.

15. Gardner DG, Hudson CD: The disturbances in odontogenesis in epidermolysis bullosa hereditaria letalis. *Oral Surg* 1975; 40:483–493.

16. Hintner H, Wolff K: Generalized atrophic benign epidermolysis bullosa. *Arch Dermatol* 1982;118:375–384.

17. Haber RM, Hanna W, Ramsay CA, et al.: Cicatricial junctional epidermolysis bullosa. *J Am Acad Dermatol* 1985;12:836–844.

18. Anton-Lamprecht I, Schnyder UW: Zur ultrastuktur der epidermolysen mit junktionaler blasenbildung. *Dermatologica* 1979; 159:377–382.

19. Tidman MJ, Eady RAJ: Junctional epidermolysis bullosa: A heterogeneous condition. *Br J Dermatol* 1983;109(suppl 24):32.

20. Tidman MJ, Eady RAJ: Junctional epidermolysis bullosa: Ultrastructural variations as demonstrated by morphometric analysis. *J Cutan Pathol* 1983;10:391.

21. Tidman MJ, Eady R: Hemidesmosome heterogeneity in junctional epidermolysis bullosa revealed by morphometric analysis. *J Invest Dermatol* 1986;86:51–56.

22. Heagerty AHM, Kennedy AR, Eady RAJ, et al.: GB3 monoclonal antibody of diagnosis for junctional epidermolysis bullosa. *Lancet* 1986;1:860.

23. Heagerty AHM, Kennedy AR, Gunner DB, et al.: Rapid prenatal diagnosis and exclusion of epidermolysis bullosa using novel antibody probes. *J Invest Dermatol* 1986;86:603–605.

24. Reed WB, College J, Francis MJO, et al.: Epidermolysis bullosa dystrophica with epidermal neoplasms. *Arch Dermatol* 1974; 110:894–902.

25. Schwartz RA, Birnkrant AP, Rubenstein DJ, et al.: Squamous cell carcinoma in dominant type epidermolysis bullosa dystrophica. *Cancer* 1981;47:615–620.

26. Briggaman RA, Wheeler CE Jr: Epidermolysis bullosa dystrophica—Recessive: A possible role of anchoring fibrils in the pathogenesis. *J Invest Dermatol* 1975;65:203–211.

27. Hanna W, Silverman E, Boxall L, et al.: Ultrastructural features of epidermolysis bullosa. *Ultrastruct Pathol* 1983;5:29–36.

28. Tidman MJ, Eady R: Evaluation of anchoring fibrils and other components of the dermal–epidermal junction in dystrophic epidermolysis bullosa by quantitative ultrastructural technique. *J Invest Dermatol* 1985;374:377.

29. Briggaman RA: Is there any specificity to defects of anchoring fibrils in epidermolysis bullosa dystrophica and what does this mean in terms of pathogenesis? *J Invest Dermatol* 1985;84:371–373.

30. Hashimoto I, Schnyder UW, Anton-Lamprecht I, et al.: Ultrastructural studies in epidermolysis bullosa hereditaria. III. Recessive dystrophic types with dermolytic blistering (Hallopeau-Siemens types and inverse type). *Arch Dermatol Res* 1976; 256:137–150.

31. Anton-Lamprecht I, Schnyder UW: Epidermolysis bullosa dystrophica dominans. Ein defekt der anchoring fibrils? *Dermatologica* 1973;147:289–298.

32. Hashimoto I, Anton-Lamprecht I, Gedde-Dahl T, et al.: Ultrastructural studies in epidermolysis bullosa hereditaria. I. Dominant dystrophic type of Pasini. *Arch Dermatol Forsch* 1975; 252:167–178.

33. Hashimoto I, Gedde-Dahl T, Schnyder UW, et al.: Ultrastructural studies in epidermolysis bullosa. II. Dominant dystrophic type of Cockayne and Touraine. *Arch Dermatol Res* 1976;255:285–295.

34. Goldsmith LA, Briggaman RA: Monoclonal antibodies to anchoring fibrils for the diagnosis of epidermolysis bullosa. *J Invest Dermatol* 1983;81:464–466.

35. Fine JD, Breathnach SM, Hintner H, et al.: KF-1 monoclonal antibody defines a specific basement membrane antigen defect in dystrophic forms of epidermolysis bullosa. *J Invest Dermatol* 1984;82:35–38.

36. Heagerty AHM, Kennedy AR, Leigh IM, et al.: Identification of an epidermal basement membrane defect in recessive forms of dystrophic epidermolysis bullosa by LH 7:2 monoclonal antibody: Use in diagnosis. *Br J Dermatol* 1986;115:125–131.

37. Roenigk HH, Ryan JG, Berfeld WF: Epidermolysis bullosa acquisita: Report of three cases and review of all published cases. *Arch Dermatol* 1971;103:1–10.

38. Kushniruk W: The immunopathology of epidermolysis bullosa acquisita. *Can Med Assoc J* 1973;108:1143–1146.

39. Nieboer C, Boorsma DM, Woerdeman MJ, et al.: Epidermolysis bullosa acquisita: Immunofluorescence, electron microscopic and immunoelectron microscopic studies in four patients. *Br J Dermatol* 1980;102:383–392.

40. Yaoita H, Briggaman RA, Lawley TJ, et al.: Epidermolysis bullosa acquisita: Ultrastructural and immunological studies. *J Invest Dermatol* 1981;76:288–292.

41. Briggaman RA, Gammon WR, Woodley DT: Epidermolysis bullosa acquisita of the immunopathologic type (dermolytic pemphigoid). *J Invest Dermatol* 1985;85(1,suppl):79s–84s.

42. Woodley DT, Briggaman RA, O'Keefe EJ, et al.: Identification of the skin basement membrane autoantigen in epidermolysis bullosa acquisita. *N Engl J Med* 1984;310:1007–1013.

43. Woodley DT, Burgeson RE, Lunstrum G, et al.: The epidermolysis bullosa acquisita antigen is the globular carboxyl terminus of type VII procollagen. *J Clin Invest*, 1988;81:683–687.

44. Sakai LY, Keene DR, Morris NP, Burgeson RE: Type VII collagen is a major structural component of anchoring fibrils. *J Cell Biol* 1986;103:1577–1586.

45. Epstein JH, Tuffanelli DL, Epstein WL: Cutaneous changes in the porphyrins. A microscopic study. *Arch Dermatol* 1973;107:689–698.

46. Harber LC, Bickers DR: Porphyria and pseudoporphyria. *J Invest Dermatol* 1984;82:207–209.

47. Zelickson AS: Phototoxic reactions with nalidixic acid. *J Am Med Assoc* 1964;190:556–557.

48. Epstein JH, Tufanelli DL, Seibert JS, et al.: Porphyria cutanea tarda-like changes induced by tetracyclic hydrochloride photosensitization. *Arch Dermatol* 1976;112:661–666.

49. Burry JN, Laurence JR: Phototoxic blisters from high furosemide dosage. *Br J Dermatol* 1976;94:495–499.

50. Gilchrest B, Rowe J, Mihm MC Jr: Bullous dermatosis of hemodialysis. *Ann Intern Med* 1975;83:480–483.

51. Poh-Fitzpatrick MB, Masullo AS, Grossman ME: Porphyria cutanea tarda associated with chronic renal disease and hemodialysis. *Arch Dermatol* 1980;116:191–195.

52. Levy R, Fisher M, Alter J: Penicillamine: Review and cutaneous manifestations. *J Am Acad Dermatol* 1983;8:548–558.

53. Beer WE, Cooke KB: Epidermolysis bullosa induced by penicillamine. *Br J Dermatol* 1967;79:123–125.

54. Katz R: Penicillamine-induced skin lesions. A possible example of human lathyrism. *Arch Dermatol* 1977;95:196–198.

55. Hashimoto K, McEvoy B, Belcher R: Ultrastructure of penicillamine-induced skin lesions. *J Am Acad Dermatol* 1981;4:300–315.

56. Muller SA, Sams WM, Dobson RL: Amyloidosis masquerading as epidermolysis bullosa acquisita. *Arch Dermatol* 1969;99:739–747.

57. Beacham BE, Greer KE, Andrews BS, et al.: Bullous amyloidosis. *J Am Acad Dermatol* 1980;3:506–510.

58. Bluhm JF III, Johnson SC, Norback DH: Bullous amyloidosis. *Arch Dermatol* 1980;116:1164–1168.

59. Westermark P, Öhman S, Domar M, et al.: Bullous amyloidosis. *Arch Dermatol* 1981;117:782–784.

60. Pearson R: Response of human epidermis to graded thermal stress. *Arch Environ Health* 1965;11:498–507.

61. Mandy S, Ackerman AB: Characteristic traumatic skin lesions in drug-induced coma. *J Am Med Assoc* 1970;213:253–256.

62. Barker DJ, Cotterill JA: Development of subepidermal bullae in the split-skin graft donor site of a psoriatic. *Dermatologica* 1980;160:311–314.

63. Baran R, Juhlin L, Brun P: Bullae in skin grafts. *Br J Dermatol* 1984;111:221–225.

SECTION VI
Pigmentary Disorders

CHAPTER 38
Hypermelanoses

T. H. Kwan

The diseases covered in this chapter are characterized by an increase in pigmentation resulting from melanin accumulation in the epidermis and/or within dermal macrophages. Melanization in these separate microscopic locations can be correlated with clinically perceived differences in pigmentation. Purely epidermal pigmentation is usually brown in normal light and accentuated when observed under ultraviolet light. Purely dermal pigmentation is said to be blue-gray in normal light and not accentuated when viewed under ultraviolet light. Although this distinction seems relatively straightforward, it may fail in clinical practice because many hypermelanoses are the result of melanization to varying degree of both the epidermis and dermis. In addition to the location of melanin, the aggregation/dispersion of melanosomes also contributes to what is perceived by the naked eye. For example, the rapid color change observed in some amphibia is correlated with pigment granule aggregation/dispersion.

A brief outline of melanin synthesis and destiny is given in Chapter 1.

Although the morphologic factors just discussed are of some importance in the classification of hypermelanoses, the most important diagnostic criteria are still clinical and laboratory data. Information obtained by light and electron microscopy of hypermelanoses is nonetheless interesting and helpful in a wide variety of situations.

A large number of lesions are due to pigments other than melanin and may be mistaken clinically for one of the hypermelanoses. Examples of these lesions are found elsewhere in this book. A large category of pigmented lesions is associated with proliferation of melanocytes, such as nevocellular nevi and melanomas, which are considered in Chapters 48 and 49.

In this chapter some of the basic hypermelanoses are highlighted. The topic of hypermelanosis is wider than the space allotted in this section. References listed at the end of this chapter will be helpful to the reader who requires greater depth and breadth.

FRECKLE (EPHELIS)

A freckle is a small (usually less than 0.5 cm across) pigmented macule of relatively uniform coloration occurring on sun-exposed skin. Freckling is usually apparent in the first 6 months of life if there is exposure to sunlight. A freckle is distinguished from other similar circumscribed hypermelanoses because it darkens in response to long-wave ultraviolet light (320–400 nm). Freckles are always multiple. Prominent freckling linked with red hair is believed to be transmitted as an autosomal dominant trait. The clinical diagnosis of a freckle is almost trivial. The primary differential diagnosis is lentigo. Lentigo can be differentiated clinically from a freckle because it does not darken appreciably after exposure to sunlight. A freckle differs from lentigo histopathologically as well.

Histologic Features

Under the microscope, a freckle discloses increased melanin, mostly within keratinocytes and usually concentrated in the more basal strata (Fig. 38–1). By electron microscopy, the number of melanocytes per unit of surface area has been found to be normal to somewhat decreased.[1] Melanocytes within the freckle also appear more active, with more branching of dendrites and numerous rod-shaped stage IV melanosomes.[1] In contrast, lentigo also discloses increased basal pigmentation, but is characterized by increased numbers of melanocytes. Rete ridge elongation is also common in lentigo. Lentigo is sometimes associated with dermal melanophages and papillary dermal fibrosis. Because melanocytes are sometimes difficult to identify in hematoxylin and eosin–stained sections, sometimes a

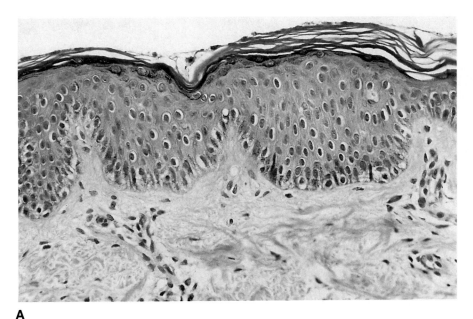

A

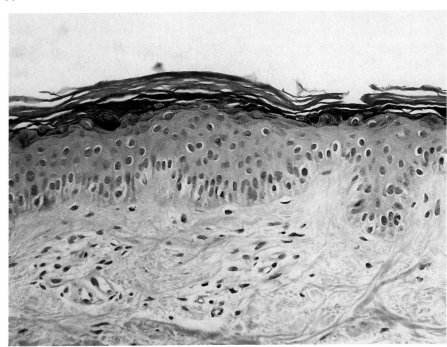

Figure 38–1.A. A. Ephelis. Note that melanization (fine granularity) is confined mostly to the basal layer. The cells with clear cytoplasm in the basal layer represent melanocytes. **B.** Normal skin from the same patient. Note that the basal layer appears less melanized than in the ephelis. (**A, B,** H&E, ×400.)

B

freckle cannot be distinguished from lentigo with certainty under the light microscope. Fortunately, electron microscopy is usually not necessary because clinical features are usually sufficient to make a diagnosis.

CAFÉ-AU-LAIT SPOT

Café-au-lait spot is a light brown (café-au-lait) macule, 1.5 to 20 cm across, circumscribed, and of uniform coloration. Its borders are often somewhat irregular. Café-au-lait spot can appear at any time of life and can occur anywhere on the skin. It has been estimated that 10% of the normal population have one to three of these spots. Six or more of these spots larger than 1.5 cm across should alert the clinician to the strong possibility of neurofibromatosis (von Recklinghausen's disease); more than 90% of neurofibromatosis patients have café-au-lait spots. These spots are also associated with Albright's, Leschke's, Watson's, and other neurocutaneous syndromes.

Histologic Features
The microscopic appearance of a café-au-lait spot is similar to that of a freckle. There is increased melanization of the basal portion of the epidermis. Melanosomes may be of normal size[2] or may be so-called macromelano-

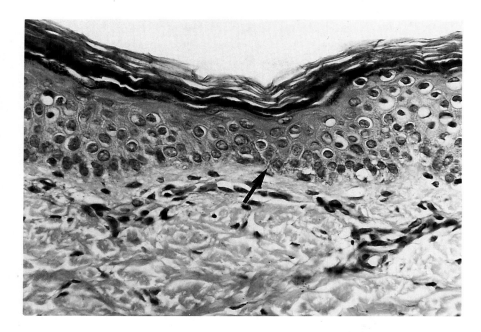

Figure 38–2. Café-au-lait spot. Note melanization of the lower strata of the epidermis and the presence of macromelanosomes (arrow). (H&E, ×640.)

somes[3,4]—so large that they can be easily visualized under the light microscope (Fig. 38–2). Macromelanosomes are found in apparently normal as well as diseased patients, and are not always associated with neurofibromatosis.[5] In the differential diagnosis between neurofibromatosis and Albright's disease, their presence in a café-au-lait spot favors the former.[6] The number of melanocytes per unit area in a café-au-lait spot appears increased compared with that of adjacent epidermis.

MELASMA (CHOLASMA, MASK OF PREGNANCY)

Melasma is a patchy hypermelanosis characterized by its location on the face, notably malar areas, but also the forehead, upper lip, and sometimes the neck. This common condition is exacerbated by light. It is more common in women and is associated with endocrine states such as pregnancy, ovarian malignancy, and ingestion of oral contraceptives. It often fades when the endocrine state returns to it prior state. It also occurs without appreciably altered endocrine states in women and men. Melanocyte-stimulating hormone levels have been described as normal.[7] Melasma has also occurred after ingestion of diphenylhydantoin and mesantoin.[8]

Histologic Features
By light microscopy melasma is associated with increased melanin within keratinocytes. Increased numbers of and increased activity of melanocytes are also reported.[9] Longstanding melasma is sometimes resistant to therapy, probably because the bleaching agents cannot reach dermal melanophages, which are almost certainly present. Ultrastructurally, melanosomes have been described as larger than normal, and a higher percentage of melanosomes in keratinocytes are dispersed singly rather than packaged together.[10]

ADDISON'S DISEASE

Diffuse hypermelanosis is associated with a variety of hormonal states of which adrenocortical insufficiency is the most common. Increased melanocyte-stimulating hormone (MSH) and adrenocorticotropic hormone (ACTH) are released from the pituitary gland as lack of feedback inhibition occurs when cortisol is deficient. Addison-like hypermelanosis has been described with administration of MSH or large doses of ACTH, and these hormones are presumed to be related to the diffuse pigmentation observed in Addison's disease.[11,12] Additional clinical findings of Addison's disease include linear hyperpigmentation of nails (a normal finding in blacks) and brown or blue macules on buccal and gingival surfaces (also a normal finding in all but lightly pigmented caucasoids). The cutaneous hyperpigmentation of Addison's disease is not necessarily uniform and may be accentuated in areas of mild trauma.

Histologic Features
The microscopic change observed consists of hyperpigmentation of the epidermis. Melanocytes are not increased in number. Melanophages are sometimes present in the dermis.[13] These histologic features are of course not specific, and the diagnosis of Addison's disease rests on clinical and laboratory findings. The precise mechanism of MSH and ACTH activity in the skin remains to be described.

POSTINFLAMMATORY HYPERPIGMENTATION

Focal (less commonly diffuse) hypermelanosis may follow any inflammatory dermatosis. The area of hyperpigmentation usually conforms to the area involved by the dermatosis.

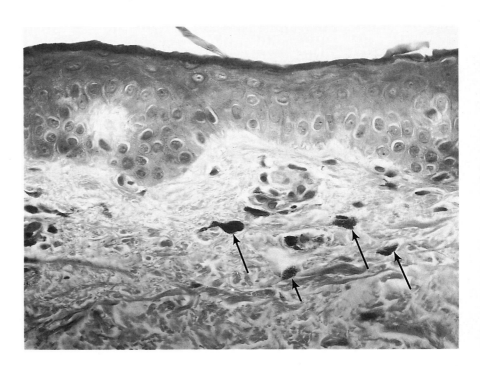

Figure 38–3. Postinflammatory hyperpigmentation. Melanin-laden macrophages (arrows) are scattered throughout the upper dermis. (H&E, ×400.)

Histologic Features

The histopathology consists of dermal melanophages (Fig. 38–3) associated with residual inflammation and changes of the primary dermatosis and sometimes fibrosis. A common component of the antecedent dermatosis is alteration of the dermoepidermal junction. The pathogenesis of postinflammatory hyperpigmentation remains to be clarified. A common speculation is that the damage to the dermoepidermal junction permits pigment to "fall" into the dermis where is ingested by macrophages. It is somewhat curious that both hyper- and hypopigmentation can follow with the same dermatosis. The mechanisms determining whether one or the other or both occurs would be of interest.

MELANIN PIGMENTATION INDUCED BY ULTRAVIOLET LIGHT (TANNING)

After exposure to ultraviolet light, two separate photoresponses occur, immediate tanning and delayed tanning.

Immediate tanning (immediate pigment darkening, Meirowsky phenomenon) occurs in response to long-wave ultraviolet (320–328 nm, UVA) light. The immediate darkening is maximal at the end of the exposure time and fades over the next 6 to 36 hours. This change is due to photooxidation of melanin, which results in a darker but less stable oxidized state. It is also associated with dispersion of microfilaments and microtubules from perinuclear to peripheral cytoplasm and to dendrites within the melanocyte. Immediate tanning is not associated with synthesis of new melanin.

Delayed tanning occurs in response to short-wave ultraviolet (290–320 nm, UVB) light and, to lesser extent, to long-wave ultraviolet and visible light.[14] Delayed tanning

is slower than immediate tanning and is perceptible 48 to 72 hours after exposure. Changes at the cellular level begin earlier: increased tyrosinase activity and formation of new melanin, increased melanization of increasing numbers of melanosomes, increased size of melanosomes, increased transfer of melanosomes to dendritic areas and to keratinocytes, changes in nuclear chromatin and nucleoli, and increasing ribosomal activity have been described.[15] The ability to tan as well as ability to retain the tan is largely under genetic control. Delayed tanning, unlike immediate tanning, is associated with melanin synthesis. Delayed tanning, but not immediate tanning, is believed to confer protection against the effects of ultraviolet light.[16]

HYPERPIGMENTATION RELATED TO DRUGS

Many drugs have been associated with hyperpigmentation. This hyperpigmentation can be epidermal and/or dermal and may be caused by substances other than melanin. Complete enumeration of drugs and their reported pigmentary features is impossible in the space allotted. The review of Granstein and Sober is recommended.[17] Some examples follow; the reader is also referred to Chapter 40.

Oil of bergamot, found in some perfumes, contains a psoralen that acts as a photosensitizing agent to stimulate epidermal melanin synthesis (berloque dermatitis). Other substances (such as found in buckwheat, buttercups, citrus peels, carrot tops, crown vetch, pigweed, and shepherd's purse, to name a few), when applied topically and exposed to light, can cause a photocontact dermatitis that is sometimes followed by postinflammatory hyperpigmentation.

The fixed drug eruption is an idiosyncratic response characterized by a circumscribed rash and/or hyperpigmentation occurring in the same cutaneous location whenever that particular drug is ingested. Phenolphthalein, phenacetin, and salicylates are some of the agents that have been associated with the features of a fixed drug eruption. The microscopic appearance of the rash is that of an interface dermatitis with vacuolization at the dermoepidermal junction, dyskeratosis, sometimes spongiosis, an upper dermal bandlike or perivascular lymphocytic infiltrate, mild exocytosis, and melanin within dermal macrophages. In the later phases, the inflammatory changes subside, leaving dermal melanophages and slight fibroplasia as the predominant changes.

Chronic use of chlorpromazine and related drugs has been associated with slate-gray or purple pigmentation of exposed areas. Chlorpromazine stimulates melanin synthesis and is associated with brown dermal pigments, which are proposed to be pigmented metabolites in the dermis; moreover, these proposed metabolites may possibly bind melanin.

Topical nitrogen mustard can cause diffuse hypermelanosis or a circumscribed pigmentation of flexural areas that tends to spread centripedally.[18] Nitrogen mustard has been associated with alterations in the aggregation/dispersion of melanosomes within keratinocytes.[19]

HEMOCHROMATOSIS

This metabolic disorder is associated with diffuse hyperpigmentation that can vary from bronze to blue-gray to brown-black. The pigmentation can also be circumscribed or accentuated in flexor creases, genital areas, areolae, and scars. Mucous membranes can also be involved. Cutaneous changes often precede the development of cardiac failure, cirrhosis, and diabetes.[20]

Histologic Features

Increased melanin is present in the epidermis and is considered to be largely, if not entirely, responsible for the pigmentation observed by the naked eye.[21] With special stains, iron in the form of hemosiderin is demonstrable within and outside of dermal macrophages, around blood vessels, and around sweat glands. Very rarely, iron can be demonstrated within basal cells of the epidermis and within sweat gland cells.[22] Iron can of course be seen in the dermis in other conditions such as trauma, the pigmentary purpuras, and stasis dermatitis, but the distribution of the iron will differ and other alterations are present in these other disorders.

It is thought that the presence of iron in the dermis stimulates the production of epidermal melanin, as the presence of other metals (such as silver and gold) in the skin is also associated with increased melanization. Although this may be true, other conditions associated with dermal hemosiderin (such as trauma and pigmentary purpuras) are not associated with epidermal melanosis. A further consideration is the occurrence of diffuse melanosis with other liver diseases such as primary biliary cirrhosis, glycogen storage disease, porphyria cutanea tarda, and Wilson's disease.

REFERENCES

1. Breathnach AS, Wyllie LM: Electron microscopy of melanocytes and melanosomes in freckled human epidermis. *J Invest Dermatol* 1964;42:389–394.
2. Silvers DN, Greenwood RS, Helwig EB: Café-au-lait spots without giant pigment granules. Occurrence in suspected neurofibromatosis. *Arch Dermatol* 1974;110:87–88.
3. Morris TJ, Johnson WG, Silvers DN: Giant pigment granules in biopsy specimens from café-au-lait spots in neurofibromatosis. *Arch Dermatol* 1982;118:385–388.
4. Jimbow K, Szabo G, Fitzpatrick TB, et al.: Ultrastructure of giant pigment granules (macromelanosomes) in the cutaneous pigmented macules of neurofibromatosis. *J Invest Dermatol* 1973;61:300–309.
5. Johnson BI, Charneco DR: Café-au-lait spot in neurofibromatosis and in normal individuals. *Arch Dermatol* 1970;102:442–446.
6. Benedict PH, Szabo G, Fitzpatrick TB, et al.: Melanotic macules in Albright's syndrome and in neurofibromatosis. *J Am Med Assoc* 1968;205:618–626.
7. Smith AG, Shuster S, Thody AJ, et al.: Chloasma, oral contraceptives, β-melanocyte-stimulating hormone. *J Invest Dermatol* 1977;68:169–170.
8. Kushe H, Krebs A: Hyperpigmentation of chloasma-type after treatment with hydantoin preparations. *Dermatologica* 1964;129:121–139.
9. Sanchez WP, Pathak MA, Sato S, et al.: Melasma: A clinical, light microscopic, ultrastructural, and immunofluorescence study. *J Am Acad Dermatol* 1981;4:698–710.
10. Konrad K, Wolff K: Hyperpigmentation: Melanosome size and distribution pattern of melanosomes. *Arch Dermatol* 1973;107:853–860.
11. Lerner AB, McGuire JS: Effect of alpha- and beta-melanocyte stimulating hormones on the skin colour of man. *Nature* 1961;189:176.
12. Lerner AB, McGuire JS: Melanocyte-stimulating hormones and adrenocorticotrophic hormone. *N Engl J Med* 1964;270:539.
13. Montgomery H, O'Leary PA: Pigmentation of the skin in Addison's disease, acanthosis nigricans, and hemochromatosis. *Arch Dermatol Syphilol* 1930;21:970–984.
14. Toda K, Shono S: Effect of UVA irradiation on the epidermal pigment darkening, in Klaus S (ed): *Pigment Cell.* Basel, Karger, 1979, vol 4, p. 318.
15. Quevedo WC, et al: Light and skin color, in Pathak MA, et al. (eds): *Sunlight and Man: Normal and Abnormal Photobiologic Responses.* Tokyo, University of Tokyo Press, 1974, p 165.
16. Willis I, Kligman A, Epstein J: Effects of long ultraviolet rays on human skin: Photoprotective or photoaugmentive? *J Invest Dermatol* 1972;59:416–420.
17. Granstein RD, Sober AJ: Drug- and heavy metal-induced hyperpigmentation. *J Am Acad Dermatol* 1981;5:1–18.
18. Doherty CStJ: Hyperpigmentation after cancer chemotherapy. Lancet 1975;2:365–366.
19. Flaxman BA, Sosis AC, Van Scott EJ: Changes in melanosome distribution in caucasoid skin following topical application of nitrogen mustard. *J Invest Dermatol* 1973;60:321–326.
20. Finch SC, Finch CA: Idiopathic hemochromatosis, an iron storage disease. A. Iron metabolism in hemochromatosis. *Medicine (Baltimore)* 1955;34:381–430.
21. Cawley EP, Hsu YT, Wood BT, et al.: Hemochromatosis of the skin. *Arch Dermatol* 1969;100:1–6.
22. Weintraub LR, Demis DJ, Conrad ME, et al.: Iron excretion by the skin. Selective localization of iron[59] in epithelial cells. *Am J Pathol* 1965;46:121–127.

CHAPTER 39
Hypomelanoses

T. H. Kwan

Hypomelanosis can be defined as decreased melanin formation with the clinical appearance of leukoderma. It is sometimes useful to distinguish hypomelanosis from amelanosis, the complete absence of melanin. The clinical classification of hypomelanoses is based largely on clinical history and clinical findings. An understanding of the sequence of melanogenesis is ultimately essential. There are many points at which melanogenesis and melanization can be perturbed, resulting in the clinical appearance of leukoderma. For example, the different disorders described in this chapter illustrate different points of disturbance in the sequence of melanogenesis/melanization. Vitiligo is related to an acquired loss of melanocytes. Piebaldism, a congenital circumscribed leukoderma, is thought to be related to a failure of melanoblast migration during embryonic life to affected areas of the skin. The halo nevus has been associated with cellular and humoral mechanisms of rejection directed at nevomelanocytes within a particular nevus or nevi. Postinflammatory hypopigmentation is not well studied, but it is likely to be related to a variety of mechanisms. Albinism is related to congenitally decreased or absent tyrosinase. The hypopigmentation of Chediak-Higashi syndrome is associated with abnormal melanosome aggregation and the lack of normal dispersion of melanosomes. It is worth noting that leukoderma is associated with the absence of melanocytes in only a few situations in dermatology: vitiligo, piebaldism, rare halo nevi, and within some traumatized areas.

A thorough discussion of hypomelanosis is beyond the scope of this chapter, and the reader should consult standard texts of dermatology for a broad overview of this largely clinical subject.

VITILIGO

Vitiligo is characterized by acquired macular depigmentation (amelanosis) and complete loss of melanocytes in depigmented areas. It is a common disorder affecting at least 1% of the population.[1] The pathogenesis of vitiligo has not been fully characterized, and has been debated exten-

sively.[2] An autoimmune process is clearly associated with loss of melanocytes.[3,4] Vitiligo is associated with a number of other disorders that are considered to be autoimmune such as atrophic gastritis, halo nevi, alopecia areata, Addison's disease, rheumatoid disease, adult-onset diabetes mellitus, thyroid diseases including Grave's disease, and Vogt-Koyanagi-Harada syndrome. A family history of vitiligo can be elicited in a significant percentage of cases. Not surprisingly, retinal pigmentary changes are present in some vitiligo patients.

Vitiligo varies widely in its presentation. It can consist of a single lesion but is usually multiple. Lesions can be measured in millimeters but are usually several centimeters across. The borders of the lesions are frequently irregular and outline abstract shapes. Occasionally, the lesions are linear or follow areas served by a single nerve segment. A fully evolved individual lesion is completely depigmented centrally. The border of the lesion may be hypopigmented, erythematous, and/or hyperpigmented. Repigmentation can occur spontaneously or with treatment. These clinical appearances can be correlated with microscopic findings.

Histologic Features

Under the microscope the depigmented area discloses a complete absence of melanocytes; Langerhans cells and indeterminate dendritic cells are present in the epidermis. The hypopigmented areas show some melanization of the epidermis and reduced numbers of melanocytes compared with normal areas (Fig. 39–1). Erythematous areas are associated with lymphocytic infiltrates, usually superficial and perivascular with variable degrees of vascular ectasia. The hyperpigmented areas can be correlated with large melanocytes whose dendrites are filled with melanin and with dermal melanophages. Some investigators have described patterns of melanocyte injury at the edges of lesions of vitiligo.[5] When compared with pigmented skin in the same individual, vitiligo skin appears to have a decreased ability to become sensitized to contactants,[6] possibly because of functional impairment of Langerhans cells.[7] Langerhans cells appear to be normal in number, but are distributed

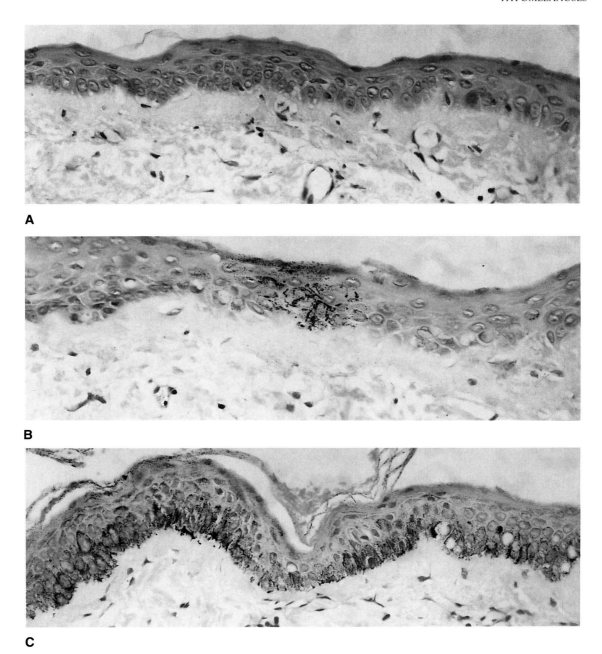

Figure 39–1. A. Vitiligo, depigmented area. Melanin and melanocytes are absent. The absence of melanocytes is difficult to judge in this preparation. **B.** Vitiligo, "trichrome" area. Partial loss of melanin. **C.** Normal skin from the vitiligo patient illustrated in A and B. Melanization is easily identified (**A–C,** Fontana-Masson, ×400.)

more basally than usual.[8] Repigmentation is associated with repopulation of amelanotic areas by melanocytes from hair follicles.

PIEBALDISM

Piebaldism (patterned leukoderma) is characterized by congenital circumscribed leukoderma. It is associated with a white forelock in over 80% of cases. Portions of the ventral surface of the body are most commonly affected. This disorder is inherited as autosomal dominant. The lesions may be either hypopigmented or depigmented and usually remain for life; some repigmentation and depigmentation are reported to occur occasionally. Within areas of leukoderma, normal or hyperpigmented areas are sometimes present. In addition, hyperpigmentation is also sometimes present in areas of normal pigmentation. Piebaldism is present in many cases of Waardenburg's syndrome (congenital deafness, lateral displacement of inner canthi, and heterochromia of irides). Heterochromic irides, deafness, and mental retardation are also rare associations. The syndrome of deafness and piebaldism is sometimes called Woolf's syndrome.[9]

Histologic Features

Areas of leukoderma disclose decreased or absent melanin and decreased numbers or absence of melanocytes.[10] Areas of hyperpigmentation show normal as well as abnormally large, spherical melanosomes that are abnormally melanized.[11] On the basis of studies in mice, failure of melanoblasts during embryonic life to populate affected areas of skin is postulated to be the basis of hypopigmented areas in piebaldism.[12,13] Mast cells have also been identified within the epidermis of hypopigmented skin in a study of a single case.[14]

HALO NEVUS

Halo nevus can be defined as acquired leukoderma surrounding a nevocellular nevus. It can occur at any age, and around one or multiple nevi.[15] Halo nevus sometimes occurs in patients who also have vitiligo and/or malignant melanoma. Most observers agree that halo nevus represents regression of a nevus. This halo phenomenon can occur around other skin lesions such as seborrheic keratosis and neurofibroma.[16] Halo nevus may remain stable, or it may progress to complete leukoderma in the area of the nevus. The leukoderma may in turn repigment. The halo phenomenon is also observed in an incomplete form adjacent to many melanomas. Knowledge of how this process (also called leukoderma acquisitum centrifugum) is regulated is, however, scant.[17]

Histologic Features

The typical microscopic picture of halo nevus is that of a nevocellular nevus heavily infiltrated with lymphocytes, histiocytes, and sometimes plasma cells[18] (Fig. 39–2). The nevocellular nevus is usually compound or dermal in type, but this phenomenon has also been observed around Spitz nevi. In later stages when fewer nevus cells are present, these cells may be missed on casual inspection. Complete leukoderma usually shows dermal fibrosis with scattered histiocytes and lymphocytes. The areas of leukoderma are usually devoid of melanocytes.[19–21]

POSTINFLAMMATORY HYPOPIGMENTATION

Leukoderma can occur secondarily to almost any inflammatory process that involves the dermoepidermal junction. It is a common finding in clinical dermatology and is particularly noted in persons of color. The location and morphologic patterns of depigmentation are often helpful in the clinical diagnosis of the primary inflammatory disorder. Histologic patterns of inflammation are also often distinctive enough for diagnosis of the primary inflammatory process. The absence of pigmentation under the microscope, however, is usually noted only if the surrounding skin is pig-

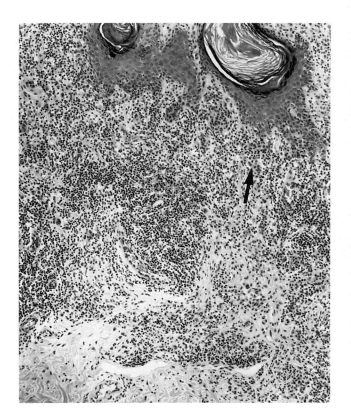

Figure 39–2. Halo nevus. A nevocellular nevus heavily infiltrated by lymphocytes is the characteristic histologic finding. The larger pale cells in this photomicrograph represent nevus cells (arrow) and the smaller cells with darkly stained nuclei are lymphocytes. (H&E, ×160.)

mented. Hence, the light microscopic findings are minimal for the clinical finding of hypopigmentation per se. With other methods of morphologic examination such as electron microscopy, the presence or absence of melanocytes, ultrastructural evidence of cellular damage, pigment dispersion, and deficiencies of melanin transport can be identified. These findings, though of some interest, are usually of limited clinical significance. It is interesting that many inflammatory disorders can also be associated with hyperpigmentation, and even occur adjacent to a hypopigmented area occasionally. The concurrence of these pigmentary opposites is sometimes called leukomelanoderma.

CHEDIAK-HIGASHI SYNDROME

A rare multisystem disorder, Chediak-Higashi syndrome is transmitted as an autosomal recessive trait and usually results in death before the teenage years. The phenotype is similar to that of tyrosinase-positive albinism, with pale skin and hair that may darken slightly with exposure to light.[22,23] The irides vary in their coloration. Translucency of the irides, photophobia, and nystagmus have also been described. These patients usually present with recurrent bacterial infections in infancy and early childhood. Seizures and other neurologic problems often begin by age 5. An "accelerated phase" consisting of pancytopenia, adenopathy, hepatosplenomegaly, gingivitis, and sloughing of buccal mucosa may herald the final stages of this syndrome. Lymphoreticular dyscrasias have been reported. Death is usually related to infection or to complications of the hematologic problems.

Histologic Features

Chediak-Higashi syndrome also has distinctive microscopic features. Melanocytes are present. Large irregular melanosomes can be seen under the light microscope as large melanin granules. These granules may be abundant in some areas of the epidermis and virtually absent in others. These same abnormal melanosomes are present in dermal macrophages.[24] Under the electron microscope, these giant melanosomes are observed to apparently fuse to form larger particles.[25] Vacuolization within melanosomes is observed. Some normal melanosomes within melanocytes are also present ultrastructurally. Transfer to keratinocytes within abnormally large phagolysosomes is observed in epidermis and hair (as well as to cells in the retina, pia-arachnoid, and choroid plexus). The phenotypic pigment dilution in these patients is thought to be caused by this abnormal packaging of melanosomes and a relative lack of the normal dispersion of melanosomes.[25] The basic problem is thought to be related to a membrane defect.

Large phagolysosome-like particles are also found in neutrophils and monocytes. These are characteristic and usually the pivotal finding in diagnosis of this syndrome. Studies have shown that bacteria are successfully incorporated into phagocytic vacuoles but that primary lysosomes are unavailable to play their role in the destruction of these microorganisms.[26] Large phagolysosome-like particles are also found in other organs of the body.

OCULOCUTANEOUS ALBINISM

Albinism is characterized by hereditary hypomelanosis or amelanosis affecting the skin, hair, and eyes with photophobia, nystagmus, and decreased visual acuity. A variety of subtypes of oculocutaneous albinism (OCA) are described. The two principal groups are tyrosinase-positive and tyrosinase-negative OCA. In the former, melanocytes possess tyrosinase and are deoxyphenylalanine (DOPA) positive, and in the latter, melanocytes lack this enzyme and are DOPA negative. The classic assay for these substances involves plucking an anagen hair and incubating it in a tyrosine or DOPA solution.[27] Darkening of hair bulbs is seen with the tyrosinase-positive variant. Both types are inherited as an autosomal recessive trait. The phenotype of both types includes decreased pigmentation of skin, hair, and ocular fundi. The tyrosinase-positive patient is able to acquire slight pigmentation with the passage of time, whereas the tyrosinase-negative patient is unable to become more pigmented. Without the protection that melanin confers, these patients are especially susceptible to short- and long-term effects of sunlight.

Under the light microscope, melanin is absent in both types, but clear cells that represent amelanotic melanocytes can be identified in their normal location in the basal layer.

Under the electron microscope, melanocytes with melanosomes can be identified in both types of OCA.[28] In the tyrosinase-positive type, stage I and II melanosomes are numerous and a few stage III and IV (melanized and more mature) melanosomes can also be found. In the tyrosinase-negative type, stage I and II melanosomes are present but not stage III and IV melanosomes. The defect in the tyrosinase-positive type is not clear; the enzyme kinetics appear to be normal. The defect in the tyrosinase-negative type can be ascribed to the complete absence of the enzyme tyrosinase.

Other forms of OCA include Hermansky-Pudlak syndrome, autosomal dominant OCA (sometimes called oculocutaneous albinoidism), yellow mutant OCA, red OCA, brown OCA, and Cross-McKusick-Breen syndrome. These disorders are all rare and, for the most part, occur in particular gene pools.

Hermansky-Pudlak syndrome is characterized by a bleeding diathesis, tyrosinase-positive OCA, and ceroid-like inclusions within macrophages of bone marrow, lymphoid tissue, spleen, and epithelial cells of the oral cavity. The nature of the bleeding defect is related to deficient platelet serotonin and ATP stored in dense bodies. Alterations in the dense bodies can be appreciated on the ultrastructural level. Platelet dysfunction is usually subclinical and may be uncovered when the patient is taking aspirin or other drugs that affect platelets. Stage I, II, III, and rare IV melanosomes are present ultrastructurally. Pheomelanosomes resembling those of normal redheads, as well as giant melanosomes, have also been described in these patients.[29,30]

Autosomal dominant OCA is phenotypically subtle compared with the other forms of OCA and may go unrecognized. These patients are healthy, they are able to tan slightly, and they are usually free of or little affected by the eye problems of other patients with albinism.

Yellow mutant, red, and brown OCA are characterized by hypopigmentation and the tints implied in their names. These patients are unable to form true melanin but are able to form other pigments to a limited extent.[31–33]

Cross-McKusick-Breen syndrome is characterized by a variety of neurologic and growth abnormalities and weakly tyrosinase-positive reactions. Microphthalmia, corneal opacity, coarse nystagmus, athetosis, marked mental and growth retardation, gingival hypertrophy, and a faint high-pitched cry have been described in this syndrome.[34]

REFERENCES

1. Lerner AB: Vitiligo. *J Invest Dermatol* 1959;32:285.
2. Lerner AB: Vitiligo. *Prog Dermatol* 1972;6:1.
3. Halder RM, Walters CS, Johnson BA, et al.: Aberrations in T lymphocytes and natural killer cells in vitiligo: A flow cytometric study. *J Am Acad Dermatol* 1986;14:733–737.
4. Grimes PE, Ghoneum M, Stockton T: T cell profiles in vitiligo. *J Am Acad Dermatol* 1986;14:196–201.
5. Murahashi M, Hashimoto K, Goodman TF Jr, et al.: Ultrastructural studies of vitiligo, Vogt-Koyanagi syndrome, and incontinentia pigmenti achromians. *Arch Dermatol* 1977;113:755–766.
6. Nordund JJ, Forget B, Kirkwood J, et al.: Dermatitis produced

by application of monobenzene in patients with active vitiligo. *Arch Dermatol* 1985;121:1141–1144.

7. Hatcome N, Aiba S, Kato T, et al.: Possible functional impairment of Langerhans cells in vitiliginous skin. *Arch Dermatol* 1987;123:51–54.

8. Birbeck MS, Breathnach AS, Everall JD: An electron microscope study of basal melanocytes and high level clear cells (Langerhans cells) in vitiligo. *J Invest Dermatol* 1961;37:51–64.

9. Woolf CM, Dolowitz DA, Aldous HE: Congenital deafness associated with piebaldness. *Arch Otolaryngol* 1965;82:244–250.

10. Breathnach AS, Fitzpatrick TB, Wyllis LMA: Electron microscopy of melanocytes in human piebaldism. *J Invest Dermatol* 1965;45:28–37.

11. Jimbow K, Fitzpatrick TB, Szabo G, et al.: Congenital circumscribed hypomelanosis: A characterization based upon electron microscopic study of tuberous sclerosis, nevus depigmentosus, and piebaldism. *J Invest Dermatol* 1975;64:50–62.

12. Mayer TC: The development of piebald spotting in mice. *Dev Biol* 1965;11:319–334.

13. Mayer TC: Temporal skin factors influencing the development of melanoblasts in piebald mice. *J Exp Zool* 1967;166:397–404.

14. Nagao S, Iijima S, Shima T: Mast cells in the epidermis of piebaldism. *Arch Dermatol Res* 1975;251:221–225.

15. Frank SB, Cohen HJ: The halo nevus. *Arch Dermatol* 1964;89:367–373.

16. Smith WE, Moseley JC: Multiple halo neurofibromas. *Arch Dermatol* 1976;112:987–990.

17. Kopf AW, Morrill SD, Silverberg I: Broad spectrum of leukoderma acquisitum centrifugum. *Arch Dermatol* 1965;92:14–35.

18. Wayte DM, Helwig EB: Halo nevi. *Cancer* 1968;22:69–90.

19. Swanson JL, Wayte DM, Helwig EB: Ultrastructure of halo nevi. *J Invest Dermatol* 1968;50:434–449.

20. Hashimoto K: Ultrastructural studies of halo nevus. *Cancer* 1974;34:1653–1666.

21. Gauthier Y, Surleve-Bazeille JE, Gauthier O, et al.: Ultrastructure of halo nevi. *J Cutan Pathol* 1975;2:71–81.

22. Blume RS, Wolff SM: The Chediak-Higashi syndrome: Studies in four patients and a review of the literature. *Medicine (Baltimore)* 1972;51:247–280.

23. Stegmaier OC, Schneider LA: Chediak-Higashi syndrome: Dermatologic manifestations. *Arch Dermatol* 1965;91:1–9.

24. Bedoya A: Pigmentary changes in Chediak-Higashi syndrome. *Br J Dermatol* 1971;85:336–347.

25. Zelickson AS, Windhorst DB, White JG, et al.: The Chediak-Higashi syndrome: Formation of giant melanosomes and the basis of hypopigmentation. *J Invest Dermatol* 1967;49:575–581.

26. Stossel TP, Root RK, Vaugh M: Phagocytosis in chronic granulomatous disease and the Chediak-Higashi syndrome. *N Engl J Med* 1972;286:120–123.

27. Kugelman TP, VanScott EJ: Tyrosinase activity in melanocytes of human albinos. *J Invest Dermatol* 1961;37:73–76.

28. Witkop CJ Jr, Hill CW, Desnick S, et al.: Ophthalmologic, biochemical, platelet and ultrastructural defects in the various types of oculocutaneous albinism. *J Invest Dermatol* 1973;60:443–456.

29. Hermansky F, Pudlak P: Albinism associated with hemorrhagic diathesis and unusual pigmented reticular cells in the bone marrow. Report of two cases with histochemical studies. *Blood* 1959;14:162.

30. Frank E, Lattion F: The melanin pigmentary disorder in a family with Hermansky-Pudlak syndrome. *J Invest Dermatol* 1982;78:141–143.

31. Quevedo WC, Witkop CJ Jr, Fitzpatrick TB: Albinism, in Stanbury JB, Wyngaarden JB, Frederickson DS (eds): *The Metabolic Basis of Inherited Disease.* New York, McGraw-Hill, 1978, p. 283.

32. Nance WE, Jackson CE, Witkop CJ Jr: Amish albinism: A distinctive autosomal recessive phenotype. *Am J Hum Genet* 1970;22:579–586.

33. King RA, Lewis RA, Townsend D, et al.: Brown oculocutaneous albinism. Clinical, ophthalmological and biochemical characterization. *Ophthalmology* 1985;92:1496–1505.

34. Cross H, McKusick J, Breen W: A new oculocerebral syndrome with hypopigmentation. *J Pediatr* 1967;70:398–406.

CHAPTER 40

Chemical and Mineral Deposition in the Skin

R. Jeffrey Herten

A number of minerals, drugs, industrial chemicals, and organic compounds may be deposited in the skin. Sometimes skin pigmentation is altered, either through hypermelanosis or as a direct result of the presence of the material in the skin.

Deposition of these materials is discussed according to the mechanisms of accumulation, including inborn errors of metabolism, abnormal storage or deposition of endogenous minerals, and deposition of exogenous chemicals.

ERRORS OF METABOLISM

Ochronosis[1–6]

History
In 1859 Bodecker first described "alkaptons": chemicals in the urine of a patient that had a strong avidity for oxygen and created a brown-black color. In 1866, Virchow designated the entity *ochronosis* for the ochre-yellow-brown granules he observed microscopically in the connective tissue of an autopsy specimen.

Clinical Features
The classic clinical triad comprises dark urine, dark skin, and arthritis. Two clinical types are recognized: hereditary and acquired.

Hereditary ochronosis is expressed as a Mendelian recessive trait and is rare (three to five per million persons). Patients are asymptomatic until the fourth decade, when alkaptonuria and ochronosis develop. Arthropathy develops a decade later.

The pigment changes that occur are blue-gray thickening of the ear cartilage and dusky blue-brown, patchy skin pigmentation (Fig. 40–1) involving principally brown nails, scleral pigment medial to the cornea, and blue tarsal plates. Cerumen may be black and sweat may be brown.

The arthritis characteristically begins with the back in the fourth decade and progresses to the knees, shoulders, and hips. Spondylosis may result in a loss of six inches of height.

The urine is dark only when alkaline and tests false positive for sugar when reducing salts are used.

The acquired type of ochronosis may be induced by exposure to chemicals that inhibit the sulfhydryl group of homogentisic acid oxidase. These include phenol, resorcin, mepacrine, and other antimalarial agents, and hydroquinone. Such patients develop skin and cartilage pigmentation, but alkaptonuria and arthropathy have not been described.

Pathophysiologic Features
Ochronosis results from a deficiency of homogentisic acid oxidase. Homogentisic acid (HGA), a breakdown product of tyrosine and phenylalanine, accumulates and polymerizes to benzoquinone acetic acid. HGA has an affinity for collagen and apparently inhibits lysyl hydroxylase, weakening the collagen by inhibiting hydroxylysine crosslinkage.

Histologic Features
The ochre-yellow to brown granules of polymerized HGA are seen free in the dermis, in macrophages, in endothelial cells, and in the basement membrane region of eccrine secretory cells. The granules first accumulate in collagen fibrils as small granules; they gradually enlarge as the surrounding collagen degenerates and form large, irregularly shaped granules (Fig. 40–1). Elastic fibers are similarly involved. Occasional foreign body giant cells may be seen surrounding the granules.

Histochemically, the granules may be difficult to distinguish from melanin. They reduce ferric ferricyanide but not acid silver nitrate, and stain black with cresyl violet or methylene blue.

Polymerized HGA can be seen deposited around individual collagen fibrils. The fibrils undergo degeneration and further deposition of HGA occurs. The HGA progressively replaces viable collagen to produce larger, irregular areas of deposition.

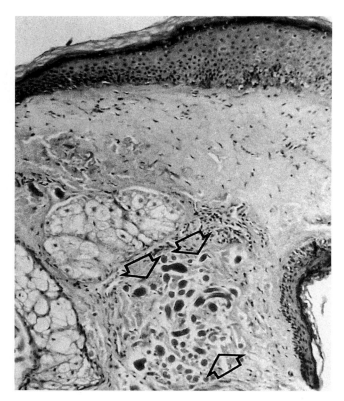

Figure 40–1. Irregularly shaped, ochre-brown granules (arrows) deposited throughout the dermis of a patient with hereditary ochronosis. (H&E, ×400.)

ABNORMAL STORAGE OR DEPOSITION OF ENDOGENEOUS MATERIALS

Hemochromatosis[7–10]

History
Hanot-Chaufford first described hemochromatosis in 1892, but the name was coined by Von Recklinghausen in 1899.

Clinical Features
Also known as "bronze diabetes," hemochromatosis is characterized by five clinical signs: cutaneous hyperpigmentation, diabetes mellitus, cirrhosis, cardiomyopathy, and arthropathy. The disease is relatively common (0.1% of large autopsy series), affects men ten times more frequently than women, and is rare under the age of 20. In most cases, onset occurs between 40 and 60 years of age.

The gold-brown hyperpigmentation may be accentuated in sun-exposed areas and is nearly universal. Mucosal pigment occurs in 5% to 25% of patients and may be more silver-gray in color as is the accentuation of pigment occurring on the genital, periareolar, flexor, and conjunctival surfaces. Scars may show hyperpigmentation.

The pigment is the first clinical sign and may precede diabetes and heart disease by years. Other clinical findings associated with hemochromatosis are ichthyosis-like derma-

titis, hair loss involving the scalp, axillary, and pubic areas, gonadal dysfunction, koilonychia, palmar erythema, spider hemangiomas, and leukonychia.

Pathophysiologic Features
Several types of hemochromatosis have been identified on the basis of etiology. The idiopathic or familial type occurs as an autosomal recessive transmitted disease and appears to be caused by a "mucosal block" resulting in increased intestinal absorption of iron. Acquired types result from increased oral intake of iron (Bantu beer brewed in iron pots and red wine) or iron overload(multiple transfusions) or are associated with entities with abnormal iron metabolism such as porphyria and hepatic cirrhosis.

Although large amounts of iron are found throughout the skin, it is clear that the pigmentation is largely melanin. Apparently, the dermal iron has a stimulatory effect on melanogenesis.

Histologic Features
The epidermis in hemochromatosis is normal in thickness, but demonstrates increased melanin in the basilar and suprabasilar layers. Hemosiderin pigment is seen free and within macrophages around the blood vessels of the superficial dermis. Hemosiderin is also present in the basement membrane of eccrine glands. Rarely, it may be seen in the epidermis and within eccrine secretory cells.

Histochemically, the hemosiderin is positive with Perls' stain.

Electron Microscopy Features
Large, irregularly shaped electron-dense granules without internal structure are seen free and within lysosomes in dermal macrophages as well as in the eccrine basement membrane. Increased melanosomes are seen in epidermal melanocytes and suprabasilar keratinocytes.

Hemosiderosis

Clinical Features
The deposition of hemosiderin in the skin is the end result of a large number of clinical entities, the majority of which have in common the disruption of the dermal capillary bed and the extravasation and destruction of erythrocytes. These entities include stasis dermatitis, sickle cell anemia, congenital hemolytic anemia, the progressive pigmented purpuric eruptions, drug eruptions, scurvy, atrophie blanche (livedo vasculitis), and acroangiodermatitis.

The initial clinical lesion in hemosiderosis is an erythematous macule that is nonblanching and gradually evolves from red through orange to ochre and then remains a tawny, orange-brown color. Dependent areas, especially over the malleolus and distal lower extremity, are predisposed. Examination with a black light intensifies the pigmentation, as most is due to hypermelanosis.

Pathophysiologic Features
Destruction of the red blood cell leaves dermal hemosiderin. As with hemochromatosis, dermal hemosiderin deposition has a stimulatory effect on melanogenesis.

Histologic Features

Hemosiderosis is identical to hemochromatosis with respect to histopathology and histochemistry. Commonly, features of the causative vascular compromise (i.e., livedo vasculitis) may be identified.

Electron microscopy yields findings similar to those in hemochromatosis.

DEPOSITION OF EXOGENOUS MATERIALS

Minocycline[11–16]

History

Basler and Kohnen first described hemosiderosis in areas of acne scarring in a patient on minocycline therapy in 1978.[13]

Clinical Features

Patients on long-term minocycline therapy may develop blue-black discoloration in areas of previous acne scarring. Gray-green discoloration at the base of teeth has been described, and an autopsy of a patient on long-term minocycline showed black discoloration of the thyroid, blue-black cartilage alteration, and some brown staining of the skull bones. Generalized gray-blue pigmentation, partially reversible with cessation of therapy, has also been reported.

Pathophysiologic Features

In experimental animals, minocycline accumulates in brain, bone, and thyroid. Evidence suggests that minocycline deposition in skin may play a role in the cutaneous pigmentation, but no explanation has been offered for the localization to areas of scarring.

Histologic Features

The epidermis is normal, but may show increased basilar and suprabasilar melanin. In the dermis, there are aggregates of brown-black granules principally within perivascular macrophages in the upper reticular dermis.

Histochemically, the granules stain positively with Perls' iron stain and with the Fontana-Masson silver method (Figs. 40–2, 40–3).

Electron-dense granules are seen within macrophages. Some are small (50–100 nm) and resemble ferritin. Larger granules (up to 1.5 nm) resembling hemosiderin and larger irregular granules, which may be minocycline related, are also seen (Fig. 40–4). The granules contain neither melanosomes nor premelanosomes.

Phenothiazines[17–22]

History

Greiner and Berry[18] first described the photoaccentuated pigmentation of patients on long-term chlorpromazine therapy in 1964. Although other phenothiazines have been implicated, chlorpromazine remains the most significant drug in this category.

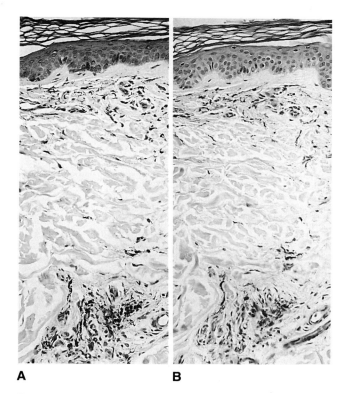

Figure 40–2. Minocycline-induced cutaneous hyperpigmentation. Pigment granules present around vessels throughout the dermis stain positively with both Fontana and Prussian blue stains. (**A,** Fontana, ×195; **B,** Prussian blue, ×195.) (*Photo courtesy of R. S. W. Basler, M.D.*)

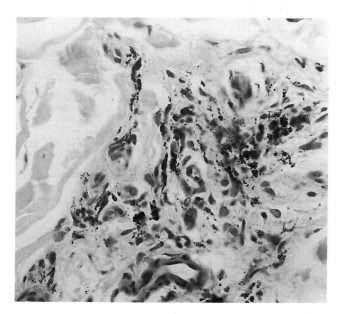

Figure 40–3. Minocycline pigmentation. Higher magnifications of biopsy specimen depicted in Fig. 40–2. (Fontana, ×400.)

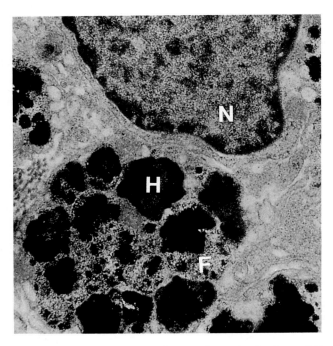

Figure 40–4. Portion of a dermal macrophage showing large, electron-dense granules of hemosiderin (H) and dispersed granules, probably ferritin (F), adjacent to macrophage nucleus (N). (×13,000.) (*Photo courtesy of R. S. W. Basler, M.D.*)

Clinical Features

Long-term chlorpromazine therapy may produce hyperpigmentation of the skin that is accentuated in sun-exposed areas. The frequency has been reported as 1% to 15% of patients on 800 to 2000 mg daily for 12 months or longer. Women are more commonly affected. The pigment varies from a violaceous hue to a blue-gray color, often described as metallic. The frontal, nasal, and malar areas are most commonly involved, and sparing of wrinkles and creases underscores the role of the sun in the production of the pigment. Involvement of sclera, cornea, and lens has been reported.

Pathophysiologic Features

Ultraviolet light produces a dechlorinated free radical of chloropromazine that polymerizes and binds to melanin. Although reversibly bound, the chlorpromazine polymer–melanin complexes are not metabolized by the body. They accumulate in the skin, in the reticuloendothelial system, and in the parenchyma of liver, lung, kidney, brain, and heart.

Histologic Features

The epidermis is normal, but an increase in basilar and suprabasilar melanin may be seen. Dark brown granules are noted within macrophages throughout the upper dermis, especially around the small capillary vessels in the upper reticular dermis. Perls' stain is negative, but the Fontana-Masson stain is positive. Dopa-positive cells are not seen in the dermis.

Ultrastructurally, there is an increased number of epidermal melanosomes. In the basal and suprabasilar layers, membrane-bound melanin granules and fine electron-dense particles are seen. The dermal macrophages show an increase in lysosomes, many of which contain melanosomes, fine electron-dense particles, and large, irregularly shaped electron-dense granules up to 3 μm in diameter (Fig. 40–5). These granules are thought to represent melanin-dechlorinated chlorpromazine polymer complexes.

Antimalarial Agents[23–27]

History

The widespread use of antimalarial agents, principally quinacrine, in the South Pacific in World War II acquainted

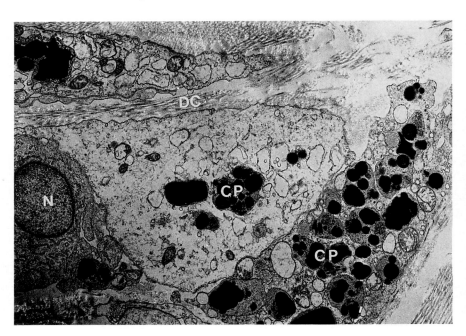

Figure 40–5. Membrane-bound granules of chlorpromazine (CP) within the cytoplasm of a dermal macrophage. DC = dermal collagen. (×12,600.) (*Photo courtesy of A. S. Zelickson, M.D.*)

physicians with the curious yellowish discoloration patients developed while taking it. Lutterloh and Shallenberger first described this discoloration in 1946.[25]

Clinical Features

Most patients taking quinacrine develop diffuse pale yellow skin coloration. Scleral involvement is absent, in contrast to jaundice. Furthermore, quinacrine and its related 4-aminoquinolones and acridines, namely, chloraquine, hydroxychloraquine, amodiaquine, and mepacrine, have been reported to produce pigmentary abnormalities in up to 25% of patients. Most commonly, pretibial patches of blue-gray pigmentation occur bilaterally. Transverse blue-black banding of the nails and palatal pigmentation have also been noted. The presence of cutaneous pigmentation increases the likelihood of retinopathy associated with these drugs. Although improvement is seen on cessation of therapy, the pigmentation does not clear completely.

Pathophysiologic Features

It appears that the antimalarial agents bind to melanin, forming a complex that is deposited in the skin and results in the pigmentation.

Histologic Features

The epidermis is normal. Yellow-brown pigment granules are present free in the dermis as well as within macrophages. The deep dermis shows the heaviest concentration of these granules.

Histochemically, Perls' stain is positive around the capillaries of the upper dermis. The Fontana-Masson method is positive throughout the entire dermis.

Clofazimine

History

A phenazine dye, variously designated as clofazimine, B 663, and Lamprene, was found to be effective in the treatment of leprosy. Early experience revealed common skin pigmentation reactions as reported by Barry et al. in 1952.

Clinical Features

Two types of pigmentation are seen in the course of treatment. The first type consists of a reddish-orange discoloration of the skin which begins within several weeks of initiation of treatment. The second type, confined to areas of lepromatous involvement, develops several months after treatment begins and consists of violaceous to blue-black patches.

Pathophysiologic Features

Clofazimine is highly fat soluble. The initial red pigmentation appears to result from accumulation of the dye in the lipids of reticuloendothelial cells of the dermis and in the lipocytes of the subcutis; internal organs with large fat accumulations or reticuloendothelial components are likewise stained. The later, dark pigmentation appears to be the result of accumulation of a ceroidlike pigment throughout the dermis which represents a complex formed by the drug

and saturated fatty acids of the leprosy bacilli. There is increased epidermal melanin and melanin incontinence which contributes to the pigmentation as well.

Histologic Features

The epidermis shows basilar and suprabasilar hypermelanosis. There is some pigment incontinence, with melanin free and within melanophages in the papillary dermis. There is diffuse brown staining of dermis and subcutis, and high-power examination reveals brown pigment in lipid vesicles within macrophages and within lipocytes in the subcutaneous fat.

Histochemically, the upper dermal pigment is positive with the Fontana-Masson method. The diffuse brown staining is acid fast; positive for lipid stains, even after fat solvent extraction; and weakly positive in the Schmorl reaction and chrom alum hematoxylin staining.

Gold (Crysoderma or Chrysiasis)[32–35]

History

Parenteral gold therapy was first used in 1917 to treat tuberculosis. The first reports of chrysiasis were published in 1928 by Hansborg.

Clinical Features

Skin pigmentation resulting from gold therapy is dose related. It is not seen in cumulative doses less than 50 mg/kg and is nearly universal in doses greater than 150 mg/kg. The pigmentation is present only in sun-exposed areas, with perioral accentuation. Skin folds are spared. The pigmentation is permanent.

Pathophysiologic Features

Gold accumulates in the dermis and its physical presence is responsible for the pigmentation, although to a lesser degree, melanin may be responsible.

Histologic Features

The epidermis may contain some increased basilar and suprabasilar melanin. In the dermis, small oval black granules are seen in macrophages in the endothelial cells of superficial dermal blood vessels and in the basement membrane of eccrine coils.

Darkfield examination shows refractive granules, larger than those of silver, in the previously mentioned locations.

Large, irregular granules 300–500 nm are seen principally in membrane-bound spaces within macrophages and coating the collagen reticulum of the eccrine basement membrane.

Silver (Argyria)[36–41]

History

Silver was used medically in the first quarter of this century as silver proteinate (Argyrol) and silver arsphenamine (Salvarsan, Neo-Silvol). Pigmentation caused by silver was first described in 1935 by Gaul and Staud.[36]

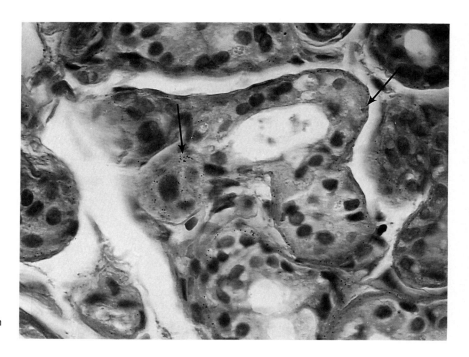

Figure 40–6. Silver granules (arrows) within an eccrine duct. (H&E, ×700.)

Clinical Features

Eight grams of silver must be ingested or absorbed to produce clinical pigmentation. The color varies from blue to slate gray and is accentuated in sun-exposed areas. The gingivae and conjunctivae are commonly involved and blue-gray discoloration of nail lunulae may be noted. The depth of pigmentation depends on the dosage of silver and the extent of sun exposure.

Pathophysiologic Features

Silver appears to react chemically with a sulfur containing organic matrix (amino acid) to produce insoluble silver sulfide. This compound may have a stimulatory effect on melanin synthesis.

Histologic Features

The epidermis may contain increased amounts of basilar and suprabasilar melanin. Small, 1-μm gray-brown granules are seen in macrophages in the basal lamina of adnexal structures, in the perineurium of peripheral nerves, and along elastic and collagen fibers (Fig. 40–6).

Histochemically, Perls' stain is negative, and the Fontana-Masson method is negative for melanin. Darkfield examination reveals brilliantly refractile granules in the locations just noted (Fig. 40–7).

Electron-dense granules are seen in macrophages, fibroblasts, elastic fibers, and lamina propria. By x-ray microanalysis, the materials are identified as silver sulfide.

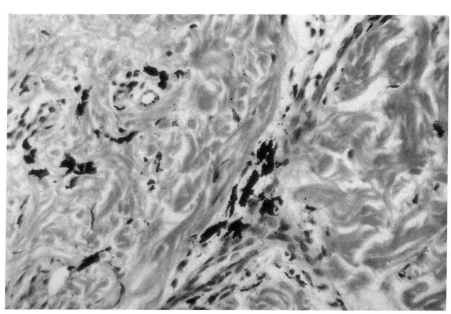

Figure 40–7. Brilliantly refractile granules of silver in the basal lamina of an eccrine coil. Darkfield microscopy, (×400).

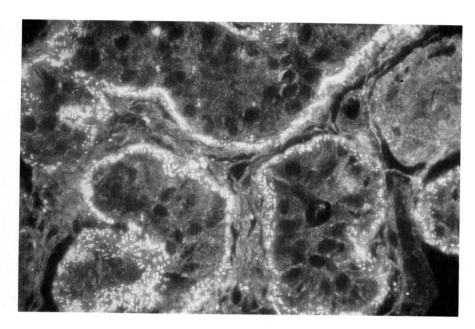

Figure 40–8. Carbon black granules within macrophages in the upper dermis. The material is chiefly perivascular but presents interstitially as well. (H&E, ×400.)

Tattoos[42–45]

History

The deliberate introduction of exogenous pigments into the skin is a ubiquitous cultural practice worldwide and dates back at least 8,000 years. Although tattooing has been practiced since ancient times, the medical complications were first recorded in 1869 by Berchon.

Clinical Features

Tattooing is performed by inoculating pigments into the skin with a needlelike device. Black is produced by using carbon, blue by using cobalt, red by using mercuric sulfide, green by using chromium, and yellow by using cadmium sulfide. Commonly, cadmium is added to mercuric sulfide to produce a brighter red and is the source of the photoreactions to red tattooed areas.

Pathophysiologic Features

The various pigments remain in the dermis, partially phagocytosed, resulting in various hues of skin pigmentation. Occasionally, sarcoidal or foreign body reactions may occur.

Histologic Features

The epidermis is normal. Granules of various sizes are seen free and within macrophages in the upper and midreticular dermis (Fig. 40–8). The pigment is concentrated principally around small dermal capillaries, but may be seen interstitially as well.

Histochemically, special stains are not helpful and darkfield examination is negative.

Electron Microscopic Features

Granules of electron-dense material are seen free in the dermis and within membrane-bound vesicles within dermal macrophages. Positive identification of the pigment can be accomplished by x-ray microanalysis.

REFERENCES

1. Bruce S, Tschen JA, Chow D: Exogenous ochronosis resulting from quinine injections. *J Am Acad Dermatol* 1986;15:357–361.
2. Hoshaw RA, Zimmerman KG, Menter A: Ochronosis-like pigmentation from hydroquinone bleaching creams in American blacks. *Arch Dermatol* 1985;121:105–108.
3. O'Brien W, Bert N, Bunim JJ: Biochemical, pathologic, and clinical aspects of alcaptonuria, ochronosis, and ochronotic arthropathy (review of world literature 1584–1962). *Am J Med* 1963;34:813–838 (353 references).
4. Phillips JI, Isaacson C, Carman H: Ochronosis in black South Africans who used skin lighteners. *Am J Acad Dermatol* 1986;8:14–21.
5. Stanbury JB, Wyngaarden JB, Frederickson DS, et al: *The Metabolic Basis of Inherited Diseases*, ed 5. New York, McGraw-Hill, 1982.
6. Woolley PB: Exogenous ochronosis. *Brit Med J* 1952;2:760.
7. Chevrant-Breton J, Simon M, Bourel M, et al.: Cutaneous manifestations of idiopathic hemochromatosis (study of 100 cases). *Arch Dermatol* 1977;113:161–165.
8. Finch SC, Finch CA: Idiopathic hemochromatosis, an iron storage disease. A. Iron metabolism in hemochromatosis. *Medicine (Baltimore)* 1955;**34**:381–430.
9. Pedrup A, Pouisen H: Hemochromatosis and vitiligo. *Arch Dermatol* 1964;90(1):34–37.
10. Tsuji T: Experimental hemochromatosis: Relationship between akin pigmentation and hemosiderin. *Acta Dermatovenereol (Stockh)* 1980;60:109–114.
11. Attwood HD, Dennett X: A black thyroid and minocycline treatment. *Br J Med* 1976;2:1109–1110.
12. Basler RSW: Minocycline therapy for acne (Letter). *Arch Dermatol* 1979;115:1391.
13. Basler RSW, Kohnen PW: Localized hemochromatosis as a sequelae of acne. *Arch Dermatol* 1978;114:1695–1697.
14. Gordon G, Sparano BM, Iatropoulos MJ: Hyperpigmentation associated with minocycline therapy. *Arch Dermatol* 1985;121:618–623.
15. McGrae JD, Zelickson AS: Skin pigmentation secondary to minocycline therapy. *Arch Dermatol* 1980;116:1262–1265.

16. Prigent F, Cavelier-Balloy B, Tollenaere C, et al.: Cutaneous pigmentation induced by minocycline: Two cases. *Ann Dermatol Venereol* 1986;113:227–233.

17. Blois MS: On chlorpromazine binding in vivo. *J Invest Dermatol* 1966;47:296–306.

18. Greiner AC, Berry K: Skin pigmentation and corneal and lens opacities with prolonged chlorpromazine therapy. *Can Med Assoc J* 1964;90:663–665.

19. Hashimoto K, Wiener W, Albert J, et al.: An electron microscopic study of chlorpromazine pigmentation. *J Invest Dermatol* 1966;47:296–306.

20. Satanou A: Pigmentation due to phenothiazines in high and prolonged dosage. *JAMA* 1965;191:263–268.

21. VanWoert MH: Isolation of chlorpromazine pigments in man. *Nature* 1968;219:1054–1056.

22. Zelickson AS, Zeller HS: A new and unusual reaction to chlorpromazine. *JAMA* 1964;188:394–395.

23. Granstein RD, Sober AJ: Drug- and heavy metal-induced hyperpigmentation. *J Am Acad Dermatol* 1981;5:1–18.

24. Levantine A, Almeyda J: Drug induced changes in pigmentation. *Br J Dermatol* 1973;89:105–112.

25. Lutterloh CC, Shallenberger PL: Unusual pigmentation developing after prolonged suppressive therapy with quinacrine hydrochloride. *Arch Dermatol Venereol* 1946;53:394–354.

26. Sams Wm, Epstein JH: The affinity of melanin for chloroquine. *J Invest Dermatol* 1965;45:482–488.

27. Tuffanelli D, Abraham RK, Dubois EI: Pigmentation from antimalarial therapy: Its possible relation to ocular lesions. *Arch Dermatol* 1963;88:419–426.

28. Conalty ML, Jackson RD: Uptake by reticulo-endothelial cells of the rimino-phenazine B663 (2-*p*-chloroanilino-5-*p*-chlorophenyl-3:5-dihydro-3-isopropyliminophenzaine). *Br J Exp Pathol* 1962;42:650–654.

29. Pettit JHS: B 663 (Lamprene) in myobacterial infections. *Br J Dermatol* 1969;81:794–795.

30. Pettit JHS, Rees RJW, Ridley DS: Chemotherapeutic trials in leprosy. 3. Pilot trial of a riminophenizine derivative B663 in the treatment of lepromatous leprosy. *Int J Lepr* 1967;35:25–33.

31. Sakurai I, Skinsnes OK: Histochemistry of B663 pigmentation: Ceroid-like pigmentation in macrophages. *Int J Lepr* 1977; 45:343–354.

32. Everett MA: Metal discolorations in dermis, in *Clinical Dermatology*, Hagerstown, Harper and Row, 1979, unit 11–14, p 3.

33. Levantine A, Almeyda J: Drug-induced changes in pigmentation. *Br J Dermatol* 1973;89:105–112.

34. Penneys NS, Ackerman AB, Gottlieb NL: Gold dermatitis, a clinical and histopathological study. *Arch Dermatol* 1974; 109:372–376.

35. Schmidt OEL: Chrysiasis. *Arch Dermatol Syphilol* 1941;44:446–452.

36. Gaul LE, Staud AH: Clinical spectroscopy: Seventy cases of generalized argyrosis following organic and colloidal silver medication, including a biospectrometric analysis of ten cases. *JAMA* 1935;104:1387–1390.

37. Hill WR, Montgomery H: Argyria with special reference to the cutaneous histopathology. *Arch Dermatol* 1941;44:588–599.

38. Marshall JP, Schneider RP: Systemic argyria secondary to topical silver nitrate. *Arch Dermatol* 1977;113:1077–1079.

39. Pariser RJ: Generalized argyria: Clinicopathologic features and histochemical studies. *Arch Dermatol* 1978;114:373–377.

40. Prose PH: An electron microscopic study of human generalized argyria. *Am J Pathol* 1963;42(3):293–303.

41. Westhoven M, Schaefer H: Generalized argyrosis in man: Neurotoxicological, ultrastructural, and x-ray microanalytical findings. *Arch Otorhinolaryngol* 1986;243(4):260–264.

42. Abel EA, Silberg I, Queen D: Studies of chronic inflammation in a red tattoo by electron microscopy and histochemistry. *Acta Dermatol Venereol* (*Stockh*) 1972;52:453–461.

43. Beerman H, Lane RAG: Tattoo: A summary of scientific literature on the medical complications of tattoos. *Am J Med Sci* 1954;227:444–465.

44. Goldstein AP: Histologic reactions in tattoos. *J Dermatol Surg Oncol* 1979;5:896–900.

45. Levy J, Sewell M, Goldstein A: A short history of tattooing. *J Dermatol Surg Oncol* 1979;5:851–856.

SECTION VII
Cysts

CHAPTER 41
Cysts

Loren E. Golitz and Somsak Poomeechaiwong

EPIDERMOID CYST (INFUNDIBULAR CYST)

Epidermoid cysts account for approximately 80% to 90% of all cutaneous cysts.[1] They are located predominantly on the face, neck, and upper trunk in a distribution similar to that of acne vulgaris. Epidermoid cysts are rare in childhood and occur predominantly in young and middle-aged adults. They are more common in individuals with a history of severe acne vulgaris. Men are affected approximately twice as often as women. Epidermoid cysts vary from 0.5 to 5 cm in diameter, may be solitary or multiple, and are often present several years before treatment is sought. Multiple epidermoid cysts are seen in Gardner's syndrome and in the nevoid basal cell carcinoma syndrome. Epidermoid cysts are relatively common on the scrotum where they have a tendency to calcify. The cysts walls may disintegrate, producing focal collections of dystrophic calcification of the scrotum known as scrotal calcinosis.[2] Clinical darkening of epidermoid cysts has been reported in individuals with hemochromatosis.[3] Skin cancer and Bowen's disease may occur in epidermoid cysts.[4] The incidence of malignancy in three studies was 1.1%,[5] 1.5%,[6] and 1.7%.[7] In MacDonald's[5] series, six of seven skin cancers were basal cell carcinomas and two thirds of these occurred in cysts located on sun-exposed skin. Molluscum contagiosum can occur within epidermoid cysts, probably as a result of localization of the virus in the ostium of hair follicles followed by obstruction and formation of a cyst.[8] In certain hereditary diseases, such as Darier's disease, the characteristic epithelial changes may also occur in the lining of epidermoid cysts. The cysts are thin walled and tend to rupture during surgical removal.

Histologic Features
The wall of epidermoid cysts is composed of stratified squamous epithelium with a well-formed granular layer (Fig. 41–1). The lumina contain a variable amount of loose keratin. Occasionally, the cysts are seen to connect to the surface of the skin through keratin-filled pores (Fig. 41–2). As the cyst wall folds back under the epidermis, the wall and epidermis appear as mirror images of each other. A variable number of bacteria may be present within the cysts. Calcification usually does not occur, although it is common in cysts that occur on the scrotum. Melanocytes and melanin pigment are usually not obvious in cysts of Caucasians. Approximately 37% of black patients have very darkly pigmented cysts;[9] 97% of darkly pigmented cysts occur in black patients.[9] In one black patient with hemochromatosis a large amount of melanin pigment was present in the keratogenous contents of an epidermoid cyst.[3] Ruptured epidermoid cysts are often associated with dermal abscess formation and a foreign body granulomatous reaction. Delicate wafers of keratin are present within the granulomatous infiltrate.

MILIUM

Primary and secondary forms of milia are recognized.[10] Primary milia occur predominantly on the face and may be seen in infants or adults. Secondary milia occur on parts of the body exposed to a variety of conditions that cause scarring, such as trauma, dermabrasion, burns, and radiation therapy. Diseases that cause subepidermal blisters, such as bullous pemphigoid, porphyria cutanea tarda, bullous lichen planus, epidermolysis bullosa, and lichen sclerosus et atrophicus,[11] may also be associated with secondary milium formation. Both forms of milia are characterized by 1- to 2-mm white to yellow papular lesions.

Histologic Features
Both forms of milia histologically resemble tiny epidermoid cysts (Fig. 41–3). Milia may connect to the epidermis or to an eccrine sweat duct or a hair follicle. Occasionally, an eccrine sweat duct may be seen to enter the wall of a milia from deeper in the dermis. The wall is composed of stratified squamous epithelium which is usually only a few cell layers thick. A granular layer is present and the cyst contains a small amount of loose keratin.

Primary milia are felt to represent cystic, keratinizing

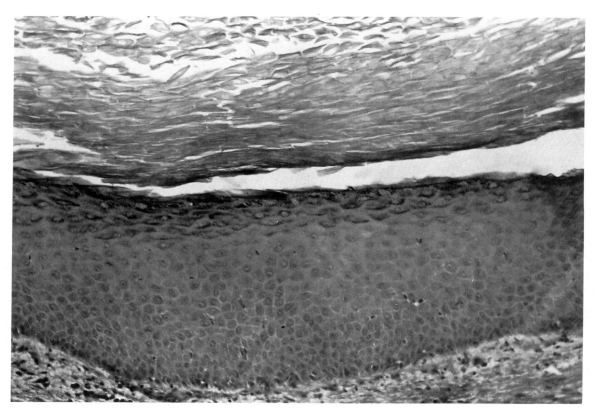

Figure 41–1. Epidermoid cyst. The cyst wall is lined by stratified squamous epithelium with a well-formed granular layer. (H&E, ×160.)

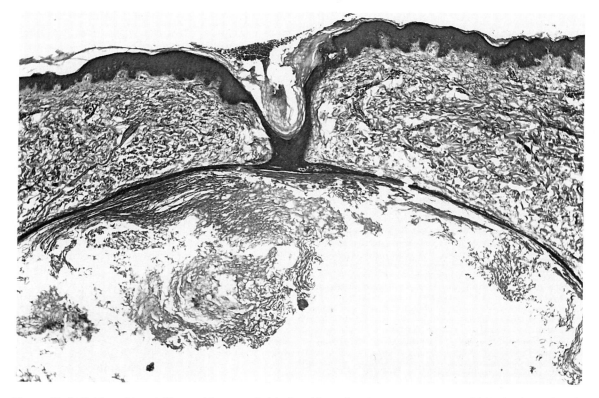

Figure 41–2. Epidermoid cyst. The cyst is connected to the skin surface by a narrow pore and contains loose keratin. (H&E, ×25.)

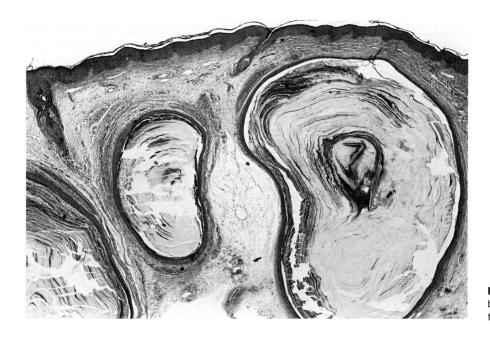

Figure 41–3. Milia. Three milia that resemble small epidermoid cysts are present in the dermis. (H&E, ×25.)

benign tumors that develop from pluripotential cells present in adnexal or epidermal epithelium.[10] Secondary milia represent small keratinizing retention cysts produced by damage to adnexal epithelium.

EPIDERMAL INCLUSION CYST (TRAUMATIC EPIDERMOID CYST)

The term *epidermal inclusion cyst* is often used incorrectly for epidermoid cysts. A true epidermal inclusion cyst occurs as the result of traumatic implantation of epidermis into the dermis.[12,13] Less than 1% of cutaneous cysts are true epidermal inclusion cysts.[6] The cysts are most common on the hands and feet; less than 10% of epidermoid cysts occur on the extremities.[14] Vulvar epidermoid cysts in the Igbos of Nigeria probably arise as a result of traumatic implantation of epithelium during ritual circumcision.[15]

Histologic Features
Epidermal inclusion cysts of acral skin resemble epidermoid cysts in that the wall is composed of stratified squamous epithelium with a well-formed granular layer. The keratin lining of the cysts, however, is thick and dense (Fig. 41–4) because of the compact nature of keratinization of acral skin. This compact pattern keratinization should not be confused with that seen in trichilemmal cysts, which occur predominantly on the scalp but never on the palms and soles.

ERUPTIVE VELLUS HAIR CYST

Hyperpigmented asymptomatic monomorphous papular lesions are found on the anterior chest, abdomen, and flexural aspects of the extremities.[16] Although usually smooth the papules may be umbilicated[17] or crusted and rough.[18]

Males and females are equally affected. Sporadic cases appear to have an onset from approximately 4 to 18 years of age. Familial cases have been reported,[18,19] with an onset from birth to early infancy. The latter cases show an autosomal dominant inheritance pattern. Approximately 25% of the reported cases spontaneously resolved, leaving either residual hyperpigmentation or small scars. It has been sug-

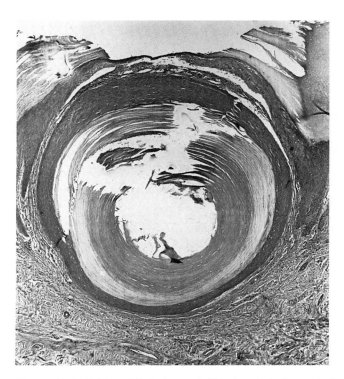

Figure 41–4. Epidermal inclusion cyst. This true inclusion cyst of acral skin was formed by the traumatic implantation of epidermis into the dermis. Note the dense keratin within the cyst. (H&E, ×25.)

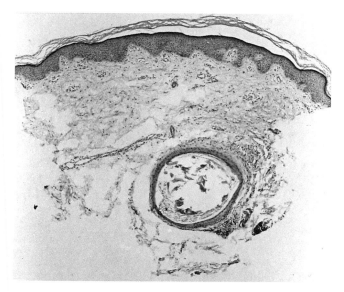

Figure 41–5. Eruptive vellus hair cyst. A tiny cyst resembling an epidermoid cyst is present in the dermis. (H&E, ×25.)

gested that spontaneous resolution occurs through the process of transepidermal elimination of the vellus hair.[17,20] Esterley et al.[16] have suggested that the condition represents a developmental anomaly of the vellus hair follicle that results in follicular plugging and subsequent deflection of the hair shaft, causing cystic dilatation of the hair follicle.

Histologic Features

Within the superficial or middermis is a small cystic structure (Fig. 41–5) lined by stratified squamous epithelium. A granular layer is present and the cyst contains loose keratin. A rudimentary telogen hair follicle may be attached to the cystic structure.[21] Within the cyst is a small nonpigmented vellus hair shaft, which appears to be coiled and cross-cut several times in sectioning (Fig. 41–6). Older lesions may show rupture of the cyst wall with granulomatous inflammation and elimination of the vellus hair shaft to the skin surface.[17]

DERMOID CYST

Dermoid cysts are usually present at birth and are most often located at the lateral aspect of the upper eyelid or eyebrow.[22] They may also be located in the midline of the nose or in the midline of the scalp or neck. Rarely, a central tuft of pigmented hair may be present. Dermoid cysts represent a developmental defect with entrapment of epithelium and adnexal structures in the subcutaneous fat during embryonic closure along the ventral midline of the body.

Histologic Features

Dermoid cysts are located in the subcutaneous fat and may be attached to the periosteum of bone.[22] The cysts are lined by stratified squamous epithelium with a granular

layer. Numerous pilosebaceous structures (Fig. 41–7) and a variable number of eccrine sweat glands empty into the lumen of the cyst. In addition to loose keratin the cyst contains numerous pigmented hair shafts. A variable amount of smooth muscle may be seen in the surrounding connective tissue. Steatocystomas differ from dermoid cysts in that they contain only single sebaceous glands and no sweat glands.

TRICHILEMMAL CYST (PILAR CYST, ISTHMUS CATAGEN CYST)

Trichilemmal cysts are the second most common type of cutaneous cyst, accounting for 15% of surgically excised cysts.[1] They are twice as common in women as men. Approximately 90% occur on the scalp.[1] These cysts occur most commonly in middle age as smooth, firm, round nodules which vary from 0.5 to 5 cm in diameter. Uncommonly, they may become inflamed and tender. Trichilemmal cysts may be inherited as an autosomal dominant trait, in which case they are often multiple and develop at a slightly earlier age.[23] The scalp hair is usually normal over the cyst and they typically do not have a visible punctum.[23] Because of their thick walls, trichilemmal cysts are usually excised intact, in contrast to epidermoid cysts which frequently rupture during surgery.

Trichilemmal cysts have historically been associated with a confusing terminology. They have been known by the common name of *wen*. In 1930, Broders and Wilson termed the cysts *sebaceous cysts* because of their strong clinical odor in comparison with epidermoid cysts.[24] McGavran recognized that the cysts were related to hair follicles and proposed the term *pilar cyst*.[1] Holmes suggested the term *trichochlamydocyst*, which indicates a cyst of the hair sheath.[25] In 1969 Pinkus coined the term *trichilemma* for the outer root sheath of the hair follicle.[26] He credited Maurer[27] with describing the type of keratinization associated with the trichilemma in 1895. It was Pinkus who proposed the term *trichilemmal cyst* to replace the term *pilar cyst*, which is less specific. Trichilemmal keratinization occurs in the follicular isthmus of normal anagen hairs and in the sack surrounding catagen hairs.[26] Because of the location of this type of keratinization the term *isthmus catagen cyst* has also been used to describe these cysts.

Histologic Features

Trichilemmal cysts (Fig. 41–8) are rarely connected to the epidermis.[28] The cyst wall is composed of stratified squamous epithelium with a palisaded outer layer resembling that of the outer root sheath of the hair follicle. The inner layer of pale-staining, keratinizing, cells shows a corrugated or scalloped appearance without a granular layer (Fig. 41–9). The content of these cells is periodic acid-Shiff positive and diastase sensitive, indicating that they contain glycogen. The keratin lining within the cysts is very dense, pink, and homogeneous in contrast to the delicate loose keratin of epidermoid cysts. Within the lumina of the cysts calcium is present in 24% and cholesterol clefts in 92%.[23] A focal,

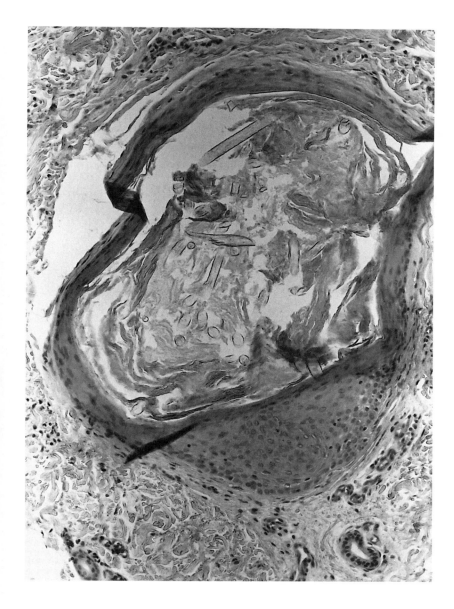

Figure 41–6. Eruptive vellus hair cyst. The cyst contains cross sections of a vellus hair shaft. (H&E, ×100.)

partial granular layer is present in 7% of trichilemmal cysts.[23] Inflammation is seen in only 15% of trichilemmal cysts in contrast to 50% of epidermoid cysts, a feature that may be related to the lack of an epidermal connection in the former.[23] The keratinizing corrugated cells lining the inner portion of the cyst can be seen to contain fine, birefringent sheaves when examined by polarized light.[1] By electron microscopy the keratinizing cells of the cyst wall contain large amounts of tonofilaments and are connected to each other by desmosomes.[29] The keratinized cells within the cyst lumen lack nuclei and cytoplasmatic organelles but, in contrast to the keratin of epidermoid cysts and to the epidermal stratum corneum, retain desmosomal connections.[29] Leppard and Sanderson noted focal budding of smaller cysts from the walls of trichilemmal cysts and proposed that trichilemmal cysts develop by budding from the outer root sheath of hair follicles at the isthmus.[28]

PROLIFERATING TRICHILEMMAL CYST (PROLIFERATING PILAR CYST, PILAR TUMOR OF THE SCALP)

The term *proliferating epidermoid cyst* was used by Wilson Jones to describe a peculiar tumor that typically involved the scalp of elderly women.[30] Women are affected twice as often as men, and in one series more than 90% of patients were over 60 years of age.[31] Patients usually seek medical advice because of enlarging scalp nodules, often associated with inflammation.[31] Brownstein noted that the sex distribution, clinical diagnosis, and location on the scalp were essentially identical for trichilemmal cysts and proliferating trichilemmal cysts.[32] Mehregan reported a case of a woman with a congenital diffuse follicular hamartoma associated with palmar pits and puntate keratoses, scarring alopecia, and multiple trichilemmal cysts and proliferating trichilemmal

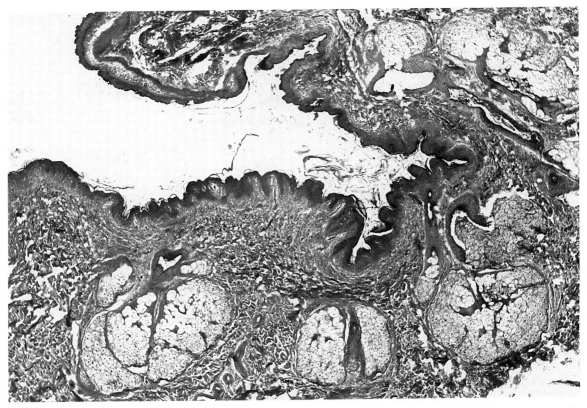

Figure 41–7. Dermoid cyst. A cyst lined by stratified squamous epithelium contains numerous pilosebaceous units in its wall. (H&E, ×25.)

cysts.[33] Proliferating trichilemmal cysts have also been reported as giant hair matrix tumor[34] and trichochlamydocarcinoma.[25]

Histologic Features

Proliferating trichilemmal cysts occur in the dermis and subcutaneous fat as well-circumscribed multilobular tumors usually 1 to 5 cm in diameter. The tumor lobules are composed of sheets of hyperplastic squamous epithelium showing central cystic change (Fig. 41–10). The cystic areas show abrupt keratinization without a granular layer. The tumor lobules contain areas of dyskeratosis with squamous eddy formation and individually dyskeratotic cells. Brownstein described a spectrum of changes (Fig. 41–11) within a single lesion, from a trichilemmal cyst with minimal hyperplasia to a fully developed proliferating trichilemmal cyst.[32] It has been proposed that trauma and inflammation may induce trichilemmal cysts to proliferate in a manner analogous to pseudoepitheliomatous hyperplasia.[28,32] Proliferating trichilemmal cysts may be more varied in their differentiation than trichilemmal cysts and may show areas of prominent nuclear atypia.[32] Malignant degeneration (Fig. 41–12) in proliferating trichilemmal cysts with metastasis has been reported rarely.[35]

HYBRID CYST

Hybrid cysts are clinically indistinguishable from trichilemmal cysts. McGavran and Binnington proposed the term *hybrid cysts* for cysts that show trichilemmal keratinization in some areas and epidermoid keratinization with a granular layer in other areas.[1] This combination of keratinizing change occurs in 7% to 10% of trichilemmal cysts but is rare in epidermoid cysts.[1] Brownstein reported seven cases of hybrid cysts in five men and two women.[36] The superficial portion of the cyst was often connected to the surface of the epidermis and showed epidermoid keratinization with a well-formed granular layer. The deeper portion of the cyst was indistinguishable from a trichilemmal cyst. He concluded that the changes in hybrid cysts supported the concept that epidermoid cysts are related to the indundibular portion of the hair follicle, whereas trichilemmal cysts are differentiated toward the follicular isthmus.[36]

STEATOCYSTOMA

Steatocystomas are uncommon cutaneous cysts that occur most often as an autosomal dominant condition known

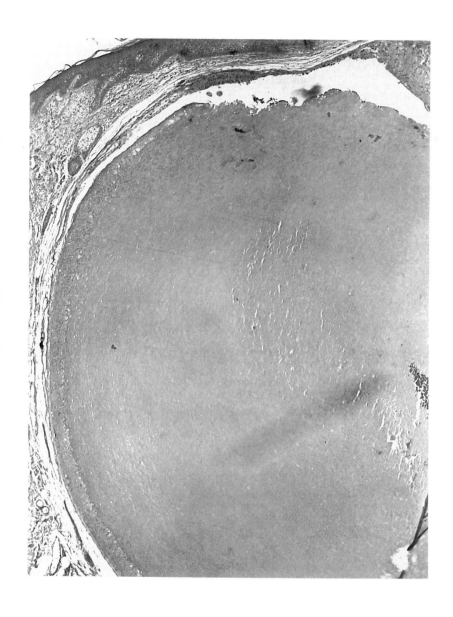

Figure 41–8. Trichilemmal cyst. The cyst lumen is completely filled by compact keratin. (H&E, ×25.)

as steatocystoma multiplex.[37,38] A family history is often but not always evident in individuals showing multiple steatocystomas.[39] Solitary, nonhereditary steatocystomas also occur.[40] Steatocystomas typically appear around the time of puberty, although onset at birth has been reported.[41] The sexes are affected equally, although in 19 nonfamilial cases of steatocystoma multiplex found in the literature, males were involved twice as often as females.[39] In men steatocystomas are typically distributed on the face, epigastrium, and back; in women they are more common on the face and in the axillae and groins.[42] The face is involved in approximately 25% of all cases.[42] Steatocystomas are usually 0.5 to 3 cm in diameter; however, cysts as large as 8 cm have been reported.[38,42] Occasionally, patients may have hundreds of lesions, and, rarely, they may become infected and painful.[39] If the cysts are lanced, a slightly yellow oily, material is discharged.

Histologic Features

Steatocystomas are located in the dermis and usually no connection to the overlying epidermis can be demonstrated.[43] They appear empty and have epithelial walls that are collapsed and folded. Occasionally, a hair shaft may be seen within the lumen. The cyst wall is composed of two to six layers of stratified squamous epithelium. The inner lining of the cyst wall is formed by a dense layer of keratin which has an undulating and hyaline appearance (Fig. 41–13). A single sebaceous gland, which may have multiple lobules, is present in the cyst wall and opens into the cyst lumen. Sometimes, the sebaceous gland may be associated with an atrophic hair follicle. Multiple hair follicles and sweat glands, which are typically seen in the wall of a dermoid cyst, are not found in steatocystomas. Some steatocystomas show focal degeneration of their epithelial walls with replacement by granulomatous inflamma-

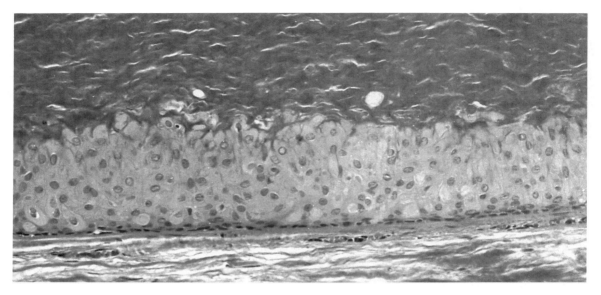

Figure 41–9. Trichilemmal cyst. The cells lining the wall are pale-staining and show a corrugated or scalloped inner layer. (H&E, ×160.)

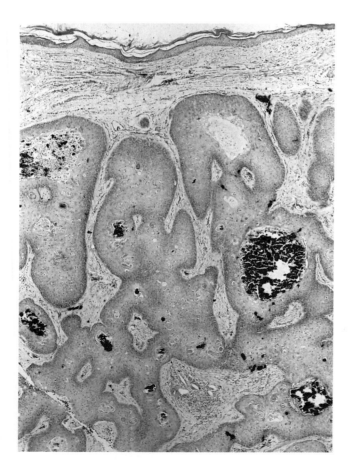

Figure 41–10. Proliferating trichilemmal cyst. The cyst lobules, which are not connected to the epidermis, show abrupt keratinization without a granular layer. (H&E, ×25.)

tion. Hashimoto et al. examined the cyst walls by electron microscopy and found the keratinization to be essentially identical to that of the epidermis.[44]

MEDIAN RAPHE CYST

Median raphe cysts most commonly occur near the ventral surface of the glans penis but may be found anywhere from the urethral meatus to the anus.[45] The cysts are usually present at birth or develop in early childhood and are typically biopsied within the first three decades of life.[46] They vary from 2 to 25 mm in diameter and most are asymptomatic. The cysts are lined by entodermal epithelium and represent defects in the embryologic development of the genitalia.[45] Cole and Helwig proposed that the cysts arise from ectopic urethral mucosa sequestered in the penile skin during embryologic development or from the epithelium of the glands of Littre.[46] Median raphe cysts may be misdiagnosed as apocrine cystadenomas.[47,48]

Histologic Features

Irregularly shaped empty cystic spaces with collapsed walls are present within the dermis without connection to the overlying surface epithelium. The cysts are lined by pseudostratified columnar epithelium, which may vary from 1 to 12 cells in thickness (Fig. 41–14). Larger cysts tend to have walls that are thinned and lined by a single layer of cells with fusiform nuclei. Occasional epithelial cells have clear cytoplasm, and in some cases numerous mucous glands are present within the cyst walls. In one study, 5 of 28 cysts had well-formed tuboalveolar mucous glands in or adjacent to their wall. The mucous glands stain positively with the periodic acid-Schiff stain and the material is diastase resistant. The cells also stain positively

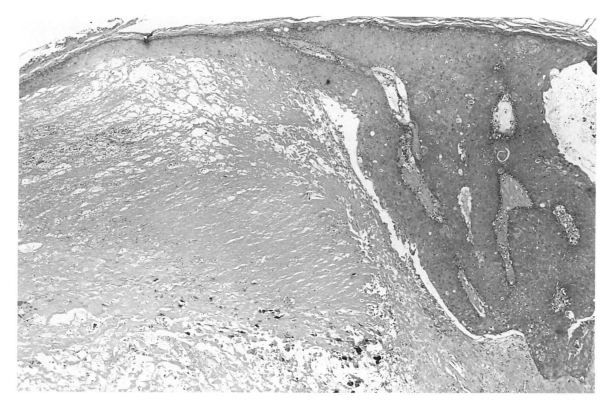

Figure 41–11. Proliferating trichilemmal cyst. This section shows the transition from an ordinary to a proliferating trichilemmal cyst. (×25.)

for acid mucopolysaccharides with the alcian blue and mucicarmine stains. As the most distal portion of the urethra is derived from ectoderm, epidermoid cysts or canals lined by stratified squamous epithelium may arise from rests containing ectodermal epithelium.[49]

BRONCHOGENIC CYST

Cutaneous bronchogenic cysts are rare, with less than 40 cases having been reported in the English-language literature by 1984.[50] The lesions are usually noted at or soon after birth as a swelling or draining sinus in the vicinity of the suprasternal notch.[51] The lesions may also occur in the lower part of the neck, the shoulders, and the chin.[52] Cutaneous bronchogenic cysts are solitary lesions that slowly increase in size and may drain a mucoid material. They rarely present as a pedunculated growth.[50] The cysts appear to represent a developmental abnormality as a result either of distant migration of sequestered epithelium from the respiratory tract or of displacement of a preformed cyst from its origin in the thorax.[51]

Histologic Features
Bronchogenic cysts are located in the dermis or subcutaneous fat and are lined by mucosa which often shows irregu-

lar folds. The lining is composed of pseudostratified columnar ciliated epithelium with goblet cells (Fig. 41–15). The lining may show areas of ciliated columnar epithelium and cuboidal epithelium and areas that are devoid of cilia. In 80% of cases, the cyst wall contains smooth muscle, and in more than 50%, it contains mucous glands. Lymphoid nodules are uncommon in the cyst wall. Cartilage was noted in only 2 of 30 cases.[51] Cutaneous bronchogenic cysts are differentiated from bronchial cleft cysts by the presence of smooth muscle and mucous glands and by the relative absence of lymphoid tissue in the former. Rarely, cutaneous bronchogenic cysts may connect to the surface epithelium.[53]

BRANCHIAL CLEFT CYST

Branchial abnormalities may appear as cysts, sinuses, fistulas, and skin tabs containing cartilage.[54] Lesions are unilateral and occur along a line from anterior to external ear to the sternum along the anterior border of the sternomastoid muscle. Sinuses and fistulas may open to the skin surface along this line or may open internally near the tonsil. Branchial cleft cysts are most commonly noted during the second and third decades of life but may be present at birth. The cysts may be associated with swelling and discomfort.

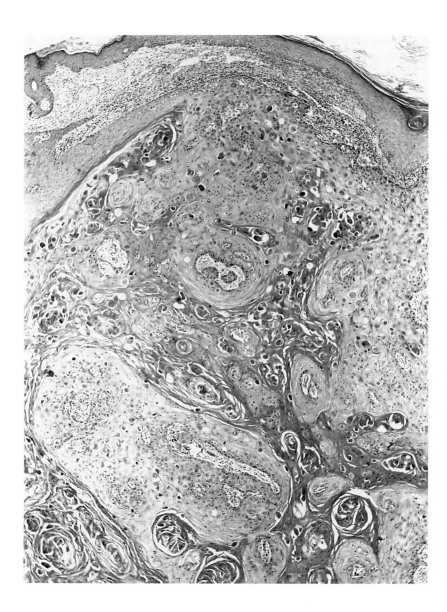

Figure 41–12. Proliferating trichilemmal cyst with squamous cell carcinoma. Shown is the transition from a proliferating trichilemmal cyst to a squamous cell carcinoma containing squamous pearls. The periphery of the tumor showed an infiltrative growth pattern. (H&E, ×25.)

Histologic Features

Branchial cleft cysts are lined by columnar epithelium, which may or may not be ciliated. Areas of squamous metaplasia are common. Sinuses and fistulas that drain to the skin surface often show a distal portion composed of stratified squamous epithelium. The epithelial wall of the cyst is often surrounded by a dense zone of lymphoid tissue (Fig. 41–16). Skin tabs frequently contain cartilage.

THYROGOSSAL DUCT CYST

Thyrogossal duct cysts typically occur in the midline of the anterior neck as cystic structures varying from 1 to 5 cm in diameter.[55] Most cysts occur during childhood. As the thyroid primordium descends into the neck, it is connected to the foramen secum by the thyrogossal duct.[56] The thyrogossal duct disappears by the eighth to tenth week of fetal development; however, a cyst may result from persistence of a portion of the embryonic duct.

Histologic Features

Thyrogossal duct cysts occur within the dermis or subcutaneous fat. They are lined by ciliated respiratory epithelium and/or stratified squamous epithelium. Unlike bronchogenic cysts, they do not contain smooth muscle or cartilage within their walls although portions of the hyoid bone[51] and thyroid follicles (Fig. 41–17) may be present.[52] Thyrogossal duct cysts should be distinguished from thymic cysts, which contain Hassall's corpuscles in or near the cyst wall and which often show cholesterol granulomas in the surrounding stroma.[56]

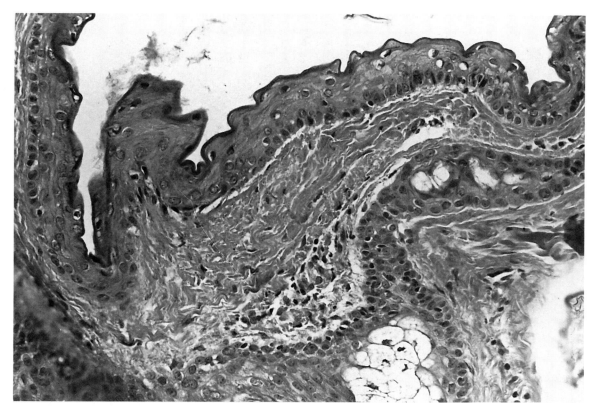

Figure 41–13. Steatocystoma. The inner lining of the cyst shows a dense keratin layer with an undulating configuration. A single sebaceous lobule is connected to the cyst by a narrow duct. (H&E, ×100.)

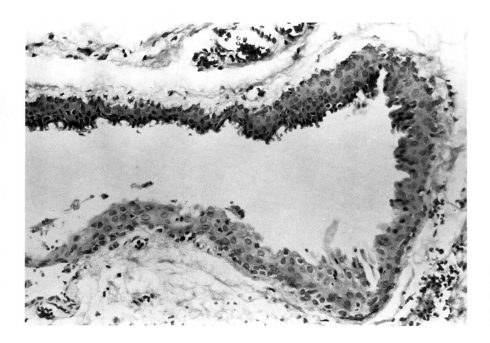

Figure 41–14. Median raphe cyst. The cyst wall is lined by pseudostratified columnar epithelium. The lining mimics the decapitation secretion characteristic of apocrine cysts. (H&E, ×100.)

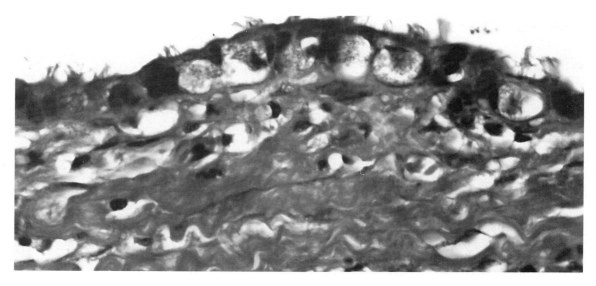

Figure 41–15. Bronchogenic cyst. The cyst wall shows ciliated epithelium with goblet cells. (H&E, ×400.)

THYMIC CYST

Thymic cysts occur either within the anterior mediastinum or in the anterior cervical triangle near the thyroid.[57] Although mediastinal cysts are usually not diagnosed until adulthood, cervical cysts are most common in children between 3 and 8 years of age.[58] More than 90% of cervical thymic cysts present as asymptomatic neck masses; however, symptoms of dyspnea, hoarseness, and dysphagia are present in about 6% of patients.[59] The majority of the thymus gland is derived from the third pharyngeal pouch. Thymic cysts appear to represent cystic remnants of thymo-

pharyngeal duct tissue sequestered in the anterior neck during development.[57,60]

Histologic Features

The cysts may be unilocular or multilocular and vary in size from 1 to 18 cm.[57] The cyst wall may show a variety of linings, from cuboidal, to columnar, to stratified squamous, to pseudostratified columnar epithelium. The wall may rupture and be replaced by granulation tissue and granulomatous inflammation. Cholesterol clefts are very common. The definitive diagnosis depends on the identification of Hassall's corpuscles within either lymphoid aggregates or lymphoid follicles adjacent to the cyst wall.

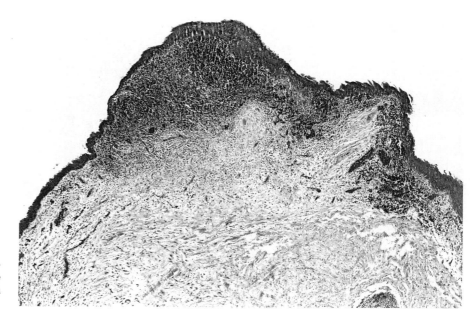

Figure 41–16. Branchial cleft cyst. A collection of lymphoid cells are present within the cyst wall which shows squamous metaplasia of columnar epithelium. (H&E, ×25.)

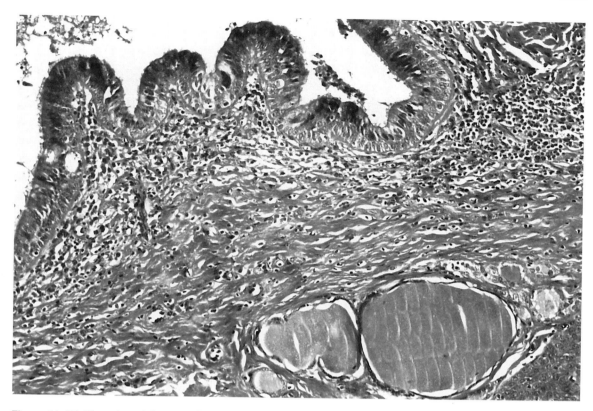

Figure 41–17. Thyroglossal duct cyst. Thyroid follicles are present adjacent to a cyst lined by ciliated epithelium. (H&E, ×100.)

CUTANEOUS CILIATED CYST

Cutaneous ciliated cysts occur on the lower extremities of women between 15 and 39 years of age.[61,62] The cysts may be painful and have been noted to increase in size during pregnancy. They are felt to represent a developmental abnormality caused by heterotopia of epithelium resembling that of the fallopian tube.[62,63] A single case has been reported in a man and it was proposed that this cyst represented metaplastic change in sweat gland epithelium.[64] Cilia

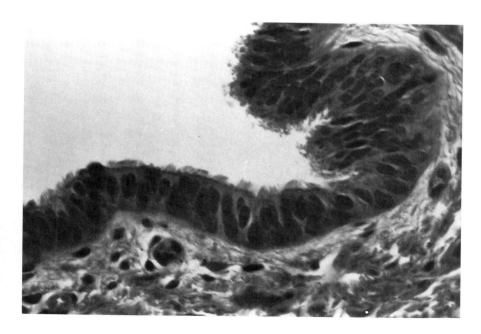

Figure 41–18. Cutaneous ciliated cyst. This cyst showing ciliated epithelium was removed from the plantar surface of a young woman. (H&E, ×400.)

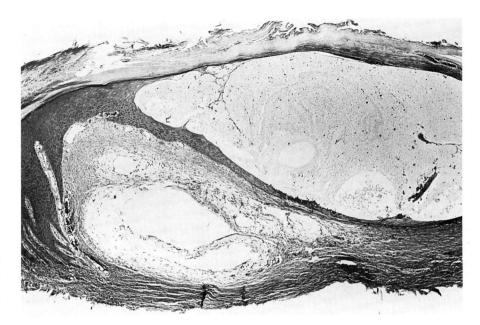

Figure 41–19. Digital mucous cyst. This traumatized cyst shows mucin free within the dermis. The epidermis has regenerated around a collection of mucin from the underlying finger joint. (H&E, ×25.)

have been demonstrated in the epithelium of eccrine sweat glands in 16-week-old embryos and focally in the ducts of an eccrine spiradenoma.[65,66]

Histologic Features

Cutaneous ciliated cysts may be unilocular or multilocular and appear empty with variable folding of their walls. The cyst lining is composed of pseudostratified ciliated co-lumnar epithelium (Fig. 41–18), which may show areas of squamous metaplasia. Mucous glands and smooth muscle are absent. The cysts are not connected to the skin surface.

DIGITAL MUCOUS CYST

Digital mucous cysts occur as firm to rubbery, translucent cysts over the dorsal aspect of a distal interphalangeal joint

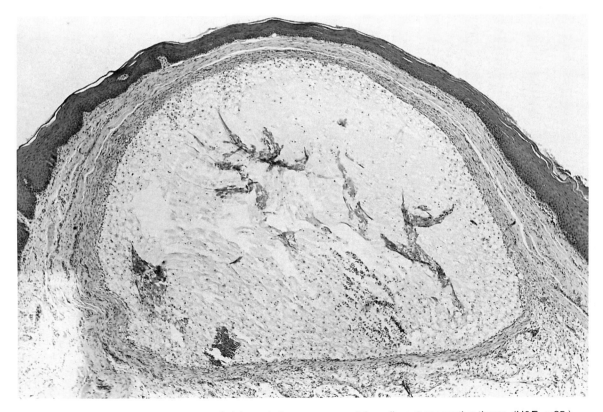

Figure 41–20. Mucocele. A collection of sialomucin has compressed the adjacent connective tissue. (H&E, ×25.)

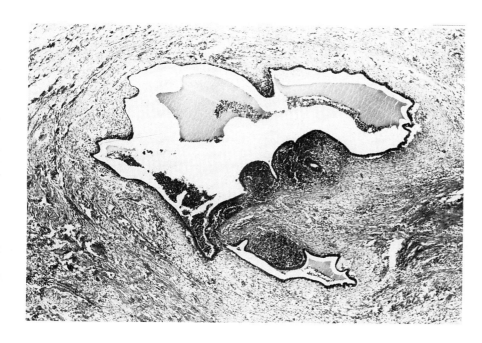

Figure 41–21. Cutaneous endometriosis. A cystic space containing red blood cells shows a lining of variable thickness. The loose stroma contains inflammatory cells and red blood cells. (H&E, ×25.)

of a finger. Women are affected more than twice as often as men and the most common sites are the middle and index fingers.[67] The cysts are usually less than 1 cm in diameter and typically occur on either side of the midline of the dorsal aspect of the finger. Approximately half of

the patients experience some tenderness or pain. If the cyst ruptures, a stringy gelatinous material is extruded. Most digital mucous cysts appear to be formed by the escape of mucin, predominantly hyaluronic acid, from the underlying joint space.[68,69] Methylene blue dye injected into the

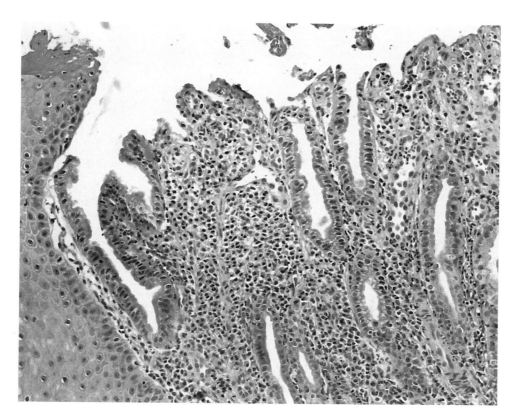

Figure 41–22. Omphalomesenteric duct cyst. A cyst lined by gastrointestinal mucosa shows an attachment to the stratified squamous epithelium of the epidermis. (H&E, ×100.)

volar aspect of the distal interphalangeal joint appears within the cyst cavity.[68] Kleinert et al. reported a visible connection during surgery between the joint space and the cyst in 100% of 30 cases.[70]

The epidermis often appears thinned and effaced by the underlying cyst. Within the dermis is pale staining mu-

Histologic Features

The epidermis often appears thinned and effaced by the underlying cyst. Within the dermis is pale staining mucinous material without a true cyst lining (Fig. 41–19). The mucin may slightly compress the adjacent connective tissue. Fusiform and stellate fibroblasts are present within the mucinous material. The material stains positive with alcian blue, colloidal iron, and mucicarmine stains.

MUCOCELE

Mucoceles occur predominantly on the mucosal surface of the lower lip, but may occasionally affect the floor of the mouth, cheek, retromolar fossae, tongue, and junction of the hard and soft palates.[71] Most mucoceles of the lower lip occur before age 40.[71] A solitary, soft cystic swelling has a translucent bluish appearance. The cyst is usually asymptomatic unless it is secondarily inflamed. Most mucoceles appear to occur secondary to traumatic rupture of a minor salivary duct, although a history of trauma is not always obtainable.

Histologic Features

A large collection of bluish, stringy or amorphous sialomucin is present within the submucosa (Fig. 41–20). The wall is composed of compressed connective tissue and a variable amount of granulation tissue and granulomatous inflammation. Occasionally, the mucosa is focally ulcerated. Inflammatory cells may be present in the cystic space. Minor salivary glands, if included in the specimen, show ductal dilatation. The mucin stains positively with alcian blue, mucicarimine, and colloidal iron stains and is removed by predigestion with sialidase.

CUTANEOUS ENDOMETRIOSIS

Cutaneous endometriosis typically occurs in cesarean section scars or other surgical scars in the umbilicus, the lower abdominal wall, or the inguinal, labial, or perineal areas.[72] Most patients are women between 20 and 50 years of age.

Histologic Features

Poorly circumscribed nodular lesions occur within the dermis or subcutaneous fat. The nodules contain multiple cystic spaces (Fig. 41–21) lined by epithelium which varies from columnar to a flattened single-cell layer. Every stage of the endometrial cycle may be exhibited and more than one stage is often present in a single specimen.[72] The stromal changes are highly variable depending on the stage of the endometrial cycle. The surrounding dermis shows a combination of inflammation, fibrosis, myxoid change, and old and recent hemorrhage.

OMPHALOMESENTERIC DUCT CYST

Omphalomesenteric duct cysts often occur as bright red papules or polyps of the periumbilical area.[73] They may feel tacky or sticky as a result of the presence of mucin, or they may discharge gas or feces. An erosive dermatitis often occurs in the surrounding skin. Approximately 20% of patients develop ileal prolapse, often within the first 2 months of life, which may be fatal.[74] Omphalomesenteric duct cysts may be associated with Meckel's diverticulum, which is the most common omphalomesenteric duct anomaly.[75]

Histologically, the cysts may be connected to the skin surface (Fig. 41–22), often contain smooth muscle within their walls, and are lined by mucosa from either small intestine (62%), stomach (33%), or colon (12%).[73]

REFERENCES

1. McGavran MN, Binnington B: Keratinous cysts of the skin: Identification and differentiation of pilar cysts from epidermal cysts. *Arch Dermatol* 1966;94:499–508.
2. Swinehart JM, Golitz LE: Scrotal calcinosis: Dystrophic calcification of epidermoid cysts. *Arch Dermatol* 1982;118:985–988.
3. Leydon JJ, Lockshin NA, Kriebel S: The black keratinous cyst: A sign of hemochromatosis *Arch Dermatol* 1972;106:379–381.
4. Shelley WB, Wood MG: Occult Bowen's disease in keratinous cysts. *Br J Dermatol* 1981;105:105–108.
5. McDonald LW: Carcinomatous change in cysts of skin. *Arch Dermatol* 1963;87:208–211.
6. Love WR, Montgomery H: Epithelial cysts. *Arch Dermatol Syphilol* 1943;47:185–196.
7. Peden JD Jr: Carcinoma developing in sebaceous cysts. *Ann Surg* 1948;128:1136–1147.
8. Aloi FG, Pippione M: Molluscum contagiosum occurring in an epidermoid cyst. *J Cutan Pathol* 1985;12:163–165.
9. Fieselman DW, Reed RJ, Ichinose H: Pigmented epidermal cyst. *J Cutan Pathol* 1974;1:256–259.
10. Epstein W, Kligman AM: The pathogenesis of milia and benign tumors of the skin.
11. Leppard B, Sneddon IB: Milia occurring in lichen sclerosus et atrophicus. *Br J Dermatol* 1975;92:711–714.
12. Wein MD, Caro MR: Traumatic epithelial cysts of the skin. *JAMA* 1934;102:197–199.
13. Yachnin SC, Summerrill F: Traumatic implantation of epithelial cysts in a phalanx. *JAMA* 1941;116:1215–1218.
14. Greer KE: Epidermal inclusion cyst of the sole. *Arch Dermatol* 1974;109:251–252.
15. Onuigbo WIB: Vulvar epidermoid cysts in the Igbos of Nigeria. *Arch Dermatol* 1976;112:1405–1406.
16. Esterley NB, Fretzin DF, Pinkus H: Eruptive vellus hair cysts. *Arch Dermatol* 1977;113:500–503.
17. Bovenmyer DA: Eruptive vellus hair cysts. *Arch Dermatol* 1979;115:338–339.
18. Steifler RE, Bergfeld WF: Eruptive vellus hair cysts: An inherited disorder. *J Am Acad Dermatol* 1980;3:425–429.
19. Piepkorn MW, Clark L, Lombardi DL: A kindred with congenital vellus hair cysts. *J Am Acad Dermatol* 1981;5:661–665.
20. Burns DA, Calnan CD: Eruptive vellus hair cysts. *Clin Exp Dermatol* 1981;6:209–213.
21. Lee S, Kim J-G: Eruptive vellus hair cyst: Clinical and histologic findings. *Arch Dermatol* 1979;115:744–746.
22. Brownstein MH, Helwig EB: Subcutaneous dermoid cysts. *Arch Dermatol* 1973;107:237–239.

23. Leppard BJ, Sanderson KV, Wells RS: Hereditary trichilemmal cysts: Herditary pilar cysts. *Clin Exp Dermatol* 1977;2:23–32.

24. Broders AC, Wilson E: Keratoma: A lesion often mistaken for sebaceous cyst. *Surg Clin North Am* 1930;10:127–130.

25. Holmes EJ: Tumors of lower hair sheath: Common histogenesis of certain so-called "sebaceous cysts," acanthomas and "sebaceous carcinomas." *Cancer* 1968;21:234–248.

26. Pinkus H: "Sebaceous cysts" are trichilemmal cysts. *Arch Dermatol* 1969;99:544–555.

27. Maurer F: *Die epidermis un ihre Abkommlinge.* Peippliz, Wilhelm Engelmann, 1895.

28. Leppard BJ, Sanderson KV: The natural history of trichilemmal cysts. *Br J Dermatol* 1976;94:379–390.

29. Kimura S: Trichilemmal cysts: Ultrastructural similarities to the trichilemmal sac. *Dermatologica* 1966;157:164–170.

30. Wilson Jones E: Proliferating epidermoid cysts. *Arch Dermatol* 1966;94:11–19.

31. Baptista, AP, Silva LGE, Born MC: Proliferating trichilemmal cyst. *J Cutan Pathol* 1983;10:178–187.

32. Brownstein, MN, Arluk DK: Proliferating trichilemmal cyst: A simulant of squamous cell carcinoma. *Cancer* 1981;48:1207–1214.

33. Mehregan AH, Hardin I: Generalized follicular hamartoma: Complicated by multiple proliferating trichilemmal cysts and palmar pits. *Arch Dermatol* 1973;107:435–438.

34. Dobska M: Grant hair matrix tumor. *Cancer* 1971;28:701–706.

35. Saida T, Oohara K, Hori Y, et al.: Development of a malignant proliferating trichilemmal cyst in a patient with multiple trichilemmal cysts. *Dermatologica* 1983;166:203–208.

36. Brownstein MH: Hybrid cyst: A combined epidermoid and trichilemmal cyst. *J Am Acad Dermatol* 1983;9:872–875.

37. Noojin RO, Reynolds JP: Familial steatocystoma multiplex: Twelve cases in three generations. *Arch Dermatol Syphilol* 1948;57:1013–1018.

38. Feinstein A, Trau H, Movshovits M, et al.: Steatocystoma multiplex. *Cutis* 1983;31:425–427.

39. Egbert BM, Price NM, Segal RJ: Steatocystoma multiplex: Report of a florid case and a review. *Arch Dermatol* 1979;115:334–335.

40. Brownstein MH: Steatocystoma simplex: A solitary steatocystoma. *Arch Dermatol* 1982;118:409–411.

41. Sachs W: Steatocystoma multiplex congenitale: Ten cases in three generations. *Arch Dermatol Syphilol* 1938;38:877–880.

42. Holmes R, Black MM: Steatocystoma multiplex with unusually prominent cysts on the face. *Br J Dermatol* 1980;102:711–713.

43. Anderson DS: Sebocystomatosis. *Br J Dermatol* 1950;62:215–220.

44. Hashimoto K, Fisher BK, Lever WF: Steatocystoma multiplex. *Hautarzt* 1964;15:299–305.

45. Asarch RG, Golitz LE, Sausker WF, et al.: Median raphe cysts of the penis. *Arch Dermatol* 1979;115:1084–1086.

46. Cole LA, Helwig EG: Mucoid cysts of the penile skin. *J Urol* 1976;115:397–400.

47. Powell RF, Palmer CH, Smith EB: Apocrine cystadenoma of the penile shaft. *Arch Dermatol* 1971;113:1250–1251.

48. Ahmed A, Jones AW: Apocrine cystadenoma: A report of two cases occurring on the prepuce. *Br J Dermatol* 1969;81:899–901.

49. Golitz LE, Robin M: Median raphe canals of the penis. *Cutis* 1981;27:170–172.

50. Miller OF III, Tyler W: Cutaneous bronchogenic cyst with papilloma and sinus presentation. *J Am Acad Dermatol* 1984;11:367–371.

51. Fraga S, Helwig EB, Rosen SH: Bronchogenic cysts in the skin and subcutaneous tissue. *Am J Clin Pathol* 1971;56:230–238.

52. Ambiavagar PH, Rosen Y: Cutaneous ciliated cyst of the chin: Probable bronchogenic cyst. *Arch Dermatol* 1979;115:895–896.

53. van der Putte SCJ, Toonstra J: Cutaneous bronchogenic cyst. *J Cutan Pathol* 1985;12:404–409.

54. Wheeler CE, Shaw RF, Cawley EP: Branchial abnormalities in three generations of one family. *Arch Dermatol* 1958;77:715–719.

55. Hawkins DB, Jacobsen BE, Klatt EC: Cysts of the thyroglossal duct. *Laryngoscope* 1982;92:1254–1258.

56. Sanusi ID, Carrington PR, Adams DN: Cervical thymic cyst. *Arch Dermatol* 1982;118:122–124.

57. Bieger RC, McAdams AJ: Thymic cysts. *Arch Pathol* 1966;82:535–541.

58. Rosai J, Levine GD: Tumor-like conditions of the thymus, in Rosai J, Levine GD (eds): *Atlas of Tumor Pathology,* Second Series, Fascicle 13. Washington, DC, Armed Forces Institute of Pathology, 1976, p 207.

59. Raines JM, Rowe LD: Progressive neonatal airway obstruction secondary to cervical thymic cyst. *Otolaryngol Head Neck Surg* 1981;89:723–725.

60. Fahmy S: Cervical thymic cysts: Their pathogenesis and relationship to branchial cysts. *J Laryngol Otol* 1974;88:47–60.

61. Farmer ER, Helwig EB: Cutaneous ciliated cysts. *Arch Dermatol* 1978;114:70–73.

62. True L, Golitz LE: Ciliated plantar cyst. *Arch Dermatol* 1980;116:1066–1067.

63. Clark JV: Ciliated epithelium in a cyst of the lower limb. *J Pathol* 1969;98:289–290.

64. Leonforte JF: Cutaneous ciliated cystadenoma in a man. *Arch Dermatol* 1982;118:1010–1012.

65. Hashimoto K, Gross BG, Lever WF: The ultrastructure of human embryo skin. *J Invest Dermatol* 1966;46:513–529.

66. Hashimoto K, Gross BJ, Nelson RG, et al.: Eccrine spiradenoma: Histochemical and electron microscopic studies. *J Invest Dermatol* 1966;46:347–365.

67. Sonnex TS: Digital myxoid cysts: A review. *Cutis* 1986;37:89–94.

68. Newmeyer WL, Kilgore ES Jr, Graham WP III: Mucous cysts: The dorsal distal interphalangeal joint ganglion. *Plast Reconstruct Surg* 1974;53:313–315.

69. Goldman JA, Goldman L, Jaffee MS, et al.: Digital mucinous pseudocysts. *Arch Rheum* 1977;20:997–1002.

70. Kleinert HE, Kutz JE, Fishman JH, et al.: Etiology and treatment of the so-called mucous cyst of the finger. *J Bone Joint Surg* 1972;54:1455–1458.

71. Cohen L: Mucoceles of the oral cavity. *Oral Surg Oral Med Oral Pathol* 1965;19:365–372.

72. Steck WD, Helwig EB: Cutaneous endometriosis. *JAMA* 1970;191:167–170.

73. Steck WD, Helwig EB: Cutaneous remnants of the omphalomesenteric duct. *Arch Dermatol* 1964;90:463–470.

74. Nix TE, Young CJ: Congenital umbilical anomalies. *Arch Dermatol* 1964;90:160–165.

75. Moore TC: Omphalomesenteric duct anomalies. *Surg Gynecol Obstet* 1956;103:569–580.

SECTION VIII
Neoplasia

CHAPTER 42
Benign Tumors of the Epidermis

Grace F. Kao

The keratinocytes of the surface epidermis and those of the acrosyringium and acrotrichium are commonly involved in benign proliferative processes. Benign epidermal tumors are composed of squamous cells found in the normal epidermis and are regarded as hyperplastic (proliferative) disorders. Benign epidermal hyperplasias can be the result of primary keratinocytic proliferation of congenital or acquired origin or of a secondary reaction to chronic inflammation or irritation. The congenital lesions usually manifest at birth or during early childhood. These lesions can be regarded as hamartomatous overgrowths or malformation of the epidermal keratinocytes and are sometimes associated with proliferation of various components of cutaneous adnexae, including sweat apparatuses and pilosebaceous structures such as those seen in nevus sebaceus.

The term *nevus* not only designates a hamartomatous proliferation of the melanocytes, such as in nevocellular nevi, but is also applied to a local or regional overgrowth of the epidermis (epidermal or epithelial nevus) and organoid nevus (nevus sebaceus of Jadassohn) that contains hyperplastic sebaceous glands and ectopic apocrine glands.

The acquired epidermal hyperplasias and neoplasias are more common in older individuals; however, those secondary to infectious causes, such as deep fungal infection, insect bite reaction, chronic irritation, or drug intake (halogenoderma) can be seen in patients of all ages. The keratinocytes in these conditions show relative normal maturation. Most epidermal hyperplasias and benign epidermal tumors show papillomatosis with papillary dermal hyperplasia and varying degrees of inflammatory infiltrate and, sometimes, entrapment of elastic and/or collagen fibers.

Benign neoplasms of other cell types of the epidermis, such as melanoctyes and Langerhans cells, are less common and are covered in other chapters.

Benign epidermal tumors show a circumscribed area of hyperplasia with relative epidermal maturation and some alteration of the normal structures. These tumors are characterized by a well-defined architecture, with superficial dermal involvement and uniformity of the proliferating cells without significant nuclear atypia or pleomorphism. In some lesions, however, foci of cytologic atypia and pleomorphism may be observed when there is intense secondary inflammation such as that seen in keratoacanthomas and inflamed (irritated) seborrheic keratoses. In these lesions, nuclear hyperchromatism and increased mitotic activity, as well as deep expansile tumor margin, may be mistaken for squamous cell carcinoma. Perineural and vascular invasion are not absolute criteria for the diagnosis of benign epidermal tumors as malignant, as some keratoacanthomas, particularly the deep and larger ones (aggressive, giant keratoacanthomas) have shown these features. Poor tumor cell–stromal relationship, infiltrative tumor margin, and malignant cytologic features are more reliable criteria for distinguishing malignant from benign tumors.

EPIDERMAL NEVUS

Clinical Features
Epidermal nevi are benign, congenital, developmental disorders of the epidermis that usually appear at birth or in infancy, but may also occur in childhood and occasionally in adult life.[1–3] Nearly 50% of patients with epidermal nevi are younger than 20 years of age. Depending on the extent of the involvement, the disease can be divided into localized and systematized forms, and several clinical variants, including nevus verrucosus, linear epidermal nevus (nevus unius lateris), systematized epidermal nevus, ichthyosis hystrix, and inflammatory linear epidermal nevus (ILVEN), are observed. About 40% of the lesions are present on the trunk, 33% in the head and neck regions, and the remaining 27% on the extremities.

The opinions or assertions contained herein are the private views of the author and are not to be construed as official or as reflecting the views of the Department of the Army or the Department of Defense.

Nevus Verrucosus. A localized type, nevus verrucosus is solitary and frequently pigmented. It varies from a few centimeters to involvement of a large area of the body. The lesions are velvety, granular, warty, or papillomatous in appearance. Some epidermal nevi may regress spontaneously.

Linear Epidermal Nevus (Nevus Unius Lateris). Linear epidermal nevi are extensive and systematized. They present as single, linear, or spiral papules or as a continuous or interrupted pattern affecting multiple sites.[4]

Systematized Epidermal Nevus. A large area of the body surface is affected by systematized epidermal nevi. The hypertrophic warty papules are frequently arranged in a pigmented, whorled pattern.

Ichthyosis Hystrix. The clinical lesions of ichthyosis hystrix show extensive, bilateral epidermal involvement by closely grouped hyperkeratotic and papillomatous papules arranged in a featherlike or marbled pattern with sheets and whorls. They appear in childhood or rarely in early adult life.[4]

Inflammatory Linear Epidermal Nevus. The lesions of inflammatory linear epidermal nevus (ILVEN) may resemble those of linear verrucous epidermal nevus. The former lesions are less verrucoid, however, and the presence of scale crusts, erythema, and pruritus may suggest the diagnosis of eczematous or atopic dermatitis. Altman and Mehregan[5] described this entity in detail. According to their study, about 12% of the patients had lesions at birth, in 50% of the patients lesions were noted at the age of 6 months, and in 25% lesions erupted between the ages of 10 and 20. The leg and thigh are the most common sites of involvement, although the buttocks and groin are also noted.[6]

Epidermal Nevus Syndrome. Epidermal nevi of the skin are associated with bony, cardiac, and central nervous system abnormalities, seizure, and brain tumors.[7]

Histologic Features

The characteristic features of epidermal nevi are marked hyperkeratosis of the surface epidermis and follicular ostia, papillomatosis, acanthosis with elongation of the rete ridges (Fig. 42–1), and varying degrees of hyperplasia of papillary connective tissue, which is responsible for the hyperkeratotic warty appearance or soft pedunculated lesions. Epidermolytic hyperkeratosis or granular degeneration of the epidermis (Fig. 42–2 and inset) are frequently observed in the systematized type, particularly ichthyosis hystrix. Acantholytic dyskeratosis, as seen in Darier's disease, may be observed in unilateral linear epidermal nevi. ILVEN lesions show hyperkeratosis, parakeratosis, psoriasiform acanthosis with fusion of the rete ridges, mild spongiosis, and dermal perivascular lymphomononuclear inflammatory infiltrate (Fig. 42–3). The histologic changes resemble those seen in atopic or eczematous dermatitis.

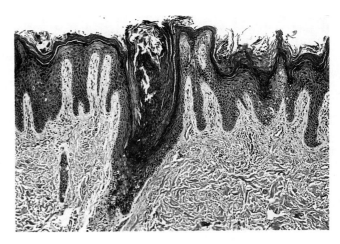

Figure 42–1. Low-power photomicrograph of a linear epidermal nevus showing hyperkeratosis of the surface epidermis and follicular ostia, acanthosis, elongation of the rete ridges, and mild papillomatosis. There is granular degeneration of the epidermis to the left of the field. (H&E, ×75.) (AFIP Neg. No. 87-7321)

Carcinoma Arising in Epidermal Nevi

Linear epidermal nevi occurring in nevus sebaceus may be associated with basal cell carcinomas.[8,9] The histopathologic features of these basal cell carcinomas are more prominent pilar differentiation and less peripheral palisading of the basaloid cells. Squamous cell carcinoma developing in epidermal nevus has been described rarely.[10]

Differential Diagnosis

Nevus Sebaceus. Verrucous epidermal nevus differs from nevus sebaceus by the lack of dermal adnexal elements and the absence of secondary development of hamartomatous (nevoid) tumor growth.

Verruca Vulgaris. The lesion has characteristic features of convergence of rete ridges, hypergranulosis, and koilocytotic vacuolated cells that are not observed in epidermal nevi.

Seborrheic Keratosis. Verrucous epidermal nevi lack the prominent horn cysts seen in most lesions of seborrheic keratosis.

Lichen Simplex Chronicus. These lesions have more prominent acanthosis, evenly elongated rete ridges, thin suprapapillary plates, and elongated papillae with dilated capillaries. The features may resemble those of ILVEN.

NEVUS SEBACEUS

Talgdrusen-naevus ("sebaceous gland nevus") was first mentioned by Jadassohn in his 1885 paper. The term *nevus sebaceus of Jadassohn* was introduced by Robinson in 1932 and subsequently adopted in the American literature. Mehregan and Pinkus[11] used the term *organoid nevus of the sebaceous type* to redefine this previously known entity. They prefer the term *organoid nevus* because the lesion represents

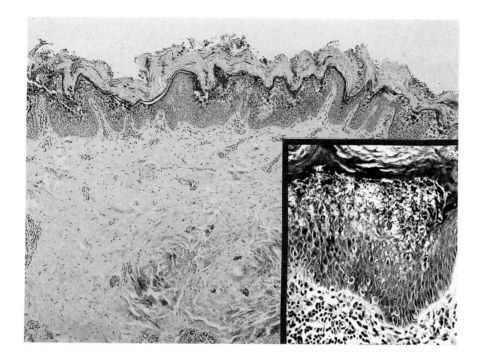

Figure 42–2. Photomicrograph of a systematized epidermal nevus displaying diffuse epidermolytic hyperkeratosis. (H&E, × 20.) (AFIP Neg. No. 85-00848) Inset: Higher magnification depicts the area of granular degeration of the epidermis as shown in the left field. (H&E, ×160.)(AFIP Neg. No. 86-4720)

a developmental abnormality of several cutaneous tissue elements, including pilosebaceous apparatuses and apocrine glands.

Clinical Features

Nevus sebaceus most frequently occurs on the scalp and face. The life history of nevus sebaceus can be divided into three phases[11–13]:

1. In the *early phase* (infancy and childhood), the typical lesion is a flesh-colored alopecic plaque on the scalp or the face. The overlying epidermis may be normal or show mild papillomatous hyperplasia.

2. The *second phase* (puberty) is the most characteristic. The alopecic area becomes a yellow, waxy papillomatous plaque as a result of the development of sebaceous and apocrine glands. The skin surface is formed by soft, yellow fibroepithelial papillomas or cysts.

3. The *third phase* is marked by development of secondary hyperplasia or neoplasia of the surface epidermis, pilosebaceous structures, and apocrine glands.

Histologic Features

Microscopic features vary in the different phases. The most constant feature is papillomatous hyperplasia of the epidermis, which is observed in more than 90% of cases. Hyperplasia is more pronounced in older lesions. Hyperkeratosis, hypergranulosis, and papillomatous acanthosis with fusion of the rete ridges are present. In some cases, the hyperplastic epidermis with underlying connective tissue containing abnormally developed hair follicles and large sebaceous glands form several pedunculated nodules above the skin surface.

Hair follicles are either absent or incompletely formed (Fig. 42–4). They are composed of cords of undifferentiated matrix cells, resembling the embryonic stage of the hair follicles. These structures resemble hair germs or hair papillae. The markedly dilated follicular infundibula containing laminated keratin resemble those of nevus comedonicus.

In the early phase, the sebaceous glands are present as small underdeveloped lobules connected to incompletely formed hair follicles. Later, the more mature sebaceous glands are present (Fig. 42–4). About 10% of nevus sebaceus lesions contain very few or no sebaceous glands.

Apocrine glands are rare in nevus sebaceus in children, but they are present in 50% of adolescent and 67% of adult patients. The morphologic and histochemical characteristics

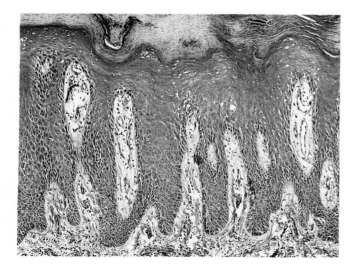

Figure 42–3. Photomicrograph of ILVEN lesion showing psoriasiform acanthosis, hyperkeratosis, parakeratosis, hypergranulosis, mild spongiosis, fusion of the rete ridges, ectasia of dermal capillaries, and mild lymphomononuclear infiltrate. (H&E, ×100.)(AFIP Neg. No. 87-7317)

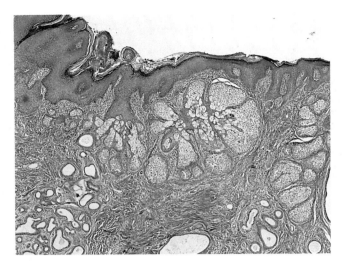

Figure 42–4. Low-power photomicrograph of a nevus sebaceus of an adolescent girl. Note epidermal hyperplasia, lobules of developing sebaceous glands associated with incompletely formed hair follicles, and numerous apocrine glands. (H&E, ×60.)

of apocrine glands in nevus sebaceus are similar to those of normal glands (Fig. 42–5). The apocrine epithelium shows decapitation secretion, and the epithelial cells contain periodic acid-Schiff (PAS)–positive, diastase-resistant secretory material as well as some iron pigment.

The dermis shows fibrosis with increased vascularity. Elastic fibers are reduced or completely absent in these areas. Diffuse deposition of hyaluronic acid in the dermis is observed in about 20% of cases.

A moderate-to-dense, chronic inflammatory infiltrate consisting of lymphocytes, plasma cells, melanophages, and some eosinophils is also seen. Endogenous foreign body, giant cell reactions to degenerating pilosebaceous structures and microcalcification are occasionally observed.

Neoplasms Associated with Nevus Sebaceus

About 40% of sebaceous nevi, particularly those that occur during the adolescent and adult phases, are associated with epithelial neoplasms of the surface epidermis and adnexal structures.[14,15] The tumors most commonly affect the scalp, rarely the forehead and behind the ear. Tumors in order of frequency are basal cell carcinoma (40%) (Fig. 42–6); adnexal and pilar tumors (40%), such as trichilemmoma, trichoepithelioma, follicular or pilar hamartoma, proliferating pilar tumor, and sebaceous adenoma; and apocrine neoplasms (20%), such as apocrine adenoma (Fig. 42–7), syringocystadenoma papilliferum, and apocrine hidrocystoma. Basal cell carcinomas associated with nevus sebaceus frequently show features of primitive hair matrix differentiation (Fig. 42–8). Eccrine sweat gland tumors such as eccrine spiradenoma, eccrine acrospiroma and microcystic adnexal (sclerosing sweat duct) carcinoma, apocrine carcinoma, squamous cell carcinoma, and poorly differentiated adnexal carcinoma arising in nevus sebaceus are rare.[14]

Differential Diagnosis

Sebaceous hyperplasia should be differentiated from nevus sebaceus. Lesions of sebaceous hyperplasia consist of central dilated, branching sebaceous ducts, and those of nevus sebaceus are composed of lobules of sebaceous gland without pilar or sebaceous ducts. Sebaceous hyperplasia lacks ectopic apocrine glands beneath the lesion, as seen in nevus sebaceus. In addition, sebaceous hyperplasia is commonly seen on the face of older individuals; in contrast, nevus sebaceus, is common in children and adolescents.

SEBORRHEIC KERATOSIS (SEBORRHEIC VERRUCA)

Seborrheic keratosis is also known as acanthosis verrucosa seborrhoica, acanthotic nevus, basal cell papilloma, keratosis pigmentosa, melanin-forming squamous cell papilloma, pigmented epithelioma, pigmented papilloma, pigmented

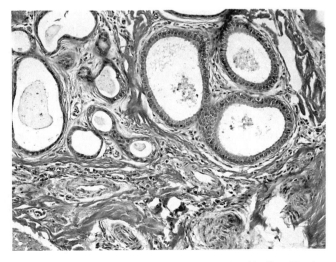

Figure 42–5. Relatively normal apocrine glands with dilated lumina, and decapitation secretion at the base of a nevus sebaceus. (H&E, ×160.)

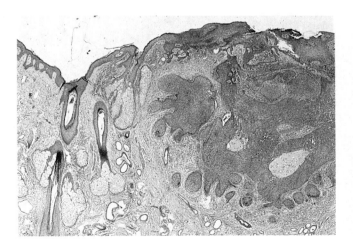

Figure 42–6. A nevus sebaceus located on the forehead of a 54-year-old man and associated with basal cell carcinoma (BCC). The BCC is connected to the overlying epidermis. A few abortive pilosebaceous structures and apocrine glands are present. (H&E, ×30.)

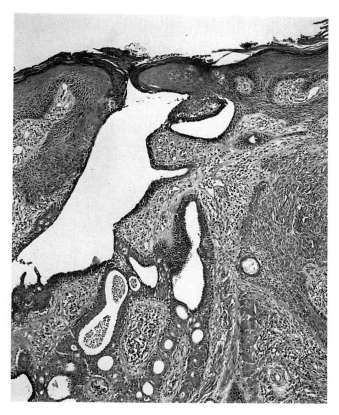

Figure 42–7. An apocrine adenoma with well-differentiated tubules associated with nevus sebaceus. The epithelium-lined ductal structure arises from the overlying epidermis, as seen in syringocystadenoma papilliferum. (H&E, ×75.)

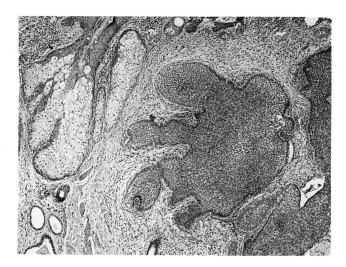

Figure 42–8. Higher magnification of Fig. 42–6 depicts a basal cell carcinoma with primitive hair follicle differentiation at the periphery (arrow). (H&E, ×75.)

verruca seborrhoica, senile warts, verruca plana seniorum, and verruca senilis.

Clinical Features

Seborrheic keratosis affects the skin of middle-aged and older individuals. The common sites of involvement include the trunk, particularly the interscapular area, the sides of the neck, the face, and the arms. The lesions appear as single or multiple brown or black patches with slightly raised and sharply demarcated borders. The surface is covered by greasy, friable scale, and the lesion has an overall "stuck on" appearance. Most lesions measure a few millimeters to several centimeters. Rarely, they may exceed 5 cm in diameter; these lesions are referred to as "giant seborrheic keratosis." The larger lesions may be mistaken for squamous cell carcinoma.

When traumatized, lesions of seborrheic keratosis become crusted and pustular, and show an erythematous inflammatory base. Occasionally seborrheic keratoses may be pedunculated, resembling fibroepithelial polyps (acrochordon). In elderly patients, eruption of multiple seborrheic keratoses within a short period may be associated with an internal malignancy (sign of Leser-Trelat).[16] Adenocarcinoma of the gastrointestinal tract is the most common associated neoplasm. Carcinoma of other organs such as the prostate, breast, ovary, uterus, liver, and lung; Sezary syndrome; and leukemia have also been reported to be associated with multiple eruptive seborrheic keratoses.

The clinical features of seborrheic keratosis may mimic those of intraepidermal epithelioma, although the latter more commonly affects the skin of the lower extremity.

Dermatosis papulosa nigra is a form of seborrheic keratosis occurring in black patients. The lesions are multiple, small, soft, round, pigmented seborrheic keratoses occurring on the face or torso of young and adult black women. Clinically, the lesions do not have the typical greasy, friable scales and "stuck on" appearance of the usual seborrheic keratoses. The microscopic features of dematosis papulosa nigra are identical to those of ordinary seborrheic keratoses, with the exception that the keratinocytes contain a large amount of melanin pigment.

Seborrheic keratoses have been regarded as a delayed type of epidermal nevus, as the lesions of dermatosus papulosa nigra begin in adolescence and progress into adulthood.

Histologic Features

At least five histologic types of seborrheic keratosis are recognized: acanthotic, hyperkeratotic, adenoidal (reticulated), clonal, and inflamed (irritated or inverted follicular). More than one type of histologic pattern can be identified in the same lesion. The common feature of all types of seborrheic keratosis is an abrupt area of hyperkeratosis, acanthosis, focal hypergranulosis, and papillomatosis adjacent to the normal epidermis. The base of the lesion in general follows a straight line from the normal epidermis at one end to the normal epidermis at the other end. Squamous and basaloid cells resembling normal epidermal basal cells constitute the bulk of the lesion. Varying amounts of melanin pigment are present in the keratinocytes and melanocytes in all types of seborrheic keratosis. Melanophages are prominent in the upper dermis in deeply pigmented

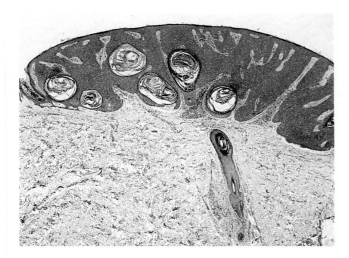

Figure 42–9. Low-power view of an acanthotic type of seborrheic keratosis showing interwoven tracts of basaloid cells arising from the epidermis, bordering horn cysts. (H&E, × 25.) (AFIP Neg. No. 86-9723)

lesions. The keratinocytes of seborrheic keratosis are believed to be of follicular infundibular origin.

Acanthotic Type. The acanthotic type (Fig. 42–9) is the most common type of seborrheic keratosis. The lesion is composed of keratinocytes arising from the surface epidermis and having the appearance of epidermal basal cells (Fig. 42–10). They form interwoven tracts bordering horn cysts and pseudohorn cysts. A bandlike lymphomononuclear inflammatory infiltrate is frequently present in the upper dermis underlying the lesion.

Hyperkeratotic Type. Hyperkeratosis and papillomatosis are pronounced, but acanthosis is not conspicuous (Fig.

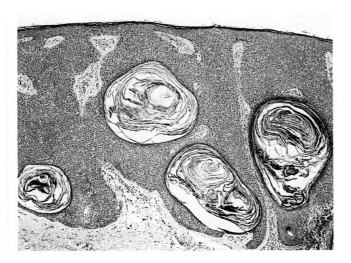

Figure 42–10. Higher magnification of Fig. 42–9 displaying basaloid cells resembling epidermal basal cells, constituting the bulk of the lesion. (H&E, ×60.) (AFIP Neg. No. 86-9724)

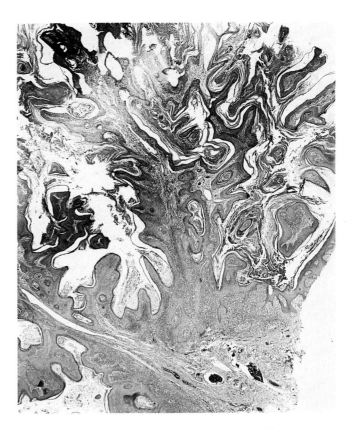

Figure 42–11. Pronounced hyperkeratosis and papillomatosis, as shown in a hyperkeratotic type of seborrheic keratosis. This lesion had the clinical appearance of a cutaneous horn. (H&E, ×75.) (AFIP Neg. No. 86-9977)

42–11), in hyperkeratotic seborrheic keratosis the epidermis consists largely of squamous cells, although small aggregates of basaloid cells may be present. This type of lesion may have the clinical appearance of cutaneous horn.

Adenoidal (Reticulated) Type. In adenoidal seborrheic keratosis, lacelike strands of basaloid cells extend from the epidermis and hair follicles (Fig. 42–12). Horn cysts and pseudohorn cysts are usually not present. This type of lesion has been shown to be closely related to lentigo senilis.

Clonal (Nesting) Type. Well-defined nests of basaloid keratinocytes are present in the epidermis (Figs. 42–13, 42–14A) in clonal seborrheic keratoses. These keratinocytes have uniform darkly stained nuclei with indistinct intercellular desmosomes. Cellular pleomorphism, atypia, or mitoses that are seen in the cell nests of intraepidermal epithelioma are not observed in those of the clonal type. It is sometimes difficult to distinguish between the two lesions, however, because of the similarity of their clinical appearance. Some authors regard the intraepidermal epithelioma lesions as a variant of the clonal type of seborrheic keratosis.

Inflamed (Irritated, Activated, or Inverted Follicular) Type. The characteristic feature in inflamed seborrheic keratosis is the presence of a large number of whorls or eddies

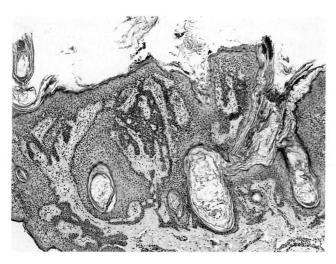

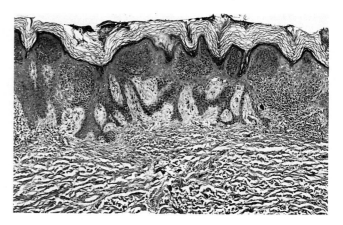

Figure 42–13. Well-defined nests of basaloid keratinocytes present in the epidermis of the clonal type of seborrheic keratosis. (H&E, ×75.) (AFIP Neg. No. 87-7319)

Figure 42–12. An adenoidal type of seborrheic keratosis displaying lacelike strands of basal cells extending from the epidermis and hair follicles. Horn cysts are also present. (H&E, ×75.) (AFIP Neg. No. 86-9974)

of flattened eosinophilic squamous cells arranged in an onion-peel fashion that resembles horn pearls (Fig. 42–15). Acantholysis, spongiosis, exocytosis of acute and chronic inflammatory cells, nuclear irregularity, focal increased mitotic activity, and marked keratinocyte hyperplasia are commonly encountered. These lesions frequently proliferate downward and break through the basal demarcation that is generally present in other types of seborrheic keratosis. The previously mentioned histologic features are also observed in giant seborrheic keratosis. These features may be mistaken for well-differentiated squamous cell carcinoma.

The entity of inverted follicular keratosis described by Helwig in 1954 and by Mehregan in 1964, as well as that

of follicular poroma designated by Duperrat and Mascaro and Grosshans and Hanau, have histologic features similar to those of seborrheic keratosis of the irritated type. These authors regard the keratin-filled invaginations in these entities as follicular infundibula and the keratinocytic proliferation arising from them.[17,18]

Melanoacanthoma[19] is regarded as a rare pigmented variant of seborrheic keratosis. This lesion differs from the more common pigmented seborrheic keratosis in that there are numerous large pigment-filled dendritic melanocytes scattered in the lesion. In contrast, the melanin pigment is present in the keratinocytes and there is a lack of melanocyte proliferation in the ordinary pigmented seborrheic keratosis.

Differential Diagnosis
Intraepidermal Epithelioma. Separation of intraepidermal epithelioma (IE) and the clonal type of seborrheic keratosis

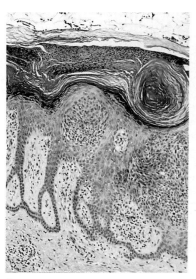

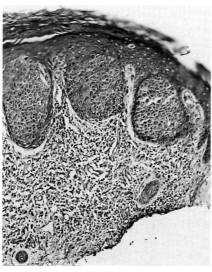

A   **B**

Figure 42–14. A split-field photomicrograph showing **(A)** indistinct nests of basaloid cells adjacent to the relatively normal epidermal keratinocytes in clonal-type seborrheic keratosis (AFIP Neg. No. 86-9975) and **(B)** well-defined cell nests with atypical keratinocytes compressing a rim of basal epidermal cells in intraepidermal epithelioma. **(A, B,** H&E, ×150.)

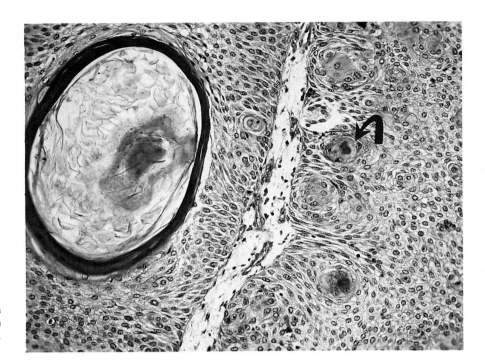

Figure 42–15. Prominent squamous eddies (curved arrow) adjacent to a horn cyst in an inflamed (irritated) seborrheic keratosis. (H&E, ×250.) (AFIP Neg. No. 83-9349)

is based solely on histologic grounds. The former lesions contain well-defined nests of atypical keratinocytes showing nuclear pleomorphism, atypia, malignant dyskeratosis, and mitoses within the epidermis (Fig. 42–14B). The epidermal cell nests tend to be larger, compressing the surrounding keratinocytes to a thin rim. The epidermal cell nests in the clonal type of seborrheic keratosis do not show significant atypia. Immunostains using anti-AE1 and AE3 have not shown an appreciable difference in the intensity of positive staining in the cell nests of both lesions. Staining with carcinoembryonic antigen (CEA) shows focal positive reactivity in the vacuolated spaces in the cell nests of IE lesions. Stains for CEA are negative in seborrheic keratosis. Stains with S-100 protein show negative reactivity in both lesions. Electron microscopic features of both lesions are of no differential diagnostic value.

The biologic behavior of IE lesions and that of seborrheic keratosis are quite different. The former lesions are regarded as premalignant, as about 9% may invade the underlying dermis and subcutaneous tissue with the development of adnexal carcinoma, whereas the latter lesions are benign.

Verruca Vulgaris. In the well-developed lesions of verrucae, the epidermal hyperplasia is both exophytic and endophytic. The epidermal collarette usually shows convergence toward the center of the lesion, and there is papillomatosis with prominent vacuolated (koilocytotic) cells in the parakeratotic layer. Lesions of seborrheic keratosis are exophytic; the base of the lesion is roughly at the level of the skin surface, and no koilocytotic cells are present.

Well-Differentiated Squamous Cell Carcinoma. The squamous eddies in squamous cell carcinoma are larger and more circumscribed than those seen in irritated seborrheic

keratosis. Keratinocyte atypia, malignant dyskeratosis, and invasion into the dermis and subcutaneous tissue are present in squamous cell carcinoma. In contrast, invasive features are not observed in lesions of seborrheic keratosis.

WARTY DYSKERATOMA

Warty dyskeratoma was first designated as isolated or solitary Darier's disease in 1954 (Helwig and Allen). Szymanski reported on two cases of similar lesions which he designated warty dyskeratoma in 1956. Graham and Helwig reported 50 cases under the term *isolated dyskeratosis follicularis* in 1958.

Clinical Features
Warty dyskeratoma occurs principally as a single lesion affecting the skin of the head and neck region, including anatomic sites rich in pilosebaceous structures such as the cheek, temple, forehead, postauricular area, and nose. The chest, back, groin, and occasionally the oral mucosa, particularly the hard palate and alveolar ridge,[20] are also involved. These lesions affect middle-aged individuals. No cases of warty dyskeratoma have been recorded in children or adolescents.

The clinical appearance of the lesion is indistinct. A variety of clinical diagnoses (sebaceous cyst, solar keratosis, basal cell carcinoma, verrucae, nevocellular nevus, and folliculitis) were suspected before a histopathologic diagnosis was rendered on the biopsied tissue. The lesions range from 1 to 10 mm in diameter, with an average of 3 to 4 mm. The clinical appearance is that of an elevated, circumscribed, brown or flesh-colored nodule or cyst with a raised border and an umbilicated or porelike center. Crusting, recurrent drainage of foul-smelling cheesy material, and

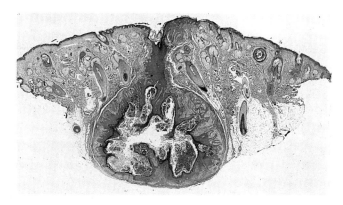

Figure 42–16. Low-power view of a warty dyskeratoma showing a typical cup-shaped invagination of a cystic, dilated hair follicle containing keratin plug. (H&E, ×2.) (AFIP Neg. No. 87-7111)

episodes of bleeding associated with trauma, itching, and a burning sensation are common symptoms.

Premalignant and malignant lesions of the skin commonly observed in older patients, such as solar keratosis, squamous cell carcinoma, basal cell carcinoma, and adnexal carcinoma, are frequently associated with lesions of warty dyskeratoma.

Histologic Features
The lesion is typically an invaginated cystic structure presenting as a markedly enlarged pilosebaceous follicle extending into the corium. On low-power examination, it has an overall cup-shaped appearance. The central cystic space contains a keratotic and a parakeratotic plug (Fig. 42–16). In general, one pilosebaceous follicle is involved, but two or three adjacent follicles may show similar changes (Fig. 42–17). The base of the lesion shows basal cell hyper-

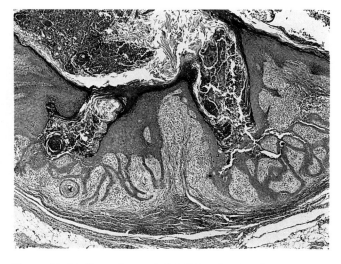

Figure 42–17. Two adjacent hair follicles showing dilatation of the infundibular ducts with suprabasal acantholysis forming clefts and keratotic lug in a warty dyskeratoma. (H&E, ×40.) (AFIP Neg. No. 87-7112)

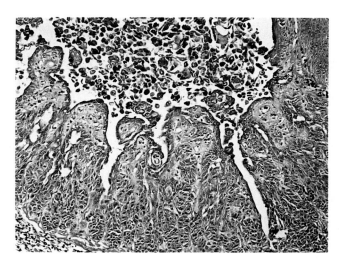

Figure 42–18. Higher magnification of Fig. 42–17 showing acantholytic and dyskeratotic cells (corps ronds and grains) in the acantholytic space. (H&E, ×150.)

plasia, suprabasal acantholysis with papillary fronds, and lacunae filled with acantholytic and dyskeratotic cells (corps ronds and grains) (Fig. 42–18). Occasionally, there are squamous whorls (eddies). Nuclear atypia and pleomorphism are not observed, but mitoses can sometimes be seen. The core of the papillae is composed of normal collagen, dilated capillaries, and a sparse lymphohistiocytic infiltrate. A zone of inflammatory infiltrate consisting of lymphocytes, plasma cells, histiocytes, and occasional eosinophils usually surrounds the lesion. The lesion has no relationship with eccrine or apocrine glands on serial sections.

A fine network of reticulum fibers, connective tissue collagen, and some acid mucopolysaccharides, i.e., hyaluronic acid, are identified in the papillae by Snook's reticulum, Masson's trichrome, and colloidal iron. Elastic fibers are present in the connective tissue sheath around the lesion but not within the lesion. The epithelial cells, like those of pilar epithelium, contain glycogen. Melanin pigment can be demonstrated in the dermal papillae. No iron pigment or amyloid is present.

Differential Diagnosis
In Darier's disease, particularly of the hypertrophic type, the acantholysis involves more than three adjacent pilosebaceous structures. In contrast, lesions of warty dyskeratoma show prominent acantholysis in one structure; rarely are two or three adjacent pilosebaceous structures involved.[21] Clinically, Darier's disease is a hereditary disease that is transmitted in an autosomal recessive pattern, whereas warty dyskeratoma is not hereditary.

CLEAR (PALE) CELL ACANTHOMA

Degos and his associates first described a benign epidermal neoplasm as *acanthome a cellules claires* in 1962. Subsequently, this lesion came to be known as clear cell tumor of the skin or clear cell acanthoma.

Clinical Features

Clear cell acanthoma typically presents as solitary, rarely multiple tumors, often localized on the leg. The lesion is asymptomatic, nontender, scaly, papular or papulonodular (Fig. 42–19), and measures 1 to 2 cm in diameter. More than 90% of lesions involve the lower extremities, particularly the leg, thigh, and knee; rarely, the arm, abdomen, and nose of adult patients are involved. More than 80% of patients are 50 years or older. Despite a rich vascular stroma and trauma-prone site of involvement, hemorrhage is uncommon. The nodule is soft, discrete, and freely movable. The clinical impressions include basal cell carcinoma, dermatofibroma, verrucae, Kaposi's sarcoma, Bowen's disease spindle cell and epithelioid cell (Spitz's) nevus, malignant melanoma, squamous cell carcinoma, eccrine poroma, and irritated seborrheic keratosis.

Histologic Features

The characteristic finding in clear cell acanthoma is an abrupt area of acanthotic epidermis containing large, pale-staining keratinocytes of the malpighian layer, bordered laterally by epidermal collarette. The basal cell layer is obscured. Three overall architectural patterns of the acanthotic epidermis are recognized: papular acanthotic (Fig. 42–20) (65%), polypoid (exophytic) (Fig. 42–19) (25%), and psoriasiform (Fig. 42–21) (10%). The acanthotic epidermis shows elongation of the rete ridges, prominent intercellular desmosomal junction between the large, pale keratinocytes, hyperkeratosis, parakeratosis, scale crust, thin or absent granular cell layer, exocytosis of neutrophils, occasional microabscess formation, and spongiosis (Fig. 42–22). The acrosyringia and acrotrichia are usually spared by the pale cells. The dermis contains prominent ectatic, tortuous capillaries and sparse mixed lymphohistiocytic infiltrate. The granular cytoplasm of the pale epidermal keratinocytes is stained intensely positive by the PAS method (Fig. 42–23), and the stain is removed by prior amylase digestion, indicating the presence of abundant intracytoplasmic glycogen.

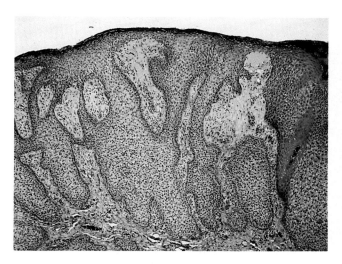

Figure 42–20. A papular acanthotic overall architectural pattern of a clear cell acanthoma. Note the large, pale-staining keratinocytes in the malpighian layer. (H&E, ×60.) (AFIP Neg. No. 86-9713)

Glycogen accumulation in clear cell acanthoma is a distinct feature of the lesion but is not pathognomonic. Wells and Wilson Jones reported that the clear cells contain low levels of phosphorylase, cytochrome oxidase, and succinic dehydrogenase.[22] This pattern of enzyme distribution and concentration differs from that found in adnexal tumors of the skin. The enzymatic histochemical findings support the concept that lesions of clear cell acanthoma most likely originated from the surface epidermis rather than the adnexal keratinocytes. Electron microscopic examination confirms that the clear cells are glycogen-filled keratinocytes of the surface epidermis.

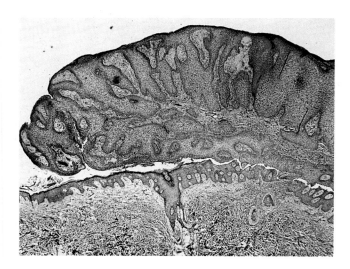

Figure 42–19. Low-power photomicrograph of an exophytic clear cell acanthoma showing the polypoid appearance. (H&E, ×25.) (AFIP Neg. No. 86-9712)

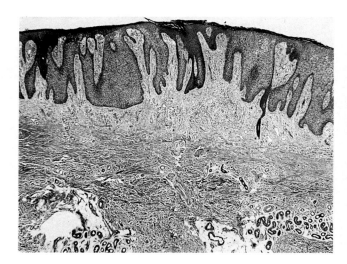

Figure 42–21. A clear cell acanthoma showing psoriasiform acanthotic pattern. Note the elongation of rete ridges and sparing of acrosyringium by the clear cells. (H&E, ×25.) (AFIP Neg. No. 86-9711)

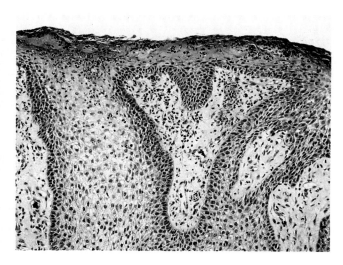

Figure 42–22. Higher magnification of Fig. 42–21 depicting prominent intercellular desmosomal junction between the clear cells, microabscesses in the scale crust, absent granular cell layer, and mild spongiosis. (H&E, ×160.) (AFIP Neg. No. 86-9714)

Differential Diagnosis

Pale cell acanthosis is a distinct reactive histologic pattern of the epidermal keratinocytes. The changes are most commonly observed diffusely in clear cell acanthomas, but they are also focally present in lesions of seborrheic keratoses and verrucae.[23]

KERATOACANTHOMA

Keratoacanthoma, also known as invasive acanthosis and invasive acanthoma, is a common benign, often self-involut-

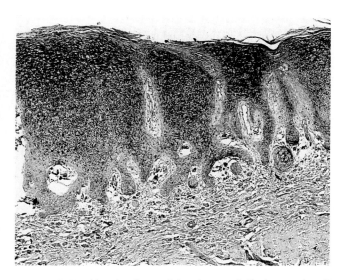

Figure 42–23. Abundant intracellular glycogen in the large pale cells of clear cell acanthoma, as shown by diffuse periodic acid–Schiff–positive, pre-diastase-digested staining methods. (Periodic acid–Schiff, ×75.) (AFIP Neg. No. 86-10158)

ing lesion. It was originally described as crateriform ulcer of the face by Sir Jonathan Hutchinson in 1889. In 1936, MacCormac and Scarff designated these lesions as "molluscum sebaceum." Other terms, verrucome and vegetating sebaceous cyst, were also encountered in the literature. The term *keratoacanthoma* was initiated by Freudenthal, and subsequently it became widely accepted.

Clinical Features

Lesions of keratoacanthoma are commonly present on sun-exposed skin and are frequently associated with solar keratoses. They usually enlarge rapidly, stabilize, and then regress partially or completely. The lesion begins as a skin-colored papule that grows to be a characteristic cup-shaped (volcanolike) nodule with a central depression within 1 week to 10 days. In 3 to 6 weeks it attains its maximum size of 2 to 3 cm in diameter. Spontaneous regression usually occurs within 6 to 12 months, leaving a slightly depressed scar. The self-limiting feature of benign biologic behavior allows a clinical diagnosis of keratoacanthoma with absolute certainty.

Rarely, keratoacanthomas may present as infiltrated plaques exceeding 5 cm in diameter, and these larger lesions may be locally aggressive with a history of multiple recurrences. Histologically, the lesion shows deep extension into the dermis, subcutaneous tissue, and sometimes the underlying bone. These lesions have been designated as "giant or aggressive keratoacanthomas."[24,25] Although only a rare case of metastasis has occurred,[26,27] some of the reported cases of aggressive keratoacanthoma are probably well-differentiated squamous cell carcinomas. Aggressive keratoacanthoma lesions should be differentiated from verrucous carcinoma of the skin (carcinoma cuniculatum).[28] The former lesions typically present with a short duration and a history of rapid growth and spontaneous regression. Keratoacanthomas are generally regarded as secondary to sun damage of the skin.[29] Multiple eruptive, small keratoacanthomas may involve the nonexposed areas of the skin.[30]

Subungual keratoacanthoma[31,32] is a distinct clinicopathologic entity. The lesions present with a history of rapid onset of pain and swelling under the nail bed, suggesting infection. X-ray film may show underlying bone erosion.[32] These lesions should be distinguished from subungual squamous cell carcinomas.

Histologic Features

The most characteristic low-power feature of keratoacanthoma is observed in a section cut through the center of a mature lesion. It shows a cup-shaped invagination of the epidermis surrounded by a mass of pseudoepitheliomatous and papillomatous proliferation of well-differentiated large, pale-staining keratinocytes adjacent to a central keratin-filled crater (Fig. 42–24) and lateral liplike extension over the sides of the crater. The base of the lesion has an irregular pushing border (Fig. 42–25), in contrast to the infiltrative growth seen in squamous cell carcinomas.

The mass of keratinocytes comprises islands of large cells containing vacuolated cytoplasm resembling those of the pilary outer root sheath and large cells with eosinophilic ground glass–like cytoplasm, as well as peripheral small cuboidal cells resembling epidermal basaloid cells. In the

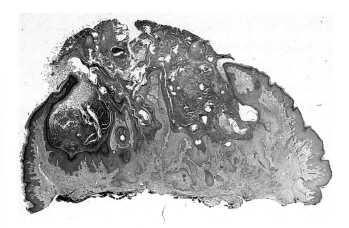

Figure 42–24. Low-power photomicrograph of a keratoacanthoma displaying a typical cup-shaped invagination of well-differentiated keratinizing squamous cells into the dermis. (H&E, ×12.) (AFIP Neg. No. 87-7325)

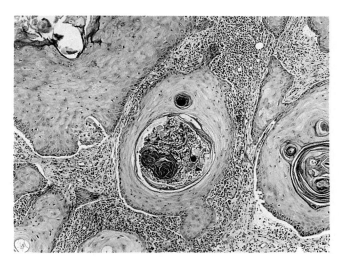

Figure 42–26. Higher magnification of a section of rapidly enlarging keratoacanthoma of several months' duration. Large islands of keratinocytes with ground-glass cytoplasm, intense stromal inflammation, and neutrophilic, eosinophilic microabscesses are present. (H&E, ×100.) (AFIP Neg. No. 86-10127)

rapidly growing lesions of keratoacanthoma, the stroma shows an intense inflammatory infiltrate. Intraepidermal eosinophilic, or neutrophilic abscesses are frequently observed (Fig. 42–26). After several months, the lesions of keratoacanthoma start to regress. The inflammation gradually subsides. About two thirds of keratoacanthomas show moderate-to-marked keratinocyte dysplasia, with large hyperchromatic nuclei, pleomorphism, and increased mitotic activity, particularly at the periphery of the squamous cell nests. Endogenous foreign body, giant cell granulomatous reaction to extruded keratin from the adjacent hair follicles is sometimes present. Subungual keratoacanthoma shows large islands of well-keratinizing squamous epithelium with numerous dyskeratotic cells, similar to those seen in resolv-

ing keratoacanthomas (Fig. 42–27). The proliferating squamous epithelium in some keratoacanthomas may invade the perineural spaces[33] (Fig. 42–28), particularly near the base of the lesion. This finding is identified in about 4% of keratoacanthomas. The squamous invaded perineural spaces are not necessarily lymphatic spaces; they are believed to be areas of dermal or subcutaneous tissue with relatively little tissue cohesion. Vascular invasion has also been observed in some keratoacanthomas.[30] The findings of perineural and vascular invasions do not adversely affect the biologic behavior and the prognosis of keratoacanthoma.

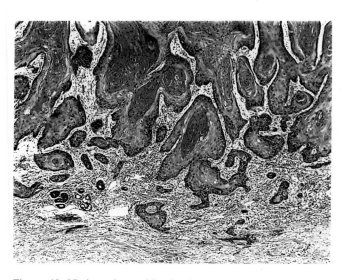

Figure 42–25. Irregular pushing border at the base of keratoacanthoma showing islands and strands of mature keratinizing squamous epithelium. There are relatively normal eccrine sweat gland lobules present in the left lower field.

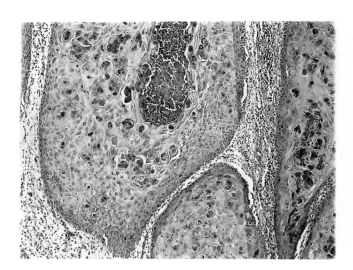

Figure 42–27. A resolving keratoacanthoma of 8 months' duration showing benign dyskeratotic cells, apoptotic cells, and civatte bodies scattered within large islands of proliferating squamous epithelium. (H&E, ×160.)

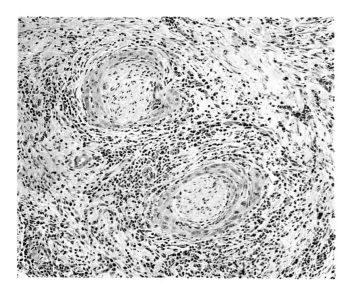

Figure 42–28. Perineural invasion by proliferating squamous epithelium seen at the base of a rapidly enlarging recurrent KA. (H&E, ×150.) (AFIP Neg. No. 86-10128)

The proliferating squamous cells disrupt dermal connective tissue fibers. The elastic and collagen bundles are trapped in the epithelial interstitium (Fig. 42–29).

In resolving keratoacanthomas, benign dyskeratotic cells, apoptotic cells, civatte bodies (Fig. 42–27), foreign body giant cells, phagocytizing necrotic epithelium, and karyorrhectic nuclei are interspersed among the dermal collagen and inflammatory cells. Acantholysis, as seen in acantholytic squamous cell carcinoma, however, is usually absent in lesions of keratoacanthoma.

Although the histologic diagnosis of keratoacanthoma is usually possible when an adequate and properly oriented biopsy specimen includes the lateral and lower margins

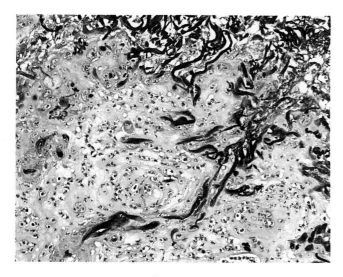

Figure 42–29. Fragments of elastic fiber trapped in islands of inflamed squamous epithelium of a keratoacanthoma. This finding is generally not seen in squamous cell carcinomas. (Movat, ×200.)

of the lesion, cases remain in which the final diagnosis has to be based on clinicopathologic correlation: a rapidly growing lesion exhibiting histologic features of a well-differentiated squamous cell carcinoma is likely to be a keratoacanthoma, whereas a slowly enlarging tumor with similar histologic features but no tendency of regression in a year or more is likely to be a squamous cell carcinoma.

The histopathologic diagnosis of keratoacanthoma can be made by examining routine hematoxylin and eosin–stained sections obtained by cutting through the center of the lesion. Special stains such as PAS, with and without prior amylase digestion, and elastic stains such as Movat's pentachrome and Verhoeff's van Gieson may be used to differentiate keratoacanthoma from well-differentiated squamous cell carcinoma in some cases. The amount of glycogen in cutaneous keratoacanthomas is reported to be significantly greater than that observed in squamous cell carcinomas arising in solar keratosis, and intraepithelial elastic fibers were found in 71% of cutaneous keratoacanthomas but in none of the squamous cell carcinomas.[34] Keratoacanthomas of the mucocutaneous junction of the lip, however, have not been shown to have significantly more glycogen than squamous cell carcinomas in the same anatomic location. The intraepithelial elastic fibers are identified in both keratoacanthomas and squamous cell carcinomas of the lip.[34] Thus, glycogen content and presence of intraepithelial elastic fibers cannot be used as definite criteria for differentiation of keratoacanthoma from squamous cell carcinoma of the mucocutaneous junction.

Electron microscopic features of keratinocytes in keratoacanthoma include clumping of short, deranged tonofilaments and lack of keratohyalin granules and sparse cytoplasmic organelles (Fig. 42–30).

Differential Diagnosis

Well-Differentiated Squamous Cell Carcinoma. Table 42–1 summarizes the differential histologic features of keratoacanthoma and well-differentiated squamous cell carcinoma (Fig. 42–31).[36–39]

Prurigo Nodularis. The lesions of prurigo nodularis show histologic features of pseudoepitheliomatous hyperplasia.[40,41] The features may mimic those of small, multiple eruptive keratoacanthomas; however, lesions of prurigo nodularis usually present with symptoms of intense pruritus. In addition, the microscopic features of hyperplasia of cutaneous nerves or neuroid structures resembling Verocay bodies and electron microscopic findings of neural proliferation involving axons and Schwann cells are encountered in some nodules of prurigo nodularis but not in lesions of keratoacanthoma. Furthermore, histologic features of lichen simplex chronicus can sometimes be observed adjacent to prurigo nodularis but not keratoacanthoma, and more than half of the lesions of prurigo nodularis show follicular involvement.[41]

Subungual Squamous Cell Carcinoma. In contrast to subungual squamous cell carcinomas, which most commonly present as protracted lesions mimicking onychomycosis, chronic paronychia, eczema, verrucae, pyogenic granuloma, subungual exostosis, or malignant melanoma, subungual keratoacanthomas are rapidly growing lesions

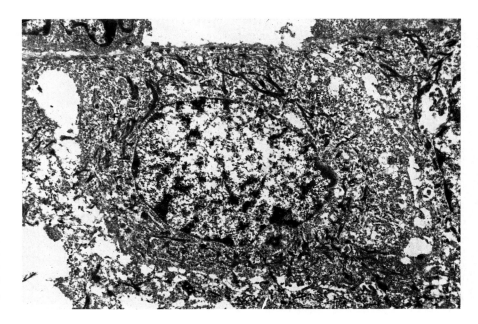

Figure 42–30. Electron micrograph of keratinocytes in keratoacanthoma showing irregular clumping of short and deranged tonofilaments (TF) and the lack of keratohyalin granules. (Uranyl acetate and lead citrate, ×22,000).

that involve the tissue under the nail bed. Microscopic examination is necessary to distinguish the two lesions. Subungual squamous cell carcinoma shows islands of poorly differentiated atypical keratinocytes with marked pleomorphism infiltrating the nail bed, rather than large islands of well-differentiated squamous cells with prominent benign dyskeratosis extending into the subungual tissue, as seen in subungual keratoacanthomas.

PSEUDOEPITHELIOMATOUS HYPERPLASIA

Pseudoepitheliomatous hyperplasia (PEH) is a benign squamous hyperplastic disorder that was initially known as "invasive acanthosis." Because, histologically, it resembles well-differentiated squamous cell carcinoma, it has also been called verrucoid epidermal hyperplasia, pseudocarcinomatous hyperplasia, and carcinomatoid hyperplasia.

Clinical Features
Lesions of PEH are benign reactive epidermal hyperplasias that appear as vegetating papillomatous plaques:

1. Adjacent to an ulcer, site of thermal or chemical burns, sinus tracts, and chronic osteomyelitis
2. In association with chronic infectious diseases such as granuloma inguinale, deep fungal infection, cutaneous leishmaniasis, atypical mycobacterial infection, and tertiary syphilis

TABLE 42–1. MICROSCOPIC FEATURES FOR THE DIFFERENTIAL DIAGNOSIS OF KERATOACANTHOMA AND SQUAMOUS CELL CARCINOMA

	Keratoacanthoma	Squamous Cell Carcinoma
Low-power architecture	Cup-shaped with central horn-filled crater, exo–endophytic, well-defined border	Primarily endophytic except for verrucous carcinoma, which has exo–endophytic growth
Epidermal ulceration	Rare	Common
Epidermal collarette	Common	None
Keratinocytes	Eosinophilic, ground-glass cytoplasm with abundant glycogen	Atypical with scanty glycogen
Intraepithelial elastic fibers	Present in 71% of cases	None
Dyskeratosis and apoptotic cells	Abundant in resolving lesions and around abscesses	Malignant dyskeratotic cells common
Acantholysis	Rare	Prominent, especially in adenoid squamous cell carcinoma
Microabscesses	Common	Rare, except for verrucous carcinoma
Inflammatory cells, foreign body and granulomatous reaction	Eosinophils, neutrophils, giant cell reaction to extruded keratin common	Plasma cells and lymphocytes dominate, granulomatous reaction uncommon

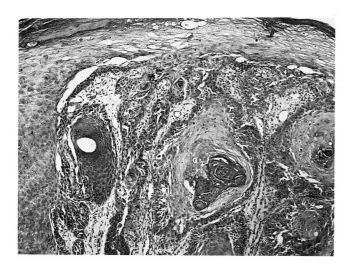

Figure 42–31. A well-differentiated squamous cell carcinoma exhibiting irregular strands and islands of atypical keratinocytes extending from the epidermis into the underlying dermis. (H&E, ×75.) (AFIP Neg. No. 87-7318)

3. Over dermal tumors such as granular cell tumor (Fig. 42–32) and, sometimes, melanocytic lesions, spindle and epithelioid cell (Spitz's) nevi, and malignant melanoma
4. In halogenoderma such as fluoroderma,[42] bromoderma, and iododerma[43,44]
5. Adjacent to verrucous carcinoma of the skin and giant keratoacanthoma

Clinically, PEH may resemble keratoacanthoma and squamous cell carcinoma; therefore, adequate biopsy and properly oriented specimens with thorough histopathologic examination are essential for an accurate diagnosis.

Histologic Features

Microscopically, PEH is similar to keratoacanthoma but without the overall cup-shaped architecture (Figs. 42–33, 42–34). There are varying degrees of hyperkeratosis, parakeratosis, and papillomatosis. The rete ridges are elongated, and the granular cell layer is prominent. The squamous keratinocytes are well differentiated with evidence of surface maturation. Although mitoses are sometimes active, significant cellular atypia or an invasive pattern, as seen in squamous cell carcinoma, is lacking. The dermis contains a mixed inflammatory infiltrate composed of acute and chronic inflammatory cells, including neutrophils, eosinophils, lymphocytes, monocytes, histiocytes, multinucleated giant cells, plasma cells, and mast cells. Intraepidermal microabscesses, tissue necrosis, and granulamatous giant cell reaction are frequently encountered in lesions of PEH associated with such infectious processes as deep fungal infection, North American blastomycosis, chromoblastomycosis, cryptococcosis, and atypical mycobacterial infection. Deeper sections and sections treated with special histochemical stains (including Brown and Hopps, PAS, Gomori's methenamine silver, acid-fast, and Warthin-Starry at pH 3.8) should be examined and microorganisms searched for, when there is suspicion of an infectious process. PEH in

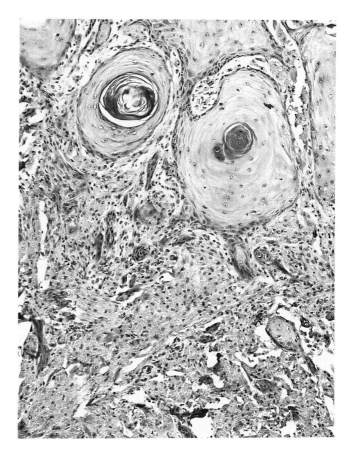

Figure 42–32. A pseudoepitheliomatous hyperplasia overlying a granular cell tumor. (H&E, ×200.) (AFIP Neg. No. 87-7323)

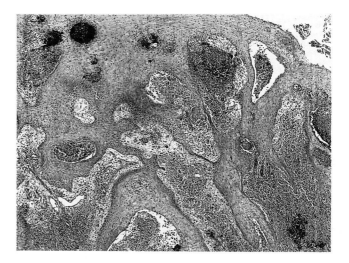

Figure 42–33. Pseudoepitheliomatous hyperplasia of the epidermis with multiple foci of microabscesses from a patient with cutaneous North American blastomycosis. (H&E, ×100.) (AFIP Neg. No. 86-10958)

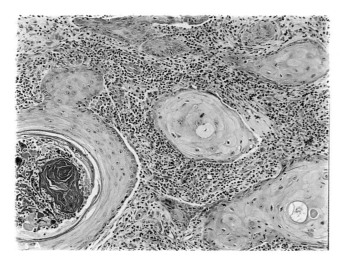

Figure 42–34. Higher magnification of pseudoepitheliomatous hyperplasia depicting nests and islands of keratinizing squamous epithelium with intense inflammation in the adjacent stroma. (H&E, ×150.)

patients with halogenoderma shows a less intense inflammatory reaction. The proliferating keratinocytes are generally connected to the surface epidermis and do not have the ground-glass appearance observed in keratoacanthomas (Fig. 42–35).

Differential Diagnosis

Squamous Cell Carcinoma. Lesions showing atypical keratinocytes with an invasive growth pattern are characteristic of squamous cell carcinoma. Benign PEH lesions display prominent intraepithelial microabscesses and a gran-

ulomatous reaction, which are lacking in squamous cell carcinomas.

Prurigo Nodularis. The microscopic features of prurigo nodularis are essentially identical to those of PEH. Clinicopathologic correlation is essential to an accurate interpretation. Prurigo nodularis lesions are associated with intense itching, and they may be associated with lichen simplex chronicus or secondary to arthropod bite reaction (20–30%). The papulonodular lesions of prurigo nodularis are frequently arranged in a linear fashion, usually along the scratching marks of the skin. In general, lesions of prurigo nodularis do not show intense inflammation and granulomatous reaction, as seen in PEH. The prominent follicular involvement and proliferation of nerve fibers at the base of the lesion are helpful features in the diagnosis of prurigo nodularis.

Keratoacanthoma. A well-developed keratoacanthoma has a characteristic cup-shaped overall architecture that is lacking in lesions of PEH; however, a resolving keratoacanthoma is indistinguishable from PEH. Clinicopathologic correlation, particularly regarding the duration, location, and history of regression, is helpful in separating the two lesions.

Halogenoderma. Ingestion of bromides and iodides and excessive application of fluoride gel to the teeth may result in the formation of papillomatous vegetating plaques of the skin.[42-44] The plaques of bromoderma are more frequently encountered on the lower extremities, and often there are pustules at the periphery of the lesions. Lesions of iododerma are similar to those of bromoderma but are more commonly seen on the face. Papules and nodules on the neck and in the preauricular regions are seen in patients with fluroderma. Microscopic sections of halogenoderma show PEH with frequent intraepidermal abscesses containing eosinophils, neutrophils, and desquamated necrotic keratinocytes. Clinicopathologic correlation with a careful history is essential in establishing the diagnosis of halogenoderma.

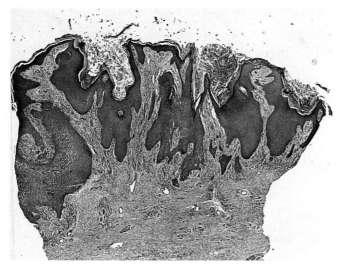

Figure 42–35. A bromoderma lesion showing pseudoepitheliomatous hyperplasia (PEH) from a patient receiving bromide-containing, over-the-counter medicine for many years. The PEH is less extensive and connected to the overlying epidermis. (H&E, ×20.) (AFIP Neg. No. 86-10955)

REFERENCES

1. Neoplastic Patterns of the Epidermis, in Hood AF, Kwan TH, Burnes DC, et al. (eds), *Primer of Dermatopathology.* Boston/Toronto, Little, Brown, 1984, chap 6, pp 79–95.
2. Hurwitz S: Epidermal nevi and tumors of the epidermal origin. *Pediatr Clin North Am* 1983;30:483–494.
3. Mehregan AH: Epidermal nevi and benign epidermoid tumors, *Pinkus' Guide to Dermatohistopathology.* E. Norwalk, Conn., Appleton-Century-Crofts, 1986, chap 34, pp 425–441.
4. Zeligman I, Pomeranz J: Variation of congenital ichthyosiform erythroderma: Report of cases of ichthyosis hystrix and nevus unius lateris. *Arch Dermatol* 1965;91:120.
5. Altman J, Mehregan AH: Inflammatory linear verrucous epidermal nevus. *Arch Dermatol* 1971;104:385–389.
6. Kennedy C: Inflammatory linear verrucous epidermal nevus (eczematous linear naevus). *Clin Exp Dermatol* 1980;5:471–473.
7. Winer LH, Levin GH: Pigmented basal cell carcinoma in verrucous nevi. *Arch Dermatol* 1961;83:960–964.
8. Horn MS, Sausker WF, Pierson DL: Basal cell carcinoma arising in a linear epidermal nevus. *Arch Dermatol* 1981;117:247.

9. Cramer SF, Mandel MA, Huler R, et al.: Squamous cell carcinoma arising in linear epidermal nevus. *Arch Dermatol* 1981; 117:222–224.

10. Levin A, Amazon K, Rywlin AM: A squamous cell carcinoma that developed in an epidermal nevus. Report of a case and a review of the literature. *Am J. Dermatopathol* 1984;6:1–55.

11. Mehregan AH, Pinkus H: Life history of organoid nevi. *Arch Dermatol* 1965;91:574–588.

12. De Lopez RMES, Hernandez-Perez E: Jadassohn's sebaceous nevus. *J Dermatol Surg Oncol* 1985;11:68–72.

13. Morioka S: The natural history of nevus sebaceus. *J Cutan Pathol* 1985;12:200–213.

14. Domingo J, Helwig EB: Malignant neoplasms associated with nevus sebaceus of Jadassohn. *J Am Acad Dermatol* 1979;1:545–556.

15. Jones EW, Heyl T: Nevus sebaceus. A report of 140 cases with special regard to the development of secondary malignant tumors. *Br J Dermatol* 1970;82:99–117.

16. Gitlin MC, Pirozzi DJ: The sign of Leser-Trelat. *Arch Dermatol* 1975;111:792–793.

17. Mehregan AH: Inverted follicular keratosis. *Arch Dermatol* 1964; 89:229–235.

18. Montgomery H: Inverted follicular keratosis, in *Dermatopathology*. New York, Harper & Row, 1967, vol 2: *Epithelial Neoplasms: Basal and Squamous Cell Neoplasms and Keratoacanthoma*, chap 31, p 954.

19. Mishima Y, Pinkus H: Benign mixed tumor of melanocytes and malpighian cells. *Arch Dermatol* 1960;1:539–550.

20. Harriest TJ, Murphy GF, Mihm MC Jr: Oral warty dyskeratoma. *Arch Dermatol* 1980;116:929–931.

21. Tanay A, Mehregan AH: Warty dyskeratoma. (Review) *Dermatologica* 1969;138:155–164.

22. Wellas GC, Wilson Jones E: Degos's acanthoma (acanthome a cellules claires). A report of five cases with particular reference to the histochemistry. *Br J Dermatol* 1967;79:249–258.

23. Fukushiro S, Takei Y, Ackerman AB: Pale cell acanthosis. *Am J Dermatopathol* 1985;7(6):515–527.

24. Pagani WA, Lorenzi G, Gorusso D: Surgical treatment for aggressive giant keratoacanthoma of the face. *J Dermatol Surg Oncol* 1986;12:3–5.

25. Walinsky S, Silvers DV, et al.: Spontaneous regression of a giant keratoacanthoma. *Cancer* 1978;41:12–16.

26. Piscioli F, Boi S, Zumiani G, et al.: A gigantic, metastasizing keratoacanthoma. Report of a case and discussion on classification. *Am J Dermatopathol* 1984;6:123–129.

27. Goldenhersh MA, Olsen TG: Invasive squamous cell carcinoma initially diagnosed as a giant keratoacanthoma. *J Am Acad Dermatol* 1984;10:372–378.

28. Kao GF, Helwig EB, et al.: Carcinoma cuniculatum (verrucous carcinoma of the skin). A clinicopathologic study of 46 cases with ultrastructural observations. *Cancer* 1982;49:2395–2403.

29. Rook A, Whimsler I: Keratoacanthoma: A thirty-year retrospect. *Br J Dermatol* 1979;100:41.

30. Reid BJ, Cheesbrough MJ: Multiple KA: A unique case and review of current classification. *Acta Dermatol Venereol (Stockh)* 1978;58:169.

31. Mehregan AH, Fabiam L: KA of nailbed: A report of two cases. *Int J Dermatol* 1973;12:149.

32. Cramer SF: Subungual KA. A benign bone-eroding neoplasm of the distal phalanx. *Am J Clin Pathol* 1981;75:425.

33. Lapins NA, Helwig EB: Perineural invasion by KA. *Arch Dermatol* 1980;37:791–792.

34. King DF, Barr RJ: Intraepithelial elastic fibers and intracytoplasmic glycogen: Diagnostic aids in differentiating keratoacanthoma from squamous cell carcinoma. *J Cutan Pathol* 1980;7:140–148.

35. Ellis GL: Differentiating keratoacanthoma from squamous cell carcinoma of the lower lip: An analysis of intraepithelial elastic fibers and intracytoplasmic glycogen. *Oral Surg., Oral Med., Oral Pathol.* 1983;56:527–532.

36. Pinkus H, Mehregan AH: *A Guide to Dermatopathology*, ed 2. New York, Appleton-Century-Crofts, 1976, p 516.

37. Wade TR, Ackerman AS: The many faces of KA. *J Dermatol Surg Oncol* 1978;4:498–501.

38. Kern WH, McCray MK: The histopathologic differentiation of keratoacanthoma and squamous cell carcinoma of the skin. *J Cutan Pathol* 1980;7:318–325.

39. Ackerman AB, Niven J, Grant-Kels JM: *Differential Diagnosis in Dermatopathology*. Philadelphia, Lea & Febiger, 1982, pp 122–125.

40. Doyle JA, Connolly SM, Hunziker N, et al.: Prurigo nodularis: A reappraisal of the clinical and histologic features. *J Cutan Pathol* 1979;6:392–403.

41. Miyauchi H, Urchara M: Follicular occurrence of prurigo nodularis. *J Cutan Pathol* 1988; 15:208–211.

42. Blasik LG, Spencer SF: Fluoroderma. *Arch Dermatol* 1979; 115:1334–1335.

43. Heydenreich G, Larsen PO: Iododerma after high dose urography in an oliguric patient. *Br J Dermatol* 1977;97:567–569.

44. Wilkin JK, Strobel D: Iododerma occurring during thyroid protective treatment. *Cutis* 1985;36:335–337.

CHAPTER 43
Precancerous Lesions and Carcinoma in Situ

Grace F. Kao

GENERAL PATHOGENESIS

Several cutaneous disorders commonly affecting the sun-exposed skin and mucocutaneous junction show characteristic histopathological features of atypical keratinocytic hyperplasia. Their natural history is often associated with the development of invasive squamous cell carcinoma and adnexal carcinoma.[1,2] These lesions are referred to as precancerous keratoses[3] or premalignant epidermal dysplasias[4] and carcinoma in situ (intraepithelial squamous cell carcinoma). These lesions may affect the epidermis and/or the pilosebaceous complexes, as well as the oral and anogenital mucous membrane and mucocutaneous junction. Each type of premalignant lesion has its characteristic clinicopathologic features and is prone to evolve into malignant tumor in a significant number of patients. The diagnosis of malignant disease is rendered on the basis of the cytological and biologic characteristics of each disorder (Table 43–1).

It is known that chronically sun-damaged skin shows keratinocytic atypia and that ultraviolet light induces epithelial changes as a result of clonal mutation[5] and damage to DNA of keratinocytes by short-wave ultraviolet (UVB) rays via a specific T-lymphocyte suppressor population.[6] It has also been suggested that unrepaired damage to DNA and to other macromolecules is partially responsible for the aging process.[6] The incidence of nonmelanoma skin cancers increases with exposure to solar radiation, particularly by UVB rays, and long-wave ultraviolet (UVA) rays can also augment the cancer-producing effects of UVB rays. Other physical agents such as thermal burn and chronic x-ray radiation may induce similar cytological changes in the surface keratinocytes and sometimes in invasive squamous cell carcinoma.

CLASSIFICATION

Cutaneous and mucosal lesions with atypical keratinocytic proliferation differ from those of carcinoma in situ by the presence of surface maturation, which is lacking in the latter. Both types of lesions are regarded as precancerous because they are capable of invading the underlying dermis and submucosa, and a squamous cell carcinoma or adnexal carcinoma may develop subsequently. Microscopically, keratinocyte atypia, nuclear pleomorphism, increased mitotic activity, and a well-preserved dermoepidermal basement membrane are observed in squamous premalignant lesions.[7]

Precancerous lesions of keratinocytes are classified as follows:

1. Solar keratosis
   a. Hypertrophic
   b. Bowenoid
   c. Atrophic
   d. Adenoid (acantholytic, pseudoglandular)
   e. Pigmented
2. Solar cheilitis
3. Radiation keratosis
4. Thermal keratosis

Carcinoma in situ includes the following entities:

1. Bowen's disease
2. Arsenical keratosis
3. Intraepidermal epithelioma
4. Erythroplasia of Queyrat

SOLAR KERATOSIS

Synonyms for solar keratosis include actinic keratosis and senile keratosis.[8]

Clinical Features

The term *solar keratosis* is more specific than *actinic keratosis*[9] because it refers to the sun as the cause whereas the adjective *actinic* refers to a variety of rays of light beyond the violet end of the spectrum. Solar keratoses develop in sun-exposed areas of aging skin, which is dry, wrinkled, and atrophic and sometimes shows hyperpigmented patches. The lesions

TABLE 43–1. TYPES AND BEHAVIOR OF PRECANCEROUS LESIONS AND CARCINOMA IN SITU OF THE SKIN AND MUCOUS MEMBRANE

Lesion	% with Carcinoma	Type of Associated Malignant Neoplasm	% With Metastasis
Solar keratosis	12–13	Squamous cell carcinoma	0
Solar keratosis-acantholysis	0.1	Adenoid squamous cell carcinoma (> 2 cm, extraorbital location)	2–3
Bowen's disease	5	Adnexal carcinoma	13
Intraepidermal epithelioma	8–9	Adnexal carcinoma	up to 6
Erythroplasia of Queyrat	30	Adnexal carcinoma	20
Solar cheilitis	50	Squamous cell carcinoma	11

are usually less than 1 cm in diameter. They are often flat, rounded, or irregularly shaped, have adherent scale, and vary from a reddish to gray-brown color. Some lesions are horny and nodular and may show a warty configuration. These lesions are more commonly multiple than single and are usually located on the face, ears, backs of the hands, and an alopecic scalp. Typical patients with solar keratosis are in their early 60s at the time of first biopsy. The lesions occur in both sexes but principally affect fair-complexioned men who have had a greater-than-average amount of sun exposure during many years. Patients with solar keratosis may also have cutaneous premalignant or malignant lesions other than solar keratosis and squamous cell carcinoma (SCC). These include lentigo maligna, basal cell carcinoma (BCC), sebaceous carcinoma, adnexal carcinoma, and malignant melanoma.[10,11]

Patients who have received combined psoralen and long-wave ultraviolet ray (PUVA) treatment for psoriasis and other disorders have also been found to develop solar keratoses and epidermal dysplasias.[6,11–13]

Histologic Features

Histologically, five types of solar keratosis can be recognized[1,2,14–17]: hypertrophic, atrophic, bowenoid, acantholytic, and pigmented.[17] The epidermis shows hyperkeratosis, parakeratosis, hypergranulosis, frequent irregular acanthosis, and sometimes atrophy. The palisaded layer of the basal epidermis and of the pilar epithelium above the sebaceous gland level is replaced by small buds, broad or elongated rete ridges containing atypical keratinocytes, sometimes associated with liquefaction degeneration (Fig. 43–1), or acantholysis. The atypical keratinocytes are characterized by hyperchromatic nuclei, prominent nucleoli, vacuolated cytoplasm, malignant dyskeratosis, multinucleated giant cells, and scattered mitotic figures (Fig. 43–2). The

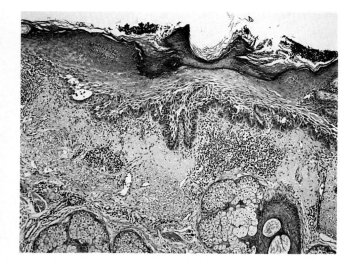

Figure 43–1. Typical histologic features of solar keratosis include hyperkeratosis, parakeratosis, and irregular basal epidermis with small buds and broad or elongated rete ridges containing atypical keratinocytes, sometimes associated with liquefaction degeneration. The upper dermis depicts solar elastosis of the collagen and a sparse lymphomononuclear infiltrate. (AFIP Neg 84-6796.) (H&E, ×160.)

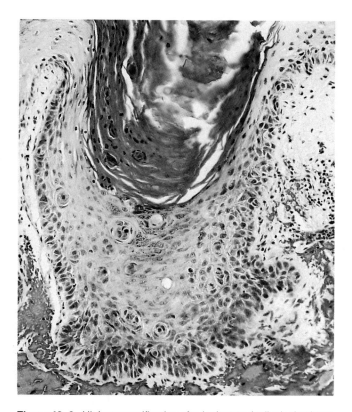

Figure 43–2. Higher magnification of solar keratosis displaying irregular basal layer with atypical keratinocytes involving the pilary epithelium. (H&E, ×250.)

atypical cells are confined by an intact dermoepidermal basement membrane. One or several layers of normal keratinocytes separate the atypical squamous cells from the horny layer. In the hypertrophic type of solar keratosis, papillomatosis is prominent, sometimes with verrucous acanthosis and cutaneous horn formation (Fig. 43–3A). The base of the lesion shows atypical keratinocytic hyperplasia (Fig. 43–3B), malignant dyskeratosis, mitosis, intact basement membrane, and sometimes acantholysis (Fig. 43–4A). Atrophic solar keratosis exhibits a thinned, atrophic epidermis with liquefaction degeneration of the dermoepidermal junction (see Fig. 43–1). The bowenoid type of solar keratosis may be difficult to distinguish from Bowen's disease. The irregular, disorganized, dysplastic cells have pale or lighter cytoplasm and frequently clumped nuclei and sometimes form a nesting pattern resembling that of intraepidermal epithelioma (IE). The atypical keratinocytes of Bowen's disease rest on dermoepidermal basement membrane. This differs from IE lesions, in which a rim of relatively normal basal cells surrounds the atypical keratinocytes. Compared with Bowen's disease, atypical keratinocytic proliferation in bowenoid solar keratosis spares the outer root sheath of the hair follicle but involves the acrotrichium. The basal epidermis in acantholytic solar keratosis shows prominent

acantholysis, with suprabasal lacunae containing malignant dyskeratotic cells (Fig. 43–4B). The acantholysis occurs in about 6 to 7% of solar keratosis lesions. Pigmented solar keratosis contains prominent pigmented, frequently spindle-shaped melanocytes in the epidermis (Fig. 43–5) and melanophages in the dermis. The epidermis in 10 to 12% of cases of solar keratosis shows features of senile lentigo. In all types of solar keratosis, the upper dermis usually shows a dense, chronic inflammatory infiltrate composed of lymphocytes, histiocytes, and plasma cells. In some instances, the infiltrate lies close to the base of the lesion and thus exhibits a lichenoid pattern.

A very rare epidermolytic variant of solar keratosis was reported by Ackerman and Reed in 1973. The histological features of this variant resemble those of epidermolytic hyperkeratosis.[15]

Solar Keratosis with Squamous Cell Carcinoma

Without treatment, 12 to 13% of patients with solar keratosis develop one or more malignant lesions that invade the underlying dermis as SCC.[1,2] The invasive lesions appear as flesh-colored to pink, red, or brown keratotic papules;

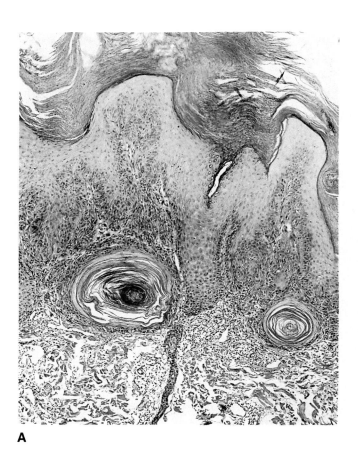

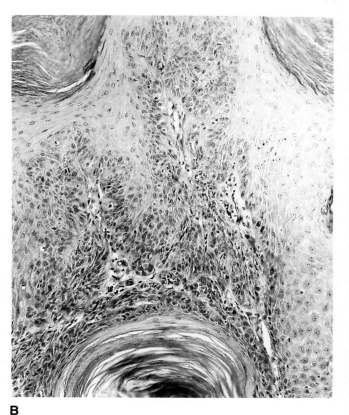

A

B

Figure 43–3. A. Hypertrophic solar keratosis shows papillomatosis with verrucous acanthosis and cutaneous horn formation on the top. (AFIP Neg 86-10145.) (H&E, ×160.) **B.** Higher magnification of Figure 43–3A showing marked keratinocyte atypia involving the lower layers of the epidermis and around the horn cyst. (AFIP Neg 86-10146.) (H&E, ×250).

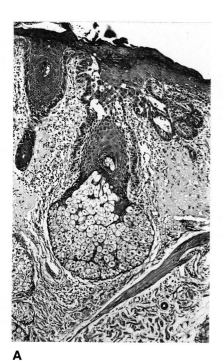

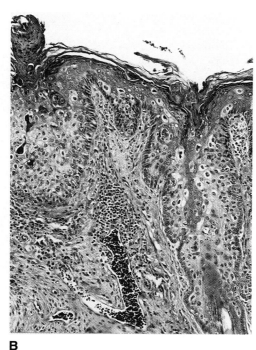

A

B

Figure 43–4. A. Acantholysis, suprabasilar separation, and lacunae formation at the dermoepidermal junction in an adenoid (acantholytic) solar keratosis. (H&E, ×60.) **B.** A bowenoid solar keratosis shows atypical keratinocytes replacing the lower layers of the epidermis. The pilar epithelium lacks full thickness of involvement by the atypical cells as seen in Bowen's disease (H&E, ×160.)

nodules, scaling, and an elevated pearly margin are seen. Common complaints include nonhealing, enlarging lesions, bleeding on trauma, pruritus, and pain. Microscopically, these lesions show disruption of the dermoepidermal basement membrane. Atypical keratinocytes can be seen to extend into the dermis to various depths, with squamous pearl formation (Fig. 43–6). The most important criterion in making the diagnosis of solar keratosis with SCC is identification of overlying epidermal changes of solar keratosis, particularly at the lateral margins of SCC. Epidermal features of senile lentigo at the lateral margins of the lesions serve as additional evidence favoring origin of the lesion in a preexisting solar keratosis. Solar keratosis with SCC is considered to be a low-grade malignancy, and studies have indicated that this type of tumor almost never metastasizes unless it is neglected and a large and deeply invasive

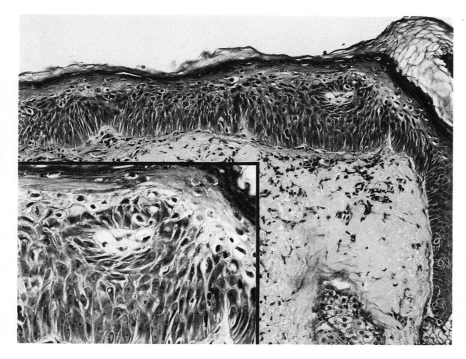

Figure 43–5. Spindle-shaped melanocytes admixed with atypical keratinocytes in a pigmented solar keratosis. Note the markedly increased cellularity at the dermoepidermal junction. (H&E, ×160). (Inset) Higher magnification showing plump atypical keratinocytes with abundant cytoplasm. Some contain melanin. (H&E, ×250.)

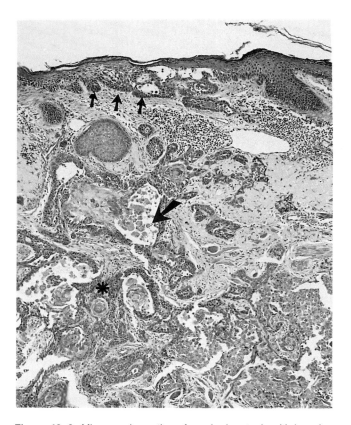

Figure 43–6. Microscopic section of a solar keratosis with invasive carcinoma (SK-SCC) depicts atypical keratinocytes invading the dermis with squamous pearl formation (*). Note the presence of acantholysis (large arrow). Features of SK (small arrows) are present in the vicinity. (H&E, ×75.)

tumor develops. Solar keratosis with acantholysis represents the precursor lesion of adenoid SCC. These tumors, like other forms of SCC, are rare in black persons. They are microscopically characterized by the presence of acantholysis with a pseudoglandular pattern (Fig. 43–7). No definite data are available regarding the percentage of patients who have lesions of solar keratosis with acantholysis who eventually develop adenoid SCC. About 2 to 3% of patients who have adenoid SCC and who have nodules 2 cm or larger show clinical and histological evidence of deep invasion with metastasis from their primary tumors.[18] However, aggressive behavior has not been observed in adenoid SCC of the eyelid and orbital areas.[19]

Differential Diagnosis

The hypertrophic type of solar keratosis should be distinguished from solar keratosis with SCC, the de novo type of SCC, keratoacanthoma, metatypical BCC, seborrheic keratosis, and lichenoid benign keratosis. SCC lacking marginal changes of solar keratosis should be classified as the de novo type. Such tumors can affect black persons but occur predominantly in white individuals, on either sun-damaged or covered areas. Data from previous studies showed that at least 8% of patients with the de novo type of SCC had evidence of regional or distant metastasis.[1,2]

Microscopically, the de novo type of SCC shows a centrally atrophic epidermis with erosion or ulcer filled with cellular debris, fragments of keratin, and necrotic tissue. The cords and columns of atypical squamous cells and stromal changes are similar to those seen in solar keratosis with SCC.

An atrophic type of solar keratosis may sometimes be mistaken for discoid lupus erythematosus, lesions of the latter type are usually reddish and have easily detachable

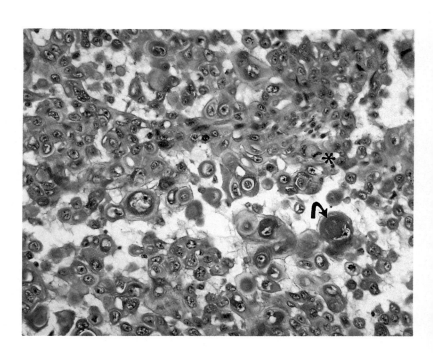

Figure 43–7. Photomicrograph of an adenoid squamous cell carcinoma showing acantholysis, nuclear pleomorphism, malignant dyskeratosis (*), mitosis (curved arrow), and a pseudoglandular pattern. (AFIP Neg 84-6810) (H&E, ×250.)

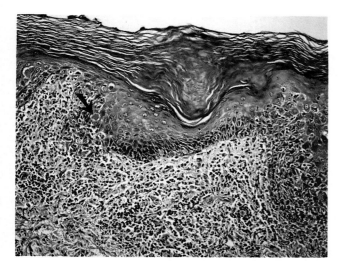

Figure 43–8. Marked spongiosis, scattered Civatte bodies (apoptotic cells) (arrows) seen in a lichenoid benign keratosis admixed with exocytosis of lymphomononuclear cells at the dermoepidermal junction. Hyperkeratosis and a dense upper dermal inflammatory infiltrate are present. (AFIP Neg 84-6089.) (H&E, ×160.)

scale. The lack of atypical keratinocytes, prominent liquefaction degeneration of the dermoepidermal junction, a patchy periappendageal lymphoplasmacytic infiltrate, and dermal mucin deposition are features in favor of the diagnosis of discoid lupus erythematosus. Localized forms of poikiloderma, atrophic lichen planus, and lichenoid drug eruption also have to be considered in the microscopic differential diagnosis. These lesions, however, do not show atypia or pleomorphism of the keratinocytes. Unlike bowenoid solar keratosis, Bowen's disease on the sun-exposed areas usually has a more irregular contour and a more erythematous base. Microscopically, full-thickness involvement of epidermal and pilar epithelium by the atypical keratinocytes is characteristic of Bowen's disease.

Acantholytic solar keratosis must be distinguished from isolated dyskeratosis follicularis (warty dyskeratoma), keratosis follicularis (Darier's disease), familial benign chronic pemphigus (Hailey-Hailey disease), transient acantholytic dermatosis, and pemphigus vulgaris. The presence of cellular pleomorphism, a disorderly arrangement of keratinocytes, malignant dyskeratosis, and an absence of corpus ronds and grains distinguish acantholytic solar keratosis from the previously mentioned conditions.

A pigmented solar keratosis may resemble lentigo maligna (melanotic freckle of Hutchinson), which is a type of precancerous, pigmented, acquired melanosis that frequently develops into lentigo maligna melanoma or desmoplastic or sometimes neurotropic malignant melanoma. Lentigo maligna usually shows more flattening of the epidermis than does pigmented solar keratosis; and, most important, atypical melanocytes but not keratinocytes are present at the dermoepidermal junction.

Lesions of lichenoid benign keratosis[20] present as a single scaly papule, most commonly on the upper arm. They may sometimes be mistaken for pigmented solar kera-

tosis, particularly when dermal melanosis is present. The lack of keratinocyte atypia, a prominent lichenoid upper dermal infiltrate with exocytosis into the epidermis, liquefaction degeneration of the dermoepidermal junction, and scattered Civatte's bodies (apoptotic cells) (Fig. 43–8), as well as the clinical presentation of a single papule on the upper extremity, distinguish lichenoid benign keratosis from solar keratosis.

SOLAR CHEILITIS

Synonyms for solar cheilitis[21] include actinic cheilitis,[22] cheilitis exfoliativa, solar cheilosis, and actinic keratosis of the lip.

Clinical Features
Solar cheilitis occurs most often on the lower lip. Two types of lesions are recognized—an acute and a chronic type. The acute form usually occurs during the summer months, after prolonged sunlight exposure. Edema, redness, fissuring, ulceration, and occasionally vesicle formation and superficial erosions characterize these lesions. The lesions persist for several days to weeks and subside when the patient is no longer exposed to the sun. However, the lesions reappear during the following summer season.

The chronic type of solar cheilitis manifests as scaling, wrinkling, or atrophy of the vermilion border and with a change in color to white-gray or brown. The wrinkles are parallel to one another and perpendicular to the long axis of the lip. Secondary infection, erosion, ulceration, and development of SCC subsequently occur.

Solar keratosis may occasionally appear as a white patch or plaque; thus, it is sometimes referred to as leukoplakia. Under this classification, the clinical differential diagnosis should include epithelial dysplasia, carcinoma in situ, lichen planus, candidiasis, and white sponge nevus. The clinical term *leukoplakia* should not be used in the histopathological diagnosis.

Histologic Features
The mucosa of the lip and the mucocutaneous junction show hyperkeratosis, parakeratosis, acanthosis, and superficial ulceration. Keratinocyte atypia, pleomorphism, frequent abnormal mitotic figures, and dyskeratosis are present. The submucosa shows solar elastosis of the collagen. A bandlike inflammatory infiltrate consists of lymphocytes, plasma cells, histiocytes, and occasional eosinophils and mast cells. The adjacent skin shows epidermal atrophy with or without keratinocyte atypia and solar elastosis of the dermal collagen.

Squamous Cell Carcinoma Arising in Solar Cheilitis

About 50% of patients with clinical lesions of solar cheilitis have histological evidence of SCC in the biopsy specimens. SCC arising in solar cheilitis is characterized by a variegated red and white blotchy appearance of the vermilion border, atrophy with focal areas of whitish thickening, persistent chapping with localized flaking and crusting, or indistinct vermilion border.

Moderately to well-differentiated or poorly differentiated SCC arises from lesions of solar cheilitis. These tumors have a more aggressive behavior than SCC with solar keratosis—that is, they have a higher rate of recurrence and metastasis to the regional lymph node. Generalized dissemination and fatality also occasionally occur.

RADIATION KERATOSIS

Synonyms for radiation keratosis include x-ray keratosis and postirradiation keratosis.

Clinical Features

Radiation keratosis may occur in a scar after radiation therapy or excessive fluoroscopy. Radiologists, radiotherapists, dentists, surgeons, and patients undergoing radiation therapy for various skin disorders, including acne vulgaris, BCC, and SCC, may be frequently exposed to small amounts of radiation and sometimes develop postirradiation keratoses. Such cases, however, are now rare. Late (chronic) radiation dermatitis and radiation keratosis occur from a few months to many years after the administration of fractional doses of radium. The affected skin shows atrophy,

telangiectasia, and irregular hyperpigmentation and hypopigmentation; ulceration and foci of hyperkeratotic scale representing radiation keratosis may sometimes be seen in the areas of atrophy. BCC or SCC may develop in these areas.[23,24]

Histologic Features

The epidermis is irregular, showing atrophy and variable areas of hyperplasia. Hyperkeratosis is present, and the squamous cells show disorderly maturation, pleomorphism with individual cell keratinization, and atypia (Fig. 43–9). Degeneration of the cells in the stratum malpighii and scanty lymphocytic exocytosis may be present.

In the dermis, the collagen bundles are enlarged and often show hyalinization (Fig. 43–10). The deep dermal blood vessels often show fibrous thickening of their walls. Some of the vessels show thrombosis and recanalization. In contrast, the upper dermal vessels may show telangiectasia. The dermal fibroblasts and endothelial cells frequently show atypia as seen in the epidermis. Lymphedema in the subepidermal region may be seen. Pilosebaceous and sweat glands are usually preserved.

Carcinoma Arising in Radiation Keratosis (Radiation Carcinoma)

SCC and BCC of the skin secondary to irradiation are relatively uncommon neoplasms. In most cases, the tumor develops either within hyperkeratotic areas of chronic radiodermatitis or in persistent ulceration. The latent period between irradiation and carcinoma is long, varying from 4 to 39 years, with a median of 7 to 12 years.[19] Before 1940, most of the reported cases of radiation carcinoma were SCC that occurred on the hands, feet, and occasionally the face. A large number of BCCs, however, have been

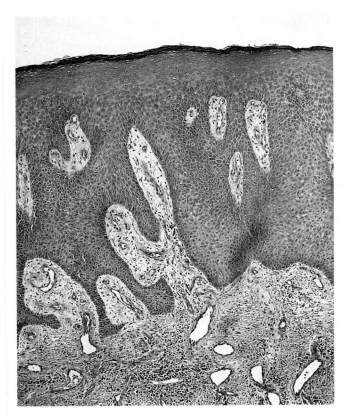

Figure 43–9. Photomicrograph of a radiation keratosis showing epidermal hyperplasia and dysplasia with irregular acanthosis. Note the upper dermal edema, ectatic capillaries, and a moderate chronic inflammatory infiltrate. (H&E, ×75.)

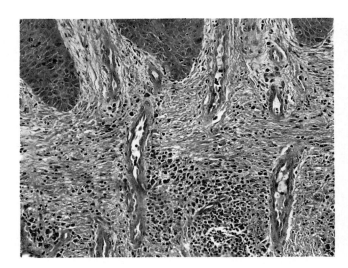

Figure 43–10. Higher magnification of Figure 43–9 displaying prominent collagen fibers with hyalinization, atypical fibroblasts, and endothelial cells lining the ectatic vessels and the perivascular lymphoplasmacytic infiltrate in the dermis of a radiation keratosis. (H&E, ×200.)

reported since 1951.[24] In radiation dermatitis, BCC develops almost exclusively in the head and neck region whereas SCC occurs most commonly in other regions. Almost all cases of radiation carcinoma encountered in recent years have been in patients treated for acne or undergoing epilation for benign skin disorders. With the development of a general awareness of the potential dangers of repeated low-dose x-ray irradiation, it can be expected that radiation carcinoma will virtually disappear in the future.

SCC arising in radiation keratosis is frequently of spindle cell type (Fig. 43–11A). Features similar to solar keratosis with SCC are frequently observed. Large columns of atypical keratinocytes are connected to the overlying epidermis, and interlacing spindle-shaped cells (Fig. 43–11B) with hyperchromatic nuclei, frequent mitotic forms, and abundant eosinophilic sometimes vacuolated cytoplasm are present. The dermal changes are similar to those in chronic radiodermatitis or radiation keratosis. The histological differential diagnosis of spindle cell SCC should include spindle cell amelanotic malignant melanoma, desmoplastic malignant melanoma, lentigo maligna melanoma, and atypical fibroxanthoma. Immunoperoxidase stain for cytokeratin is usually positive in the tumor cells of spindle cell SCC, and electron microscopic demonstration of cytoplasmic tonofilaments arising from intercellular desmosomes (Fig. 43–12) confirms the diagnosis.

THERMAL KERATOSIS

Clinical Features

Prolonged exposure of the skin to heat may result in histopathological changes similar to those in solar keratosis.[25,26]

Several clinical presentations have been identified in this group of diseases: Kangri basket cancers of the thighs and lower abdomen in the Kashmiris, Kang cancers of the skin over the greater trochanters in Chinese and Tibetans, Kairo cancers of the abdomen in Japanese, carcinoma of the hard palate associated with reverse smoking, and carcinoma of the lower legs associated with erythema ab igne in Britain and Ireland.[27] Erythema ab igne presents as a reticular, telangiectatic, and pigmented dermatosis occurring most commonly on the lower legs after prolonged exposure to infrared radiation that is insufficient to produce a thermal burn.[28] Because of the histopathologic similarities between the heat-induced lesions and solar keratosis, the former have been referred to as thermal keratoses. The reported cases suggest that heat may induce epithelial changes as a result of clonal mutation in the same way that ultraviolet light produces atypical epithelial changes.[13]

Histologic Features

The microscopic features of thermal keratosis are similar to those seen in solar keratosis, solar cheilitis, and radiation keratosis. The atypical keratinocyte hyperplasia in thermal keratosis tends to spare the achrotrichium and acrosyringium, whereas in solar keratosis and radiation keratosis keratinocyte atypia as a rule involves the adnexal epithelium. Although vascular ectasia is a common finding in thermal keratosis, atypical reactive endothelial cells and fibroblasts as seen in radiation keratosis are generally not observed.

SCC arising in thermal keratosis is rare. Although these lesions are believed to be less aggressive than other forms of SCC and to biologically resemble those arising in solar keratosis, some metastasize.[23]

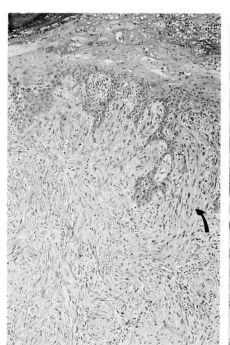
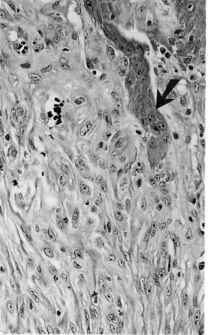

A   **B**

Figure 43–11. A split-field photomicrograph of radiation keratosis with invasive spindle cell squamous carcinoma. **A.** Keratinocyte atypia similar to solar keratosis present in the overlying epidermis; focally, the spindle-shaped tumor cells extend from the epidermis into the dermis (arrow). (H&E × 75.) **B.** Higher magnification of Figure 43–15A showing a thin column of atypical keratinocytes (arrow) surrounded by spindle-shaped tumor cells. (H&E, ×250).

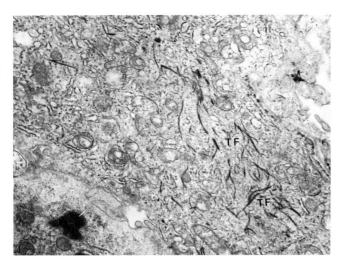

Figure 43–12. Electron micrograph of a spindle cell squamous carcinoma showing bundles of tonofilaments (TF) arising from desmosomes. (Uranyl acetate and lead citrate, ×6000.)

BOWEN'S DISEASE

Synonyms for Bowen's disease include squamous cell carcinoma in situ, bowenoid dysplasia, and bowenoid carcinoma in situ.

Clinical Features
Bowen's disease occurs in both sexes but predominantly in fair-complexioned Caucasian men. About 20% of the patients are women. The average age at onset of the disease is 48 years, and the average age at first biopsy is 55 years. The lesions occur equally on covered and exposed skin. About one third of the cases occur in the head and neck areas, particularly the face.[1,2]

Bowen's disease manifests as a slowly enlarging, erythematous, round to irregular, lenticular, polycystic, pigmented, scaly, keratotic, fissured, crusty, nodular, eroded plaque. The plaques are devoid of hair and usually appear sharply demarcated from the surrounding normal skin. Areas of normal-appearing skin may occur within the boundaries of larger lesions of Bowen's disease. The average duration of the lesions is 6.4 years. Lesions occur in the anogenital area and, particularly in women, may appear verrucoid or polypoid and are frequently pigmented. The decision to classify BD as a precancerous lesion should be based on the microscopic features of carcinoma in situ involving the epidermis and the pilosebaceous epithelium. The presence of an extracutaneous malignant neoplasm in a patient with Bowen's disease was initially recorded by Bowen in 1920.[29] That patient died of gastric carcinoma after having had lesions of Bowen's disease for 34 years. Similar observations were made by Kao,[30] Graham,[10] Callen and Headington,[31,32] Braverman,[33] Miki and co-workers,[34] and King and associates.[35] At least 25% of patients with BD reported by Graham and Helwig in 1961 had primary extracutaneous cancers.[10] From 100 cases of carcinoma arising in Bowen's disease selected from the Armed Forces Institute of Pathology (AFIP) file, 19 of the patients showed evidence of cutaneous and extracutaneous malignant neoplasm.[1,2,30] Although evidence of association of BD and internal malignancies exists, there is still controversy regarding the statistical findings of this association.[36]

Histologic Features
The typical microscopic features of Bowen's disease are hyperkeratosis, parakeratosis, hypergranulosis, plaquelike acanthosis, and a chronic inflammatory infiltrate in the upper corium. The epidermis exhibits total or focal loss of normal polarity and progression of keratinocyte maturation. The loss of normal epidermal architecture is characterized by a windblown appearance of atypical keratinocytes, hyperchromatism, vacuolated cells, multinucleated cells, malignant dyskeratosis, and abnormal mitosis. These changes occur at all epidermal levels (Fig. 43–13), but may be focal, and are confined by an intact dermoepidermal basement membrane. Examination of multiple and serial sections of Bowen's disease lesions from hair-bearing areas invariably shows involvement of the pilary acrotrichium, infundibulum, and sebaceous gland (Fig. 43–14). The atypical cellular proliferation involves all levels of the outer root sheath and eventually replaces the sebaceous gland cells. In some lesions, most of the atypical epithelial cells appear vacuolated and sometimes are contrasted with hyperchromatic undifferentiated keratinocytes that replace the epidermal basal layer and the pilary outer root sheath, giving the appearance of cellular nesting. The acrosyringium generally is not involved. The inflammatory infiltrate of lymphocytes, histiocytes, and sometimes plasma cells is seen in the upper corium subjacent to the Bowen's disease lesion. A common feature in the upper dermis is capillary-endothelial proliferation and some ectatic small vessels. Lesions located on the sun-exposed areas of the body show prominent solar elastosis.

The atypical vacuolated keratinocytes are routinely negative for cytoplasmic mucin; some, however, contain glycogen. Melanin pigment is present in the atypical cells in Bowen's disease lesions. The abnormal keratinizing cells are intensely reactive with glucose-6-phosphate dehydrogenase (Table 43–2).[10]

Ultrastructural changes of Bowen's disease include abnormal cell division of malignant dyskeratotic cells, abnormal mitotic figures, decrease in tonofilament-desmosomal attachments, absence of keratohyalin granules, and aggregate tonofilaments and nuclear substances (Fig. 43–15).

Bowen's Disease with Invasive Adnexal Carcinoma[30]

About 3 to 5% of patients with Bowen's disease develop invasive carcinoma (see Table 43–1).[1,2] The common presenting features include a rapidly growing ulcerating tumor occurring in a preexisting scaly, erythematous, or pigmented patch of many years duration. In a study of 100 such cases from the AFIP files, the patients' ages ranged from 29 to 91 years, with a male:female ratio of 3:1 and a white:black ratio of 20:1. The extremities, face, and anogenital areas were common sites of involvement. The size of

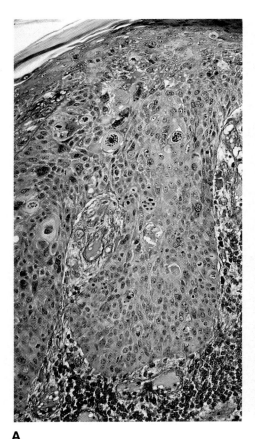 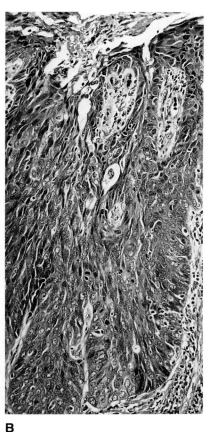

A   **B**

Figure 43–13. Photomicrographs of Bowen's disease showing full thickness of epidermal keratinocyte atypia. **A.** Note hyperkeratosis, hypogranulosis, scattered bizarre, anaplastic nuclei, abnormal mitotic structures, and a dense dermal plasmacytic infiltrate. (AFIP Neg. No. 82-8030.) (H&E ×250.) **B.** Many of the atypical keratinocytes are spindle shaped with high nucleus-to-cytoplasm ratio. The lack of maturation qualifies these lesions as carcinoma in situ. (AFIP Neg 82-8014) (H&E, ×250).

the tumors varied from 1 to 12 cm in diameter. Histopathological evidence of Bowen's disease involving the epidermis or pilosebaceous epithelium was identified in tissue sections from Bowen's disease with invasive adnexal carcinoma.

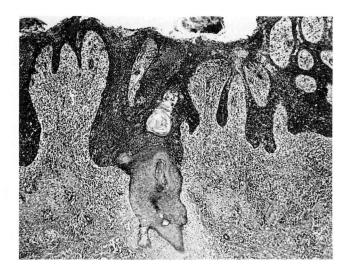

Figure 43–14. Malignant adnexal keratinocytes in Bowen's disease replaced the acrotrichium and follicular infundibulum (AFIP Neg 81-16766) (H&E, ×160).

The cytological changes showed basaloid, squamous, pilar, pilosebaceous (Fig. 43–16), and occasionally glandular differentiations (Fig. 43–17), favoring interpretation of the invasive lesion as a form of adnexal carcinoma. Mitosis and malignant dyskeratosis are commonly seen. At least 19% of patients had evidence of cutaneous and extracutaneous malignant neoplasms, including BCC, SCC, carcinoma of the gastrointestinal tract, respiratory tract, and genitourinary tract; and malignant melanoma.

Differential Diagnosis

Lesions of bowenoid solar keratosis show atypical keratinocytes similar to those seen in Bowen's disease. However, the former lesions are smaller, occurring almost exclusively on sun-exposed areas, and microscopically the epidermis shows surface maturation and the atypical keratinocytes do not involve the entire thickness of the epidermis or pilary epithelium such as seen in Bowen's disease.

Lesions of bowenoid papulosis show some histological similarity to Bowen's disease, but the characteristic clinical presentation of the former includes multiple pigmented papules or small nodules on the external genitalia and anogenital region,[37] whereas the latter presents a single plaque on the sun-exposed or nonexposed skin. The presence of superficial keratinocyte maturation in lesions of bowenoid papulosis further differentiates the lesions from those of Bowen's disease, which show full thickness of epidermal and pilosebaceous epithelial involvement by the atypical

TABLE 43–2. DIFFERENTIAL DIAGNOSIS OF LESIONS WITH INTRAEPIDERMAL NESTING PATTERN

Diagnosis	Cell Type and Characteristic Features	Histochemistry
Intraepidermal epithelioma	Atypical, multipluripotential cells, sharply demarcated cell nests	Glycogen, amount variable; carcinoembryonic antigen focal weak +
Inflamed seborrheic keratosis	Basal keratinocytes, prominent squamous eddies	Some glycogen
Bowen's disease	Adnexal keratinocytes, full thickness of epidermis, and pilar epithelial atypia	Some glycogen; glucose-6-phosphate dehydrogenase 4+
Mammary, extramammary Paget's disease	Ductal epithelial cells, adnexal (apocrine) cells forming ducts	Sialomucin; some glycogen; carcinoembryonic antigen 4+
Nevocellular nevus	Melanocytes	Melanin
Precancerous melanosis	Atypical melanocytes, pagetoid spread	Melanin

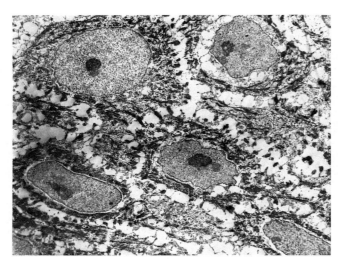

Figure 43–15. Electron micrograph of the surface atypical keratinocytes of Bowen's disease shows abnormal maturation. Note the lack of keratohyalin granules, decreased tonofilament-desmosomal attachment, and aggregated tonofilaments (AFIP Neg 81-14203) (uranyl acetate and lead citrate, ×9000).

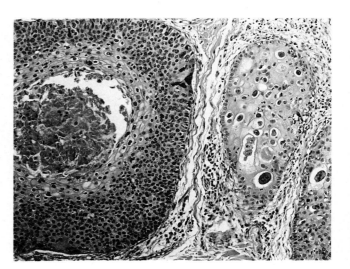

Figure 43–16. Invasive carcinoma arising in Bowen's disease shows various histological differentiation: Squamous, basaloid, pilar, and pilosebaceous (AFIP Neg 84-5535) (H&E, ×160).

keratinocytes (Fig. 43–18). The immunoperoxidase staining method using specific and pooled antibodies to human papillomavirus (HPV) has demonstrated positive staining in lesions of bowenoid papulosis[38,39] but not in those of Bowen's disease. Ikenberg and colleagues demonstrated HPV type 16-related DNA in six of ten cases of Bowen's disease and eight of ten cases of bowenoid papulosis.[40]

The Paget's cells in mammary and extramammary Paget's disease contain sialomucin and stain diffusely and strongly positive with carcinoembryonic antigen. They differ from the vacuolated cells of Bowen's disease, which contain glycogen. Paget's cells frequently form glandular structures at the dermoepidermal junction, a feature lacking in Bowen's disease.

The cellular nesting of vacuolated pagetoid cells in some lesions of Bowen's disease can cause histological confusion with malignant melanoma of the superficial spreading type (so-called pagetoid melanoma) and intraepidermal epithelioma. In malignant melanoma, the melanoma cell nests in-

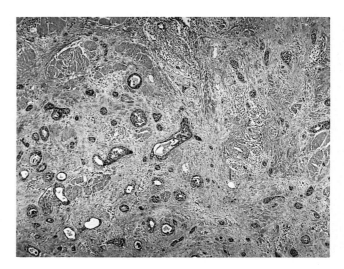

Figure 43–17. Bowen's disease with occasional ductal differentiation, qualifying as an adnexal carcinoma (AFIP Neg 82-8026) (H&E, ×60).

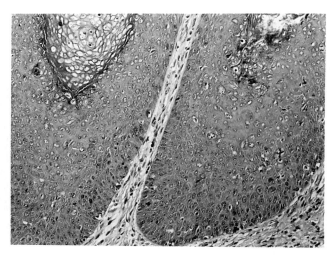

Figure 43–18. Scattered dyskeratotic cells in an orderly background of maturing keratinocytes and the presence of surface maturation differentiate lesions of bowenoid papulosis from those of Bowen's disease. Note koilocytotic cells in the subcorneal region (double arrow) (H&E, ×150).

volve the dermoepidermal junction and are scattered in the epidermis. In contrast, the vacuolated cells in Bowen's disease generally spare the dermoepidermal junction and are present in the malpighian and granular cell layers. In lesions of IE, the atypical keratinocyte cell nests are surrounded by relatively normal keratinocytes; however, the atypical keratinocytes totally replace the epidermis in Bowen's disease.

ARSENICAL KERATOSIS AND ARSENICAL CARCINOMA

Clinical Features
Clinically, arsenical keratosis frequently presents as punctate, cornlike, papulonodular keratotic lesions, more profuse on the extremities and characteristically affecting the palms and soles.[1,2,41] The trunk and other parts of the extremities are also affected.

Histologic Features
The microscopic features of arsenical keratosis and carcinoma arising in arsenical keratosis are indistinguishable from Bowen's disease and adnexal carcinoma arising in Bowen's disease.[1,2] More than 50% of patients with history of chronic arsenicism develop Bowen's disease and multiple cutaneous malignant neoplasms such as squamous cell carcinoma and basal cell carcinoma.[41] It has been postulated that arsenical keratosis and Bowen's disease may represent the same disease, and because of the clinical, histopathological, histochemical, chemical, and carcinogenic similarities between the two diseases, it is suggested that arsenic is probably a common causative agent.[9,41,42]

Differential Diagnosis
Clinically, lesions of arsenical keratosis must be differentiated from various types of punctate keratosis, such as dis-

seminated punctate keratoderma, which usually appears in early life. Darier's disease and lichen planus usually have characteristic lesions elsewhere, in addition to those present on the acral skin. Plantar warts differ from arsenical keratosis in that the former lesions are papillomatous, and microscopic evidence of viral inclusions confirm the diagnosis of verrucae.

INTRAEPIDERMAL EPITHELIOMA[43,44]

Synonyms for intraepidermal epithelioma (IE) include Montgomery's superficial epitheliomatosis,[45] intraepidermal basal cell epithelioma,[46] intraepidermal nevus,[47] hidracanthoma simplex,[48,49] intraepidermal epithelioma of Borst-Jadassohn,[50–53] intraepidermal acanthoma,[54] and intraepidermal eccrine poroma.[55]

Clinical Features
Lesions of IE share many clinical features with Bowen's disease and in most instances are indistinguishable. IE occurs as a single gray to tan-brown, keratotic, scaly, flat, sometimes verrucous, round to irregularly shaped papule, plaque, or nodule varying from 0.5 to 10 cm in diameter. The plaques usually are sharply demarcated from the adjacent normal-appearing skin. Papillary lesions are uncommon, and erosion and ulceration sometimes occur. Lesions occur on all parts of the body except the palms and soles. About 45% of the lesions are on the lower extremities; 25% are located on the head and neck areas, particularly the face (17%); and the remainder are found on the buttocks, chest, back, upper extremities, abdomen, and feet, in decreasing order of frequency. The disease affects predominantly fair-complexioned individuals in the fifth through eighth decades of life and is encountered more often in women than in men. The lesions are generally slow growing. The duration varies from less than 1 month to more than 30 years, with more than half of the lesions present less than 3 years. Because of the controversy over the exact cell type in the epidermal nests and the pathogenesis, lesions of IE have been reported under various classifications as listed under the synonyms.[43–55]

In the past, IE has been considered by some observers to represent intraepidermal basal cell epithelioma[46] or a combined intraepidermal basosquamous carcinoma. Most of the published reports refer to this cutaneous keratotic disease under the terminology of Borst-Jadassohn epithelioma.[50–53] However, it is believed that Borst described an invasive SCC of the lip that showed nesting of the surface epithelium; if this is true, his name should be excluded from the diagnosis IE. Some observers conclude that the lesion represents a benign epidermal proliferation such as seborrheic keratosis or epithelial nevus.[47] Others classify the IE lesion as a primary epidermal acanthoma[54] with differentiating potentialities. Based on the histopathological features, the lesion is best regarded as a variety of carcinoma in situ arising from keratinocytes of the eccrine acrosyringium or multipluripotential adnexal cells.

Histologic Features
Sections of IE lesions show hyperkeratosis, spotted parakeratosis, hypergranulosis, horn cysts (sometimes), plaquelike

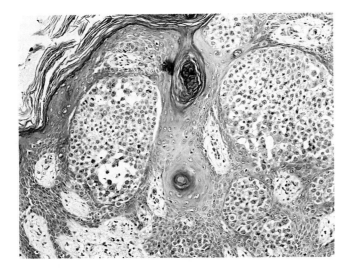

Figure 43–19. The epidermal cell nests of intraepidermal epithelioma are separated from the dermoepidermal junction by a rim of compressed, relatively normal epidermal keratinocytes. Note prominent loss of cell cohesion and sparing of the acrotrichium (H&E, ×150).

acanthosis, and discrete nests of uniform to dysplastic, or atypical, keratinocytes composed of basaloid or squamous cell types within the stratum malpighii (Fig. 43–19). Some lesions show prominent papillomatosis and verrucous acanthosis. Spindle-shaped and pigmented cells are sometimes present. Individual keratinocytes within the discrete nests are connected by intercellular desmosomes. Keratinocytes within the discrete nests involve superficial epidermal levels with focal disruption of the granular cell layers; one or more layers of normal-appearing to compressed malpighian cells separate the nests of keratinocytes from the dermoepi-

dermal junction (Fig. 43–20). Serial sections show involvement of the acrosyringium, and, rarely, there are discrete keratinocyte nests in the acrotrichium, follicular infundibulum, and sebaceous glands. Some keratinocytes in the cell nests form squamous eddies, a feature that is reminiscent of an inflamed seborrheic keratosis, inverted follicular keratosis, and epidermal nevus. The keratinocytes within the discrete nests contain variable amounts of glycogen. Some cells contain nonsulfated, hyaluronidase-resistant sialomucin. Immunoperoxidase stains show diffusely positive cytokeratin (AE1/AE3) and focally positive carcinoembryonic antigen. Enzyme stains performed on frozen sections are positive for phosphorylase and succinic dehydrogenase. The presence of lumenlike structures in some of the cell nests and occasional association with underlying dermal sweat gland tumors, as well as the histochemical and enzyme stains, are features supporting eccrine histogenesis.[55] The pigmented IE lesions show melanin pigment associated with discrete nests of keratinocytes, and pigment granules are free or within melanophages in the papillary dermis. The upper corium usually shows a mild to moderate lymphohistiocytic infiltrate. Capillary-endothelial proliferation, vascular ectasia, and fibrosis are present in the upper dermis of most lesions. In more than 90% of IE lesions, the dermoepidermal basement membrane remains intact for long periods of time. Long-term follow-up of patients with IE shows that about 15% developed local recurrences, in most cases secondary to incomplete removal of the lesions.

Intraepidermal Epithelioma with Invasive Carcinoma (Malignant Hidracanthoma Simplex)[56-59]

Eight to 9% of patients with IE show clinical and microscopic evidence of invasive carcinoma in their primary lesions (see Table 43–1).[1,2,9,44] In general, lesions of IE with invasive

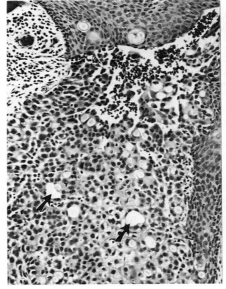
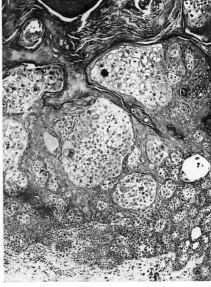

Figure 43–20. A split-field photomicrograph of an intraepidermal epithelioma. **A.** An invasive adnexal carcinoma adjacent to the area shown in Figure 43–20B. Note the disorganized patterns and the tendency of tumor cells to form ductular structures in the carcinoma (arrows) (H&E, ×150). **B.** Well-nested atypical keratinocytes in the acanthotic epidermis.

A   **B**

carcinoma are larger than those of IE, and they appear as papillary areas with epidermal erosion or ulceration. Histologic sections show intraepidermal cell nests with marked cellular atypia, pleomorphism, malignant dyskeratosis, vacuolated cells, mitotic figures, and occasionally multinucleated cells, disruption of the dermoepidermal basement membrane, and atypical keratinocytes invaded into the dermis (Figs. 43–20*B* and 43–21).

The tumor cells infiltrating the dermis and those at metastatic sites show some tendency of nesting, as seen in the epidermis. Anaplastic keratinocytes located in the corium adjacent to primary lesions and at the metastatic site show some disposition for ductal arrangement (Fig. 43–21). Carcinoma arising in IE should be regarded as a form of adnexal carcinoma, although the terms *malignant hidracanthoma simplex*[56] and *squamous cell carcinoma developing in the Jadassohn phenomenon*[58] were designated in the reported cases. Metastasis occurs in 6% of the patients. The biologic potential for distant spread is a feature that places the lesions of IE in the category with other cutaneous premalignant diseases. In comparison with Bowen's disease, the IE lesion is more prone to invade the underlying dermis as carcinoma, but there is less biologic potential for metastasis (see Table 43–1).

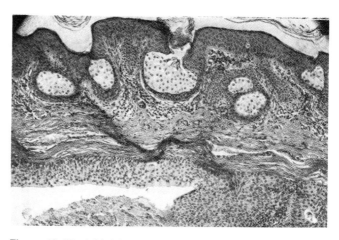

Figure 43–22. A bladder carcinoma that metastasized to the skin shows epidermotropism. The nesting pattern is similar to that seen in intraepidermal epithelioma; however, the tumor cell nests are connected to the dermal tumor cells (From Fig. 43–16*B*: *Cancer* 1964; 17:609–636. Courtesy of Amir H. Mehregan, M.D.).

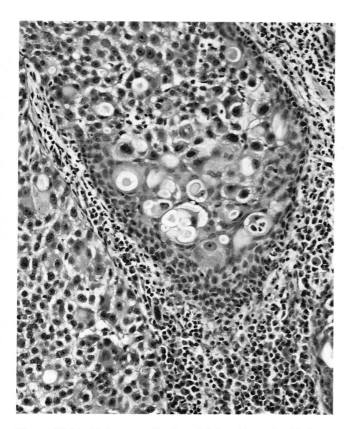

Figure 43–21. Higher magnification of intraepidermal epithelioma with invasive carcinoma depicts squamoid differentiation of the tumor cells and ductular formation. A dense chronic inflammatory infiltrate is seen in the surrounding stroma (AFIP Neg 87-6894) (H&E, ×250).

Differential Diagnosis

Cutaneous epithelial neoplasms that show cellular nesting (see Table 43–2) must be differentiated from IE lesions; the former group includes seborrheic keratosis, epidermal nevus, inverted follicular keratosis, lichenoid benign keratosis, Bowen's disease, mammary and extramammary Paget's disease, nevocellular nevus, malignant melanoma of the superficial spreading type, solar keratosis, and squamous cell carcinoma. Seborrheic keratosis show prominent squamous eddy formation within the epidermal cell nests, when they become inflamed, and these epidermal lesions are the greatest source of microscopic confusion with IE. The cell nests in seborrheic keratosis, epidermal nevus, lichenoid benign keratosis, and nevocellular nevus do not show nuclear atypia or pleomorphism as seen in IE lesions. In some lesions of Bowen's disease, areas of anaplastic cell nests are surrounded by normal-appearing epidermis, but other areas of the tumor show typical replacement of the entire thickness of the epidermis and pilosebaceous epithelium by the atypical keratinocytes. The presence of sialomucin and positive staining by carcinoembryonic antigen of the Paget's cells provide differentiation of Paget's disease from IE lesions. Pagetoid malignant melanoma cells almost always stain positive for S-100 protein and negative for cytokeratin. IE cells, however, stain negative for S-100 protein but positive for cytokeratin (AE1/AE3). The epidermotropic cell nests from metastatic carcinomas such as that of the breast and urinary tract can be distinguished from IE cells by the presence of sialomucin and the involvement of the dermoepidermal junction, as well as continuity of the epidermal cell nests from the underlying dermal tumor (see Fig. 43–22). On the basis of the gross features, typical microscopic cytological changes, immunopathologic findings,[59] and the occurrence of invasive carcinoma in some lesions, IE lesions can be distinguished from other skin lesions showing a cellular nesting pattern.

ERYTHROPLASIA OF QUEYRAT

Synonyms for erythroplasia of Queyrat include carcinoma in situ and Bowen's disease of the glans penis.

Clinical Features

Erythroplasia of Queyrat is a distinct clinicopathologic entity.[2,60] It is a carcinoma in situ involving the penile skin, mucosa, and mucocutaneous junction of the glans penis. The clinical and pathologic features are similar to those of Bowen's disease, particularly involvement of the anogenital regions. The disease occurs almost exclusively in uncircumcised men. It typically appears as an asymptomatic, well-demarcated, red, velvety plaque with yellow crusted flecks on the glans penis, in the coronal sulcus, or on the inner surface of the prepuce. Ulceration, crusting, and erosion are sometimes observed. The disease more commonly affects middle-aged and older individuals. The average duration to diagnosis is about 3 years, and the median size of the lesion is 1.0 cm.

Histologic Features

Erythroplasia of Queyrat is marked by thickening of the penile skin, mucocutaneous junction, and glans penis mucosa, with increased cellularity, hypokeratosis, and focal erosion. The microscopic features are those of carcinoma in situ. No surface keratinocyte maturation is present. All layers of the normal keratinocytes are replaced by nonkeratinizing basaloid cells with mild nuclear hyperchromatism and pleomorphism (Fig. 43–23A). The dermis and submucosa display a dense lymphoplasmacytic infiltrate. The adjacent adnexal structures are usually spared of the epithelial dysplasia.

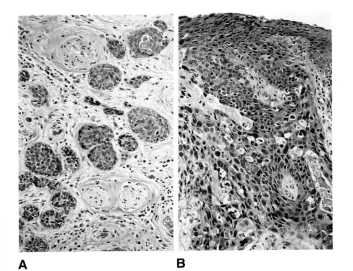

A   **B**

Figure 43–23. A split-field photomicrograph of erythroplasia of Queyrat (EQ) with invasive carcinoma. **A.** An adnexal carcinoma arising in EQ showing squamoid cells forming nests and ductal structures (H&E, ×160). **B.** Features of carcinoma in situ seen in a plaque of EQ involving the penile mucosa (H&E, ×150). Note squamous carcinoma cells extending from the mucosa into the submucosa.

Adnexal Carcinoma Arising in Erythroplasia of Queyrat

Without adequate treatment, as many as 30% of patients may develop invasive carcinoma, which shows various histological differentiation, including squamous, basaloid, and ductal features (Fig. 43–23B). The neoplasm is identical to that observed in adnexal carcinoma arising in Bowen's disease. Areas of invasive dermal or submucosal neoplastic cells in continuity with the overlying epithelium are frequently observed. About 20% of patients with invasive carcinoma develop metatasis.[60]

Differential Diagnosis

Bowenoid papulosis can be distinguished from erythroplasia of Queyrat by the presence of surface epidermal and mucocutaneous epithelial maturation as well as koilocytotic cells suggesting human papillomavirus infection. The characteristic clinical appearances of the two diseases also are distinct.

EXTRAMAMMARY PAGET'S DISEASE

Clinical Features

Extramammary Paget's disease as a clinical entity was initially described by Radcliffe Crocker in 1889. It is an uncommon tumor occurring on the vulva, male genitalia, perineum, perianal region and less frequently in the axilla.[61–64] Rare cases have been reported involving the external auditory canal[65] and oral mucosa.[66] Extramedullary Paget's disease occurs predominantly in the 6th and 7th decades, with females affected more than males. The lesions are typically erythematous patches or plaques, usually greater than 3 cm in diameter, and have a hyperkeratotic, crusted or eroded surface. It is frequently initially misdiagnosed as a dermatitis or mucositis. Pruritus, pain, tenderness, and bleeding are common symptoms. Multiple lesions are common and different noncontiguous anatomic sites may be involved.

Extramammary Paget's disease may remain localized to the epidermis and adnexal structures, may be associated with local cutaneous adnexal carcinoma, particularly that of sweat gland origin or may be associated with regional visceral malignancy, including lower GU and GI tract carcinoma. There does not appear to be a significant latent period to the development of an associated carcinoma.[61] The frequency of associated carcinomas has been variably reported from less than 2% in vulvar disease[64] to 45% in anogenital disease.[61] Lesions associated with adnexal or visceral carcinomas have a high frequency of tumor metastasis.[61]

Histologic Features

Extramammary Paget's disease has a distinctive microscopic appearance (Fig. 43–24). The tumor is composed of large, variable-sized, pale, vacuolated cells occurring singly, in clusters, or in an acinar array. The cells are most numerous in the lower half of the epidermis and may involve the basal cell layer and extend down the rete and adnexal structures. Eccrine, apocrine, and hair follicle epithelium may

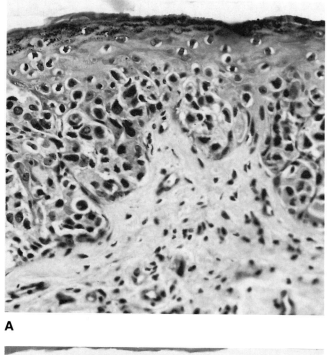

A

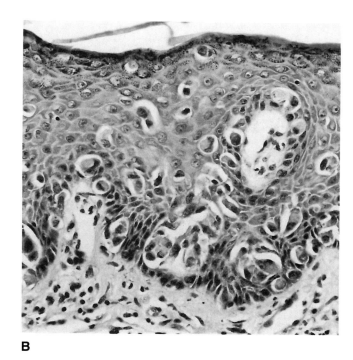

B

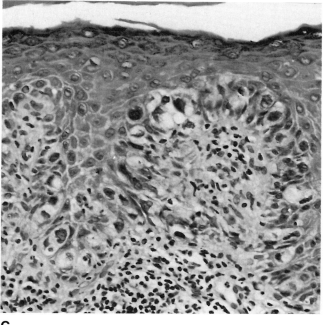

C

Figure 43–24. Extramammary Paget's disease. Large, atypical cells with abundant pale cytoplasms, occur in nests (**A&B**), singly (**B**), and in a linear (**C**) array within the epidermis (H&E, ×280).

be involved. Paget's cells have a pale to vesicular nucleus that is often compressed laterally by the abundant clear, bluish or granular cytoplasm forming a signet ring pattern. Nucleoli are often prominent and mitoses may be present. Paget cells may invade the dermis and subcutis.[62] Accompanying epidermal changes include hyperkeratosis, parakeratosis, and acanthosis. A variably intense dermal infiltrate of lymphocytes, histiocytic cells, and plasma cells may occur

associated with fibrosis, vascular proliferation, and ectasia.

The Paget cells stain positive for sialomucin using PAS with diastase digestion, mucicarmine, and colloidal iron with hyaluronidase digestion. They are Fontana positive and dopa negative, indicating transfer of melanosomes from melanocytes.[61] Paget cells also contain or express keratin, carcinoembryonic antigen[59] and gross cystic fluid protein[63] by immunoperoxidase staining.

Differential Diagnosis

Extramammary Paget's disease must be differentiated from in situ squamous cell carcinoma (Bowen's disease), erythroplasia of Queyrat, and melanoma. Staining for sialomucin and immunoperoxidase staining for carcinoembryonic antigen, keratin and gross cystic fluid protein should differentiate most cases.[59]

REFERENCES

1. Kao GF, Graham JH: Premalignant cutaneous disorders of the head and neck. In: *Otolaryngology*. England GM ed. Vol 5. Philadelphia, Pa: Harper & Row; 1986:1–20.
2. Goldes JA, Kao GF: Premalignant lesions of the skin. In: *Principles of Dermatologic Surgery*. Roenigk RK and Roegnigk HH, Jr., eds. New York, NY: Marcel Dekker; 1989:563–590.
3. Pinkus H, Mehregan AH: Epidermal precancerous, squamous cell carcinoma and pseudocarcinoma. In: *A Guide to Dermatopathology*. Mehregan AH ed. New York, NY: Appleton-Century-Crofts; 1976:443–460.
4. Reed RJ: Neoplasms of the skin. In: Steven G. Silverberg, ed. *Principles and Practices of Surgical Pathology*. Vol 1. New York, NY: John Wiley and Sons; 1982:164–166.
5. Reed RJ, Leone P: Porokeratosis: a mutan clonal keratosis of the epidermis. *Arch Dermatol*. 1970;101:340–347.
6. Epstein JH: Photocarcinogenesis, skin cancer, and aging. *J Am Acad Dermatol*. 1983;9:487–502.
7. Neoplastic patterns of the epidermis. In: *Primer of Dermatopathology*. Hood AF, Kwan TH, Burnes DC, Mihm MC Jr, eds. Boston, Mass: Little, Brown & Co; 1984:79–95.
8. Pinkus H: Keratosis senilis. *Am J Clin Pathol*. 1958;29:193–207.
9. Brownstein MH, Rabinowitz AD: The precursors of cutaneous squamous cell carcinoma. *Int J Dermatol*. 1979;18:1–16.
10. Graham JH: Selected precancerous skin and mucocutaneous lesions. In: *Neoplasms of the Skin and Malignant Melanoma*. Chicago, Ill: Year Book Medical Publishers; 1976:86–99, 118–121.
11. Holman CD, Armstrong BK, Evans PR, et al: Relationship of solar keratosis and history of skin cancer to objective measures of actinic skin damage. *Br J Dermatol*. 1984;110:129–138.
12. Abel EA, Cox AJ, Farber EM: Epidermal dystrophy and actinic keratoses in psoriasis patients following oral psoralen photochemotherapy (PUVA): follow-up study. *J Am Acad Dermatol*. 1982;7:333–340.
13. Niemi KM, Niemi A, Kanerva L: Morphologic changes in epidermis of PUVA-treated patients with psoriasis with or without a history of arsenic therapy. *Arch Dermtol*. 1983;119:904–909.
14. Lever WF, Schaumburg-lever G: Tumors and cysts of the epidermis. In: Lever WF, Schaumburg-Lever G, eds. *Histopathology of the Skin*. Philadelphia, Pa: JB Lippincott; 1983:489–493.
15. Ackerman AB, Reed RJ: Epidemolytic variant of solar keratosis. *Arch Dermatol*. 1973;107:104–106.
16. Wade TR, Ackerman AB: The many faces of solar keratoses. *J Dermatol Surg Oncol*. 1978;4:730–734.
17. Subert P, Jorizzo JL, Apisarnthanarax P: Spreading pigmented actinic keratosis. *J Am Acad Dermatol*. 1983;8:63–67.
18. Johnson WC, Helwig EB: Adenoid squamous cell carcinoma (adenoacanthoma). *Cancer*. 1966;19:1639–1650.
19. Caya JG, Hidayat AA, Weiner JM: A clinicopathologic study of 21 cases of adenoid squamous cell carcinoma of the eyelid and periorbital region. *Am J Ophthalmol*. 1985;99:291–297.
20. Berger TG, Graham JG, Goette DK: Lichenoid benign keratosis. *J Am Acad Dermatol*. 1984;11:635–638.
21. Cataldo E, Doku HC: Solar cheilitis. *J Dermatol Surg Oncol*. 1981;7:989–995.
22. Picasia DD, Robinson JK: Actinic cheilitis: A review of the etiology, differential diagnosis, and treatment. *J Am Acad Dermatol*. 1987;17:255–264.
23. Moschella SL: Reactions to physical agents. In: Moschella SL, Pillsbury DM, Hurley HJ, eds. *Dermatology*. Philadelphia, Pa: WB Saunders Co; 1975:1452–1455.
24. Anderson NP, Anderson HE: Development of basal cell epithelioma as a consequence of radiodermatitis. *Arch Dermatol Syphilol*. 1951;63:586–596.
25. Arrington JH III, Lockman DS: Thermal keratoses and squamous cell carcinoma in situ associated with erythema ab igne. *Arch Dermatol*. 1979;115:1226–1228.
26. Wilkinson DS: Cutaneous reactions to mechanical and thermal injury. In: Rook A, Wilkinson DS, Enling JFG, eds. *Textbook of Dermatology*. 2nd ed. Oxford, England: Blackwell Scientific Publications; 1972:435–436.
27. Cross F: On a turf (peat) fire cancer: malignant change superimposed on erythema ab igne. *Proc R Soc Med*. 1967;60:1307–1308.
28. Shahrad P, Marks R: The wages of warmth changes on erythema ab igne. *Br J Dermatol*. 1977;97:179–186.
29. Bowen JT: Precancerous dermatoses: the further course of 2 cases previously reported. *Arch Dermatol Syphilol*. 1920;1:23–24.
30. Kao GF: Carcinoma arising in Bowen's disease. *Arch Dermatol*. 1986;122:1124–1126. Editorial.
31. Callen JP, Headington J: Bowen's and nonBowen's squamous intraepidermal neoplasia of the skin. *Arch Dermatol*. 1960;116:422–426.
32. Callen JP: *Cutaneous Aspects of Internal Disease*. Chicago, Ill: Year Book Medical Publishers, 1981:209–212.
33. Braverman IM: *Skin Signs of Systemic Disease*. 2nd ed. Philadelphia, Pa: WB Saunders Co; 1981:67–77.
34. Miki Y, Kawatsu T, Matsuda K, et al: Cutaneous and pulmonary cancers associated with Bowen's disease. *J Acad Dermatol*. 1982;6:26–31.
35. King CM, Yates VM, Dave VK: Multicentric pigmented Bowen's disease of the genitalia associated with carcinoma in situ of the cervix. *Br J Vener Dis*. 1984;60:406–408.
36. Arbesman H, Ransohoff, DF: Is Bowen's disease a predictor for the development of internal malignancy? A methodological critique of the literature. *JAMA*. 1987;257:516–518.
37. Patterson JW, Kao GF, Graham JH et al: Bowenoid papulosis: a clinicopathologic study with ultrastructural observations. *Cancer*. 1986;57:823–836.
38. Farmer ER, Braun L, Shah KV: Immunologic staining for human papilloma virus in cutaneous dysplasia. *Arch Dermatol*. 1980;116:1389. Abstract.
39. Penneys NS, Molollon RJ, Nadji M, et al: Papillomavirus common antigens: papillomavirus antigen in verruca, benign paillomatous lesions, trichilemmoma, and bowenoid papulosis: an immunoperoxidase study. *Arch Dermatol*. 1984;120:859–861.
40. Ikenberg H, Gissmann L, Gross G, et al: Human papillomavirus type 16 related NDA in genital Bowen's disease and in bowenoid papulosis. *Int J Cancer*. 1983;32:563–565.
41. Yeh S: Cancer in chronic arsenism. *Hum Pathol*. 1973;4:469–485.
42. Bettley FR, O'Shea JA: The absorption of arsenic and its relation to carcinoma. *Br J Dermatol*. 1975;92:563–568.
43. Mehregan AH, Pinkus H: Intraepidermal epithelioma: a critical study. *Cancer*. 1964;17:609–636.
44. Berger P, Baughman R: Intraepidermal epithelioma. *Br J Dermatol*. 1974;90:343–349.
45. Montgomery H: Superficial epitheliomatosis. *Arch Dermatol*. 1979;20:338–357.
46. Sims CF, Parker RL: Intraepidermal basal cell epithelioma. *Arch Dermatol*. 1949;59:45–49.
47. Sachs W: Intraepidermal nevus. *Arch Dermatol*. 1952;65:110.

48. Smith JLS, Coburn JS: Hidroacanthoma simplex: an assessment of a selected group of intraepidermal basal cell epithelioma and of their malignant homologues. *Br J Dermatol*. 1956;68:400–418.

49. Mehregan AH, Levson DN: Hidroacanthoma simplex. *Arch Dermatol*. 1969;100:303–305.

50. Goltz RW, Fusaro RM, Sweitzer SE: Borst-Jadassohn epithelioma: a reevaluation. *Arch Dermatol*. 1957;75:117–122.

51. Siegel JM: Intraepidermal epithelioma of Jadassohn. *Arch Dermatol*. 1974;110:478.

52. Cook MG, Ridgeway HA: The intraepidermal epithelioma of Jadassohn: a distinct entity. *Br J Dermatol*. 1979;101:659–667.

53. Steffen C, Ackerman AB: Intraepidermal epithelioma of Borst-Jadassohn. *Am J Dermatopathol*. 1985;7:5–24.

54. Haber H: Intraepidermal acanthoma: recent observation on Borst-Jadassohn epithelioma. *Dermatologica*. 1958;117:304–316.

55. Holubar K, Wolf K: Intraepidermal eccrine poroma: a histochemical and enzyme histochemical study. *Cancer*. 1969;23:626–635.

56. Ishikawa K: Malignant hidracanthoma simplex. *Arch Dermatol*. 1971;104:529–532.

57. Kitamura K, Kinehara M, Tamura, N, et al: Hidracanthoma simplex with invasive growth. *Cutis*. 1983;32:83–88.

58. Mitchell RE: Squamous cell carcinoma developing in the Jadassohn phenomenon: a case report. *Aust J Dermatol*. 1975;16:79–82.

59. Guldhammer B, Norgaard T: The differential diagnosis of intraepidermal malignant lesions using immunohistochemistry. *Am J Dermatopathol*. 1986;8:295–301.

60. Graham JH, Helwig EB: Erythroplasia of Queyrat. *Cancer*. 1973;32:1396–1414.

61. Helwig EB, Graham JH: Anogenital extramammary Paget's disease: A clinicopathologic review. *Cancer*. 1963;16:387–403.

62. Jones RE, Austin C, Ackerman AB: Extramammary Paget's disease: A critical reexamination. *Am J Dermatopathol*. 1979;1:101–132.

63. Merot Y, Mazoujian G, Pinkus G, et al: Extramammary Paget's disease of the perianal and perineal regions. *Arch Dermatol*. 1985;121:750–752.

64. Wick MR, Goellner JR, Wolfe JT III, Su WP: Vulvar sweat gland carcinomas. *Arch Pathol Lab Med*. 1985;109:43–47.

65. Fliegiel Z, Kaneko M: Extramammary Paget's disease of the external ear canal in association with ceruminous gland carcinomas. *Cancer*. 1975;36:1072–1076.

66. Threaker JM: Extramammary Paget's disease of the oral mucosa with in situ carcinoma of minor salivary gland ducts. *Am J Surg Pathol*. 1988;12:890–895.

CHAPTER 44

Malignant Tumors of the Epidermis

Mark R. Wick

Carcinomas of the skin are the most frequently seen malignancies in clinical medicine. Indeed, regardless of their realm of specialty practice, most physicians encounter patients with such lesions regularly.

In this chapter, the pathologic features of two common skin cancers, basal cell carcinoma (BCC) and squamous cell carcinoma (SCC), are outlined. In addition, a relative "newcomer" to dermatopathology, primary neuroendocrine carcinoma of the skin (PNCS), is discussed.

"Histogenesis" is a nebulous term, as it is virtually impossible to determine the cellular derivation of any neoplasm in vivo. Hence, I do not expend much effort on a consideration of this topic. Rather, the lines of *differentiation* toward target cell types in BCC, SCC, and PNCS are elucidated in the following discussion.

The three specified neoplasms occur in a spectrum of clinical settings, and the latter are briefly enumerated as well. Finally, histopathologic differential diagnoses are considered, with commentaries on the use of specialized techniques in difficult cases.

BASAL CELL CARCINOMA

History

Although Krompecher is generally accorded recognition for having given certain cutaneous carcinomas ("epitheliomas") the designation of "basal cell," with the implication that their constituent elements resembled the basal cells of the epidermis,[1] these neoplasms had been well characterized as distinct clinicopathologic entities for some time previously. In Hyde and Montgomery's text on diseases of the skin, published in 1897,[2] basal cell carcinoma is easily recognized, as described under the appellations "superficial epithelioma" and "rodent ulcer" (clinical) or "tubular epithelioma" (histopathologic). It is also notable that the behavior and treatment of BCC were accurately understood at that time.

In the intervening 90 years, a great deal of literature has accrued on the growth and postulated origins, as well as the variant microscopic patterns, of this tumor. Accordingly, it is now generally accepted that "basal cell carcinoma" exhibits a spectrum of biologic behavior,[3,4] and that the latter can be related to histopathologic features with a modicum of efficacy.

Histologic Features

As true of many carcinomas, BCC displays a considerable diversity of appearances under the microscope. These may be divided into nodulocystic, superficial, adenoid, morpheaform, infiltrative, keratotic, and pigmented forms, as well as rarer variants.[5,6]

Nodulocystic BCC. Nodulocystic BCC is the most frequent (approximately 70% of cases), and is composed of rounded or bluntly branched lobules of small hyperchromatic cells, which are connected to the overlying epidermis by narrow cords or broad trabeculae. These cellular clusters vary slightly to moderately in size and shape; however, they are typified by the roughly parallel alignment of peripheral nuclei at right angles to those in the center of the nodules—the so-called "peripheral palisading" (Fig. 44–1). The tumor cells themselves are uniform in size and polygonal in shape, with generally oval nuclei and inconspicuous nucleoli. Exceptionally, spindle or "giant" dysplastic nuclear forms may be observed; these appear to have no prognostic significance.[7] Cytoplasm is scanty and amphophilic, and mitotic activity is variable. From 0 to 2 division figures are typically seen per high-power ($\times$ 400) field, but up to 10 may be observed in selected neoplasms. The stroma in this form of BCC is fibromyxoid, and characteristically exhibits a retraction from tumor cell clusters, in specimens fixed in formalin. Peritumoral actinic elastosis is almost invariably seen in the surrounding dermis.

Not uncommonly, centrilobular necrosis in nodular BCCs accounts for their "cystic" quality, both clinically and microscopically. Necrotic areas in adjacent cellular lobules may become confluent, yielding broad areas of anucleate debris. The overlying epidermis may or may not be ulcerated.

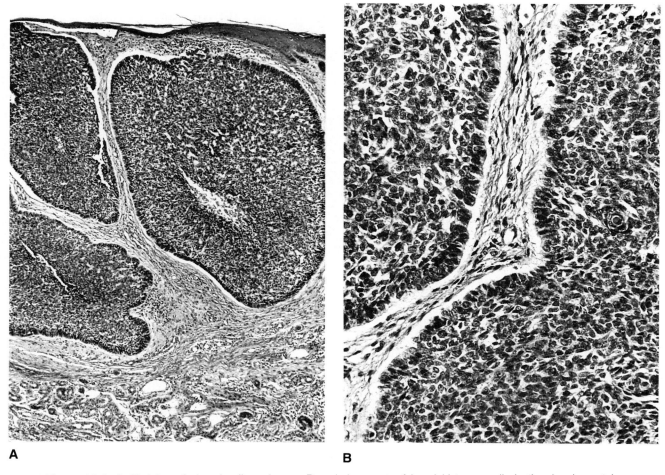

Figure 44–1. A. Nodulocystic basal cell carcinoma. Rounded masses of basaloid tumor cells in the dermis contain small central foci of cystic necrosis. **B.** Peripheral nuclear palisading in cellular nests of nodulocystic basal cell carinoma.

Superficial BCC. Superficial BCC differs from the foregoing description in being multifocal in a high percentage of cases, and in showing a downward, budlike growth of tumorous lobules from the basal epidermis (Fig. 44–2). These seldom extend more deeply than the papillary dermis, but have a cellular composition similar to that of nodulocystic lesions. The surrounding stroma is less likely to manifest fibromyxoid change in superficial multifocal BCC, but dermal elastosis is again common. Overlying ulceration is infrequently observed, but epidermal atrophy is often seen. Although acantholysis is generally uncommon in BCC, Mehregan has suggested that the superficial subtype is most likely to demonstrate this finding.[8]

Adenoid BCC. Roughly 20% of basal cell carcinomas display a reticulated and glandlike growth pattern within tumor cell clusters (Fig. 44–3). Not all cellular lobules show such changes, but a pseudoglandular appearance should be readily apparent on low-power microscopy to classify a BCC as "adenoid." The spaces formed in these lesions may contain an amorphous, granular, or colloidlike material; alternatively, they may consist only of fibromyxoid stroma. Connections between the dermal tumor mass and

the overlying epidermis are invariably present in adenoid BCC, but they are more focal than in other variants; step-sections may be required through the paraffin-embedded specimen to document their locations. The most helpful features in distinguishing this form of basal cell carcinoma from true glandular tumors of the skin are its retention of peripheral nuclear palisading and the presence of stromal retraction.

Morpheaform BCC. Morpheaform BCC accounts for approximately 15% of all basal cell carcinomas. This variant is so named because of the intense stromal fibrous proliferation (morphea-like) that is an integral part of its growth. Tumor cells are thereby compressed into narrow cords, which are commonly branched; however, linear single-cell profiles also are frequently observed in such neoplasms (Fig. 44–4). Because of these features, peripheral nuclear palisading is not readily apparent, and stromal retraction is likewise inconspicuous. Again, step-sections may be required to demonstrate a connection between the tumor and the epidermis, as they are usually focal. Morpheaform BCC is characterized by its deep invasion of the dermis; indeed, the subcutis is involved in many cases. The overly-

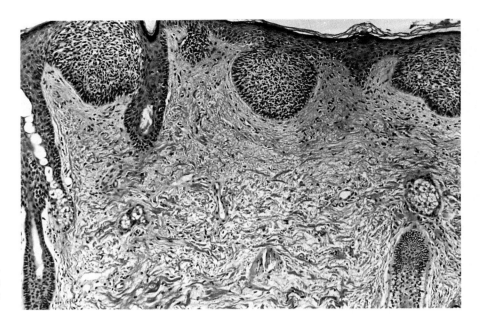

Figure 44–2. Superficial basal cell carcinoma. Three separate nests of tumor cells are seen "budding" from the epidermis in this photomicrograph.

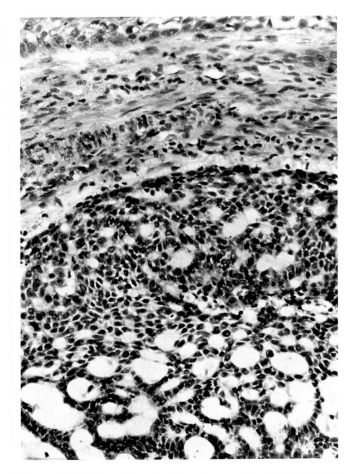

Figure 44–3. Adenoid basal cell carcinoma. Basaloid tumor cells enclose pseudoglandular spaces that are filled with hypodense stromal material.

ing skin surface may be atrophic, ulcerated, or relatively normal in appearance.

Infiltrative BCC. Infiltrative BCCs are "hybrids" of the nodulocystic and morpheaform varieties, in that they show a combination of expansile solidly cellular, branched, sharply angulated, and linear cell groupings.[9] The irregular and acutely tapered profiles of tumor cells in this lesion have been described as "spiky" by Jacobs et al.[10] Deep dermal invasion is typical, and epidermal ulceration is not infrequent. The stroma is more fibrous than that of nodulocystic BCC, but less so than in morphea-like tumors (Fig. 44–5). Infiltrative BCC is perhaps the best in vivo example of the growth-related interdependency between the tumor cells and stroma in this epithelial neoplasm. The latter component consists of a more cellular, fibroblast-rich population than seen in other variants, and it is more intimately attached to basaloid cell clusters. As a result, artifactual stromal retraction is not particularly notable in such lesions.

Keratotic BCC. Some basal cell carcinomas that are otherwise identical to the nodulocystic variety contain keratinaceous ("horn") cysts and clusters of parakeratotic cells, which are interspersed throughout these tumors (Fig. 44–6). The parakeratotic element possesses more abundant and eosinophilic cytoplasm than that of the basaloid tumor cells, and often surrounds the accumulations of anucleate keratin, which may become densely calcified. There are no granular keratinocytes between the horn cysts and parakeratotic cells in this form of BCC. The contents of the cysts often assume a concentrically lamellated, whorled appearance, and are commonly apparent on low-power examination. In light of these features, keratotic BCC is also known as "pilar" basal cell carcinoma, because of a similarity between the complexes just mentioned and developing hair

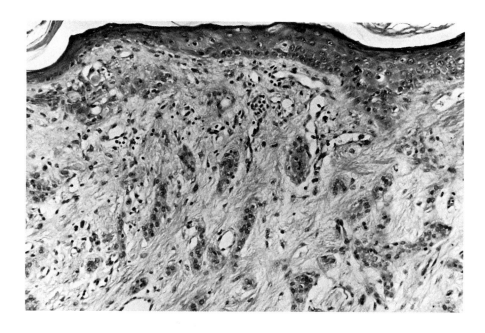

Figure 44–4. Morpheaform (desmoplastic) basal cell carcinoma. Small linear profiles of tumor cells are embedded in a dense collagenous stroma in the dermis.

follicles. This contention is also supported by the presence of citrulline in keratotic BCC[11]; the latter moiety is evident in pilar keratin, but not in surface epidermal keratin.

Pigmented BCC. An additional special feature of some basal cell carcinomas with a nodulocystic growth pattern is the presence of abundant intratumoral melanocytes[5,12] (Fig. 44–7). These are apparently an integral part of such neoplasms, and may reflect "divergent differentiation" in BCC. The melanocytic elements are usually evenly admixed with nonpigmented tumor cells, but have more dendritic individual profiles. In addition, pigment-containing melanophages are numerous in the stroma; indeed, they account

for most of the gross coloration noted clinically in these lesions, as the melanocytes themselves contain only a scanty amount of finely granular melanin.[12]

"Basosebaceous" BCC. Rare examples of BCC express another line of ectodermal differentiation: the presence of mature sebaceous cells (Fig. 44–8). These are abruptly interposed among otherwise typical basaloid cell nests, without transitional forms. Neoplasms displaying this morphological pattern are otherwise most like nodulocystic BCCs.[13] In fact, it has been postulated that some examples of the latter possess their partially cystic character as a result of the spontaneous lysis of sebaceous elements. Basoseba-

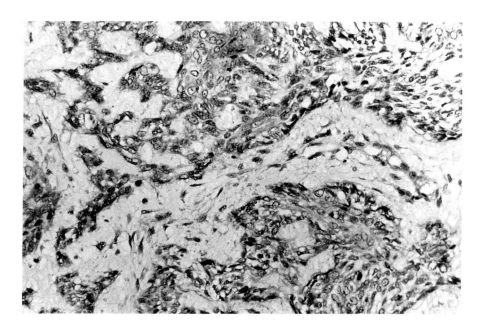

Figure 44–5. Infiltrative basal cell carcinoma. Tumor cells are spindle-shaped, and have an intimate relationship with the supporting stroma.

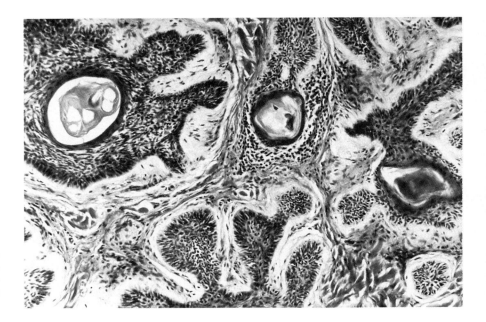

Figure 44–6. Keratotic (pilar) basal cell carcinoma. Well-defined foci of pilar-type keratinization are interspersed throughout the lesion. These tumors are difficult to distinguish from trichoepithelioma in selected cases.

ceous BCC should not be confused diagnostically with true sebaceous carcinoma, which characteristically displays global nuclear atypia in its sebaceous elements and has a more aggressive biologic potential.[13,14]

"Eccrine" BCC. Several reports have appeared on cutaneous neoplasms that were composed of tubular arrays of basaloid cells in a densely fibrous stroma, and in which the luminal cells of the tubular spaces exhibited "eccrine" enzymatic activity and ultrastructural evidence of glandular differentiation.[15] These have been categorized as eccrine epitheliomas, implying that true sudoriferous elements were present within otherwise typical basal cell carcinomas. My opinion, however, is that many reported examples of

these lesions are actually cases of adenoid cystic sweat gland carcinoma,[16] rather than BCC. This contention is based on the knowledge that their tubular profiles lack a connection with the epidermis, contain material that stains with the periodic acid-Schiff (PAS) and colloidal iron methods (unlike adenoid BCC), and are devoid of peripheral nuclear palisading. Also, the composition of the stroma in the two tumors is dissimilar; adenoid cystic carcinoma displays a densely collagenous matrix, rather than the loose, elastotic, fibromyxoid interstitium of BCC.

These points notwithstanding, I have indeed observed extremely rare cases of basal cell carcinoma with verifiable glandular (apparently eccrine) differentiation by simple cuboidal tumor cells. In such lesions, the latter feature is

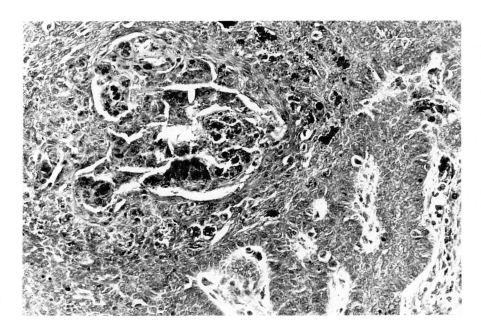

Figure 44–7. Pigmented basal cell carcinoma. Scattered neoplastic cells contain dark, coarse melanin pigment.

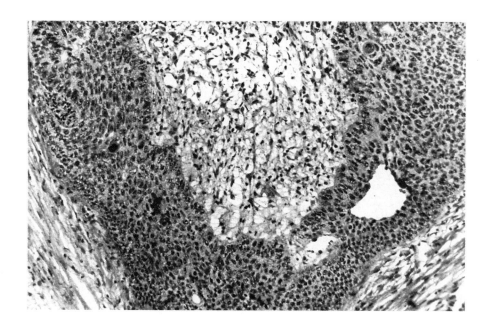

Figure 44–8. Basosebaceous basal cell carcinoma. The central portion of this tumor cell nest is occupied by finely vacuolated cells showing sebaceous differentiation.

evident focally in the center of solid cellular lobules, in otherwise typical nodulocystic tumors. Special staining procedures reveal the presence of alcian blue–reactive material in the gland spaces of eccrine BCC, whereas the remainder of constituent cells are nonreactive. Perineural infiltration is a common finding in cutaneous adenoid cystic carcinoma; however, BCC may exhibit this feature as well,[17] making it noncontributory to a distinction between the two.

"Apocrine" BCC. In analogy to the foregoing discussion, apocrine epitheliomas are represented by purported basal cell carcinomas with focal apocrine glandular differentiation.[18] The existence of these variants has again been supported by the results of enzyme histochemistry and conventional special stains, especially for mucin. Apocrine glands are usually typified by the presence of luminal "teat" formation and decapitation secretion, neither of which has been well documented in BCC; however, some examples of nodulocystic and adenoid tumors are punctuated by signet ring cells, which contain neutral epithelial (mucicarmine-positive) mucins (Fig. 44–9). Inasmuch as the latter products appear to be confined to apocrine glands in normal skin, it would seem that such signet ring basal cell carcinomas do indeed manifest differentiation toward these structures.

"Fibroepitheliomatous" BCC. A peculiar cutaneous tumor that manifests the combined features of intracanalicular fibroadenoma of the breast, seborrheic keratosis of the skin, and superficial BCC has been given the name of *fibroepithelioma*. It is now generally accepted that lesions having such attributes are variants of basal cell carcinoma.[5] They are characterized by elongated, branched, and trabecular strands of basaloid cells, with connections to the epidermis, which may contain "horn cysts" (Fig. 44–10). Fibromyxoid matrix is enclosed by these cellular arrays in a geographic pattern, yielding a reticulated appearance. Nuclear palisad-

ing is not a conspicuous finding in fibroepitheliomatous BCC, nor is stromal retraction prominent. Profiles of tumor cells in this variant seldom extend past the midreticular dermis.

"Adamantinoid" BCC. Lerchin and Rahbari have documented several examples of a BCC subtype with a resemblance to adamantinoma of long bones or ameloblastoma of the jaws.[19] This variant is characterized by solid, nodular masses of basaloid cells in the corium, with epidermal attachments and peripheral palisading, like banal BCC. The proliferating cells are stellate rather than polygonal, however, and are attached to one another by thin connecting bridges, enclosing an amorphous, amphophilic intercellular material. The remainder of the stroma is fibromyxoid, and shows retraction from the epithelial cell clusters. Histologic aspects of this form of BCC do not appear to represent merely a degenerative change, as alcian blue, PAS, and aldehyde fuchsin stains are reactive with the intercellular matrix.[19]

"Basosquamous" BCC. There is some controversy in the literature on BCC as to which tumors of this type should be classified as "basosquamous." Some authors include cases that show a gradual transition between basaloid elements and cell nests with more abundant eosinophilic cytoplasm, larger nuclei, and a concentric arrangement ("pearls"), whereas others restrict the term to lesions with distinct but admixed components of BCC and overt squamous carcinoma.[20–24] My preference is toward the latter approach, as the distinction between the former description and that of keratotic or metatypical BCC is otherwise unclear. In keeping with this premise, the squamous carcinomatous element of basosquamous carcinoma should demonstrate nuclear anaplasia, dyskeratosis, nucleolar prominence, and mitotic activity, to avoid confusion with areas of simple squamous metaplasia in BCC (Fig. 44–11).

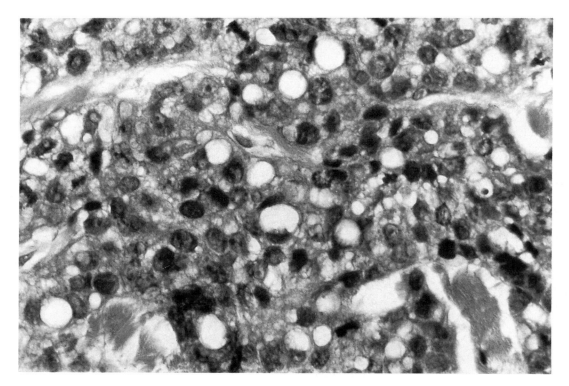

Figure 44–9. Basal cell carcinoma containing signet ring cells.

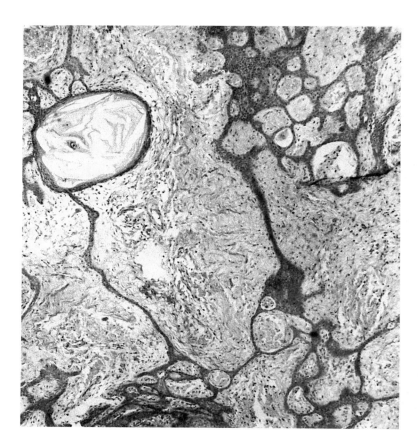

Figure 44–10. Fibroepitheliomatous basal cell carcinoma (of Pinkus). Elongated cords of tumor cells are punctuated by microcystic formations.

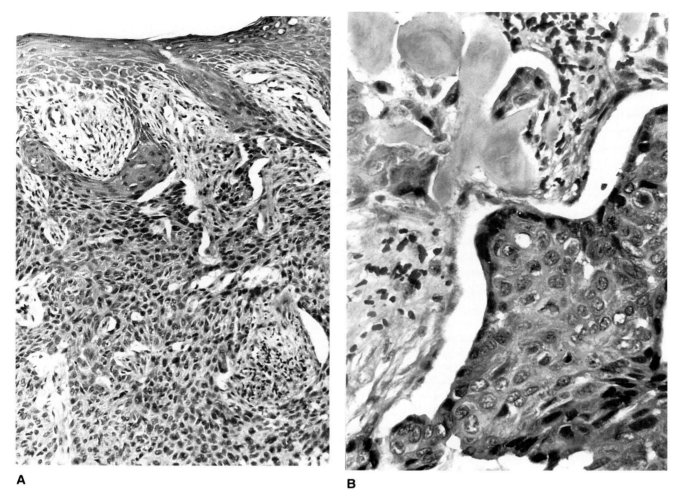

Figure 44–11. Basosquamous carcinoma. **A.** Superficial basal cell carcinoma is seen to blend with deeper cells having overtly squamous characteristics **(B)**. **B.** Note also stromal amyloid, which is a feature of basal cell carcinoma of the skin but not squamous tumors.

The basocellular component of such neoplasms may exhibit nodulocystic, adenoid, superficial, or infiltrative growth patterns. This variant of BCC is quite rare (less than 0.5% of all cases), if the foregoing criteria are observed.

"Metatypical" BCC. Similarly, "metatypical" BCC has been defined in various fashions by several authors.[5,20,21,25] In my view, this term is intended to describe variants of basal cell carcinoma that lack peripheral palisading within cellular lobules; have larger nuclei and more abundant, eosinophilic cytoplasm; and display a bluntly spindle cell growth pattern with focally prominent intercellular bridges. Cell nests are more elongated than those in nodulocystic BCC, and the stroma is variably fibroblastic (Fig. 44–12). Hence, metatypical BCC integrates certain features of the infiltrative and adamantinoid subtypes; in addition, De Faria has suggested that metatypical BCC is cytologically intermediate to nodulocystic BCC and squamous carcinoma.[21] Perineural and lymphatic permeation is seen more commonly in cases of metatypical BCC, relative to other variants.

"Dedifferentiated" (Carcinosarcomatous) BCC. Quay et al.[26] and Dawson[27] have reported two cases of basal cell carcinoma that were intimately associated with malignant mesenchymal tissues, within the same tumor masses. Each exhibited the presence of fibrosarcoma and osteosarcoma in addition to nodulocystic BCC, and one patient manifested chondrosarcomatous and synoviosarcomatous growth as well.[26] In analogy to "dedifferentiation" of chondrosarcoma, squamous carcinoma, and other tumors, repeated recurrence appears to be an etiologic factor in the clonal divergence of some BCCs.

BCC in Association With Other Lesions

Basal cell carcinoma has been reported to arise in transition from, or in contiguity with, several other cutaneous lesions, including nevus sebaceus of Jadassohn, dermatofibroma, congenital nevus, linear epidermal nevus, onchocercoma, and seborrheic keratosis.[28–33] These concurrences are rare (with the possible exception of nevus sebaceus), and may represent the simple coincidence of a relatively common

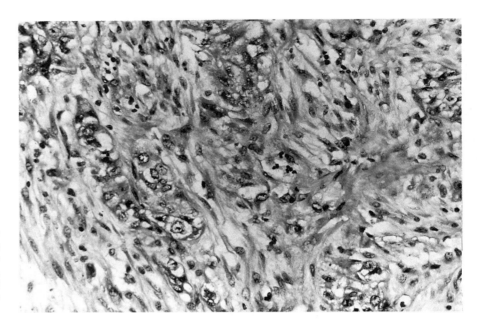

Figure 44–12. Metatypical basal cell carcinoma. Tumor cells are spindled, and some possess vesicular nuclei with discernible nucleoli, like squamous carcinoma; however, the overall growth pattern in such cases is like that of conventional basal cell carcinomas.

neoplasm (BCC) with other cellular proliferations of the skin. With respect to dermatofibroma, Goette and Helwig have indicated that many overlying BCC-like lesions actually represent basaloid forms of pseudoepitheliomatous hyperplasia.[30] Nonetheless, they also reported several indisputable examples of true basal cell carcinoma in this context.

Specialized Pathologic Studies

Because of the prevalence of basal cell carcinoma and its corresponding familiarity to most pathologists and dermatologists, specialized pathologic studies are not usually necessary for diagnosis. Nevertheless, occasional cases of BCC may simulate adnexal carcinomas of the skin, such as adenoid cystic carcinoma of eccrine glands[16] and basaloid sebaceous carcinoma.[14] In such circumstances, conventional special stains, electron microscopy, or immunohistochemistry can be employed to resolve interpretative difficulties.

Conventional Special Stains. Basal cell carcinoma contains a negligible amount of glycogen, as demonstrated by relative nonreactivity with the PAS stain. The mucicarmine reaction is seen focally in examples of "apocrine" BCC, as well as in tumors containing signet ring cells; the same neoplasms display diastase-resistant PAS positivity. Similarly, the colloidal iron technique can be used to label the epithelium-related mucosubstance in adenoid BCC; it also stains the stroma of most basal cell carcinomas faintly. Hyaluronidase digestion abolishes the latter but not the former of these reactivities. The Movat stain also labels the contents of pseudoglandular profiles in adenoid neoplasms, but they are PAS negative. This constellation of results differs from that of true glandular tumors of the skin. Lipid stains (oil-red-O and Sudan IV) are nonreactive with conventional BCC, but amyloid can be detected by the Congo red, Lieb, and thioflavine-T techniques in up to 70% of such neoplasms.[34–36] The latter finding appears to be independent of histologic subtype, and may be related to a relatively high degree of tumor cell apoptosis.

Electron Microscopy. BCC tumor cells have been divided into three types by some authors on the basis of ultrastructural features—so-called "light," "intermediate," and "dark."[37] It seems that little would be gained by this approach, because it is likely that relative cellular densities in most neoplasms are intimately dependent on the efficacy of fixation and the respective viability of cellular constituents.

Nevertheless, a heterogeneous population of cells can indeed be discerned in such tumors, by electron microscopy. These cells form a continuum, ranging from elements with a paucity of intracytoplasmic organelles (rough endoplasmic reticulum, Golgi bodies, lysosomes, mitochondria, broad keratin filaments ["tonofibrils"], and keratohyaline granules) to cells with an abundance of cellular contents[38] (Fig. 44–13). Likewise, the density of pericellular basal lamina and desmosomal attachments between tumor cells varies greatly within the same lesion.[39] Cytoplasmic lipid and true microvillous modifications of plasmalemmae are not evident in BCC lacking additional differentiation.

Ishibashi and colleagues[38] implied that the presence of amorphous granular accumulations within the rough endoplasmic reticulum of BCC cells could be correlated with the presence of extracellular mucopolysaccharide, in a secretory relationship. There have been no immunoultrastructural corroborations of this contention, however. Rupec et al.[39] observed that "sphaeridia"-like intranuclear inclusions are seen less often in BCC than in normal basal epidermal cells, and concluded that this finding could be correlated with the lesser protein synthesis by the neoplastic cells. In keeping with the light microscopic observation of amyloid in BCC, Hashimoto and Brownstein have confirmed the ultrastructural presence of this protein in the stroma of basal cell carcinomas.[34] Finally, Kobayasi has described abnormalities in the basement membrane of the epidermis overlying such tumors.[39a]

An interesting subset of basal cell carcinomas has been identified ultrastructurally by Dardi et al.[40] and Eusebi and

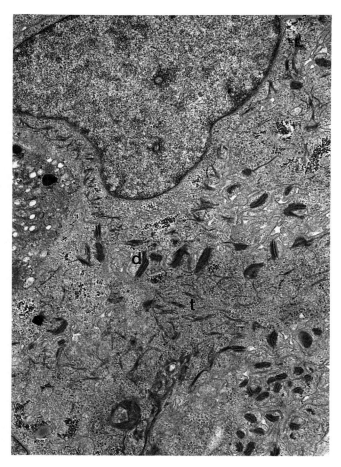

Figure 44–13. Electron photomicrograph of basal cell carcinoma. Numerous cytoplasmic tonofilaments (T) are evident, many of which insert into well-formed desmosomes (D).

co-workers.[41] These investigators demonstrated the presence of clustered neurosecretory granules (as seen in "neuroendocrine" neoplasms) within the cytoplasm of some BCC cells. Such inclusions were correlated with positive results of silver impregnation stains (e.g., the Grimelius technique) at the light microscopic level; in addition, some of these neoplasms showed immunoreactivity for neuropeptides or biogenic amines.[40]

Aside from the latter observations, the electron microscopic attributes of most BCCs are generally similar to those of embryonic basal epidermal cells.[42] As discussed subsequently, these primitive features are helpful in differential diagnosis with selected other basaloid tumors of the skin.

Immunohistochemistry. Among all malignant neoplasms of the skin, those showing cellular differentiation toward keratinocytes (BCC and squamous cell carcinoma) are immunohistochemical "have nots." They lack most specialized determinants other than cytokeratin polypeptides (the basic cytoskeletal proteins of epithelial cells and neoplasms)[43] and a restricted group of cell membrane–related cell products. Specifically, epithelial membrane antigen, other human milk fat globule proteins, Leu MI, salivary-type amy-

lase, S100 protein, and carcinoembryonic antigen are not observed in basal cell carcinomas.[16,44]

Thomas and colleagues have demonstrated that normal epidermal basal cells and BCC cells display selective immunoreactivity for low-molecular-weight (40 to 46 kDa [kDa]) keratin proteins.[45] In contrast, other keratinocytes, pilar tumors, and squamous carcinomas exhibit staining for a broad spectrum of cytokeratins (45 to 65 kDa). These observations may be useful in separating trichoepithelioma or small cell squamous carcinoma (see later) from BCC; however, they do not allow for a similar distinction between basal cell carcinomas and sudoriferous or sebaceous tumors, as these adnexal lesions also have a typically restricted (low-molecular-weight) keratin profile.[14,43,46] Immunostains for the other cell products listed in the previous paragraph attain their value in the latter differential diagnosis. It is of interest that the intratumoral amyloid seen in many cases of BCC is apparently of keratinaceous origin, as documented immunocytochemically.[36] This finding further supports the premise that BCC amyloid is related to apoptosis and degeneration of cytoskeletal protein.

Additional cell membrane determinants that have been detected in BCC are of little diagnostic use. These include transferrin receptor proteins (which are merely markers of active cellular proliferation),[44] and β_2-microglobulin (B2M), a component of human histocompatibility locus antigens.[16,46] A proposal has been made that malignant tumors lacking B2M are more likely to exhibit an aggressive clinical course.[47] In general, this premise has not proven to be valid; in specific reference to BCC, B2M has no relationship whatever to biologic behavior.[48]

The aforementioned ability of BCC to display partial neuroendocrine differentiation can be correlated immunohistochemically to the expression of appropriate cell markers. I have observed several examples of this tumor with diffuse reactivity for neuron-specific enolase, and focal chromogranin positivity has also been evident in such cases. Although suitable specimens for electron microscopy were not available, it may be presumed that these lesions would have shown the presence of neurosecretory granules ultrastructurally, as discussed earlier.

"Eccrine" BCC may express S100 protein in the tubular profiles corresponding to adnexal differentiation, but carcinoembryonic antigen is absent in such lesions. The presence of gross cystic disease fluid protein-15 (a marker for apocrine differentiation)[49] has not yet been assessed in "apocrine" BCC.

As a final note on this topic, it is of interest that many basal cell carcinomas incite an inflammatory response in the surrounding dermis. Reactive hematopoietic cells consist primarily of lymphocytes, which have been shown to manifest a predominance of T-cell immunophenotypes.[50] More specific subclassification of these elements (as suppressor or helper cells) has not yet been accomplished.

Clinical Spectrum of Basal Cell Carcinoma: Correlations Between Histology and Biology

Several clinical subtypes of BCC are well known to dermatologists, including papulonodular, pigmented, morphea-like, fibroepitheliomatous, and superficial forms.[51] These correspond well to the histologic variants described earlier. The term *horrifying* also has been introduced in recent years in connection with huge or mutilating basal cell carcinomas;[4] these most often assume nodulocystic or infiltrating microscopic patterns. Kuflik has introduced yet another designation, keratopurpuric BCC, to describe lesions with a central scale and peritumoral blush on clinical examination.[52] Histologically, such neoplasms show abundant overlying parakeratosis and a peritumoral network of granulation tissue-like stroma.

Although BCC is seen overwhelmingly in sun-exposed skin, numerous reports have documented its occurrence in protected cutaneous sites in some patients.[53–55] Some, but not all, of these individuals had had prior radiotherapy to the tumor site for unrelated conditions. Other rare clinical presentations include the bilateral, symmetric growth of multiple basal cell carcinomas, and associations with hidradenitis suppurativa, stasis dermatitis, smallpox vaccinations, amputation stumps, lupus vulgaris, cutaneous gummata, and onchocerciasis.[5,28,56,57]

Recent publications have attempted to identify histologic features that can be correlated with frequent recurrence and tenacious growth of BCC, so that appropriately extirpative surgery can be undertaken from the outset.[3,10,58,59] Lang and Maize[58] and Jacobs et al.[10] showed that tumors with an infiltrative or micronodular pattern at first excision often pursued an aggressive clinical course. In addition, basal cell carcinomas in which peripheral nuclear palisading was irregular or absent manifested a tendency to recur in several series.[3,58,59] The same propensity has been associated with basosquamous carcinomas; moreover, these tumors appear to metastasize more frequently than other subtypes of BCC.[20,21]

With respect to the last point, it would appear that approximately 0.1% of all basal cell carcinomas lacking squamous differentiation exhibit distant spread beyond the skin.[60] Regional lymph nodes, lungs, and bones are most frequently involved in such cases, fewer than 200 of which may be found in the literature.[25,54,60–62] Although numerous attempts have been made to relate clinical or histologic features of conventional BCC to its risk of metastasis, these activities have proven less than fruitful; however, it would appear that large, neglected lesions are most likely to display metastatic behavior, especially if they occur in immunocompromised or malnourished patients.[60] Lymphatic, hematogenous, and interstitial ("in transit") routes for distant spread have been proposed, all of which probably pertain to selected cases.

Basal cell carcinoma is also included among cutaneous neoplasms with a potential for perineural invasion, both clinically and histopathologically.[17] This tendency may result in neoplastic neuropathies, in cases where the tumor infiltrates major motor or sensory nerve trunks.

On the other hand, approximately 5% of basal cell carcinomas demonstrate spontaneous regression, as reported by Curson and Weedon.[63] This is rarely if ever complete, and is associated with heavy peritumoral lymphocytic infiltration and abundant apoptosis, microscopically.

BCC is an essential diagnostic element of the basal cell nevus syndrome.[64–65] This complex features multiple cutaneous basal cell lesions, multifocal keratocysts of the jawbones, bifid ribs, neurologic abnormalities (including

neoplasms of the central nervous system), cutaneous epidermoid inclusion cysts, palmar and plantar "pits," and a characteristic facies.[66] It is inherited in an autosomal dominant fashion with variable expressivity. Although basal cell carcinoma rarely occurs de novo in children and adolescents,[67] many cases of this neoplasm in preadult patients are attributable to the basal cell nevus syndrome; hence, BCC in a pediatric patient should prompt a thorough examination of the familial pedigree. As noted by Lindeberg and Jepsen,[65] histologic examination of a single BCC in patients with this constellation shows no microscopic features unique to basal cell nevus syndrome.

Bazex syndrome, linear unilateral basal cell nevus syndrome and the xeroderma pigmentosum syndrome are additional "seed beds" for BCC.[5,68,69] The first of these disorders features hypotrichosis, follicular atrophoderma, and hypohidrosis. The second is typified by a congenital, unilateral, zosteriform eruption of papulonodular BCCs, accompanied by comedones and irregular cutaneous atrophy. The last involves hypersensitivity to actinic skin damage, because of the genetically determined cellular deficiency of a restriction endonuclease.

Differential Diagnosis

Several other primary cutaneous neoplasms enter into differential diagnosis with basal cell carcinoma variants. These include conventional trichoepithelioma (which resembles keratotic BCC), desmoplastic trichoepithelioma (with similarities to morpheaform BCC),[70] small cell squamous carcinoma[71] and basaloid sebaceous carcinoma[14] (which mimic nodulocystic BCC), and adenoid cystic eccrine carcinoma (simulating adenoid or "eccrine" BCC).[16]

In general, trichoepitheliomas exhibit a much more organoid growth pattern than BCC, with more equally sized cellular lobules (Fig. 44–14A). Also, broad connections to the epidermis are rare in dermal hair sheath tumors (except via pilosebaceous units), whereas they are regularly observed in cases of BCC. Finally, the fibromyxoid stroma of basal cell carcinoma is not recapitulated by the fibrous matrix of trichoepithelioma, nor is cellular retraction as prominent a feature of the latter tumor. In difficult cases, immunohistochemical determinations of cytokeratin profiles may be employed diagnostically to separate these lesions, as described earlier.[45]

Desmoplastic trichoepithelioma can be distinguished from morphea-like BCC by the uniform observation of horn cysts in the former, along with an absence of expansile cell nests and the nearly universal presence of epidermal hyperplasia (Fig. 44–14B). Also, desmoplastic trichoepithelioma occurs in a younger patient population than typical cases of morpheaform BCC.[70]

Small cell squamous carcinoma is devoid of nuclear palisading, as well as the fibromyxoid stroma of BCC. Moreover, tumor cell nuclei in small cell squamous carcinoma are vesicular with prominent nucleoli, as opposed to the generally compact, anucleolated forms seen in basal cell carcinomas.[71]

Basaloid sebaceous carcinoma must be distinguished from "basosebaceous" BCC. This separation is particularly difficult, as the distribution of obvious areas of sebaceous differentiation in both lesions may be similar, and each

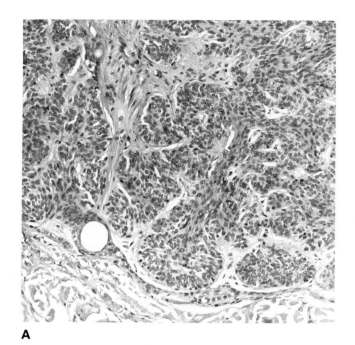

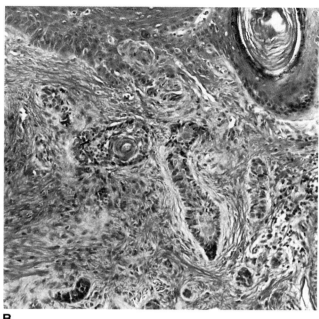

A   **B**

Figure 44–14. Trichoepithelioma. **A.** Tumor cells are basaloid, but do not exhibit the retraction artifact from surrounding stroma that characterizes basal cell carcinoma. A focus of pilar keratinization is apparent at lower left portion of photograph. **B.** Desmoplastic trichoepithelioma. Narrow cords of tumor cells, one containing pilar keratinization (top left), are embedded in a fibrogenic stroma. This lesion may be confused with sclerosing basal cell carcinoma.

has the capacity for nuclear palisading.[14] Pagetoid involvement of the epidermis favors an interpretation of sebaceous carcinoma, but is not invariably present. Diagnosis may be facilitated by lipophilic stains on frozen tissue or immunostains for epithelial membrane antigen in difficult cases.[14] Sebaceous carcinomas display diffuse positivity with both of these techniques,[13,46] whereas basosebaceous BCC is reactive only in areas of obvious sebaceous differentiation. Ultrastructural studies reveal the widespread presence of intracytoplasmic lipid droplets in only the first of these two lesions.[14]

Adenoid cystic sweat gland carcinoma lacks the epidermal connections of adenoid or "eccrine" BCC. Nonetheless, the distinction between these entities is extremely challenging, accounting for the fact that several reported examples of "eccrine" BCC actually appear to represent adenoid cystic carcinomas. The reverse of this situation holds true as well. Immunostains for carcinoembryonic and epithelial membrane antigens are extremely helpful in this context, as they are consistently positive in adenoid cystic carcinoma and negative in BCC.[16,46] In addition, electron microscopy demonstrates true glandular (microvillous) differentiation in adenoid cystic eccrine tumors, which is not apparent in BCC.

SQUAMOUS CELL CARCINOMA

History
Like BCC, squamous cell carcinoma (SCC) has been recognized as a distinctive entity for several decades. Early publi-

cations on this neoplasm gave it the clinical designation of deep, papillary, or tubercular epithelioma; pathologically, it was known as lobular epithelioma.[2] The ability of SCC to metastasize to lymph nodes, as well as its tendency to invade deeply into fascia, muscle, and other structures underlying the skin, has been well known for many years.

Histologic Features
Squamous cell carcinoma of the skin is capable of assuming a diversity of histologic growth patterns, again like BCC. These include conventional, adenoid, spindle-pleomorphic, small cell, clear cell, and verrucous variants.[5,71–82] Also, this neoplasm can be graded according to its level of nucleocytoplasmic differentiation and depth of dermal invasion.[83,84] Lastly, SCC in situ (Bowen's disease) has a distinctive clinicopathologic appearance, but may be confused with a number of other dermatopathologic entities.[83]

Bowen's Disease of the Skin. SCC in situ usually appears clinically in middle age or adulthood, as an irregular, reddish, and scaly thickening of the skin.[85] Both sun-exposed and protected cutaneous areas may be affected by this proliferation. When it occurs on the glans penis, Bowen's disease is traditionally referred to as erythroplasia of Queyrat.[86]

Histologically, Bowen's disease is characterized by global epidermal atypia, acanthosis, and elongation of the rete ridges. There is little or no maturation of neoplastic keratinocytes within the epidermis, and their nuclear-to-cytoplasmic ratios are greatly increased. The basement membrane is intact, but the atypical proliferation may involve the follicular infundibula fairly deeply. Nuclear chromatin is either hyperchromatic and uniformly distributed, or vesicular; nucleoli are often prominent (Fig. 44–15). Tumor cell size varies significantly from case to case, and even within the same lesion. One of the hallmarks of this lesion is the irregular dispersal of dyskeratotic cells throughout the epidermis; these often show an artifactual retraction from their "neighbors," and contain hypereosinophilic cytoplasm and pyknotic nuclei. Also, random mitoses that are not uncommonly atypical in shape are regularly observed. The horny layer of the skin is moderately thickened and parakeratotic.[85]

Some cases of Bowen's disease show nests of atypical keratinocytes in an otherwise unremarkable epidermis, and still others manifest cytoplasmic clarity in the neoplastic cells.[85,87] The first of these patterns was formerly included in the now-defunct concept of intraepidermal epithelioma of Borst-Jadassohn.[88] Strayer and Santa Cruz also have described atrophic, psoriasiform, verrucous, and metaplastic forms of Bowen's disease.[85] The latter variant features intraepidermal amyloid, mucinous cells, or foci of sebaceous differentiation.[89]

Invasive SCC has eventuated from Bowen's disease in less than 1% to 11% of cases, in various reports on this entity.[85,86,90,91] When this occurs, the infiltrative component often appears, cytologically, more well differentiated than that present above the basement membrane. Foci of dermal fibrosis and chronic inflammation beneath apparently intraepidermal SCC should prompt examination of stepsections, to detect areas of microinvasion.

Conventional SCC. Conventional SCC features the interanastomosing growth of cords and nests of polygonal cells, with eosinophilic or amphophilic cytoplasm, and enlarged nuclei (Fig. 44–16). The latter contain generally vesicular chromatin and prominent nucleoli; mitotic activity is variable, and mitoses may be atypical in shape. Dyskeratotic cells, along with parakeratosis of the horny layer, are regularly present.

Well-differentiated neoplasms (Broders' grade 1)[83] have abundantly keratinized, glassy eosinophilic cytoplasm and intercellular "bridges" on high-power microscopy. Tumor cells are often arranged focally in a concentric fashion, enclosing masses of anucleate keratin—the so-called "keratin pearls." Invasive growth extends downward into the dermis in a jagged fashion, and usually extends no deeper than the midreticular layer. Fibrosis and lymphoplasmacytic inflammation typically are evident at the interface between corium and tumor, but necrosis is unusual. The level of nucleocytoplasmic differentiation in these lesions roughly approximates that of the normal keratinocyte.

Moderately differentiated SCC (Broders' grades 2 and 3)[83] shows less propensity for pearl formation, is more deeply invasive, has less eosinophilic cytoplasm, and manifests more nuclear hyperchromasia and mitotic activity. Regional necrosis within cell nests makes its appearance at this level of differentiation, and invasion of blood vessels and perineural sheaths may be appreciated. Tumoral lobules tend to be less uniform in shape and size than those of well-differentiated SCC, and have a more irregular outline.

Poorly differentiated squamous carcinoma (Broders' grade 4)[83] commonly infiltrates the subcutis, and has little if any obvious keratinization. Cytoplasm is amphophilic, nuclei are more pleomorphic and hyperchromatic, and mitoses are abundant. Necrosis is typically prominent, and cellular lobules often become confluent and have extremely irregular borders. Lymphatic and perineurial invasion may be observed in roughly 50% of cases.

Surface ulceration becomes more likely as the level of

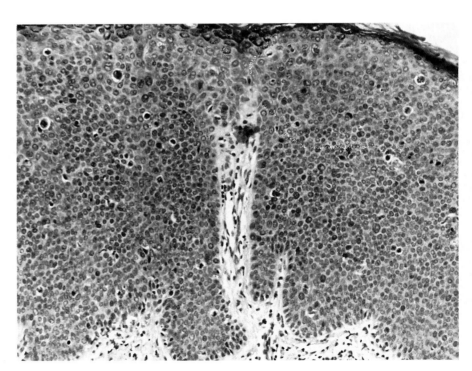

Figure 44–15. Bowen's disease of the skin (intraepithelial squamous carcinoma). Atypical keratinocytes occupy the entirety of the epidermis. Scattered, large dyskeratotic cells are evident.

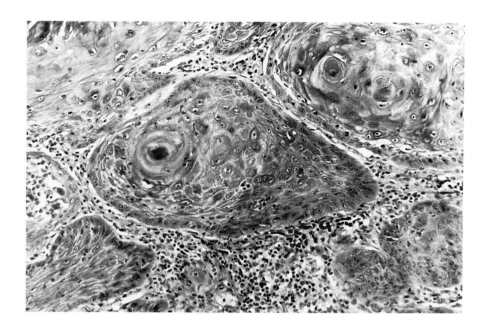

Figure 44–16. Well-differentiated squamous carcinoma of the skin. Cytologic anaplasia is only slight, and keratinization is abundant.

differentiation lessens. Conversely, residual actinic keratosis-like changes in the surrounding epidermis are usually seen in well-differentiated tumors of sun-exposed skin areas. Regardless of grade, the SCC in such locations is associated with prominent elastosis of the contiguous dermis.

Adenoid SCC. In 1947, Lever described a neoplasm showing an apparent combination of glandular and squamous differentiation, which he termed *adenoacanthoma*.[80] It was originally felt to represent an adnexal carcinoma, but subsequent studies have shown this lesion to be a variant of SCC.[76]

As a result of acantholysis, the tumor cells of adenoid squamous carcinoma lose their cohesiveness (Fig. 44–17). This results in the formation of tubular and alveolar profiles, simulating the true glands of sweat gland carcinoma or the vascular spaces of epithelioid angiosarcoma. In the first of these three tumors, however, pseudoglandular arrays are lined by PAS-negative keratinizing cells, in contrast to sweat gland carcinomas; neoplastic keratinocytes are also present within the ''lumina'' of adenoid SCC, whereas true glandular spaces are acellular and vascular spaces contain erythrocytes. Lastly, a continuity between invasive tumor and the epidermis is virtually always evident in adenoid SCC, whereas this finding is not made in angiosarcoma and is apparent in only a minority of duct-forming sweat gland carcinomas.

Adenoid SCC is often associated with solar keratoses.[76] Accordingly, the face and neck are favored sites for its occurrence.

Spindled and Pleomorphic Cell SCC. Some examples of grade 4 SCC are composed exclusively of fusiform and giant pleomorphic cells, with little or no keratinization[72,75,81,84] (Fig. 44–18). Necrosis is variable, but mitotic activity is regu-

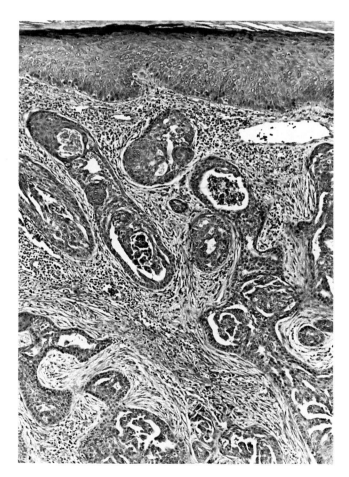

Figure 44–17. Adenoid squamous carcinoma. Nests of keratinocytes are dispersed throughout the dermis in this field, with internal pseudolumen formation. This appearance may lead to confusion with a glandular adnexal tumor.

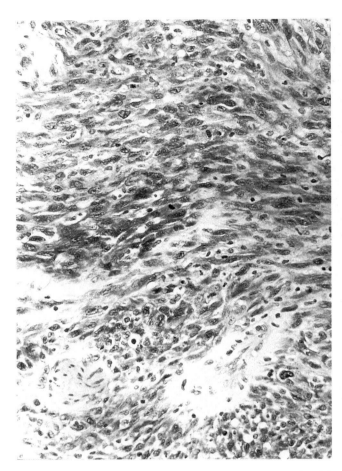

Figure 44–18. Spindle cell variant of squamous carcinoma. Keratinization is inapparent in this example; special studies such as electron microscopy or immunohistology may be necessary for correct diagnosis.

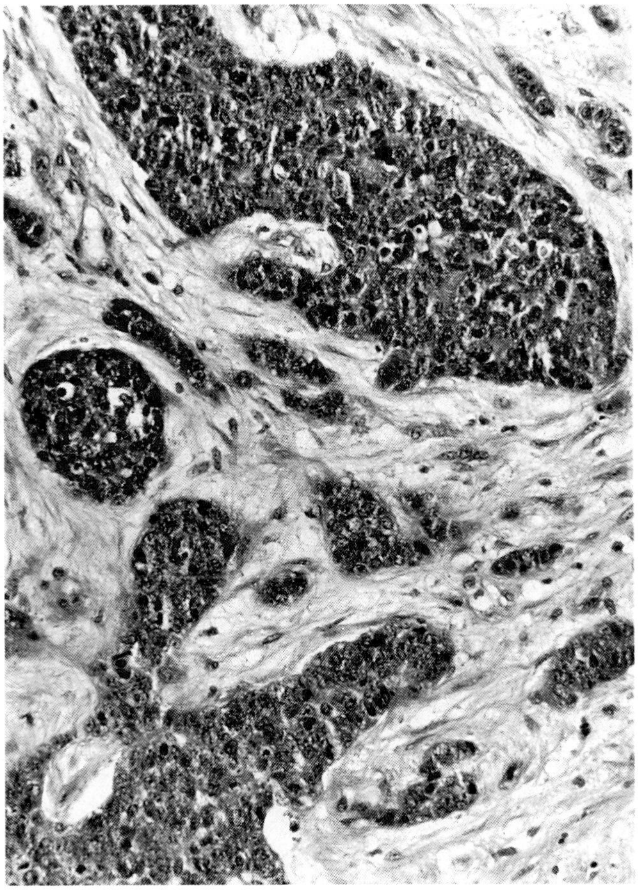

Figure 44–19. Small cell variant of squamous carcinoma. Although keratinization is lacking, the abundant desmoplastic stroma seen here distinguishes small cell squamous carcinoma from other small cell tumors of the skin.

larly evident and focally atypical. The surrounding dermis often shows edema rather than fibrosis, and peritumoral inflammation may or may not be apparent. Continuity between these neoplasms and an intact overlying epidermis is observed in a minority of cases; most manifest surface ulceration.

Spindle cell and pleomorphic SCC characteristically occur in sun-damaged skin. In common with other poorly differentiated cutaneous squamous neoplasms, deep infiltration of the dermis, subcutis, and underlying fascia is frequently observed.[84]

Small Cell SCC. Rare cases of poorly differentiated cutaneous squamous carcinoma manifest a purely small cell appearance, superficially resembling one of the variants of Merkel cell carcinoma (see later)[71] (Fig. 44–19). This likeness is heightened by the fact that both neoplasms may contain foci of keratinization and may be associated with overlying Bowen's disease[92,93]; however, the cells of small cell SCC typically contain more abundant cytoplasm, and have more vesicular nuclei with prominent nucleoli. Regional necrosis and abundant mitotic activity may be present in either small

cell SCC or Merkel cell carcinoma. Involvement of the epidermis by the small cell proliferation favors a diagnosis of SCC, as this feature is seen in less than 10% of Merkel cell carcinomas.[71]

Clear Cell (Hydropic) SCC. Kuo was the first to call attention to a variant of SCC composed of clear, nonvacuolated cells[78] (Fig. 44–20). At first glance, this neoplasm may be confused with clear cell eccrine carcinoma or sebaceous carcinoma.

Any of these three lesions may contain foci of keratinization. Nevertheless, invasive clear cell SCC usually has broad connections to the epidermis, in contrast to eccrine or sebaceous carcinomas. Because it appears that the cytoplasmic clarity in the first of these tumors is due to the degenerative accumulation of intracellular fluid, clear cell squamous carcinoma is also known as "hydropic" SCC.

Verrucous SCC. Squamous carcinomas that grossly simulate giant condylomata or verrucae have been diversely described as giant condyloma of Buschke and Loewenstein,[94] carcinoma cuniculatum,[77] or verrucous carci-

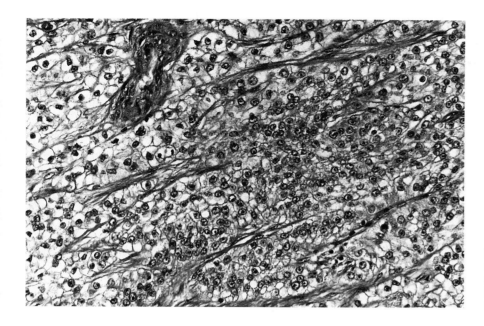

Figure 44–20. Clear cell (hydropic) squamous carcinoma. Tumor cells in such lesions are typically nonreactive for glycogen and lipid, in contrast to other clear cell cutaneous neoplasms.

noma[73,95] based on their anatomic locations. Basically, all of these lesions are identical and can be considered as a group.

Verrucous SCC is characterized by marked papillomatosis and acanthosis, with "church spiring" of the neoplastic epidermis (Fig. 44–21). As a rule, cytologic atypia is only slight in this neoplasm, mitotic activity is scant, and dyskeratosis is less marked than in other forms of SCC.[77] Infiltration of the dermis occurs in broad, blunt cellular tongues, rather than the jagged profiles seen in conventional squamous carcinoma. Reactive fibrosis and inflammation are minimal. Vascular and perineural invasion are seen only rarely.

The criteria just given should be rigorously met before a squamous carcinoma is labeled as verrucous, because other forms (such as conventional SCC) occasionally demonstrate verrucoid growth, but do not behave as indolently as true verrucous carcinoma. In particular, tumors displaying marked cellular atypia and abnormal mitotic figures should not be classified as verrucous SCC.

SCC Associated with Other Cutaneous Lesions

Squamous carcinoma may arise in association with several other cutaneous disorders, including linear epidermal nevus, nevus sebaceus of Jadassohn, epidermodysplasia verruciformis, epidermolysis bullosa, xeroderma pigmento-

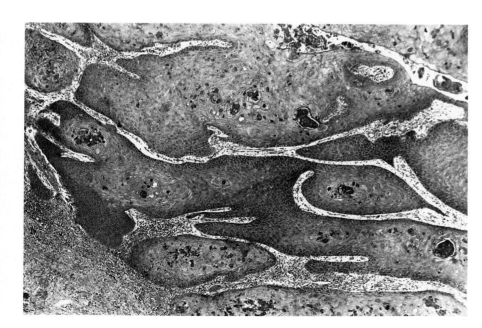

Figure 44–21. Base of infiltrative verrucous carcinoma of the skin. Broad tongues of neoplastic keratinocytes form a blunt interface with the underlying dermis.

sum, seborrheic keratosis, verruca vulgaris, hidradenitis suppurativa, condyloma accuminatum, lichen planus, discoid lupus erythematosus, actinic porokeratosis, extramammary Paget's disease, epidermoid inclusion cysts, and lupus vulgaris.[5,29,96–101]

Moreover, it is now generally accepted that sites of chronic epithelial regeneration, resulting from recalcitrant infections, radiodermatitis, or burn scars, carry a definite risk of malignant transformation to SCC.[5] With respect to sinuses draining underlying foci of osteomyelitis, the name *Marjolin's ulcers* has been appended to carcinomas originating in this context. Although they are well differentiated histologically, these tumors may pursue an aggressive clinical course.

Special Pathologic Studies

Conventional Special Stains. Conventional histochemical staining methods are of limited use in the diagnostic definition of SCC. The PAS method yields variable reactivity with this neoplasm; however, if a clear cell cutaneous tumor *fails* to contain glycogen, metastatic renal cell carcinoma and eccrine carcinoma may be excluded from consideration, and hydropic SCC assumes greater importance in differential diagnosis.[78] Mucin stains are nonreactive with SCC, as are the alcian blue and colloidal iron techniques. These methods may be of some assistance in discriminating between adenoid squamous carcinoma and sweat gland tumors.

Electron Microscopy. Ultrastructural studies of SCC have shown that this tumor possesses the features of developing keratinocytes.[30,72,75,77,78,81,102] These include prominent desmosomal intercellular attachments, tonofibrils, keratohyaline granules, and rough endoplasmic reticulum. Cytoplasmic lipid droplets, glycogen pools, neurosecretory granules, and glandular differentiation are uniformly lacking. It is true that the density of intracellular organelles decreases with increasing tumor grade, but careful analysis of electron microscopic specimens invariably demonstrates the presence of diagnostic features of SCC, even in poorly differentiated lesions.

Immunohistochemistry. As noted earlier under Basal Cell Carcinoma, squamous cell carcinoma of the skin demonstrates reactivity for medium- and high-molecular-weight cytokeratins.[45] Poorly differentiated tumors typically express low-molecular-weight keratin as well[46] (Fig. 44–22). Spindle cell and pleomorphic squamous carcinomas manifest the facultative ability to reexpress vimentin, the intermediate filament seen in virtually all embryonic cells and in mature mesenchymal tissues.[46] Thus, reliance on vimentin immunostains alone is not a valid means of separating spindle cell carcinomas from true sarcomas. Similarly, α_1-antichymotrypsin, which has been touted as a marker for "fibrohistiocytic" neoplasms, is also present in pleomorphic SCC and should not be used exclusively in diagnosis in the absence of intermediate filament stains.[46]

An interesting trend in immunoreactivity may be seen with antibodies to epithelial membrane antigen (EMA), in the analysis of SCC of varying grades. Well-differentiated cutaneous tumors lack EMA, moderately differentiated SCCs express it patchily, and high-grade neoplasms are diffusely positive for this determinant.[46,79] The significance of these findings is unclear at a molecular level, but it appears likely that EMA immunostains may have some role in prognostication of the clinical behavior of SCC.

Other antigens of interest in dermatopathology, such as S100 protein, carcinoembryonic antigen, neuron-specific enolase, and salivary-type amylase, are absent in squamous carcinoma of the skin regardless of grade.[46] The differential diagnostic use of these reactants is discussed subsequently. Also, recent publications on SCC have considered the expression of molecular moieties usually associated with normal keratinocytes. These include involucrin, filaggrin, and

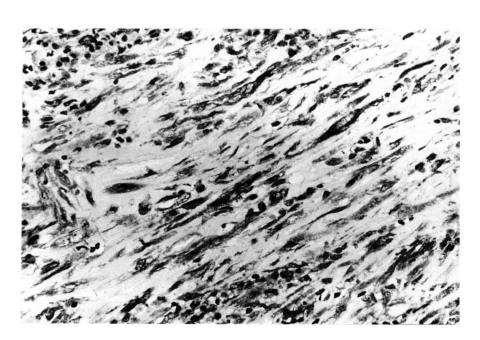

Figure 44–22. Immunoreactivity for cytokeratin in spindle cell squamous carcinoma of the skin.

peptidylarginine deiminase.[103] As expected, such proteins are expressed in a progressively diminishing fashion, as tumor differentiation lessens. Also, they appear to have little utility in the diagnostic separation of pseudoepitheliomatous hyperplasia and keratoacanthoma from well-differentiated squamous carcinoma.

Clinical Features

The likelihood that squamous carcinoma of the skin will recur locally or metastasize is directly related to its anatomic location, association with other cutaneous disorders, histologic grade, and depth of invasion, and to the immunocompetence of the host.[5,83,84] Bowen's disease without an infiltrative component never metastasizes, but may recur if inadequately excised. It should be noted that considerable attention has been given to the premise that Bowen's disease may be a cutaneous marker for internal malignancy[91]; however, recent publications have concluded that this relationship is not statistically significant.[90]

Squamous carcinomas arising from solar keratoses metastasize only rarely (0.5%),[104] whereas histologically identical tumors associated with burn scars, draining sinuses, and radiodermatitis show distant spread in 20% to 30% of cases.[105] In like manner, SCCs located at the vermilion border of the lower lip and other "modified" skin sites (vulva, glans penis, etc.) demonstrate more aggressive behavior than actinic SCCs. Squamous carcinomas in immunosuppressed patients exhibit inexorable growth and metastasis in many cases, despite a low-grade appearance.

Evans and Smith[84] showed that the clinical courses of spindle cell and pleomorphic forms of SCC are intimately related to depth of invasion. Those lesions involving the deep dermis and subcutis metastasized much more frequently than others with superficial invasion of the corium. This trend is generally true of *all* cutaneous squamous carcinomas with Broders' grades higher than 2.

Verrucous squamous carcinoma rarely metastasizes, although this possibility is not unknown.[82] Rather, verrucous SCC is typified by repeated recurrence and locally destructive growth. A report by Perez-Mesa et al. documented the "dedifferentiation" of verrucous carcinoma after radiation therapy.[95] The latter modality of treatment has been proscribed ever since, but the actual incidence of such transformations is unknown.

Differential Diagnosis

Because of its potential to vary in appearance, SCC of the skin may be confused microscopically with several other cutaneous neoplasms and pseudoneoplastic proliferations, including extramammary Paget's disease, pseudoepitheliomatous hyperplasia, keratoacanthoma, sweat gland carcinoma, epithelioid angiosarcoma, atypical fibroxanthoma, spindle cell amelanotic melanoma, Merkel cell carcinoma, basal cell carcinoma, basaloid sebaceous carcinoma, and small cell eccrine carcinoma.[5,14,71,74–76,87,106–108] The distinguishing points between these differential diagnostic considerations and SCC variants are outlined in Tables 44–1 to 44–5.

TABLE 44–1. DIFFERENTIAL DIAGNOSIS OF WELL DIFFERENTIATED SQUAMOUS CELL CARCINOMA

Histologic Feature	WDSCC[a]	PEH	KA
Horn-filled central crater	0	0	+
Intraepithelial abscesses	0	0	+
Cytoplasmic lucency	0	0	+
Mitotic activity	V	0	V
Cellular atypia	V	0	V
Apoptosis and dyskeratosis	+	0	V
Sharply angulated cell profiles at lesion base	+	V	0
Dermal fibrosis and chronic inflammation	V	V	V[b]
Perineural invasion in dermis	V	0	V[b]

[a] WDSCC, well-differentiated squamous cell carcinoma; PEH, pseudoepitheliomatous hyperplasia; KA, keratoacanthoma.
+, consistently present; 0, consistently absent; V, variably present.
[b] Regressing keratoacanthomas may demonstrate perilesional fibrosis; rare examples are neuroinvasive.

TABLE 44–2. DIFFERENTIAL DIAGNOSIS OF CUTANEOUS BOWEN'S DISEASE

Histologic Feature	Pagetoid BD[a]	EPD
Acantholysis involving atypical intraepidermal cells	0[b]	+
Cytoplasmic lucency	V	+
Dyskeratosis and apoptosis	+	0
Global atypia of keratinocytes	+	0
Immunoreactivity for carcinoembryonic antigen and/ or gross cystic disease fluid protein-15	0	+

[a] BD, Bowen's disease; EPD, extramammary Paget's disease.
[b] See Table 44–1 for explanation of symbols.

TABLE 44–3. DIFFERENTIAL DIAGNOSIS OF CUTANEOUS TUMORS CONTAINING GLANDULAR OR PSEUDOGLANDULAR SPACES

Histologic Feature	ASCC[a]	EAS	SGC
Continuity of cells in glandlike spaces with epidermis	+[b]	0	V (Rare +)
Erythrocytes in glandlike spaces	0	+	0
Mucin/PAS positivity	0	0	+
Keratin immunoreactivity	+	0	+
Binding of *Ulex europaeus* I lectin	V	+	V
Immunoreactivity for carcinoembryonic antigen, S100 protein, amylase, or Leu-M1	0	0	+

[a] ASCC, adenoid squamous cell carcinoma; EAS, epithelioid angiosarcoma; SGC, sweat gland carcinoma.
[b] See Table 44–1 for explanation of symbols.

TABLE 44–4. DIFFERENTIAL DIAGNOSIS OF SPINDLE CELL AND PLEOMORPHIC SQUAMOUS CELL CARCINOMA

Histologic Feature	SC-PSCC[a]	MM	AFX
Continuity of tumor cells with epidermis	V[b]	V	0
Junctional melanocytic atypia	0	+	0
Immunoreactivity for keratin	+	0	0
Immunoreactivity for vimentin	V	+	+
Immunoreactivity for S100 protein	0	+	0
Immunoreactivity for α_1-antichymotrypsin	V	V	+

[a] SC-PSCC, spindle cell and pleomorphic squamous cell carcinoma; MM, malignant melanoma; AFX, atypical fibroxanthoma.
[b] See Table 44–1 for explanation of symbols.

TABLE 44–5. HISTOLOGIC DIFFERENTIAL DIAGNOSIS OF SMALL CELL SQUAMOUS CARCINOMA OF THE SKIN

Histologic Feature	SCSCC[a]	SCSGC	SCMM	PNCS	BCC	BSC
Continuity of tumor with epidermis	+	0	V	0[b]	+	V
Junctional melanocytic atypia	0	0	+	0	0	0
Formation of keratin "pearls"	V	0	0	V	V	V
Vesicular nuclear chromatin	+	+	V	0	0	+
Nucleolar prominence	+	+	V	0	0	V
Focal glandular differentiation	0	V	0	V	V	0
Peripheral nuclear palisading	0	0	0	0	+	V
Argentaffinity	0	0	+	0	0	0
Lipophilia	0	0	0	0	0	+

[a] SCSCC, small cell squamous cell carcinoma; SCSGC, small cell sweat gland carcinoma; SCMM, small cell malignant melanoma; PNCS, primary neuroendocrine carcinoma of the skin (Merkel cell carcinoma); BCC, basal cell carcinoma; BSC, basaloid sebaceous carcinoma.
[b] Ten percent of PNCS cases show focal involvement of epidermis.
[c] See Table 44–1 for explanation of symbols.

PRIMARY NEUROENDOCRINE CARCINOMA OF THE SKIN ("MERKEL CELL" CARCINOMA)

Since its relatively recent recognition, primary neuroendocrine carcinoma of the skin has been the subject of intensive clinicopathologic study. Because this neoplasm demonstrates neuroepithelial differentiation, like that of normal Merkel cells of the skin ("Tastzellen"), the alternative term *Merkel cell carcinoma* is also widely used.

History
In 1972, Toker described a small cell cutaneous neoplasm that tended to occur in sun-exposed skin areas in elderly patients.[109] It resembled malignant lymphoma or metastatic oat cell carcinoma microscopically, and had been so diagnosed in the past; however, local recurrence, regional lymph node metastasis, and a lengthy survival in some cases made it evident that the lesion was primary in the skin.

Because he observed a ribboning growth pattern in some instances, Toker designated this neoplasm as trabecular carcinoma. In the interim, various other diagnostic labels have been applied to it, such as those just mentioned, as well as "small cell carcinoma of the skin,"[110] "endocrine carcinoma of the skin,"[93] and "undifferentiated carcinoma of the skin."[111]

The premise that such lesions exhibit Merkel cell differentiation is based on indirect morphologic and immunohis-

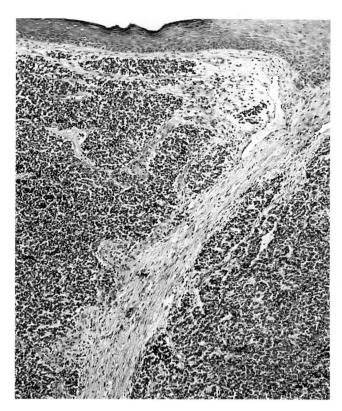

Figure 44–23. Merkel cell carcinoma of the skin. Small, lymphocyte-like tumor cells are disposed in a medullary fashion in the dermis. *From Ref. 118.*

tochemical data. Warner et al.[112] have outlined the ultra-structural similarities between primary neuroendocrine carcinoma of the skin and normal Merkel cells; in addition, Hartschuh and colleagues[113] and Sibley and Dahl[114] demonstrated that certain secretory cell products (e.g., vasoactive intestinal polypeptide) are common to both. Nevertheless, the anatomic distribution of normal Merkel cells (epidermal; predominantly in the digits[112,115]) is not recapitulated by the topography of PNCS.[71] Moreover, one of the intermediate filament polypeptides, neurofilament protein, is often present in PNCS[114,116] but is not seen in normal merkelocytes.[117]

Therefore, the nomenclature attending this neoplasm is arbitrary. Accordingly, it is best to list the diagnostic synonyms for PNCS in pathologic reports to avoid confusion on the part of attending physicians.

Histologic Features

Typical PNCS is characterized by the medullary, organoid, or trabecular growth of small oval cells in the corium, with various degrees of intercellular cohesion (Fig. 44–23). A "grenz" zone is usually present between the tumor and the epidermis; however, the latter structure may be involved focally in approximately 10% of cases. Dermal appendages are usually spared, but permeative growth into the subcutis is often apparent. Adipocytes may be entrapped by tumor cells, simulating lymphoma cutis in appearance (Fig. 44–24). Regional coagulative necrosis and apoptosis are common within PNCS.[71,93,120]

Nuclei are round to oval, with evenly dispersed chromatin, inconspicuous nucleoli, and abundant mitoses (up

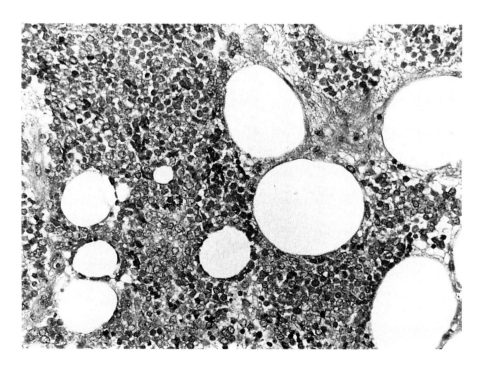

Figure 44–24. Permeation of subcuticular adipose tissue by Merkel cell carcinoma. This growth pattern may lead to confusion with lymphoma cutis.

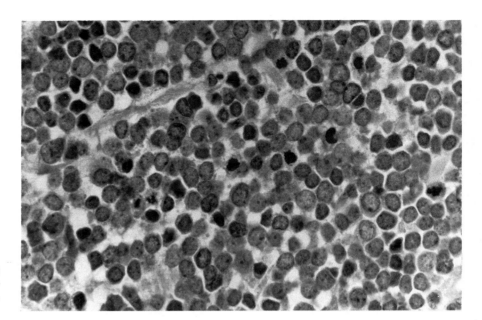

Figure 44–25. Cytologic detail of Merkel cell carcinoma. Tumor cells contain evenly distributed chromatin and show a high mitotic rate. *From Ref. 119.*

to 12 per high-power field) (Fig. 44–25). Cytoplasm is scanty and amphophilic, and cellular borders are indistinct. The stroma of PNCS may be sclerotic focally (sometimes mimicking the appearance of amyloid), and is richly endowed with capillary- or venule-sized vessels, which may be dilated. Lymphatic invasion is apparent in 20% of cases, and variably intense stromal lymphoplasmacytic inflammation is evident in most examples.[93]

Variations on the histopathologic description just given include lesions showing scattered uninucleated tumor "giant" cells, formation of Homer-Wright rosettes, myxoid stroma, spindle cell growth, and foci of squamous or glan-dular differentiation.[71,93] Another subtype of PNCS is the "oat cell" variant, displaying nests of small, hyperchromatic, partially crushed tumor cells with prominent nuclear molding.[93] The microscopic similarities between the latter and metastatic pulmonary small cell neuroendocrine carcinoma are obvious[116,121]; however, I have never observed the Azzopardi phenomenon (DNA encrustation of intratumoral blood vessels) in PNCS, whereas it is common in metastatic oat cell carcinoma of the lung (Fig. 44–26).

Gould et al. have documented a spectrum of differentiation in PNCS, including intermediate and large cell subtypes.[122] It is probable that the cases of "primary cutane-

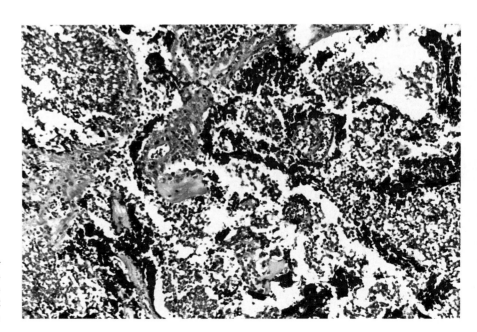

Figure 44–26. Condensation of nuclear chromatin around intratumoral vessels ("Azzopardi effect"), in metastatic small cell carcinoma of the skin. This appearance is not observed in primary Merkel cell carcinomas.

ous carcinoid" reported by van Dijk and Ten Seldam[123] and Smith and Chappell[124] fall into the second of these categories.

PNCS Associated With Other Skin Lesions

The association between PNCS and squamous carcinoma is now well recognized[92] (Fig. 44–27). Roughly 25% of patients with neuroendocrine skin cancer have had squamous carcinoma in the same cutaneous region, either metachronously or synchronously with the former lesion.[93] Both invasive SCC and Bowen's disease have been documented in this context. In addition, Silva et al. described a case in which overt sweat gland carcinoma and PNCS were admixed.[93]

I have observed one example of cutaneous neuroendocrine carcinoma arising in a background of hypohidrotic ectodermal dysplasia; the patient also had multifocal basal cell carcinomas and trichoepitheliomas in the same skin field.[125] Moreover, in the M. D. Anderson Hospital experience with this neoplasm, 9 of 67 cases showed the concurrence of PNCS and adjacent BCC.[93] Nevertheless, a histologic admixture of these two neoplasms has not been reported to date. Another example of PNCS in my files occurred in a large congenital nevus, and one patient mentioned by Silva and colleagues had had a noncontiguous malignant melanoma.[93]

Special Pathologic Studies

Conventional Special Stains. The PAS method may demonstrate scanty glycogen in the cells of PNCS, but this reactivity is seen in less than 15% of cases. The mucicarmine stain is consistently negative, but alcian blue and colloidal iron techniques sometimes result in labeling of the tumoral stroma. Argyrophil stains (e.g., Grimelius, Churukian-

Schenk) are positive in less than 10% of cutaneous neuroendocrine carcinomas that have been formalin fixed, but preservation in Bouin's solution yields silver reactivity in the majority of cases.[115] Argentaffin and amyloid stains are uniformly negative.

Electron Microscopy. Ultrastructurally, tumor cells in PNCS are invested focally by basal lamina and bound to one another by macula adherens–type junctions (Fig. 44–28). Nuclear chromatin is evenly distributed, with small chromocenters. Cytoplasmic contents include scanty glycogen, small numbers of mitochondria, free ribosomes, focally prominent Golgi bodies, occasional lysosomes, and short profiles of rough endoplasmic reticulum.[93]

The diagnostic electron microscopic elements in this neoplasm are twofold. First, dense-core neurosecretory granules are evident in the cytoplasm, both within cell bodies and in blunt cellular extensions; these inclusions measure 80 to 120 nm in diameter. Second, paranuclear whorls and skeins of intermediate filaments, in which neurosecretory granules may be enmeshed, are consistently detectable[71,110] (Fig. 44–29).

Rare intracellular microlumina have been described in PNCS by Silva et al.,[93] but I have not observed such structures in my case material. By light microscopy, cytoplasmic tonofilaments are not evident in neoplasms lacking squamous differentiation, but may be apparent in combined neuroendocrine/squamous tumors. Premelanosomes are always absent.

Immunohistochemistry. PNCS is typified by consistent reactivity for cytokeratin, in one of two patterns—diffuse or globular/paranuclear.[110,116,126] The second of these is *diagnostic* of neuroendocrine differentiation in a cutaneous small cell tumor, but is seen in only 40% to 50% of cases[126] (Fig.

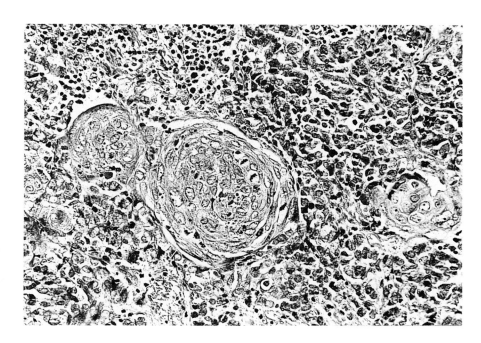

Figure 44–27. Focal squamous carcinomatous differentiation in Merkel cell carcinoma. *From Ref. 118.*

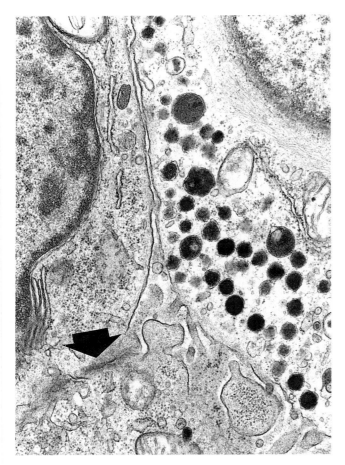

Figure 44–28. Macular intercellular junction (arrowhead) between two adjacent Merkel cell carcinoma cells. Numerous lysosomes and neurosecretory granules are seen in the cell at the right of the photograph.

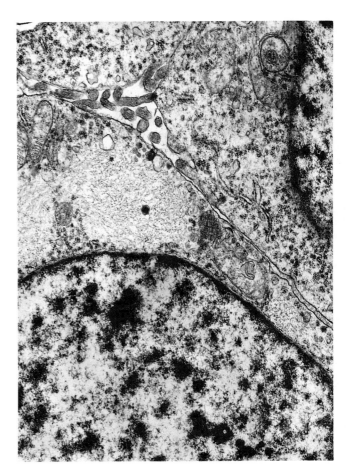

Figure 44–29. Perinuclear whorl of intermediate filaments, in which a neurosecretory granule is enmeshed, in Merkel cell carcinoma cell. *From Ref. 118.*

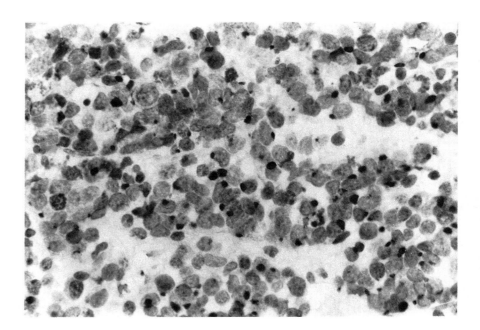

Figure 44–30. Perinuclear immunoreactivity for cytokeratin polypeptides, in Merkel cell carcinoma. This pattern of staining is pathognomonic of neuroendocrine differentiation in cutaneous carcinomas.

44–30). Concomitant positivity for neurofilament protein can be detected in 33%,[114,116] with a similar cytoplasmic distribution.

Additional evidence for the epithelial differentiation of cutaneous neuroendocrine carcinomas is represented by immunopositivity for epithelial membrane antigen.[127] This determinant is less ubiquitous than cytokeratin in such tumors, but it is apparent in more than 75% of cases.

The most sensitive "endocrine" marker for PNCS is neuron-specific enolase (NSE), the γ–γ dimer of 2-D-phosphoglycerate hydrolase[46,71,126] (Fig. 44–31). Although NSE is seen in all tumors of this type, it is not specific for PNCS. As mentioned previously, occasional basal cell carcinomas express this protein as well, and I have also observed it in sweat gland carcinomas. The latter finding is not unexpected, since Haimoto et al. have demonstrated NSE in normal eccrine glands.[128] Chromogranin, a very specific indicator of neuroendocrine differentiation,[46] is seen in 33% of PCNS cases[116]; in addition, 5% to 30% exhibit focal reactivity for vasoactive intestinal polypeptide, calcitonin, pancreatic polypeptide, ACTH, gastrin, insulin, or somatostatin.[93,114,127,129] S100 protein, carcinoembryonic antigen, and salivary-type amylase are consistently lacking in PNCS.[46,114,129]

Although neuroendocrine carcinoma of the skin does not display leukocyte common antigen,[127] as seen in malignant lymphomas, it may express reactivity for other determinants commonly associated with hematopoietic cells (OKT9, Leu-7, and BA1). OKT9 corresponds to the transferrin receptor,[127] seen in virtually all replicative cells[44]; Leu-7 and BA1 are shared by several neuroendocrine cells and tumors, and are nonspecific for topographic origins.[130,131]

Clinicopathologic Correlation

PNCS is an aggressive neoplasm, with a cumulative mortality of up to 50% in some series.[93,120] Several pathologic features have been identified by Silva and co-workers that putatively predict those lesions at risk of pursuing an untoward clinical course. These include a gross size greater than 2 cm, more than 10 mitoses per high-power field, lymphatic invasion, and presence of the "oat cell" PNCS growth pattern.[93]

In such cases, prophylactic regional lymphadenectomy is recommended subsequent to primary tumor removal. If the resected lymph nodes contain tumor, adjuvant radiotherapy to the tumor bed and remaining local lymphoid tissue is indicated.[93]

Multifocality has been documented at initial diagnosis in 12 patients with PNCS.[93,125,132] Because such a clinical presentation is much more suggestive of metastasis *to* the skin of a visceral carcinoma,[121] great caution should be exercised before a diagnosis of PNCS is accepted in cases with more than one lesion.

Spontaneous regression of cutaneous neuroendocrine carcinoma has been described by O'Rourke and Bell.[133] In the light of the large number of recognized cases of PNCS, this phenomenon must be extremely rare; moreover, the biologic mechanisms underlying it are unknown.

Differential Diagnosis

The differential diagnosis of small cell neoplasms of the skin is extensive. Small cell SCC, eccrine carcinoma, and malignant melanoma must be included in this group, as should malignant lymphoma, metastatic neuroendocrine carcinoma from visceral sites, peripheral neuroepithelioma, and Ewing's sarcoma.[71]

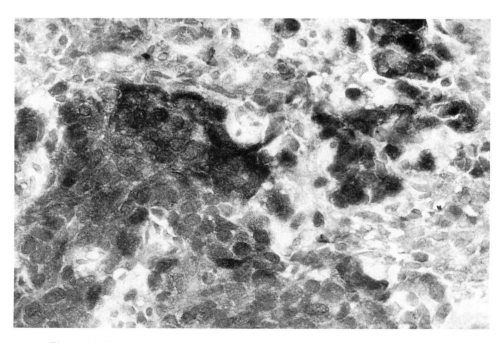

Figure 44–31. Immunoreactivity of neuron-specific enolase in Merkel cell carcinoma.

TABLE 44–6. ELECTRON MICROSCOPIC AND ULTRASTRUCTURAL DIFFERENTIAL DIAGNOSIS OF CUTANEOUS SMALL CELL TUMORS

Diagnostic Feature	PNCS[a]	SCSCC	ML	SCMM	SCSGC	MNEC	PNE	ES
Ultrastructural								
Cytoplasmic extensions	+[b,c]	0	0	0	0	+[c]	+[d]	0
Macula adherens	+	+	0	V	+	+	+	+
Neurosecretory granules	+	0	0	V	0	+	+	0
Glycogen pools in cytoplasm	0	V	0	0	V	0	0	+
Perinuclear whorls of microfilaments	+	0	0	0	0	V[e]	0	0
Microglandular spaces	0	0	0	0	+	0	0	0
Immunohistochemical Reactivity								
Keratin	+[f]	+	0	0	+	+	0	0
S100 protein	0	0	0	+	V	0	0	0
Neurofilaments	V	0	0	0	0	V	V	0
Vimentin	0	0	V	+	0	0	V	+
Neuron-specific enolase	+	0	0	+	V	+	+	V
Leukocyte common antigen	0	0	+	0	0	0	0	0

[a] PNCS, primary neuroendocrine carcinoma of skin; SCSCC, small cell squamous cell carcinoma; ML, malignant lymphoma; SCMM, small cell malignant melanoma; SCSGC, small cell sweat gland carcinoma; MNEC, metastatic neuroendocrine carcinoma of skin; PNE, peripheral neuroepithelioma; ES, Ewing's sarcoma.
[b] See Table 44–1 for explanation of symbols.
[c] Blunt cytoplasmic extensions.
[d] Elongated cytoplasmic extensions.
[e] Perinuclear filament whorls are rare in MNEC.
[f] Perinuclear globular reactivity.

Ultrastructural and immunohistochemical studies are extremely useful in this context. The results of these specialized techniques are summarized in Table 44–6.

REFERENCES

1. Krompecher E: *Der Basalzellenkrebs.* Jena, Fischer, 1903.
2. Hyde JN, Montgomery FH: *Diseases of the Skin,* ed 4. Philadelphia, Lea Brothers, 1897, pp 669–688.
3. Dellon AL: Host–tumor relationships in basal cell and squamous cell cancer of the skin. *Plast Reconstruct Surg* 1978;62:37–48.
4. Hauben DJ, Zirkin H, Mahler D, et al: The biologic behavior of basal cell carcinoma: Part I. *Plast Reconstruct Surg* 1982;69:103–116.
5. McGibbon DH: Malignant epidermal tumors. *J Cutan Pathol* 1985;12:224–238.
6. Wade TR, Ackerman AB: The many faces of basal cell carcinoma. *J Dermatol Surg Oncol* 1978;4:23–28.
7. Okun MR, Blumenthal G: Basal cell epithelioma with giant cells and nuclear atypicality. *Arch Dermatol* 1964;89:598–602.
8. Mehregan AH: Acantholysis in basal cell epithelioma. *J Cutan Pathol* 1979;6:280–283.
9. Siegle RJ, MacMillan J, Pollack SV: Infiltrative basal cell carcinoma: A nonsclerosing subtype. *J Dermatol Surg Oncol* 1986;12:830–836.
10. Jacobs GH, Rippey JJ, Altini M: Prediction of aggressive behavior in basal cell carcinoma. *Cancer* 1982;49:533–537.
11. Holmes EJ, Bennington JL, Haber SL: Citrulline-containing basal cell carcinomas. *Cancer* 1968;22:663–670.
12. Ono T, Fallas VH, Higo J: Basal cell epithelioma with dermal melanocytes. *J Dermatol* 1986;13:63–66.
13. Rulon DB, Helwig EB: Cutaneous sebaceous neoplasms. *Cancer* 1974;33:82–102.
14. Wolfe JT III, Wick MR, Campbell RJ: Sebaceous carcinomas of the oculocutaneous adnexa and extraocular skin, in Wick MR (ed): *Pathology of Unusual Malignant Cutaneous Tumors.* New York, Marcel Dekker, 1985, pp 77–106.
15. Hanke CW, Temofeew RK: Basal cell carcinoma with eccrine differentiation (eccrine epithelioma). *J Dermatol Surg Oncol* 1986;12:820–824.
16. Wick MR, Swanson PE: Primary adenoid cystic carcinoma of the skin. *Am J Dermatopathol* 1986;8:2–13.
17. Morris JGL, Joffe R: Perineural spread of cutaneous basal and squamous cell carcinomas. The clinical appearance of spread into the trigeminal and facial nerves. *Arch Neurol* 1983;40:424–429.
18. Sakamoto F, Ito M, Sato S, et al: Basal cell tumor with apocrine differentiation (apocrine epithelioma). *J Am Acad Dermatol* 1985;13:355–363.
19. Lerchin E, Rahbari H: Adamantinoid basal cell epithelioma: A histological variant. *Arch Dermatol* 1975;111:586–588.
20. Borel DM: Cutaneous basosquamous carcinoma. Review of the literature and report of 35 cases. *Arch Pathol* 1973;95:293–297.
21. DeFaria JL: Basal cell carcinoma of the skin with areas of squamous cell carcinoma: A basosquamous cell carcinoma? *J Clin Pathol* 1985;38:1273–1277.
22. Gertler W: Zur Epithelverbundenheit der Basaliome. *Dermatol Wochenschr* 1965;151:673–677.
23. Montgomery H: Basal squamous cell epithelioma. *Arch Dermatol Syphilol* 1928;18:50–73.
24. Schuller DE, Berg JW, Sherman G, et al: Cutaneous basosquamous carcinoma of the head and neck: A comparative analysis. *Otolaryngol Head Neck Surg* 1979;87:420–427.
25. Farmer ER, Helwig EB: Metastatic basal cell carcinoma: A clinicopathologic study of seventeen cases. *Cancer* 1980;46:748–757.
26. Quay SC, Harrist TJ, Mihm MC Jr: Carcinosarcoma of the skin: Case report and review. *J Cutan Pathol* 1981;8:241–246.

27. Dawson EK: Carcinosarcoma of the skin. J R Coll Surg Edinb 1972;17:242–246.

28. Abram H, Barsky S: Pigmented basal cell epithelioma arising in the scar of an onchocerciasis nodule. *Int J Dermatol* 1984;23:658–660.

29. Domingo J, Helwig EB: Malignant neoplasms associated with nevus sebaceus of Jadassohn. *J Am Acad Dermatol* 1979;1:545–556.

30. Goette DK, Helwig EB: Basal cell carcinomas and basal cell carcinoma-like changes overlying dermatofibromas. *Arch Dermatol* 1975;111:589–592.

31. Goldberg HS: Basal cell epitheliomas developing in a localized linear epidermal nevus. *Cutis* 1980;25:295–299.

32. Mikhail GR, Mehregan AH: Basal cell carcinoma in seborrheic keratosis. *J Am Acad Dermatol* 1982;6:500–506.

33. Rosenblum GA: Large basal cell carcinoma in a congenital nevus. *J Dermatol Surg Oncol* 1986;12:166–168.

34. Hashimoto K, Brownstein MH: Localized amyloidosis in basal cell epitheliomas. *Acta Dermatol (Stockh)* 1973;53:331–339.

35. Looi LM: Localized amyloidosis in basal cell carcinomas: A pathologic study. *Cancer* 1983;52:1833–1836.

36. Masu S, Hosokawa M, Seiji M: Amyloid in localized cutaneous amyloidosis: Immunofluorescence studies with anti-keratin antiserum, especially concerning the difference between systemic and localized cutaneous amyloidosis. *Acta Dermatol (Stockh)* 1981;61:381–384.

37. Brody I: Contributions to the histogenesis of basal cell carcinoma. *J Ultrastruct Res* 1970;33:60–79.

38. Ishibashi A, Kasuga T, Tsuchiya E: Electron microscopic study of basal cell carcinoma. *J Invest Dermatol* 1971;56:298–304.

39. Rupec M, Kint A, Himmelmann GW: On the occurrence of sphaeridia in basalioma cells and the basal cells of the overlying epidermis. *Arch Dermatol Res* 1976;256:33–37.

39a. Kobayasi T: Dermo-epidermal junction in basal cell carcinoma. *Acta Dermatol (Stockh)* 1970;50:401–411.

40. Dardi LE, Memoli VA, Gould VE: Neuroendocrine differentiation in basal cell carcinomas. *J Cutan Pathol* 1981;8:335–341.

41. Eusebi V, Mambelli V, Tison V, et al: Endocrine differentiation in basal cell carcinoma. *Tumori* 1979;65:191–199.

42. Kumakiri M, Hashimoto K: Ultrastructural resemblance of basal cell epithelioma to primary epithelial germ. *J Cutan Pathol* 1978;5:53–67.

43. Miettinen M, Lehto VP, Virtanen I: Antibodies to intermediate filament proteins: The differential diagnosis of cutaneous tumors. *Arch Dermatol* 1985;121:736–741.

44. Gatter KC, Pulford KAF, Van Stapel MJ, et al.: An immunohistological study of benign and malignant skin tumours: Epithelial aspects. *Histopathology* 1984;8:209–227.

45. Thomas P, Said JW, Nash G, et al.: Profiles of keratin proteins in basal and squamous cell carcinomas of the skin: An immunohistochemical study. *Lab Invest* 1984;50:36–41.

46. Wick MR, Kaye VN: The role of diagnostic immunohistochemistry in dermatology. *Semin Dermatol* 1986;5:136–147.

47. Dahl M: Beta-2-microglobulin in skin cancer. *J Am Acad Dermatol* 1981;5:698–699.

48. Kallioinen M, Dammert K: Beta-2-microglobulin in benign and malignant adnexal skin tumors and metastasizing basocellular carcinomas. *J Cutan Pathol* 1984;11:27–34.

49. Mazoujian G, Pinkus GS, Haagensen DE Jr: Extramammary Paget's disease—Evidence for an apocrine origin. An immunoperoxidase study of gross cystic disease fluid protein-15, carcinoembryonic antigen, and keratin proteins. *Am J Surg Pathol* 1984;8:43–50.

50. Claudy AL, Viac J, Schmitt D, et al.: Identification of mononuclear cells infiltrating basal cell carcinomas. *Acta Dermatol (Stockh)* 1976;56:361–365.

51. Kuflik EG: Clinical variants of basal cell carcinoma. *Cutis* 1981;28:403–408.

52. Kuflik EG: Basal cell carcinoma: An unusual clinical and histologic variant. *J Dermatol Surg Oncol* 1980;6:730–732.

53. Mehregan AH: Aggressive basal cell epithelioma on sunlight-protected skin: Report of eight cases, one with pulmonary and bone metastases. *Am J Dermatopathol* 1983;5:221–229.

54. Perrone T, Twiggs LB, Adcock LL, et al.: Vulvar basal cell carcinoma: An infrequently metastasizing neoplasm. *Int J Gynecol Pathol*, in press.

55. Robins P, Rabinovitz HS, Rigel D: Basal cell carcinomas on covered or unusual sites of the body. *J Dermatol Surg Oncol* 1981;7:803–806.

56. Black MM, Walkden VM: Basal cell carcinomatous changes on the lower leg: A possible association with chronic venous stasis. *Histopathology* 1983;7:219–227.

57. Peled IJ, Wexler MR: Symmetric basal cell carcinoma of the auricles. *J Dermatol Surg Oncol* 1985;11:164.

58. Lang PG Jr, Maize JC: Histologic evolution of recurrent basal cell carcinoma and treatment implications. *J Am Acad Dermatol* 1986;14:186–196.

59. Sloane JP: The value of typing basal cell carcinomas in predicting recurrence after surgical excision. *Br J Dermatol* 1977;96:127–132.

60. Domarus HV, Stevens PJ: Metastatic basal cell carcinoma: Report of five cases and review of 170 cases in the literature. *J Am Acad Dermatol* 1984;10:1043–1060.

61. Menz J, Sterrett G, Wall L: Metastatic basal cell carcinoma associated with a small primary tumor. *Aust J Dermatol* 1985;26:121–124.

62. Scanlon EF, Volkmer DD, Oviedo MA, et al.: Metastatic basal cell carcinoma. *J Surg Oncol* 1980;15:171–180.

63. Curson C, Weedon D: Spontaneous regression in basal cell carcinomas. *J Cutan Pathol* 1979;6:432–437.

64. Donatsky O, Hjorting-Hansen E, Philipsen HP, Fejerskov O: Clinical, radiologic, and histopathologic aspects of 13 cases of nevoid basal cell carcinoma syndrome. *Int J Oral Surg* 1976;5:19–28.

65. Lindeberg H, Jepsen FL: The nevoid basal cell carcinoma syndrome: Histopathology of the basal cell tumors. *J Cutan Pathol* 1983;10:68–73.

66. Southwick GJ, Schwartz RA: The basal cell nevus syndrome. *Cancer* 1979;44:2294–2305.

67. Rahbari H, Mehregan AH: Basal cell epithelioma (carcinoma) in children and adolescents. *Cancer* 1982;49:350–353.

68. Bleiberg J, Brodkin RH: Linear unilateral basal cell nevus with comedones. *Arch Dermatol* 1969;100:187–190.

69. Plosila M, Kiistala R, Niemi KM: The Bazex syndrome: Follicular atrophoderma with multiple basal cell carcinomas, hypotrichosis, and hypohidrosis. *Clin Exp Dermatol* 1981;6:31–37.

70. Brownstein MH, Shapiro L: Desmoplastic trichoepithelioma. *Cancer* 1977;40:2979–2986.

71. Wick MR, Scheithauer BW: Primary neuroendocrine carcinoma of the skin, in Wick MR (ed): *Pathology of Unusual Malignant Cutaneous Tumors*. New York, Marcel Dekker, 1985, pp 107–180.

72. Battifora H: Spindle-cell carcinoma: Ultrastructural evidence of squamous origin and collagen production by the tumor cells. *Cancer* 1976;37:2275–2282.

73. Brownstein MH, Shapiro L: Verrucous carcinoma of skin: Epithelioma cuniculatum plantare. *Cancer* 1976;38:1710–1716.

74. Eusebi V, Ceccarelli C, Piscioli F, et al.: Spindle-cell tumours of the skin of debatable origin: An immunocytochemical study. *J Pathol* 1984;144:189–199.

75. Feldman PS, Barr RJ: Ultrastructure of spindle-cell squamous carcinoma. *J Cutan Pathol* 1976;3:17–24.

76. Johnson WC, Helwig EB: Adenoid squamous cell carcinoma. *Cancer* 1966;19:1639–1650.

77. Kao GF, Graham JH, Helwig EB: Carcinoma cuniculatum (verrucous carcinoma of the skin): A clinicopathologic study of 46 cases with ultrastructural observations. *Cancer* 1982;49:2395–2403.

78. Kuo TT: Clear-cell carcinoma of the skin: A variant of the squamous cell carcinoma that simulates sebaceous carcinoma. *Am J Surg Pathol* 1980;4:573–583.

79. Kuwano H, Hashimoto H, Enjoji M: Atypical fibroxanthoma distinguishable from spindle-cell carcinoma in sarcoma-like skin lesions. *Cancer* 1985;55:172–180.

80. Lever WF: Adenoacanthoma of sweat glands. *Arch Dermatol Syphilol* 1947;56:157–171.

81. Lichtiger B, Mackay B, Tessmer CF: Spindle-cell variant of squamous cell carcinoma. A light and electron microscopic study of 13 cases. *Cancer* 1970;26:1311–1320.

82. McKee PH, Wilkinson JD, Corbett MF, et al.: Carcinoma cuniculatum: A case metastasizing to skin and lymph nodes. *Clin Exp Dermatol* 1981;6:613–618.

83. Broders AC: Squamous cell epithelioma of the skin. *Ann Surg* 1921;73:141–160.

84. Evans HL, Smith JL: Spindle-cell squamous carcinomas and sarcoma-like tumors of the skin: A comparative study of 38 cases. *Cancer* 1980;45:2687–2697.

85. Strayer DS, Santa Cruz DJ: Carcinoma in situ of the skin: A review of histopathology. *J Cutan Pathol* 1980;7:244–259.

86. Graham JH, Helwig EB: Erythroplasia of Queyrat, in Graham JH, Johnson WC, Helwig EB (eds): *Dermal Pathology*. Hagerstown, Harper & Row, 1972, pp 597–606.

87. Jones RE Jr, Austin C, Ackerman AB: Extramammary Paget's disease: A critical reexamination. *Am J Dermatopathol* 1979;1:101–132.

88. Steffen C, Ackerman AB: Intraepidermal epithelioma of Borst-Jadassohn. *Am J Dermatopathol* 1985;7:5–24.

89. Fulling KH, Strayer DS, Santa Cruz DJ: Adnexal metaplasia in carcinoma *in situ* of the skin. *J Cutan Pathol* 1981;8:79–88.

90. Callen JP, Headington JT: Bowen's disease and non-Bowen's squamous intraepidermal neoplasia of the skin. *Arch Dermatol* 1980;116:422–426.

91. Graham JH, Helwig EB: Bowen's disease and its relationship to systemic cancer. *Arch Dermatol* 1959;80:133–159.

92. Gomez LG, DiMaio S, Silva EG, et al.: Association between neuroendocrine (Merkel cell) carcinoma and squamous carcinoma of the skin. *Am J Surg Pathol* 1983;7:171–177.

93. Silva EG, Mackay B, Goepfert H, et al.: Endocrine carcinoma of the skin (Merkel cell carcinoma). *Pathol Annu* 1984;19(2):1–30.

94. Balazs M: Buschke-Loewenstein tumour: A histologic and ultrastructural study of six cases. *Virchow's Arch Pathol Anat* 1986;410:83–92.

95. Perez-Mesa CA, Kraus FT, Evans JC, et al.: Anaplastic transformation in verrucous carcinoma of the oral cavity after radiation therapy. *Radiology* 1966;86:108–115.

96. Chernosky ME, Rapini RP: Squamous cell carcinoma in lesions of disseminated superficial actinic porokeratosis: A report of two cases. *Arch Dermatol* 1986;122:853–854.

97. Davidson TM, Bone RC, Kiessling PJ: Epidermoid carcinoma arising from within an epidermoid inclusion cyst. *Ann Otol Rhinol Laryngol* 1976;85:417–418.

98. Garrett AB: Multiple squamous cell carcinomas in lesions of discoid lupus erythematosus. *Cutis* 1985;36:313–316.

99. Grussendorf EI, Gahlen W: Metaplasia of a verruca vulgaris into spinocellular carcinoma. *Dermatologica* 1975;150:295–299.

100. Levin A, Amazon K, Rywlin AM: A squamous cell carcinoma that developed in an epidermal nevus: Report of a case and review of the literature. *Am J Dermatopathol* 1984;6:51–55.

101. Peralta OC, Barr RJ, Romansky SG: Mixed carcinoma in situ: An immunohistochemical study. *J Cutan Pathol* 1983;10:350–358.

102. Fisher ER, McCoy MM, Wechsler HI: Analysis of histopathologic and electron microscopic determinants of keratoacanthoma and squamous cell carcinoma. *Cancer* 1972;29:1387–1397.

103. Kvedar JC, Fewkes J, Baden HP: Immunologic detection of markers of keratinocyte differentiation in neoplastic and preneoplastic lesions of skin. *Arch Pathol Lab Med* 1986;110:183–188.

104. Fukamizu H, Inoue K, Matsumoto K, et al.: Metastatic squamous cell carcinomas derived from solar keratoses. *J Dermatol Surg Oncol* 1985;11:518–522.

105. Moller R, Reymann F, Hou-Jensen K: Metastases in dermatological patients with squamous cell carcinoma. *Arch Dermatol* 1979;115:703–705.

106. Chalet MD, Connors RC, Ackerman AB: Squamous cell carcinoma vs. keratoacanthoma: Criteria for histologic differentiation. *J Dermatol Surg* 1975;1:16–17.

107. Kern WH, McCray MK: The histopathologic differentiation of keratoacanthoma and squamous cell carcinoma of the skin. *J Cutan Pathol* 1980;7:318–325.

108. Matsuo K, Sakamoto A, Kawai K, et al.: Small cell carcinoma of the skin: "Non-Merkel cell type." *Acta Pathol Jpn* 1985;35:1029–1036.

109. Toker C: Trabecular carcinoma of the skin. *Arch Pathol* 1972;105:107–110.

110. Kuhajda FP, Olson JL, Mann RB: Merkel cell (small cell) carcinoma of the skin: Immunohistochemical and ultrastructural demonstration of distinctive perinuclear cytokeratin aggregates and a possible association with B-cell neoplasms. *Histochem J* 1986;18:239–244.

111. Stern JB: "Murky cell" carcinoma (formerly trabecular carcinoma). *Am J Dermatopathol* 1982;4:517–519.

112. Warner TFCS, Uno H, Hafez R, et al.: Merkel cells and Merkel cell tumors. Ultrastructure, immunocytochemistry, and review of the literature. *Cancer* 1983;52:238–245.

113. Hartschuh W, Weihe E, Yanihara N, Reinecke M: Immunohistochemical localization of vasoactive intestinal polypeptide (VIP) in Merkel cells of various animals: Evidence for a neuromodulator function of the Merkel cell. *J Invest Dermatol* 1983;81:361–364.

114. Sibley RK, Dahl D: Neuroendocrine (Merkel cell?) carcinoma of the skin. II. An immunohistochemical study of 21 cases. *Am J Surg Pathol* 1985;9:109–116.

115. Frigerio B, Capella C, Eusebi V, et al.: Merkel cell carcinoma of the skin: The structure and function of normal Merkel cells. *Histopathology* 1983;7:229–249.

116. Battifora H, Silva EG: The use of antikeratin antibodies in the immunohistochemical distinction between neuroendocrine (Merkel cell) carcinoma of the skin, lymphoma, and oat-cell carcinoma. *Cancer* 1986;58:1040–1046.

117. Saurat JH, Didierjean L, Skalli O, et al.: The intermediate filament proteins of rabbit normal epidermal Merkel cells are cytokeratins. *J Invest Dermatol* 1984;83:431–435.

118. Wick MR (ed): *Pathology of Unusual Malignant Cutaneous Tumors.* New York, Marcel Dekker, 1985.

119. Wick MR: Primary neuroendocrine carcinoma and small-cell malignant lymphoma of the skin: a discriminant immunohistochemical comparison. *J Cutan Pathol* 1986;13:347–358.

120. Sibley RK, Dehner LP, Rosai J: Neuroendocrine (Merkel cell?) carcinoma of the skin. I. Clinicopathologic and ultrastructural study of 43 cases. *Am J Surg Pathol* 1985;9:95–108.

121. Wick MR, Millns JL, Sibley RK, et al.: Secondary neuroendocrine carcinomas of the skin: An immunohistochemical comparison with primary neuroendocrine carcinomas of the skin

("Merkel cell carcinomas"). *J Am Acad Dermatol* 1985;13:134–142.

122. Gould VE, Moll R, Moll I, et al.: Neuroendocrine (Merkel) cells of the skin: Hyperplasias, dysplasias, and neoplasms. *Lab Invest* 1985;52:334–349.

123. Van Dijk C, Ten Seldam REJ: A possible primary cutaneous carcinoid. *Cancer* 1975;36:1016–1020.

124. Smith PA, Chappell RH: Another possible primary carcinoid tumor of skin? *Virchow's Arch Pathol Anat* 1985;408:99–103.

125. Wick MR, Thomas JR III, Scheithauer BW, et al.: Multifocal Merkel's cell tumors associated with a cutaneous dysplasia syndrome. *Arch Dermatol* 1983;119:409–414.

126. Hoefler H, Kerl H, Rauch HJ, et al.: New immunocytochemical observations with diagnostic significance in cutaneous neuroendocrine carcinoma. Am J Dermatopathol 1984;6:525–530.

127. Drijkoningen M, DeWolf-Peeters C, Van Limberger E, et al.: Merkel cell tumor of the skin: An immunohistochemical study. *Hum Pathol* 1986;17:301–307.

128. Haimoto H, Takahashi Y, Koshikawa T, et al.: Immunohisto-chemical localization of gamma-enolase in normal human tissues other than nervous and neuroendocrine tissues. *Lab Invest* 1985;52:257–263.

129. Layfield L, Ulich T, Liao S, et al.: Neuroendocrine carcinoma of the skin: An immunohistochemical study of tumor markers and neuroendocrine products. *J Cutan Pathol* 1986;13:268–273.

130. Linder J, Wilson RB, Armitage JO: B-lymphocyte monoclonal antibody reactivity with neuroendocrine tumors. (Abstract) *Lab Invest* 1985;52:39A.

131. Tsutsumi Y: Leu 7 immunoreactivity as a histochemical marker for paraffin-embedded neuroendocrine tumors. *Acta Histochem Cytochem* 1984;17:15–22.

132. Katenkamp D, Watzig V: Multiple neuroendocrine carcinomas (so-called Merkel cell tumors) of the skin: Report on two cases with unique clinical course. *Virchow's Arch Pathol Anat* 1984;404:403–411.

133. O'Rourke MGE, Bell JR: Merkel cell tumor with spontaneous regression. *J Dermatol Surg Oncol* 1986;12:994–1000.

CHAPTER 45
Tumors of Hair Follicle Differentiation

John T. Headington

FOLLICULAR HAMARTOMAS

Hamartomas of hair germ (Table 45–1) are benign epithelial or epithelialstromal proliferations that are inappropriate for a reparative or reactive response. Although, theoretically, they may be derived from any germinative epithelium, they characteristically differentiate toward follicular structures to some degree. If there is sufficient differentiation for recognition of the various derivatives of hair matrix, an inductive stromal component is invariably present. Hamartomas with limited differentiation can be classified separately from those in which matrix cell or outer sheath cell differentiation predominates and from generalized follicular hamartomas (Table 45–1).

THE NEVUS SEBACEOUS COMPLEX

Follicular hamartomas may be found as a component of the mature nevus sebaceous complex (Fig. 45–1). Wilson Jones and Heyl[1] in a study of 140 cases found occasional basaloid proliferations suggesting abortive follicular differentiation. Similar findings were described in another large study of 150 cases.[2]

BASAL CELL HAMARTOMA

Basal cell hamartoma with follicular differentiation[3] is characterized by symmetric periorbital papules that are clinically similar to syringomas. Histologically, there is a subepidermal platelike proliferation of basal cells with varying degrees of limited follicular differentiation, including abortive hair bulbs.

BASAL CELL NEVUS

Basal cell nevus most commonly presents as linear and unilateral patches and plaques.[4-8] Some are slightly hypopigmented. Most are hairless and a few include small comedones. Two cases are reported with small areas of alopecia of the scalp in addition to other lesions.

Histologic studies of basal cell nevi have found thin strands of basaloid epithelium in focal continuity with epidermis or follicular infundibula. With the investing stroma, these proliferating basaloid foci form small budding nodules that expand the papillary dermis. Follicular differentiation, if present, does not go beyond the formation of immature hair buds. A review of reported cases suggests a morphologically and clinically heterogeneous group with such diverse features as basal cell carcinoma in some lesions and suggestion of fibroepithelioma in others (Pinkus).

TRICHOEPITHELIOMA

Trichoepitheliomas are benign cutaneous epithelial-mesenchymal hamartomas best classified as tumors of hair germ with limited differentiation.[9] Although the entire histogenetic sequence is certain, serial sections of individual lesions may demonstrate multiple points of epithelial continuity with both epidermis and outer hair sheath. Using glucose-6-phosphate dehydrogenase (G6PD) mosaicism as a tracer in a study of multiple hereditary trichoepitheliomas, Gartler and others[10] determined that trichoepitheliomas from a G6PD heterozygote were composed of both normal and enzyme-deficient epithelial cells. These findings suggest that tumor induction affects a large target cell population having potentially different clonal characteristics (e.g., epidermis and outer hair sheath).

Clinical Features
Clinical onset may occur during childhood or adult life, and a conspicuous increase in the number of lesions can

TABLE 45–1. FOLLICULAR HAMARTOMAS

Localized hamartomas with limited differentiation
    Hamartomas of the nevus sebaceus complex
    Basal cell harmartoma
    Solitary, unclassified
    Basal cell nevus
Trichoepithelioma
    Desmoplastic variant
    Trichoadenoma
Localized hamartomas with advanced differentiation
    Trichofolliculoma
    Congenital vellus hamartoma
    Solitary, unclassified
Generalized hamartomas without differentiation
Generalized hamartomas with differentiation

occur during puberty. Multiple familial lesions, inherited as an autosomal dominant trait,[11] appear as small, discrete, grouped, skin-colored nodules and papules with a tendency to congregate on the upper lip and nasolabial folds. Trichoepitheliomas may also be distributed on the scalp, ears, upper extremities, and trunk. Individual tumors on the face and neck usually do not exceed 0.5 cm, but may be larger elsewhere. Growth is limited and a stationary size is generally reached after a few years. Solitary trichoepitheliomas clinically present as nondescript asymptomatic papules or nodules with predilection for the face and neck, as do the multiple tumors. The solitary trichoepithelioma commonly simulates basal cell carcinoma, nevocellular nevus, or other benign-appearing lesions.

Genetic studies have suggested that the well-known coexistence of dermal eccrine cylindromas and trichoepitheliomas in the same patient is due to a single autosomal dominant gene capable of phenotypic dimorphism and vari-

able penetrance.[12] A possible variant syndrome comprises trichoepitheliomas, cylindromas, and milia.[13] There have also been described two patients with the SST syndrome (skin and salivary tumors), who have dermal eccrine cylindromas, trichoepitheliomas, and membranous monomorphic adenomas of salivary gland.[14,15] The membranous adenomas of salivary gland are close morphologic analogs of dermal eccrine cylindroma. Malignant dermal eccrine cylindroma and malignant salivary gland tumors may supervene in the SST syndrome. Carcinoma of the breast has also been reported in a patient with multiple trichoepitheliomas[16] but may represent a chance occurrence.

The Rombo syndrome,[17] described in a single Scandinavian family, is a disorder characterized by vermiculate atrophoderma, milia, hypotrichosis, trichoepitheliomas, basal cell carcinomas, and peripheral vasodilatation with cyanosis. A case of generalized trichoepitheliomas with alopecia and myasthenia gravis has been recorded.[18]

Histologic Features

Histologically, trichoepithelioma occurs as a combined epithelial-mesenchymal proliferation. The investing tumor-associated stroma frequently circumscribes the epithelial component within the dermis so that after tissue fixation and processing, some retraction of the tumor nodule from normal dermal collagen may be found (Figs. 45–2, 45–3). The fibroblastic stroma is generally fibrotic rather than myxoid. Budding epithelial islands of poorly specialized basophilic keratinocytes present in a variety of histologic patterns: solid, microcystic, radiate, or trabecular. Epithelial islands are frequently marginated by a peripheral nuclear palisade. Focal epithelial continuity with epidermis or outer hair sheath is common, as are small keratinous microcysts. The small keratinous cysts are lined by flattened squamous cells containing keratohyaline granules with an abrupt zone

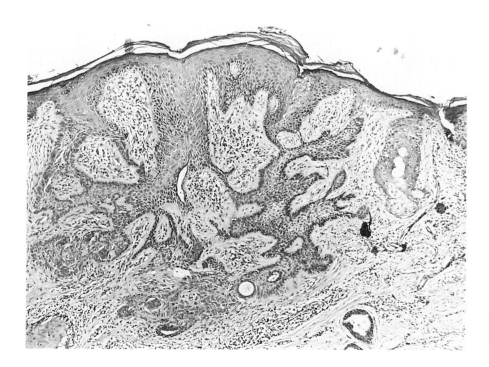

Figure 45–1. Follicular hamartoma in nevus sebaceus. Differentiation is usually limited. Types vary considerably. (H&E, ×16.)

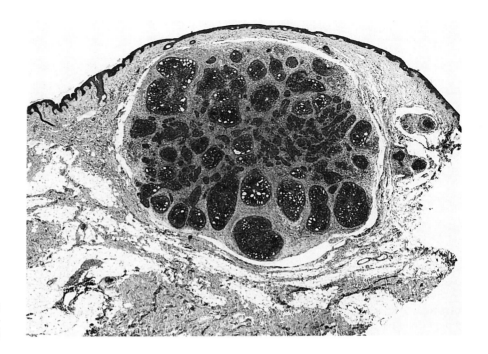

Figure 45–2. Trichoepithelioma. A basaloid undifferentiated tumor. Note retraction of entire tumor nodule from dermis. (H&E, ×16.)

of keratinization. On occasion, keratotic debris undergo dystrophic calcification. Intracellular melanin may be present and tonofibrils within epithelium can be demonstrated with polarized light and by electron microscopy.

Electron Microscopy

The ultrastructural details of trichoepithelioma include increased intracellular glycogen, a continuous or discontinuous basal lamina, and the presence of hemidesmo-

somes at the periphery of tumor lobules. In addition to keratinocytic tumor cells, there is a heterogeneous indigenous population of Langerhans cells, Merkel cells, and melanocytes.[19,20] Curious banded endoplasmic reticulum has been found in one solitary trichoepithelioma.[21]

Histologic variants of trichoepithelioma include tumors composed exclusively of small nonkeratinizing basophilic cells, tumors composed predominantly of cystic spherical nodules of well-differentiated keratinocytes, rare tumors

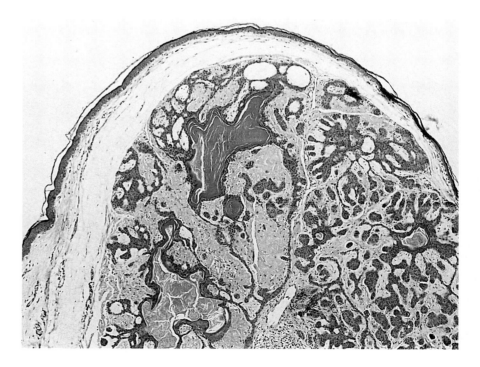

Figure 45–3. Trichoepithelioma. A radiate pattern, with keratin filling irregular cystic spaces. Note retraction of entire tumor nodule from dermis. (H&E, ×16.)

showing advanced stromal induction of hair follicules, and rare tumors containing well-differentiated sebaceous and apocrine epithelium.

Desmoplastic Trichoepithelioma

Desmoplastic trichoepithelioma[22] (sclerosing epithelial hamartoma[23]) is a lesion of putative follicular origin with distinctive clinicopathologic features. The tumor generally occurs as a solitary morpheaform plaque, usually somewhat annular in contour. Borders are slightly elevated and the center depressed—often vaguely white or yellow in hue. Small milia may be seen in the central area. The lesion occurs most frequently on the cheek and is uncommon in other areas of the head and neck or elsewhere. Women are affected in about 85% of cases and about one half of patients are under 30. Lesions may occur in children. Duration is frequently prolonged; a clinical history of several years is commonplace. Familial occurrence has been recorded.[24] The clinical appearance is obviously quite different from that of the usual nodular solitary trichoepithelioma with conventional histology.

Histologic Features

The most important microscopic findings for diagnosis of desmoplastic trichoepithelioma are (1) delicate strands or columns of small basaloid tumor cells; (2) keratinizing microcysts with or without dystrophic calcification; and (3) a densely sclerotic fibroblastic tumor–associated stroma (Figs. 45–4, 45–5). In addition to the frequent small calcific deposits, occasional foreign body granulomas are found, probably in response to extruded keratin. The overall architectural pattern is a rather poorly delineated intradermal epithelial proliferation. Several points of tumor cell continuity with epidermis are commonly present; in contrast, extension of the tumor into the subcutis generally is not seen. There is negligible nuclear atypia, and mitoses as well as apoptotic cells are rare.

The major histologic findings that suggest a relationship to the conventional trichoepithelioma are a fibroblastic tumor–associated stroma and the formation of keratinous microcysts. In contrast to some basal cell carcinomas, the basement membranes have been found to be continuous around most of the epithelial components of desmoplastic trichoepithelioma, except around large keratinizing cysts and calcific foci.[24]

Differential Diagnosis

Problems in diagnosis occasionally arise in differentiation of desmoplastic trichoepithelioma from syringoma and desmoplastic basal cell carcinomas. The small microcystic structures in syringoma rarely undergo squamous transformation; small cysts in syringomas are usually lined by large pale, somewhat foamy-appearing cells frequently forming PAS-positive cuticular layers. Desmoplastic basal cell carcinomas readily penetrate the boundary of dermis and subcutis, and are often associated with a hyaluronic acid–rich stroma. Some forms of microcystic adnexal carcinoma (syringoid carcinoma) can also stimulate desmoplastic trichoepithelioma.

Trichoadenoma

Trichoadenoma is an uncommon variant form of trichoepithelioma characterized by intradermal cystic nodules of well-differentiated keratinocytes enclosed within a fibrocellular stroma (Figs. 45–6, 45–7). The cuticular mode of keratinization is suggestive of the pilary canal above the level of the entrance of the sebaceous duct. All lesions reported thus far have been solitary, from 3 to 15 mm in diameter, and there has been a predilection for the facial area.[25]

TRICHOFOLLICULOMA

Trichofolliculoma is a morphologically complex hamartoma of the pilosebaceous unit characterized by one or more large cystic follicles with smaller radiating follicular structures.[26,27] Earlier names for this lesion include folliculoma and hair follicle nevus.

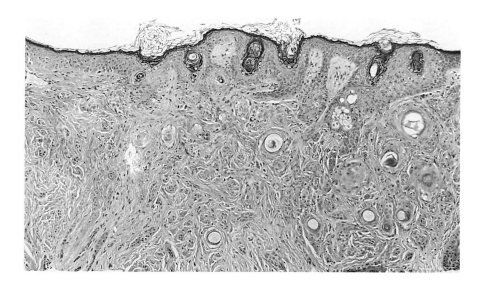

Figure 45–4. Desmoplastic trichoepithelioma. Epidermis may be flattened but is not eroded by tumor. The tumor is circumscribed, usually confined to the dermis. (H&E, ×16.)

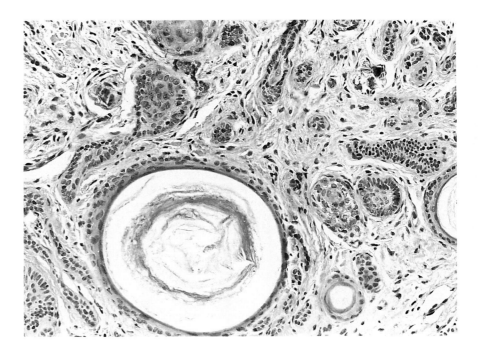

Figure 45–5. Desmoplastic trichoepithelioma. Basal cells differentiate to form keratinous microcysts. There is no cytologic atypia. Apoptotic cells and mitoses are rare. Tumor-associated stroma is collagenous not myxoid. (H&E, ×64.)

Clinical Features

The clinical manifestation is usually a small elevated plaque or flattened nodule with a central pore or depression. Occasionally, a comedo or a sebumlike exudate has been noted. A tuft of small short hairs, either white or pigmented, or a woollike wisp of trichoidal keratin may protrude from the lesion and serves as a reliable sign for clinical recognition. In reported cases, trichofolliculoma has been limited to the head and neck, and is most commonly located on the face. Unusual locations are the margin of the eyelid and the external auditory canal. Although data for age and sex distribution are probably biased by a large series of cases reported from the Armed Forces Institute of Pathology,[27] random reports indicate a preponderance in adult males. Trichofolliculomas have been found in both black and white patients.

Histologic Features

The characteristic histologic pattern is a large dilated or cystic follicle within the upper dermis that frequently com-

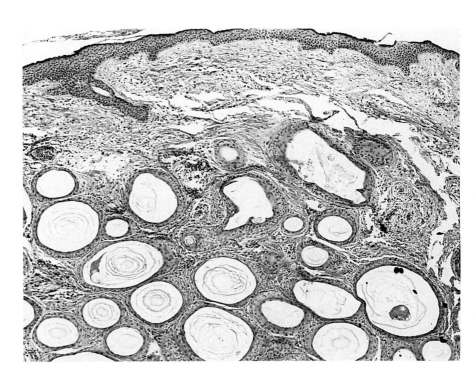

Figure 45–6. Trichoadenoma. A circumscribed intradermal tumor nodule is composed of aggregated small keratinous microcysts. (H&E, ×16.)

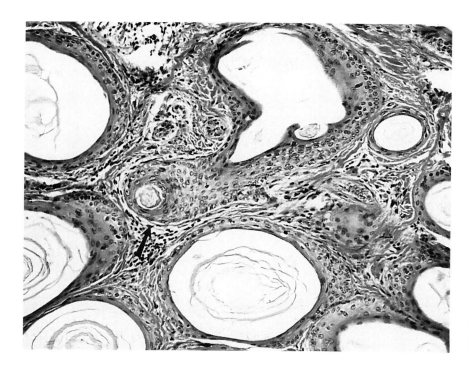

Figure 45–7. Trichoadenoma. Follicular differentiation, if present, is very limited (arrow). The mode of keratinization is cuticular. (H&E, ×64.)

municates to the skin surface. The keratinous epithelium of the cystic space usually features a distinct granular layer and exfoliates loose lamellar keratin similar to the normal follicular infundibulum. Other follicles or follicle-like structures, with or without dermal papillae, branch or radiate from the primary epithelium, sometimes arborizing to form secondary or tertiary units (Figs. 45–8, 45–9). When hair shafts or masses of hair keratins are formed, they are projected centripetally or beyond the skin surface. Well-formed sebaceous elements may be found in association with fol-

licular induction. A distinctive subset or variant form has been termed *sebaceous trichofolliculoma.*[28] This lesion is largely composed of radiating lobules of sebaceous epithelium with the formation of acini and ducts. Small vellus hair follicles are in attendance but represent an unobtrusive component.

An investing fibrocellular tumor-associated stroma is present in all cases of trichofolliculoma in which there is follicular induction. Occasionally, however, trichofolliculoma may show very limited follicular induction. In such lesions, the distinction between trichofolliculoma and pilar

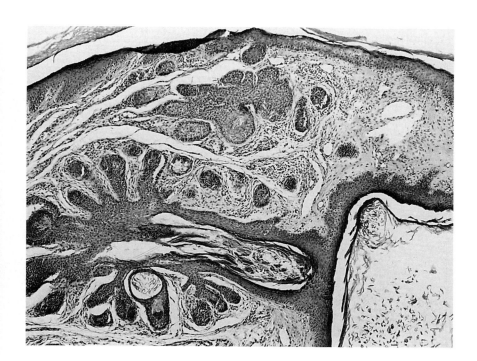

Figure 45–8. Trichofolliculoma. Budding follicular structures extend outward from a central dilated follicular infundibulum. (H&E, ×64.)

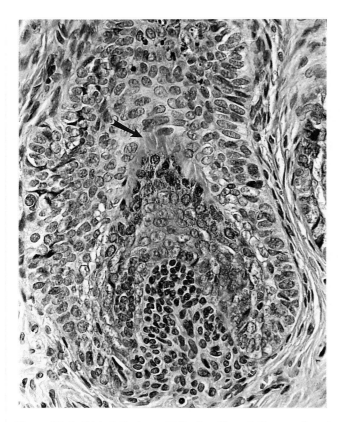

Figure 45–9. Trichofolliculoma. Follicular differentiation may be advanced or limited. Note dermal papilla and inner sheath differentiation (arrow). (H&E, ×260.)

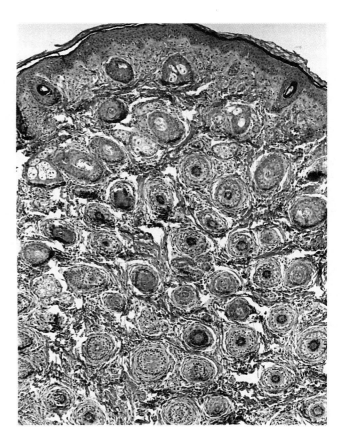

Figure 45–10. Congenital vellus hamartoma. Numerous closely packed vellus follicles are normally differentiated. They group to form a small nodule. (H&E, ×16.)

sheath acanthoma is not clear. A morphologic continuum between well-differentiated trichofolliculoma and pilar sheath acanthoma can be demonstrated.

To date, all reported examples of trichofolliculomas have been clinically benign. There is a solitary report of trichofolliculoma showing perineural invasion,[29] but this report is difficult to evaluate: a tumor-associated stroma was not well illustrated in the paper and induction of follicular structures was absent. The features described suggest that this tumor may be an endophytic variant or botryoid form of keratoacanthoma.

CONGENITAL VELLUS HAMARTOMA

The congenital vellus hamartoma is a small cutaneous tumor nodule composed of well-formed vellus hair follicles.[30–32] The rare reported cases have all been on the head and neck, with two on the eyelid.

The number of follicles is strikingly in excess of the expected density for normal skin (Fig. 45–10). It is notable that the arrector pili muscle is absent. The congenital vellus hamartoma is probably a result of localized excessive proliferation of primary hair germ during an early stage of development. Normal differentiation then follows.

SOLITARY UNCLASSIFIED HAMARTOMAS

Solitary unclassified hamartomas with limited differentiation may be found at any site but are most common as lesions of the head and neck.

GENERALIZED HAMARTOMAS

Generalized hamartomas of hair germ somewhat resembling trichoepitheliomas without follicular differentiation are reported in a unique case with aminoaciduria and progressive alopecia.[33] Generalized hamartomas of hair germ with advanced differentiation have not yet been reported.

TUMORS OF HAIR GERM

Tumors of hair germ (Table 45–2) are defined as a group of primary cutaneous neoplasms composed of basaloid epithelial and/or mesenchymal elements which by their size, location, and histologic and cytologic features are readily separable from other tumors of the hair follicle.[34] The germinal epithelium component is possibly derived from telogen hair germ and may undergo variable histodifferentiation as a result of stromal induction when tumor-associated stroma is present as part of the neoplasm.

The classification of tumors of hair germ is based on a close analogy with the more common odontogenic tumors and can similarly be divided into two primary groups: epithelial and mesenchymal. Epithelial trichogenic tumors are further subdivided into tumors that are purely epithelial and epithelial tumors with mesenchymal components that may or may not cause inductive differentiation. Pure epithelial neoplasms are termed *trichoblastomas*. Mixed epithelial-mesenchymal neoplasms in which inductive differentiation varies from nil to the formation of complete hair follicles are termed *trichoblastic fibromas*. An older term for fully differentiated tumors, trichogenic trichoblastoma, is now included in trichoblastic fibroma to simplify the classification.

TRICHOBLASTIC FIBROMA

The trichoblastic fibroma[34] is a mixed epithelial mesenchymal neoplasm of hair germ that is localized to skin and subcutis. The odontogenic analog is the ameloblastic fibroma. The fibroblastic stromal component is potentially inductive and histodifferentiation toward follicular structures varies from nil to the formation of complete hair follicles.

Clinical Features

Trichoblastic fibromas may be located either within the dermis (dermal type) or within the subcutis. Clinical findings therefore vary with location, but individual tumors are always nodular and well localized. Tumors within the subcutis generally "shell out." Tumors vary from less than 1 cm to as large as 8 cm in diameter and weigh 249 g.[35] Site is quite variable and includes the thigh, shoulder, buttock, and arm as well as the head and neck. Very similar tumors occur in canines. All reported trichoblastic fibromas have been in adults, with about equal occurrence in males and females.

Histologic Features

The histologic finding in trichoblastic fibroma is a very sharply circumscribed tumor within either the dermis or the subcutis (Fig. 45–11). Three-dimensionally complex lobules and strands of basaloid epithelial cells are contained within a variable fibrocellular matrix which also circumscribes the tumor. The epithelial component is also variable, but distinctive and characteristic features include interconnecting double-layered strands of epithelium and the formation of primary germinal buds, which recapitulate the primitive budding of primary hair germ from the embryonic periderm (Fig. 45–12). Stromal inductive effects further modify the epithelium. Small keratinous microcysts are common and larger keratinous cysts are occasionally encountered (Fig. 45–13). Focal hair matrix cell formation may occur, and further differentiation of matrix cells can result in inner hair sheath formation and even complete hair follicle development. With advanced follicle formation, outer hair sheath differentiation is also found. Lobular sebaceous differentiation can occur with advanced follicle development, and numerous small foci of sebocytes may be found in some less differentiated tumors.

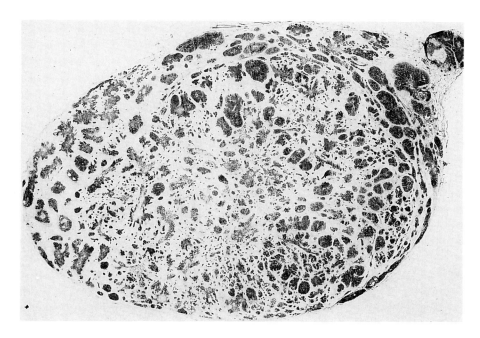

Figure 45–11. Trichoblastic fibroma. Solitary tumors are found in dermis and subcutis. They are well circumscribed with a peripheral stromal envelope. (H&E, ×8.)

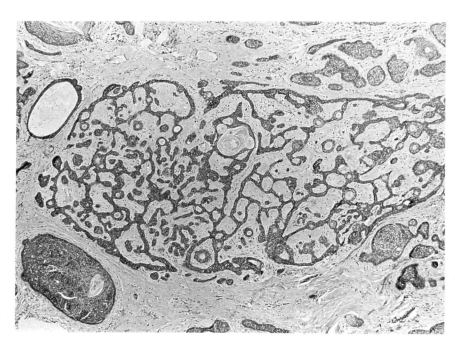

Figure 45–12. Trichoblastic fibroma. Epithelium is frequently arranged in thin strands with an investing fibrocellular stroma. (H&E, ×8.)

Differential Diagnosis

The histologic differential diagnosis is largely confined to solitary trichoepithelioma. The small intradermal tricho-blastic fibroma in the skin of the head and neck closely simulates trichoepithelioma and, undoubtedly, some tricho-blastic fibromas are incorrectly diagnosed as solitary tri-choepitheliomas. Differences are partly in the level of differentiation: trichoepitheliomas tend to be less differentiated and often are in focal continuity with epidermis. The usual fibroblastic fibroma is, however, removed from subcutis without attachment to epidermis and is not usually a tumor of the head and neck. Trichoblastic fibromas are solitary,

acquired tumors and there is no evidence for an autosomal dominant hamartomatous disease as with trichoepithelioma.

TUMORS OF HAIR MATRIX

HAMARTOMAS OF HAIR MATRIX

A classification of tumors of hair matrix is given in Table 45–3.

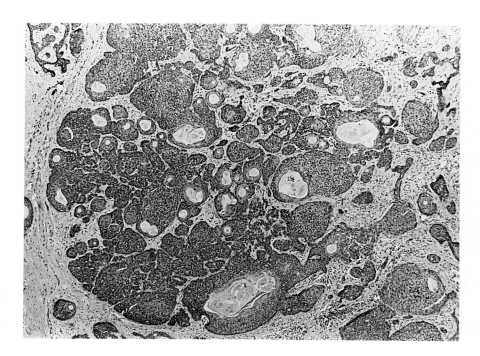

Figure 45–13. Trichoblastic fibroma. More solid epithelial areas may be encountered. Keratinous microcysts may be frequent in such areas. (H&E, ×16.)

Benign cutaneous tumors that have hamartomatous features in which hair matrix cells predominate but that are clearly different from trichomatricoma are occasionally encountered. One such reported case features an intradermal epidermoid cyst with somewhat organoid differentiation of matrix cells as part of the proliferation.[36]

TRICHOMATRICOMA

Trichomatricoma [pilomatrixoma, calcifying epithelioma (Malherbe)][37,38] is a benign tumor of pilar keratinocytes in which there is limited cytodifferentiation toward cells of hair matrix, the hair cortex, and cells of the inner hair sheath.

Clinical Features

When solitary, about 50% of all tumors are found on the head and neck; another 25% on the arms, and the remainder are distributed over the trunk and lower extremities. No cases have been reported on the palms or soles. Characteristically a tumor of the young, 40% of trichomatricomas are diagnosed by age 10, 50% before age 20.[39] An association with Gardner's syndrome has been noted[40,41] and some of the epidermoid cysts found in Gardner's syndrome may contain epithelium suggesting focal matrix cell differentiation. Familial occurrence of trichomatricomas has been repeatedly described. Trichomatricomas may also be a clinical cutaneous sign of myotonic dystrophy. A review of tricho-matricomas and myotonic dystrophy[42] reports that these tumors are multiple in 75% of patients with the associated disorders: 16 separate tumors were found in one patient. Trichomatricoma in association with Goldenhar's syndrome and in a patient with multiple tumors and hypercalcemia has been reported.[43]

Clinically, trichomatricoma appears as a small cutaneous tumor nodule that is very firm to palpation but movable over deep structures. Although the skin is usually normal in appearance, red or blue colors may be seen. On rare occasions, the tumor contents may be extruded to the skin surface through superficial erosions. Eruptive onset of multiple tumors has been noted.

Histologic Features

Small tumors are sharply circumscribed and cystlike, with a perimeter of uniform small dark cells that closely resemble normal hair matrix. In proliferative areas, mitoses may be numerous and nucleic acid synthesis has been demonstrated in vitro.[44] With further growth, some tumors become multilobular and more complex in outline (Fig. 45–14). Matrix cell differentiation may be either toward hair cortex, with formation of dense translucent hyaline protein resembling hard keratin, or toward large squamoid keratinocytes with prominent trichohyaline granules suggestive of prekeratinizing inner sheath cells (Fig. 45–15). Necrobiosis of undifferentiated matrix cells results in masses and columns of distinctive anucleate shadow cells. More complete necrosis forms acellular debris.

Polariscopy reveals a characteristic pattern of coarse intracytoplasmic anisotropic fibrils in shadow cells. Fully organized hair shafts are not found. Dystropic calcification of epithelium frequently occurs, and osseous metaplasia of stroma is occasionally found with formation of both lamellar and woven bone (Fig. 45–16). Small amounts of intracel-

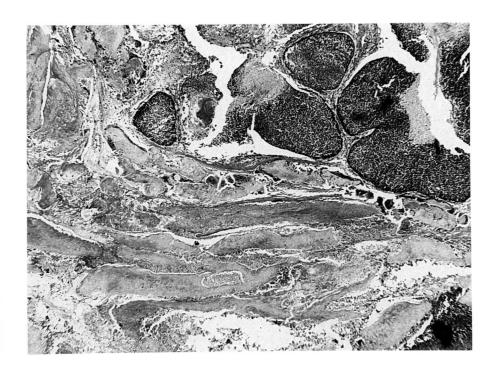

Figure 45–14. Trichomatricoma. Basaloid mature cells form circumscribed islands. Undifferentiated hair keratins form thick lamellar sheets. (H&E, ×40.)

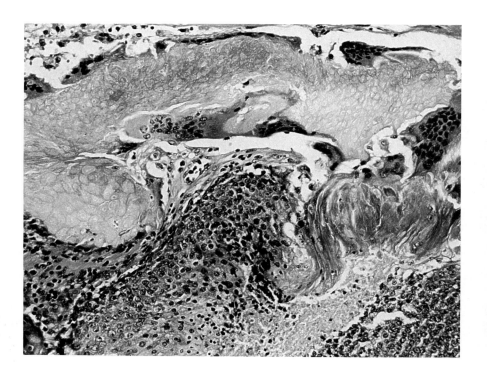

Figure 45–15. Trichomatricoma. Basaloid matrical keratinocytes terminally differentiate to form shadow cells. Keratin acts as a foreign body. Note foreign body giant cells. (H&E, ×162.)

lular melanin can be found in 10% to 15% of trichomatricomas. Stromal amyloid has been found by conventional stains and documented by electron microscopy. A tumor-associated stroma is an inconspicuous element of trichomatricoma and the epithelial elements are very poorly vascularized. A prominent mononuclear phagocytic "foreign body" response with multinucleate giant cell formation is frequent, probably in response to naked keratins.

Minor histologic variants of trichomatricoma include

tumors with abundant melanin[45] and tumors with extensive osseous metaplasia. Occasional tumors may feature large thin-walled vascular spaces. The end-stage tumor contains no viable epithelium, with only keratotic and inflammatory remnants as clues to the precursor lesion.

The available histochemical and ultrastructural evidence supports the histogenetic postulate that the proliferate compartment of the trichomatricoma differentiates as does hair matrix. The most important histochemical findings

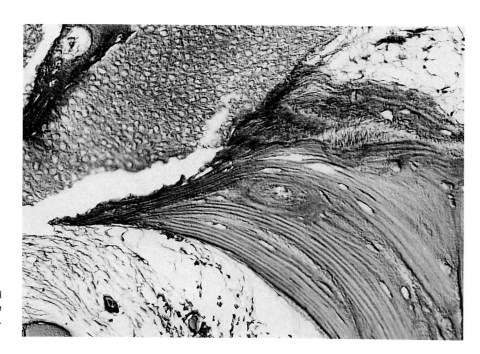

Figure 45–16. Trichomatricoma. Stromal changes include osseous metaplasia. Note lamellar bone adjacent to shadow cells. (H&E, ×162.)

are similarities in intensity and distribution of the –SH and –SS groups as found in the sulfur-rich protein of the shadow cell precursors when compared with the normal cells of hair cortex.[46] In addition, a homologous pattern of distribution of citrulline is found in some areas of lamellar tumor keratin and keratin of the inner hair sheath.[47] Ultrastructurally, most of the keratinizing cells of the trichomatricoma contain filamentous x-keratin but not epidermoid keratohyaline granules.[48] The pattern of keratinization in tumor cells is similar to that of the normal hair cortex but is unlike that of the epidermis.

An immunohistochemical study of 13 tumors found high-molecular-weight keratins in 10 of 13 but no low-molecular-weight keratins. A few tumors were positive for β_2-microglobulin, epithelial membrane antigen, and peanut agglutinin binding.[49]

Nosologically, the trichomatricoma is best considered to be a hamartoma of the hair follicle. Not encountered as congenital lesions, trichomatricomas are probably acquired as rare isolated faults in normal follicular histogenesis, possibly beginning as failure of stromal induction during anagen. Proliferating matrix cells might then fail to normally organize, and although some limited cytodifferentiation occurs, histodifferentiation does not. In the absence of adequate stromal induction well-formed hair shafts are never seen. The trichomatricoma is a benign tumor of limited growth that characteristically undergoes spontaneous involution, a feature shared with few other neoplasms but consistent with a genetically programmed limited proliferative capacity of the matrix cells. It may be that the proliferative potential for matrix cells of the trichomatricoma is approximately the same as the normal anagen time of the follicle from which it was derived.

TUMORS OF THE EXTERNAL HAIR SHEATH

The outer hair sheath, the tricholemma, is a specialized derivative of the primary hair germ. Above the level of the sebaceous duct the outer sheath forms the epithelium of the pilary canal. In this area, there is a zone of gradual epithelial transition from the lower tricholemmal keratinization characteristic of the outer sheath to the upper epidermoid keratinization characteristic of the follicular infundibulum near the epidermal surface.

One important biologic feature of tricholemmal keratinization is that proliferation and subsequent desquamation are subtly restrained—the pilary canal does not fill with desquamated outer sheath keratin. Another important biologic feature of tricholemmal keratinization is that differentiation apparently does not require the presence of hair matrix cells, which form only hair shaft and inner sheath keratins.

Theoretically, tricholemmal differentiation can occur from any proliferating epithelial component of the integument, including the epidermis. There is, therefore, the probability that some tricholemmal tumors originate from primary or secondary hair germ, as well as the possibility of focal tricholemmal differentiation directly from the epidermis.

There is one final but important consideration relevant to tricholemmal differentiation which is concerned with epithelial involution of the telogen bulb. Normally, during telogen, there is progressive volumetric reduction of outer sheath epithelium below the level of the sebaceous duct as hair matrix proliferation is shut down with the onset of the resting phase of the hair cycle. This volumetric reduction is accomplished by a normal noninflammatory mode of individual cell death termed *apoptosis*. The process of volumetric involution is thereafter carried to completion after the club hair is lost, when the follicle settles into resting telogen or as new follicle is restructured from telogen germ. From the preceding, it can be appreciated that an important potential source of keratinizing tricholemmal epithelium is residual to telogen hair bulb epithelium if normal involution is not completed. It is extremely likely that telogen bulb epithelium is the source of both tricholemmal (pilar) cysts and proliferating tricholemmal tumors (pilar tumors), whether or not proliferating tumors originate in cysts.

The classification in Table 45–4 is fully consistent with benign and malignant tricholemmal tumors originating from epidermis, normal outer sheath epithelium, primary and secondary hair germ, or remnants of the tricholemmal bulb of the telogen follicle.

TRICHOLEMMAL HAMARTOMAS

Tricholemmal hamartomas appear to exist in at least two different clinical settings. One form is an integral part of a unique disseminated cutaneous abnormality characterized as a generalized follicular hamartoma complicated by multiple proliferating tricholemmal cysts and palmar pits.[50] Small solid and cystic epithelial lesions featuring tricholemmal differentiation are found within deep reticular dermis.

The other form of tricholemmal hamartoma is the papular epithelial hamartoma found as part of Cowden's disease.[51] Multiple facial tricholemmal hamartomas constitute one of several epithelial and mesenchymal hamartomatous manifestations of Cowden's disease. In addition to skin and mucous membrane, other organs may be involved, particularly the breasts, thyroid gland, gastrointestinal tract, and female genital tract. A very high incidence of breast cancer in females with Cowden's disease[52] makes it especially important to identify such patients.

The histologic and cytologic details of the papular tricholemmal hamartomas of Cowden's disease are not remarkably different from those of solitary sporadic tricholemmomas, with the possible exception that the epithelium of some small lesions may appear to be a more integral component of contiguous epidermis than are the more bul-

TABLE 45–4. TUMORS OF EXTERNAL HAIR SHEATH (TRICHOLEMMOMA)

Cystic tricholemmal hamartomas

Papular tricholemmal hamartomas (Cowden's disease)

Solitary tricholemmomas

Tricholemmal keratosis

Proliferating tricholemmal tumors

Tricholemmal carcinoma

bous intradermal tricholemmomas encountered as solitary tumors.

TRICHOLEMMOMA

Tricholemmoma is a benign neoplasm of the hair follicle and is derived from outer sheath or infundibular epithelium.[53] Differentiation and keratinization follow a tricholemmal mode.

Clinical Features

Tricholemmoma is generally found as a small, solitary, nondescript skin-colored keratotic papule. Over 90% of lesions occur on the head and neck. There is a predilection for the upper lip and nose as well as the skin around the eye, including the lid margin. There is probably no significant difference in prevalence according to sex; the age at time of diagnosis ranges widely from the second to the ninth decade. Clinically, a tricholemmoma is often confused for verruca vulgaris, actinic keratosis, seborrheic keratosis, keratotic basal cell carcinoma, or nevocellular nevus.

Histologic Features

The histologic pattern of tricholemmoma is a sharply circumscribed lobulated epithelial neoplasm, often in continuity with the epidermis or outer sheath epithelium at several points (Fig. 45–17). Individual tumors tend to be both exo- and endophytic; the overlying epidermis is often irregular in contour and may also be focally hyperkeratotic. Peripheral reserve cells of the lobule tend to palisade and are associated with a prominent basement membrane reminiscent of the vitreous sheath of the normal follicle (Fig. 45–18). Small squamous eddies may occasionally be observed. Large lobules may have keratinous microcysts containing lamellar keratin debris.

A cytologic hallmark of the tricholemmoma is some degree of clear cell change resulting from abundant cytoplasmic glycogen. Glycogen content, as histochemically determined by diastase digestion, diminishes in zones of transition between tumor lobules and adjacent follicular epithelium or epidermis. An intermediate cellular phenotype containing little excess glycogen may dominate the cytologic appearance of some tumors. Individual tumor cells are smaller than the average epidermal keratinocyte, are vaguely polygonal in outline, and have small, somewhat homogeneous nuclei with small but distinct nucleoli. The presence of anisotropic tonofibrils is easily demonstrated in intermediate or transitional cells.

An indigenous and characteristic feature of the tumor-associated stroma of the tricholemmoma is formation of dense homogeneous-appearing collagenous bands. With polarization microscopy, these smudgy eosinophilic areas resolve into fine fibrillar collagen; they do not take stains for amyloid.

Differential Diagnosis

In large tricholemmomas in which clear cells predominate, the most troublesome lesions to exclude is the clear cell variant form of eccrine acrospiroma (clear cell hidradenoma). The lobular growth and focal epidermal continuity of acrospiroma may closely simulate tricholemmoma, but the acrospiroma does not have a peripheral cellular palisade or a prominent basement membrane. The reserve cell of the acrospiroma tends to lie adjacent to the stromal vessels and is not always arrayed at the periphery of the lobule.

In small lesions where intermediate cells may predominate, differentiation from the so-called irritated seborrheic keratosis (inverted follicular keratosis) may be difficult. Occasionally, small palisading basal cell carcinomas with areas of clear cells resulting from accumulation of lipid or glycogen can also be mistaken for small tricholemmomas.

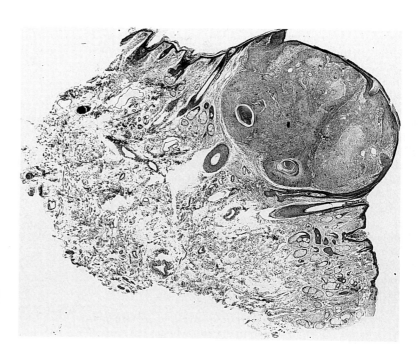

Figure 45–17. Tricholemmoma. A sharply circumscribed tumor nodule is in focal continuity with epidermis. Small keratinous microcysts may occur. Tumor-associated stroma is frequently dense and hyalinized. (H&E, ×4.)

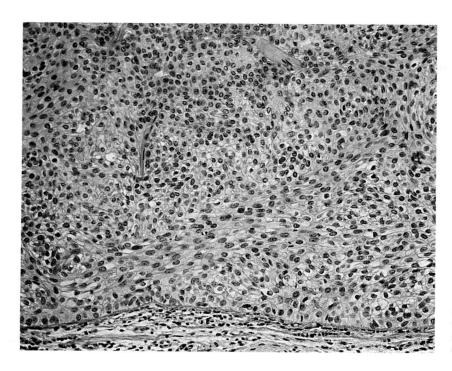

Figure 45–18. Tricholemmoma. Tumor lobules are well marginated and membrane bound. Basal palisading is often present. Increased cystoplasmic glycogen results in clear cell change. (H&E, ×162.)

TRICHOLEMMAL KERATOSIS

Tricholemmal keratosis is an uncommon keratinizing tumor of the epidermis that resembles a cutaneous horn or hyperkeratotic actinic keratosis.[34]

Although clinical data are meager, distribution appears to be varied; solitary lesions have been reported from the extremities, head, neck, and back.[54] Lesions are probably as common in males as in females, with a wide age range at the time of diagnosis.

The histologic pattern is generally a verrucous epidermal hyperplasia with striking orthokeratotic hyperkeratosis. Intradermal epithelial growth occurs in the form of rounded lobules of large pale-staining keratinocytes. Within the epidermis there is often an abrupt transition between epidermal and tricholemmal keratinization (Fig. 45–19). The pattern of keratinization of the epithelium of the keratosis is similar to that seen within the normal follicular *isthmus* or telogen bulb. Tumor lobules within the dermis closely simulate those found in proliferating tricholemmal tumors and on occasion may form small cystic structures as a deep component of the keratosis.

It is most probable that this lesion represents a proliferative as well as a phenotypic change of the epidermal or infundibular keratinocyte. The histologic differential diagnosis includes other hyperkeratotic lesions that clinically feature a cutaneous "horn," particularly the actinic keratosis and some variant forms of seborrheic keratosis.

PROLIFERATING TRICHOLEMMAL TUMORS

Proliferating tricholemmal tumors (pilar tumors) are uncommon neoplasms of outer sheath cells, which often result in a distinctive clinicopathologic picture.[55] Frequently quite large (up to 25.0 cm) and exophytic, these neoplasms are most commonly found on the scalp and back of the neck, but they can occur elsewhere. They are approximately five times more common in women. While the age range of subjects is from the fourth to the ninth decade, the mean age is about 65 years. Prolonged duration is characteristic. Proliferating tricholemmal tumors are often clinically misdiagnosed as squamous cell carcinomas.

Histologic Features

The histologic features, although they vary from tumor to tumor, are nevertheless sufficiently distinctive to be diagnostic. These include a sharply circumscribed pattern of convoluted lobules with pushing margins (Fig. 45–20), frequent continuity with the epidermis, extensive areas of tumor cell necrosis, and tricholemmal keratinization with abrupt transition to dense keratin but without formation of a granular layer. Reserve cell differentiation is generally toward large polygonal keratinocytes. Basal or reserve cell orientation to a prominent hyaline PAS-positive basement membrane is occasionally found but is not a constant feature. Cellular disarray is a common observation (Fig. 45–21).

The stroma is loose and poorly vascularized. Occasional granulomatous foreign body reactions similar to those seen in trichomatricomas are encountered. Polariscopic examination is characteristic: in those tumors with peripheral epithelial cell organization similar to that found in the tricholemmal cysts, prominent tonofibrils are oriented vertically to the epithelial-keratinous interface. Throughout the epithelial lobules, the anisotropic tonofilamentous pattern exhibits individual cell keratinization without formation of lamellar keratin. In some tumors, extensive areas of tumor cell necrosis are found with formation of amorphous debris.

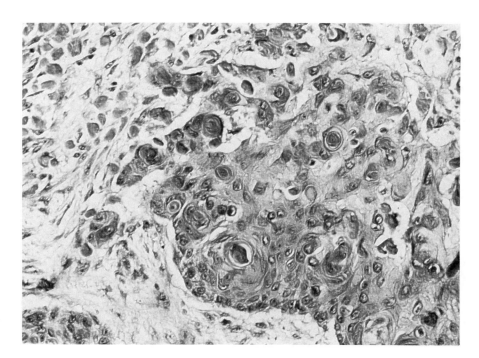

Figure 45–19. Tricholemmal keratosis. Epidermis is hyperplastic in a verrucous pattern. Dense keratin forms vertical spires. Cytodifferention of epidermis is focally tricholemmal. (H&E, ×260.)

Cytologic variants include clear cell types suggestive of giant tricholemmomas as well as spindle forms and dyskeratotic forms suggestive of lobular acantholytic squamous cell carcinoma. The lobular growth pattern and tendency for centripetal keratinization of large trichomatricomas can simulate proliferating tricholemmal tumors, but the trichomatricomas can be differentiated by recognition of matrix cells and by polariscopy (viable matrix cells contain no or few anisotropic tonofibrils).

Histologic patterns of aggressive growth are occasionally present, and substantial cytologic atypism may be encountered. Regional node metastasis is rarely reported, however, and a microscopic diagnosis of carcinoma in this neoplasm should be made with restraint.[56]

Terminology has been confused and histogenesis uncertain. These tumors were first grouped as an entity under the term *proliferating epidermoid cysts*.[57] Almost simultaneously, a separate study independently described this neoplasm as invasive pilomatrixoma.[58] An additional series was subsequently reported as trichochlamydocarcinoma, which was believed to originate from the lower external sheath.[59] A more recent report of giant hair matrix tumor reaffirmed matrical origin.[60] Synonyms include pilar tumor, hydatidiform keratinous cyst, and tricholemmal pilar tumor.

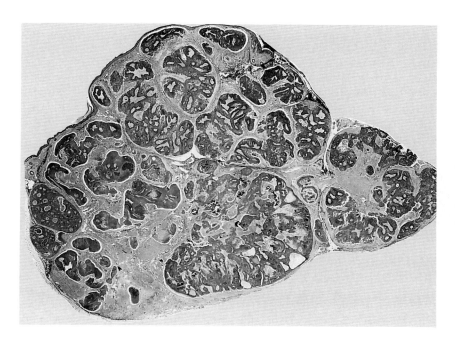

Figure 45–20. Proliferating tricholemmal tumor. Note distinctive complex lobular arrays. Cytodifferentiation is centripetal. (H&E, ×4.)

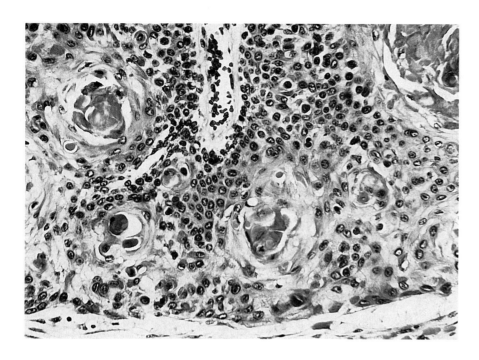

Figure 45–21. Proliferating tricholemmal tumor. Basal cells differentiate to form large and small masses of keratin against a background of cellular disarray. Clear cell changes may predominate. (H&E, ×162.)

Proliferating epithelial foci are not exceptional in tricholemmal cysts, and cystic tumors of a type intermediate between tricholemmal cysts and fully developed proliferating tricholemmal tumors are occasionally encountered. A key factor in proliferation may be vascularization of cyst epithelium, possibly secondary to focal injury. Histochemical and ultrastructural details strongly favor hair sheath origin. The malignant variant should be termed *malignant proliferating tricholemmal tumor* in distinction to tricholemmal carcinoma, which is the malignant form of tricholemmoma.

TUMORS OF THE INTRAEPIDERMAL FOLLICLE AND INFUNDIBULUM

The various tumors related to the intraepidermal follicle and follicular infundibulum are listed in Table 45–5.

NEVUS COMEDONICUS

Nevus comedonicus is a localized cystic hamartoma of the follicular infundibulum. The clinical lesion is found in an aggregate of dilated follicular openings often containing pigmented keratinous plugs. The distribution may be a

TABLE 45–5. TUMORS OF THE INTRAEPIDERMAL FOLLICLE AND INFUNDIBULUM

Nevus comedonicus
Dilated pore
Tumor of follicular infundibulum
Pilar sheath acanthoma
Fibrofolliculoma

small agminate patch or plaque, but linear, segmental, or randomly distributed lesions may also occur.

Histologic examination of the advanced lesion reveals a somewhat tubular dilatation of the follicular infundibulum and pilary canal to the level of the sebaceous duct, often with attenuation of the outer sheath epithelium.[61] Comedonal contents include normal-appearing lamellar keratin, whereas hairs are usually absent. Inflammatory changes may be superimposed but secondary neoplastic phenomena are not encountered. Nevus comedonicus should be distinguished from acquired comedones as well as from familial dyskeratotic comedones.[62]

DILATED PORE

The dilated pore[63] is clinically and histologically a large comedo-like structure that opens directly to the skin surface. Only a few such lesions have been described in detail, but most appear to be found as solitary lesions on the face in men. The upper lip and cheek are common sites.

Histologically, the lesion apparently originates from the follicular infundibulum: the epithelium of the cyst keratinizes in an epidermal mode, with the formation of loose lamellar flaky keratin. The wall is usually hyperplastic with digitate or clavate patterns (Fig. 45–22).

TUMOR OF FOLLICULAR INFUNDIBULUM

Tumors of the follicular infundibulum[64,65] are found as small solitary plaquelike, skin-colored lesions of the face.

The histologic appearance is a fenestrated sheetlike subepidermal proliferation of benign squamous epithelium in continuity with both the epidermis and the upper outer

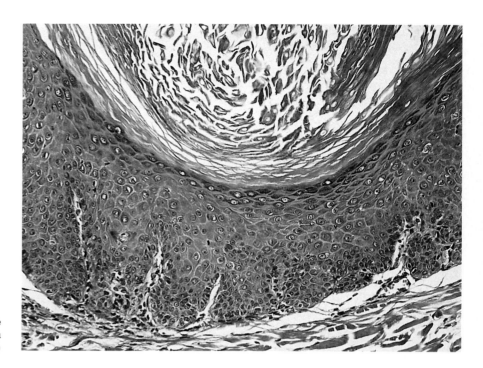

Figure 45–22. Dilated pore: Detail of the deep cystic area shows a digitate hyperplasia with epidermal differentiation. (H&E, ×64.)

hair sheath. This lesion is topographically similar to the multiple superficial basal cell hamartomas with focal follicular differentiation, although tumors of follicular infundibulum characteristically have been single lesions without follicular differentiation.

PILAR SHEATH ACANTHOMA

Pilar sheath acanthoma[66] is a benign follicular hamartoma in which epithelial lobules suggesting infundibular differentiation radiate from a central cystic space in the dermis.

Only a small number of lesions have been described thus far, but there appears to be an unusual predilection for the upper lip. The lesion may clinically simulate a small epidermoid cyst with a prominent epidermal pore. Males and females are about equally involved.

The histologic appearance is a dilated, somewhat flask-shaped cystic lesion that opens directly to the skin surface (Fig. 45–23). The epithelium lining the central cavity differentiates in an epidermal mode. Bulbous epithelial lobules that radiate into adjacent reticular dermis feature a peripheral basal layer and usually some element of tumor-associated adventitia. Abortive hair bulbs are occasionally found as an element of the radiate lobules.

Pilar sheath acanthoma and trichofolliculoma share several clinical and histologic characteristics. It is reasonable to suggest that these two lesions represent a continuum of change in which the differentiating feature is sufficient stromal induction of epithelium to promote recognizable follicular differentiation.

The clinical and histologic differential diagnosis includes trichofolliculoma and dilated pore. Follicular differentiation separates trichofolliculoma (see earlier); the hyperplastic epithelium of the dilated pore may be digitate or clavate but the pilar sheath acanthoma is patterned as radiate lobules.

FIBROFOLLICULOMA

Fibrofolliculoma is a fibroepithelial hamartoma related to the follicular infundibulum.

Inherited as an autosomal dominant trait,[67] fibrofolliculomas appear as small pale or skin-colored, dome-shaped or comedonal papules. They are found mainly on the head, neck, and upper extremities.[67–70] Individual lesions may be scattered or aggregated as sheets or plaques. The age of onset appears to be postadolescence. In two families, some individuals have also had trichodiscomas and acrochordons.[67,69]

Fibrofolliculomas are organized as small, circumscribed, fibroepithelial proliferations. Although usually in the upper reticular dermis, single lesions can be pedunculated. The lesions are follicular and centered, with narrow elongate strands of infundibular epithelium extending as an irregular mantle into the surrounding fibrocellular mesenchyme. The epithelial component may be complex in the three-dimensional aspect with several points of continuity with the infundibulum, whereas adjacent follicles may be involved as well. Small lesions may simply exaggerate mantle hairs with an expanded nodule of follicular adventitia. In fibrofolliculomas described thus far, there has been no apparent inductive effect of the tumor-associated stroma and no secondary follicular structures are formed.

The differential diagnosis includes both the solitary

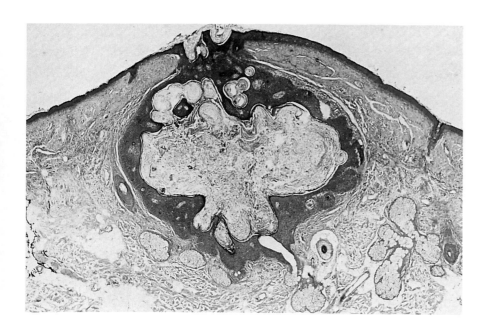

Figure 45–23. Pilar sheath acanthoma. Epithelial lobules radiate from a flask-shaped cystic lesion. Advanced follicular differentiation does not occur. See trichofolliculoma. (H&E, ×8.)

acquired and the multiple familial forms of perifollicular fibromas. Perifollicular fibromas lack the epithelial mantle. A small trichofolliculoma with little or no stromal induction (pilar sheath acanthoma) might simulate fibrofolliculoma, but the latter lacks the central dilated infundibulum.

Histologically, individual lesions are expansile sessile nodules in the papillary dermis composed of loosely aggregated collagenous and elastic fibers in a hyaluronidase-sensitive myxoid matrix. Small vessels may be prominent, and stellate stromal cells with phagocytosed melanin granules have been found. Prominent myelinated nerves and hair follicles are often in close proximity.

REFERENCES

1. Wilson Jones E, Heyl T: Naevus sebaceous. A report of 140 cases with special regard to the development of secondary malignant tumors. *Br J Dermatol* 1970;82:99–117.
2. Mehregan AH, Pinkus H: Life history of organoid nevi. Special reference to nevus sebaceus of Jadassohn. *Arch Dermatol* 1965;91:574–588.
3. Johnson WC, Hookerman BJ: Basal cell hamartoma with follicular differentiation. *Arch Dermatol* 1972;105:105–106.
4. Carney RG: Linear unilateral basal cell nevus with comedones. Report of a case. *Arch Dermatol* 1952;65:571–576.
5. Bleiberg J, Brodkin RH: Linear unilateral basal cell nevus with comedones. *Arch Dermatol* 1969;100:187–190.
6. Anderson TE, Best PV: Linear basal cell nevus. *Br J Dermatol* 1962;74:20–23.
7. Kraus Z, Vortel V: Unilateral indolent basal cell nevus with comedones. *Exp Med Sec XIV Dermatol Venerol* 1961;51:121–124.
8. Mehregan AH, Baker S: Basaloid follicular hamartoma: Three cases with localized and systematized unilateral lesions. *J Cutan Pathol* 1985;12:55–65.
9. Gray HR, Helwig EB: Epithelioma adenoides cysticum and solitary trichoepithelioma. *Arch Dermatol* 1963;87:102–114.
10. Gartler SM, Ziprkowski L, Krakowski A, et al.: Glucose-6-phosphate dehydrogenase mosaicism as a tracer in the study of hereditary multiple trichoepithelioma. *Am J Hum Genet* 1966;18:282–287.
11. Gaul LE: Heredity of multiple benign cystic epithelioma: "The Indiana Family." *Arch Dermatol Syphilol* 1953;68:517–524.
12. Welch JP, Wells RS, Kerr CB: Ancell-Spiegler cylindromas (turban tumors) and Brooke-Fordyce trichoepitheliomas: Evidence for a single genetic entity. *J Med Genet* 1968;5:29–35.
13. Rasmussen JE: A syndrome of trichoepitheliomas, milia and cylindromas. *Arch Dermatol* 1975;111:610–614.
14. Headington JT, Batsakis JG, Beals TF, et al.: Membranous basal cell adenoma of parotid gland, dermal cylindromas, and trichoepitheliomas. Comparative histochemistry and ultrastructure. *Cancer* 1977;39:2460–2469.
15. Reingold IM, Keasbey LA, Graham JH: Multicentric dermal-type cylindromas of the parotid glands in a patient with florid turban tumor. *Cancer* 1977;40:1702–1710.
16. Sandbank M, Bashan D: Multiple trichoepithelioma and breast cancer. *Arch Dermatol* 1978;114:1230.
17. Michaelsson G, Olsson E, Westermark P: The Rombo syndrome: A familial disorder with vermiculate atrophoderma, milia, hypotrichosis, trichoepitheliomas, basal cell carcinomas and peripheral vasodilatation with cyanosis. *Acta Dermatovenereol* 1981;61:497–503.
18. Starink TM, Lane EB, Meijer CJL: Generalized trichoepitheliomas with alopecia and myasthenia gravis: Clinicopathologic and immunohistochemical study and comparison with classic and desmoplastic trichoepithelioma. *J Am Acad Dermatol* 1986;15:1104–1112.
19. Hirone T, Eryu Y, Otsuki N, et al.: Light and electron microscopic studies of trichoepithelioma and papulosum multiplex, in Kobori T, et al. (eds): *The First International Symposium. Biology and Disease of Hair.* Tokyo, University of Tokyo Press, 1975, pp 397–407.
20. Ueda K, Komore Y, Maruo M, et al.: Ultrastructure of trichoepithelioma papulosum multiplex. *J Cutan Pathol* 1981;8:188–198.
21. Ono T, Sakazake Y, Jono M, et al.: Banded structure in solitary trichoepithelioma. *Acta Dermatovenereol* 1981;62:687–692.
22. Brownstein MH, Shapiro L: Desmoplastic trichoepithelioma. *Cancer* 1977;40:2979–2986.

23. Macdonald DM, Wilson Jones E, Marks R: Sclerosing epithelial hamartoma. *Clin Exp Dermatol* 1977;2:153–160.

24. Kallioinen M, Twomi M-L, Dammert K, et al.: Desmoplastic trichoepithelioma: Clinicopathologic features and immunohistochemical study of basement membrane proteins, laminin and type IV collagen. *Br J Dermatol* 1984;111:571–577.

25. Rahbari H, Mehregan A, Pinkus H: Trichoadenoma of Nikolowski. *J Cutan Pathol* 1977;4:90–98.

26. Kligman AM, Pinkus H: The histogenesis of nevoid tumors of the skin: The folliculoma-a hair-follicle tumor. *Arch Dermatol* 1960;81:922–930.

27. Gray FHR, Helwig EB: Trichofolliculoma. *Arch Dermatol* 1962;86:619–625.

28. Plewig G: Sebaceous trichofolliculoma. *J Cutan Pathol* 1980; 7:394–403.

29. Stern JB, Stout DA: Trichofolliculoma showing perineural invasion. *Arch Dermatol* 1979;115:1003–1004.

30. Fessler A: Angeborene Haargeschwulst. *Arch Dermatol Syphilol* 1924;146:411–414.

31. Doxanas MT, Green WR, Arentsen JJ, et al.: Lid lesions of childhood: A histopathologic survey at the Wilmer Institute (1923–1974). *J Pediatr Ophthalmol* 1976;13:7–39.

32. Hendricks WM, Taub S, Hu C-H: Congenital vellus hamartoma. *Cutis* 1981;27:67–68.

33. Brown AC, Crounse RG, Winkelmann RK: Generalized hair-follicle hamartoma. *Arch Dermatol* 1969;99:478–493.

34. Headington JT: Tumors of the hair follicle. A review. *Am J Pathol* 1976;85:480–505.

35. Czernobilsky B: Giant solitary trichoepithelioma. *Arch Dermatol* 1972;105:587–588.

36. Wilson Jones E, Schellander FG: Multifocal pilomatrixoma. Part of a follicular malformation. *Trans St Johns Hosp Dermatol Soc* 1972;58:182–185.

37. Forbis R Jr, Helwig EB: Pilomatrixoma (calcifying epithelioma). *Arch Dermatol* 1961;83:606–618.

38. Booth JC, Kramer H, Taylor KB: Pilomatrixoma: Calcifying epithelioma (Malherbe). *Pathology* 1969;1:119–127.

39. Moehlenbeck FW: Pilomatrixoma (calcifying epithelioma): A statistical study. *Arch Dermatol* 1973;108:532–534.

40. Piffaretti PG, Foroglou G: Syndrome de Gardner. *Schweiz Med Wochenschr* 1965;95:1096–1101.

41. Braillon G, Chapuis H, Boulanger JP: A propos du syndrome de Gardner. *Lyon Chir* 1972;68:382–383.

42. Runne V, Childf E-N, Zentner J: Multiple pilomatrixome als symptom der Myotonia dystrophica Curschmann-Steinert. *Hautarzt* 1982;33:271–275.

43. Guegen MH: [Multiple mummified Malherbe's tumors with hypercalcemia and skull dysostosis.] *Bull Soc Fr Dermatol Syphil* 1969;76:858–859.

44. DeLa Brassinne M, Lachappelle JM: Etude autoradiographique de la synthése des acides nucléique dans l'épithelioma calcifié de Malherbe. *Dermatologica* 1972;144:325–331.

45. Cazers JS, Okun MR, Pearson SH: Pigmented calcifying epithelioma: Review and presentation of a case with unusual features. *Arch Dermatol* 1974;110:773–774.

46. Hashimoto K, Nelson RG, Lever WF: Calcifying epithelioma of Malherbe. Histochemical and electron microscopic studies. *J Invest Dermatol* 1966;46:391–408.

47. Holmes EJ: A histochemical test for citrulline: Adaptation of the carbamido diacetyl reaction to histologic sections with positive results in pilomatrixoma (calcifying epitheliomas). *J Histochem Cytochem* 1968;16:136–146.

48. McGavran MH: Ultrastructure of pilomatrixoma (calcifying epithelioma). *Cancer* 1965;18:1445–1456.

49. Manivel C, Wick MR, Muka K: Pilomatrix carcinoma: An immunohistochemical comparison with benign pilomatrixoma and other benign cutaneous lesions of pilar origin. *J Cutan Pathol* 1986;13:22–29.

50. Mehregan AH, Hardin T: Generalized follicular hamartoma. Complicated by multiple proliferating tricholemmal cysts and palmar pits. *Arch Dermatol* 1973;107:435–438.

51. Brownstein MH, Mehregan AH, Bikowski JB, et al.: The dermatopathology of Cowden's syndrome. *Br J Dermatol* 1979;100:667–673.

52. Brownstein MH, Wolf M, Bikowski JB: Cowden's disease: A cutaneous marker of breast cancer. *Cancer* 1978;41:2393–2398.

53. Brownstein MH, Shapiro L. Tricholemmoma: Analysis of 40 new cases. *Arch Dermatol* 1973;107:866–869.

54. Brownstein MH: Trichilemmal horn: Cutaneous horn showing tricholemmal keratinization. *Br J Dermatol* 1979;100:303–309.

55. Bloch PH, Muller HD. Pilartumor der Kopfhaut. Fallbericht and Studie uber 59 Falle. *Hautarzt* 1979;30:84–88.

56. Batman PA, Evans JHR. Metastasizing pilar tumor of scalp. *J Clin Pathol* 1986;39:757–760.

57. Wilson Jones E. Proliferating epidermoid cysts. *Arch Dermatol* 1966;94:11–19.

58. Reed RJ, Lamar LM: Invasive hair matrix tumors of the scalp: Invasive pilomatrixoma. *Arch Dermatol* 1966;94:310–316.

59. Holmes EJ: Tumors of lower hair sheath: Common histogenesis of certain so-called "sebaceous cysts," acanthomas and "sebaceous carcinomas." *Cancer* 1968;21:234–248.

60. Dabska M: Giant hair matrix tumor. *Cancer* 1971;28:701–706.

61. Nabai H, Mehregan AH: Nevus comedonicus. A review of the literature and report of twelve cases. *Acta Dermatol Venereol* 1973;53:71–74.

62. Carneiro SJC, Dickson J, Knox J. Familial dyskeratotic comedones. *Arch Dermatol* 1972;105:249–251.

63. Winer LH: The dilated pore, a trichoepithelioma. *J Invest Dermatol* 1954;23:181–188.

64. Mehregan AH, Butler JD: A tumor of follicular infundibulum: Report of a case. *Arch Dermatol* 1961;83:924–927.

65. Mehregan AH: Tumor of follicular infundibulum. *Dermatologica* 1971;142:177–183.

66. Mehregan AH, Brownstein MH: Pilar sheath acanthoma. *Arch Dermatol* 1978;114:1495–1497.

67. Birt AR, Hogg GR, Dube WJ: Hereditary multiple fibrofolliculomas with trichodiscomas and acrochordons. *Arch Dermatol* 1977;113:1674–1677.

68. Weintraub R, Pinkus H: Multiple fibrofolliculomas (Birt-Hogg-Dube) associated with a large connective tissue nevus. *J Cutan Pathol* 1977;4:289–299.

69. Fujita WH, Barr RJ, Headley JL: Multiple fibrofolliculomas with trichodiscomas and acrochordons. *Arch Dermatol* 1981;117:32–35.

70. Foucar K, Rosen T, Foucar E, et al.: Fibrofolliculoma. A clinicopathologic study. *Cutis* 1981;28:429–432.

CHAPTER 46

Tumors of Sebaceous Gland Differentiation

Walter H. C. Burgdorf

Sebaceous neoplasms share many features with the normal sebaceous gland. They typically arise in association with hair follicles, have a lobular pattern, and progress from basaloid peripheral cells to central foamy lipid-rich cells that decay, emptying into a central duct. Sebaceous neoplasms are categorized on the basis of their similarity to the normal sebaceous gland. As the growths deviate from the norm, they tend to be biologically more aggressive and histologically more difficult to identify. Figure 46–1 is a "shadow" depiction of the main variants of sebaceous neoplasms, which, in addition to a normal sebaceous gland, include the following:

- *Sebaceous adenoma:* Normal sebaceous structure with basaloid periphery less than two to three cells thick; more than 50% of cells are foamy.
- *Sebaceous epithelioma:* More than 50% of cells are basaloid; some loss of lobular structure.
- *Sebaceous carcinoma:* Cytologic atypia and pleomorphism, mitoses present, loss of lobular pattern.

History

The watershed paper in cutaneous sebaceous proliferations is that of Rulon and Helwig.[1] They proposed a widely used classification identical to the preceding scheme, except that "sebaceous epithelioma" was replaced by "basal cell carcinoma with sebaceous differentiation." Although both terms are acceptable, I prefer sebaceous epithelioma because the alternate term is also used to describe typical basal cell carcinomas with focal sebaceous change. Several older reviews are still valuable sources of clinical and microscopic information; unfortunately, their utility is clouded by highly variable terminology.[2–6]

Identification

Modern histochemical staining techniques have added little to the identification of sebaceous proliferations, especially those that are poorly differentiated and/or are processed by formalin fixation and paraffin embedding. The following approaches are available.

Fat Stains. If frozen tissue or formalin-fixed, unembedded tissue can be obtained, a fat stain such as oil-red-O or Sudan IV can be used to identify lipid in the cytoplasm of sebaceous cells.

PAS Stain With and Without Diastase. Sebaceous tumors typically lack glycogen, whereas metastatic renal cell carcinomas and clear cell eccrine tumors are variably positive for glycogen.

Mucicarmine and PAS With Diastase. These stains may help separate metastatic adenocarcinomas, which often contain mucin, from sebaceous tumors, which do not. Some adenocarcinomas, such as those arising in the kidney and prostate, are often mucicarmine negative, so this stain has limited utility.

Immunohistochemical Studies. No antibody clearly identifies sebaceous cells to the exclusion of other tumors. Anticytokeratin and antiepithelial membrane antibody stains may separate poorly differentiated sebaceous growths from mesenchymal and hematopoietic malignancies. An S100 antibody may be helpful in separating malignant melanoma from sebaceous carcinoma; the former is generally positive, the latter negative.

Electron Microscopy. If properly fixed tissue is available, intracytoplasmic lipids can be seen, confirming the identity of sebaceous cells. It is evident that light microscopic examination of hematoxylin and eosin-stained sections of tissue remains the mainstay for diagnosing sebaceous lesions.

In evaluating a tumor suspected of being sebaceous in origin, particular attention should be paid to the following points.

Appreciation of Basic Anatomy. Most sebaceous proliferations can be correlated with part of the normal sebaceous apparatus. In addition, an appreciation of normal anatomy in other animals may be helpful. For example, dog anal glands typically have mixed apocrine and sebaceous compo-

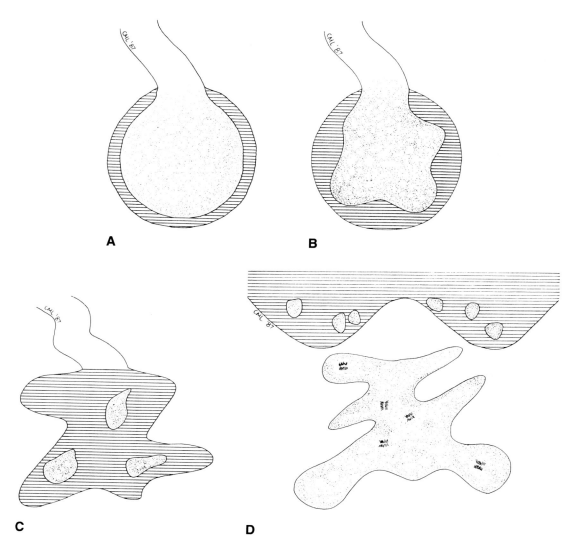

Figure 46–1. Diagrammatic representation of the different types of sebaceous proliferations. **A.** Normal sebaceous gland with two to three layers of basaloid cells at periphery and central foamy cells in a uniform lobule emptying into a duct. **B.** Sebaceous adenoma with more basaloid cells, some loss of structure, but still a lobular pattern duct. **C.** Sebaceous epithelioma. More than 50% of the cells are basaloid. There are still islands of sebaceous differentiation. The lobular pattern is more irregular but there is often a ductal connection. **D.** Sebaceous carcinoma. There is cytologic atypia, including occasional mitoses with loss of a lobular pattern and often loss of a ductal connection. There may be intraepidermal spread of sebaceous cells. (Illustrations by Curt M. Littler, M.D., San Diego, California.)

nents, as do some human adnexal proliferations. Similarly, avian epidermis contains sebokeratinocytes; perhaps not all sebaceous cells in the epidermis represent spread from a gland; some may be normal.[7]

Pattern. A lobular configuration suggests benign behavior, whereas an infiltrative pattern is more worrisome.

Differentiation. Both the ratio of basaloid to foamy cells and their distribution peripherally and centrally are helpful. Generally, the basaloid cells should be peripheral and not more than two to three cell layers thick.

Follicular Orientation. All but the most poorly differentiated sebaceous neoplasms show some follicular inclination.

Manifestations may include central necrosis (also known as comedo formation), duct formation, and focal keratinization.

Intraepidermal Spread. Sebaceous carcinomas of the eyelid are particularly likely to spread intraepidermally in a pagetoid fashion; this feature should be searched for in neoplasms of possible sebaceous origin.

Cytologic Atypia. Cytologic atypia remains the gold standard for identification of sebaceous carcinoma; mitoses can be found in the peripheral or basaloid areas of many sebaceous proliferations. More central or abnormal mitoses, multiple nucleoli, and variation in cell size and shape are all useful clues.

MUCOSAL SEBACEOUS GROWTHS

Normal sebaceous glands can be seen as tiny yellow papules on the lips (Fordyce spots), mucosal surface of eyelids (Meibomian gland), genitalia, and nipples (Montgomery's tubercles). The nodules occasionally become inflamed, but otherwise are asymptomatic. On histologic examination, all show an identical picture, with sebaceous lobules feeding a central duct that opens onto a mucosal surface (Fig. 46–2). Adjacent structures may give a clue as to the site of biopsy, i.e., interweaving muscle from lip, smooth muscle from nipple. The only "abnormal" features are mucosal epithelium and lack of associated hair follicles; the glands themselves are entirely normal.

SEBACEOUS HYPERPLASIA

Sebaceous hyperplasia (unfortunately designated senile sebaceous hyperplasia) is a common finding far before the onset of senility. Clinicians easily recognize the tiny yellow papules grouped about a follicular opening. Lesions may be removed for cosmetic reasons, because of extreme size, or rarely because of lack of familiarity with the clinical entity. Histologically, sebaceous hyperplasia is a straightforward diagnosis. Numerous sebaceous glands are arranged around a central follicle. There is little if any variation in either pattern of cytology; instead, there are simply too many normal glands for the central, single follicle (Fig. 46–3).

SEBACEOUS ADENOMA

Sebaceous adenoma has few clinically distinctive features. Tumors are usually dermal nodules and less likely to have the distinct yellow color of sebaceous hyperplasia. Microscopically, an almost normal sebaceous gland is found with a lobular pattern, but often with a less clear relation to hair follicles. The basaloid zone may be three to four layers thick, but less than 50% of cells are basaloid and the rest are clear cells with varying degrees of duct formation and keratinization (Fig. 46–4). In one scheme,[8] sebaceous adenomas were subclassified into three types: solid or lobular, cystic or "comedo," and keratoacanthoma-like. Although the subdivision is perhaps unnecessary, it emphasizes the relationship of the adenomas to normal structures, with solid tumors resembling the sebaceous gland; cystic, the duct; and keratoacanthoma-like, the follicle opening.

SEBACEOUS EPITHELIOMA

Clinically, sebaceous epithelioma presents as a papule or nodule, most often on the head or neck. It is unlikely to

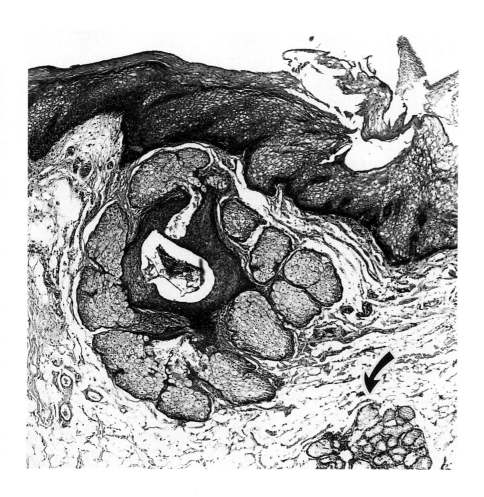

Figure 46–2. Fordyce gland. Normal sebaceous glands are arranged around a central follicle. The overlying mucosa with acanthosis with focal parakeratosis, the absence of other appendages, and the minor salivary gland (arrow) suggest that the tissue is from the oral mucosa. (H&E, ×40.)

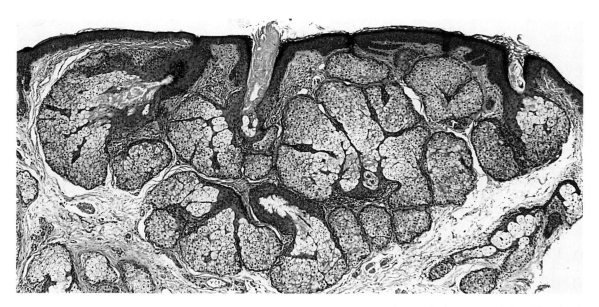

Figure 46–3. Sebaceous hyperplasia. Numerous sebaceous glands are grouped around a large central duct. The glands themselves are entirely normal. The duct is rather large and has too many glands for a normal hair follicle. (H&E, ×60.)

have the yellowish color of better differentiated sebaceous neoplasms. Histologically, the lesions are predominantly basaloid but still may be lobular. They are dominated by basaloid cells, and may have only small foci of clear cells[9] (Figs. 46–5, 46–6). They lack features of an ordinary basal cell carcinoma, such as peripheral palisading or clefting.

SEBACEOUS CARCINOMA

Sebaceous carcinoma[10] is generally divided into two subtypes based on site: ocular and extraocular. The ocular le-

sions are far more common, arising primarily in the eyelid, but also involving other ocular adnexa. Several types of sebaceous glands are seen in eyelids: (1) on the inner surface, the Meibomian glands empty onto the mucosal surface; (2) the glands of Zeis are associated with eyelash follicles; and (3) other glands are associated with the fine hairs of the outer eyelid. The eyebrows, of course, also have sebaceous glands. Nonocular sebaceous carcinoma may arise anywhere where sebaceous glands and hair are found; thus, the distribution is widespread but favors the head and neck.[11–13]

Clinically, the ocular lesions are frequently misdiag-

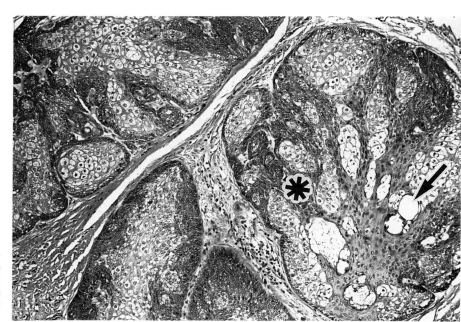

Figure 46–4. Sebaceous adenoma. The basaloid layer is frequently more than three cells thick and there are strands of basaloid cells across the entire section (*). There is also duct formation (arrow). Normal foamy cells can still be seen. (H&E, ×125.)

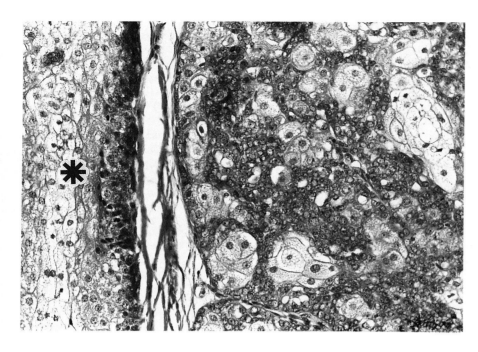

Figure 46–5. Sebaceous epithelioma. On the left is a normal sebaceous gland (*); on the right is a sebaceous epithelioma showing widely dispersed clear cells with some cytologic atypia and with greater than 50% basaloid cells not confined to the periphery. (H&E, ×400.)

nosed as chalazions, as well as a variety of tumors. The nonocular lesions are generally described simply as a mass or nodule with no unique features.[14] Both lesions are aggressive with a significant risk of local recurrence exceeding 33%, coupled with lower risks of metastatic disease (15% to 33%) and death (less than 10%). All these parameters have markedly improved in the past decade, presumably because of earlier and more accurate recognition.[15]

Sebaceous carcinomas must be identified as sebaceous on the basis of the preceding criteria and as carcinoma by cellular atypia. Both the degree of differentiation and the degree of infiltration (Figs. 46–7, 46–8) have some predictive value in assessing metastasis and recurrence. A unique histologic feature of eyelid sebaceous carcinomas is pagetoid or intraepidermal spread of atypical foamy sebocytes[16] (Figs. 46–9, 46–10). In some series, more than 75% of ocular sebaceous carcinomas show this feature; it is much less common in extraocular lesions but does occur.

When sebaceous carcinomas are primarily basaloid, they have been designated "small cell variant"[1] and fall into the differential of small blue tumors in the skin, to include neuroendocrine (Merkel cell or trabecular) carci-

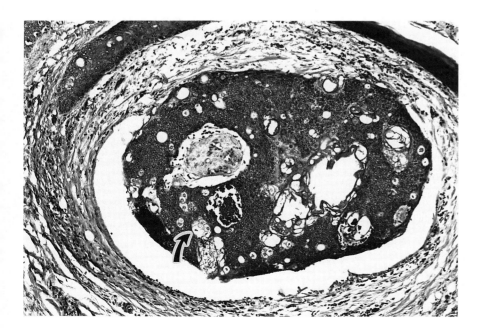

Figure 46–6. An almost exclusively basaloid sebaceous proliferation. Only occasional foamy cells are seen (arrow). In some terminologies this would be called a sebaceoma. (H&E, ×125.)

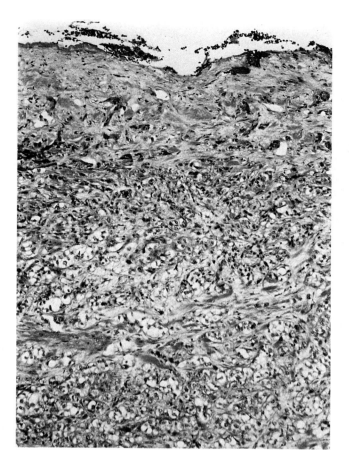

Figure 46–7. Sebaceous carcinoma. A pleomorphic infiltrate extends between strands of collagen, much as might be seen in a metastatic tumor. Even at low power, the cells are shown to be clear cell in nature, but there is no evidence of a follicular orientation or of a lobular structure. This tumor arose on the skin of a forehead. (H&E, ×125.)

noma, metastatic neuroendocrine tumor, basal cell carcinoma, and hematopoietic infiltrates. Lipid-rich cells are hard to identify except by ultrastructure (Fig. 46–11).

MISCELLANEOUS SEBACEOUS PROLIFERATIONS

Several other less common but perhaps distinct sebaceous lesions have been identified. If the more standard sebaceous neoplasms are visualized as variations on the lobular sebaceous gland, the following growths can be best perceived as arising more exclusively from the ductal and infrafollicular part of the sebaceous apparatus.

Infundibular Adenoma. In a survey of 68 inverted follicular keratoses, six with sebaceous and apocrine differentiation were identified.[17] Presumably the sebaceous and apocrine ducts give rise to these elements, amidst the basaloid follicular proliferation, although sebocytes can occur in any epidermis, independent of follicles. Many observers might include such tumors as inverted follicular keratoses without further subdivision.

Mixed Sebaceous–Apocrine Adenoma. A single tumor with poroma-like features but showing both apocrine and sebaceous areas has been described.[18] This lesion from the abdomen of a middle-aged female most resembled an eccrine poroma with broad lobules and a sharp dividing line between normal and neoplastic growth. In the lobules there were both sebaceous elements and "canaliculi" with apocrine-like areas.

Superficial Epithelioma With Sebaceous Differentiation. A benign superficial basaloid proliferation, superficial epithelioma with sebaceous differentiation is characterized by a platelike proliferation in the papillary dermis with broad

Figure 46–8. Sebaceous carcinoma. This pleomorphic, non-ocular sebaceous carcinoma demonstrates a wide variation in cytologic size and shape and an infiltrated pattern, with little to suggest that it is sebaceous in origin except for the numerous foamy cells. (arrow) (H&E, ×400.)

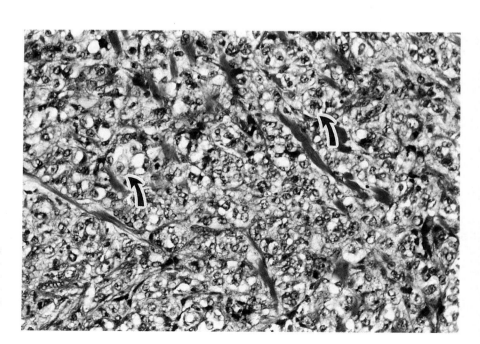

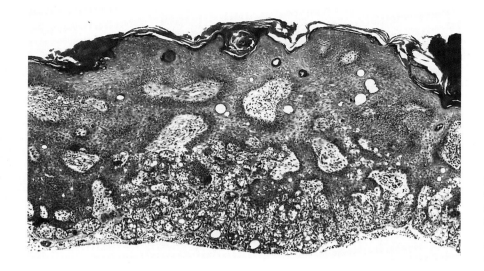

Figure 46–9. Sebaceous carcinoma on the eyelid. Sections from an eyelid tumor show a foamy proliferation impinging on the epidermis with intraepidermal spread of clear cells. (H&E, ×40.) (*Histologic material courtesy of W. Richard Green, M.D., Baltimore, Maryland.*)

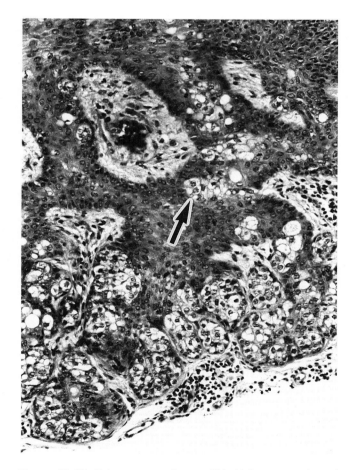

Figure 46–10. Sebaceous carcinoma. This higher-power view of Fig. 46–9 shows atypical clear cell proliferation at the base with intraepidermal spread (arrow) (H&E, ×400.) (*Histologic material courtesy of W. Richard Green, M.D., Baltimore, Maryland.*)

areas of attachment to the epidermis.[19,20] Focal accumulations of sebaceous cells are seen (Fig. 46–12). This lesion is most analogous to an infundibular sebaceous adenoma; the plate is reminiscent of hair follicle infundibular tumors. Although the name implies overlap with superficial basal cell carcinoma (epithelioma), the main similarity is the plate-like epidermal attachment. The lesions are nonaggressive.

Sebaceous Trichofolliculoma. Trichofolliculomas from sebaceous-rich areas may have a striking sebaceous component.[21] These tumors may be a variant of dorsal nasal cysts with follicular proliferation and normal sebaceous glands.[22,23]

The age-old lumper-vs-splitter question has always been applicable to sebaceous growths. My view is that sebaceous adenoma, sebaceous epithelioma, and sebaceous carcinoma allows identification of the vast bulk of solitary proliferations. There is striking variation between lobules of a single sebaceous proliferation, so efforts should be concentrated on not missing a sebaceous carcinoma that requires more radical surgical intervention than its benign counterparts.

MULTIPLE SEBACEOUS TUMORS

For patients with multiple sebaceous neoplasms, the utility of histologic classification lessens. Nonetheless, tumors from these patients are most important to identify, because they may be the first marker of an internal malignancy. Torre[24] and Muir et al.[25] almost simultaneously described individuals with multiple sebaceous neoplasms, multiple keratoacanthomas, and multiple internal malignancies. Such patients have been identified as having Torre syndrome, Muir syndrome, or permutations thereof.[26–29]

A number of generalizations can be made about the

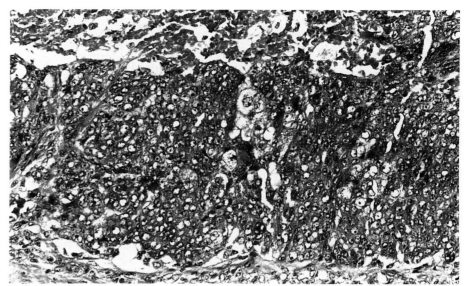

Figure 46–11. Sebaceous carcinoma. This murky small cell variant of sebaceous carcinoma has no unique features except for an occasional large clear cell amidst a background of small blue nondescript cells. (H&E, ×125.)

Torre syndrome. First, skin findings precede internal malignancies in about half the patients. Second, there is often a striking family history of cancer. In two cancer family syndrome pedigrees, patients with multiple sebaceous neoplasms and multiple keratoacanthomas have been found,[30,31] suggesting that the phenotype of multiple sebaceous neoplasms may be a part of the cancer family syndrome. Third, patients with Torre syndrome tend to have multiple internal malignancies, developing them at an early age, but having a far longer survival than control patients with similar sporadic tumors. Gastrointestinal carcinomas are most frequent, with pulmonary and genitourinary tumors also common.

Sebaceous growths from patients with Torre syndrome create two problems for a dermatopathologist: (1) The histologic appearance often does not fit the accepted categories.

(2) The correlation between histologic picture and clinical behavior is less reliable than in sporadic lesions. For example, a wide variety of unusual cystic structures, peculiar overlaps between follicular and sebaceous growths, and striking intralesional variation have been described in Torre syndrome patients.[32]

Several other interesting situations arise. In one review, three cases of Torre syndrome were described in which a single sebaceous carcinoma was associated with internal malignancy. It is unclear if these patients are correctly identified as Torre-Muir syndrome, but one should be aware of a possible association, even with a single tumor.[33] Finally, Torre syndrome has been described in a patient with a difficult-to-manage and difficult-to-characterize sebaceous lesion of the eyelid.[34]

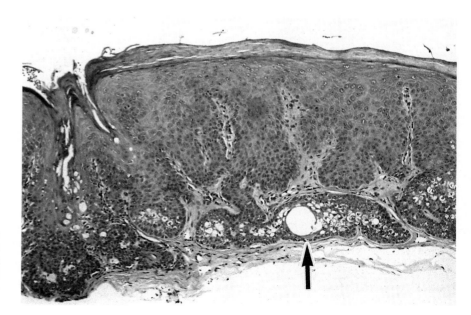

Figure 46–12. Superficial epithelioma with sebaceous differentiation. There is a platelike proliferation just beneath the epidermis that is rich in foamy cells (arrow). (H&E, ×125.) (*Histologic material courtesy of Kenneth J. Friedman, MD, Baltimore, Maryland.*)

SEBACEOUS MISTAKES

At least three lesions are almost always mistakenly called "sebaceous" proliferations. A "sebaceous cyst" is a keratinous or epidermoid cyst, with no sebaceous glands in its wall; it, as well as the true sebaceous cysts (steatocystoma and dermoid), are covered in Chapter 41. Nevus sebaceous is an organoid or hamartomatous growth, reflecting excessive proliferation of many epithelial elements in addition to sebaceous glands. Finally, adenoma sebaceum is an angiofibroma amidst the rich sebaceous gland background of the nasolabial fold in tuberous sclerosis patients.

The differential diagnosis of sebaceous proliferations takes many forms.

When a lobular proliferation with foamy cells is present, the main problems is the overlaps between normal and adenoma, adenoma and epithelioma, and, rarely, epithelioma and carcinoma. Only the latter distinction is crucial, and then one should rely on cytologic atypia and infiltrative pattern.

With intraepidermal clear cells, especially on the eyelid, sebaceous carcinoma must be separated from squamous cell carcinoma in situ, pagetoid malignant melanoma, and extramammary Paget's disease. Identification of lipids is most discriminating.

For small blue cell tumors, the differential here is legion; if focal sebaceous areas are not found, ultrastructure is usually needed to show intracellular lipids or glycogen.

In malignant clear cell tumors, when a sebaceous carcinoma lacks a lobular pattern and is dominated by clear cells, the differential includes metastatic adenocarcinoma, clear cell squamous cell carcinoma, malignant melanoma, and eccrine carcinoma.[35] Identification of lipids as discussed under special stains, coupled with a thorough history and knowledge of other primary tumors, should resolve this issue.

REFERENCES

1. Rulon DB, Helwig EB: Cutaneous sebaceous neoplasms. *Cancer* 1974;33:82–102.
2. Warren S, Warvi WN: Tumors of sebaceous glands. *Am J Pathol* 1943;19:441–459.
3. Urban FH, Winkelmann RK: Sebaceous malignancy. *Arch Dermatol* 1961;84:113–122.
4. Zackheim HS: The sebaceous epithelioma: A clinical and histologic study. *Arch Dermatol* 1964;89:711–724.
5. Miller RE, White JJ Jr: Sebaceous gland carcinoma. *Am J Surg* 1967;114:958–961.
6. Holmes EJ: Tumors of lower hair sheath. *Cancer* 1968;21:234–248.
7. Wrench R, Hardy JA, Spearman RIC: Sebokeratocytes of avian epidermis—With mammalian comparisons, in Spearman RIC, Riley PA (eds): *The Skin of Vertebrates*. London, Academic Press, 1978, pp 47–56.
8. Banse-Kupin L, Morales A, Barlow M: Torre's syndrome: Report of two cases and review of the literature. *J Am Acad Dermatol* 1984;10:803–817.
9. Troy JL, Ackerman AB: Sebaceoma: A distinctive benign neoplasm of adnexal epithelium differentiating toward sebaceous cells. *Am J Dermatopathol* 1984;6:7–13.
10. Wolfe JT, Wick MR, Campbell RJ: Sebaceous carcinoma of the oculocutaneous adnexa and extraocular skin, in Wick MR (ed): *Pathology of Unusual Malignant Cutaneous Tumors*. New York, Marcel Dekker, 1985, pp. 77–106.
11. Pricolo VE, Rodil JV, Vezeridis MP: Extraorbital sebaceous carcinoma. *Arch Surg* 1985;120:853–855.
12. Wick MR, Goellner JR, Wolfe JT, et al.: Adnexal carcinomas of the skin. II. Extraocular sebaceous carcinomas. *Cancer* 1985;56:1163–1172.
13. Graham RM, McKee PH, McGibbon D: Sebaceous carcinoma. *Clin Exp Dermatol* 1984;9:466–471.
14. Wolfe JT, Campbell RJ, Yeatts RP, et al.: Sebaceous carcinoma of the eyelid: Errors in clinical and pathologic diagnosis. *Am J Surg Pathol* 1984;8:597–606.
15. Doxanas MT, Green WR: Sebaceous gland carcinoma: Review of 40 cases. *Arch Ophthalmol* 1984;102:245–249.
16. Russell WG, Page DL, Hough AJ, et al.: Sebaceous carcinoma of meibomian gland origin: The diagnostic importance of pagetoid spread of neoplastic cells. *Am J Clin Pathol* 1980;73:504–511.
17. Grosshans E, Hanau D: L'adenome infundibulaire: Un porome folliculaire a differenciation sebacee et apocrine. *Ann Dermatol Venereol (Paris)* 1981;108:59–66.
18. Hanau D, Grosshans E, Laplanche G: A complex poroma-like adnexal adenoma. *Am J Dermatopathol* 1984;6:567–572.
19. Rothko K, Farmer ER, Zeligman I: Superficial epithelioma with sebaceous differentiation. *Arch Dermatol* 1980;116:329–331.
20. Friedman KJ, Boudreau S, Farmer ER: Superficial epithelioma with sebaceous differentiation. *J Cutan Pathol* 1987;14:193–197.
21. Plewig G: Sebaceous trichofolliculoma. *J Cutan Pathol* 1980;7:394–403.
22. Silva LGE: Tricofoliculoma sebaceo. *Med Cut ILA* 1982;10:51–54.
23. Brownstein MH, Shapiro L, Slevin R: Fistula of the dorsum of the nose. *Arch Dermatol* 1974;109:227–229.
24. Torre D: Multiple sebaceous tumors. *Arch Dermatol* 1968;98:549–551.
25. Muir EG, Yates Bell AJ, Barlow KA: Multiple primary carcinomata of the colon, duodenum, and larynx associated with kerato-acanthomata of the face. *Br J Surg* 1967;54:191–195.
26. Rulon DB, Helwig EB: Multiple sebaceous neoplasms of the skin: An association with multiple visceral carcinomas, especially of the colon. *Am J Clin Pathol* 1973;60:745–753.
27. Housholder MS, Zeligman I: Sebaceous neoplasms associated with visceral carcinomas. *Arch Dermatol* 1980;116:61–64.
28. Fahmy A, Burgdorf WHC, Schosser RH, et al.: Muir-Torre syndrome: Report of a case and reevaluation of the dermatopathologic features. *Cancer* 1982;49:1898–1903.
29. Finan MC, Connolly SM: Sebaceous gland tumors and systemic disease: A clinicopathologic analysis. *Medicine* 1984;63:232–242.
30. Lynch HT, Lynch PM, Pester J, et al.: The cancer family syndrome: Rare cutaneous phenotypic linkage of Torre's syndrome. *Arch Intern Med* 1981;141:607–611.
31. Anderson DE: An inherited form of large bowel cancer: Muir's syndrome. *Cancer* 1980;45:1103–1107.
32. Burgdorf WHC, Pitha J, Fahmy A: Muir-Torre syndrome. Histologic spectrum of sebaceous proliferations. *Am J Dermatopathol* 1986;8(3):202–208.
33. Graham R, McKee P, McGibbon D, et al.: Torre-Muir syndrome: An association with isolated sebaceous carcinoma. *Cancer* 1985;55:2868–2873.
34. Jakobiec FA: Sebaceous adenoma of the eyelid and visceral malignancy. *Am J Ophthalmol* 1974;78:952–960.
35. Kuo T: Clear cell carcinoma of the skin: A variant of the squamous cell carcinoma that stimulates sebaceous carcinoma. *Am J Surg Pathol* 1980;4:573–583.

CHAPTER 47
Tumors of Sweat Gland Differentiation

Daniel J. Santa Cruz

Adnexal neoplasms, in general, and sweat gland neoplasms, in particular, exhibit wide and overlapping histologic variation. Sweat gland neoplasms have traditionally been rigorously classified as either eccrine or apocrine; however, to better represent the entire spectrum of their differentiation these neoplasms should be classified as follows:

• *Secretory:* Containing either eccrine and apocrine differentiation
• *Myoepithelial:* A poorly documented form, and often only as a partial component of adnexal tumors
• *Ductal:* The most common type

In fact, with the possible exceptions of mucinous carcinoma and papillary eccrine adenoma, all of the "eccrine" tumors display ductal differentiation. It is not possible to distinguish between apocrine and eccrine ducts, other than the anatomic relation to hair follicles observed in apocrine ducts. Some neoplasms defy classification, for example, dermal cylindroma, and are, by convention, placed in the chapter on sweat gland tumors. Others express multidirectional differentiation toward more than one adnexal structure, as seen in mixed tumors.

Most adnexal neoplasms are benign (Table 47–1). Sweat gland carcinomas are rare and offer a similar complex spectrum of their benign counterparts. No single diagnostic criterion differentiates the benign and malignant forms. The usual criteria of malignancy, i.e., infiltrative growth, necrosis, nuclear atypia, and high mitotic rate, are useful but not always reliable markers. Thus, mitotic figures may be seen with some frequency in adenomas and be rare in some variants of carcinomas.[1] On the other hand, there is a rare but definite malignant potential in some sweat gland adenomas;[2,3] this is often heralded by an abrupt growth in a long-standing stable tumor.

ECCRINE NEVI AND MALFORMATIONS

Malformations of eccrine sweat glands are both rare and varied.[4] Goldstein reported a patient with hiperhidrosis in a localized area of skin in which the eccrine glands were morphologically normal but hyperplastic.[5] Pippione et al. described a 32-year-old woman with a congenital lesion that histologically consisted of solid cords and immature glands; they termed this malformation an *eccrine nevus.*[6] In their textbook, Pinkus and Mehregan reported by the same name a lesion with an increased number of histologically normal sweat gland coils.[7]

Several curious combinations of angiomatous and sweat gland proliferations have been reported. Some of these contained other hamartomatous anomalies as well, and some presented with hyperhidrosis.[8–11]

Abell and Read reported an interesting case of hamartomatous sweat ducts in a 3-year-old child who presented with a warty lesion on the sole of one foot. Histologic examination revealed dilation of the upper part of the eccrine sweat ducts with thick cornoid lamallae in the central portion.[12] Marsden et al. described a lesion they called a comedo nevus.[13] Histologically, it consisted of widely dilated eccrine sweat ducts filled with parakeratotic keratin. Leppard and Marks reported similar cases.[14]

A curious lesion described as acrosyringeal nevus was reported by Weedon and Lewis.[15] The lesion presented as a verrucous plaque composed of poroma-like cells that formed an interconnecting network between the undersurface of the epidermis and adjacent sweat ducts.

ECCRINE HIDROCYSTOMA

Hidrocystomas are commonly single cystic lesions localized most commonly on the face. There is a slight female prevalence.[16]

Hidrocystomas have classically been divided into eccrine and apocrine types based on their cyst linings. The eccrine type is lined by one or two rows of flat cuboidal epithelium (Fig. 47–1). The apocrine form, in contrast, is lined by an outer layer of myoepithelial cells and an inner layer of secretory apocrine cells. The entire lesion has the appearance of dilated, often multilocular, sweat glands.

TABLE 47–1. BENIGN SWEAT GLAND TUMORS

Eccrine tumors

Eccrine nevi and malformations
Eccrine hidrocystoma
Eccrine acrospiroma
    Intraepidermal (hidroacanthoma simplex)
    Juxtaepidermal (eccrine poroma)
    Intradermal
        Cystic acrospiroma
        Solid or solid cystic acrospiroma (nodular hidradenoma)
        Clear cell acrospiroma
        Acrospiroma with small nodules (dermal duct tumor)
        Pigmented acrospiroma
        Acrospiroma with features of an eccrine poroma
Syringoma
Eccrine spiradenoma
Cylindroma
Mixed tumor (chondroid syringoma)
Papillary eccrine adenoma

Apocrine tumors

Apocrine nevus
Apocrine cystadenoma
Papillary hidradenoma
Tubular apocrine adenoma
Papillary syringoadenoma
Nipple adenomatosis

The so-called eccrine variant sometimes coexists with an apocrine component, and the observer is left with the impression that the eccrine hidrocystoma is a proliferative change of the sweat duct and not of the secretory epithelium.[17] To avoid futile subclassification attempts, the simple name of *hidrocystoma* may be more fitting.[18,19]

ECCRINE ACROSPIROMA

Johnson and Helwig coined the term *eccrine acrospiroma* to describe a distinctive clinicopathologic but morphologically

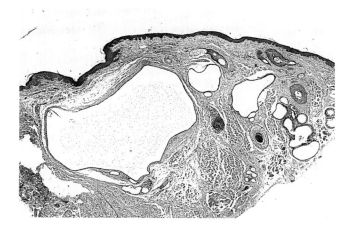

Figure 47–1. Eccrine hidrocystoma. Multiple thin-lined cysts appear to connect with the eccrine glands below.

complex group of neoplasms showing what they believed was differentiation toward the distal (ductal) part of the sweat gland.[20] By extension of this concept, there are three tumor subtypes of eccrine acrospiroma, each of which has a distinctive but sometimes variable histologic pattern: (1) intraepidermal (hidroacanthoma simplex); (2) juxtaepidermal (eccrine poroma); and (3) intradermal (dermal ductal tumor, nodular hidradenoma). The name *acrospiroma* is sometimes used only for the third subtype. Frequently, a neoplasm has features of more than one subtype, which makes precise classification impossible.

Intraepidermal Acrospiroma (Hidroacanthoma Simplex)

History

A highly controversial neoplasm, intraepidermal acrospiroma was first described by Smith and Coburn in 1956 as hidroacanthoma simplex.[21] The term *intraepidermal epithelioma of Borst-Jadassohn* (or simply Jadassohn) was used previously to describe a variety of lesions that had in common the development of basaloid nests of cells within the epidermis. These included a variety of conditions ranging from squamous cell carcinoma to seborrheic keratosis.[22,23] Smith and Coburn also concurrently described a lesion that they named *plane variety*; however, this lesion differs histologically from the current concept of hidroacanthoma simplex.[21]

Holubar and Wolff, on the basis of enzyme histochemical studies, concluded that this tumor had eccrine differentiation and renamed it intraepidermal eccrine poroma.[24]

Cook and Ridgway attempted to revive the concept of Jadassohn's epithelioma and described 40 cases of their own. Invasive growth was present in five cases, and one metastasized.[25] The interpretation, however, has been strongly contested.[26,27]

Clinical Features

The lesions of hidroacanthoma simplex are usually flat or slightly elevated, irregularly verrucous plaques with a brown decoloration and a greasy appearance, resembling flat seborrheic keratoses.[28] They are more commonly present in older women, on the lower extremities.

Histologic Features

The histology of hidroacanthoma simplex is confusing, primarily because of the controversy of what should be included under this name. We prefer to follow Smith and Coburn's original description.[21]

The lesions of hidroacanthoma simplex are flat superficial lesions located in an acanthotic, hyperkeratotic, and sometimes verrucous epidermis. Within the epidermis, there are rounded masses of small basaloid cells which are often situated in the lower part and bulge into the dermis (Fig. 47–2). Eccrine poromas and lesions described as poroepitheliomas occasionally have similar intraepidermal nests. Occasionally, the nests are higher in the epidermis and produce lenticular accumulations of parakeratotic keratin. Larger nodules have a central cavity containing an amorphous proteinaceous content. Mitoses are rare. Sweat ducts lose their identifying features as they enter

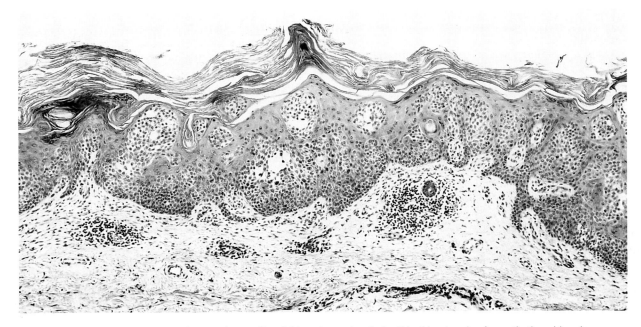

Figure 47–2. Intraepidermal acrospiroma. Basaloid nests are located within thin strands of acanthotic epidermis.

and merge with these tumors. The tumor cells are strongly PAS-positive and diastase labile, indicating the presence of abundant intracytoplasmic glycogen.[29]

The tumor cells are similar by electron microscopy to those of the eccrine poroma and contain large amounts of cytoplasmic glycogen. They also have a ring-shaped perinuclear distribution of tonofilaments and underdeveloped desmosomes. Melanocytes have been found among tumor cells.[30]

Histogenesis

Although the histogenesis and differentiation of many adnexal tumors are controversial, there is considerable controversy as to whether hidroacanthoma simplex is an adnexal neoplasm at all.[22,23,29–32] Because of its morphologic spectrum with lesions of eccrine poroma and acrospiromas, an intraepidermal duct origin for hidroacanthoma simplex is likely.[35,36] Certainly, intraepidermal basaloid nests are found in conditions other than hidroacanthoma simplex. Carcinoma in situ of the skin sometimes can have such a growth pattern,[22,23,33] and the controversy would be compounded if a malignant form of hidroacanthoma simplex were accepted.[34]

The question also arises as to whether hidroacanthoma simplex is a form of seborrheic keratosis, a condition that it resembles both clinically and histologically.[32] Histogenetically, both are epidermal tumors.

We believe there is enough evidence to support a poral, sweat gland differentiation for the hidroacanthoma simplex. Other lesions with intraepidermal nesting enter into the differential diagnosis.[23,37]

Most lesions of hidroacanthoma simplex have a benign course. It is unclear exactly how many are or become malignant, as there is so much confusion in the literature as to what actually constitutes this lesion. Depending on which entities are included under this name, the prognosis varies. Poroepitheliomas, which belong to the group of acrospiromas, have a good prognosis.[38,39] Those classified as porocarcinomas tend to follow an aggressive course. These tumors have been recognized by some authors as malignant hidroacanthoma simplex, or malignant eccrine poroma, respectively.[34,38]

Juxtaepidermal Acrospiroma (Eccrine Poroma)

History

Pinkus et al. described the eccrine poroma in 1956.[40] Eccrine poromas are fleshy, dome-shaped nodules that arise most frequently on the sole of the foot (69%). The remainder are distributed over the remaining body surface. The age of presentation ranges from 15 to 83 years. They occur in all races, and the sexual distribution is about equal.

Clinical Features

Although eccrine poromas are usually asymptomatic, the most common presenting complaint is bleeding. Trauma appears to precede the tumor in a substantial number of cases.[41]

Histologic Features

Eccrine poromas characteristically present as soft, nontender, pink or red nodules. They are usually sessile, but are occasionally pedunculated. Those located on the plantar and palmar surfaces often appear to be partially sunken into the surrounding epidermis, forming a keratotic collarette with a groove around the tumors. They vary from 4 to 30 mm, but most are about 1 cm or less in diameter.

The large majority of eccrine poromas are solitary; however, Goldner described a patient with more than 100 plantar and palmar eccrine poromas, a condition he termed eccrine *poromatosis*.[42] Another example of widespread poromatosis was reported by Wilkinson et al. in a case of hidrotic ectodermal dysplasia.[43] Ogino reported as *linear eccrine poromas* a linear lesion of the lower extremity with histological features of eccrine poroma.[44]

Clinically, eccrine poromas may be mistaken for pyogenic granulomas, amelanotic melanomas, dermatofibromas, scars, hemangiomas, and verruca vulgares.

On gross examination of a cross section, eccrine poromas have a sessile polypoid configuration. Microscopically, large masses of basaloid cells proliferate from the epidermis into the dermis (Fig. 47–3). The tumor cells often replace the whole thickness of the epidermis, but sometimes individual tumor nodules are separated by normal epidermis in a pattern reminiscent of hidroacanthoma simplex.[1]

The tumor cells are small and uniform in appearance with scant cytoplasm and oval nuclei with dispersed chromatin. The cells of an eccrine poroma do not palisade at the periphery of the tumor, and there is a sharp contrast with the surrounding epidermis. Although ductlike structures may occasionally be prominent, there is often little, if any, lumen formation.

Some tumors have pronounced areas of fibrosis with a hyalinized stroma. Others have numerous blood vessels and strikingly resemble pyogenic granulomas. Occasional eccrine poromas have variable amounts of melanin pigmentation. When this occurs, the pigment is more abundant in the superficial layers, and the melanin is usually evenly distributed within the poroma cells, but occasionally may be present in numerous dendritic melanocytes.

Very rarely, eccrine poromas have keratin cysts: when these are present, the tumors strongly resemble seborrheic keratoses.

The tumor cells of eccrine poroma are strongly positive for amylophosphorylase, succinic dehydrogenase, and cytochrome oxidase.[45] In addition to these enzymes, Hashimoto and Lever described strong reactions to branching enzyme and malic dehydrogenase.[46]

Ultrastructurally, the cells contain abundant glycogen.

Numerous tonofilaments show an annular configuration around the nuclei, and the tumor cells have a tendency to form intracellular lumens. Hashimoto and Lever compared the ultrastructural characteristics to the outer cells of the embryonic acrosyringium and the cells of the sweat duct ridge.[46]

Histogenesis

Most authors agree that eccrine poromas are differentiated toward the intraepidermal eccrine duct unit. This hypothesis is supported by the frequent location of the tumor on the plantar surface, an area devoid of hair follicles. Whether eccrine poromas actually originate from the acrosyringium is more difficult to assess, but their close association with the epidermis suggests an origin in that area of the skin.

Eccrine poromas are neoplasms with a fairly well-defined set of histologic criteria. There is, however, a spectrum between an eccrine poroma and its more superficial form, which is often referred to as hidroacanthoma simplex. Similarly, some tumors display a spectrum of growth pattern within the same lesion; they resemble eccrine poromas in the superficial aspects and acrospiromas in the deep dermis.[47]

Differential Diagnosis

Histologically, eccrine poromas can be confused with basal cell carcinomas. The latter often are devoid of glycogen and the peripheral cells tend to display a palisaded arrangement with dermoepidermal cleft formation. Basal cell carcinomas almost always have apoptotic cells in the midst of their masses. The location of basal cell carcinomas on volar skin is extremely unusual, whereas it is the favorite location for eccrine poromas.

The differentiation of extraplantar eccrine poromas from seborrheic keratoses can be difficult. Unlike eccrine poroma, seborrheic keratoses characteristically have numerous horn cysts and an exophytic growth pattern above the surface of the skin.

Some cases of eccrine poroma can be difficult to differentiate from pyogenic granuloma as some eccrine poromas

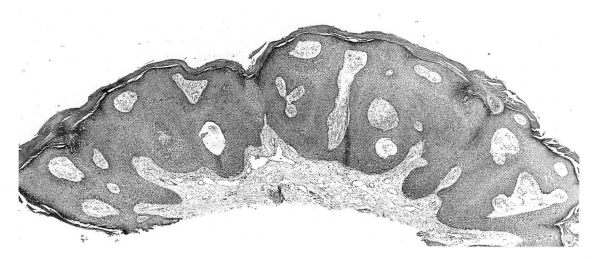

Figure 47–3. Juxtaepidermal acrospiroma. There are proliferations of basaloid cells with multiple epidermal contacts.

have extensive vascular proliferation within their stromas and only a thin layer of proliferating epithelium. The high glycogen content of eccrine poromas is often a helpful diagnostic clue.

Intradermal Acrospiroma

History

Lever first recognized this intradermal acrospiroma in 1948[48,49] and suggested the name *myoepithelioma*. Liu described similar cases in 1949, and believed that these tumors were a form of low-grade malignancy that originated in the hair follicle.[50] Stout and Conley hypothesized that they were of sweat gland origin.[51] Johnson and Helwig, in 1969, reported 319 tumors, reviewed 74 neoplasms from the literature, and coined the term *acrospiroma*.[20]

Clinical Features

The varied clinical and histologic presentations of acrospiromas explain the numerous names used in the past. The neoplasms typically present as cystic or solid dermal nodules, and sometimes as a combination of both. They usually measure about 1 cm, but can be as large as 10 cm.

The median duration of the tumor before excision in Johnson and Helwig's series was 2 years, with a range from weeks to 64 years.[20] The median age of patients at the time of excision was 35 years, with a range of 3 to 93 years. They appear to be slightly more common in women than men, occur in all races, and may arise on all parts of the body. There is some pain on pressure in about 20% of patients, and some spontaneous oozing occurs in 16%.[20,52]

Histologic Features

Grossly, the tumors are sharply circumscribed, and consist of lobules of various size that lie in the dermis and subcutaneous tissue. Although most tumors are solid, some have cystic cavities filled with serous or gelatinous material (Figs. 47–4 and 47–5). Sinus tracts that open onto the epidermis may be present.

Histologically, there are pronounced variations of patterns and cell types, many of which are often present within a single tumor. Some acrospiromas involve or replace the epidermis in a manner similar to eccrine poromas. Others have no epidermal contact, and are situated entirely within the dermis (Fig. 47–6).

Macroscopic and microscopic cyst and lumen formation may be present within a single tumor. These cavities usually have either a cuboidal or cylindric epithelial cell lining; focally, these cells can have mucinous (goblet cell) differentiation. The cystic spaces contain amorphous, proteinaceous eosinophilic material.

The tumors with epidermal contact often comprise solid sheets of small cuboidal cells with uniform nuclei and scant basophilic cytoplasm. Similar cell types also predominate in mostly intradermal solid tumors. Occasionally, moderate to heavy melanin pigmentation is present.[53]

Large polygonal cells with abundant eosinophilic cytoplasm and squamoid features are also common, and tend to occur in aggregates in a concentric fashion, producing whorls. These cells often form a central lumen with cuticular differentiation. Sometimes there is cytoplasmic vacuolization, which represents intracytoplasmic lumen formation and recapitulates the embryogenesis of the eccrine sweat ducts (Fig. 47–7).

Occasional acrospiromas have sheets of polygonal cells with abundant clear cytoplasm, centrally located nuclei,

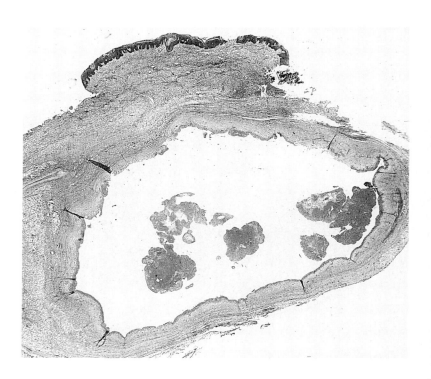

Figure 47–4. Dermal acrospiroma. A predominantly cystic lesion that also has solid areas.

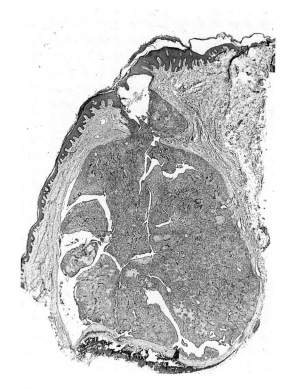

Figure 47–5. Dermal acrospiroma. A largely solid lesion with epidermal contact.

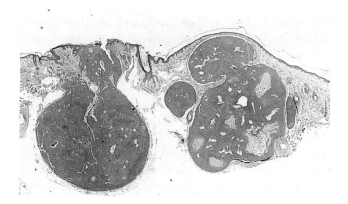

Figure 47–6. Dermal acrospiroma. A multilobulated neoplasm that has features of both juxtaepidermal and dermal tumors.

and distinct cell membranes. This cell type can constitute either a small part or the majority of a tumor (Fig. 47–8).

The stroma characteristically contains eosinophilic hyalinized collagen and, less often, delicate collagen fibers. Rarely, an inflammatory infiltrate accompanies the periph-

eral tumor lobules. Some tumors have small, centrally located areas of necrosis.

Although the nuclei are usually vesicular with finely granular chromatin, some tumors occasionally have cells with large, moderately atypical nuclei; this may arouse concern. This change, however, is almost always limited to a few cells, and does not seem to have prognostic significance.[54] Mitotic figures are not rare, and are abundant in some eccrine acrospiromas.[1]

Occasionally, some tumors display a pattern of small, thin cords and nests. Others have rounded nests of small, regular basaloid cells, with a poroma-like intraepidermal component. Frequently, as noted earlier, tumor nodules have a central cystic, lumenlike cavity filled with eosinophilic, granular material; this subtype of acrospiroma is known as a dermal duct tumor[55–57] or poroepithelioma.[38,39]

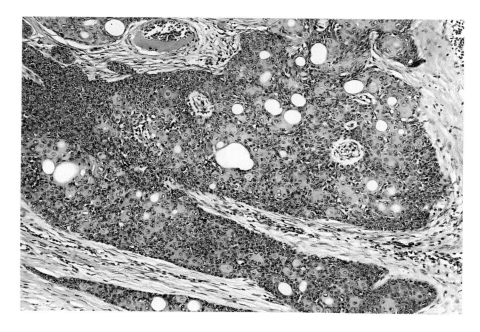

Figure 47–7. Dermal acrospiroma. A basaloid and squamoid neoplasm that exhibits extensive intra- and extracellular lumen formation.

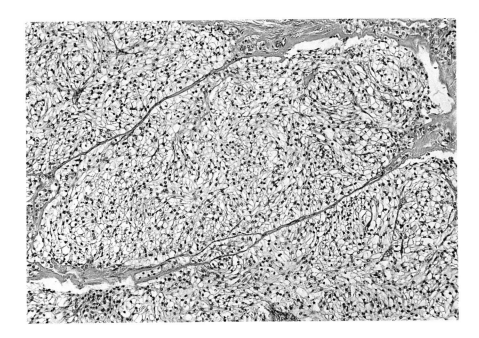

Figure 47–8. Dermal acrospiroma. The clear cell variant has abundant clear cytoplasm and prominent cell membranes.

In summary, the following patterns may occur alone or in any combination in an eccrine acrospiroma:

- Cystic acrospiroma (a largely cystic tumor)
- Solid or solid cystic acrospiroma with squamoid features (also known as nodular hidradenoma)
- Clear cell acrospiroma
- Acrospiroma with small nodules (also known as dermal duct tumor or poroepithelioma)
- Pigmented acrospiroma
- Acrospiroma with features of eccrine poroma

Thirty-eight examples of recurrent acrospiromas studied by Johnson and Helwig[20] showed histologic features essentially similar to those of the original primary neoplasm. The tumors were located deeper in the dermis, and did not show any aggressive growth pattern or atypical cytologic features. Interestingly, some recurrent tumors were more characteristic of eccrine acrospiromas than the primary lesions.

The information on the histochemistry and enzyme histochemistry of these tumors is somewhat fragmentary and applies to two main variants. The clear cell type shows abundant cytoplasmic glycogen demonstrated by PAS positivity and diastase digestion. A variable amount of cells also contain sialomucins.

The enzyme histochemistry favors sweat gland differentiation with controversial findings as to what part of the segment.[28,57–60]

Histogenesis

Few adnexal neoplasms have generated so much controversy as the acrospiroma.[61,62] This is due mostly to the varied histologic patterns and cell types that this neoplasm is capable of producing. Although there is general agreement that the most superficial forms (eccrine poroma and dermal duct tumor) show ductal differentiation, the clear cell type has remained controversial. Currently, most au-

thors believe that the clear cell type is an eccrine neoplasm. In the past, some favored myoepithelial differentiation,[48,49] and others, pilar origin.[50] Mascaro hypothesizes that the clear cell variety has different histogenetic origins, such as sweat glands, pilar apparatus, sebaceous glands, and epidermis.[63]

Johnson and Helwig, who represent most current thinking, believe that the clear cell type is of ductal differentiation.[20] Although apocrine and eccrine ducts are essentially identical, an eccrine differentiation and/or origin is supported.

Some authors, based on electron microscopic and immunohistochemical evidence, support a differentiation toward the intraepidermal eccrine duct (acrosyringium) for eccrine acrospiromas.[38,39,53] Hashimoto et al. found, in addition, some evidence for secretory differentiation in the clear cell type.[59] Winkelman and co-workers' studies on the dermal duct tumor gave more support to its differentiation towards the dermal portion of the eccrine duct.[55,56] O'Hara et al., however, felt that the clear cell type had features similar to those of the light cells of the secretory portion of the eccrine sweat glands.[58,62] We believe that the bulk of information on eccrine acrospiromas favors a ductal differentiation.

Differential Diagnosis

Histologically, the varied architectural and cytologic patterns pose different sets of diagnostic problems. The clear cell type should be differentiated from other lesions that can also comprise clear cells, such as sebaceous tumors and balloon cell melanoma and nevi.[64]

Tricholemmoma can pose a particularly difficult differential diagnosis. They are small, often measuring less than 0.5 cm, and are located almost exclusively on the face. Histologically, most tricholemmomas are integrally related to the epidermis. Occasionally, a small cystic space is found in the center of the tumor lobule. A thickened basement membrane and peripheral palisading of tumor cells are also characteristic features of tricholemmomas. Both tricholemmomas and clear cell hidradenomas have abundant glycogen-rich cytoplasm.

Metastatic renal cell carcinoma can at times be difficult to distinguish from clear cell acrospiromas. Acrospiromas are commonly multilobulated, and have a hyaline stroma, as well as glandular lumens and numerous areas with sialic acid–containing cytoplasmic mucin. Renal cell carcinoma, on the other hand, presents as a single nodule with a highly vascular stroma. The cells are arranged in papillary and alveolar patterns and contain intracytoplasmic lipid droplets.

The variant known as dermal duct tumor can be confused with a basal cell carcinoma and other adnexal neoplasms composed of small, basophilic cells such as a cylindroma and spiradenoma.

Tumors with squamoid differentiation (epidermoid hidradenoma)[65] must be differentiated from proliferative tricholemmal tumors with scant keratinization. A diligent search, however, reveals foci of pilar-type keratinization, which are not present in acrospiromas.

Differentiation of benign from malignant acrospiromas seldom poses a problem. The malignant neoplasms characteristically have a high mitotic rate, atypical mitoses, and areas of necrosis. The cells also display marked cytologic atypia. An inflammatory infiltrate accompanies the malignant tumors. Benign acrospiromas may occasionally have isolated, nuclear irregularities, with rare large, irregular hyperchromatic nuclei.[54]

Glomus tumors, especially those located under the nail, may show a lobulated solid pattern with a striking resemblance to acrospiromas. Glomus tumors often have abundant stromal mucin. The location under the nail, the characteristic pain, and the vascular lumina usually make differentiation between the two neoplasms straightforward.

SYRINGOMA

History
Syringomas were first described in 1876 by Kaposi who, like his contemporaries, believed these tumors were of vascular origin. Unna in 1894 was the first to call them syringomas.[66]

Clinical Features
Syringomas have different clinical presentations, but they most commonly manifest as multiple bilateral small papules on the lower eyelids. They are usually flesh-colored, tan, red, or brown. Syringomas are often clinically inapparent, and may be found incidentally in surgical specimens from excisions of xanthelasmas and basal cell carcinomas of the eyelids. Other sites where these tumors occur are the side of the neck and anterior thorax.

A second form of presentation is the eruptive type in which numerous crops of syringomas appear. They often start at puberty or adolescence, and spread to most parts of the body, although they have a marked preference for the ventral skin.[67–69]

Vulvar[70–72] and penile[73] lesions have been described

both as solitary tumors and as part of a more extensive involvement. A linear unilateral lesion[74] and an acral (dorsum of the hand) lesion[75] have also been reported. A highly unusual presentation is a patch of alopecia on the scalp.[76–79]

Syringomas often appear in the third and fourth decades of life and increase in number with age. Women are affected twice as commonly as men, and Japanese women have an unusually high incidence.[80]

Familial syringomas have been described, but the pattern of inheritance is not yet clear in the few cases reported in the literature.[81–83]

Butterworth et al. found syringomas in 19% of the mongoloids in a state hospital. Their incidence is similar to that of the Simian crease, and the presence of syringomas has been proposed as an additional diagnostic criterion for mongolism.[80,84]

Syringomas may be under hormonal influence as they proliferate at puberty, occur more commonly in women, and increase in size during both pregnancy and the premenstrual period.[85]

Histologic Features
The histology of syringomas is highly characteristic. Nests, cords, and small cystic structures lie within dense collagenous tissue in the upper half of the dermis (Fig. 47–9). The cystic lumina are small, and are lined by one or two layers of cuboidal cells. Sometimes, a lateral taillike projection is present, the so-called "comma tail." The epithelial elements seldom have epidermal contact, but if they do, it is often in connection with small keratinizing cystic structures.

Some tumors have only sparse epithelial structures, whereas others have numerous hyperplastic cystic structures with luminal, lamellar keratinization. Rupture of cysts with foreign body reaction to keratin occurs frequently.

The walls of the cystic structures often consist of cells with a clear, vacuolated cytoplasm that can be mistaken for sebaceous cells. A rare variant, known as clear cell syringoma, displays larger, glandlike nests of clear cells with abundant glycogen[86–88] (Fig. 47–10).

All the semiquantitative studies of tumor enzymes are largely in agreement.[68,86,89–91] The ultrastructural features of syringomas and eruptive hidradenomas are similar.[68] Similar to optical microscopy, electron microscopy shows abundant lumen formation, and the luminal cells have blunt, round microvilli, and abundant tonofilaments with well-developed desmosomes and terminal bars. The tonofilaments are often disposed in a ringlike fashion in a paraluminar location. Multivesicular bodies (lysosomes) and keratohyaline granules are often present. Rare myoepithelial cells are noted. The external cells, which are abundant, lack multivesicular bodies and the bandlike disposition of the tonofilaments. Collagen bundles lie between tumor cells and in the glandular lumina. Langerhans cells are present.[68,89]

Histogenesis
Most investigators agree that syringomas are eccrine sweat gland tumors. It is curious that all reported cases are from hair-bearing sites, whereas they have only rarely been de-

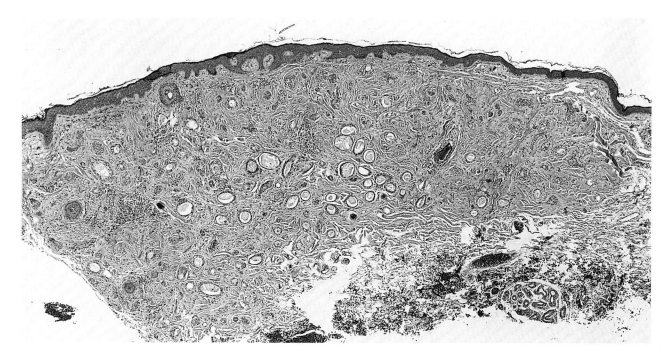

Figure 47–9. Syringoma. Multiple regular lumina are present in the middermis.

scribed in areas exclusively containing eccrine sweat glands, such as the palms and soles. Therefore, some have favored an apocrine[92] or sebaceous gland origin.[93] Current evidence overwhelmingly favors ductal differentiation.

Apocrine and eccrine ducts are, however, quite similar and share many morphologic and physiologic features.[94–96] The continuity of syringomas with follicular structures and not with eccrine glands, when examined by serial sectioning, lends support to an apocrine duct histogenesis.[66,97]

Differential Diagnosis

Histologically, the most common differential diagnosis is with desmoplastic trichoepithelioma. Both tumors consist of small keratinizing cysts and cords of epithelium. Desmoplastic trichoepithelioma differs by being a solitary lesion that clinically has a rolled border and depressed center. Histologically, a desmoplastic trichoepithelioma displays numerous concentrically keratinized cystic structures. The remainder of the tumor comprises thin cords of epithelium immersed in a dense desmoplastic stroma without lumen formation.

Syringomas, in contrast, have fewer keratinizing structures. Many of the cords have small glandular lumina, and the collagenous stroma is compact, with increased amounts of clumped elastic fibers.

A recently described low-grade glandular neoplasm, the microcystic carcinoma, has histologic features similar to those of syringomas and desmoplastic trichoepitheliomas. It probably represents a malignant syringoma.[98,99]

ECCRINE SPIRADENOMA

History

The first example of eccrine spiradenoma was reported by Sutton in 1934.[100] Kersting and Helwig in 1956 provided the definitive description of eccrine spiradenomas, based on their study of 136 cases.[101]

Clinical Features

Eccrine spiradenomas are usually solitary but occasionally multiple tumors.[102,103] They lie within the dermis or subcutaneous tissue and commonly arise in the second to fourth decades. Seventy-nine percent of Kersting and Helwig's patients presented with ventral nodules, and three-quarters (76%) were situated on the upper half of the body. When multiple, the lesions tend to be grouped; however, disseminated tumors, most often in a linear arrangement, have been described.[100,103–105] Individual tumors average 1 cm, but some in Kersting and Helwig's series measured up to 5 cm.[101]

Eccrine spiradenomas are rounded, often deeply seated nodules that have a spongy or cystic consistency. They are covered by an intact, usually normal epidermis; however, one third have a bluish discoloration.

The majority of the tumors in the Armed Forces Institute of Pathology series (91%) were symptomatic. Fifty-two percent were described as painful and 39% as tender.[101] The pain may be spontaneous but is often stimulated by light pressure, such as from clothing. Sometimes the pain is severe or paroxysmal, and radiates to other parts of the

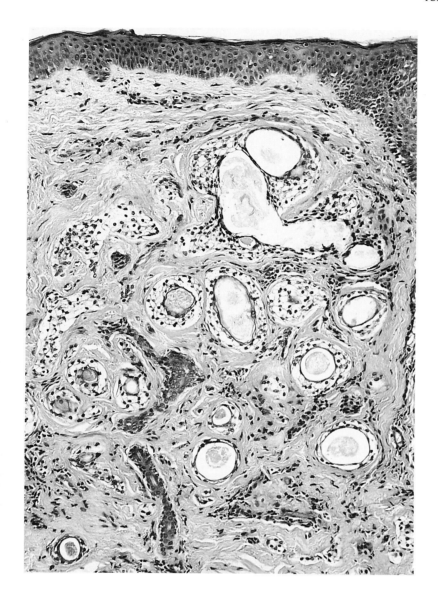

Figure 47–10. Syringoma. The clear cell variant displays similar architectural features with prominent cuticular luminal differentiation.

body. Pain has also been produced experimentally by cold and needle puncture. Injection of acetylcholine produces a severe pain, which can be prevented or abolished by a prior or subsequent injection of atropine.[106]

Histologic Features

Eccrine spiradenomas consist of one or more distinct lobules that are usually oval or round, located in the deep dermis or the subcutaneous tissue. On low magnification, they appear homogeneously basophilic with a well-defined fibrous capsule, and at first glance are reminiscent of a lymph node (Fig. 47–11). Occasional tumors, often the larger ones, are partially or almost wholly cystic; the cystic contents are either an eosinophilic proteinaceous material or red blood cells, mimicking a vascular neoplasm. Some neoplasms have extensive areas of fibrosis, distorting the usually monotonous architecture.

The nodules of an eccrine spiradenoma consist of tightly packed cells arranged in a diffuse "alveolar" or pseudorosette formation. Commonly, two cell types can be recognized. One cell type has a large vesicular nucleus with granular chromatin and often a prominent nucleolus; and scant cytoplasm. The smaller cells have a denser, smaller nucleus; these cells are often located peripherally to the larger cells (Fig. 47–12). Some tumors have a variable component of cells arranged in tubules that are often located at the periphery of the lesions. These cells have a larger, eosinophilic cytoplasm.

Eccrine spiradenomas can display profound degenerative changes, fibrosis, and cyst formation. Some of the larger tumors are partially or totally necrotic and have only a thin rim of cell nests[107] (Fig. 47–13). Thrombosis can be associated with the vascular eccrine spiradenomas.

In some tumors, extensive deposits of eosinophilic, basement membrane–like material surround the atrophic glandular lobules. This material is PAS positive and resem-

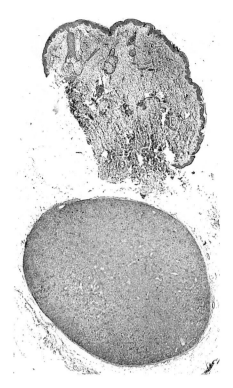

Figure 47–11. Spiradenoma. Well-circumscribed subcutaneous nodule.

bles the hyaline present in cylindromas. Because of this feature, Kersting and Helwig believed that some tumors share features of both cylindromas and eccrine spiradenomas.[101] Enzyme histochemistry did not favor a specific line of differentiation.[108–110] Several groups have studied the ultrastructural features of spiradenomas. These reports fail to conclusively demonstrate a specific line of differentiation.[109,111,112]

Histogenesis

As is the case with many adnexal tumors, the histogenesis and differentiation of spiradenomas is controversial. In two cases studied by serial sectioning, Kersting and Helwig and Blanchard et al. found that the tumor nodules were continuous with eccrine sweat glands.[101,105]

On the other hand, Nodl described a patient with multiple lesions, some of which were connected to follicular structures.[103] This finding was intriguing, as spiradenomas have been observed in association with cylindromas and trichoepitheliomas.[113,114] Castro and Winkelmann regarded spiradenomas as having a basal cell (basaloid) differentiation similar to that of cylindromas and trichoepitheliomas.[109] Hashimoto et al. favored a ductal differentiation because of the lumen formation, cuticular differentiation, and tonofilaments.[108] The currently available information appears to support an eccrine sweat gland histogenesis which produces a poorly differentiated adnexal neoplasm.

Differential Diagnosis

Histologically, a differential diagnosis with cylindroma can occasionally be extremely difficult if not impossible.[101,115] The tumor nodules of a spiradenoma tend to be rounded. When cystic, an eccrine spiradenoma must be differentiated from a vascular neoplasm or a lymphangioma.

Cases of malignant transformation have been reported; however, this occurrence appears to be exceedingly rare.[3,116]

CYLINDROMA

History

Ancell in 1842 is credited with the first description, and Billroth in 1859 coined the term *cylindroma.* There is

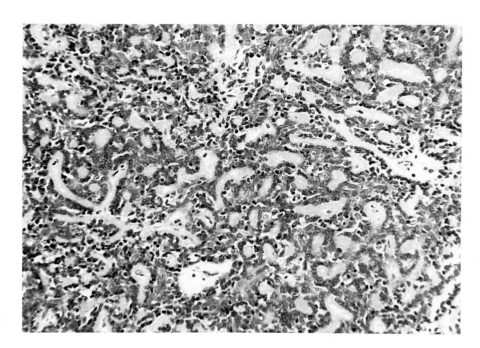

Figure 47–12. Spiradenoma. Cords of small and large cells with hyalinized stroma.

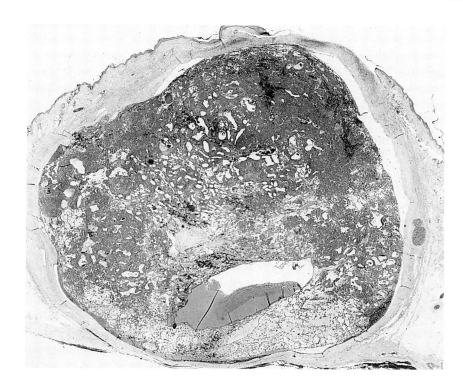

Figure 47–13. Spiradenoma. A large tumor showing necrosis and vascular transformation of the central portion.

considerable confusion with the usage of the term *cylindroma*, as it is also used to describe a malignant neoplasm usually of salivary gland origin that is better known today as adenoid cystic carcinoma.[115] Cutaneous cylindromas most commonly present as solitary nodules on the scalp and face, but multiple tumors also occur frequently. They range in size from a few millimeters to several centimeters.

Clinical Features

A relatively rare, but highly recognizable form of presentation is that of multiple tumors covering most of the scalp and large areas of the face and upper trunk; these are commonly known as turban tumors.[115]

An association with other adnexal neoplasms, most frequently trichoepitheliomas, is relatively common.[117–119] A peculiar combination of dermal cylindromas and parotid basal cell adenomas, a tumor with remarkably similar histology, has been reported in several patients.[119–121]

Some cylindromas are familial and are inherited in an autosomal dominant fashion.[117] They may occur at any age, but most commonly arise in the third and fourth decades. Women are affected at least twice as often as men.[115] Although cylindromas are generally regarded as painless tumors, 35% of the patients in Crain and Helwig's series described some type of painful sensation.[115]

Black and Wilson Jones reported two patients who developed their tumors 40 to 50 years after x-ray epilation of the scalp.[122]

Histologic Features

Histologically, the tumor nodules are well defined but not encapsulated, and have a tendency to coalesce. The individual nodules consist of epithelial islands and cords that vary considerably in size and composition (Fig. 47–14). Commonly, they are made up of rounded nests of basaloid cells, which sometimes interlock with the adjacent nests to form a jigsawlike pattern (Fig. 47–15). Although some nests are largely solid, others have an extensive lumen and pseudolumen formation. Two cell types are often described: a small dark cell, often located in the periphery of the tumor lobules, and a larger lighter cell, which makes up the central portion of the cords.

A characteristic feature of cylindroma is the thick, eosinophilic, "hyaline" basement membrane material that surrounds the individual tumor lobules. This material is also found inside the tumor lobules as "globules," and represents invaginations of the peripheral thickened basement membrane. It is strongly PAS positive, and resistant to diastase.

The histology of the lobules appears to vary with the age of the individual lesions. In older lesions, the hyaline material often makes up most of the tumor nodules.

The histology of irradiated tumors shows large areas of acellular hyaline material as well as large areas of glandular lumen formation resembling syringomas.[115,122]

Focally, some tumors have basaloid, thin proliferations of cells with a cribriform pattern resembling adenoid cystic carcinoma.

The tumor nodules contain acid mucopolysaccharides demonstrable by alcian blue and colloidal iron stains. The combination alcian blue-PAS stain demonstrates a multilayered PAS-positive basement membrane with pockets of acid mucopolysaccharides which are stained by the alcian blue.[115]

Enzyme histochemistry studies were not helpful.[119,125] The hyaline areas consist under the electron microscope

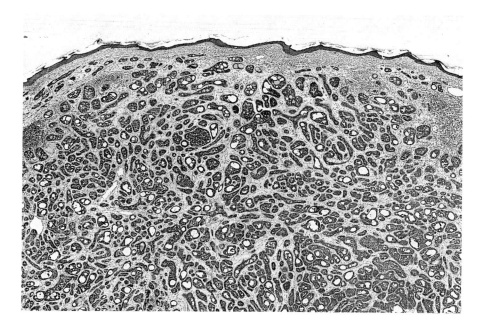

Figure 47–14. Cylindroma. Solid proliferations of basaloid cords with microcystic appearance.

of a multilayered basal lamina material with interstitial small collagen fibers and numerous anchoring fibrils attached to the different levels of the basal lamina. The hyaline material located inside the tumor nodules has an identical configuration.[126] Reynes et al described two types of tumor cells: light and dark. The later had interdigitations and lined the ductal lumens.[127] The cell population was divided into four basic types: secretory, indeterminate, tonofilamentous,

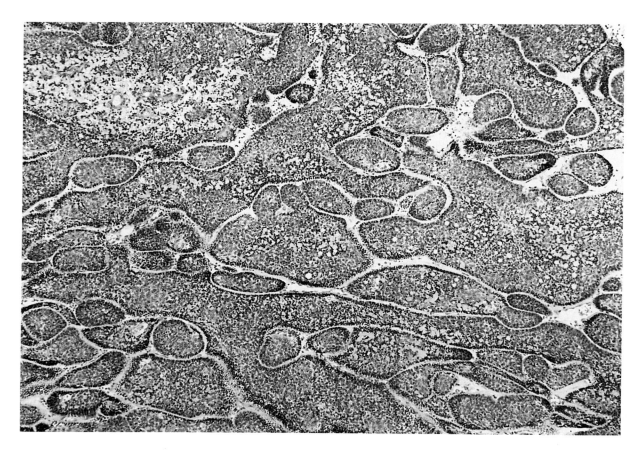

Figure 47–15. Cylindroma. Solid basaloid cords interconnect like a jigsaw puzzle. Note the thickened basement membrane.

and basaloid.[119] Langerhans cells have been described in tumor nodules.[119,126]

Histogenesis

With respect to histogenesis and differentiation, cutaneous cylindroma is one of the most controversial of all adnexal neoplasms. Eccrine,[115,128] apocrine,[126] and pilar[7] differentiation have been claimed by different authors.

The eccrine theory is in part supported by the continuity of some tumors with eccrine sweat glands. Some tumors have extensive tubular (glandular) differentiation, and postradiation tumors resemble syringomas. Electron microscopy, although largely inconclusive, shows cuticular differentiation and secretory features similar to those of eccrine secretory cells. Additional support is found in the similarity with and the rare coexistence of spiradenomas,[113,114] a tumor assumed to be of eccrine origin and/or differentiation. Recently, immunocytochemical findings supportive of eccrine differentiation were reported.[128]

The apocrine theory rests on similar grounds. Glandular differentiation with cuticular features can also be seen in the apocrine duct. Additional weight is given to the observation that these tumors occur in apocrine (or pilar) territory. No case has ever been reported on the palms and soles.

The pilar origin is supported by the exclusive occurrence of cylindromas in hair-bearing skin and their common association with the also dominantly inherited trichoepithelioma, a tumor with indisputable pilar differentiation. The thick basement membrane so characteristic of cylindromas is similar to the glassy membrane of hair follicles. The occurrence of cutaneous and parotid tumors with similar histology undoubtedly adds complexity to this speculation. The balance of all the facts presented does not favor conclusively any specific line of differentiation.

Differential Diagnosis

Histologically, a differential diagnosis with basal cell carcinoma is occasionally difficult. A peripheral palisaded arrangement of the cells, numerous apoptotic cells, induced stroma, and lack of the thick hyaline membrane are features of basal cell carcinoma.

Spiradenomas can bear a striking similarity to cylindromas. Syringomas and adenoid cystic carcinomas are less likely to be confused.

MIXED TUMOR (CHONDROID SYRINGOMA)

History

Nasse in 1892 is generally credited with the first report of a cutaneous mixed tumor.[129] Prior to 1959, the cases described in the literature, in addition to their own, were reviewed by Lennox et al.,[130] Greeley et al.,[131] and Morehead.[132] Stout and Gorman in 1959 reported the first large series, which included their own 39 cases as well as 95 additional cases from the literature.[133]

Headington in 1961 divided the mixed tumors into eccrine and apocrine types.[129] That same year Hirsch and Helwig reported 188 cases from the files of the Armed Forces Institute of Pathology, and coined the term *chondroid syringoma* for this neoplasm.[134]

Clinical Features

Mixed tumors of the skin are dermal or subcutaneous nodular tumors. They are twice as common in men as women, and the large majority of the tumors arise in the head and neck area (80%), the most frequent site being the central part of the face.

Grossly, cutaneous mixed tumors are spherical or lobulated, and well encapsulated. The cut surface is fibrous or glistening in appearance, and cystic cavities may be present.

Histologic Features

Histologically, there are circumscribed tumor nodules within the dermis or subcutaneous tissue; epidermal connections are absent (Fig. 47–16). Hirsch and Helwig found epidermal attachments in only 2 of 188 tumors.[134]

Cutaneous mixed tumors comprise a mixture of epithelial structures which are immersed in a cellular stroma. The epithelium is arranged in two basic patterns: microtubular and tubulobranching.

Mixed tumors with a microtubular pattern, consisting of small tubular lumina lined by cuboidal epithelium, were described as eccrine mixed tumors.[129] These are usually located in the dermis, and are the rarer of the two main forms. The stroma usually displays a chondroid or frank cartilaginous differentiation, and occasionally a mucoid or myxoid matrix is present. These tumors have abundant elastic fibers around the glands. Focally, the epithelial component may have a flat, cribriform pattern in a mucoid stroma, highly reminiscent of adenoid cystic carcinoma of salivary glands.

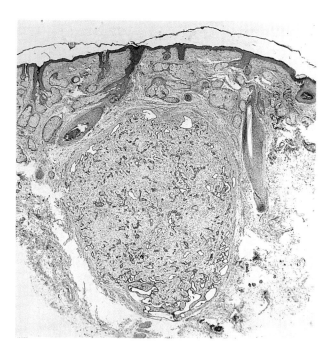

Figure 47–16. Mixed tumor. A well-circumscribed dermal nodule, composed of both stromal and glandular components.

The more common type of cutaneous mixed tumor has a tubulobranching pattern. These show a wide degree of pattern variation. The glandular component has an irregular, complex system of interconnecting glandular lumina, which are lined by one or two layers of cells. The luminal cells are cuboidal or cylindrical. This glandular component may be either evenly distributed throughout the tumor, arranged in a nodular pattern, or present mostly at the periphery. Areas of squamous differentiation are not rare, and keratinizing microcysts may occur.

It is usually not possible to ascribe a clear apocrine differentiation to most of these neoplasms as they appear to be largely of ductal differentiation. In the eyelids,[135] eyebrows, and external ear canal, however, these tumors often have frank apocrine cell differentiation. The luminal cells are tall with eosinophilic cytoplasm, supranuclear Golgi, and parabasal nuclei. They display the characteristic "pinched off" decapitation secretion, and rest on myoepithelial cells. The tumors of the external ear canal clearly belong to the spectrum of ceruminomas, and are discussed in more detail elsewhere.

Some cutaneous mixed tumors located on the scalp have areas of a combination of basophilic and shadow cells, and are strongly reminiscent of pilomatricomas.[134] Other tumors we have studied have follicular differentiation with hair papilla formation, and even immature Huxley and Henle's layers with trichohyalin. These often have a more squamous appearance with numerous keratinous cysts and a less conspicuous glandular component. Melanin is commonly found in the epithelial structures of these tumors, and the stroma is often more fibroblastic or myxoid rather than chondroid. In some respects, these neoplasms are similar to the tumors of the hair germ (trichoblastomas). Mixed tumors, therefore, may have epithelial components that reproduce eccrine, apocrine, and follicular structures. In the two basic architectural patterns, the microtubular and tubulobranching types, there are clusters of small cells with

an epithelioid appearance. These cells often have laterally displaced vesicular nuclei, and ample amorphous eosinophilic cytoplasm. They appear to gradually incorporate themselves into the mucoid or chondroid matrix, and it may be tempting to try to trace intermediate cells all the way to typical chondrocytes.

The stroma often composes half of the tumor bulk. It varies from fibroblastic to mucoid, myxoid, or chondroid, and rarely is frankly osteoid or with mature adipocytes. Sometimes it has an eosinophilic, keloidal appearance (Fig. 47–17). In the microtubular pattern of cutaneous mixed tumor, the stroma has a homogeneous, mucoid appearance. In the tubulobranching pattern, the stroma is heterogeneous in composition, with areas of loosely myxoid connective tissue and chondroid matrix.

Rarely, the chondroid stroma compresses most of the tumor, with only a few atrophic glands in the periphery. If this does occur, this tumor may be easily confused with a chondroma.

The epithelial tumor cells occasionally show mucinous metaplasia having the properties of sialomucins. The stroma has large amounts of acid glycosaminoglycans with a high content of hyaluronic acid.

Histogenesis

Hernandez described the ultrastructural features in two cases.[136] The epithelial component had largely a ductal differentiation with tonofilaments. No myoepithelial cells were identified. The stromal cell had ultrastructural features of fibroblasts and chondrocytes. Some stromal cells had tonofilaments, a feature of epithelial cells. Hernandez believed that there was a continuum of differentiation between the epithelial and stromal components, with no participation by myoepithelial cells. Mills and Cooper's findings were similar and their conclusions were the same.[137]

In contrast, based on their study of one tumor, Varela-Duran et al. found evidence of ductal and myoepithelial

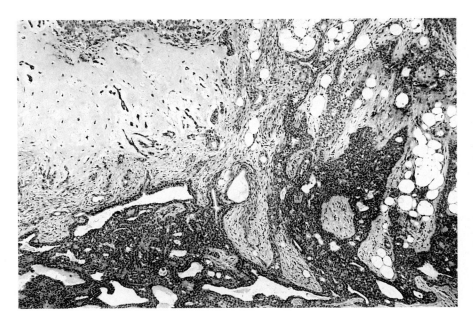

Figure 47–17. Mixed tumor. The neoplasm is composed of epithelial cords, adipose, and chondroid stromas.

differentiation. According to their interpretation, the stromal cells are derived from the other two cell types and are not true chondrocytes.[138]

Few neoplasms have attracted as much interest as mixed tumors, and the source of the cartilaginous stroma has long been a puzzle. Two major theories have evolved. Proponents of the first believe that the chondroid cells are derived from the epithelial elements. If this is true, the question arises as to the cell of origin. For a long time it was thought to be the myoepithelial cells. These cells share some properties with epithelial and muscle cells; however, documentation of the role of myoepithelial cells in the formation of mixed tumors has been minimal for both the salivary glandular[141] and the dermal types.[137] The probability of ductal cell participation in the formation of the stromal cells is more convincing.[137,139] It is possible, however, that both myoepithelial and ductal cells may be the origin of stromal cells, given the wide range of morphologic variation in mixed tumors.

The other hypothesis maintains that the chondroid matrix is an expression of a tumor-associated stroma that is histogenetically independent from its epithelial component. This position has less morphologic support. The question, therefore, is whether the stromal cells are true chondrocytes or metaplastic epithelial cells.

The matter of differentiation, or histosimilarity, is somewhat simpler. It appears clear that most cutaneous mixed tumors are neoplasms with ductal differentiation, based on the presence of tonofilaments and absence of secretory features. The myoepithelial cells belong, however, to the secretory portion of the sweat glands. Neither the ductal nor the myoepithelial cells have different characteristics in either apocrine or eccrine glands. Therefore, most cutaneous mixed tumors cannot be thought of as differentiating toward either gland. It is also apparent that some rare tumors provide convincing evidence of secretory apocrine and pilar differentiation.

PAPILLARY ECCRINE ADENOMA

History
Rulon and Helwig first described the papillary eccrine adenoma.[140] They studied 14 cases, and subsequently several additional examples have been reported.[141–143]

Clinical Features
Most tumors occurred on the extremities, and appear to be more common in women. Papillary eccrine adenomas present as dome-shaped, red, brown, or gray nodules which average about 1 cm in diameter.

Histologic Features
Microscopically, the tumors are often well circumscribed, nonencapsulated, dermal neoplasms located just below the epidermis (Fig. 47–18). They consist of dilated tortuous ducts of variable caliber. The ducts have a prominent, papillated appearance, and the cells lining the lumina are uniformly cuboidal and are arranged in a double layer. The ducts are surrounded by fibrocollagenous stroma, and their lumina occasionally contain granular or amorphous eosino-

philic material. The nuclei of the cuboidal lining cells are oval or round, and the nucleoli are small. Mitoses are either rare or absent (Fig. 47–19).

Differential Diagnosis
Microcystic carcinoma may have papillary areas that resemble those of papillary eccrine adenoma. In addition, there is a cystic component superficially and a small cell nesting pattern. Perineural invasion and invasive growth are very prominent in microcystic carcinoma.[98,99]

Although unlikely, there may be a problem differentiating a papillary eccrine adenoma from tumors with apocrine differentiation, such as papillary hidradenoma and papillary syringadenoma. The classic apocrine differentiation with tall columnar cells with parabasal nuclei, prominent supranuclear Golgi, and iron-positive cytoplasmic granules is not found in papillary eccrine adenomas.

Tubular apocrine adenoma can pose an especially difficult differential diagnosis.[144,145] These neoplasms are intradermal, and have tubular structures and papillation of the tumor cells which can resemble papillary eccrine adenoma. In the two cases of tubular adenoma in which electron microscopy was performed, the cells had the typical secretory features of apocrine cells. One tumor had, in addition, structures with ductal features: paraluminal ringlike disposition of tonofilaments and lack of secretory granules.[7,8] A conspicuous feature of tubular adenomas is the connection with the epidermis by one or more ductlike structures.

Civatte et al. described four tubular adenomas with features remarkably similar to those of papillary eccrine adenoma.[146]

APOCRINE NEVUS

Clinical Features
Although hamartomatous collections of apocrine glands are sometimes seen with either a nevus sebaceus of Jadassohn or a syringocystadenoma papilliferum, pure apocrine gland nevi are extremely rare. These mature circumscribed collections of apocrine glands are asymptomatic, occur in the second and third decades in both sexes, and may be solitary or multiple.[147–149] They have been described in the scalp, axillae, and presternum.

Apocrine nevi vary from a few millimeters to as much as 8 cm, and except for a dome-shaped configuration resulting from the underlying tumor, the surface of the skin is uninvolved. On cross section, they had a lobulated, yellowish, lipomalike appearance.[147]

Histologic Features
Histologically, these lesions are not encapsulated and comprise sheets of mature apocrine glands with no papillary infolding or cystic dilatation. The luminal cells have characteristic apocrine features, and rest on myoepithelial cells and hyaline basement membrane. Intracytoplasmic iron may be present in small amounts.[147]

Civatte et al. reported two cases of what they termed apocrine nevi, with such severe basaloid proliferation of the epithelium overlying the apocrine nevi that they resembled basal cell carcinomas.[150] Both of their cases occurred

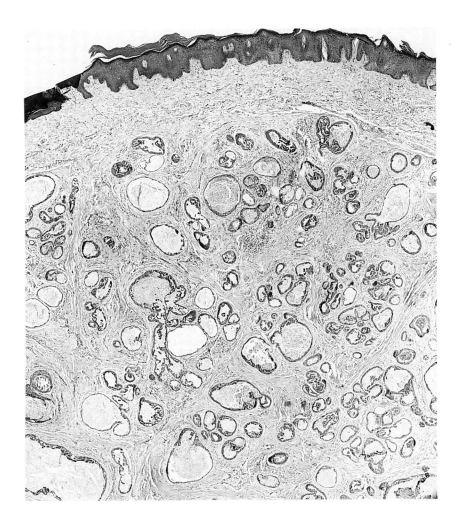

Figure 47–18. Papillary eccrine adenoma. The neoplasm has a papillary glandular arrangement within a dense fibrous stroma.

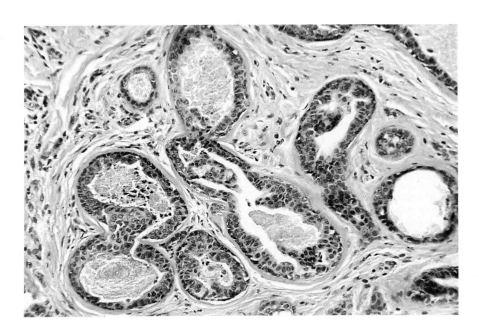

Figure 47–19. Papillary eccrine adenoma. The glands generally have a two-cell layer with intraluminal papillations.

on the scalp, however, and were also associated with pilose-baceous agenesis and stromal abnormalities, and we believe that they might be better classified along with the nevus sebaceus of Jadassohn as organoid hamartomas.

APOCRINE CYSTADENOMA

History

We view apocrine hidrocystomas and cystadenomas as variants of the same pathologic entity. Some reserve the term *apocrine hidrocystoma* for fluid-filled cystic structures lined by mature apocrine glandular epithelium with few if any papillary infoldings, and refer to neoplasms comprising both cystic and solid structures of apocrine glandular epithelium as *apocrine cystadenomas*. Others use the terms interchangeably. Clinically they do not differ, and histologically there is a broad spectrum of tumors between them.

Mehregan states that the hidrocystoma is a true organoid growth and not a simple retention cyst. He supports his hypothesis with these observations: (1) the hidrocystoma is lined by high-columnar apocrine secretory epithelium that shows no evidence of having been flattened as would be expected in a retention cyst; (2) the cyst walls have areas of papillomatous hyperplasia that project into the central cavity; and (3) the cysts are surrounded by well-organized fibrous stroma.[151] This epithelium and mesenchymal interrelation is characteristic of all cutaneous adnexal tumors.[152]

For simplicity's sake and to avoid confusion, we refer to this group of neoplasms as cystadenomas, and use the term *hidrocystoma* only when the tumor is predominantly a solitary cystic cavity with relatively little glandular epithelium.

Clinical Features

Apocrine hidrocystomas and cystadenomas may present as skin-colored, bluish, bluish-black, black, or brown, slightly translucent papules or nodules.[152,153] Approximately 50% are pigmented.[151,154] The tumors are asymptomatic and usually measure less than 15 mm, although Holder et al. described one that meaured 5 × 7 cm.[155] The age of the patients is usually over 30.

They occur most commonly on the face. Less frequently, they are seen in other areas of the head and neck, especially ears, eyelids, and scalp, and may occasionally be associated with a nevus sebaceus of Jadossohn. Rarely, they are found in other sites which include the anal region,[156,157] the penis,[158,159] and the thoracic area.[155,160–162] Von Seebach et al. described several cases. One tumor presented as a polyp at the anal ring, three were found incidentally in hemorrhoidectomy specimens, and two were discovered on gynecologic examination, one of which was at the anorectal junction and the other 6 cm up the rectum.[156] Ahmed and Jones reported two which occurred on the prepuce,[158] and Armijo et al. described an apocrine cystadenoma of the urethral meatus.[163]

For those tumors on the head and trunk, the sexual distribution is about equal. As Kruse et al. have noted, however, all reported cases on the genitalia have been in men, whereas all cases of genital hidradenoma papilliferum

have occurred in women.[154] They speculate that the histogenesis is similar, and that the expression differs when these tumors occur on the genitalia. This possible distinction obviously does not apply to the anorectal area, as all six of the patients reported by von Seebach were women.[156]

In practically all cases, apocrine cystadenomas are solitary; however, multiple tumors have occurred. Grinspan et al. described a patient with six lesions,[164] and Smith and Cernosky reported one patient with four, one with three, and three patients with two lesions.[160] Kruse et al. described a 56-year-old man with approximately 40 apocrine cystadenomas on the face and ears.[154]

Histologic Features

The tumors are well circumscribed, and the cystic spaces are lined by apocrine gland–type epithelium. This lining consists of a layer of high-columnar cells with abundant eosinophilic granular cytoplasm and a round basally situated nucleus; decapitation secretion is often present.

Usually, there are papillary infoldings into the cystic cavity. These projections consist of a stalk of vascular connective tissue covered by apocrine-type epithelium. Rarely, the lining epithelium may form a cribriform pattern. Other areas may be lined by cuboidal cells with no secretory activity, and occasional areas may have a ductlike lining.[151]

Myoepithelial cells generally lie beneath the epithelial layer, although these have not been observed in all cases.[158] A basement membrane separates the cystic structure from the adjacent stroma. This characteristic stroma is composed of well organized, loosely woven fibrous tissue and often contains accumulations of extravasated erythrocytes.

The epithelial secretory cells contain a large number of PAS-positive, diastase-resistant granules as well as aldehyde-fuchsin– and methlene blue–positive granules in their apical portions. Occasional cells contain pigmented granules; these are neither hemosiderin nor melanin, and likely represent lipofuscin.

By electron microscopy, the epithelial cells have features seen in mature apocrine glands. Well-formed micrivilli project into the lumina, and the apical caps contain many secretory granules, and numerous vesicles and vacuoles.[165] The cytoplasmic organelles indicate considerable secretory activity, and the endoplasmic reticulum is highly developed.[165] The secretory cells contain a variety of granules of apocrine secretory epithelium and others contain lamellar structures.[166]

PAPILLARY HIDRADENOMA

History

Papillary hidradenomas are benign neoplasms that occur almost exclusively in the female anogenital region. First described by Werth in 1878,[167] this tumor is relatively uncommon although more than 300 cases have been reported.

Clinical Features

Two major series have been compiled. Woodworth et al. studied 69 tumors in 65 patients seen over a 60-year period at the Mayo Clinic,[168] and Meeker et al. reported 65 tumors in 63 patients from the Armed Forces Institute of Pathology

(AFIP).[169] All of their patients were white women between the ages of 25 and 69. The Mayo Clinic group studied only vulvar tumors and found three patients with multiple papillary hidradenomas, one having three and the others two.[168] In the AFIP series, two patients had two tumors each, the remainder being solitary. Seventy-eight percent of their tumors were genital and twenty-two percent, perianal.[169] Most were on the labium majus. Rarely, papillary hidradenomas have been found elsewhere.[170]

Typically, a patient notices a dome-shaped nodule, which may occasionally be associated with bleeding or pain. Four of the patients described by Meeker et al. and one by Woodworth et al. noted changes in their tumors during menstruation.[168,169]

Histologic Features

The lesions are circumscribed, may feel either solid or cystic, and measure about 0.5 cm, although they may range up to 3 cm.[168] Most are in the middermis; however, a small number communicate with the epidermis, and an occasional tumor presents as an exophytic, raspberry-like lesion which simulates a pyogenic granuloma.[171] Clinically, most are misdiagnosed and are usually thought to be cysts or, if perianal, hemorrhoids.

Papillary hidradenomas bear a striking resemblance to mammary intraductal papillomas. Both Meeker et al. and Woodworth et al. compared the papillary hidradenomas they studied to intraductal papillomas.[168,169] Meeker et al. found that the mammary neoplasms tended to be larger, less circumscribed, and irregular in outline. In addition, the mammary tumors often comprised multiple nodules that involved more than one duct, and extensive fibrosis often replaced large portions of the tumors.[169] Woodworth et al. also noted that the amount of breast involved was frequently greater as a result of the extensive papillomatosis within multiple ducts. In their study, the degree of fibrosis was more extensive than in papillary hidradenomas, but it varied markedly.[168]

Papillary hidradenomas are generally well circumscribed, spherical middermal nodules that measure between 0.3 and 1 cm and that on cross section have a grayish color and firm consistency. Many lie within cystic spaces. Occasionally, they communicate with the surface epidermis, and rarely they present as an exophytic mass.

Microscopically, a pseudocapsule formed by compression of the adjacent stroma is often present. The tumors characteristically comprise both papillary and glandular elements (Fig. 47–20). In the series reported by Meeker et al., the papillary pattern predominated in 68%, the glandular pattern in 7%, and in 21% the distribution of the two patterns was about equal.[169]

The epithelial lining may be either one or two cells thick. Typically, the luminal cells are tall, columnar, apocrine-type cells with abundant granular eosinophilic cytoplasm, a round basilar nucleus, and apical decapitation (Fig. 47–21). These may or may not rest on smaller, cuboidal cells which are myoepithelial cells. Occasionally, the luminal cells are somewhat flattened. Meeker et al. have also observed areas in which the epithelial lining is composed of cells without decapitation and that resemble those seen in apocrine metaplasia of the breast.[169]

In the papillated portion, the epithelial layer rests on

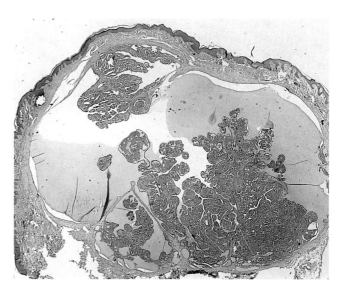

Figure 47–20. Papillary hidradenoma. Cystic tumor partially filled by multicystic papillary fronds.

slender fibrovascular stalks. The adjacent stroma is sparse, and occasionally there may be focal fibrosis. The overlying epidermis may be hyperplastic or atrophic. Unless a tumor is ulcerated or has been traumatized, no inflammatory infiltrate is present. Meeker et al. found minute focal calcification in two lesions and squamous metaplasia in one.[169] Occasional mitoses may be seen.

Similar to apocrine glandular epithelium, the tall columnar luminal cells of hidradenoma papilliferum are PAS positive and diastase resistant. The intraluminal material is weakly positive with the mucicarmine stain.

TUBULAR APOCRINE ADENOMA

History

In 1972, Landry and Winkelmann described a tubular apocrine adenoma that arose in a nevus sebaceus on the scalp of a 66-year-old woman.[144] Subsequently, similar neoplasms have been reported.[144–146]

Clinical Features

Tubular apocrine adenomas are rare, occur mainly in women between the ages of 18 and 76, and have usually been apparent for several years by the time the patient seeks medical attention. The tumors present as asymptomatic solitary nodules and have a pinkish-red coloration; their surfaces may be either irregular and cerebriform or smooth. They may or may not occur in an organoid nevus, and have been found on the leg, back, anogenital area, and axilla as well as the scalp.

Most of these neoplasms range from 1 to 2 cm in diameter; however, they may be considerably larger, and one measuring 7 × 4 cm has been reported.[144]

Histologic Features

By light microscopy, tubular apocrine adenomas are moderately well circumscribed intradermal neoplasm that may

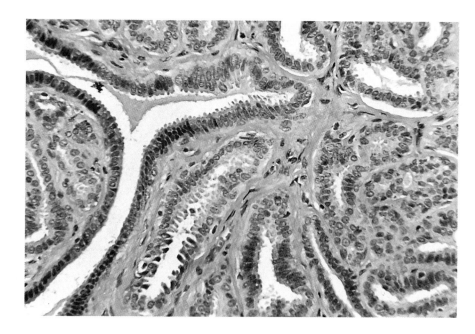

Figure 47–21. Papillary hidradenoma. The apocrine differentiation with pinched-off apical cytoplasm is evident.

extend into the subcutis. They have a lobular pattern surrounded by a fibrous stroma. These lobules comprise multiple tubular structures, which usually have double but which may have single- or many-layered epithelial linings, and frequently have papillary infoldings or projections into the lumina. The tubules vary markedly in size, and dilatation is a prominent feature. The cells lining the lumina show apocrine differentiation. The nuclei are uniform, nucleoli are not prominent, and mitotic figures are rare.

The overlying epidermis may be hyperplastic or atrophic, and occasional ducts may empty onto its surface. A sparse infiltrate of mast and plasma cells may be present.

Histogenesis

Histochemical studies support an apocrine differentiation.[145] By electron microscopy, the cells have microvilli and nipple-like cytoplasmic projections into the lumina, but are not identical to normal secretory apocrine epithelium.[144,145] Myoepithelial cells have not been seen, and there are no features of eccrine differentiation.

Differential Diagnosis

A tubular apocrine adenoma can be differentiated from an apocrine nevus because a nevus consists of mature apocrine glandular structures, whereas an adenoma is characterized by loss of architectural features of normal apocrine glands. Papillary hidradenoma differs by its papillary architecture, and a cystadenoma typically has a prominent cystic component. It can be difficult to distinguish a tubular apocrine adenoma from a papillary eccrine adenoma.

PAPILLARY SYRINGADENOMA

History

Papillary syringadenoma has been grouped with the tumors of the apocrine gland apparatus although it has many hamartomatous features and might more justifiably be classified as a nevus or hamartoma. We believe that the vast majority of these lesions differentiate more toward the apocrine than the eccrine gland, but this opinion is not universally accepted.

Peterson in 1892[173] and Elliot in 1893[174] first described this tumor. It was Werther in 1913, however, who termed it *syringadenoma papilliferum* and whose name is most often associated with it.[175]

Clinical Features

Papillary syringadenoma is an uncommon solitary growth that clinically presents itself as a fleshy, hairless plaque or nodule, and which may occasionally be pedunculated[176,177] or linear.[178,179] It is gray or brown, often moist and oozing, and its surface has a papillated verrucoid appearance. Usually, they are asymptomatic, but there may occasionally be crusting or bleeding. Most measure about 2 to 3 cm, but the variation in size is considerable.

In the largest published series of papillary syringadenoma, Helwig and Hackney reported 100 cases from the Armed Forces Institute of Pathology.[180] All were solitary. Seventy-six of their cases were confined to the head and neck; of these, 55 were on the scalp, and 11 on the forehead or temple. Those tumors not in the head or neck region were mainly on the trunk. Of the 100 patients, 91 were male; however, this likely reflects a bias resulting from the predominantly male composition of the armed forces. In 45 of their patients, the lesions were thought to have been congenital, and in an additional 13, the tumor arose before age 10; the incidence lessened with each decade. For those lesions that occurred in the early age groups, it is not known whether the tumor was in fact a papillary syringadenoma or a nevus sebaceus of Jadassohn or some other abnormality.[180] Of the 30 patients with syringocystadenoma papilliferum reported by Pinkus in 1954, however, 15 had the lesions at birth and an additional 8 developed them in infancy or childhood.[176]

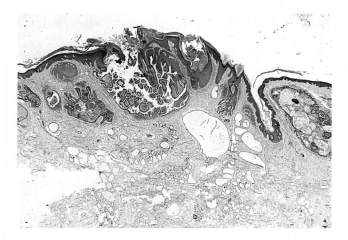

Figure 47–22. Papillary syringadenoma. The papillary fronds have wide epidermal connections. The dermis displays numerous apocrine glands.

Frequently, papillary syringadenoma is associated with a nevus sebaceus of Jadassohn. Of the 140 cases of nevus sebaceus reported by Wilson Jones and Heyl, 27 had within the nevus a papillary syringadenoma.[181] Of these 27, there was a nearly equal male-to-female ratio, and their ages ranged widely; 6 were between one and 19 years old, 11 between 20 and 39, and 10 were over age 40. Mehregan and Pinkus found eight papillary syringadenomas in their 150 cases of nevus sebaceus of Jadassohn, and seven of these were in adults.[182]

Histologic Features
On cross section under low magnification, a papillary syringadenoma consists of vertically oriented papillary projections, which are often multiple and which lead into one or more cystic invagination (Fig. 47–22). Near the surface, the lining is usually keratinizing squamous epithelium and it is similar to the adjacent epidermis. Further into the in-

vagination, the lining is composed of two epithelial cell layers: a luminal low-columnar layer, and an outer layer of flattened or cuboidal cells. At the base of the cystic invaginations, the lining usually comprises an inner tall-columnar layer and an underlying cuboidal row. The tall-columnar cells have a round or oval nucleus situated in the middle or basal portion of the cell, slightly eosinophilic cytoplasm, and, frequently, "decapitation" secretion.

The epithelial portion of this tumor is surrounded by a fibrous connective tissue stroma. Plasma cells are commonly present and tend to be congregated in the upper portion of the lesion, especially in the papillary processes (Fig. 47–23). Polymorphonuclear leukocytes, lymphocytes, and mast cells are not as characteristic but may be seen.

In their series of 100 cases, Helwig and Hackney found several common variations.[180] The luminal lining cell of the cystic invagination may be small with meager cytoplasm or disposed in multiple layers. Sometimes the squamous-lined ducts formed cysts filled, or partly filled, with keratin. The epidermis at the margin of the lesion may be hyperplastic and at times papillomatous.[180]

Melanocytes may be present, and rarely nests of melanocytic nevus cells may be seen.[175,176,183]

Histogenesis
There is no general agreement whether the differentiation of papillary syringadenoma is toward apocrine or eccrine structures. In support of eccrine differentiation, Helwig and Hackney pointed out that 90% occur in areas in which apocrine glands do not normally exist.[180] The validity of this argument is questionable, however, as not all neoplasms with apocrine features occur predominantly in the so-called apocrine areas. The frequent association of the papillary syringadenoma with nevus sebaceus of Jadassohn, which characteristically has an apocrine glandular component, suggests a relationship between the two, and further supports apocrine differentiation of the papillary syringadenoma.[184] The two published ultrastructural studies have yielded contradictory interpretations.[185,186]

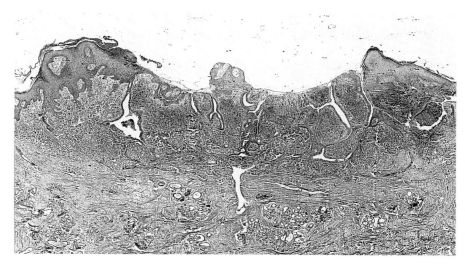

Figure 47–23. Papillary syringadenoma. This lesion is associated with a dense inflammatory stroma.

NIPPLE ADENOMATOSIS

History
Nipple adenomatosis is a rare benign mammary neoplasm, the importance of which lies in its ability to mimic Paget's disease clinically and ductal carcinoma of the breast histologically. Jones (1955) was the first to formally describe this lesion and he termed it *florid papillomatosis of the nipple ducts* in his series of five patients.[187] A review of the older literature, however, reveals reports of similar cases by Miller and Lewis (1923)[188] and Haagensen et al. (1951).[189]

Clinical Features
Nipple adenomatosis usually presents with a sanguineous, serous, or serosanguineous discharge.[190–193] The nipple is often sore, enlarged, and crusted. Frequently, the patient feels an underlying lump. Rarely, it is found incidentally. The eczematous or erosive appearance closely mimics mammary Paget's disease with which it is usually confused clinically.

Over 200 cases of nipple adenomatosis have been published.[194] The larger series are those of Perzin and Lattes at Columbia-Presbyterian Medical Center (65 cases),[193] Taylor and Robertson from the Armed Forces Institute of Pathology (29 cases),[195] Nichols et al. of the Mayo Clinic (16 cases),[190] and Doctor and Sirsat in Bombay (11 cases).[192]

This lesion occurs predominantly in middle-aged women with a peak incidence in the fourth and fifth decades, although there have been reports of its occurrence as early as age 9[196] and as late as age 72.[190] Civatte et al. described nipple adenomatosis that arose in a supernumerary nipple,[197] and rarely cases have occurred in men,[195,196,198,199] one in a man who received diethylstilbestrol therapy.[200]

Histologic Features
Grossly, the nipple may appear enlarged and eroded, and on cross section it contains a moderately circumscribed 0.7- to 1.5-cm nodule, which often reaches the nipple surface. The area of ulceration is usually the tumor itself. Large surface papillary projections, which are reminiscent of those of a papillary syringadenoma,[195–199] are lined by squamous epithelium at their tips and columnar or cuboidal tumor epithelium below.

The bulk of the neoplasm comprises a nonencapsulated dense proliferation of ductlike structures running in all directions (Fig. 47–24). These vary greatly in size, ramify ex-

tensively in the nipple stroma, and may simulate infiltrating mammary duct carcinoma. The ducts are lined by an outer flattened or cuboidal myoepithelial layer and an inner tall-columnar or cuboidal layer.[20] The double-layered epithelium is a key to the benign nature of this lesion. Sometimes the epithelium is focally squamous.[191]

Papillary proliferation is generally present and may be a conspicuous feature. For this reason, Perzin and Lattes thought the term *papillary adenoma* was more appropriate.[193] Focally, it may be so marked as to produce almost solid plugging of the ducts. Occasional cysts lined by squamous epithelium may be present.

Intraductal papillomas, usually deep to the nipple adenomatosis, may be present, and were seen in 12 of the 65 cases described by Perzin and Lattes.[193] They performed serial sections on two specimens, and demonstrated intraductal papillomas in both.

Apocrine-type lining may be seen,[192,193,195,201] and when present is usually inconspicuous. In one instance, nipple adenomatosis lined completely by apocrine-type cells was described.[202]

The stroma is moderately dense and fibrous, and at times there may be a marked similarity to sclerosing adenomatosis.[203] Taylor and Robertson reported an inflammatory infiltrate composed primarily of lymphocytes and an appreciable number of plasma cells in over half of their cases with a papillary component.[195]

Histogenesis
Nipple adenomatosis apparently arises from lactiferous ducts. Its similarity to the papillary syringadenoma is not surprising when one remembers that the breast is a highly differentiated modified sweat gland apparatus.

SWEAT GLAND CARCINOMAS

Sweat gland carcinomas are rare and troublesome neoplasms. Most reports treat sweat gland carcinomas as a homogeneous entity. Only a few authors have attempted to separate these neoplasms into distinct entities with corresponding histologic findings. Several well-defined clinicopathologic entities do exist and can be sorted out from the apparently confusing and overlapping histologic patterns. This approach has therapeutic and prognostic value, as tumors of high and low malignant potential can then be identified. Some sweat gland carcinomas such as micro-

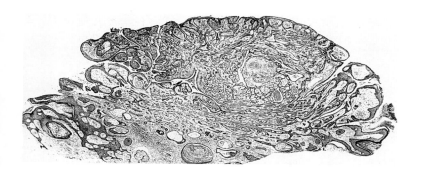

Figure 47–24. Nipple adenomatosis. The nipple has been replaced by a very complex ductal proliferation.

TABLE 47–2. SWEAT GLAND CARCINOMAS: CLASSIFICATION BY MALIGNANT POTENTIAL

Low

 Microcystic carcinoma
 Adenoid cystic carcinoma
 Eccrine epithelioma
 Mucinous carcinoma
 Extramammary's Paget's disease

Intermediate

 Ductal adenocarcinoma
 Aggressive digital papillary adenocarcinoma
 Malignant acrospiroma (polypoid & desmoplastic)

High

 Malignant acrospiroma
  Malignant hidroacanthoma
  Malignant eccrine poroma
  Clear cell hidroadenocarcinoma
 Malignant mixed tumor
 Malignant spiradenoma
 Malignant cylindroma
 Apocrine carcinoma

Unknown[a]

 Signet ring cell carcinoma
 Malignant papillary syringadenoma
 Mucoepidermoid carcinoma

[a] Insufficient number of cases to evaluate biologic behavior.

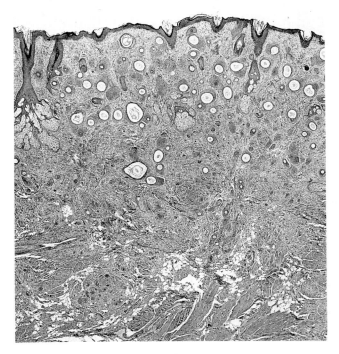

Figure 47–25. Microcystic carcinoma. The tumor is composed of multiple superficial cysts of benign appearance, but invades the skeletal muscle at the deepest portion.

cystic and mucinous carcinomas, for example, have mostly locally invasive potential. Others such as malignant acrospiroma pose a definite threat for metastatic disease. The most useful classification of adnexal carcinomas uses criteria similar to those for benign adnexal neoplasms (Table 47–2).

MICROCYSTIC CARCINOMA (SCLEROSING SWEAT DUCT CARCINOMA)

Clinical Features

This neoplasm is of recent recognition.[98] Seventy-five percent are located on the face, with preference on the upper lip. There is a wide range (20 to 76 years; mean 47 years) and about equal sex distribution.[98,99,204–210]

The tumor presents as ill-defined induration, firm plaque, or discrete nodules. The neoplasms grow slowly, from 1 to 17 years on the average; in one case the tumor evolved over 30 years.[208] The epidermal surface is smooth or crusted and yellowish or flesh-colored.

Histologic Features

The histology is highly characteristic; a variety of histologic patterns exist. In untreated lesions, the histologic features are somewhat stratified (Fig. 47–25). The most superficial part is made up of small keratinous cysts with well-developed lamellar keratin. Alternating with the cysts are solid strands of the epithelium formed by small basaloid cells with scant eosinophilic cytoplasm. Some of the strands may develop small lumina and calcification. At the midlevel of the lesion, the solid strands prevail, but they become smaller. Small glandular lumina lined by cuboidal cells are also present (Fig. 47–26). The cords may have rounded or

larger branching lumina with small solid papillation of cuboidal cells. The presence of this component is very irregular, being almost nonexistent in some tumors but making up one third or more in rare ones. Deeper in the dermis, the cell nests become smaller, diminishing to clusters of only two or three cells. The stroma becomes increasingly fibrous, and the neoplasm now has a frankly scirrhous, infiltrative growth. The tumor invades the striated muscle and, in a few cases, manifests itself in the corium of the buccal mucosa. At the deeper levels there is extensive perineural invasion. The lesion lacks cytologic atypia and mitotic figures are rare. Some histologic variants present pronounced papillated lumen formation, extensive clear cell change, branching tubules, or solid cords.

Differential Diagnosis

Several conditions enter into the differential diagnosis of microcystic carcinoma. The most likely lesion for it to be confused with it is desmoplastic trichoepithelioma. Syringoma and papillary eccrine adenoma may also pose differential diagnosis problems.

ADENOID CYSTIC CARCINOMA

History

True adenoid cystic carcinoma of the skin is a very rare lesion. Only rare examples are reported.[130,211–217] These tumors have a wide distribution, with the scalp being the

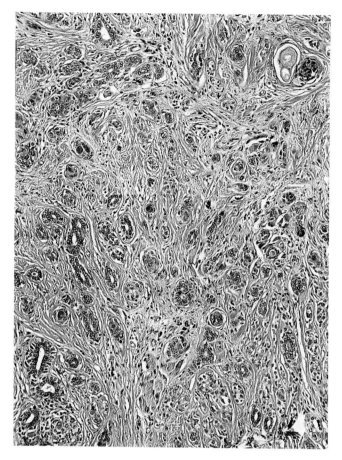

Figure 47–26. Microcystic carcinoma. Small solid cords and glands are associated with a dense fibrous stroma.

preferential location. They have an indolent but progressive course of up to 14 years. Metastases were reported in only one case.[215] The tumor presents as crusted verrucous plaques or deep-seated nodules.

Histologic Features

Adenoid cystic carcinoma presents histologically as dermal nodules without epidermal contact. The tumor lobules, as its name indicates, are made up of largely cystic islands with areas of solid nests. The predominant cell type is a small, basophilic cell with scant cytoplasm. Some of the tumor masses have central small cavitations giving the lobules a cribriform appearance (Fig. 47–27).

Cysts and cell interstices have abundant basophilic, mucinous material. The cells have granular chromatin, prominent nucleoli, and rare mitotic figures. The stroma is fibrous with numerous fibroblasts and variable lymphocytic infiltrate. Thin sleeves of tumor cells surround the dermal nerves. The tumor has a generally infiltrative growth extending deep into the dermis and even the subcutaneous tissue.

Histogenesis

Histologically, adenoid cystic carcinoma poses a difficult differential with the so-called "adenoid cystic" variant of basal cell carcinoma. Mucin histochemistry is of no help, as both have similar hyaluronic acid–rich "stromal" mucins. The epidermal origin of basal cell carcinoma is helpful as is, of course, the perineural invasion common in adenoid cystic carcinoma.

ECCRINE EPITHELIOMA

History/Clinical Features

Eccrine epithelioma was described by Freeman and Winkelmann in 1969.[219] A total of 12 cases has been reported.[219–227] It affects males and females in equal numbers.

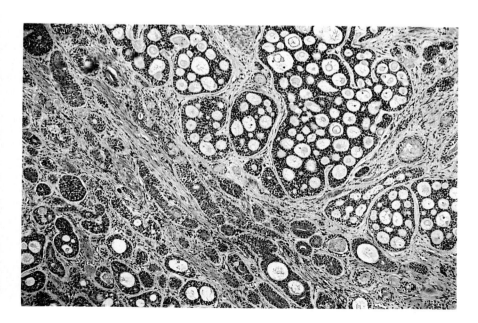

Figure 47–27. Adenoid cystic carcinoma. The two classical patterns are present: cribriform and tubular.

The neoplasm is recognized in a wide age range, from 25 to 70 years (mean 49). It often has a long course that ranges between 2 and 40 years, with an average of 13 years. The scalp is more frequently involved (nine times) than other sites. Some tumors have attained a large size; more than half of the eccrine epitheliomas were 5 cm in diameter or larger. The largest tumor reached 15 × 17 cm. Clinically, the neoplasm presents as a slowly enlarging, long-standing, crusted ulcerative process with a rolled, pearly border. The tumor size is often underestimated clinically, resulting in multiple recurrences. Three patients had three recurrent neoplasms, one had six, and another patient had "several" recurrences. In one patient eccrine epithelioma developed in a site irradiated 25 years earlier (for a "birthmark" at age 10). This tumor also invaded the outer skull table.[226] One patient experienced local lymph node metastasis after a 3.5-year course.[223]

Histologic Features

The tumors are composed of basophilic staining cuboidal cells arranged in luminal, alveolar, or cystic arrays. Some solid masses have a cribriform appearance. The tumor nests extend through the dermis and sometimes invade the subcutaneous tissue in more advanced or recurrent lesions. The tubular lumina contain granular eosinophilic material. The cribriform structures have a distinct PAS-stainable basement membrane that encloses both the periphery of the nests and the luminal membrane. The stroma is composed of dense collagenous tissue, with numerous fibroblasts. Areas resembling basal cell carcinoma may be found.

Differential Diagnosis

Eccrine epithelioma has to be differentiated from basal cell carcinoma syringoma and microcystic carcinoma.

MUCINOUS CARCINOMA

History/Clinical Features

Mucinous carcinoma is one of the most common adnexal carcinomas of the skin.[130,212,228–239] Although other carcinomas of adnexal origin may be muciparous, the name *mucinous carcinoma* is reserved for this neoplasm, which produces abundant mucinous lakes and, morphologically, is highly similar to colloid carcinoma of the breast. The use of the term *adenocystic* in association with this neoplasm is a poor choice. It may lead to confusion with a totally different lesion, the adenoid cystic carcinoma, found only rarely in the skin, but more frequently in the salivary glands.

Mendoza and Helwig described 14 cases, established the diagnostic criteria, and delineated its clinical features.[231] Headington reported the ultrastructural and enzyme histochemical features.[235] Wright and Font described 21 cases located in the eyelids, a site of predilection for mucinous carcinomas.[238]

The tumor presents as nodules less than 3 cm in size. It is usually flesh-colored, but sometimes is tan, gray, red, or blue. These tumors often can be transilluminated. The tumor has a soft, spongy consistency, but may feel firm or hard.

The large majority of the tumors are located on the face. Twenty-four were on the eyelid area (lower lid, 12; upper lid, 6; inner canthus, 3). Ten tumors were on the other areas of the face (cheek, 5; chin, 2; ear, 1). Eight cases were on the scalp, 6 were on the axilla, 3 were on the trunk, and there was one each on the neck and foot.

The tumor affects twice as many males as females (35:14). These statistics could be biased, as they are based on two larger series published from the Armed Forces Institute of Pathology, an institution with a historically predominant male population of patients.[231,238] Curiously, 14 of the patients were black, a race in whom cutaneous tumors, epithelial or melanocytic, are generally rare.

Most tumors presented between the ages of 50 and 70 (mean 60); however, they have been observed in patients from 8 to 84 years old.

Recurrence is common, with 19 cases recurring (12 recurred once; 3 twice; 2 three times; and 2 had "several" recurrences). The recurrence is often after a few years, with an average lapse of 4 years.

Mucinous carcinoma is a tumor with low metastasizing potential. Only seven tumors metastasized, five of them to the local lymph nodes. Two patients had extensive metastatic disease. One tumor invaded local structures (bone and transverse sinus).[228] One other patient was alive with disease 8 years after the excision.

In summary, mucinous carcinoma often affects middle-aged to older males. It is relatively common in blacks. It involves predominantly the head and, conspicuously, the eyelids. This tumor has a high recurrence rate and low metastatic potential.

Grossly, the tumor shows a lobulated mucoid, glistening appearance.

Histologic Features

Histologically, the neoplasm is composed of cords and lobules of epithelial cells, floating in large pools of slightly basophilic mucin, separated by thin fibrovascular septa (Fig. 47–28). Larger lobules of tumor cells have several lumina, conferring a cribriform pattern. The cells are cuboidal or polygonal, with moderate to ample eosinophilic cytoplasm (Fig. 47–29). The cytoplasm is homogeneous or slightly vacuolated. The nucleus is vesicular and isomorphic. On occasion, "light" and "dark" cells can be identified in the tumor lobules.

Most tumors are made of lobules that grow in an expansile fashion. Invasive growth is also found more rarely. There is practically no stromal or inflammatory reaction in primary tumors. Mitoses are rare. Focal hemorrhage and hemosiderin-laden macrophages are common findings. No necrosis is found.

Though rare, some tumors can develop a mostly solid pattern. One of the cases I studied was diagnosed as a benign acrospiroma. The two consecutive recurrences showed the classic mucinous lakes of mucinous carcinoma. On review of the primary lesion, numerous lumina filled with mucicarmine-positive material were found. It is not clear if this represented an example of an acrospiroma evolving into a mucinous carcinoma, or in fact, if it had been a mucinous carcinoma from the onset.[237] On occasion, the recurrent tumors have a more solid pattern than the primary neoplasm.

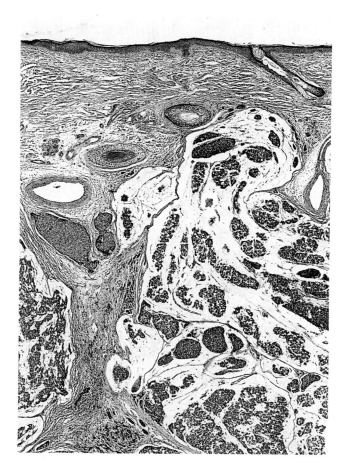

Figure 47–28. Mucinous carcinoma. Nests of epithelial cells are immersed in mucinous pools. Note the solid islands at center left.

Differential Diagnosis

The most important differential diagnosis includes metastatic mucinous carcinoma. A morphologic distinction with a mammary colloid carcinoma may be impossible. It must be borne in mind, however, that cutaneous mucinous carcinoma has an indolent course with local recurrences. Progression to widespread metastatic disease is unlikely. Therefore, clinical history is of utmost importance in settling the problem.

Metastatic mucinous carcinoma, mostly from the gastrointestinal tract or ovary, may closely mimic primary cutaneous mucinous carcinoma. The mucin histochemistry is, however, distinctive and would allow a correct diagnosis. Three types of mucins are present in gastrointestinal carcinomas: neutral mucins, sialomucins, and sulfomucins. Most commonly, the tumor has a mixture of these, with one or two prevailing. The presence of sulfomucins is highly distinctive of carcinomas of gastrointestinal origin.[240] Sulfomucins, like sialomucins, are acid mucins. It is possible to distinguish them by alcian blue stain at pH 1.0 in which sulfomucins are positive but sialic mucins are not. Electron microscopy, in addition, could provide additional differentiating features.[241]

Some basal cell carcinomas, such as the so-called "adenoid cystic" basal cell carcinoma, may have large areas of mucinous material. The mucinous material, however, is hyaluronidase sensitive and sialidase resistant (the reverse from mucinous carcinoma), when stained with alcian blue.

MALIGNANT ACROSPIROMA

As most malignant neoplasms of sweat glands are difficult to classify, those tumors with close epidermal contact and poorly differentiated squamous features pose an additional

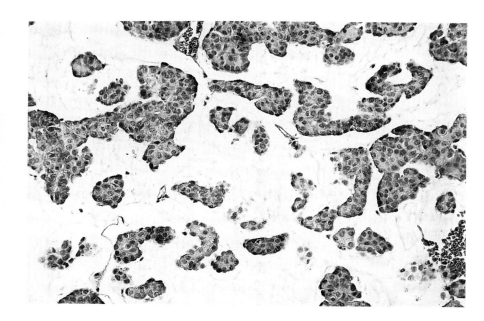

Figure 47–29. Mucinous carcinoma. The small cords of tumor cells are devoid of cellular atypia.

problem. They have to be differentiated from tumors of squamous differentiation, both epidermal squamous cell carcinoma and poorly differentiated metastatic visceral carcinomas.

Authors have tried to compare these malignant neoplasm with their benign counterparts. Therefore, cases reported as malignant hidroacanthoma simplex, malignant eccrine poroma, or malignant acrospiroma are published. In our review of the handful of well-documented cases, it became obvious that a clear distinction between a malignant version of hidroacanthoma simplex (a lesion already controversial in itself) and a malignant eccrine poroma was an extremely difficult, if not impossible task, given the extreme histologic overlap of the few cases reported under either name. We have chosen the name *malignant eccrine poroma* to designate all these cases. Subdivision of these cases may be necessary in the future as more cases are accumulated and their characteristics are identified.

Malignant eccrine poromas are sufficiently different from malignant acrospiromas to warrant separation of the two. As with their benign counterparts, there is considerable overlap of morphologic features between the two groups. In general, malignant eccrine poromas have a relatively large number of intraepidermal components, whereas malignant acrospiromas are largely dermal neoplasms.

Malignant Eccrine Poroma

History
Malignant eccrine poroma was described by Pinkus and Mehregan in 1963 as epidermotropic eccrine carcinoma.[242] Few sporadic case reports have been published since then.[39,243–252] Two large series reporting 27 and 18 cases, respectively, were recently published.[253,254] About 55 cases were published by 1983.

Clinical Features
The tumor presents as a verrucous plaque with a variable but often lengthy duration (from 2 months to 40 years). In at least 15 cases the neoplasms were present for 10 years or longer. The tumor has an almost equal sexual distribution. It presents commonly in older age groups. It has been described in patients from 19 to 90 years old (average 65 years). Its most common location is the lower extremities (60% or 30 cases), followed by the head (20% or 10 cases), upper extremities (16% or 8 cases), and trunk (6% or 3 cases). Patients with tumors located on the head are usually younger than patients whose neoplasms are on the extremities.

The lesion is usually a nodule or a noduloulcerative or infiltrated plaque with verrucous features. It usually measures 1 to 5 cm in diameter, reaching up to 10 cm. A peculiar mode of presentation observed in four patients, including the original case of Pinkus and Mehregan, is the dissemination of numerous cutaneous tumor nodules distributed in a fashion suggesting a lymphangitic spread.[242,243,250,251] In three patients the neoplasms were intraepidermal. Recurrences were frequent after attempts at local destruction or excision (20% or 11 cases). Metastases were present in similar numbers (20% or 11 cases). Most of the metastatic spread

was to local lymph nodes. All four patients with disseminated cutaneous metastasis just mentioned presented metastatic lymph node spread, and for three of them, death was attributable to the tumor. Diffuse intraabdominal metastatic disease was found in one patient who underwent autopsy. The fourth patient had a very short follow-up.

Histologic Features
The neoplasms have a plaquelike growth with a characteristic intraepidermal component of nests and islands of small cells sharply demarcated from the surrounding epidermal keratinocytes (Fig. 47–30A). The cells may have regular vesicular nuclei and scant cytoplasm. The tumor cells located near sites of dermal invasion often display a greater degree of cytologic atypia. There is no tendency for the cells to undergo keratinization. Those nests that occupy the whole thickness of the epidermis produce a parakeratotic scale that contrasts with the orthokeratotic epidermis. Dyskeratosis or apoptosis is not found. An inflammatory infiltrate located in the superficial dermis is found in association with more anaplastic areas of the neoplasm.

Several changes supervene when the tumor invades the dermis. The tumor masses with similar but often larger cells have a wide epidermal contact. Although some nodules have cytologic features nearly identical to those of the intraepidermal component (i.e., small regular cells with scant cytoplasm), others present a striking variation of pattern. Some of the cells of the tumor nodules, especially at the deeper portions, display cytoplasmic vacuolization with formation of intracellular lumina (Fig. 47–30B). These multiple vacuoles may coalesce to form ductal lumina. These cells are often larger and have ample eosinophilic cytoplasm. Central necrosis may be found in larger tumor nodules present in the dermis. On occasion, a variable part of the tumor may display extensive sheaths of cells with clear cytoplasm. These areas often have more anaplastic features, a high mitotic rate, and extensive areas of necrosis, strongly resembling a malignant clear cell acrospiroma. Both perineural invasion and lymphatic embolization may be seen.

One curious property of this neoplasm that is seen particularly in the peculiar epidermotropic type is the invasion of the epidermis from a dermal metastatic nodule. The resulting histologic picture is indistinguishable from primary lesions that started in the epidermis and later invaded the dermis (Fig. 47–17). This phenomenon may be extensive, as seen in four cases reported in the literature.[242,243,250,251]

Metastatic nodules in lymph nodes appear as anaplastic nonkeratinizing carcinomas made up of cells with large atypical vesicular nuclei and ample clear cytoplasm. Necrosis and high mitotic rates are common.

Differential Diagnosis
Malignant eccrine poromas have to be differentiated from a variety of benign and malignant tumors. The intraepidermal phase must be distinguished from hidroacanthoma simplex, carcinoma in situ, and Paget's disease. In the invasive phase, the most difficult differential diagnosis is with the nonkeratinizing squamous cell carcinomas arising in Bowen's disease and metastatic disease.

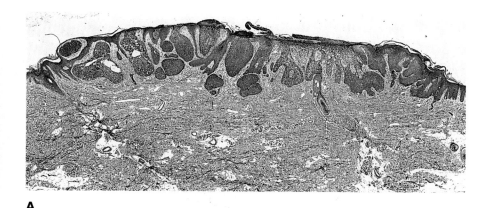

A

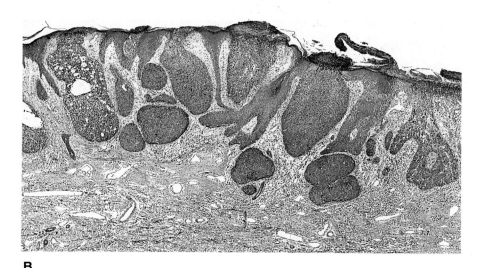

B

Figure 47–30. Malignant eccrine poroma: **A.** Plaquelike tumor. **B.** Lobules of basaloid cells invade superficial dermis. Some ductal differentiation is present on the left.

Malignant Acrospiroma

Clinical Features

The tumor was located on the face in 11 cases (cheek, 5; temple, 2; nose, 2; scalp, 1; eyelid, 1); were on the extremities in 6 cases (hand, 3; sole, 2; wrist, finger, and leg, 1 each); and on the axilla,[33,60–69] in 1 case.

The patients were 10 men and 5 women. Most were in the sixth decade (mean 61); two patients were in the second decade. One tumor was present at birth. It grew slowly for 15 months and then accelerated downhill; the patient died in 4 months.[261] The tumors present as large, ulcerated masses or nodules. Metastatic disease occurred in 10 of the 15 patients. In 8 cases, local and regional lymph node involvement was noted. Three patients had metastatic disease in the lung, diagnosed by chest x-ray, and three had metastases to bones.[52,211,256–264]

Follow-up information in the literature either is brief or simply does not exist. At least 6 patients have died of the disease. One patient was alive but had extensive pulmonary metastases, and another had disseminated disease at the time their cases were reported.

Histologic Features

Malignant acrospiroma has three specific forms.

- *Polypoid Type:* These tumors produce fleshy polypoid exophytic growths. There is adjacent intraepidermal carcinoma in situ with characteristic clear cell formation. The tumor grows in solid lobules.
- *Sclerosing Type:* These tumors present as an infiltrated plaque. The central portion often shows intense fibrosis, and the tumor lobules exhibit infiltrative but well-delimited growth into the surrounding dermis.
- *Comedo Type:* This type produced large lobulated dermal masses with central necrosis. The tumor lobules may approach the epidermis from below to produce intraepidermal invasion as nested tumor cells that are sharply distinguished from the surrounding epidermal keratinocytes.

The tumor lobules are made up of polygon-shaped, pale to clear cytoplasm with distinct cell membranes (Fig. 47–31). Areas of smaller, more basophilic cells, often at the periphery of the lobules, can also be observed.

Most tumors are made of solid sheets. Acinar or ductal-type lumen formation is very rare. A common finding,

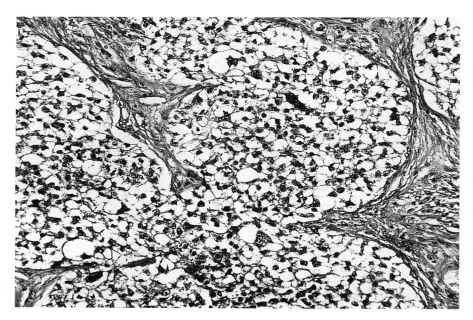

Figure 47–31. Malignant acrospiroma: This neoplasm is made up of lobules of atypical clear cells.

however, and an important feature for diagnosis is intracellular lumen formation. Intracellular lumina appear as cytoplasmic vacuoles that tend to push the nuclei peripherally. In more advanced intracytoplasmic lumen formation, a peripheral eosinophilic ring of tonofilaments is observed. These features can be enhanced by polarization microscopy as a refractile periluminal ring. This finding is termed *cuticular differentiation* and is characteristic of tumors of ductal differentiation.

Occasionally, a dense peripheral inflammatory infiltrate is present. Melanocytes may be seen in the midst of the tumor lobules and in the metastases.

The cytologic features vary from tumor to tumor. Although some have deceptively benign cytology indistinguishable from benign acrospiromas, others have numerous mitoses and pronounced nuclear pleomorphism.

Some malignant acrospiromas may have a small basophilic cell component similar to malignant eccrine poromas. Tumors made up of eosinophilic polyhedral cells with an epidermoid appearance can also be found. Benign eccrine acrospiromas may display atypical nuclear changes and increased mitotic activity. These changes are usually focal and may not have prognostic significance; however, in a study of 18 cases, Mambo[267] found 5 cases that recurred. Three of them were felt to be malignant, and one metastasized to a local lymph node. These tumors may have been carcinomas from the onset.[52]

Features suggestive of malignancy are infiltrative growth, necrosis, large size, recent growth, confluent cytologic atypia, high mitotic rate, and peripheral inflammatory reaction. Sebaceous carcinomas are equally rare neoplasms that display large areas of clear cells. In general, these tumors have a bubbly cytoplasm because of the lipid vacuoles. The clear cell change is often more limited. Lipid stains, when possible, provide the correct diagnosis. A useful clue is the presence of xanthomatous cells next to tumor lobules,

reacting to the lipid spillage from cell necrosis often seen in sebaceous neoplasms.

MALIGNANT MIXED TUMOR

Clinical Findings
Malignant adnexal tumors of the skin with associated chondroid stroma are very rare. At least 18 well-documented cases have been reported. Most tumors were diagnosed after the third decade; three exceptions were two 15-year-olds and one 14-year-old.[134,265–274] The patients consisted of 11 women and 3 men. Most of the tumors were located on the extremities. Four patients had tumors on the upper extremities (two on the upper arm, and one each on the wrist and palm); five tumors were on the lower extremities (three on the sole, and one each on the thigh and groin); three tumors were on the head (one each on the scalp, face, and external auditory meatus); one patient had a tumor on the sacral area and on the back.

Some tumors appear to arise in previously benign lesions[265] as juxtaposed areas of benign and malignant tissue were observed. Another appeared to have arisen in association with a spiradenoma.[271] Three tumors were accompanied by cytologic atypia, but did not metastasize or recur after excision. Another eight patients had local recurrences, from 6 months to 4 years after excision. Five of these patients presented with synchronous or metachronous metastatic disease.

Eleven of fifteen patients had local or distant metastases. Five tumors metastasized to the regional lymph nodes, four to the lungs, and one to the kidney; three had local soft tissue metastases. In one case metastatic disease developed, but only after 16 years. Another patient had widespread metastases.

Five patients died from the tumor. Follow-up was unavailable on two other patients with extensive metastatic disease.

Most tumors appear to be larger than the average benign mixed tumor. They often present as cystic structures with a mucoid consistency. Infiltrative growth is common; therefore, these tumors do not enucleate out as the benign counterparts.

Histologic Features

Histologically, the tumors can be similar to benign mixed tumors. Benign and malignant areas can be seen side by side. One tumor was associated with a spiradenoma. Four tumors presented with areas of ossification.

Most neoplasms presented with variable degrees of cellular atypia, mitotic figures, and areas of poorly differentiated epithelial structures. These were inconsistent and unreliable prognostic indicators, as some tumors with similar features followed a benign course. Recurrent tumors often become cytologically increasingly atypical.

Morphologic features suggestive of malignancy are cytologic atypia, high mitotic rate, infiltrative growth pattern, and an associated lymphocytic inflammatory infiltrate.

Differential Diagnosis

The most important differential diagnostic problem is with benign mixed tumors. Important diagnostic criteria include large size of the tumor, cytologic atypia, high mitotic rate, infiltrative growth, and associated inflammatory infiltrate. Malignant mixed tumors can also be confused with myxopapillary ependymomas.[275,276] Soft tissue tumors, such as extraskeletal myxoid chondrosarcoma[277] and its close relative chordoid sarcoma,[278] may also have peripheral nests and cords of cells with a distinctive epithelioid appearance.

MALIGNANT SPIRADENOMA

Whereas most adnexal carcinomas are sufficiently distinctive, the diagnosis of malignant spiradenoma requires the histologic identification of an associated benign spiradenoma. This is due to the relative lack of differentiating features of the tumor cells of benign spiradenoma, on the one hand, and the variable histology of the malignant tumor originating from them, on the other.

To date, 11 examples of adnexal carcinomas associated with spiradenomas have been reported.[271,279–283] No sex predilection is noted. Patients ranged between 26 and 85 years in age. The usual history was that of a long-standing nodule that had recently grown rapidly. The tumor had been present from 15 to 50 years. Its location was variable: three were on the digits; three on the back; two on the legs; and one each on the palm, neck, and chest. One patient had a regional lymph node metastasis that was excised. After 7 years of follow-up, no metastases or recurrences were noted.[280] Another patient had a local recurrence that was treated; she was disease free 2 years later.[271] A third patient had a rapid downhill course and died 11 months after her last surgical procedure. Autopsy revealed numerous metastases in the brain and bone, and a single pulmonary metastasis.[279]

The histologic changes in this handful of cases are re-

markably regular. In all 11 cases, in some of them only after a careful search, a benign spiradenoma was found. The malignant tumor had variable histology ranging from a solid nonkeratinizing tumor to a carcinoma with squamous and adenocarcinomatous features.[279,280] Some carcinomas had a sarcomatoid or osteoclastic-like cytologic character.[279] One neoplasm had histologic features of a malignant mixed tumor with cartilaginous stroma.[271] Direct contiguous transformation from the benign spiradenoma to the malignant part of the neoplasm was documented in 7 of the 11 cases.

No ultrastructural or histochemical features have as yet been reported in these exceedingly rare neoplasms.

Their diagnosis depends exclusively on identifying the benign spiradenoma. This diagnosis should be suspected in any high-grade cutaneous carcinoma arising in a long-standing, deep-seated nodule.

MALIGNANT CYLINDROMA

Clinical Features

Eleven cases of malignant cylindromas have been reported.[284–293] The patients were between 59 and 96 years of age. Men and women were equally afflicted.

In seven of the cases, the carcinomatous growth arose on the scalp or face in association with long-standing tumors identified clinically and histologically as cylindromas. One patient had had multiple scalp tumors for 22 years. After biopsy, these were felt to be solid carcinomatous growths with some features of cylindroma; however, no areas of classic benign cylindroma were identified.[291] In another case, a tumor of 2 months' duration was present in the thigh of a 96-year-old woman. This lesion was felt, by the authors, to be histologically a malignant cylindroma.[290]

The malignant cylindromas often have a very aggressive course with widespread metastases. Visceral, lymph nodal, and bony metastases are reported.

Histologic Features

The tumors have some similarity to dermal cylindromas with nests and cords of basaloid cells. The tumor cells display a considerable degree of atypia with focal necrosis. Thick, homogeneous hyaline, as seen in the benign counterpart, is often not found.

Histologic examination commonly identifies a benign cylindroma component. It is debatable if a diagnosis of malignant cylindroma can be made in the absence of the benign counterpart, or in a site other than the scalp which is an exclusive location for the form known as multiple cylindromas (turban tumor).

Differential Diagnosis

The same concepts discussed for malignant spiradenoma apply to malignant cylindroma. The malignant components lack sufficient differentiating features per se.

Ideally, a case diagnosed as malignant cylindroma should possess the following characteristics:

1. Family history (cylindromas are often inherited in an autosomal dominant pattern.)
2. Long-standing history of benign cylindromas histologically documented

3. Histologic evidence of a malignant neoplasm (Cylindromas may follow an aggressive growth on the scalp without necessarily becoming biologically malignant.)
4. Metastases

It is clear that all these criteria are very stringent and may not be met in most instances.

As was emphasized earlier, the diagnosis of malignant cylindroma can be made if both malignant and benign areas are documented. As most malignant cylindromas reported arose in the form known as turban tumor, special care should be exercised in following these patients for the rare possibility of malignant conversion. This malignant transformation appears to be multifocal and part of well-orchestrated biologic changes in the tumor.[294,295]

APOCRINE ADENOCARCINOMA

History

Apocrine adenocarcinoma is a rare entity. Because reports in the literature of apocrine adenocarcinoma have been few and sporadic, and many cases of obviously benign tumors have been incorrectly interpreted as malignant,[296] it is difficult to establish an accurate clinical profile. In addition, many cases have been reported as "sweat gland carcinomas" without adequate descriptions of their differentiation; we interpret most of them as "eccrine." In this section, malignant neoplasms that resemble either syringomas or cylindromas are excluded, as it is believed that their differentiation most resembles that of eccrine glands.[230]

Clinical Features

Most apocrine gland carcinomas arise in the axillary or anogenital regions,[297] the axilla being the most frequent.[298] Less commonly, they have occurred on the scalp, face, and trunk.[298–300] With rare exceptions, these neoplasm are solitary.[301,302]

In the series of 10 apocrine adenocarcinomas of the axilla reported from the Armed Forces Institute of Pathology by Warkel and Helwig, the average age was 57.9 years, and all patients were older than 25.[298] This leads to speculation that full apocrine maturity following puberty might be an important factor. Rarely have they arisen in adolescence.[303] There appears to be no distinct sex predominance, and the duration of an adenocarcinoma has frequently been reported to be over 10 years and rarely as long as 30 years.[211,304] Slow growth often accompanied by late anaplastic change is characteristic.

According to Warkel and Helwig, these neoplasm do not have distinctive clinical findings that would enable an accurate preoperative diagnosis.[298] Patients may experience some discomfort but usually no pain. The tumors may be single or multinodular, firm or cystic, and the overlying skin is red to purple with occasional ulceration. In the Armed Forces Institute of Pathology series, the size ranged from 1.5 to 8 cm.[298]

On cross section, apocrine adenocarcinomas are usually reddish, circumscribed, firm, and solid with occasional cystic or hemorrhagic foci.[298]

Histologic Features

Microscopically, they are nonencapsulated, and are usually intradermal but may extend into the epidermis and subcutis. Their histologic pattern may very considerably from normal-appearing, easily recognizable apocrine glandlike structures to relatively undifferentiated neoplasms. They may be papillary, tubular, or solid. In two cases, Warkel and Helwig could identify a transition from normal-appearing apocrine structures to a malignant neoplasm.[298] Decapitation secretion, an important criterion for apocrine differentiation, is usually but not always present.[299] Warkel and Helwig noted that mitotic figures ranged from few to four per high-power field, and used a combination of features, including the degree of cellular pleomorphism, hyperchromasia, mitotic activity, and the presence of stromal invasion, to separate the adenocarcinomas from adenomas.[298]

Within the fibroblastic stroma, usually a dense lymphocytic infiltrate often contains plasma cells. Warkel and Helwig were unable to demonstrate myoepithelial cells with the PTAH stain.[298]

Differential Diagnosis

Histologically, the distinction between an apocrine adenoma and an adenocarcinoma can be extremely difficult because of the often subtle histologic features that distinguish these two entities. As with most neoplasms, infiltration of nerves or vessels, when present, is a key criterion; stromal invasion is less so and often difficult to determine in apocrine neoplasms. Cellular pleomorphism and mitotic activity are also useful. Special care should be exercised to differentiate those tumors with apocrine differentiation from those ductal tumors with eosinophilic cells and pinched off luminal cytoplasm reminiscent of decapitation secretion of apocrine glands.

MISCELLANEOUS RARE TUMORS

Few adnexal carcinomas still defy precise classification. This is due both to the relative lack of histologic differentiation and to the rarity of the tumors so that their clinical and histologic characteristics are not understood.

Some sweat gland carcinomas are morphologically distinctive enough to suggest that if sufficient cases are collected, they may produce well-defined clinicopathologic entities. One such neoplasm is the *signet ring cell carcinoma* that is characteristically located on the eyelids.[305,306] It has a bland, single-cell infiltrating pattern. The cells have vesicular nuclei and ample bubbly cytoplasm and have a strong resemblance to histiocytes (Fig. 47–32). The clinical course is protracted. As they are often confused with metastases, a diligent search for primary tumor is usually nonproductive. The tumor cells are positive for sialic acid–containing mucins (PAS, alcian blue, and mucicarmine stains are removed by sialidase) and for carcinoembryonic antigen. Similar histologic findings have been reported in breast carcinomas metastatic to the eyelids.[307]

Another neoplasm with distinctive features is the *malignant form of the papillary syringadenoma*, of which only a few cases have been reported.[308,309] These tumors also lack precise morphologic definition, but some appear to have

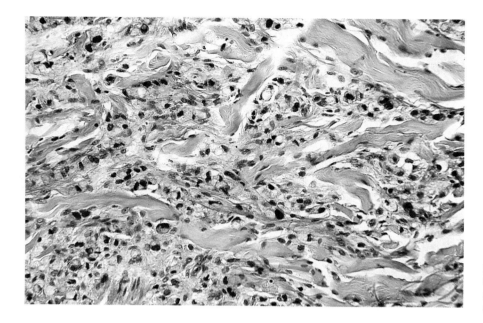

Figure 47–32. Signet ring cell carcinoma. Sheets of small cells invade between collagen bundles. The signet ring tumor cells resemble histiocytes.

a remarkable yet cytologically malignant similarity to their benign counterpart.

Very rare neoplasms have both mucin production and squamous differentiation. These tumors are known as *mucoepidermoid carcinomas.*[239,310–313]

A most interesting form of sweat gland carcinoma, and perhaps a relatively common one, is the *ductal adenocarcinoma.* The tumor presents as a schirrous, radiating lesion in the dermis, composed of branching papillated tumor strands embedded in a dense fibrous and inflammatory stroma (Fig. 47–33). The neoplastic cells show variable degree of atypia and ample eosinophilic cytoplasm. The cells have a pinched off luminal appearance, highly reminiscent of apocrine cells. It is very likely that ductal adenocarcino-

mas are confused with apocrine carcinomas; however, electron microscopic studies demonstrate abundant periluminal tonofilament characteristic of the cuticular differentiation. Ductal adenocarcinoma has to be differentiated from the glandular form of microcystic carcinoma and the aggressive digital papillary adenoma.

Aggressive digital papillary adenoma has a preference for the digits and adjacent tissue of the palms and soles (Fig. 47–34). It affects older individuals. It has a tendency for local recurrence and deep soft tissue infiltration. Fifteen percent of the patients had metastatic disease. It is very difficult to differentiate those tumors that are locally aggressive from those that may metastasize.[314]

From the preceding conclusion, it is clear that sweat

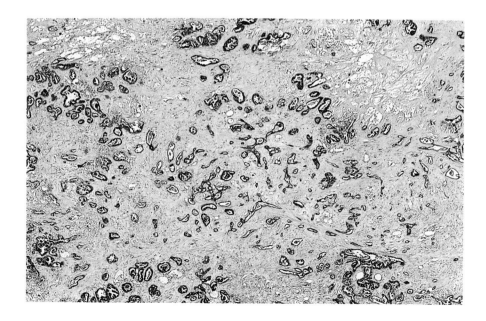

Figure 47–33. Ductal adenocarcinoma. Numerous branching glandular lumina, some showing intraluminal papillations, are embedded in a fibrous stroma.

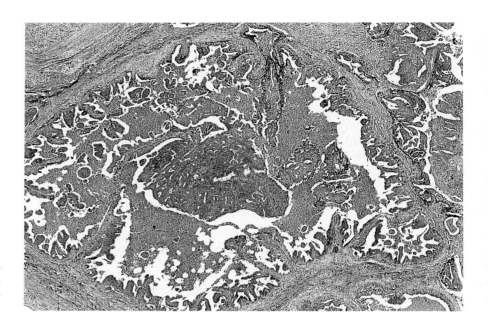

Figure 47–34. Aggressive digital papillary adenoma. This is a recurrent neoplasm exhibiting the characteristic papillary cystic pattern.

gland carcinomas constitute a hetereogeneous group of neoplasms with variable biologic behavior. The appropriate classification is of crucial importance to institution of an appropriate treatment modality. Most sweat gland carcinomas are well-defined clinicopathologic entities even when only small numbers are properly studied. We have currently established a registry for these neoplasms with the purpose of better understanding these fascinating and rare adnexal tumors.

REFERENCES

1. Cooper PH: Mitotic figures in sweat gland adenomas. *J Cutan Pathol* 1987;14:10–14.
2. Galadari E, Mehregan AH, Lee KC: Malignant transformation of eccrine tumors. *J Cutan Pathol* 1987;14:15–22.
3. Santa Cruz DJ: Sweat gland carcinomas: A comprehensive review. *Semin Diagn Pathol* 1987;4:38–74.
4. Takahashi S, Sato T: The first case of eccrine nevus in Japan, and with reference to review of the original literatures on this nevus and the nosologic study. *Nippon Hifuka Gakkai Zasshi* 1978;88:715–719.
5. Goldstein CN: Epihidrosis (local hyperhidrosis) nevus sudoriferous. *Arch Dermatol* 1967;96:67–68.
6. Pippione M, Depaoli MA, Sartoris S: Naevus eccrine. *Dermatologica* 1976;152:41–46.
7. Pinkus H, Mehregan AH: *A Guide to Dermatohistopathology,* ed 3. E. Norwalk, Conn, Appleton-Century Crofts, 1981.
8. Domonkos AN, Suarez LS: Sudoriparous angioma. *Arch Dermatol* 1967;96:552–553.
9. Hyman AB, Harris H, Brownstein MH: Eccrine angiomatous harmartoma. *NY State J Med* 1968;68:2813–2816.
10. Zeller DJ, Goldman RL: Eccrine-pilar angiomatous harmartoma. *Dermatologica* 1971;143:111–114.
11. Challa VE, Jona J: Eccrine angiomatous harmartoma: A rare skin lesion with diverse histological features. *Dermatologica* 1977;155:216—219.
12. Abell E, Read SI: Porokeratotic eccrine ostial and dermal duct nevus. *Br J Dermatol* 1981;113:435–441.
13. Marsden RA, Fleming K, Dawber RPR: Comedo naevus of the palm—A sweat duct naevus *Br J Dermatol* 1981;111:717–722.
14. Leppard B, Marks R: Comedone nevus: A report of nine cases. *Trans St John's Hosp Dermatol Soc* 1973;59:45–51.
15. Weedon D, Lewis J: Acrosyringeal nevus. *J Cutan Pathol* 1977;4:166–168.
16. Smith JD, Chernosky ME: Hidrocystomas. *Arch Dermatol* 1973;108:676–679.
17. Hassan MO, Khan MA: Ultrastructure of eccrine cystadenoma. A case report. *Arch Dermatol* 1979;115:1217–1221.
18. Bures FA, Kotynek J: Differentiating between apocrine and eccrine hidrocystoma. *Cutis* 1982;9:616–619.
19. Sperling LC, Sakas EL: Eccrine hidrocystomas. *J Am Acad Dermatol* 1982;7:763–770.
20. Johnson BL, Helwig EB: Eccrine acrospiroma. A clinico-pathologic study. *Cancer* 1969;23:641–657.
21. Smith JLS, Coburn JG: Hidroacanthoma simplex. An assessment of a selected group of intraepidermal basal cell epitheliomata and of their malignant homologues. *Br J Dermatol* 1956;68:411–418.
22. Mehregan AH, Pinkus H: Intraepidermal epithelioma: A critical study. *Cancer* 1964;17:619–636.
23. Mehregan AH: Intraepidermal epithelioma, in Andrade et al. (eds): *Cancer of the Skin.* Philadelphia, Saunders, 1976, pp. 713–714.
24. Holubar K, Wolff K: Intraepidermal eccrine poroma. A histochemical and enzyme-histochemical study. *Cancer* 1969;23:626–635.
25. Cook MG, Ridgway HA: The intra-epidermal epithelioma of Jadassohn: A distinct entity. *Br J Dermatol* 1979;101:659–667.
26. Holubar K: Intraepidermal epithelioma of Jadassohn. *Br J Dermatol* 1981;113:461–462.
27. Pinkus H: Intraepidermal epithelioma of Jadassohn. *Br J Dermatol* 1981;113:462–463.
28. Mehregan AH, Levson DN: Hidroacanthoma simplex. A report of two cases. *Arch Dermatol* 1969;111:313–315.
29. Goltz RW, Fusaro RM, and Sweitzer SE: Borst-Jadassohn epithelioma. A re-evaluation. *Arch Dermatol* 1957;75:117–122.
30. Oka K, Morohashi M, Nitto H: Hidroacanthoma simplex: An ultrastructural study and comparison with eccrine poroma. *J Dermatol* 1975;2:69–78.

31. Haber H: Intraepidermal acanthoma. Recent observations on Borst-Jadassohn epithelioma. *Dermatologica* 1958;117:314–316.

32. Morales A, Hu F: Seborrheic verruca and intraepidermal basal cell epithelioma of Jadassohn. *Arch Dermatol* 1965;91:342–344.

33. Strayer DS, Santa Cruz DJ: Carcinoma in situ of the skin: A review of histopathology. *J Cutan Pathol* 1981;7:244–259.

34. Ishikawa K: Malignant hidroacanthoma simplex. *Arch Dermatol* 1971;114:529–532.

35. Rahbari H: Hidroacanthoma-simplex: A review of 15 cases. *Br J Dermatol* 1983;109:219–225.

36. Rahbari H: Syringoacanthoma: Acanthotic lesion of the acrosyringium. *Arch Dermatol* 1984;120:751–756.

37. Rahbari H: Acervate epidermal tumors. *Semin Dermatol* 1984;3:62–68.

38. Mishima Y: Epitheliomatous differentiation of the intraepidermal eccrine sweat duct. Eccrine poroepithelioma revealed by electron microscopy. *J Invest Dermatol* 1969;52:233–246.

39. Mishima Y, Morioka S: Oncogenic differentiation of the intraepidermal eccrine sweat duct: Eccrine poroma, poroepithelioma and porocarcinoma. *Dermatologica* 1969;138:238–251.

40. Pinkus H, Rogin JR, Goldman P: Eccrine poroma. Tumors exhibiting features of the epidermal sweat duct unit. *Arch Dermatol* 1956;74:511–521.

41. Hyman AB, Brownstein MH: Eccrine poroma. An analysis of forty-five new cases. *Dermatologica* 1969;138:29–38.

42. Goldner R: Eccrine poromatosis. *Arch Dermatol* 1971;101:606–608.

43. Wilkinson RD, Schopflocher P, Rozenfeld M: Hidrotic ectodermal dysplasia with diffuse eccrine poromatosis. *Arch Dermatol* 1977;113:472–476.

44. Ogino A: Linear eccrine poroma. *Arch Dermatol* 1976;112:841–844.

45. Sanderson KV, Ryan EA: The histochemistry of eccrine poroma. *Br J Dermatol* 1963;75:86–88.

46. Hashimoto K, Lever WF: Eccrine poroma. Histochemical and electron microscopic studies. *J Invest Dermatol* 1964;43:237–248.

47. Pinkus H: The discovery of eccrine poroma. *Dermatology* 1979;2:26–38.

48. Lever WF: Myoepithelial sweat gland tumor: Myoepithelioma. *Arch Dermatol* 1948;57:332–347.

49. Lever WF, Castleman B: Clear cell myoepithelioma of the skin. *Am J Pathol* 1952;28:691–699.

50. Liu Y: The histogenesis of clear cell papillary carcinoma of the skin. *Am J Pathol* 1949;25:93–103.

51. Stout AP, Cooley SGE: Carcinoma of sweat glands. *Cancer* 1951;4:521–536.

52. Hernandez-Perez E, Cestoni-Parducci R: Nodular hidradenoma and hidradenocarcinoma. A 10-year review. *J Am Acad Dermatol* 1985;12:15–20.

53. Wilson Jones E: Pigmented nodular hidradenoma. *Arch Dermatol* 1971;104:117–123.

54. Mambo NC: The significance of atypical nuclear changes in benign acrospiromas: A clinical and pathological study of 18 cases. *J Cutan Pathol* 1984;11:35–44.

55. Winkelmann RK, McLeod WA: The dermal duct tumor. *Arch Dermatol* 1966;94:50–55.

56. Faure M, Colomb D: Dermal duct tumor. *J Cutan Pathol* 1979;6:317–322.

57. Hu CH, Marques AS, Winkelmann RK: Dermal duct tumor. A histochemical and electron microscopic study. *Arch Dermatol* 1978;114:1659–1664.

58. O'Hara JM, Bensch K, Ioannides G, et al.: Eccrine sweat gland adenoma clear cell type. A histochemical study. *Cancer* 1966;19:1438–1450.

59. Hashimoto K, DiBella RJ, Lever WF: Clear cell hidradenoma. Histological, histochemical, and electron microscopic studies. *Arch Dermatol* 1967;96:18–38.

60. O'Hara JM, Bensch KG: Fine structure of eccrine sweat gland adenoma, clear cell type. *J Invest Dermatol* 1967;49:261–272.

61. Winkelmann RK, Wolff K: Solid-cystic hidradenoma of the skin. Clinical and histopathologic study. *Arch Dermatol* 1968;97:651–661.

62. Azzopardi JG: Clear cell hidradenoma. *J Pathol Bacteriol* 1958;76:379–382.

63. Mascaro JM: Considerations sur L'histogenese des tumeurs a cellules claires de la peau. *Bull Soc Fr Dermatol* 1963;70:506–511.

64. Civatte J: Clear-cell tumors of the skin, a histopathologic review. *J Cutan Pathol* 1984;11:165–175.

65. Stanley RJ, Sanchez NP, Massa MC, et al.: Epidermoid hidradenoma. A clinico-pathologic study. *J Cutan Pathol* 1982;9:293–302.

66. Haensch R, Aretz G, Hornstein OP: Zur Histotopie und Histogenese der multiplen Syringome. *Arch Derm Forsch* 1971;241:245–258.

67. Woringer F, Eichler W: Constatations et reflexions au sujet dun cas d'hidradenomes eruptifs. *Ann Dermatol* 1951;78:152–164.

68. Hashimoto K, DiBella RJ, Borsuk GM, et al.: Eruptive hidradenoma and syringoma: Histological, histochemical, and electron microscopic studies. *Arch Dermatol* 1967;96:511–519.

69. Dupre A, Carrere S, Bonafe JL, et al.: Syringomes eruptifs generalises, grains de milium et atrophodermie vermiculee. Syndrome de Nicolau et Balus. *Dermatologica* 1981;162:281–286.

70. Brown SM, Freeman RG: Syringoma limited to the vulva. *Arch Dermatol* 1971;114:331.

71. Isaacson D, Turner ML: Localized vulvar syringomas. *J Am Acad Dermatol* 1979;1:352–356.

72. Young AW Jr, Herman EW, Tovell HMM: Syringoma of the vulva: Incidence, diagnosis and cause of pruritus. *Obstet Gynecol* 1981;55:515–518.

73. Zalla JA, Perry HO: An unusual case of syringoma. *Arch Dermatol* 1971;113:215–217.

74. Yung CW, Soltani K, Bernstein JE, et al.: Unilateral linear nevoidal syringoma. *J Am Acad Dermatol* 1981;4:412–416.

75. Hughes PSH, Apisarnthanarax P: Acral syringoma. *Arch Dermatol* 1977;113:1435–1436.

76. Dupre A, Andrieu H, Fontan, et al.: Hidradenomes eruptifs generalises avec atteinte du cuir chevelu et acne conglobata. *Bull Soc Fr Dermatol* 1975;82:166–167.

77. Shelley WB, Wood MG: Occult syringomas of scalp associated with progressive hair loss. *Arch Dermatol* 1981;116:843–844.

78. Dupre A, Bonafe JL, Christol B: Syringomas as a causative factor for cicatricial alopecia. *Arch Dermatol* 1981;117:315.

79. Trozak DJ, Wood C: Occult eccrine sweat duct hamartoma and cicatricial scalp alopecia. *Cutis* 1984;34:475–477.

80. Butterworth T, Strean LP, Beerman H, et al.: Syringoma and mongolism. *Arch Dermatol* 1964;91:483–487.

81. Yesudian P, Thambiah A: Familial syringoma. *Dermatologica* 1975;151:32–35.

82. Baden HP: Hereditary syringoms. *Arch Dermatol* 1977;113:1133.

83. Hashimoto K, Blum D, Fukaya T, et al.: Familial syringoma. Case history and application of monoclonal anti–eccrine gland antibodies. *Arch Dermatol* 1985;121:756–760.

84. Dupre A, Bonafe JL: Syringomes, mongolisme, maladie de Marfan et Syndrome D'Ehlers-Danlos. Nouvelle entite posant les rapport des syringomes avec les maladies hereditares du tissu conjonctif. *Ann Dermatol Venereol* 1977;114:224–231.

85. Goltz RW: Syringoma (syringocystadenoma), in Demis J, Dob-

son RL, McGuire J (eds): *Clinical Dermatology.* Hagerstown, Harper & Row, 1979, vol 4.

86. Headington JT, Koski J, Murphy PJ: Clear cell glycogenenosis in multiple syringomas. Description and enzyme histochemistry. *Arch Dermatol* 1972;116:353–356.

87. Feibelman CE, Maize JC: Clear cell syringoma. A study by conventional and electron microscopy. *Am J Dermatopathol* 1984;6:139–150.

88. Furue M, Hori Y, Nakabayashi Y: Clear cell syringoma. Association with diabetes mellitus. *Am J Dermatopathol* 1984;6:131–138.

89. Hashimoto K, Gross BG, Lever WF: Syringoma. Histochemical and electron microscopic studies. *J Invest Dermatol* 1966;46:151–166.

90. Mustakallio KK: Succinic dehydrogenase activity of syringomas. *Acta Dermato-Venereol* 1959;39:318–323.

91. Winkelmann RK, Gottlieb BF: Syringoma: An enzymatic study. *Cancer* 1963;16:665–669.

92. Pinkus H, Mehregan AJ: Sweat apparatus tumors, in *A Guide to Dermatohistopathology,* ed 3. East Norwalk, Conn, Appleton-Century-Crofts, 1987.

93. Kwittken J: The sebaceous duct adenoma (so-called syringoma). *Mt Sinai J Med* 1976;43:553–557.

94. Hashimoto K, Gross BG, Lever WF: Electron microscopic study of the human adult eccrine gland. In the duct. *J Invest Dermatol* 1966;46:172–185.

95. Kurosumi K: Fine structure of the human sweat ducts of eccrine and apocrine types. *Arch Histol Jap* 1977;41:213–224.

96. Tani M, Yamamoto K, Mishima Y: Apocrine acrosyringeal complex in the human skin. *J Invest Dermatol* 1981;75:431–435.

97. Daicker VB: Das Lidsyringom. Studien uber seinen geweblichen Bau and Seine Histogenese. *Dermatologica* 1964;128:417–463.

98. Goldstein DJ, Barr RJ, Santa Cruz DJ: Microcystic adnexal carcinoma. A distinct clinicopathologic entity. *Cancer* 1982;50:566–572.

99. Cooper PH, Mills SE, Leonard DD, et al.: Sclerosing sweat duct (syringomatous) carcinoma. *Am J Surg Pathol* 1985;9:422–433.

100. Sutton RL: A rare sweat gland tumor. Syringocystadenoma nodularis. *Arch Dermatol* 1934;30:195–206.

101. Kersting DW, Helwig EB: Eccrine spiradenoma. *Arch Dermatol* 1956;72:199–227.

102. Mambo NC: Eccrine spiradenoma: Clinical and pathologic study of 49 tumors. *J Cutan Pathol* 1983;10:312–320.

103. Nodl F: Zur Histogenese der ekkrinen Spiradenome. *Arch Klin Exp Dermatol* 1965;221:323–335.

104. Tsur H, Lipskier E, Fisher BK: Multiple linear spiradenomas. *Plast Reconstruct Surg* 1981;68:100–102.

105. Blanchard L, Hodge SJ, Owen LG: Linear eccrine nevus with comedones. *Arch Dermatol* 1981;117:357–359.

106. Berghorn BM, Munger BL, Helwig EB: Eccrine spiradenoma: A pharmacologic study. *Arch Dermatol* 1961;84:434–438.

107. Cotton DWK, Slater DN, Rooney N, et al.: Giant vascular eccrine spiradenomas: A report of two cases with histology, immunohistology and electron microscopy. *Histopathology* 1986;10:1093–1099.

108. Hashimoto K, Gross BG, Lever WF: Eccrine spiradenoma. Histochemical and electron microscopic studies. *J Invest Dermatol* 1966;46:347–365.

109. Castro C, Winkelmann RK: Spiradenoma. Histochemical and electron microscopic study. *Arch Dermatol* 1974;109:40–48.

110. Winkelmann RK, Wolff K: Histochemistry of hidradenoma and eccrine spiradenoma. *J Invest Dermatol* 1967;49:173–180.

111. Munger BL, Berghorn BM, Helwig EB: A light and electron-microscopic study of a case of multiple eccrine spiradenoma. *J Invest Dermatol* 1962;38:289–297.

112. Lauret P, Boullie MC, Thomine E, et al.: Spiradenome eccrine geant. *Ann Dermatol Venereol* 1977;104:485–487.

113. Magnin PH, Duhm G, Casas JG: Espiroadenoma, cilindroma cutaneo y tricoepiteliomas multiples y familiares, in *Temas De Dermatologia.* Buenos Aires, Eudeba, 1977, vol 5, p 35.

114. Gottschalk HR, Graham JH, Aston EE: Dermal eccrine cylindroma, epithelioma adenoides cysticum of Brooke and eccrine spiradenoma. *Arch Dermatol* 1974;110:473–474.

115. Crain RC, Helwig EB: Dermal cylindroma (dermal eccrine cylindroma). *Am J Pathol* 1961;35:504–515.

116. Evans HL, Su WPD, Smith JL, et al.: Carcinoma arising in eccrine spiradenoma. *Cancer* 1979;43:1881–1884.

117. Welch JP, Wells RS, Kerr CB: Ancell-Spiegler cylindromas (turban tumours) and Brooke-Fordyce trichoepitheliomas: Evidence for a single genetic entity. *Med Genet* 1968;5:29–35.

118. Rasmussen JE: A syndrome of trichoepitheliomas, milia, and cylindromas. *Arch Dermatol* 1975;111:610–614.

119. Headington JT, Batsakis JG, Beals TF, et al.: Membranous basal cell adenoma of parotid gland, dermal cylindromas, and trichoepitheliomas. *Cancer* 1977;39:2460–2469.

120. Reingold IM, Keasbey LE, Graham JH: Multicentric dermal-type cylindromas of the parotid glands in a patient with florid turban tumor. *Cancer* 1977;40:1702–1710.

121. Batsakis JG, Brannon RB, Sciubba JJ: Monomorphic adenomas of major salivary glands: A histologic study of 96 tumours. *Clin Otolaryngol* 1981;6:129–143.

122. Black MD, Wilson Jones E: Dermal cylindroma following X-ray epilation of the scalp. *Br J Dermatol* 1971;85:70–72.

123. Munger BL, Graham JH, Helwig EB: Ultrastructure and histochemical characteristics of dermal eccrine cylindroma (turban tumor). *J Invest Dermatol* 1962;398:577–595.

124. Urbach F, Graham JH, Goldstein J, et al.: Dermal Eccrine Cylindroma. A histochemical, electron microscopic and therapeutic (x-ray) study. *Arch Dermatol* 1963;88:880–894.

125. Holubar K, Wolff K: Zur Histogenese des Cylindrom Eine Enzymhistochemische Studie. *Arch Klin Exp Dermatol* 1976;229:205–216.

126. Hashimoto K, Lever WF: *Appendage Tumors of the Skin.* Springfield, Ill, CC Thomas, 1968.

127. Reynes M, Puissant A, Delanoe J, et al.: Ultrastructural study of cylindroma (Poncet-Spiegler tumor). *J Cutan Pathol* 1976;3:95–101.

128. Cotton DNK, Braye SG: Dermal cylindromas originate from the eccrine sweat gland. *Br J Dermatol* 1984;111:53–61.

129. Headington JT: Mixed tumors of the skin: Eccrine and apocrine types. *Arch Dermatol* 1961;84:989–996.

130. Lennon B, Piarse AGE, Richards HGH: Mucin secreting tumors of the skin: With special reference to the so-called mixed salivary tumour of the skin and its relation to hidradenoma. *J Path Bacteriol* 1952;64:865–880.

131. Greeley PW, Gleason MC, Curtin JW: Mixed cell tumors of the skin. *Plast Reconstruct Surg* 1956;181:427–435.

132. Morehead RP: Mixed tumors of the skin. Report of cases, with a consideration of the histogenesis of mixed tumors of organs derived from ectoderm. *Arch Pathol* 1945;40:107–113.

133. Stout AP, Gorman JG: Mixed tumors of the skin of the salivary gland type. *Cancer* 1959;12:537–543.

134. Hirsch P, Helwig EG: Chondroid syringoma. Mixed tumor of the skin salivary gland type. *Arch Dermatol* 1961;84:835–847.

135. Daicker B, Gafner E: Apocrine mixed tumor of the lid. *Ophthalmologica* 1975;170:548–553.

136. Hernandez FJ: Mixed tumors of the skin of the salivary gland type: A light and electron microscopic study. *J Invest Dermatol* 1976;66:49–52.

137. Mills SE, Cooper PH: An ultrastructural study of cartilaginous zones and surrounding epithelium in mixed tumors of salivary glands and skin. *Lab Invest* 1981;44:6–12.

138. Varela-Duran J, Diaz-Florez L, Varela Nunez R: Ultrastructure of chondroid syringoma. Role of the myoepithelial cell in the development of the mixed tumor of the skin and soft tissues. *Cancer* 1979;44:148–156.

139. Dardick I, Van Nostrand AWP, Phillips MJ: Histogenesis of salivary gland pleomorphic adenoma (mixed tumor) with an evaluation of the role of the myoepithelial cell. *Hum Pathol* 1982;13:62–75.

140. Rulon DB, Helwig EB: Papillary eccrine adenoma. *Arch Dermatol* 1977;113:596–598.

141. Elpern DJ, Farmer ER: Papillary eccrine adenoma. (*Letter*) *Arch Dermatol* 1978;114:1241.

142. Sina B, Dilaimy M, Kallayee D: Papillary eccrine adenoma. *Arch Dermatol* 1980;116:719–720.

143. Falck VG, Jordaan HF: Papillary eccrine adenoma. A tubulo-papillary hidradenoma with eccrine differentiation. *Am J Dermatopathol* 1986;8:64–72.

144. Landry M, Winkelmann RK: An unusual tubular apocrine adenoma. *Arch Dermatol* 1972;105:869–879.

145. Umbert P, Winkelmann, RK: Tubular apocrine adenoma. *J Cut Pathol* 1976;3:75–87.

146. Civatte J, Belaich S, Lauret P: Adenome tubulaire apocrine. *Ann Dermatol Venereol* 1979;106:665–669.

147. Rabens SF, Naness JI, Gottlieb BF: Apocrine gland organic hamartoma (apocrine nevus). *Arch Dermatol* 1976;112:520–522.

148. Vakilzadeh F, Happle R, Peters P, et al.: Fokale dermale hypoplasie mit apokrinen naevi und streifenformiger anomalie der knochen. *Arch Dermatol Red* 1976;256:189–195.

149. Mehregan AH, Rahbari H: Benign epithelial tumors of the skin. IV. Benign apocrine gland tumors. *Cutis* 1978;21:53–56.

150. Civatte J, Tsoitis G, Preauz J: Le naevus apocrine. Etude de 2 cas. *Ann Dermatol Syphilol* 1974;101:251–261.

151. Mehregan AH: Apocrine cystadenoma. A clinicopathologic study with special reference to the pigmented variety. *Arch Dermatol* 1964;90:274–279.

152. Mehregan AH, Pinkus H: Organoid tumors of the skin, in *Proceedings of the XII International Congress of Dermatology, 1963*, vol 2, pp 1597–1599.

153. Mehregan AH, Rahbari H: Benign epithelial tumors of the skin. IV. Benign apocrine gland tumors. *Cutis* 1978;21:53–56.

154. Kruse TV, Khan MA, Hassan MO: Multiple apocrine cystadenomas. *Brit J of Dermatol* 1979;100:675–681.

155. Holder WR, Smith JD, Mocega EE: Giant apocrine hidrocystoma. *Arch Dermatol* 1971;104:522–523.

156. Von Seebach HB, Stumm D, Misch P, et al.: Hidrocystoma and adenoma of apocrine anal glands. *Virchow's Arch A Pathol Anat Histol* 1980;386:231–237.

157. Weigand DV, Burgdorf WHC: Perianal apocrine gland adenoma. *Arch Dermatol* 1980;116:1051–1053.

158. Ahmed A, Jones AW: Apocrine cystadenoma. *Br J Dermatol* 1969;81:899–901.

159. Powell RF, Palmer CH, Smith EB: Apocrine cystadenoma of the penile shaft. *Arch Dermatol* 1977;113:1250–1251.

160. Smith JD, Chernosky ME: Apocrine hidrocystoma (cystadenoma). *Arch Dermatol* 1974;109:700–702.

161. Benich B, Peison B: Apocrine hidrocystoma of the shoulder. *Arch Dermatol* 1977;113:71–72.

162. Ter Poorten HJ: Apocrine hidrocystoma of the right scapula. (Letter) *Arch Dermatol* 1977;113:1730.

163. Armijo M, DeUnamuno P, Herrera E: Cystadenome apocrine. A propos de 3 observations dont une de siege balanique. *Ann Dermatol Venereol (Paris)* 1978;105:411–414.

164. Grinspan D, Abulafia J, Jaimovich L, et al.: Hidrocystoma. *Dermatol Ibero Latino-Americana* 1968;10:397–408.

165. Hassan MO, Khan MA, Kruse TV: Apocrine cystadenoma. An ultrastructural study. *Arch Dermatol* 1979;115:194–200.

166. Hashimoto K, Lever WF: *Appendage Tumors of the Skin.* Springfield, Ill, CC Thomas, 1968, p 52.

167. Werth R: Anatomy of cysts of the vulva. *Zentralbl Gynakol* 1878;22:513–516.

168. Woodworth H, Dockerty MD, Wilson RB, et al.: Papillary hidradenoma of the vulva: A clinicopathologic study of 69 cases. *Am J Obstet Gynecol* 1971;110:501–508.

169. Meeker JH, Neubecker RD, Helwig EB: Hidradenoma papilliferum. *Am J Clin Pathol* 1962;37:182–195.

170. Santa Cruz DJ, Prioleau PG, Smith ME: Papillary hidradenoma of the eyelid. *Arch Dermatol* 1981;117:55.

171. Anderson NP: Hidradenoma of the vulva. *Arch Dermatol Syphilol* 1950;62:873–892.

172. Tappeiner J, Wolff K: Hidradenoma papilliferum. Eine enzymhistochemische and elektronemikroskopische studie. *Hautarzt* 1968;19:101–109.

173. Peterson W: Ein Fall von multiplen Knaueldrusen-geschwulsten dem Bilde eines Navus verrucosus unius lateris. *Arch Dermatol Syphilis* 1892;24:919–930.

174. Elliot GT: Adeno-cystoma intracanaliculare occurring in a naevus unius lateris. *J Cutan Genito-Urinary Dis* 1893;11:168–173.

175. Werther L: Syringoadenoma papilliferum (naevus syringadenomatosus papilliferus). *Arch Dermatol Syphilis* 1913;116:865–870.

176. Pinkus H: Life history of Naevus syringadenomatosus papilliferus. *Arch Dermatol Syphilol* 1954;69:305–322.

177. Thyresson N: Naevus syringo-cystadenomatosus papilliferus with structures of epithelioma adenoides cysticum. *Acta Dermatovenereol* 1951;31:290–292.

178. Rostan SE, Waller JD: Syringocystadenoma papilliferum in an unusual location. *Arch Dermatol* 1976;1122:835–836.

179. Appel B: Nevus syringadenomatosus papilliferus. *Arch Dermatol Syphilol* 1950;61:311–318.

180. Helwig EB, Hackney VC: Syringadenoma papilliferum. *Arch Dermatol Syphilol* 1955;71:361–372.

181. Wilson Jones E, Heyl T: Naevus sebaceus. *Br J Dermatol* 1970;82:99–117.

182. Mehregan AH, Pinkus H: Life history of organoid nevi. *Arch Dermatol* 1965;91:574–588.

183. Sachs W, Lewis GM: Naevus syringadenomatosus papilliferus (Werther). *Arch Dermatol Syphilol* 1934;30:1202–1209.

184. Grund JL: Syringocystadenoma papilliferum and nevus sebaceus (Jadassohn) occurring as a single tumor. *Arch Dermatol Syphilol*

185. Hashimoto K: Syringocystadenoma papilliferum. An electron microscopic study. *Arch Dermatol Forsch* 1972;245:353–369.

186. Niizuma K: Syringocystadenoma papilliferum: Light and electron microscopic studies. *Acta Dermatovenereol (Stockh)* 1976;56:327–336.

187. Jones DB: Florid papillomatosis of the nipple ducts. *Cancer* 1955;8:315–319.

188. Miller EM, Lewis D: The significance of a serohemorrhagic or hemorrhagic discharge from the nipple. *JAMA* 1923;81:1651–1657.

189. Haagensen CD, Stout AP, Phillips JS: The papillary neoplasms of the breast. *Ann Surg* 1951;133:18–36.

190. Nichols FC, Dockerty MB, Judd ES: Florid papillomatosis of the nipple. *Surg Gynecol Obstet* 1958;107:474–480.

191. Handley RS, Thackray AC: Adenoma of the nipple. *Br J Cancer* 1962;16:187–194.

192. Doctor VM, Sirsat MV: Florid papillomatosis (adenoma) and other benign tumours of the nipple and areola. *Br J Cancer* 1971;25:1–9.

193. Perzin KH, Lattes R: Papillary adenoma of the nipple (florid papillomatosis, adenoma, adenomatosis). A clinicopathologic study. *Cancer* 1972;29:966–1002.

194. Smith NP, Wilson Jones E: Erosive adenomatosis of the nipple. *Clin Exp Dermatol* 1977;2:79–84.

195. Taylor HB, Robertson AG: Adenomas of the nipple. *Cancer* 1965;18:995–1002.

196. Miller G, Bernier L: Adenomatose erosive du mamelon. *Can J Surg* 1965;8:261–266.

197. Civatte J, Restout S, Delomenie DC: Adenomatose erosive sur mamelon surnumeraire. *Ann Dermatol Venereol (Paris)* 1977;104:777–779.

198. Richards AT, Jaffe A, Hunt JA: Adenoma of the nipple in a male. *S Afr Med J* 1973;47:581–583.

199. Shapiro L, Karpas CM: Floris papillomatosis of the nipple. First reported case in a male. *Am J Clin Pathol* 1965;41:155–159.

200. Waldo ED, Sidhu GS, Hu AW: Florid papillomatosis of male nipple after diethylstilbestrol therapy. *Arch Pathol* 1975;100:364–366.

201. Azzopardi JG: Adenoma of the nipple, in Bennington JL (ed): Vol. 11 in series *Major Problems in Pathology*. London, Saunders, 1979, vol II: *Problems of Breast Pathology*, pp 260–266.

202. Costa A: Una variante non conosciuta di adenoma puro della ghiandola mammaria: L'adenoma puro a cellule apocrine. *Arch Vecchi Perl Anat Patol Med Clin* 1974;60:394–401.

203. McDivitt RW, Stewart FW, Berg JW: Subareolar duct papillomatosis, in *Tumors of the Breast*. Washington, DC, Armed Forces Institute of Pathology, 1968, pp 138–139.

204. Cooper PH: Sclerosing carcinomas of sweat ducts (microcystic adnexal carcinoma). *Arch Dermatol* 1986;122:261–264.

205. Glatt HJ, Proia AD, Tsoy EA, et al.: Malignant syringoma of the eyelid. *Ophthalmology* 1984;91:987–990.

206. Lipper S, Peiper SC: Sweat gland carcinoma with syringomatous features: A light microscopic and ultrastructural study. *Cancer* 1979;44:157–163.

207. Cooper PH, Robinson CR, Greer KE: Lowgrade clear cell eccrine carcinoma. *Arch Dermatol* 1984;120:1076–1078.

208. Lupton GP, McMarlin SL: Microcystic adnexal carcinoma. Report of a case with 30 year follow-up. *Arch Dermatol* 1986;122:286–289.

209. Fleischmann HE, Roth RJ, Wood C, Nickoloff B: Microcystic adnexal carcinoma treated by microscopically controlled excision. *J Dermatol Surg Oncol* 1984;10:873–875.

210. Nickoloff BJ, Fleishmann HE, Carmel J: Microcystic adnexal carcinoma. Immunohistologic observations suggesting dual (pilar and eccrine) differentiation. *Arch Dermatol* 1986;122:290–294.

211. Stout AP, Cooley SGE: Carcinoma of sweat glands. *Cancer* 1951;4:521–536.

212. Miller WL: Sweat-gland carcinoma. *Am J Clin Pathol* 1967;47:763–780.

213. Boggio R: Adenoid cystic carcinoma of the scalp. *Arch Dermatol* 1975;111:793–794.

214. Headington JT, Teears R, Niederhuber JE, et al.: Primary adenoid cystic carcinoma of the skin. *Arch Dermatol* 1978;114:421–424.

215. Sanderson KV, Batten JC: Adenoid cystic carcinoma of the scalp with pulmonary metastasis. *Proc R Soc Med* 1975;68:649–650.

216. Cooper PH, Adelson GL, Holthaus WH: Primary cutaneous adenoid cystic carcinoma. *Arch Dermatol* 1984;120:774–777.

217. Wick MR, Swanson PE: Primary adenoid cystic carcinoma of the skin. A clinical, histological, and immunocytochemical comparison with adenoid cystic carcinoma of salivary glands and adenoid basal cell carcinoma. *Am J Surg Pathol* 1986;8:2–13.

218. Perzin KH, Gullane P, Conley J: Adenoid cystic carcinoma involving the external auditory canal. A clinicopathologic study of 16 cases. *Cancer* 1982;50:2873–2883.

219. Freeman RG, Winkelmann RK: Basal cell tumor with eccrine differentiation (eccrine epithelioma). *Arch Dermatol* 1969;100:234–242.

220. Shmunes E, Izumi A, Beerman H: Syringeal hidradenoma— An unusual eccrine tumor. *Acta Dermatovenereol* 1971;51:460–466.

221. Baer RL, Robbins P, Menn HW: Ekkrines Epitheliom Behandlung mittels Chemochirurgie nach Mohs. *Hautarzt* 1971;22:241–244.

222. Degos R, Garabiol B, Bonvalet D: Tumeur sudorale du cuir chevelu avec envahissement osseux. *Bull Soc Fr Dermatol Syphilol* 1973;80:624–625.

223. Gomez Orbaneja J, Sanchez Yus E, Diaz Flores L, et al.: Adenocarcinom der ekkrinen Schweissdrusen. Klinische, histopathologische, histoenzymatische and ultrastructurelle Unterschung eines falles. *Hautarzt* 1973;24:197–202.

224. Cramer: Zur kenntnis der Hidradenome der haut. Synoptische Betrachtungen zum syringealen Hidradenome, ekkrinen Epitheliom und ekkrinen Basaliom. *Zentralbl Allg Pathol Anat Dtsch* 1976;120:193–198.

225. Noble JP, Lessana-Leibowitch M, Sedel D, et al.: Syringome du cuir chevelu surmonte par une plaque alopecique sclerolichenoide. *Ann Dermatol Venereol* 1979;106:275–277.

226. Cottel WI: Eccrine epithelioma: Case report. *J Dermatol Surg Oncol* 1982;8:610–611.

227. Sanchez NP, Winkelmann RK: Basal cell tumor with eccrine differentiation (eccrine epithelioma). *J Am Acad Dermatol* 1982;6:514–518.

228. Wolfe JJ, Segerberg LH: Metastasizing sweat gland carcinoma of the scalp involving the transverse sinus. Report of a case. *Am J Surg* 1954;88:849–851.

229. Lund HZ: Tumors of the skin, in *Atlas of Tumor Pathology*. Washington, DC, Armed Forces Institute of Pathology, 1957, sect 1, fasc 2, pp 120.

230. Berg JW, McDivitt RW: Pathology of sweat gland carcinoma. *Pathol Annu* 1968;3:123–144.

231. Mendoza S, Helwig EB: Mucinous (adenocystic) carcinoma of the skin. *Arch Dermatol* 1971;103:68–78.

232. Rodriguez MM, Lubowitz RM, Shannon GM: Mucinous (adenocystic) carcinoma of the eyelid. *Arch Ophthalmol* 1973;89:493–494.

233. Metz J, Filipp N, Metz G: Mucinoses carcinom der ekkrinen schweissdrusen. *Z Hautkr* 1974;49:964–974.

234. Grossman JR, Izuno GT: Primary mucinous (adenocystic) carcinoma of the skin. *Arch Dermatol* 1974;110:274–276.

235. Headington JT: Primary mucinous carcinoma of skin. Histochemistry and electron microscopy. *Cancer* 1977;39:1055–1063.

236. Yeung K-Y, Stinson JC: Mucinous (adenocystic) carcinoma of sweat glands with widespread metastasis. Case report with ultrastructural study. *Cancer* 1977;39:2556–2562.

237. Santa Cruz DJ, Meyers JH, Gnepp DR, et al.: Primary mucinous carcinoma of the skin. *Br J Dermatol* 1978;68:645–653.

238. Wright JD, Font RL: Mucinous sweat gland adenocarcinoma of eyelid. A clinicopathologic study of 21 cases with histochemical and electron microscopic observations. *Cancer* 1979;44:1757–1768.

239. Dissanayake RVP, Salm R: Sweat gland carcinomas: Prognosis related to histological type. *Histopathology* 1980;4:445–466.

240. Filipe MI: Mucins in the human gastrointestinal epithelium: A review. *Invest Cell Pathol* 1979;2:195–216.

241. Salto A, Maie O, Kato T: Ultrastructure of signet ring cells in cutaneous metastases of gastric carcinoma. *Arch Dermatol Forsch* 1973;247:99–109.

242. Pinkus H, Mehregan AH: Epidermotropic eccrine carcinoma. A case combining features of eccrine poroma and Paget's dermatosis. *Arch Dermatol* 1963;88:597–606.

243. Miura Y: Epidermotropic eccrine carcinoma. *Jap J Dermatol (Ser B)* 1968;78:226–230.

244. Hadida E, Sayag J, Sayag J, et al.: Poro-epithelioma avec metastases ganglionaires. *Bull Soc Fr Dermatol* 1972;79:271–272.

245. Kawamura T, Ikeda S, Mori S, et al.: Three cases of epidermotropic carcinoma. *Jap J Dermatol (Ser B)* 1968;78:239–243.

246. Bardach H: Hidroacanthoma simplex with in situ porocarcinoma. A case suggesting malignant transformation. *J Cutan Pathol* 1978;5:236–248.

247. Berger P, Baughman R: Intra-epidermal epithelioma. Report of a case with invasion after many years. *Br J Dermatol* 1974;90:343–349.

248. Isikawa K: Malignant hidroacanthoma simplex. *Arch Dermatol* 1972;104:529–532.

249. Diaz-Flores L, Aneiros J, Camacho F, et al.: Poroma ecrino de comportamiento maligno. Estudio optico y ultrastructural en sus fases intraepidermica, dermica y metastasica. *Morfol Norm Patol (Sec B)* 1978;2:579–589.

250. Grosshans E, Vetter JM, Capesius C: Poromes eccrines malins (poro-epitheliomas, porocarcinomes). *Ann Anat Pathol* 1975; 20:381–394.

251. Turner JJ, Maxwell L, Bursle GA: Eccrine porocarcinoma: A case report with light microscopy and ultrastructure. *Pathology* 1982;14:469–475.

252. Krinitz K: Malignes intraepidermales ekkrines Porom. *Z Haut Geschl Kr* 1972;47:9–17.

253. Shaw M, McKee PH, Howe D, et al.: Malignant eccrine poroma: A study of twenty-seven cases. *Br J Dermatol* 1982;107:675–680.

254. Mehregan AH, Hashimoto K, Rahbari H: Eccrine adenocarcinoma. A clinicopathologic study of 35 cases. *Arch Dermatol* 1983;119:104–114.

255. Altmeyer P: Kutane Metastasen eines Bronchialkarzinoms unter dem histologischen bild des ekkrinen Porokarzinoms. *Hautarzt* 1977;28:661–663.

256. Keasbey LE, Hadley GG: Clear-cell hidradenoma. Report of three cases with widespread metastases. *Cancer* 1954;7:934–952.

257. MacKenzie DH: A clear-cell hidradenocarcinoma with metastases. *Cancer* 1957;10:1021–1023.

258. Kersting DW: Clear cell hidradenoma and hidradenocarcinoma. *Arch Dermatol* 1963;87:323–333.

259. Santler R, Eberhartinger C: Malignes Klarzellen-Myoepitheliom. *Dermatologica* 1965;130:340–347.

260. Meijer AH, Rijsbosch JKC: Sweat gland carcinoma with regional lymph node metastasis. *Arch Chir Neerland* 1975;27:77–84.

261. Hernandez-Perez E, Cruz FA: Clear cell hidradenocarcinoma. Report of an unusual case. *Dermatologica* 1976;153:249–252.

262. Loup J, Bouissou H: Hidradenome malin de la main. *Ann Dermatol Venereol* 1978;105:537–539.

263. Headington JT, Niederhuber JE, Beals TF: Malignant clear cell acrospiroma. *Cancer* 1978;41:641–647.

264. Czarnecki DB, Aarons I, Dowling JP, et al.: Malignant clear cell hidradenoma: A case report. *Acta Dermatovenereol* 1982;62:173–176.

265. Sharvill DE: Mixed salivary-type tumour of the skin with malignant recurrence. *Br J Dermatol* 1962;74:103–104.

266. Gubareva AV: Mixed tumors of the skin. *Ark Patol* 1963;25:17–24.

267. Rosborough D: Malignant mixed tumours of the skin. *Br J Surg* 1963;50:697–699.

268. Matz LR, McCully DJ, Stokes BAR: Metastasizing chondroid syringoma: A case report. *Pathology* 1969;1:77–81.

269. Hilton JMN, Blackwell JB: Metastasising chondroid syringoma. *J Pathol* 1973;109:167–170.

270. Webb JN, Stott WG: Malignant chondroid syringoma of the thigh. Report of a case with electron microscopy of the tumour. *J Pathol* 1975;116:43–46.

271. Lucas GL, Nordby EJ: Sweat gland carcinoma of the hand. *Hand* 1974;6:98–102.

272. Botha JBC, Kahn LB: Aggressive chondroid syringoma. Report of a case in an unusual location and with local recurrence. *Arch Dermatol* 1978;114:954–955.

273. Redono C, Rocamora A, Villoria F, et al.: Malignant mixed tumor of the skin. Malignant chondroid syringoma. *Cancer* 1982;49:1690–1696.

274. Ishimura E, Iwamoto H, Kobashi Y, et al.: Malignant chondroid syringoma. Report of a case with widespread metastasis and review of the pertinent literature. *Cancer* 1983;52:1966–1973.

275. Anderson MS: Myxopapillary ependymomas presenting in the soft tissue over the sacrococcygeal region. *Cancer* 1966;19:585–590.

276. Stern JB, Helwig EB: Ultrastructure of subcutaneous sacrococcygeal myxopapillary ependymoma. *Arch Pathol Lab Med* 1981;105:524–526.

277. Enzinger FM, Shiraki M: Extraskeletal myxoid chondrosarcoma. An analysis of 34 cases. *Hum Pathol* 1972;3:421–435.

278. Martin RF, Melnick PJ, Warner NE, et al.: Chordoid sarcoma. *Am J Clin Pathol* 1973;59:623–635.

279. Dabska M: Malignant transformation of eccrine spiradenoma. *Pol Med J* 1972;11:388–396.

280. Evans HL, Su DWP, Smith JL, et al.: Carcinoma arising in eccrine spiradenoma. *Cancer* 1979;43:1881–1884.

281. Mambo NC: Eccrine spiradenoma: Clinical and pathologic study of 49 tumors. *J Cutan Pathol* 1983;10:312–320.

282. Yaremchuck MJ, Elias LS, Graham RR, et al.: Sweat gland carcinoma of the hand: Two cases of malignant eccrine spiradenoma. *J Hand Surg* 1984;9A:910–914.

283. Cooper PH, Frierson HF, Morrison AG: Malignant transformation of eccrine spiradenoma. *Arch Dermatol* 1985;121:1445–1448.

284. Luger A: Das cylindrom der Haut und seine maligne Degeneration. *Arch Dermatol Syphilol* 1949;188:155–180.

285. Lausecker H: Beitrag zu den Naevo-Epitheliomen. *Arch Dermatol Syphilol* 1952;194:639–662.

286. Gertler W: Spieglersche, Tumoren mit ubergang in matastasierendes spinaliom. *Dermatol Mschr* 1953;128:673–674.

287. Zontschew P: Cylindroma capitis mit maligner Entartung. *Zentralbl Chir* 1961;86:1875–1879.

288. Lyon JB, Rouillard LM: Malignant degeneration of turban tumour of scalp. *Trans St John's Hosp Dermatol Soc* 1961;46:74–77.

289. Korting GW, Hoede N, Gebhardt R: Kurzer Bericht uber eine maligne entarteten Spiegler-Tumor. *Dermatol Mschr* 1970; 156:141–147.

290. Bondeson L: Malignant dermal eccrine cylindroma. *Acta Dermatovenereol* 1979;59:92–94.

291. Tsambaos D, Greither A, Orfanos CE: Multiple malignant Spiegler tumors with brachydactyly and racket nails. *J Cutan Pathol* 1979;6:31–41.

292. Bourlond A, Clerens A, Sigard H: Cylindrome malin. *Dermatologica* 1979;158:203–207.

293. Greither A, Rehrmann A: Spiegler-Karzinome Mit Assoziierten Symptomen. *Dermatologica* 1980;160:361–370.

294. Urbanski SJ, From L, Abramowicz A, et al.: Metamorphosis of dermal cylindroma: Possible relation to malignant transformation. *J Am Acad Dermatol* 1985;12:188–195.

295. Pierard-Franchimont C, Pierard GE: Developpement et progression neoplasique des cylindromes cutanes benins et malins. *Ann Dermatol Venereol* 1984;111:1093–1098.

296. McDonald JR: Apocrine sweat gland carcinoma of the vulva. *Am J Clin Pathol* 1941;11:890–897.

297. Aurora AL, Luxenberg MN: Case report of adenocarcinoma of glands of Moll. *Am J Ophthalmol* 1970;70:984–990.

298. Warkel RL, Helwig EB: Apocrine gland adenoma and adenocarcinoma of the axilla. *Arch Dermatol* 1978;114:198–203.

299. Baes H, Suurmond D: Apocrine sweat gland carcinoma: Report of a case. *Br J Dermatol* 1970;83:483–486.

300. Okun MR, Finn R, Blumental G: Apocrine adenoma versus apocrine carcinoma. *J Am Acad Dermatol* 1980;2:322–326.

301. Futrell JW, Krueger GR, Chretien PB, et al.: Multiple primary sweat gland carcinomas. *Cancer* 1971;28:686–691.

302. Tavani E, Giardini R: Carcinoma apocrino pluricentrico. *Pathologica* 1979;71:111–114.

303. Futrell JW, Krueger GR, Morton DL, et al.: Carcinoma of sweat gland in adolescents. *Am J Surg* 1972;123:594–597.

304. Saigal RK, Khanna SD, Chandler J: Apocrine gland carcinoma in axilla: Report of a case. *Indian J Dermatol* 1971;37:177–180.

305. Rosen Y, Kim B, Yermakov VA: Eccrine sweat gland tumor of clear cell origin involving the eyelids. *Cancer* 1975;36:1034.

306. Grizzard WS, Torczynski E, Edwards WC: Adenocarcinoma of the eccrine sweat glands. *Arch Ophthalmol* 1976;94:2112.

307. Hood CI, Font RL, Zimmerman LE: Metastatic mammary carcinoma in the eyelid with histiocytoid appearance. *Cancer* 1973;31:793.

308. Maier T: Autoptisch Gesichertes Metastatasierendes Schweissdrusenkarzinom auf dem Bodes eines Naevus syringoadenomatosus papilliferus. *Allg Pathol* 1949;85:377.

309. Seco Navedo MA, Fresno Forcelledo M, Orduna Domingo A, et al.: Syringocystadenome papillifere a evolution maligne. Presentation d'un cas. *Ann Dermatol Venereol* 1982;109:685.

310. Gallager HS, Miller GV, Grampa G: Primary mucoepidermoid carcinoma of the skin. Report of a case. *Cancer* 1959;12:286–288.

311. Vogel MH: Mucoepidermoid carcinomas of the lid. A clinicopathologic report of two cases. *Ophthalmologica* 1976;174:171–175.

312. Wenig BL, Sciubba JJ, Goodman RS, et al.: Primary cutaneous mucoepidermoid carcinoma of the anterior neck. *Laryngoscope* 1983;93:464–467.

313. Weidner N, Foucar E: Adenosquamous carcinoma of the skin. An aggressive mucin and gland forming squamous cell carcinoma. *Arch Dermatol* 1985;121:775–779.

314. Kao GF, Helwig EB, Graham JH: Aggressive digital papillary adenoma and adenocarcinoma. A clinicopathological study of 57 patients, with histochemical, immunopathological, and ultrastructural observations. *J Cutan Pathol* 1987;14:129–146.

CHAPTER 48
Benign Melanocytic Tumors

Michael J. Imber and Martin C. Mihm, Jr.

CHARACTERISTICS OF MELANOCYTES

The diagnosis of benign melanocytic disorders requires familiarity with the normal developmental biology of the human melanocyte. An understanding of the spectrum of benign proliferative patterns is a prerequisite to the study of the aberrant histologic and cytologic features of malignant melanoma and precursor lesions.

Melanocytes originate from neural crest precursor cells, which also give rise to peripheral neurons and Schwann cells.[1] In experimental studies of avian neural crest tissue, cells migrating from the neural crest may initially differentiate along melanocytic or neural pathways.[2,3] Subsequently, cell populations destined to become either peripheral neurons or "supportive cells" emerge. These supportive cell precursors may evolve into either Schwann cells or melanocytes.[4,5] Cellular interaction between melanocyte precursors and epithelial cells may be necessary for further differentiation. Migration of precursor cells occurs along mesenchymal pathways lined by fibronectin.[6,7] Neural crest cell differentiation in mouse embryo studies suggests that the in vitro developmental potential of neural crest precursors is similar in avian and mammalian systems.[8,9]

In humans, cells destined to become epidermal melanocytes migrate to the periderm, where they ultimately develop the dendritic morphology and ultrastructural characteristics of mature melanocytes. The cytokinetic behavior of melanocytes during embryogenesis and their developmental relationship to other cells of the peripheral nervous system are likely basic factors underlying the morphologic spectrum of benign melanocytic lesions. The existence of pigmented neurofibromas and melanocytic schwannomas, the association of leptomeningeal melanocytosis in association with giant congenital melanocytic nevi, and the commonly observed phenomenon of schwannian differentiation or neurotization in acquired melanocytic nevi underscore this point.[10] Experimentally induced pigmented lesions in Syrian golden hamsters also display ultrastructural and histochemical features suggestive of neural origin.[11] These include nonspecific cholinesterase activity within tumor cells and the proliferation of melanocytes within nerve fascicles.

These properties suggest that criteria used for distinguishing benign from malignant melanocytic proliferations and for identifying precursor and borderline lesions must necessarily be different from those applied to epithelial proliferations.[12,13] The melanocyte is after all a migratory cell. Its usual location dispersed among the basal keratinocytes of the epidermis is quite stable, and evidence of migration and mitotic activity is rare. Proliferation and migration of melanocytes may be seen in regenerating epidermis and in repigmenting areas of vitiligo.[14] Melanocytes normally dispersed along the basal layer of hair follicles are likely the principal reservoir for melanocytes repopulating reepithelialized epidermis.[15]

Migration of melanocytes across the basement membrane zone of the epidermis and into the papillary dermis is part of the normal development of many benign melanocytic lesions, including most acquired melanocytic nevi. In addition, upward or lateral migration of melanocytes within the epidermis may also be seen in a number of benign lesions including the spindle and epithelioid cell nevus and the pigmented spindle cell nevus. Therefore, the isolated histologic observation of invasive behavior does not necessarily denote malignancy in a melanocytic lesion, as this finding usually suggests in an epithelial tumor.[16,17]

CHARACTERISTICS OF BENIGN MELANOCYTIC PROLIFERATIONS

Most benign lesions that originate from epidermal melanocytes display various combinations of three proliferative patterns readily apparent under low-power microscopic examination. Lentiginous hyperplasia describes a pattern of crowded single-cell melanocytic growth along the dermoepidermal junction. This pattern is often seen in compound nevi and lentigines. Nested proliferation describes the clonal growth of numerous microanatomically discrete clusters of melanocytes. The distribution of such nests or theques of cells within the epidermis or along the junction is often quite characteristic of certain specific types of melanocytic nevi, including pigmented spindle cell nevi and spindle and epithelioid cell nevi. Finally, pagetoid proliferation describes the pattern of discohesive single-cell growth throughout the entire epidermis. Although commonly associated with melanoma, pagetoid spread may be observed in Spitz nevi, pigmented spindle cell nevi, and in common acquired nevi occurring in acral locations.

The cytologic characteristics of benign melanocytes or nevus cells are often quite variable. It is helpful to compare the nuclear features of melanocytes with adjacent normal keratinocyte or endothelial cell nuclei as internal references for nuclear size and detail. Normal melanocytes residing within the basal layer of the epidermis typically have a nucleus somewhat smaller and slightly more hyperchromatic than nearby keratinocytes.[18] The chromatin pattern is uniform, and no nucleoli are evident. The nuclear contour often appears polygonal or indented, and the cell cytoplasm appears clear as a result of artifactual retraction.

Benign melanocytic lesions do not display anaplastic cytological characteristics. A wide spectrum of atypical nuclear change may be seen in such lesions, but these changes generally represent reactive, degenerative, or senescent phenomena rather than true anaplastic atypia characteristic of malignant transformation. True hyperchromasia and coarse nuclear membrane and chromatin clumping are rarely encountered in benign pigment cell lesions. Certain morphologies seem to be represented in most benign lesions, whereas other cytologic patterns are typical of specific lesions such as Spitz nevi or pigmented spindle cell nevi.

A symmetric pattern of growth and ultimately of involution is characteristic of benign melanocytic proliferations. Histologic symmetry from left to right is readily apparent at low power and includes congruent development of the epidermal component to the dermal component. Simply stated, a junctional melanocytic proliferation synchronously migrates across the dermoepidermal junction and establishes a dermal component over a lateral dimension equal to that of the original epidermal component. The presence of a so-called shoulder of junctional melanocytic hyperplasia lateral to the bulk of an otherwise benign compound lesion reflects aberrant development. Such apparent histologic asymmetry may reflect the asynchronous migration of the junctional melanocyte population into the papillary dermis or the resumption of junctional melanocytic proliferation in what had otherwise been a normally evolving lesion.

An apparent vertical gradient of cytological development usually referred to as maturation is present in benign melanocytic proliferations. Cellular pleomorphism and atypical nuclear features are more evident near the epidermal origin of the tumor, with deeper cells becoming smaller and more cytologically banal. Histologic maturation is likewise evident by the progressively smaller size of nevus cell nests or their replacement by discohesively infiltrating single cells at the base of the lesion.

Subsequent involution is symmetric and proceeds from top to bottom, with replacement of dermal nevomelanocytes with normal dermal connective tissue. A wide spectrum of histologic patterns of senescence may be seen in benign melanocytic lesions. These include schwannian differentiation or neurotization, lipomatous degeneration, and inflammatory regression. Various cytologic patterns of senescence may also be observed, including giant cell transformation and balloon cell formation. In all cases, however, such histologic patterns of senescence appear uniform and symmetric.

ACQUIRED MELANOCYTIC NEVI

Common acquired melanocytic nevi or moles are the most common melanocytic tumors in humans. The histopathogenetic relationship of nevus cells with melanocytes is supported by ultrastructural demonstration of melanosomes, and the immunohistochemical demonstration of cytoplasmic S-100 protein in nevus cells.[19,20] Studies of nevus cells cultured in vitro reveal similar patterns of growth and surface antigen expression as displayed by melanocytes in tissue culture.[21–28] The experimental induction of melanocytic tumors in animals with chemical carcinogens also supports the concept of a developmental framework of tumor progression starting with epidermal melanocytes.[29,30]

With increasing age, most individuals will develop varying numbers of nevi. These usually appear as brown pigmented lesions, less than 0.6 cm in diameter, and may occur anywhere on the skin surface. Common sites include the head and neck and sun-exposed portions of the trunk and extremities. Nevi may first appear early in childhood, with increasing numbers observed through adulthood. Thereafter, the observed incidence of nevi declines with advancing decades.[31] This may reflect the self-limited growth pattern observed in most common acquired nevi: a proliferative phase, in which a clinically observable pigmented lesion results from the orderly growth and migration of nevomelanocytes from the dermoepidermal junction; followed by a senescent phase, in which the lesion is replaced by connective tissue stroma and either clinically disappears or evolves into a common skin tag.[32] Although most individuals acquire a small number of common nevi at different times and anatomic locations during their lives, the rapid eruption of widespread multiple benign nevi has also been described.[33]

Three major histologic groupings exist, representing stages in the developmental progression of benign nevi and often corresponding to characteristic gross morphologies: junctional, compound, and dermal nevi. The histopathologic alterations observed in these lesions predominantly affect the epidermis and papillary dermis.

Junctional, Compound, and Dermal Nevi

Junctional nevi represent the earliest stage of intraepidermal melanocytic proliferation (Fig. 48–1). Nevomelanocytes are dispersed in multiple discrete nests along the dermoepidermal junction, although lentiginous melanocytic hyperplasia may be present as well. Junctional nevi appear clinically as small, slightly raised and deeply pigmented lesions. *Compound* melanocytic nevi include both a junctional component and apparent infiltration of the dermis by nevus cells distributed singly and in nests (Fig. 48–2). Clinically,

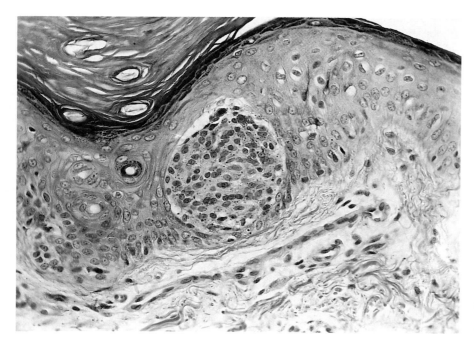

Figure 48–1. Junctional nevus. The intradermal nest of junctional nevus cells contains a uniform population of coarsely melanized, type A nevus cells (H&E, ×313).

such lesions appear elevated or dome shaped and are less intensely pigmented than junctional nevi. *Dermal nevi* no longer display a junctional component; nevomelanocytes are confined to the dermis and are often associated with varying degrees of senescent histologic change. Clinically they appear flesh colored or lightly pigmented and are dome shaped or pedunculated.

The designations junctional, dermal, and compound do not refer to discrete melanocytic entities but rather to histologically characteristic stages in the natural progression of common acquired melanocytic nevi. Apparent intermediate forms are routinely encountered. The compulsive search, however, for a rare junctional nest of nevus cells for the sake of labeling what is predominantly a dermal nevus, a compound nevus instead, is wasteful and overlooks the significance of a developmental spectrum.[34]

Recent ultrastructural studies suggest that many apparent compound nevi may, in fact, be completely intraepidermal. Three-dimensional reconstruction of nevi based on multiple serial sections demonstrated that discrete dermal

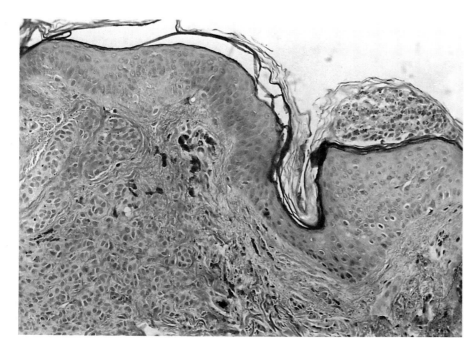

Figure 48–2. Compound nevus. There is transepidermal elimination of an intraepidermal nevus cell nest. This occasional finding in benign nevi should not be mistaken as a sign of malignancy (H&E, ×125).

nests observed in one histologic section were always in continuity with junctional nevus nests observed in other sections.[35] Furthermore, basement membrane zone material was observed originating from the dermoepidermal junction adjacent to dermal nevus cell nests and reflected over the deepest extent of the nevus in contact with dermal connective tissue.[36,37] No basement membrane zone material was observed between basilar epidermis and immediately subjacent nevus cell nests. Although the precise relationships between acquired nevus cell growth patterns, the dermoepidermal basement membrane zone, and underlying papillary dermal connective tissue remain to be elucidated, an origin for acquired nevi from intraepidermal melanocytic precursors is supported by these observations.[38]

Certain cytologic features are characteristic of stages in the evolution of melanocytic nevi. The intraepidermal nevus cell, referred to as the epithelioid melanocyte or type A nevus cell, contains a round to oval nucleus that is slightly smaller than the nuclei of adjacent keratinocytes. The nucleus contains finely dispersed chromatin similar to neuroendocrine cells and occasionally a single inconspicuous nucleolus. The cytoplasm is prominent and often contains moderately coarse melanin granules.

The lymphocyte-like or type B melanocyte is usually part of the dermal component of compound nevi. The nucleus is small, round to oval, and contains uniformly dispersed chromatin with no apparent nucleoli. The nuclear contours may appear undulating and grooved. Scant nonpigmented cytoplasm is evident. Type B cells are usually distributed in dense array without apparent cytoplasmic borders.

The neural or type C nevus cell is often present at the base of melanocytic lesions. This cell is often spindle shaped and contains a somewhat smaller, oval nucleus with a banal chromatin pattern. These fusiform cells come to rest at or singly infiltrate superficial reticular dermal collagen bundles.

Different patterns of epidermal hyperplasia may be seen in association with melanocytic nevi.[39] Acanthotic epidermal proliferation with pseudohorn cyst formation may clinically and histologically mimic seborrheic keratoses. Extensive reticulated epidermal retiform hyperplasia is common in some pedunculated dermal nevi. Rarely, alterative mesenchymal changes including bone formation and amyloid deposition may be observed in nevi.[40]

Senescent Transformation

Long-term clinical observation of benign nevi reveals that most lesions undergo gradual involution.[41,42] Residual dermal nevus cells are replaced by fibrous stroma. The subsequent fibrous papule or fibroepithelial polyp may contain no histologic evidence of a preexisting pigmented lesion. Melanocytic nevi on occasion display histologic and cytologic variations that reflect senescence. Prominent among histological senescent patterns is *neurotization,* or *schwannian differentiation,* with formation of neuroid structures in loose connective tissue, often simulating a neurofibroma (Figs. 48–3 and 48–4).

A second pattern of senescent transformation often observed in nevi from the buttocks or thighs is *lipomatous degeneration* with apparent infiltration of dermal nevi by fat cells (Figs. 48–5 and 48–6). Complete replacement of the nevus by adipose tissue may simulate the histology of nevus lipomatosus superficialis, a mesenchymal hamartoma that is often observed in the same body location. The two entities may be discriminated histologically if exaggerated fatty tissue growth is observed in continuity with adnexal adventitia, a feature not observed in nevi displaying lipomatous degeneration.

The *fibrous papule of the face,* or *melanocytic angiofibroma,* may represent a senescent pattern of dermal nevus transformation unique to this anatomic location (Figs. 48–7

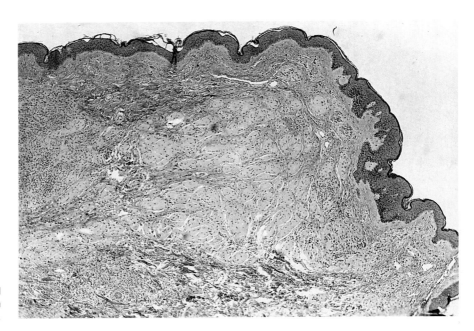

Figure 48–3. Dermal nevus. The dermal component displays extensive neurotization or schwannian differentiation (H&E, ×50).

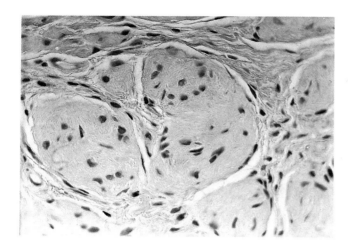

Figure 48–4. Dermal nevus (same case as Fig. 48–3). Nests of neurotized dermal nevus cells may resemble peripheral neural structures such as the Wagner-Meissner corpuscle (H&E, ×500).

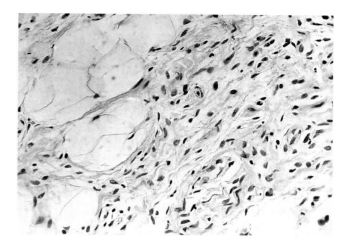

Figure 48–6. Dermal nevus (same case as Fig. 48–5). Areas of lipomatous transformation (left) display features of adipocytes with eccentric nuclei and clear cytoplasm (H&E, ×313).

and 48–8).[43–46] Histological features include replacement of normal dermal collagen and elastic fibers with delicate, hyalinized bands of connective tissue. Prominent ectatic vessels are usually observed, as are typical pleomorphic stellate or giant cells dispersed within the lesion stroma. Hyperplasia of epithelioid melanocytes or type A nevus cells is seen along the basal layer of the overlying epidermis in most lesions.[47] Considerable debate has been provoked regarding the origin of this lesion from melanocytic versus fibrohistiocytic precursors.[48–52] The simultaneous observation of dermal nevus cell nests and the histochemical demonstration of enzyme patterns reflecting nevomelanocytic origin in the stromal stellate cells suggests that at least some fibrous papules evolve from precursor nevi.

Balloon Cell Nevus

Various cytologic presentations that may reflect senescence include the presence of balloon cells or nevus giant cells. Such unusual histologic and cytologic patterns may also occur in melanoma and should therefore never be used solely to discriminate benign from malignant melanocytic tumors.

Balloon cell nevi are observed infrequently and are clinically indistinguishable from common acquired nevi.[53–55] Balloon cell nevi have been reported to occur most frequently on the head and neck in individuals during the first three decades. Histologically, these lesions are composed of a mixture of characteristic vacuolated balloon cells

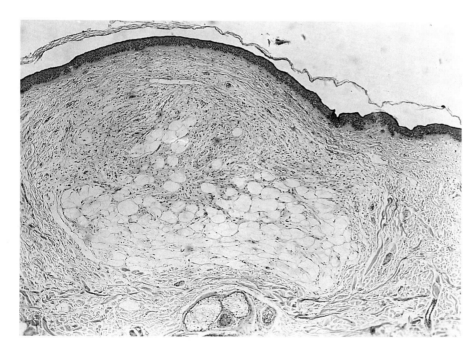

Figure 48–5. Dermal nevus. Extensive lipomatous transformation of dermal nevus cells is present (H&E, ×50).

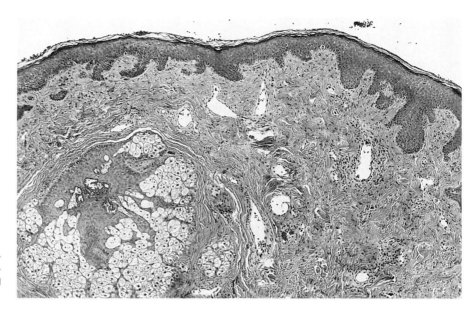

Figure 48–7. Melanocytic angiofibroma. Nevus cells are scattered within reticular dermis displaying ectatic vascular channels and periadnexal fibrosis (H&E, ×50).

and normal-appearing nevus cells (Figs. 48–9 and 48–10). Rarely are such lesions composed entirely of balloon cells. The histologic differential diagnosis may include granular cell tumor, xanthoma, or a metastatic clear cell tumor. Ultrastructural studies have demonstrated that the characteristic cytoplasmic appearance of balloon cells results from the coalescence and subsequent degeneration of nonmelanized melanosomes.[56]

The presence of varying numbers of nevus giant cells has been observed in balloon cell nevi. Nevus giant cells may also be seen in histologically unremarkable common acquired nevi (Fig. 48–11). This characteristic pattern of cytologic senescence may at times microscopically mimic a xanthomatous/granulomatous process. The coalescence or overlapping of multiple nevus giant cell nuclei in routine histologic sections may simulate the appearance of individual anaplastic nuclei characteristic of melanoma or dysplas-

tic nevi. The lack of additional microscopic features of melanocytic dysplasia and the presence of banal nevus giant cells elsewhere throughout the lesion should permit the correct interpretation.

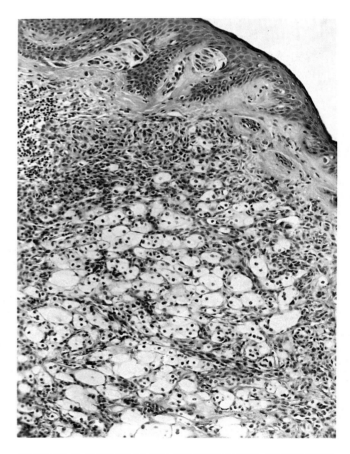

Figure 48–9. Compound nevus. Extensive balloon cell transformation is present throughout the dermal component (H&E, ×125).

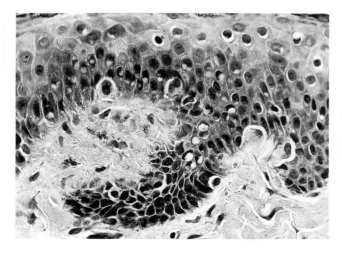

Figure 48–8. Melanocytic angiofibroma (same case as Fig. 48–7). Prominent epithelioid, often binucleate, type A nevomelanocytes are distributed along the basal layer (H&E, ×500).

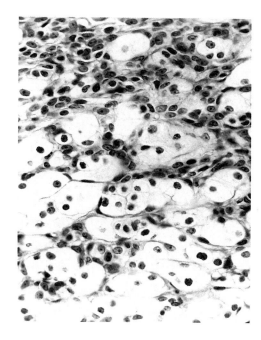

Figure 48–10. Compound nevus (same case as Fig. 48–9). Nevus cells displaying balloon cell transformation may superficially resemble sebaceous epithelium. The cytoplasm is clear or slightly foamy, with centrally placed nuclei displaying typical features of type A nevus cells (H&E, ×500).

Halo Nevus

The presence of a host inflammatory cell response in a pigmented lesion may represent various phenomena. External trauma to a nevus may result from excoriation or pluck-ing of hairs. The presence of focal epidermal necrosis, impetiginization, or a foreign body response to keratinous debris suggests such causes. A chronic inflammatory cell infiltrate at the base of the lesion is often observed in malignant melanoma and dysplastic melanocytic nevi. In such cases, the presence of such an infiltrate reflects an immune response to the expression of new cell surface antigens associated with malignant transformation. Regression of the primary proliferative lesion may occur subsequent to such an immune response, with resulting foci of hypopigmentation. A benign melanocytic tumor that displays this microscopic pattern of cellular immune response and clinical hypopigmentation is the halo nevus.

Halo nevi are most often multiple and occur frequently on the back in young individuals.[57] Normal-appearing acquired melanocytic nevi develop a centripetally enlarging peripheral rim of hypopigmentation. During a period of several months, the preexisting nevus may disappear completely, leaving a macular area of hypopigmentation. The so-called halo phenomenon, or leukoderma acquisitum centrifigum, is characteristic of halo nevi but has been reported in association with other primary cutaneous tumors of neuroectodermal origin including malignant melanomas, neurofibromas, and blue nevi.[58] This uncommon form of symmetric inflammatory regression may be in part genetically determined, as the familial occurrence of halo nevi has been reported. The possible contribution of an autoimmune response to nevomelanocyte antigens is suggested by coexisting vitiligo in as many as 25% of individuals with halo nevi. The halo phenomenon on a slower scale may participate with other mechanisms of senescence in the gradual involution of common acquired nevi with advancing age.

Microscopically, halo nevi feature diffuse infiltration of the nevus by lymphocytes and histiocytes with subsequent destruction of pigment-containing cells (Fig. 48–12).[59,60] Residual nevus cell nests may display reactive cyto-

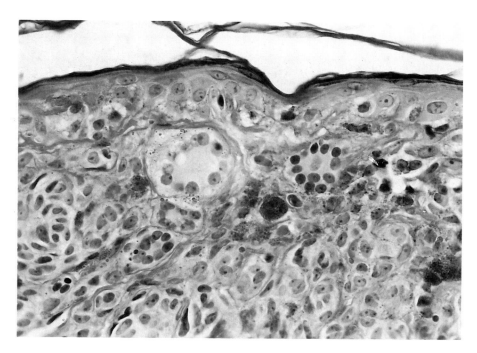

Figure 48–11. Compound nevus. Extensive nevus giant cell formation is present (H&E, ×250).

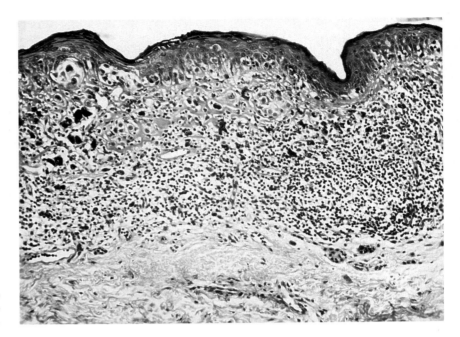

Figure 48–12. Halo nevus. A dense lymphohistiocytic infiltrate is present, with extensive stromal melanophage accumulation (H&E, ×160).

logic atypia with prominent eosinophilic nucleoli and nuclear clearing. This appearance may simulate melanoma, especially in the presence of a brisk lymphocytic response. The absence of outright anaplastic nuclear features or atypical mitoses should facilitate the correct interpretation. The epidermis from hypopigmented areas displays complete absence of melanocytes and appears identical to the epidermis of vitiliginous skin.

Recurrent Nevus

Incomplete surgical excision of acquired melanocytic nevi by shave excision or curettage may result in later proliferation of residual nevomelanocytes.[61–63] The subsequent recurrent nevus may display an atypical clinical distribution of pigment and scar formation.[64] The anatomic distribution of recurrent nevi reflects that of primary nevi. Most recurrent nevi appear within 6 months of the initial excision.[65]

Most recurrent nevi display prominent junctional melanocytic hyperplasia in both nested and lentiginous arrays, with underlying dermal scar formation (Fig. 48–13). Beneath the region of scar fibrosis, residual nests of dermal nevus cells may be present. Papillary dermal migration of type A nevus cells in association with dermal scar may simulate the appearance of a dysplastic nevus or lentigo maligna melanoma. Although the term *pseudomelanoma* has been used to describe the histological appearance of some recurrent nevi, the actual incidence of anaplastic cytologic features in such lesions is quite low.

CONGENITAL MELANOCYTIC NEVI

Congenital melanocytic nevi occur in approximately 1% of neonates.[66] Although some are similar in size to common acquired melanocytic nevi, these clinically distinct lesions

are larger and more irregular in contour than acquired nevi and are often hair bearing. A clinical distinction is often drawn between nongiant and giant congenital melanocytic nevi. There is some evidence to suggest that congenital melanocytic nevi may be at greater risk to evolve into melanoma than other benign melanocytic proliferations.[67,68] Whether this reflects unique biologic properties of congenital nevus cells or simply the presence of greater numbers of potential transformable nevomelanocytes is yet unresolved.

Histologically, compound and dermal patterns are seen. Some congenital nevi are indistinguishable from benign acquired nevi under the microscope. In histologically identifiable lesions, the distribution of nevus cells through-

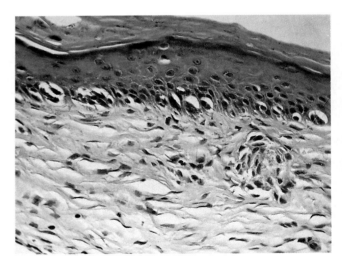

Figure 48–13. Recurrent nevus. Lentiginous melanocytic hyperplasia is present in attenuated epidermis. Sclerotic dermis is present, entrapping a solitary nest of dermal nevus cells (H&E, ×320).

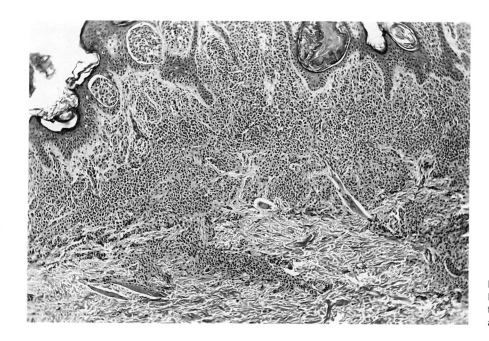

Figure 48–14. Congenital compound nevus. Nevus cells are present deep within the reticular dermis and in close association with appendages (H&E, ×79).

out the dermis is more extensive than in acquired nevi, typically involving a lower two thirds of the reticular dermis and often infiltrating the subcutaneous fat (Fig. 48–14).[69] The presence of nevus cells within cutaneous structures including sebaceous lobules, multiple arrector pili muscles, and the perineurium of peripheral nerves is characteristic of congenital nevi and is not seen in acquired nevi (Figs. 48–15 through 48–18). Morphologic studies of congenital nevi obtained from children less than 1 year of age suggest that appendageal infiltration by nevus cells may not be a common feature of very young congenital nevi and may require increasing age to develop.[70] The cytologic features of congenital melanocytic nevus cells and their patterns of maturation and senescence differ little from features already described for acquired nevi.

SPINDLE AND EPITHELIOID CELL NEVUS (SPITZ NEVI)

Spindle and epithelioid cell nevi are of tremendous diagnostic importance because of their histological similarity to malignant melanoma. This entity had in the past received the confusing title "benign juvenile melanoma," which nevertheless summarized its clinically benign yet histologically menacing status.[71,72] Often referred to today as Spitz nevi, these benign melanocytic lesions may occur at all ages, although they are usually observed in children and young adults. Common sites include the head, neck, and upper extremities. Clinically, this nevus presents as a small, solitary, dome-shaped dermal nodule. The presence of a prominent vascular component to the tumor stroma and a relative

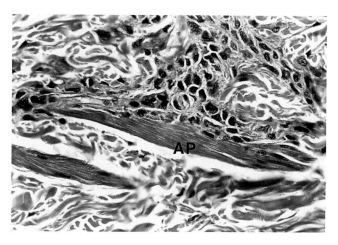

Figure 48–15. Congenital compound nevus (same case as Fig. 48–14). Nevus cells (arrow) are present within a sebaceous lobule (H&E, ×313).

Figure 48–16. Congenital compound nevus (same case as Fig. 48–14). Nevus cells are seen infiltrating an arrector pili (AP) muscle (H&E, ×313).

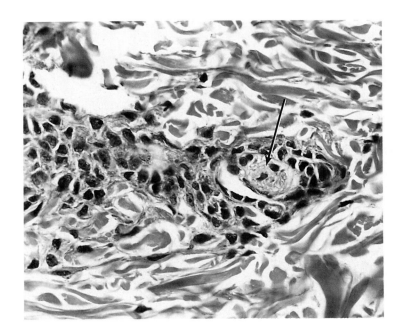

Figure 48–17. Congenital compound nevus (same case as Fig. 48–14). Nevus cells are present around a peripheral nerve twig (arrow) (H&E, ×313).

lack of melanin pigmentation results in its frequent clinical misdiagnosis as a hemangioma or pyogenic granuloma. An incompletely excised Spitz nevus may recur as a nodular lesion.[73]

Histologic Features

The histologic distribution of nevus cells in Spitz nevi mirrors that of common acquired nevi, displaying junctional, compound, and dermal forms.[74,75] However, Spitz nevi, like many congenital nevi, usually have a very prominent dermal component. The overall architecture of the lesion is symmetric with abrupt attenuation of junctional nests at the lateral borders. The nevi are composed of various proportions of spindle and epithelioid melanocytes (Figs. 48–19 and 48–20). Spindle cells are usually present in fascicles arrayed perpendicular to the epidermis, whereas epithelioid cells are dispersed individually throughout the le-

sion (Fig. 48–21). The overall histologic pattern is often discohesive and infiltrative, as opposed to the confluent and expansile growth pattern of malignant melanoma. The cells taper from a broad base superficially to a narrow point in the deep dermis, architecturally resembling an inverted, imperfect triangle. Also, the nevus cells mature by becoming smaller from the superficial to the deep part of the tumor.

The atypical cytologic features of spindle and epithelioid cell nevi often result in histopathologic confusion with melanoma. An extreme degree of cellular pleomorphism, particularly of epithelioid melanocytes, may be seen (Figs. 48–22 and 48–23). The nuclei of these cells may be quite large and irregular in contour, and contain prominent eosinophilic nucleoli, but are otherwise open or vesicular in appearance and lacking the coarse anaplastic features characteristic of malignant cells. Often present are eosinophilic cytoplasmic invaginations or nuclear pseudoinclusions. The presence of mitotic figures and occasional pagetoid epidermal spread of epithelioid melanocytes may mimic melanoma. The overwhelming majority of the cells, however, have a benign cytologic appearance that is highlighted by the atypical cells. It is the background of benignity that allows for the correct interpretation of the lesion.

Those nevi that contain predominantly spindle melanocytes arranged in fascicles are usually more readily diagnosed than lesions consisting largely of pleomorphic epithelioid cells. A number of rather unique histologic features are regularly seen in Spitz nevi. These include the deposition of eosinophilic globules of hyalin-like material near the dermoepidermal junction and artifactual separation of papillary dermal nests from the overlying epidermis.[76,77] The tumor stroma may appear quite vascular and edematous. Lymphocytic infiltration is not uncommon, and long-standing lesions may display a densely sclerotic stroma with scattered individual tumor cells trapped amidst dermal collagen.[78]

Histologic differentiation from melanoma may usually be made based on the overall symmetry of the lesion and the apparent cytologic maturation of nevus cells at the base

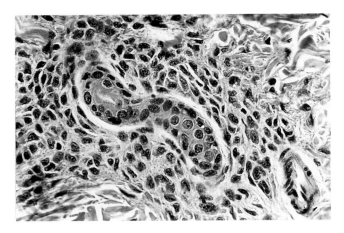

Figure 48–18. Congenital compound nevus (same case as Fig. 48–14). Nevus cells are present infiltrating the perieccrine adventitia (H&E, ×313).

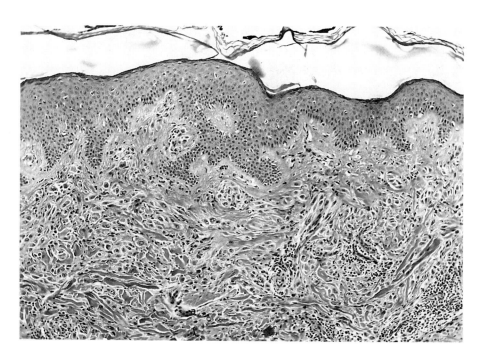

Figure 48–19. Spindle and epithelioid cell nevus, predominantly dermal. This nevus is composed of both spindle cells arranged in characteristic fascicles and individual epithelioid cells infiltrating the dermis (H&E, ×79).

of the lesion. Spindle and epithelioid cell nevi may rarely be precursors of melanoma. Careful cytologic study for truly anaplastic nuclear features, bizarre mitoses, and aberrant or asymmetric proliferation should be made in borderline cases.

PIGMENTED SPINDLE CELL NEVUS

Regarded as a variant of the Spitz nevus by some authors, the pigmented spindle cell nevus has quite distinctive clinical and histopathologic features that justify its recognition as a separate entity.[79,80] This lesion usually occurs as a small (less than 1 cm), solitary, deeply pigmented yet well circumscribed maculopapule on the extremities or trunk. Women are more frequently affected than men, and the median age of diagnosis is in the third decade. The intense pigmentation results in its frequent clinical misdiagnosis as superficial spreading melanoma. Unlike Spitz nevi, pigmented spindle cell nevi rarely involve the head and neck.

Histologic Features
Like other benign nevomelanocytic proliferations, pigmented spindle cell nevi display histologic symmetry and

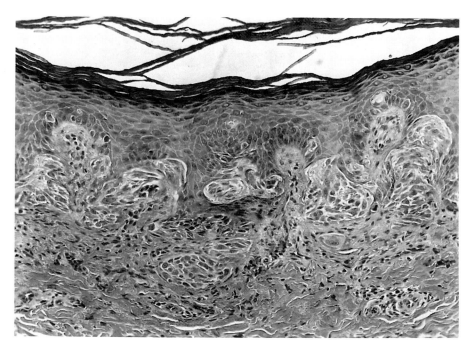

Figure 48–20. Spindle and epithelioid cell nevus, compound. This predominantly spindle cell nevus displays characteristic fascicles of amelanotic cells along the dermoepidermal junction and infiltrating the papillary dermis (H&E, ×125).

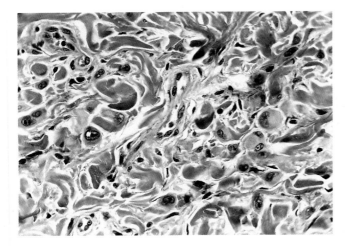

Figure 48–21. Spindle and epithelioid cell nevus (same case as Fig. 48–19). A mixture of pleomorphic, atypical epithelioid cells and small, banal-appearing cells infiltrate reticular dermis in a discohesive pattern (H&E, ×313).

cytologic maturation. The histologic appearance is quite characteristic.[81] Nests and fascicles of spindle melanocytes arrayed parallel to the long axis of the epidermis are distributed along the dermoepidermal junction and within dermal papillae to form a confluent plaque of tumor growth (Figs. 48–24, 48–26, 48–28).[82] Junctional and compound varieties are exclusively seen. The base of the lesion usually extends no deeper than the superficial reticular dermis. The overall histologic pattern is one of expansile growth as opposed to the infiltrative pattern seen at the base of Spitz nevi.

The nevus cells contain abundant melanin pigment (unlike Spitz nevus cells) and are often associated with

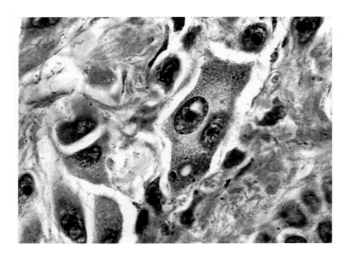

Figure 48–22. Spindle and epithelioid cell nevus (same case as Fig. 48–19). Cytologically atypical binucleate epithelioid nevus cell resembling a Reed-Sternberg cell is present in the reticular dermis (H&E, ×500).

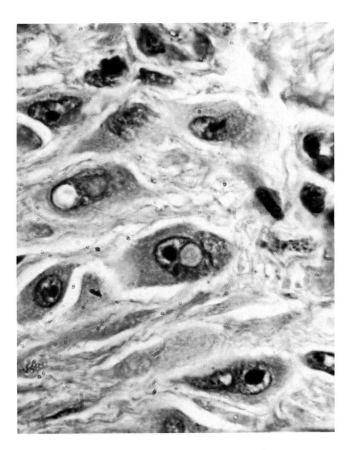

Figure 48–23. Spindle and epithelioid cell nevus (same case as Fig. 48–19). Cytologically atypical epithelioid nevus cells with prominent nucleoli and cytoplasmic nuclear invaginations are present in the reticular dermis (H&E, ×500).

dense melanophage accumulation. The nuclear characteristics are usually monomorphous throughout the lesion. A curious cytologic trait of the pigmented spindle cell nevus is the close resemblance of the nevus cell nuclei to the nuclei of nearby epidermal keratinocytes (Figs. 48–25, 48–27, 48–29). The nuclei of these nevus cells generally appear larger and more open than junctional cells of common acquired melanocytic nevi. One or more prominent small nucleoli are typically present. A lymphocytic response may be seen at the base of the lesion. Mitotic figures are uncommon. Reactive nuclear atypia and single-cell intraepidermal spread of nevomelanocytes may simulate melanoma in some lesions (Figs. 48–28 and 48–29). Although the spectrum of senescent patterns has not been fully described in these lesions, transepidermal elimination of entire junctional nests of nevus cells may be observed (Fig. 48–26).

DERMAL MELANOCYTOSES

Certain acquired and congenital pigmented lesions represent proliferative disorders of dermal melanocytes.[83] Such dermal melanocytes may be derived from ectopic rests of

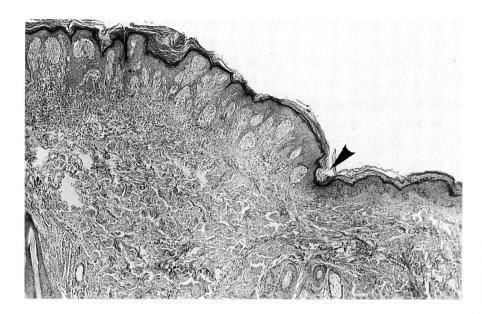

Figure 48–24. Pigmented spindle cell nevus. Nests of nevus cells are distributed in a plaque along the dermoepidermal junction and within dermal papillae. Note the sharp lateral margin (arrowhead) (H&E, ×50).

migratory neural crest cells. These lesions include the common and cellular blue nevus, the Mongolian spot, the nevus of Ota, and the nevus of Ito. All feature the presence of delicate spindle cells containing melanin granules dissecting between bundles of reticular dermal collagen. The density and distribution of such dermal melanocytes, the degree of melanin pigmentation, and the presence of associated melanophage deposition usually allow histologic discrimination of these entities. Clinically, the dermal melanocytoses display a blue or gray color that results from the absorption of long visible light wavelengths by dermal melanin and reflection of the shorter blue wavelengths.

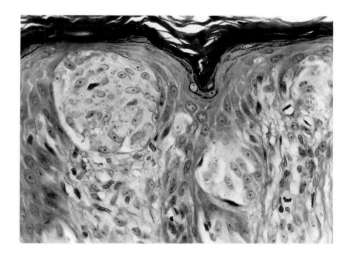

Figure 48–25. Pigmented spindle cell nevus (same case as Fig. 48–24). Junctional and papillary dermal nests are composed of spindle cells with coarse melanin pigment and nuclei similar in appearance to adjacent keratinocyte nuclei (H&E, ×313).

Common Blue Nevus

Common blue nevi are solitary, small, less than 1.0 cm, slightly elevated or dome-shaped lesions often occurring on the dorsa of the hands and feet. They are acquired lesions, usually seen in adults. The intense dark pigmentation may clinically simulate melanoma. Eruptive multiple blue nevi may occur rarely.[84]

Histologic examination at low power reveals a dense, well-circumscribed area of pigment deposition within the dermis (see Fig. 48–30).[85] Most of the pigment is present within melanophages, often obscuring the background distribution of dermal melanocytes. The melanocytic proliferation and pigment deposition may occupy the entire reticular dermis and occasionally the subcutaneous fat. The cells are often distributed in the periadnexal arrangement.

Blue nevi may histopathologically resemble sclerosing hemangiomas, dermatofibromas, or pigmented spindle cell nevi. They may occur in other organs in addition to the skin.[86,87]

Cellular Blue Nevus

Cellular blue nevi usually occur on the lower back or buttocks and present as a bluish dermal nodule or plaque measuring greater than 1.5 cm in diameter.

On microscopic examination, the lesions display a well-circumscribed cellular mass of interweaving fascicles of unpigmented spindle cells (Fig. 48–31).[88] The histological differential diagnosis may include other cellular spindle cell tumors such as a dermatofibroma or leiomyoma. Close examination reveals the presence of melanin-containing fusiform dermal melanocytes interspersed throughout the lesion (Fig. 48–32).

The rare identification of nevus cells in the subcapsular

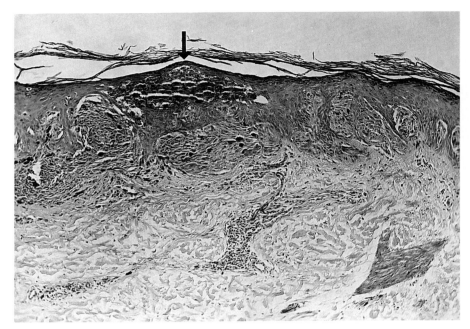

Figure 48–26. Pigmented spindle cell nevus. Dense melanin pigment deposition and transepidermal elimination of a junctional nest (arrow) may result in confusion with superficial spreading melanoma (H&E, ×79).

sinuses of regional lymph nodes probably reflects benign migration of cellular blue nevus cells into cutaneous lymphatics with subsequent deposition in regional nodes.[89–91]

Mongolian Spot

A Mongolian spot is a congenital disorder possibly resulting from the aberrant development or migration of epidermal melanocytic precursors. The lesion appears clinically as a diffuse area of macular blue-black uniform pigmentation over the lower back or buttocks.[92] Ectopic Mongolian spots may occur at other body sites as well. These lesions are present in more than 90% of Oriental infants less than 1 year old and usually regress within several years. Approximately 4% of young Oriental adults have persistent Mongolian spots.[93]

Biopsy specimens of involved skin appear normal at low power. High-power study reveals the presence of rare elongate dermal melanocytes containing fine melanin pigment granules. The melanocytes are usually present in the lower two thirds or one half of the reticular dermis and are not associated with melanophage accumulation.

Nevus of Ota and Nevus of Ito

Nevus of Ota and nevus of Ito are uncommon pigmented lesions that are acquired hamartomas of dermal melanocytes, usually occurring in the first or second decades. They are most frequently observed in Orientals but may also occur in Hispanics, Afro Americans and American Indians. They appear clinically as agminated and irregular confluent macular areas of blue–gray pigmentation.[94] Nevus of Ota, also known as nevus fusoceruleus ophthalmomaxillaris, occurs in periorbital and temporal skin in the distribution of the first and second branches of the trigeminal nerve.[95] Many individuals display bluish scleral discoloration in addition to ipsilateral skin findings. The skin of the eyelids is usually most affected, with fading toward the zygomatic and maxillary regions.[96] Most cases are unilateral. The nevus of Ito occurs over supraclavicular and scapular skin in the distribution of the lateral supraclavicular and brachial nerves. The skin changes appear clinically similar to those observed in the nevus of Ota.[97]

Histologic Features

These lesions appear histologically distinct from the Mongolian spot. Low-power examination reveals deeply pigmented cells scattered sparsely, usually throughout the entire reticular dermis but sometimes limited to the upper

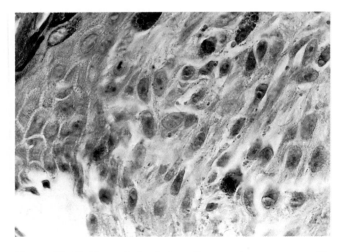

Figure 48–27. Pigmented spindle cell nevus (same case as Fig. 48–26). Close examination reveals banal cytologic appearance often obscured by coarse melanin pigment deposition (H&E, ×313).

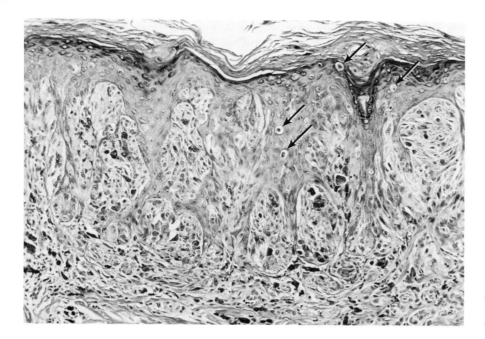

Figure 48–28. Pigmented spindle cell nevus. Single cell infiltration of the epidermis (arrows) may result in histologic confusion with melanoma (H&E, ×125).

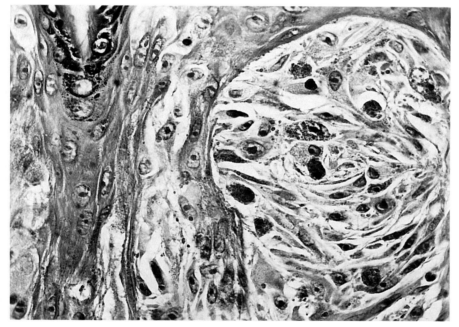

Figure 48–29. Pigmented spindle cell nevus (same case as Fig. 48–28). Close examination reveals reactive nuclear changes in both nevus cells and keratinocytes. Note the similar size and overall appearance of nevus cell and keratinocyte nuclei (H&E, ×313).

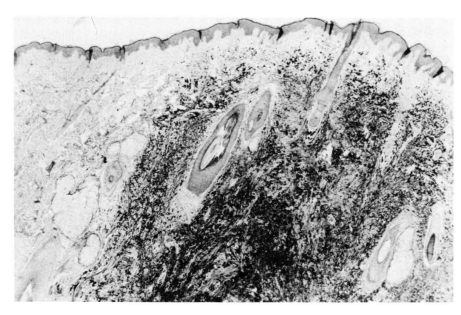

Figure 48–30. Common blue nevus. Dense melanin pigment deposition is present in a nodular aggregate throughout the reticular dermis. Most of the pigment is present within melanophages (H&E, ×79).

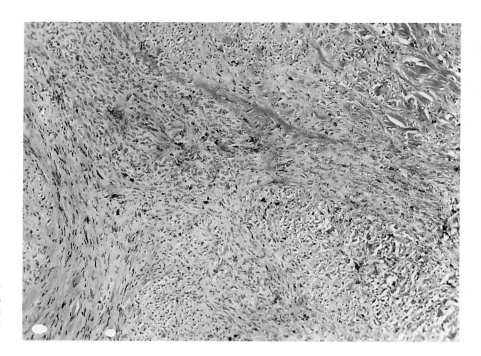

Figure 48–31. Cellular blue nevus. Interweaving fascicles of amelanotic spindle cells contain foci of melanin pigment deposition in both melanophages and dermal melanocytes (H&E, ×79).

third (Fig. 48–33). Fusiform or wavy dermal melanocytes with delicate melanin pigment granules are present in association with melanophages, often in a perivascular and periadnexal distribution (Fig. 48–34).

MISCELLANEOUS NEVOMELANOCYTIC LESIONS

Combined Nevus

On occasion, elements of two different types of both dermal and/or epidermal melanocytic proliferations may be present in the same pigmented lesion.[98] These so-called combined nevi most commonly include acquired melanocytic nevus and common blue nevus components (Figs. 48–35 and 48–36).[99] Rarely, Spitz nevus cells may be present as well. Combined nevi may display an aberrant histological pattern of maturation with pigmented epithelioid type A nevus cells present at the base of the lesion instead of at the dermoepidermal junction. Such variants should be considered in cases that otherwise appear cytologically and architecturally benign. Such inverted type A cells should be recognized as such and not mistaken for malignant degeneration simply because they are pigmented and ectopically located.

Lentigo

Common lentigo or *lentigo simplex* may be a counterpart to acquired junctional nevi, differing in the pattern of melanocytic proliferation. These are acquired lesions, often occurring during childhood, and appear as sharply circumscribed, uniformly dark brown macules measuring less than 3 mm in diameter. They may occur anywhere on the skin but show a predilection for acral and sun-exposed sites.

Microscopic examination reveals lentiginous melanocytic hyperplasia, usually distributed along the tips of rete ridges (Fig. 48–37). Hyperpigmentation of adjacent keratinocytes is usually present and often obscures the background melanocytic hyperplasia. The extensive melanin deposition in keratinocytes is responsible for the dark appearance. Also present are various degrees of epidermal rete hyperplasia. The histopathologic features are distinguished from acquired melanocytic nevi by the absence of nested melanocytic hyperplasia and lack of infiltration of the papillary dermis by nevomelanocytes.[100]

Solar lentigo is a variant occurring on sun-exposed skin

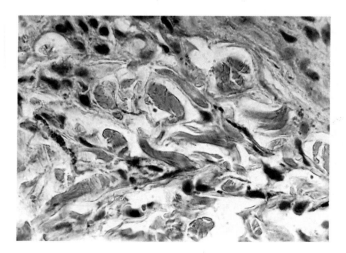

Figure 48–32. Cellular blue nevus (same case as Fig. 48–31). Delicate melanin-containing dendritic cells are present between reticular dermal collagen bundles (H&E, ×600).

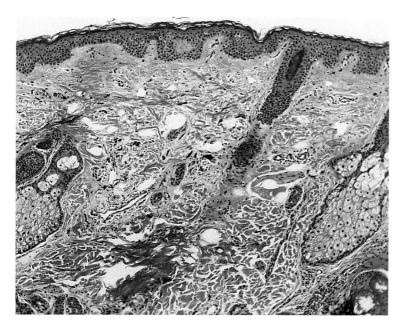

Figure 48–33. Nevus of Ota. Scattered deposits of dense melanin pigment are observed throughout the reticular dermis (H&E, ×50).

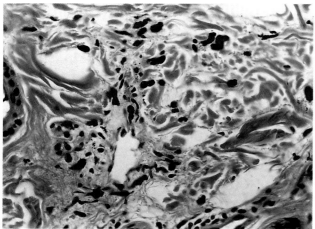

Figure 48–34. Nevus of Ota (same case as Fig. 48–33). Melanin pigment is present in both delicate spindled dermal melanocytes and melanophages (H&E, ×313).

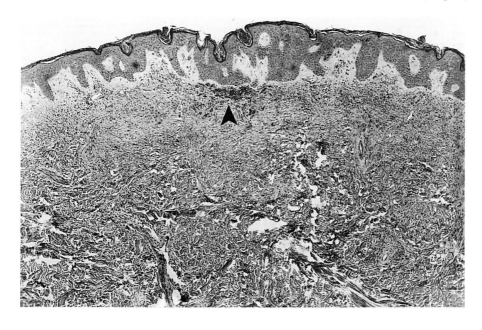

Figure 48–35. Combined dermal/blue nevus. A solitary central focus of dense pigment deposition (arrowhead) is present amidst dermal nevus cells (H&E, ×50).

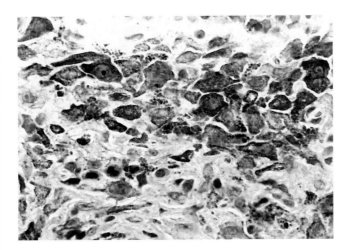

Figure 48–36. Combined dermal/blue nevus (same case as Fig. 48–35). Melanin deposition is present within melanophages, scattered amidst fusiform dermal melanocytes (H&E, ×313).

of older individuals. These lesions appear as multiple, often poorly circumscribed areas of macular hyperpigmentation and may vary in size up to 1 cm or more in diameter.[101] Histologically, lentiginous melanocytic hyperplasia is seen in association with marked secondary epidermal rete hyperplasia, sometimes simulating the appearance of a reticulated seborrheic keratosis. At times, however, there may be a mixture of epidermal atrophy alternating with areas of epidermal hyperplasia.

Melanoacanthoma

Melanoacanthoma is an uncommon lesion that may simply be a histological variant of a seborrheic keratosis or it may represent a combined hyperplasia of keratinocyte and melanocytes. Melanoacanthoma may masquerade clinically as a pigmented seborrheic keratosis, pigmented basal cell carcinoma, or malignant melanoma.[102–104]

Histologically, these lesions appear to be seborrheic keratoses with prominent, dendritic melanocytes engorged with melanin granules. The melanocytes and their dendritic processes are usually quite obvious on routinely stained sections and are scattered individually throughout the lesion, the dendritic array giving rise to a spindle cell appearance of the lesion. An apparent block in melanin pigment transfer exists, because little if any melanin is observed in keratinocytes.

Café au Lait Macule

Café au lait macules are well-circumscribed, uniformly pigmented tan macules measuring between 1 and 20 cm in diameter. They display irregular, often jagged contours and occur on any skin surface. Although these lesions are most often incidental findings in otherwise normal individuals, they may occur in association with von Recklinghausen's neurofibromatosis (VRNF).[105] Café au lait macules occur in approximately 10 to 20% of healthy individuals as isolated lesions. Nearly all healthy individuals with isolated macules have fewer than three lesions.[106] Café au lait macules occur in more than 90% of patients with VRNF, and most of those patients have more than six lesions.[107]

Microscopic study of café au lait macules demonstrated increased melanin pigment deposition in both melanocytes and basilar keratinocytes (Fig. 48–38). Increased numbers of melanocytes are present within lesions relative to adjacent normal-appearing skin. This disorder may reflect both a local melanocytic hyperplasia and elevated melanin synthesis production and transfer. The observed hyperplasia of normal melanocytes and increased pigmentation may not be diagnostic in the absence of normal skin for comparison.

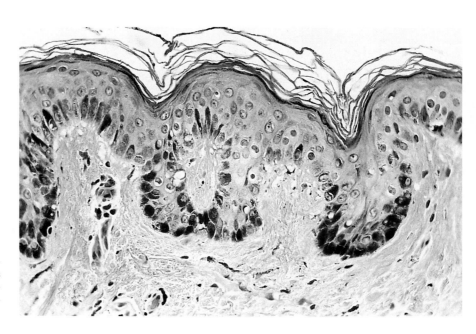

Figure 48–37. Lentigo simplex. Dense melanin deposition in basilar keratinocytes is observed primarily along rete ridges. Lentiginous melanocytic hyperplasia may be obscured by the pigment (H&E, ×125).

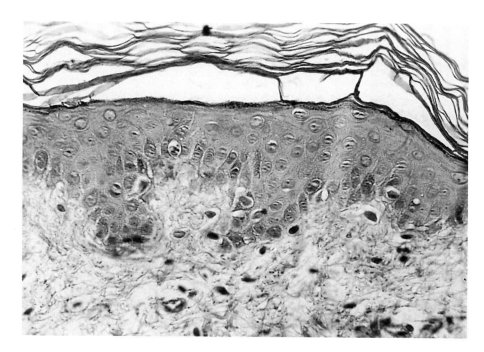

Figure 48–38. Café au lait spot, von-Recklinghausen's neurofibromatosis. Slight lentiginous melanocytic hyperplasia and basilar keratinocytic hyperpigmentation is evident only on comparison with normally pigmented skin (H&E, ×125).

The café au lait macules of VRNF often display abnormally large melanin pigment globules with both melanocytes and keratinocytes.[108] These deposits, variously referred to as macromelanosomes or melanin macroglobules, are quite evident on routinely stained sections when present. Their presence is not diagnostic of VRNF, and they may occasionally be seen in other pigmented lesions including dysplastic nevi and lentigines.

REFERENCES

1. Le Douarin NM. Cell line segregation during peripheral nervous system ontogeny. *Science*. 1986;231:1515–1522.
2. Ciment G, Glimelius B, Nelson DM, et al. Reversal of a developmental restriction in neural crest-derived cells of avian embryos by a phorbol ester drug. *Dev Biol*. 1986;118:392–398.
3. Sieber-Blum M, Cohen AM. Clonal analysis of quail neural crest cells: they are pluripotent and differentiate in-vitro in the absence of noncrest cells. *Dev Biol*. 1980;80:96–106.
4. Nichols DH, Weston JA. Melanogenesis in cultures of peripheral nervous tissue. I: the origin and prospective fate of cells giving rise to melanocytes. *Dev Biol*. 1977;60:217–225.
5. Nichols DH, Kaplan RA, Weston JA. Melanogenesis in cultures of peripheral nervous tissue. II: environmental factors determining the fate of pigment-forming cells. *Dev Biol*. 1977;60:226–237.
6. Thiery JP, Duband JL, Rocher S, et al. Adhesion and migration of avian neural crest cells: an evaluation of the role of several extracellular matrix components. *Prog Dev Biol*. 1986;217B:155–168.
7. Rovasio RA, Delouvee A, Yamada KM, et al. Neural crest cell migration: requirements for exogenous fibronectin and high cell density. *J Cell Biol*. 1983;96:462–473.
8. Ito K, Takeuchi T. The differentiation in-vitro of the neural crest cells of the mouse embryo. *J Embryol Exp Morphol*. 1984;84:49–62.
9. Quevedo WC, Fleischmann RD. Developmental biology of mammalian melanocytes. *J Invest Dermatol*. 1980;75:116–120.
10. Slaughter JC, Hardman JM, Kempe LG, et al. Neurocutaneous melanosis and leptomeningeal melanomatosis in children. *Arch Pathol*. 1969;88:298–304.
11. Nakai T, Rappaport H. A study of the histogenesis of experimental melanotic tumors resembling cellular blue nevi: the evidence in support of their neurogenic origin. *Am J Pathol* 1963;43:175–199.
12. Reed RJ, Ichninose H, Clark WH, et al. Common and uncommon melanocytic nevi and borderline melanomas. *Semin Oncol*. 1975;2:119–147.
13. Reed RJ, Clark WH Jr, Mihm MC. Premalignant melanocytic dysplasias. In: Ackerman AB, ed. *Pathology of Malignant Melanoma*. New York, NY: Masson; 1981. pp 159–183.
14. Breathnach AS. Melanocytes in early regenerated human epidermis. *J Invest Dermatol*. 1960;35:245–251.
15. Staricco RG. Mechanism of migration of the melanocytes from the hair follicle into the epidermis following dermabrasion. *J Invest Dermatol*. 1961;36:99–104.
16. Ainsworth AM, Folberg R, Reed RJ, et al. Melanocytic nevi, melanocytomas, melanocytic dysplasias, and uncommon forms of melanoma. In: Clark WH, Goldman LI, Mastrangelo MJ, eds. *Human Malignant Melanoma*. Orlando, Fla: Grune & Stratton; 1979:167–208.
17. McGovern VJ. Pigmented cutaneous lesions: the difficult case. *Pathol Ann*. 1978;13:415–442.
18. Hu F. Melanocyte cytology in normal skin, melanocytic nevi, and malignant melanomas: a review. In: Ackerman AB, ed. *Pathology of Malignant Melanoma*. New York, NY: Masson; 1981:1–21.
19. Gottlieb B, Brown AL, Winkelmann RK. Fine structure of the nevus cell. *Arch Dermatol*. 1965;92:81–87.
20. Paul E, Wen DR, Cochran AJ. Variations in S-100 protein expression in naevocellular naevi may be related to metabolic activity. *Br J Dermatol*. 1987;116:371–378.
21. Herlyn M, Thurin J, Balaban G, et al. Characteristics of cultured human melanocytes isolated from different stages of tumor progression. *Cancer Res*. 1985;45:5670–5676.

22. Herlyn M, Herlyn D, Elder DE, et al. Phenotypic characteristics of cells derived from precursors of human melanoma. *Cancer Res.* 1983;43:5502–5508.

23. Houghton AN, Eisinger M, Albino AP, et al. Surface antigens of melanocytes and melanomas: markers of melanocyte differentiation and melanoma subsets. *J Exp Med.* 1982;156:1755–1766.

24. Albino AP, Houghton AN. Cell surface antigens of melanocytes and melanoma. *Cancer Surv.* 1985;4:185–211.

25. Real FX, Houghton AN, Albino AP, et al. Surface antigens of melanomas and melanocytes defined by mouse monoclonal antibodies: specificity analysis and comparison of antigen expression in cultured cells and tissues. *Cancer Res.* 1985;45:4401–4411.

26. Houghton AN, Cordon-Cardo C, Eisinger M. Differentiation antigens of melanoma and melanocytes. *Int Rev Exp Pathol.* 1986;28:217–248.

27. Gilchrest BA, Treloar V, Grassi AM, et al. Characteristics of cultivated adult human nevocellular nevus cells. *J Invest Dermatol.* 1986;87:102–107.

28. Halaban R, Ghosh S, Duray P, et al. Human melanocytes cultured from nevi and melanomas. *J Invest Dermatol.* 1986;87:95–101.

29. Pawlowski A, Lea PJ. Nevi and melanoma induced by chemical carcinogens in laboratory animals: similarities and differences with human lesions. *J Cutan Pathol.* 1983;10:81–110.

30. Pawlowski A, Haberman HF, Menon IA. Skin melanoma induced by 7,12-dimethylbenzanthracene in albino guinea pigs and its similarities to skin melanoma of humans. *Cancer Res.* 1980;40.

31. Maize JC, Foster G. Age-related changes in melanocytic naevi. *Clin Exp Dermatol.* 1979;4:49–58.

32. Clark WH, Elder DE, Guerry D, et al. A study of tumor progression: the precursor lesions of superficial spreading and nodular melanoma. *Hum Pathol.* 1984;15:1147–65.

33. Eady RAJ, Gilkes JJH, Wilson Jones E. Eruptive naevi: report of two cases. *Br J Dermatol.* 1977;97:267–278.

34. Masson P. My conception of cellular nevi. *Cancer.* 1951;4:9–38.

35. Lea PJ, Pawlowski A. Human melanocytic naevi. I: electron microscopy and 3-dimensional computer reconstruction of naevi and basement membrane zone from ultrathin serial sections. *Acta Derm Venereol (Stockh).* 1986;127(suppl):5–15.

36. Lea PJ, Pawlowski A. Human melanocytic naevi. II: depth of dermal protrusion: comparative measures of the basement membrane zone and diameters of intracellular microfibrils using a microcomputer analysis system. *Acta Derm Venereol (Stockh).* 1986;127(suppl):17–21.

37. Lea PJ, Pawlowski A. Human melanocytic naevi. III: immunofluorescence and immunoelectron microscopy of the basement membrane zone. *Acta Derm Venereol (Stockh).* 1986;127(suppl):23–30.

38. Stenback F, Wasenius VM. Occurrence of basement membranes in pigment cell tumors of the skin, relation to cell type and clinical behavior. *J Cutan Pathol.* 1986;13:175–186.

39. Bentley-Phillips CB, Marks R. The epidermal component of melanocytic naevi. *J Cutan Pathol.* 1976;3:190–194.

40. Weedon D. Unusual features of nevocellular nevi. *J Cutan Pathol.* 1982;9:284–292.

41. Stegmaier OC. Natural regression of the melanocytic nevus. *J Invest Dermatol.* 1959;32:413–419.

42. Lund HZ, Stobbe GD. The natural history of the pigmented nevus. Factors of age and anatomic location. *Am J Pathol.* 1949;25:1117–1147.

43. Graham JH, Sanders JB, Johnson WC, et al. Fibrous papule of the nose: a clinicopathological study. *J Invest Dermatol.* 1965;45:194–203.

44. McGibbon DH, Wilson Jones E. Fibrous papule of the face (nose): fibrosing nevocytic nevus. *Am J Dermatopathol.* 1979;1:345–348.

45. Reed RJ, Hairston MA, Palomeque FE. The histologic identity of adenoma sebaceum and solitary melanocytic angiofibroma. *Dermatol Int.* 1966;5:3–11.

46. Saylan T, Marks R, Wilson Jones E. Fibrous papule of the nose. *Br J Dermatol.* 1971;85:111–118.

47. Reed RJ. Fibrous papule of the face: melanocytic angiofibroma. *Am J Dermatopathol.* 1979;1:343–344.

48. Meigel WN, Ackerman AB. Fibrous papule of the face. *Am J Dermatopathol.* 1979;1:329–340.

49. Ragaz A, Berezowsky V. Fibrous papule of the face: a study of five cases by electron microscopy. *Am J Dermatopathol.* 1979;1:353–355.

50. Santa Cruz DJ, Prioleau PG. Fibrous papule of the face: an electron-microscopic study of two cases. *Am J Dermatopathol.* 1979;1:349–352.

51. Kwan TH, Smoller BR, Schneider DR. Alpha-1-antitrypsin and lysozyme in fibrous papules and angiofibromas. *J Am Acad Dermatol.* 1985;12:99–101.

52. Spiegel J, Nadji M, Penneys NS. Fibrous papule: an immunohistochemical study with an antibody to S100 protein. *J Am Acad Dermatol.* 1983;9:360–362.

53. Schrader WA, Helwig EB. Balloon cell nevi. *Cancer.* 1967;20:1502–1514.

54. Goette DK, Doty RD. Balloon cell nevus. *Arch Dermatol.* 1978;114:109–111.

55. Jones EW, Sanderson KV. Cellular naevi with peculiar foam cells. *Br J Dermatol.* 1963;75:47–54.

56. Hashimoto K, Bale GF. An electron microscopic study of balloon cell nevi. *Cancer.* 1972;30:530–540.

57. Wayte DM, Helwig EB. Halo nevi. *Cancer.* 1968;22:69–90.

58. Kopf AW, Morrill SD, Silberberg I. Broad spectrum of leukoderma acquisitum centrifugum. *Arch Dermatol.* 1965;92:64–68.

59. Findlay GH. The histology of Sutton's nevus. *Br J Dermatol.* 1957;69:389–394.

60. Swanson JL, Wayte DM, Helwig EB. Ultrastructure of halo nevi. *J Invest Dermatol.* 1968;50:434–437.

61. Schoenfeld RJ, Pinkus H. The recurrence of nevi after incomplete removal. *Arch Dermatol.* 1958;78:30–35.

62. Cox AJ, Walton RG. The induction of junctional changes in pigmented nevi. *Arch Pathol.* 1965;79:428–434.

63. Imagawa I, Endo M, Morishima T. Mechanism of recurrence of pigmented nevi following dermabrasion. *Acta Derm Venereol (Stockh).* 1976;56:353–359.

64. Kornberg R, Ackerman AB. Pseudomelanoma: recurrent melanocytic nevus following partial surgical removal. *Arch Dermatol.* 1975;111:1588–1590.

65. Park HK, Leonard DD, Arrington JH, et al. Recurrent melanocytic nevi: clinical and histologic review of 175 cases. *J Am Acad Dermatol.* 1987;17:285–292.

66. Silvers DN, Helwig EB. Melanocytic nevi in neonates. *J Am Acad Dermatol.* 1981;4:166–175.

67. Rhodes AR, Sober AJ, Day CL, et al. The malignant potential of small congenital nevocellular nevi: an estimate of association based on a histologic study of 234 primary cutaneous melanomas. *J Am Acad Dermatol.* 1982;6:230–241.

68. Rhodes AR. Pigmented birthmarks and precursor melanocytic lesions of cutaneous melanoma identifiable in childhood. *Pediatr Clin North Am.* 1983;30:435–463.

69. Mark GJ, Mihm MC, Liteplo MG, et al. Congenital melanocytic nevi of the small and garment type: clinical, histologic and ultrastructural studies. *Hum Pathol.* 1973;4:395–418.

70. Kuehnl-Petzoldt C, Volk B, et al. Histology of congenital nevi during the first year of life: a study by conventional and electron microscopy. *Am J Dermatopathol.* 1984;6(suppl):81–88.

71. Spitz S. Melanomas of childhood. *Am J Pathol.* 1948;24:591–609.

72. Allen AC. Juvenile melanomas of children and adults and melanocarcinomas of children. *Arch Dermatol.* 1960;82:325–335.

73. Omura EF, Kheir SM. Recurrent Spitz's nevus. *Am J Dermatopathol.* 1984;6(suppl):207–212.

74. Weedon D, Little JH. Spindle and epithelioid cell nevi in children and adults: a review of 211 cases of the Spitz cell nevus. *Cancer.* 1977;40:217–225.

75. Paniago-Pereira C, Maize JC, Ackerman AB. Nevus of large spindle and/or epithelioid cells (Spitz's nevus). *Arch Dermatol.* 1978;114:1811–1823.

76. Kamino H, Misheloff E, Ackerman AB, et al. Eosinophilic globules in Spitz's nevi: new findings and a diagnostic sign. *Am J Dermatopathol.* 1979;1:319–324.

77. Kamino H, Jagirdar J. Fibronectin in eosinophilic globules of Spitz's nevi. *Am J Dermatopathol.* 1984;6(suppl):313–316.

78. Barr RJ, Morales RV, Graham JH. Desmoplastic nevus: a distinct histologic variant of mixed spindle cell and epithelioid cell nevus. *Cancer.* 1980;46:557–564.

79. Ainsworth AM, Folberg R, Reed RJ, et al. Pigmented spindle cell tumor. In: Clark WH, Goldman LI, Mastrangelo MJ, eds. Human Malignant Melanoma. Orlando, Fla: Grune & Stratton; 1979:179.

80. Sau P, Graham JH, Helwig EB. Pigmented spindle cell nevus. *Arch Dermatol.* 1984;120:1615.

81. Sagebiel RW, Chinn EK, Egbert BM. Pigmented spindle cell nevus: clinical and histologic review of 90 cases. *Am J Surg Pathol.* 1984;120:1615.

82. Smith NP. The pigmented spindle cell tumor of Reed: an underdiagnosed lesion. *Semin Diagn Pathol.* 1987;4:75–87.

83. Mevorah B, Frenk E, Delecretaz J. Dermal melanocytosis. *Dermatologica.* 1977;154:107–114.

84. Hendricks WM. Eruptive blue nevi. *J Am Acad Dermatol.* 1981;4:50–53.

85. Dorsey CS, Montgomery H. Blue nevus and its distinction from Mongolian spot and the nevus of Ota. *J Invest Dermatol.* 1954;22:225–236.

86. Jao W, Fretzin DF, Christ ML, et al. Blue nevus of the prostate gland. *Arch Pathol.* 1971;91:187–191.

87. Qizilibash AH. Blue nevus of the uterine cervix. *Am J Clin Pathol.* 1973;59:803–806.

88. Rodriquez HA, Ackerman LV. Cellular blue nevus: clinicopathologic study of forty-five cases. *Cancer.* 1968;21:393–405.

89. Lambert WC, Brodkin RH. Nodal and subcutaneous cellular blue nevi: a pseudometastasizing pseudomelanoma. *Arch Dermatol.* 1984;120:367–370.

90. Johnson WT, Helwig EB. Benign nevus cells in the capsule of lymph nodes. *Cancer.* 1969;23:747–753.

91. Ridolfi RL, Rosen PP, Thaler H. Nevus cell aggregates associated with lymph nodes: estimated frequency and clinical significance. *Cancer.* 1977;39:164–171.

92. Kikuchi I, Inoue S. Natural history of the Mongolian spot. *J Dermatol.* 1980;7:449–450.

93. Hidano A. Persistent Mongolian spot in the adult. *Arch Dermatol.* 1971;103:680–681.

94. Hidano A, Kajima H, Ikeda S, et al. Natural history of nevus of Ota. *Arch Dermatol.* 1967;95:187–195.

95. Ota M, Tanino H. A type of nevus frequently seen in our country: the naevus fusco-caeruleus ophthalmo-maxillaris and its relationship to pigmentary changes of the eye. *Tokyo Med J.* 1939;63:1243–1245.

96. Kopf AW, Weidman A. Nevus of Ota. *Arch Dermatol.* 1962;85:195–208.

97. Mishima Y, Mevorah B. Nevus Ota and Nevus Ito in American Negroes. *J Invest Dermatol.* 1961;36:133–154.

98. Fletcher V, Sagebiel RW. The Combined Nevus. In: Ackerman AB, ed. *Pathology of Malignant Melanoma.* New York, NY: Masson; 1981:273–283.

99. Leopold JG, Richards DB. The interrelationship of blue and common nevi. *J Pathol.* 1968;95:37–43.

100. Hirone T, Eryu Y. Ultrastucture of giant pigment granules in lentigo simplex. *Acta Derm Venereol (Stockh).* 1978;58:223–229.

101. Mehregan AH. Lentigo senilis and its evolution. *J Invest Dermatol.* 1975;65:429–433.

102. Mishima Y, Pinkus H. Benign mixed tumor of melanocytes and melpighian cells. *Arch Dermatol.* 1960;81:539–550.

103. Schlappner OLA, Rowden G, Phillips TM, et al. Melanoacanthoma: ultrastructural and immunological studies. *J Cutan Pathol.* 1978;5:127–141.

104. Matsuoka LY, Glasser S, Barsky S. Melanoacanthoma of the lip. *Arch Dermatol.* 1979;115:1116–1117.

105. Benedict PH, Szabo G, Fitzpatrick TB, et al. Melanotic macules in Albright's syndrome and in neurofibromatosis. *JAMA.* 1968;205:618–626.

106. Johnson BI, Charneco DR. Cafe-au-lait spots in neurofibromatosis and in normal individuals. *Arch Dermatol.* 1970;102:442–446.

107. Crowe FW, Schull WJ. Diagnostic importance of cafe-au-lait spot in neurofibromatosis. *Arch Intern Med.* 1953;91:758–766.

108. Jimbow K, Szabo G, Fitzpatrick TB. Ultrastructure of giant pigment granules (macromelanosomes) in the cutaneous pigmented macules of neurofibromatosis. *J Invest Dermatol.* 1973;61:300–309.

CHAPTER 49
Dysplastic Nevi and Malignant Melanoma

Wallace H. Clark, Jr., David E. Elder, and DuPont Guerry, IV

The known inductive agents and mechanisms of the neoplastic system affecting human epidermal melanocytes do not, as a rule, directly induce a lesion that is malignant melanoma* from its inception.[1–3] In humans and experimental animals, the evident initial lesions attesting to the induction of melanocytic neoplasia constitute a diverse class of benign, proliferative lesions that may rarely progress to malignant melanoma. This chapter discusses the nature and histology of these initial responders to known and unknown carcinogenic stimuli, with emphasis on dysplastic nevi, lesions that have been demonstrated to be precursors of and risk markers for melanoma. The discussion of melanoma itself will include the following topics:

1. The biologic forms of melanoma.
2. The clinical and histologic features of primary melanoma, including its radial (nontumorigenic) and its vertical (tumorigenic) growth phases.
3. The prognostic attributes that indicate the likelihood of a primary melanoma in the vertical growth phase giving rise to clinically evident metastatic disease.
4. Some aspects of the biology of metastasis.
5. The pathology of the uncommon forms of melanoma.
6. The matter of histologic differential diagnosis.

NEOPLASTIC DEVELOPMENT AND TUMOR PROGRESSION

In this chapter, the definition of tumor progression encompasses all of the apparent, sequential lesions of a neoplastic system, including the myriad potential precursor lesions that only rarely actually progress.[4–6] By inference, such a definition also includes other and inapparent events in neoplasia, such as initiation and promotion. Farber, Sarma, Cameron, and their associates at the University of Toronto have carefully studied the development of cancer in a rat liver model.[7,8] These studies may be rightfully regarded as illuminating continuations of the pioneering work on tumor progression by the late Leslie Foulds.[9] These workers restrict the term tumor progression to "the process whereby one or more focal proliferations, such as papillomas, polyps, and nodules, undergo a slow cellular evolution to malignant neoplasm. Included in this term are the series of changes which a malignant neoplasm may undergo as it becomes more malignant, and more prone to show invasion and then to metastasize."[8] As noted later, this restricted definition of tumor progression is used to define its distal events as cancer. Thus, *distal tumor progression* includes the events related to the development of overt cancer and the changes that occur within an evolving lesion by which it acquires the properties of invasion and finally metastasis ("changes which a malignant neoplasm may undergo as it becomes more malignant, and more prone to show invasion and then to metastasize"[8]). Such properties are acquired seriatim, but the path from an intraepidermal lesion, disposed entirely above the basement membrane zone, to fully evolved metastatic malignancy is not inexorably followed.

One cannot comfortably use our general definition of tumor progression without defining its distal lesions: cancer. Although there is no generally accepted definition of this term, there is some agreement that one property of a cancer is persistent growth. Such growth is at least partially autonomous and without temporal restriction.[10] The early lesions of neoplastic development (proximal lesions in tumor progression) grow relatively independently of the host, but differing from cancer, their growth ceases after a time: It is temporally restricted. Beyond in vivo autonomous growth, some would require the capacity for metastasis before using the term *cancer*. This requirement need not be accepted, for it would leave us without a name for most primary cancers. Many of these primary lesions, at the

---

*The term is not used consistently: Some use it synonymously with cancer; others use it for all new growths, benign and malignant. The authors use the term in the latter sense to include all focal new growths that continue to grow after the stimuli that initiated them cease. Such persistence in growth distinguishes neoplasia from hyperplasia.

From The Pigmented Lesion Study Group, and the Departments of Dermatology, Pathology, Medicine (Hematology-Oncology) and the Cancer Center, University of Pennsylvania School of Medicine Philadelphia, Penn. 19104.

time of removal, are not associated with metastatic disease, and metastases at a later date are the exception rather than the rule. With these constraints in mind, our definition of cancer, after Foulds, Farber and Sarma, and others, is a focal collection of cells with an autonomous, temporally unrestricted, selective growth preference over surrounding cells. Such growths are probably clonal and have a strong tendency to undergo progressive change, thereby serially acquiring the properties of invasion and metastasis.[11] It should be emphasized that this appreciable potential for progressive change (distal tumor progression) is a part of our definition of cancer. This definition of cancer does not include the beginnings of the neoplastic system, *proximal tumor progression*.

The initial lesions of neoplastic development, the lesions of proximal tumor progression, have the following properties:

1. Selective, preferential growth, over surrounding normal cells, which is temporally restricted (self-limited).
2. A tendency to evolve serially into histologically heterogeneous lesions. The earliest lesions are structurally benign and the later lesions abnormal in form, but these express only some, not all, of the histologic characteristics of cancer.
3. The lesions tend to regress along a programmed pathway of differentiation.
4. A rare, histologically abnormal lesion will become cancer.
5. Progression from one lesion to the next in the precursor stages of neoplasia is a rare and nonobligatory event. This single property is the overriding characteristic distinguishing the series of initial lesions of neoplastic development from the series of lesional events occurring within a given cancer—events that tend to be inexorable.

From the foregoing it follows that the complete system of neoplasia—all of the new growths affecting a given cellular system—may be divided into two large groups: (1) the *proximal* or *precursor lesions* and (2) the *distal lesions*, or *cancer*. All of the lesions of cancer and its precursor lesions are characterized by *inappropriate cell proliferation*, again borrowing a term from Farber and Sarma. The inappropriate cell proliferation is so designated because a stimulus for the proliferation is rarely apparent or necessarily continuously operative. In one sense, our discussion of tumor progression is an exposition of the various inappropriate cell proliferations constituting the panoply of neoplastic events. It is important in management of precursor lesions to emphasize the biologic meaning of the term. Only a rare lesion proceeds to cancer. This statement is based on epidemiologic evidence. Clinicopathologic features, in general, do not permit one to recognize that a given lesion has a high probability of developing cancer. Some of the precursor lesions have atypical cells, structurally indistinguishable from some cells in established cancers. It has become customary to call such lesions premalignant. We are in agreement with Foulds that such terms are to be avoided. "Without being accurately descriptive they are unreliably prophetic."[12] The avoidance of such terms as *premalignant* is not to satisfy a semantic fetish. The term's implicit meaning usually leads to ablative therapy. Such therapy is rarely indicated for clinically stable precursor lesions. Precursor lesions are, however, of bio-

logic and clinical importance. Biologically they delineate one pathway of neoplasia and clinically they indicate a risk, albeit variable and often small, for the development of cancer. Thus knowledge of neoplastic development and tumor progression is singularly germane to the appropriate management of benign and malignant lesions of cutaneous melanocytic origin.

THE ETIOLOGY AND EPIDEMIOLOGY OF NEVI AND MALIGNANT MELANOMA

Any discussion of the etiology of cancer necessarily contains imprecision and the seeds of controversy. For example, is a suspect initiating agent causative of the precursor lesions? Is it also causative of cancer in an induced neoplastic system? Are other causes required for the development of cancer in addition to those responsible for induction? It is beyond the scope of this chapter to attempt a discussion of the etiology of melanoma with all of its inherent complexities. As one looks critically at the nature of cancer, an ever stronger suspicion emerges: The search for a simple etiology in this complex chronic disease, in a manner analogous with the designation of a certain strain of *Streptococcus* as the causative agent of scarlet fever, is quixotic. Although we shall discuss the possible multiple roles that light plays in the entire system of melanocytic neoplasia, light is neither necessary nor sufficient as the explicator of melanoma etiology. At the outset, keep in mind that melanoma, differing from all of the common forms of cutaneous cancer, occurs in people of all races and colors, dispersed at all latitudes and longitudes. The disease also may be located at anatomic sites "where the sun never shines." Also noteworthy, with regard to the role of light in induction and progression of melanoma, is the prevalence of the disease in the animal kingdom. It is probably ubiquitous, certainly from fish to higher forms of life. Light would not seem to play an important role in animal melanoma. There are forms in some fish that seem to be entirely heritable.[13] In experimental systems, melanoma and its precursors may be readily and consistently induced by chemical carcinogens as well as by light (e.g., in the South American opossum, *Monodelphis domestica*) (Ley, RD. Personal communication).[14] In spite of these various confounding factors, light clearly plays an important part in the human disease, perhaps the dominant role in the currently impressive rise in incidence of melanona in humans. Our discussion of etiology consequently focuses only on light.

Etiologic Agents and Inductive Mechanisms

Holman and colleagues have discussed the relationship of melanoma to individual sunlight-exposure habits.[15] One should also refer to the studies by Kopf and associates, as well as the studies from the Danish Cancer Registry and the National Cancer Institute (Environmental Epidemiology Branch of the Division of Cancer Etiology).[16–18] The evidence for the inductive role of sunlight is summarized in the paragraphs that follow.

Higher Incidence in Fair-Skinned People. Ninety-eight percent of melanomas occur in whites. Within the white population there is, again, a higher incidence in lighter-skinned individuals.

Higher Incidence in Lower Latitudes. The incidence and mortality rates for melanoma are higher in those white populations living close to the equator, and the incidence and mortality gradient correlate with progressively lower latitudes.

Gender Differences in Anatomic Site Distribution. There are anatomic site-specific gender differences in melanoma. The disease is nine times more common on the legs (primarily the calf) of women than on the legs of men and is more frequent on the breasts of men than the breasts of women. Such differences may be related to different light exposure, in turn related to different clothing styles.

Skin Reaction to Sun. There is an increased risk of melanoma associated with increasing skin sensitivity to sunlight. This generality is doubtless of significance, but must be tempered by knowledge that the association does not always persist after correction for red hair and fair skin color. The association may also be confounded by assiduous avoidance of sun exposure by persons with the most sensitive skin.

History of Sunburn. A history of multiple severe sunburns is difficult to consider as a single risk factor. The significance of severe sunburns is confounded by extreme sun sensitivity; heavy vacation and recreational sun exposure; absence of an obvious anatomic relationship between the site of the burn and the subsequent melanoma; hair and eye color; sun-induced freckling; and the coincidence of sun-induced freckles and moles. Together, these last two confounding factors have been said to confer a 29-fold relative risk for melanoma when compared with the risk in the absence of either trait.[19] Nevertheless, the combination of high sun sensitivity and multiple severe sunburns confers, regardless of the other factors, a two to threefold increased risk for the development of melanoma.[20-22] Rhodes and his associates have discussed the complex interrelationships of these various factors.[20]

Sun Exposure in the First 10 Years of Life. Exposure to a high level of sunlight in early childhood seems to be a crucial event in establishing an increased risk of malignant melanoma and is associated with an increased number of nevi.

Sun Exposure in Young Adulthood. Studies have detected an increased risk of melanoma associated with high levels of sun exposure in young adulthood. In addition to the significance of the age (under 10 years) of immigrants to western Australia, Holman and colleagues also demonstrated that high levels of light exposure in age-groups 10 to 24 years and 25 to 39 years resulted in an increased melanoma risk.[15,23] In western Canada, Elwood's group found no significance for occupational sun exposure, but

high levels of recreational exposure were associated with increased melanoma risk.[24] Their studies suggest that intermittent exposure of susceptible skin to sunlight in young adult life is an important risk factor for melanoma.

Actinic Skin Damage. Holman and Armstrong have studied the relationship of actinic skin damage using cutaneous microtopography, a method more sensitive than the assessment of actinic cutaneous damage by histologic methods alone. Increasing actinic damage was associated with increased risk of melanoma. The odds ratio is 4.37 for lentigo maligna melanoma (Hutchinson's melanotic freckle) and 2.68 for all histogenetic types of melanoma. This kind of evidence is particularly important because it reflects the actual amount and biologic effect of ultraviolet (UV) light delivered to the region of the basement membrane zone, the anatomic site of melanoma histogenesis.[25]

Increased Number of Normal Nevi Related to Sun Exposure. An increased number of palpable nevi on the arms seems to be related to sun exposure during the first decade of life.[23] In turn, increasing numbers of nevi are related to melanoma.[26] This relationship is discussed in some detail later in this chapter. The relationship of light to melanocytic nevi and melanoma is by no means a simple dose-response relationship. In fact, Rampen and associates have stated that the prevalence of common acquired nevi and dysplastic nevi is not related to ultraviolet exposure.[27] In their study, however, they ignored sun exposure in prepuberty and puberty, the ages deemed to be of greatest importance in epidemiologic studies.[23] Observations in the Pigmented Lesion Clinic of the University of Pennsylvania suggest that excessive amounts of light seem to confer an increased risk of melanoma in certain cutaneous phenotypes without the induction of a single melanocytic nevus. In other kinds of skin, the melanocarcinogenic effects of light seem to be mediated through melanocytic nevi, with and without dysplasia. In an occasional individual, one may see rather dramatic evidence of the diversity of the effects of light. Where light exposure has been prolonged and excessive there may be numerous small freckles and no moles. Those body areas with much less light exposure may show scattered melanocytic nevi and no freckles.

Increased Number of Normal Nevi Related to the Presence of Dysplastic Nevi. Just as an increasing number of normal nevi is related to melanoma, such an increase is also related to the presence of dysplastic nevi. The evidence for this will be discussed subsequently.

Epidemiology of Malignant Melanoma

In the United States, melanoma represents 3% of all incident cancers, excluding other skin cancers. The rate of increase of incidence of melanoma is rising more rapidly than that of any other cancer in North America and is estimated to be 10% annually for whites in a non-Sunbelt area and 34% in the Sunbelt.[28] This phenomenon is ubiquitous in white populations. In the United States, 27,300 new cases are expected in 1988, and the probability that an individual born in 1985 will develop melanoma is 1%.[29] That such data do not simply reflect biases in ascertainment is indicated by a burgeoning mortality, estimated as increasing by 3 to 5% per year in white populations. The number of deaths from melanoma expected in the United States in 1988 is 5800 (2% of cancer deaths in men and 1% in women). These deaths will occur mainly in a relatively young adult population. Despite these alarming trends, the case fatality rate is falling (from 40% in 1960–1963 to 20% in 1979–1984), presumably because of detection and treatment of biologically early disease.[30] The epidemic of melanoma poses problems for several constituencies.

For the General Population. Until recently, the term *malignant melanoma* and its significance were known by relatively few people outside the profession. Current and proposed educational programs will reverse this state of ignorance.[31] The initial response by the public will likely be the presentation to the physician of virtually all pigmented lesions, innocuous to malignant and all gradations between. This welcome change in public knowledge is rapidly altering the responsibilities and burden of clinicians and pathologists with regard to pigmented lesions. Such responsibilities will precipitously increase over the next 15 years or so before leveling off, after having significantly altered the practice of medicine.

For Clinicians. Careful and knowledgeable examination and management of cutaneous pigmented lesions will be within the purview of a wide variety of medical disciplines. Dermatologists will or should be in the forefront of this expanding knowledge base. A major part of their effort, after their own proper education in these matters, should be the education of other physicians in diagnosis and appropriate therapy.[32] The sheer quantity of the effort should prevent pigmented lesion provincialism. It is beyond the scope of this chapter to extensively discuss clinical management. One must state, however, that a complete physical examination includes, as a standard, the examination of the entire skin, with the scalp, genitalia, buttocks, volar, and subungual sites not exempted.[32]

For Pathologists. The problems falling to pathologists as a result of this explosion of interest in such lesions are perhaps the greatest of all. Biopsy of an ever increasing number of small and new pigmented lesions has and will outstrip not only their methods, but the necessary precision of language required for communication about them. The vast majority of lesions begin as proliferations of intraepidermal melanocytes, and even at this beginning point there is no general nosologic agreement. The earlier a melanocytic proliferation is removed the greater is the likelihood of that growth pattern being ill-defined and rigorously resisting classification. Such a state can generate chaos as pathologist after pathologist applies his or her own querulous prejudices and fetishes without regard for the literature and scientific discipline. It is far better to handle pigmented lesions descriptively when characteristic histologic features are lacking than to force them into a diagnostic entity simply to dismiss them from the mind and the microscope. The incorrect use of terms is already generating confusion, as will be discussed under problems with nomenclature.[32]

DEVELOPMENT AND EVOLUTION OF MELANOCYTIC NEVI

It has been customary, almost to the point of conventional wisdom, to discuss the histogenesis of noncongenital melanocytic nevi as following a programmed pathway of evolution that begins as an intraepidermal proliferation of melanocytes. In all likelihood, such proliferations differ from hyperplasia in being clonal (though this has yet to be proved in ordinary nevi). Without such proof, however, it is obvious that a common acquired nevus is qualitatively different from hyperplasia. Melanocytic hyperplasia is coeval in time and place with its inductive mechanism. A melanocytic nevus is not. A diffuse nevus does not emerge ubiquitously correspondent with the impact site of light on the skin, but is a focal event. A nevus that has been induced experimentally does not disappear if its inductive agent is removed.[1] It persists. It has also been widely accepted to classify nevi into four entities: lentigo, junctional nevus, compound nevus, and dermal nevus. Chronologically, these lesions seem to follow one upon the other, each merging gradually with the following pattern of nevic histology. If one accepts this pathway of development, there would be but one common nevus presenting at a given time a different histological face beckoning us to assign a new name. While discussing the principles of this histogenetic pathway, it should be emphasized that even if such a pathway is ultimately deemed correct, it is not an inexorable pathway. Apparently, the evolving melanocytic lesions, regardless of their position in the course of development, may become stable and remain in any given histologic state.[4] We will frequently return to lack of inexorability in the various lesions and steps of a neoplastic system. Although the pathway is programmed, it is not an imperative.

The Initial Lesions: Lentigo

The earliest acquired melanocytic nevi usually appear between the 6th and 18th months of life. When first recognized, they are small, tan dots less than 1 mm in diameter. Their color is uniform, and they are flat and cannot be felt. New melanocytic lesions continue to appear with varying frequency during the first two decades of life, and as far as is known, these lesions are similar in appearance and evolution to the first pigmented lesions of the early months of life. All developing pigmented lesions may become stable and remain as indolent, flat brown spots some 2 to 3 mm in diameter or they may evolve through a pathway of differentiation. This differentiation pathway encompasses the histological pictures we have come to call junctional nevi, compound nevi, and dermal nevi, to be presently described. The initial melanocytic lesions, regardless of the age when they are recognized, show an increase in basilar epidermal pigment associated with an increased number of basilar melanocytes that may or may not be in nests. Similar lesions may appear in the fourth or fifth decades of life.[4] These late appearing lesions do not evolve through a differentiation pathway, as far as we know.

Junctional Nevus, Compound Nevus, Dermal Nevus

Junctional, compound, and dermal nevi are described elsewhere in this book. Although those lesions are completely benign and most are stable for life except for their tendency to differentiate and disappear, they constitute the first step of a nonobligate tumor progression pathway that may lead to melanoma (lesional step 1 of tumor progression, discussed later). Here we shall make only a few salient points about the relationship of these lesions to dysplastic nevi. Aside from those lesions located on glabrous skin, junctional nevi and compound nevi are not sharply delimited from each other. Pure junctional nevi are rare. As they develop they tend to extend into the dermis, forming a plaque of nevic tissue with the odd nest or two of melanocytes in the epidermis. Most characteristic junctional nevi are found after arduously searching the files for a reproducible picture that conforms with a traditional description. A classic compound nevus is almost as uncommon as the pristine junctional nevus. Dermal nevi are common. An important question is raised by the progressive cellular events of the melanocytic nevus: By what mechanism do the nevic cells enter the dermis from their original intraepidermal location? Before extension into the dermis, the intraepidermal cells tend to migrate to the tips of rete ridges, where they have the appearance of melanocytic nests in routine histological preparations. Serial sections of the skin parallel to the epidermal surface give some evidence that the nests are tubes (or a single serpentine tube) extending along the tips of the rete. [One would hardly expect a clone of cells to be arrayed in multiple, discrete nests.] The cells extend from the tips of the rete into the dermis as individual cells or as small clusters. This process is accompanied by the formation of a basement membrane zone around each nevic cell or cluster of cells.[33] For the most part, the dermal nevic cells are separated from their dermal environment by the newly formed basement membrane zone. This nevic mechanism of extension into the dermis may be different from the mechanism by which melanoma cells invade from epidermis into dermis. The cells of melanoma traverse the basement membrane zone through the conjoint action of many molecular species, including laminin receptor, type IV collagenase, and tissue plasminogen activator.[34]

Differentiation Within a Dermal Nevus

Dermal nevi are of particular interest because of their fascinating tendency to differentiate and disappear. This is apparently accomplished by differentiation along schwannian lines and has been described in detail elsewhere.[4] This tendency for nevi to disappear is analogous with similar events in other neoplastic systems.[7]

THE DYSPLASTIC NEVUS: DYSREGULATED GROWTH

The hallmark of a dysplastic nevus is the development of a new period of inappropriate cell proliferation, characterized by the development of asymmetry of form. It is within this area of asymmetric cell proliferation that some atypical melanocytes appear. With their appearance, the term *melanocytic dysplasia* is applied. The new period of cell proliferation, with or without atypical melanocytes, is temporally restricted: It is not persistent in time, not autonomous. The histologic diagnosis of dysplastic nevi is confusing. Some would require only an abnormal pattern of intraepidermal melanocytic growth. This results in overdiagnosis of a well-defined clinicopathologic entity. One reason for the confusion, as has been pointed out by Mackie,[35] lies in the promiscuous application of terminology. The same term, *dysplastic nevus,* is used for the clinical presentation *and* for the distinctive histology, as we have described it, *and* for varying patterns of abnormal intraepidermal melanocytic architecture.[35] A patient may have clinically obvious dysplastic nevi, but many of the nevi on such a patient are *not* dysplastic histologically, by the criteria set forth here. Some lesions from such patients may be ordinary nevi, but other lesions show an abnormal pattern of intraepidermal melanocytic growth and, because of their clinical setting, may be erroneously interpreted as dysplastic nevi. Nevi with only an abnormal pattern (architecture) of their intraepidermal melanocytes usually represent lesional step 2 of melanocytic tumor progression (melanocytic nevus with persistent lentiginous melanocytic hyperplasia . . . aberrant differentiation), but are not step 3: melanocytic dysplasia (Table 49–1). Step 2 lesions, those with only aberrant differentiation manifested by an abnormal architecture of intraepidermal melanocytes, are frequently seen as lesions

TABLE 49–1. TUMOR PROGRESSION

Melanocytic Lesions	Generic Lesions
1. Common acquired melanocytic nevus	1. Selective focal proliferation of structurally normal cells (a benign tumor)
2. Melanocytic nevus with persistent (but ultimately limited) lentiginous melanocytic hyperplasia (aberrant differentiation)	2. Abnormal pattern of hyperplasia (aberrant differentiation)
3. Melanocytic nevus with persistent lentiginous melanocytic hyperplasia (aberrant differentiation) and melanocytic nuclear atypia: melanocytic dysplasia	3. Abnormal pattern of hyperplasia and random cytologic atypia (aberrant differentiation and the appearance of cells with nuclear atypia)
4. Radial growth phase of primary melanoma (nontumorigenic melanoma)	4. Primary cancer without competence for metastasis
5. Vertical growth phase of primary melanoma (tumorigenic melanoma)	5. Primary cancer with competence for metastasis
6. Metastatic melanoma	6. Metastatic cancer

in patients with and without clinically dysplastic nevi. The diagnosis of dysplastic nevus is unwarranted in those lesions with an abnormal melanocytic architecture. If one makes such unwarranted diagnoses, the concept of dysplastic nevi and the dysplastic nevus syndrome becomes ill defined and of unclear biologic significance. The histologic term *dysplastic nevus* should only be used by strictly defined criteria, to be presently described, if it is to serve as a guideline for appropriate clinical management.[32]

The present difficulties in clinical, histologic, and biologic characterization of dysplastic nevi are compounded by familial (and, in all likelihood, heritable) factors. There is no question that some dysplastic nevi are familial, as are some melanomas. The familial dysplastic nevus syndrome may be defined as a constellation of traits that confer an increased relative risk for melanoma on a given individual. The traits are (1) a distinctive clinical appearance of abnormal melanocytic nevi;[36–38] (2) unique histological features including an abnormal architectural pattern of intraepidermal melanocytes, cytologically atypical intraepidermal melanocytes, connective tissue changes, and a lymphocytic infiltrate[4,39]; (3) an autosomal dominant inheritance has been mapped to chromosome 1p36[40]; and (4) hypermutability of fibroblasts and lymphoblasts.[41–43]

The evidence is also strong that dysplastic nevi occur sporadically.[44] The sporadic dysplastic nevus syndrome is defined by the same clinical and histologic characteristics as are seen in the familial form of the disease. However, hypermutability studies in patients with sporadic dysplastic nevi have not yet been reported. No one has yet made a careful attempt to distinguish familial and sporadic dysplastic nevi by histological, clinical, or other means, except for family history. Further, methods for making precise decisions about the presence or absence of the dysplastic nevus syndrome and dividing the syndrome into various subsets are not available. We continue to be surprised at the power of good histology in nosology, but cells can only do a few things, restricting the usefulness of histology in this and other disorders. Until there are tests that supplement histology and clinical observations, confusion is likely to surround the nature of dysplastic nevi and the dysplastic nevus syndrome. It is possible that the studies of Sanford[43] and associates may be used as a test for melanocytic dysplasia. They have shown enhanced G_2 chromatid radiosensitivity in individuals with dysplastic nevi (familial) or hereditary cutaneous malignant melanoma with dysplastic nevi.[43] Until such studies have been extended, one must rely on histology, and uncritical use of the term *dysplastic nevus syndrome* should be avoided. Thus, a particular affected patient should be described as having dysplastic nevi, clinically or histologically confirmed, with or without a family (or personal) history of melanoma and with or without a family history of dysplastic nevi, as the case may be.

CLINICAL LESION

The details of the clinical presentation of dysplastic nevi have been presented in several publications.[32,36,37] Certain features of individual lesions are important, especially with regard to methods of biopsy and histologic interpretation.

Virtually all dysplastic nevi have some component that is macular and asymmetric. The flat part of these lesions usually has not only an irregular outline, but a border that is hazy, lacking sharp delimitation from the surrounding skin. This distinctive portion of the lesion as a rule presents the characteristic histologic features. Diagnostic biopsies, by scalpel excision with a narrow border of normal skin, should always include the macular component of the lesion. The pathologist should make sure that this component is studied microscopically.

HISTOLOGIC LESION

The most distinctive and most frequently encountered histologic pattern of melanocytic dysplasia is seen at the periphery of a melanocytic nevus—junctional, compound, or dermal—that is not itself dysplastic. The changes are usually seen in a limited area of the periphery, an ectopic shoulder of dysplasia. This combination of features, remnants of a banal nevus with peripheral areas of dysplasia, suggests that the lesion was not, ab initio, dysplastic. Other lesions, seen less often, may show the histology of dysplasia, to be presently described, in the epidermis alone or as dermo-epidermal dysplasia without evidence of a precursor ordinary nevus. These could be dysplastic, ab initio.

Pattern of Growth of the Intraepidermal Melanocytic Component
A new round of inappropriate melanocytic growth, the second clinically apparent one in neoplastic development affecting the melanocytic system, forms the abnormal architectual pattern and creates the ectopia. It may simulate the very beginnings of melanocytic neoplasia, showing basilar melanocytic proliferation similar to that of a lentigo. Thus one may see a junctional, compound, or dermal nevus with an area of basilar melanocytic proliferation extending from a limited area of its border (Fig. 49–1). This melanocytic growth is only a partial expression of the fully developed melanocytic dysplasia, a portent of the events to come. One may also see a more profuse form of melanocytic growth in the basilar region associated with elongation of the rete ridges (Fig. 49–2). Here the basal layer is composed of melanocytes, not keratinocytes. Such melanocytes are larger than normal and may show a curious bridging from one rete to the next. Less commonly, the abnormal architectural growth pattern may be manifested by an increased number of large epithelioid melanocytes, disposed either singly or in a pattern of small nests (Fig. 49–3). The two flawed patterns of melanocytic growth just described may stand alone or may be seen admixed with each other.

Melanocytic Nuclear Atypia Within the Pattern of Abnormal Intraepidermal Growth
The cytologically atypical melanocytes have the same features as cytologically atypical cells in any neoplastic system. Such cells are larger than normal melanocytes or the intraepidermal melanocytes of an ordinary melanocytic nevus. Their nuclei are large, and this characteristic permits one to identify them in the area of ectopic proliferation or to identify them as isolated cells in the basal layer of the epider-

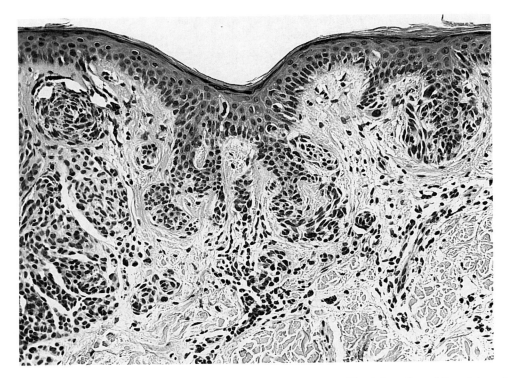

Figure 49–1. Compound nevus with melanocytic dysplasia at the shoulder. The left portion of the picture shows a compound nevus. Extending to the right from the nevus, the architecture of melanocytic growth is abnormal and atypical melanocytic nuclei are evident. A sparse lymphocytic infiltrate is present.

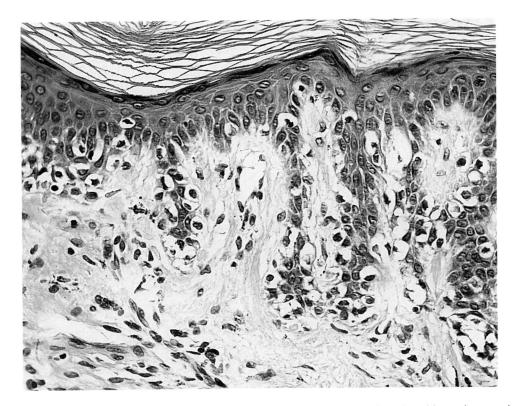

Figure 49–2. Lentiginous melanocytic dysplasia. The rete are elongated and largely replaced by an increased number of melanocytes, most of which show a cytoplasmic retraction artifact.

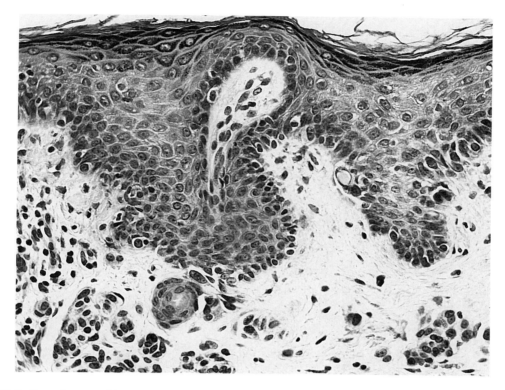

Figure 49–3. Dermal nevus with epithelioid melanocytic dysplasia. A small dermal nevus is seen in the lower left. The adjacent epidermis shows large and variably atypical epithelioid melanocytes.

mis quite separate from their seemingly normal parent nevus. Such large nuclei may be no darker than the nuclei of surrounding melanocytes. These nuclei have an increased amount of chromatin but do not, as a rule, have prominent nucleoli (Figs. 49–4 and 49–5). Some atypical cells may show nuclear hyperchromatism and, consequently, are quickly identified. Hyperchromatism is not, however, a requirement for atypia in this setting. The large epithelioid cells, with or without hyperchromatic nuclei, are similar in their individual cellular form to the cells that are seen in melanoma, especially superficial spreading melanoma. These cells are identical with the giant and nontheque basal epithelioid melanocytes described in an excellent study by Aronson and associates (Figs. 49–6 and 49–7).[45] Such large and atypical melanocytes reacted in paraffin-embedded tissues with a monoclonal antibody (AFH1), produced using a human melanoma cell line (A375) as an immunogen. The reactivity of 72.6% of these cells is almost identical with the 78% reactivity of intraepidermal melanoma cells.[45] Though similar in form, their size is smaller, being intermediate between the cells of superficial spreading melanoma and the melanocytes of normal skin and normal nevi. The melanocytes dispersed individually in dysplastic nevi average 48.3 μm^2; in superficial spreading melanoma, 72.1 μm^2; in ordinary nevi, 25.3 μm^2; and normal melanocytes 27.3 μm^2.[46] The nuclei of these same cells show a parallel variation in cross-sectional area.

The pattern of growth and distribution of intraepidermal melanocytes in dysplastic nevi is different from that in superficial spreading melanoma. In the dysplastic nevus,

they tend to be more or less separate from each other. Contiguous atypical growth and upward growth in the epidermis, characteristically seen in superficial spreading melanoma, are either totally absent or minimal in dysplastic nevi. Exceptions to this statement result in a histologically borderline lesion having many features suggesting melanoma. This problem occurs with some frequency in scalp lesions and may be prominent in lesions of the female breast. The cytologic atypia of dysplastic nevi is, in our opinion, relatively mild. Severe or startling atypia is rarely seen, and mitoses are quite uncommon. When such findings are observed, they should rouse the serious consideration of melanoma, calling for a careful evaluation of the size, growth pattern, and host epithelial and lymphocytic responses of the lesion.

Requirement for Histologic Diagnosis of Dysplastic Nevus. We have insisted that the histologic diagnosis of melanocytic dysplasia of the type seen in the dysplastic nevus syndrome include an abnormal pattern of melanocytic growth *and* melanocytic nuclear atypia. Other histologic findings are usually seen in dysplastic nevi, but abnormal growth pattern and nuclear atypia of melanocytes are presented as the imperatives.

If one strictly adheres to the foregoing description of melanocytic pathology, overdiagnosis of melanocytic dysplasia is not likely to occur. It is of importance that the diagnosis be made with precision and consistency. Such a histologic diagnosis may cause the affected individual to be examined for a lifetime, with the appropriately atten-

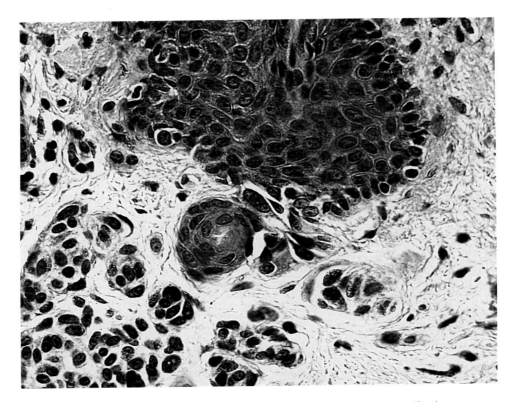

Figure 49–4. The same lesion as shown in Figure 49–3 at higher magnification.

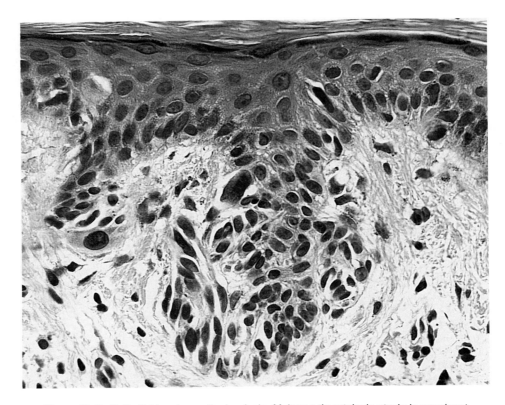

Figure 49–5. Epithelioid melanocytic dysplasia. Melanocytic cytologic atypia is prominent.

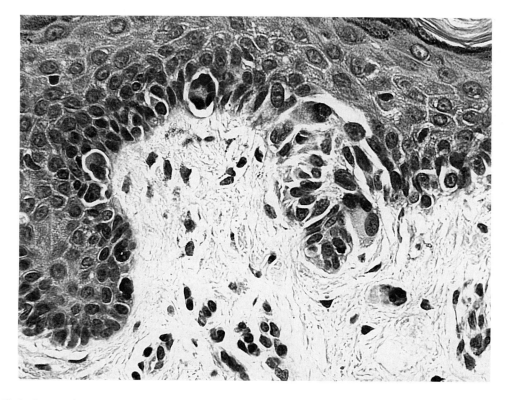

Figure 49–6. A nest of abnormal melanocytes in epithelioid melanocytic dysplasia. The nest is interretial in location; the cells are variable in form, and some are quite large. Compare with a normal nest of a compound nevus shown in Figure 49–7.

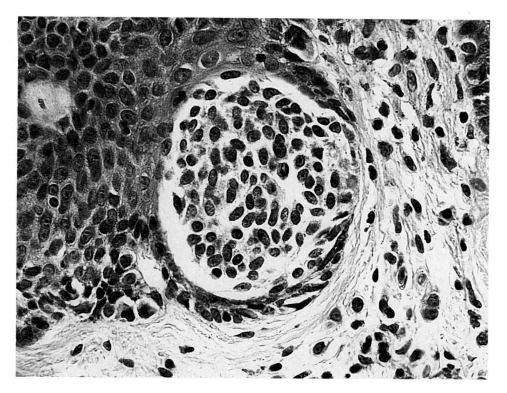

Figure 49–7. A normal nest within a compound nevus. The cells are uniform. Their cytoplasm is scanty, and there is some retraction of the entire nest.

dant anxieties generated by visits to a physician and the divulged risk for the development of melanoma. In addition, a histologic diagnosis is a hollow exercise unless its clinical significance is known. The clinical significance of melanocytic dysplasia was at first based on the work of Greene and Kraemer.[36,37] They determined this significance by studies of melanoma risk conferred by familial and sporadic melanocytic dysplasia after the lesions had been classified as dysplastic by the histologic criteria just described. Therefore, if one wishes to know that the diagnosis of melanocytic dysplasia indicates a melanoma risk 10 or 200 or 400 times greater than the unaffected (depending on the familial setting), the histologic criteria, as set forth, must be used.

Such a rigid stance may not be justified. There is no question that the lesion referred to as a melanocytic nevus with lentiginous melanocytic proliferation (aberrant differentiation) is an abnormal melanocytic nevus. Doubtless it is of *some* significance in the histogenesis of melanoma. This significance has not yet been established, and the classification of such lesions as dysplastic nevi only adds confusion. The use of melanocytic nuclear atypia as a criterion should prevent overdiagnosis, which we believe should be assiduously avoided. We therefore recommend that the histologic characteristics herein set forth be applied in the routine histologic evaluation of dysplastic nevi. It should also be borne in mind that studies of all aspects of dysplastic nevi are remarkably young for any inquiry into a particular of the biology of a chronic disease evolving over some two thirds of the human life span, as does melanoma (and most forms of cancer). Until patients with dysplastic nevi are followed prospectively for 30 years or more, the quiddity of these lesions will remain partially unknown. Shifts in emphasis and interpretation of dysplastic nevi in the future are to be expected and are welcome, for proper science is self-corrective based on evolution in observation and interpretation.

Analogies Between Melanocytic and Keratinocytic Neoplasia. We are further informed about the importance and significance of nuclear atypia in neoplastic development by an analogy with keratinocytic neoplasia. The practicing cutaneous pathologist every day sees many examples of keratinocytic proliferation and hyperkeratosis that defy codification into a precise entity in the spectrum of keratinocytic neoplasia. Such bits of keratinocytic debris are usually dismissed as benign keratosis. Admixed with the lot of this are doubtless examples of abnormal ("inappropriate") keratinocytic hyperplasia analogous to the abnormal pattern of melanocytic hyperplasia (step 2 of melanocytic tumor progression—see the foregoing discussion) that is the first manifestation of what is to become a dysplastic nevus. If one were to diagnose these nonspecific keratinocytic hyperplasias as actinic keratoses, it would be all but impossible to detect a relationship between the thus defined actinic keratosis and squamous cell carcinoma. However, if the actinic keratosis is defined by keratinocytic nuclear atypia, the relationship with squamous cell carcinoma becomes apparent.

Lymphocytic Infiltrate

A lymphocytic infiltrate is a routine part of the pathology of a dysplastic nevus (Fig. 49–8). It is usually sparse to moderately dense and immediately deep to the area of abnormal melanocytic growth. One may commonly see cytologic atypia of melanocytes immediately above the small patches of lymphocytes. Rarely the infiltrate is quite dense and bandlike, but this finding is more commonly associated with melanomas.

Connective Tissue Changes

Two alterations in connective tissue are observed in many dysplastic nevi. Such changes are not unique to dysplastic

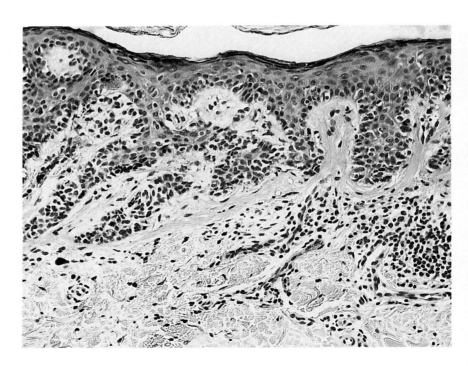

Figure 49–8. Concentric eosinophilic fibroplasia. The right portion of the photomicrograph shows a band of compact, relatively acellular fibrous tissue outlining the rete, flowing from one to the next. A patchy lymphocytic infiltrate is present below the fibroplasia.

nevi but are so frequently associated with them that they are valuable microscopic markers indicating the likely presence of melanocytic dysplasia. The first change, concentric eosinophilic fibroplasia, presents as a bright eosinophilic band some 3 to 5 μm in thickness, parallel with the outline of a rete ridge (see Fig. 49–8). The pink band may surround several adjacent retes and is readily seen. The second change, lamellar fibroplasia, is less common, more subtle, and more interesting. It is found subjacent to and blending with the base of a melanocytic nest (Fig. 49–9). Such a nest may be at the tip of a rete. Lamellar fibroplasia consists of remarkably attenuated melanocytes, appearing as elongated threadlike structures frequently containing small beads of melanin. The thin, long cells are stacked on each other and separated by similarly thin layers or small plates of collagen. The lamillated structure narrows at its base, forming a small cup attached to the base of a rete and well delimited from the surrounding dermal mesenchyme. The alternate stacks of melanocytes and thin collagen layers suggest that the attenuated melanin-containing cells are derived from the melanocytes in the overlying nest and at the same time such cells are synthesizing collagen. Such an interpretation is reasonable in light of the known formation of a variety of mesenchymal tissues by neural crest-derived cells. As a matter of fact, one third of the cephalad mesenchyme of the body, including the tracheal cartilages, is of neural crest origin. Further, in desmoplastic melanoma, it has been shown that the same cell may simultaneously synthesize collagen and melanin.[47]

Associated Normal Nevic Tissue

Melanocytic dysplasia apparently may occur de novo, but in most instances it is associated with some form of a melanocytic nevus, junctional, compound, or dermal. Thus at one margin of a compound nevus one may see the features of melanocytic dysplasia (Fig. 49–1). Such interfaces are favorable areas for comparing the appearance of melanocytes in normal nevi with those of dysplasia.

Histologic Features

Controversy surrounds the histologic diagnosis of dysplastic nevi. The histologic diagnosis is not difficult if the following principles are kept in mind. The changes are usually focal and associated with some form of ordinary nevus. The focal changes are commonly somewhere at the margin of the nevus. All of the histologic characteristics except classic lamellar fibroplasia, which is highly distinctive but uncommon, are present in aggregate. Abnormal melanocytic architecture, large melanocytes, scattered uncommon atypical melanocytes, concentric eosinophilic fibroplasia, and a patchy lymphocytic infiltrate are the congeries that form the diagnostic picture (see Fig. 49–1).

Differential Diagnosis

Acquired Lentiginous Melanocytic Nevi of the Back Commonly Appearing in Adulthood. Adults acquire small lentigines or lentiginous melanocytic nevi. These are common on the trunk, especially the back, and are usually no more

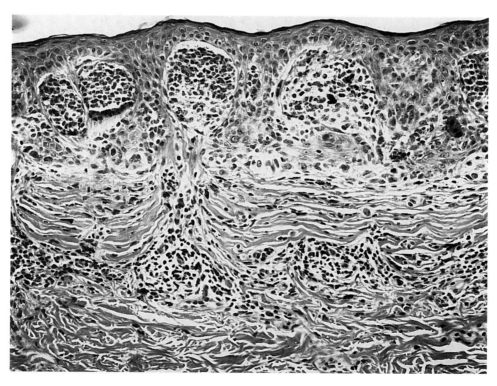

Figure 49–9. Lamellar fibroplasia. A broad area of thin layers of fibrous tissue, stacked one on the other, is below the epidermis. These layers tend to blend with the melanocytes extending from the epidermis into the outer portion of the dermis.

than 2 to 3 mm wide. This very size is of importance. All of the histologic features of a true dysplastic nevus are usually present in significantly larger lesions (4 to 7 mm). Casual microscopic examination tempts one to call these lesions dysplastic. There is concentric eosinophilic fibroplasia, elongation of rete, a prominent increase in the number of basilar melanocytes, and even occasional melanocytic bridging from one rete to the next. Rare, small patches of lymphocytes are occasionally seen. Atypical melanocytes are not seen, or such atypia is minimal and borderline. The entire substance of the lentiginous melanocytic nevus has the histologic characteristics just described, whereas true dysplasia is most often a focal or ectopic change within an ordinary nevus. This is the most important feature distinguishing the lentiginous melanocytic nevus from a nevus with dysplasia. De novo melanocytic dysplasia is not common but would, by definition, show dysplastic changes throughout its substance. However, these may be distinguished rather easily from the lentiginous melanocytic nevus. The de novo dysplastic nevi are not characterized by regular elongation of rete, but the random scattering of nests of melanocytes along the dermoepidermal interface, associated with singly disposed large melanocytes. Melanocytic nuclear atypia is usually prominent, as is the lymphocytic infiltrate. If there is any question that a given lesion may not be a dysplastic nevus of the type seen in the dysplastic nevus syndrome, the diagnosis should not be rendered on the basis of the questionable histology. One should then resort to careful clinicopathologic correlation, the underlying principle of all pathology, and biopsies of other pigmented lesions for histologic diagnosis with reasonable certitude.

Malignant Melanoma. This discussion concerns the histologic features useful in distinguishing the early stages of the radial growth phase of malignant melanoma of the superficial spreading type from melanocytic displasia (Table 49–2). Lentigo maligna may be confused with a dysplastic nevus, as discussed later in this chapter. As a rule, dysplastic nevi do not give rise to lentigo maligna melanoma or to acral lentiginous melanoma. However, distinguishing dysplastic nevi from the radial growth phase of these forms of melanoma is a problem occasionally encountered in practice.

Initial development of the radial growth phase of superficial spreading melanoma is characterized by the contiguous growth of melanocytes that are uniformly atypical. Nuclei are large, and nucleoli are usually prominent or at least readily seen. Dysplastic nevi, in contrast, do not show the contiguous growth of atypical melanocytes. Their atypical melanocytes appear as individual cells standing alone or admixed with smaller neoplastic basilar melanocytes; they are randomly scattered throughout the lesion and are rarely numerous. Macronucleoli in these atypical cells are uncommon or inconspicuous.

Atypical melanocytes of superficial spreading melanoma are commonly disposed throughout all layers of the epidermis including the granular layer. This array may present the cells in nests or as individual cells. Such diffuse growth throughout the epidermis is quite characteristic of melanoma (Fig. 49–10). Some upward growth may be seen in a dysplastic nevus, but if this is more than sparse and focal, the lesion is probably melanoma.

When dermal invasion occurs in superficial spreading melanoma it may be along a relatively broad front. One then sees small clusters of melanoma cells in the papillary dermis, along with a scattering of individual melanoma cells. Atypical melanocytes of dysplastic nevi are uncommonly found in the papillary dermis. This does not mandate a diagnosis of melanoma. When atypical melanocytes are present in the dermis in dysplastic nevi, they are not associated with a broad area of overlying contiguous atypical cells as seen in superficial spreading melanoma. Further, it is likely that the dermal atypical cells of dysplastic nevi traverse the basement membrane zone in an entirely different way than the cells of melanoma. The invasion of radial growth phase melanoma may be similar to the traverse seen in nevi or may be accomplished by the dissolution of the basement membrane zone, and then a lamina densa does not surround the dermal melanoma cells.[34] In dysplastic nevi (as in ordinary nevi), extension into the dermis is not associated with basement membrane dissolution and the cells in the dermis form a lamina densa.

Where melanoma develops, the rete ridges are frequently effaced; a relatively straight line replaces the usual undulation of the dermal-epidermal interface. This does not occur with melanocytic dysplasia; the interface retains its undulation, or it may even be exaggerated.

TABLE 49–2. HISTOLOGIC DIFFERENTIAL—RADIAL GROWTH PHASE SSM AND MELANOCYTIC DYSPLASIA

Radial Growth Phase-SSM	Melanocytic Dysplasia
Contiguous growth of atypical melanocytes at dermoepidermal interface	Atypical melanocytes sparse, separate, randomly dispersed
Melanoma cells dispersed at all epidermal strata	Atypical melanocytes usually basilar, rarely higher
When invasive, usually along a relatively broad front	Only protrusion of a few cells in focal areas into dermis
Rete ridges may be effaced	Rete not effaced
Connective tissue changes of dysplastic nevi absent or rare	Concentric eosinophilic fibroplasia or lamellar fibroplasia seen
Brisk lymphocytic infiltrate	Patchy, sparse to moderate lymphocytic infiltrate

SSM, superficial spreading melanoma.

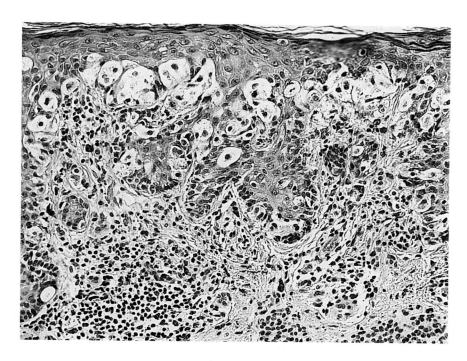

Figure 49–10. Malignant melanoma, superficial spreading type, radial growth phase. The large epithelioid melanocytes are present above the basal layer of the epidermis. Their cytoplasm is abundant and tan and dusty when viewed with the microscope. The cells are more numerous than the variably atypical melanocytes characteristic of melanocytic dysplasia. Compare with Figures 49–3, 49–4, and 49–5.

Concentric eosinophilic fibroplasia and lamellar fibroplasia are quite uncommon in melanoma but are hallmarks of the dysplastic nevus. Such changes are occasionally seen beneath characteristic melanoma in the epidermis, a finding that leads to speculation that a preexisting dysplasic nevus may have been overgrown by the melanoma.

Lymphocytic infiltrate of the radial growth phase of superficial spreading melanoma is brisk, even before invasion. In the dysplastic nevus it is patchy and sparse, but there are exceptions to this statement.

Atypical Melanocytic Nevi of the Genital (Vulvar) Type. Melanocytic dysplasia of the type seen in the dysplastic nevus syndrome may be seen on the vulva and, less commonly, on the male genitalia. This condition is not being discussed in this section on differential diagnosis. What *is* being discussed is a form of atypical melanocytic growth occurring in the intraepidermal component of a nevus; it simulates malignant melanoma somewhat more closely than melanocytic dysplasia but may be distinguished from melanoma.[48,49] The lesions are more common in females and usually develop in the reproductive years, but they occur in childhood and after the menopause. These lesions are described in some detail in the differential diagnosis of melanoma. One must be painfully careful in the histological assessment of these lesions. Overdiagnosis may lead to destructive surgery, vastly diminishing the quality of a life for its duration. Clinical information about these lesions is critical. The lesions resemble benign nevi, albeit dark. In histologic consultation, we have seen lesions that have been called melanoma, usually to the great surprise of the clinician. Melanomas of the vulva are similar to those anywhere—their greater size, border irregularity, and pigment variation, with black color usually prominent.

Malignant melanoma of the vulva is a disease of older women, occurring at a median age of 65 years. Its occurrence in a young woman is truly rare. A rare superficial spreading melanoma may occur in a relatively young woman. These are on the outer aspect of the labia majora as a rule, and in clinical and histologic appearance they are identical to similar lesions occurring on the nonglabrous skin of other parts of the body. We would like to emphasize the rarity of such melanomas in young women. They have been seen in consultation, but not in our melanoma data base. Our data base of 1651 cases contains 6 vulvar melanoma cases (0.36%); their age range is 49.4 years to 72.6 years (median = 65.3 years). In addition, the vulvar melanomas are usually of the mucosal lentiginous type. The radial growth phase is typically quite lentiginous in pattern; it is large and should not be confused with the atypical melanocytic hyperplasia being discussed. Nodular melanomas may occur on the vulva but do not present difficulty in histologic differentiation from the atypical nevi: Nodular melanomas are almost the obverse in histology, as the dermal component is entirely melanoma and abnormal epidermal melanocytes may be inconspicuous. Careful attention to histology and consideration of clinical information should prevent catastrophic misdiagnoses of these atypical melanocytic nevi of the genital type.

Intraepidermal Component of Congenital Melanocytic Nevi (Not in the Neonatal Period). Giant hairy nevi may show some quite remarkable and alarming melanocytic proliferations and may also develop melanomas. These do not resemble dysplastic nevi and will be discussed in the appropriate section of this chapter. Small and medium-sized congenital melanocytic nevi usually show intraepidermal melanocytic proliferation. The pattern is usually abnormal. Rete are elongated and narrow, routinely presenting an increase in large melanocytes. At a glance, the picture is a bit disturbing, but there is no upward growth and no true atypia. A lymphocytic infiltrate is uncommon. In a patient affected by the dysplastic nevus syndrome, there will occasionally be dysplasia somewhere along the rim of the nevus. This does not differ in any way from dysplasia adjacent to a noncongenital melanocytic nevus. Sometimes this phenomenon is isolated—there are no acquired dysplastic nevi elsewhere. The significance of this finding in terms of melanoma risk is unknown.

Relationship of Melanocytic Nevi and Dysplastic Nevi to Melanoma

Melanocytic Nevi

Historically, junctional nevi were regarded as premalignant for melanoma. Recent evidence does not support the separation of junctional nevi from other melanocytic nevi for the purposes of assignment of risk factors for malignant melanoma. The total number of melanocytic nevi is, however, a major risk factor for melanoma. The relative risk for individuals with 11 to 25 nevi is 1.6, but for those having more than 100 the relative risk is 9.8. Melanoma patients have, on average, 97 normal nevi and appropriately matched controls only 36. These figures are from the recent and careful study by Holly and colleagues.[26] Their assessment of risk was based on total body count of nevi. In common practice, it seems likely that risk assessment will be based on the counting of nevi on the arms and trunk (possibly only the back will be necessary), sites readily available for evaluation. In studying the relationship of dysplastic nevi to sporadic melanoma, to be presently discussed, Guerry and associates noted that patients with dysplastic nevi had more melanocytic nevi than patients without dysplastic nevi.[50] One of the most interesting studies relating melanocytic nevi to malignant melanoma is that by Cooke and colleagues.[51] They compared counts of nevi in a defined adult population at three different times: the early 1950s, the early 1970s, and the mid-1980s. This study has shown that the number of melanocytic nevi are increasing over time as the incidence of melanoma has increased. These results are compelling evidence linking the number of melanocytic nevi to melanoma.

Sporadic Dysplastic Nevi

The evidence relating dysplastic nevi, both as a risk factor and histogenetically, to *familial* malignant melanoma is convincing and essentially consistent in a number of reports. Familial cancer of any given cell system does not differ in any substantive way from nonfamilial or sporadic cancer. The sequential events are the same in both forms of the disease. The only important difference is that the events in the familial disease, including the appearance of the final cancers, occur at a younger age: Heritability telescopes the timing of the neoplastic process. It is, therefore, to be expected that dysplastic nevi are significantly related to *sporadic* melanoma. The adjusted relative risk of malignant melanoma in patients bearing one to five dysplastic nevi is 3.8, and for those with more than six dysplastic nevi the relative risk is 6.3.[26] Holly and colleagues have also shown that the higher the number of nondysplastic nevi

in melanoma patients, the larger the number of dysplastic nevi. Similarly, Guerry and associates found that patients with sporadic melanoma and dysplastic nevi had a higher count of nondysplastic melanocytic nevi than those with melanoma alone (34 versus 15). Of these 105 patients with sporadic melanoma, 49% had dysplastic nevi: 23% of the patients had such nevi away from the primary site; 19% had both noncontiguous and contiguous lesions; and the remaining 7% had only a single, contiguous dysplastic nevus.[50] The studies by Holly and colleagues, Guerry and associates, and Kraemer and co-workers[52] have led to the conclusion that the presence of dysplastic nevi on a patient without a family history of melanoma increases the risk of development of melanoma when compared with patients who lack these lesions or who have very few of them. This risk is not great however, being between 4 and 10 times depending on the number of dysplastic nevi and on how they are assessed. Histology confirms the clinical diagnosis of dysplastic nevi outside the context of hereditary melanoma in some 83% of patients and 70% of lesions.[50]

Familial Dysplastic Nevi with Hereditary Melanoma

Dysplastic nevi were first described in association with hereditary melanoma kindreds—families in which two or more melanomas have occurred. The early studies found dysplastic nevi to be present in virtually all of the cases of melanoma, and in about 50% of their adult blood relatives. This finding suggested that melanoma risk was associated with the dysplastic nevus phenotype and that transmission of dysplastic nevi was hereditary. Later, formal studies confirmed these hypotheses. A segregation analysis confirmed that the trait (for both melanoma and dysplastic nevi) was inherited as an autosomal dominant.[40,53] An 8-year longitudinal follow-up study of 401 members of 14 of these hereditary melanoma families revealed a lifetime melanoma risk approaching 100%.[54] In this study, 127 primary melanomas were documented in 69 family members, including 39 new primary melanomas diagnosed in 22 members during follow-up. The melanomas arose in a putative precursor dysplastic nevus in 70% of cases (92% of cases where melanomas were found in prospective follow-up), and dysplastic nevi were identified in about 50% of the blood members of each of the 14 kindreds. Thus, hereditary melanoma was highly associated with the dysplastic nevus phenotype. The 39 newly diagnosed primary melanomas occurred only in family members with dysplastic nevi, so that dysplastic nevi were a perfect marker of risk for prospective melanomas. The prospective age-adjusted incidence of melanoma was 1430 per 100,000 person-years of follow-up, with a cumulative melanoma risk of 7.2% at 8 follow-up years. The mean thickness of the newly diagnosed cases was only 0.76 mm, compared with 1.86 mm for the index cases (the first two melanomas that occurred in each family). This important finding suggests that the type of education and follow-up care that was offered to these families can result in the diagnosis of melanomas in their early, curable stages.

These findings are confirmed by additional observations (unpublished) from the Pigmented Lesion Study Group at the University of Pennsylvania. During the past 10 years or so, we have seen more than 500 members of over 200 hereditary melanoma kindreds. Among these people, 188 have dysplastic nevi and 127 have normal skin. A review of these cases is now in progress. To date, 123 charts have been reviewed of patients seen at the clinic and known to have dysplastic nevi. These patients have been followed a total of 558.65 patient-years and have developed nine newly diagnosed melanomas, for a melanoma incidence of 1611.01 per 100,000 person-years of follow-up. Among our patients who had dysplastic nevi and a prior melanoma, the incidence was 2101.13 per 100,000, and in patients with no prior melanoma, one newly diagnosed melanoma has occurred, for an incidence of 562.09 per 100,000. Thus, prior melanoma appears to be a risk factor for additional melanomas in patients with dysplastic nevi, though this difference tends to disappear in our data when corrected for age. No new melanomas have occurred in the 85 members of these families who have no dysplastic nevi on their skin. The total follow-up time for these family members is 121.77 years. Thus, again, dysplastic nevi are a marker for heightened melanoma risk in this large series of hereditary melanoma kindreds.

Studies with Monoclonal Antibodies

During the past decade, a large number of monoclonal antibodies have been raised against human tumors. Most of these antibodies have been produced in murine hybridoma systems, although a few hybridomas of human origin have been described. With few exceptions, the antibodies have been screened in systems using living cells as targets. Many of the antibodies produced in this way have also exhibited reactivity in frozen sections of unfixed human tumors. Such preparations afford the ability to distinguish reactivity of cells from different compartments of the lesions, to avoid selection biases that may occur in culture systems, and to study cell types that are impossible to maintain in culture. A major goal of tumor immunology has been the identification of tumor-specific antigens—antigens that might be expressed only on malignant tumors or on particular stages of tumor progression. Such antigens, if they exist, would be useful in tumor diagnosis, and identification of the biochemical nature of these antigens might elucidate mechanisms of attributes of the neoplastic phenotype. However, few if any antigens that correlate specifically with "malignancy" have been identified, as judged either by histologic diagnosis or by biologic behavior (inexorable growth, invasion or metastasis). Nevertheless, several groups have produced antibodies that do show relative specificity for melanoma compared with nevi.[46,55,56] Most of these antibodies have also reacted with a few nonmalignant lesions, especially dysplastic nevi. We have obtained similar data from a study of more than 40 monoclonal antibodies produced by Herlyn and colleagues at the Wistar Institute.[57] From these antibodies, 16 were selected on the basis of their reactivity with various categories of melanocytic lesions. Eight of these antibodies reacted with common and dysplastic nevi, with radial and vertical growth phase melanomas, and with metastases. The other eight show partial specificity for the later stages of tumor progression, reacting more frequently with melanomas than dysplastic nevi, and reacting with virtually 100% of cases of vertical growth

phase and metastasis. These data offer the encouraging possibility that antibodies may be developed for use in making the important diagnostic distinction between melanomas with competence for metastasis and biologically benign lesions, and the data certainly support the hypothesis of melanocytic tumor progression outlined earlier in this chapter.

In Vitro Studies of Cells Derived from Dysplastic Nevi in Comparison with Normal Melanocytes and the Cells from Melanocytic Nevi Without Dysplasia

As a rule, the cells derived from the sequential lesions of melanocytic neoplastic development are different in appearance from each other and have different growth requirements in tissue culture (Table 49–3).[58] Progression from a nevus without melanocytic dysplasia through dysplastic nevi, to the various steps of distal tumor progression in established melanomas is generally reflected by less dependency on additions to a basic culture medium. At this time, however, one cannot make any generalizations about cells derived from dysplastic nevi. Although one does see *in vitro* growth from dysplastic nevi, it is not known whether the growing cells are from the areas of true histologic dysplasia. In our experience, the cells that grow may be similar to the diploid cells of ordinary nevi, may show chromosomal abnormalities, or may have clonal karyotypic abnormalities.

Fine Structural Studies

As lesions evolve toward cancer, proximal to distal, along the evolutionary biologic pathway that is tumor progression, attributes of dysplastic nevi (clinical, histologic, epidemiologic, antigenic, and in vitro) characterize the lesions as intermediate between a banal nevus and the radial growth phase of melanoma of the superficial spreading type. Fine structural studies precisely confirm this intermediate nosologic niche of dysplastic nevi. This has been clearly shown by Takahashi and colleagues[59] and by the meticulous study of Rhodes and associates.[60] In the latter study, the authors described three abnormal melanosomal forms: *abortive* (disorganized melanofilaments in nonparallel array), *granular* (finely dispersed electron-dense granules without melanofilaments), and *peripheral deposition of melanin* (melanin along delimiting membrane, sparing the central portion of the melanosome). They compared the solitary basal unit melanocytes (individually dispersed) from normal skin, acquired nevomelanocytic nevi, dysplastic melanocytic nevi, and superficial spreading melanoma in relationship to the number of abnormal melanosomes and various other quantitative cellular parameters. Rhodes'[60] study showed a significant difference between the melanocytes in each of the four categories studied. On average, the number of abnormal melanosomes per cell was as follows: **normal skin**—0.7, **nevomelanocytic nevus**—3.5, **dysplastic melanocytic nevus**—40.9, and **superficial spreading melanoma**—70.2. Other quantitative parameters also distinguished between the study groups.

TABLE 49–3. TISSUE CULTURE GROWTH CHARACTERISTICS OF MELANOCYTES FROM NORMAL SKIN, MELANOCYTIC NEVI, AND DYSPLASTIC NEVI

Characteristic	Normal	Melanocytic Nevus[*]	Dysplastic Nevus
Success rate for growth in culture	90%	80%	?[†]
Life span—growth rate			
Newborn	Survival to 50 doubling times (2–4 days)		
Adult	Survival to 10 doubling times (7–14 days)	Survival to 20–50 doubling times (20 hours–7 days)	Prolonged but not indefinite life span
Growth requirements	2% fetal calf serum with insulin, Ca^{++}, TPA[‡], pituitary extract needed	2% fetal calf serum with insulin, Ca^{++}, TPA[‡], pituitary extract *not* needed	2% fetal calf serum with insulin, Ca^{++}, pituitary extract *not* needed
Antigen expression	p145[§], p98[§], p120[§] p97[‖], proteoglycan[‖] acetyl GD_3[‖], GD_3[‖]	p145[§], p98[§], p120[§] p97[‖], proteoglycan[‖] acetyl GD_3[‖], GD_3[‖] HLA-DR	p145[§], p98[§], p120[§] p97[‖], proteoglycan[‖] acetyl GD_3[‖], GD_3[‖] HLA-DR

[*] Acquired and congential nevi without dysplasia.
[†] Success rate similar to melanocytic nevi without dysplasia. It is not known whether there is outgrowth from the area of histological dysplasia.
[‡] Phorbal ester.
[§] Nevic antigens.
[‖] Melanoma antigens.

MELANOMA

TUMOR PROGRESSION WITHIN ESTABLISHED PRIMARY MELANOMAS

Concept of the Radial Growth Phase (Nontumorigenic Melanoma)

The radial growth phase (lesional step 4 of the tumor progression pathway) of a primary melanoma may be defined as a distinctive stage in the evolution of primary melanomas, which is not associated with metastatic disease. It includes both in situ melanoma and a form of invasive, nontumorigenic melanoma apparently lacking competence for metastasis.[4–6,57,61] The earliest attempts to determine outcome of melanoma patients as judged by histologic characteristics emphasized that superficial tumors had a better prognosis. Attempts to quantitate superficiality culminated in the mensural technique of Breslow: The maximum thickness of a tumor is measured with an ocular micrometer.[62] Such emphasis on increasing thickness as an adverse prognostic attribute generated a simplistic hypothesis concerning the nature of cancer. This inadvertently derived hypothesis posits that a primary malignant tumor has a set of properties, such as the ability to invade and metastasize, that are ever more likely to be expressed with enlargement of the neoplasm. The application of such thinking to a primary cancer tends to cause one to overlook qualitative changes that occur in most primary melanomas (and most primary cancers) after they have been growing for about 1 to 5 years.

The initial developmental stages of most primary melanomas are characterized by a period of growth of abnormal melanocytes in the epidermis and, after a variable length of time, invasion into the papillary dermis. The primary melanoma at this stage of development enlarges slowly along the radii of an imperfect circle and, consequently,

has been called the radial growth phase. It is to be emphasized that this is a clinical term describing the net direction of growth of the lesion. The clinical term has histologic corollaries that vary from one biologic type of melanoma to the next. These corollaries will be described under the specific biologic forms of primary melanoma as they define, in part, these forms. The term *radial growth* does not define a growth direction of specific melanoma cells; during radial growth, cells grow upward, downward, and toward the periphery of the tumor. The *net* clinical enlargement is radial. In addition, the transformed cells of this step in tumor progression do not form a cohesive mass or nodule; they do not form a tumor. The essence of the radial growth phase is the incapacity to form tumor nodules in the dermis. Thus the radial growth phase may also be called nontumorigenic. Further, although invasion is commonly present, metastasis does not occur—*the* important attribute of this stage in the evolutionary biology of a primary melanoma. From this it follows that one may differentiate between the properties of invasion and metastasis: Cells that can invade do not necessarily have the ability to metastasize. One can investigate stages of tumor progression distinguished from each other by the presence or absence of competence for metastasis. Obviously, and of paramount importance, the designation in a pathology report of the presence of the radial growth phase and the absence of the vertical growth phase indicates 100% survival in relationship to melanoma. Thus, the growth phase of a primary melanoma becomes its single most important prognostic attribute. The *clinical* term *radial growth* and its counterpart, the *vertical growth* of the next phase of tumor progression, may be confusing when applied to two-dimensional pathology slides. We therefore propose here a time-honored pathology term, *microinvasive*, for those tumors in the radial growth phase that are invasive. Radial growth phase or nontumorigenic melanoma thus encompasses two pathologic states, in situ and microinvasive melanoma. In the latter state there is invasion but no tumorigenic growth (see the next section). The cells have the capacity for invasion of the dermis and for survival but not proliferation in that nonepidermal tissue.

Radial growth phase melanomas are distinguished from vertical growth disease by more than clinical and histologic characteristics. The antigenic and in vitro properties are quite different. The most obvious and possibly the most important difference in vitro between radial and vertical growth phase melanoma is the great difficulty in growing radial growth phase melanoma cells in culture. In spite of numerous attempts, we have but two cell lines derived from primary melanomas entirely within the radial growth phase. However, studies of DNA content by flow cytometry of radial growth phase cells derived from paraffin-embedded material have shown these cells to be euploid.[63] The in vitro characteristics of radial growth phase cells are summarized in Table 49–4.

Reed has classified melanomas differently from the system presented in this chapter.[64,65] Our categories are conceptually histogenetic, and thus the different kinds of melanoma are recognized by the clinical and histological characteristics of the early stages of the melanoma: radial growth (nontumorigenic) phase melanoma. Although Reed recognizes the histogenetic types presented here (in fact, he and Arrington and colleagues are largely responsible for the description of acral lentiginous melanoma),[66] his perception of the varied histologies and cytologies differs from ours in three important ways.

First he believes that the classic histology of one intraepidermal pattern of growth of melanocytes (pagetoid growth of large intraepidermal, epithelioid melanocytes, disposed indiviually or in small clusters, with or without dermal invasion of similar cells) is a final common pathway of severe dysplasia occurring in all forms of melanoma that initially present in the radial growth phase. He does not believe that this histology is largely limited to melanoma of the superficial spreading type. It may occur near the periphery of superficial spreading melanoma and does not occur at the marginal limits of acral lentiginous melanoma and lentigo maligna melanoma, and this point is useful in distinguishing the various melanomas.

Second, Reed does not specify as melanoma the different kinds of radial growth phases we have described but calls them (1) a "final common pathway of severe dysplasia"; (2) lentigo maligna (including those cases with nontu-

morigenic invasion into the papillary dermis), or (3) severe dysplasia, acral variant (again, including those cases with nontumorigenic invasion of the papillary dermis). Reed does not assign the term *melanoma* to a lesion unless there is tumorigenic dermal invasion (a phenomenon we call the vertical growth phase). His designations are clearly prescient, as it is now known that the nontumorigenic stages in the evolution of the primary melanomas are not associated with metastasis. However, the use of "severe dysplasia" in this context confounds the nosology of cancer. Perhaps it is more accurate to state that the nature of cancer confounds the nosologic efforts of the pathologist. Stated another way, "When, in a system of neoplastic cellular evolution (tumor progression), is the term *cancer* to be applied?" In part, the answer to the question depends on whether cancer is to be defined in biologic terms or humanistic ones, a problem discussed at the end of this chapter. Suffice it to say, for the present, that Reed has selected a *humanistic* point in neoplasia for designating a step in tumor progression as cancer (a step with *some* level of established metastatic potential). We have attempted to use *biologic* guidelines for incriminating a phase in tumor progression as cancer (the histologic characteristics of the first *clinical* step showing persistent autonomous growth).

Third, Reed has emphasized the importance of various cytological and histologic patterns occurring in the vertical growth phase (tumorigenic melanoma). When these appearances differ significantly from the classic histology of vertical growth phase, Reed designates the lesions as some form of minimal deviation melanoma. This aspect of his work is discussed later in the chapter.

Another approach to melanoma classification is that proposed by Ackerman.[67] For invasive melanomas, he records the thickness. Melanomas are not further classified. The approach is simple and readily used. Presently available information suggests, however, that other information is useful in determining prognosis and something of the nature of the disease. Lentigo maligna melanoma and acral lentiginous melanoma are at opposite epidemiologic and demographic poles in the spectrum of melanomas. Knowledge of biologic type of melanoma and data of prognostic import should be included in pathology reports, in our opinion.

Concept of the Vertical Growth Phase (Tumorigenic Melanoma)

The final stage of evolution of primary melanomas (lesional step 5 in the tumor progression pathway; see Table 49–1) is manifested by acquisition of competence for metastasis, a competence expressed by about 30% of melanomas that have entered the vertical growth phase. Vertical growth phase is tumorigenic melanoma, a primary lesion in which a focal subpopultion of transformed cells has acquired and expressed the capacity for forming one or several cohesive nodules or plaques in the dermis.

Vertical Growth Phase

The vertical growth phase is a stage in the evolution of a primary melanoma when a population of cells is selected during intraepidermal growth for its capacity to replicate in the dermis and form a mass or tumor at that mesenchymal

TABLE 49–4. CELLS OF DYSPLASTIC NEVI AND RADIAL GROWTH PHASE PRIMARY MELANOMAS: IN VITRO CHARACTERISTICS

Morphologically "transformed" phenotype

No growth stimulation by phorbol ester

Random chromosomal abnormalities

Rarely tumorigenic in nude mice

Prolonged but not indefinite life span

Expression of nevus and melanoma-associated antigens, including GD_2 and GD_3

Stimulation of autologous T cells

Possible acquisition of tumorigenicity in vitro

Cells are euploid

site. We therefore propose the term *tumorigenic melanoma* as a descriptive modifier of the vertical growth phase.

Definition

The vertical growth phase is, by definition, the appearance of a population of cells within the primary neoplasm that has not been previously manifest in the neoplastic system. The cells of the vertical growth phase are usually different in appearance and form, and certainly different in their growth properties from the cells of the radial growth phase (Table 49–5).

Progression into the Vertical Growth Phase

Progression into the vertical growth phase is manifested by a shift in the dominant site of tumor growth from the epidermis to a focus in the dermis. In many instances, this dermal growth site simulates the growth pattern of a metastasis; the formation of such a spheroidal nodule is a portent of its metastatic potential—the capacity for *discontinuous* growth as a nodule.

Direct Tumor Progression

Some malignant melanomas called nodular melanomas show, from the outset, a dominant growth site of tumor cells in the dermis. These uncommon melanomas undoubtedly originate from intraepidermal melanocytes, but no prolonged period of intraepidermal growth ensues. The cells of nodular melanoma invade the dermis early. Thus, this becomes the primary focus of tumor growth, virtually from the outset of the manifest cancer.[5]

COMMON BIOLOGIC FORMS OF PRIMARY MELANOMAS

MELANOMA OF THE SUPERFICIAL SPREADING TYPE

Clinical Features

This form of melanoma is the most common form of the disease in Caucasians and constitutes about 70% of the disease in the United States. The lesions may occur any-

where on the skin, but most are seen on the trunk and extremities, proximal to the wrists and ankles. Lesions on the face and scalp are occasionally seen in young adults, but this kind of melanoma is quite uncommon on the hands and feet. The classic clinical lesion is, as a rule, larger than a melanocytic nevus or a dysplastic nevus, commonly being 1 to 2 cm in diameter when first recognized. The margin is irregular and may or may not be palpable. The shape is variably asymmetric. Tan, brown, and black are almost invariably present. Pink, blue, and blue-white are common, the latter two hues indicating regression. Smaller lesions, in the range of 0.5 to 0.8 cm, may be indistinguishable from dysplastic nevi. Clinical diagnosis of *small* malignant melanomas of the superficial spreading type is frequently not accurate. If serial clinical observations with baseline photography are available, such lesions are most often excised because of a documentation of growth or color change.

Histologic Features

Radial Growth Phase. Histologic recognition of the radial growth phase is the single most important determinant of prognosis in melanoma. As will be discussed under prognostic attributes, patients whose primary lesions are solely in the radial growth phase (have not entered the vertical growth phase) have a projected survival that approaches 100%. Further, variations in the histology of the radial growth phase constitute the primary basis for the classification of melanoma into its different biologic forms. As a matter of fact, the determination of whether or not a given lesion is or is not melanoma usually depends on the proper evaluation of the detailed histology of the radial growth phase. When a tumor has entered the vertical growth phase, the diagnosis of melanoma is rarely problematic. It is the radial growth phase that must be distinguished from the many atypical lesions that have some of the features of melanoma, yet are not.

The classic histology of the radial growth phase of superficial spreading melanoma is readily recognized. The cells grow at all levels of the epidermis including the granular layer (Figs. 49–10 and 49–11). Individual cells and small inspissated nests of cells may even be seen in the stratum corneum. In the nucleated epidermal layers, the cells are disposed in large nests that may occasionally bridge the entire epidermal thickness. As a rule, individual cells are more prominent than the nests, being arrayed in a fashion that simulates Paget's disease of the breast. It is uncommon to see this distinctive pattern of melanoma without invasion. The invasive component associated with the foregoing intraepidermal pathology shows individual cells and small clusters of cells dispersed in the papillary dermis. The cells are of the same form as those in the epidermis, and no nest of cells seemingly has a growth preference over other nests (Fig. 49–12). With rare exceptions, the dermal nests are smaller than any in the epidermis. Mitotic figures are rare in the dermal component of these lesions. One gets the impression that the growth of melanoma in the radial growth phase is in the epidermis. The cells have the properties necessary to traverse the basement membrane zone, but having reached the dermis do not grow there (are not tumorigenic). No dominant tumor nodules are formed. A brisk lymphocytic infiltrate is usually associated with the

---

TABLE 49–5. CELLS OF VERTICAL GROWTH PHASE PRIMARY MELANOMAS: IN VITRO CHARACTERISTICS

Morphological similarities with metastatic melanoma

Tumorigenicity in nude mouse

Cells are commonly aneuploid and show nonrandom chromosomal abnormalities involving chromosomes 1, 6, and 7

Permanent cell lines

Production of platelet-derived growth factor (PDGF)

Epidermal growth factor (EGF) and insulin required for growth

Growth to low densities with relatively long doubling times

No expression of nevus-associated antigens

No stimulation of autologous T cells

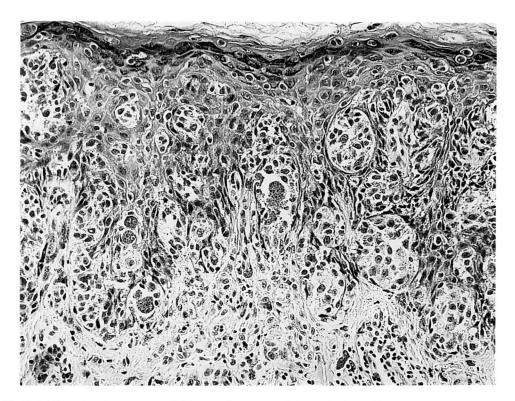

Figure 49–11. Malignant melanoma, superficial spreading type, radial growth phase. The melanocytes are present at all layers of the epidermis, including the granular layer. Microinvasion is present.

melanoma cells in the dermis. The melanoma cells forming this classic histology are large and epithelioid, without demonstrable dendrites. The cytoplasm is abundant and dusty tan. The nuclei are large. Macronucleoli are frequently seen,

in contrast to the cells of dysplastic nevi. In spite of the cells being large and clearly different from the melanocytes of nevi and from normal melanocytes, they are rather uniform in relationship to each other. Pleomorphism

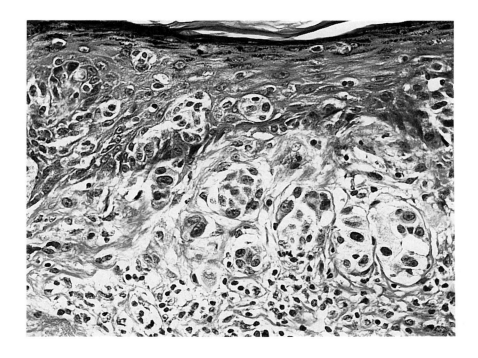

Figure 49–12. Malignant melanoma, superficial spreading type, radial growth phase. The pattern of invasion of the dermis characteristic of the radial growth phase is illustrated. Small nests are shown. No nest has a growth preference over other nests.

TABLE 49–6. CLINICAL AND HISTOLOGIC DIFFERENCES BETWEEN RADIAL AND VERTICAL GROWTH PHASE MALIGNANT MELANOMA

Radial Growth Phase—SSM	Vertical Growth Phase—SSM
Flat or slightly elevated plateaulike lesion of variegated color.	Focal, elevated nodule, uniform in color—red or black within the radial growth phase.
Dominant site of cell proliferation is within the epidermis.	Dominant site of cell proliferation is in the dermis.
Cells usually grow at all epidermal strata and extend into papillary dermis.	Cells grow initially in a single nodule or plaque in the dermis.
Cells in dermis arrayed individually or as small nests, 5–10 cells wide.	Dermal growth is larger than epidermal nests and has growth preference over small cell nests of radial growth.
Epithelioid melanocytes with a tan, dusty cytoplasm.	Cells usually different from those of radial growth phase. Amelanotic or more melanotic. Cell form different.
Brisk lymphocytic response usually present.	Lymphocytic response may be absent or sparse. Occasionally brisk.

SSM, superficial spreading melanoma.

is not a usual part of this histology (Tables 49–2 and 49–6).

One important variant histology of this particular radial growth phase lacks the distinctive pattern of pagetoid intraepidermal growth. One may see a few foci of upward growth, but the melanoma cells are usually seen as a layer of contiguous cells at the dermoepidermal interface. The cells may form a row only one cell thick. More commonly there is a layer of cells two to four cells thick separating the keratinocytic epidermis, above, from the dermis, below. Such areas of plaquelike growth at the dermoepidermal interface are frequently associated with effacement of the rete ridges. In such instances, the interface, when viewed at low power, tends to be a straight line populated by a layer of melanoma cells somewhat smaller than those of the classic histologic picture. The invasive cells in the papillary dermis are not the classic large epithelioid melanocytes, but are somewhat smaller. The host lymphocytic response is usually brisk and may be so when the lesion is not invasive. This variant pattern is commonly, but not exclusively, seen in lesions of the lower limbs.

Vertical Growth Phase. The well-developed vertical growth phase is obvious even on casual inspection of a histologic preparation (Fig. 49–13). It is manifested by a focus of growth of melanoma cells in the dermis. This is usually in the papillary dermis, which is filled and widened by the cells of the vertical growth phase. It is to be emphasized that the vertical growth phase is a focal phenomenon, a single focus at its inception. Except in neglected primaries, the radial growth phase is not replaced by the vertical growth phase. The dominant site of growth of the tumor is shifted from the epidermis to a single collection of cells in the dermis, and these now show a growth preference over the other epidermal and dermal components of the tumor. The vertical growth phase is characterized by a spherical nodule or plaque of tumor cells larger than any other collection of tumor cells in the primary. The cells are frequently, but not always, different from those of the

radial growth phase: They may be amelanotic as opposed to melanin containing, smaller or larger, or of different form. In contrast to the radial growth phase, the host response of lymphocytes, macrophages, and other cells of the immune and inflammatory systems may be absent in the vertical growth phase. When those cells are present, depending on their density and configuration in relationship to the tumor cells, the host response may be of significant prognostic importance. The detailed histology of the host response to the tumor as related to prognosis will be described under prognostic attributes.

The Problem of the Early Vertical Growth Phase. If one accepts the premise that the cells of the vertical growth phase represent a new population of tumor cells not previously apparent in the primary cancer, it follows that there must be the limiting case in which the vertical growth phase is but a single cell, having properties different from those of the radial growth phase. Obviously, that single cell cannot be recognized by the microscopist. Even if it had expanded as a new subclone of cells into a small cluster, it might be quite similar to the surrounding radial growth phase. There is compelling evidence that the vertical growth phase represents the acquisition of competence for metastasis. Consequently, recognition of this phase, even when early and thin, becomes an imperative. Early vertical growth phase should be reported when one or more of the following features are present in the dermis: (1) a nest of cells larger than any epidermal nest; (2) a nest of cells that is clearly larger than the other dermal cell clusters of the radial growth phase; (3) a nest of cells that is different in form or pigment content from the cells of the radial growth phase; or (4) any contiguous collection of cells, spheroid, plaquelike, or of nondescript outline that tends to fill the papillary dermis, impinging on the reticular dermis (Figs. 49–14 and 49–15). A rule of thumb: If there is a suspicion that the vertical growth phase is present, report it as "probable early growth phase." We have been following this rule for some years and have not, thus far, seen metastases from early vertical

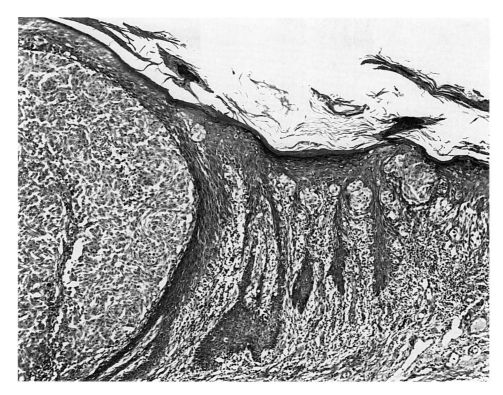

Figure 49–13. Malignant melanoma, superficial spreading type, radial growth phase and vertical growth phase. A prototypic example of radial growth phase (right) and vertical growth phase (left) is depicted.

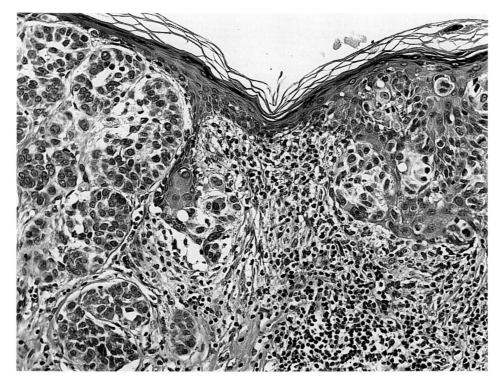

Figure 49–14. Malignant melanoma, superficial spreading type, radial growth phase and vertical growth phase, early. The left part of the illustration shows a small nest of early but definite vertical growth phase. The nidus of growth is in the dermis, no longer the epidermis, as is the case in the radial growth phase.

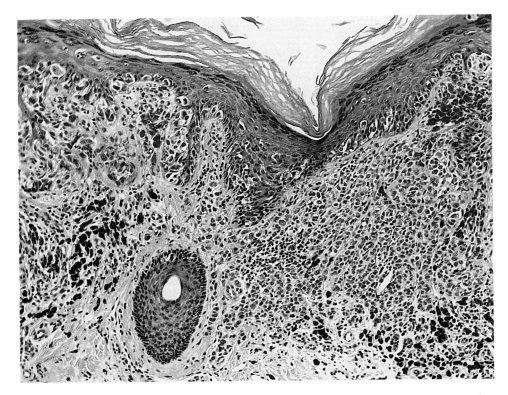

Figure 49–15. Malignant melanoma, superficial spreading type, radial growth phase and vertical growth phase, early. On the right, a plaque of cells is present in the dermis. Again the focus of growth has shifted into the dermis, the hallmark of the vertical growth phase.

growth phase. Nevertheless, when there is doubt, one should still err on the side of reporting the presence of an early vertical growth phase.

MELANOMA OF THE LENTIGO MALIGNA TYPE

Clinical Features

Lentigo maligna melanoma develops in an indolent manner over the course of many years on the face, neck, backs of the hands, and rarely at other cutaneous sites. As a rule, the vertical growth phase develops after 5 to 10 or more years of growth of the radial growth phase. This growth phase, as a consequence, may be several centimeters in width when the patient initially presents for examination. Such lesions are characteristically flat, irregular in outline, and colored by rich shades of tan, brown, and black. As in superficial spreading melanoma, regression may be present and, at times, extensive. The regressed areas are blue-white or white and may actually cause the primary tumor to appear broken apart as if formed by disparate areas of pigmentation separated by the whiteness of regression.

Histologic Features

Radial Growth Phase. The abnormal cells tend to lie in or near the basilar region of the epidermis, which may be of normal thickness, or atrophic, reflecting the cutaneous phenotype, solar damage, and the age of patients who develop this form of melanoma. The tumor cells are disposed in small nests, which extend down from the epidermis into the papillary dermis without overt invasion (Fig. 49–16). The cells composing the nests tend to be small, slightly pleomorphic, and exhibit diminished cohesiveness (Fig. 49–17). In between the nests individual cells are disposed, largely in the basal layer. Such cells may be numerous and almost contiguous but are often moderate in number and clearly separate from each other. There may be some upward growth of cells, but their dominant disposition is in the basilar epidermal area. This pattern is in contrast to many examples of superficial spreading melanoma, which tend to grow at all epidermal levels. A frequent histologic feature is a tendency to involve the external root sheath of hair follicles. This involvement may be extensive, and invasion of the surrounding dermis is at times a result of this pilar involvement. If there is no invasion, the foregoing histologic picture is called lentigo maligna, not lentigo maligna melanoma. By convention, invasion is required before such lesions are designated melanoma. Conceptually, however, some such lesions may be regarded as examples of in situ melnoma. We are most concerned with this diagnosis when the lesional cells, though exclusively above the basement membrane zone, show moderate or severe atypia that is uniform (involves 50% or more of the lesional melanocytic cell population). When invasion is present, it differs from that of superficial spreading melanoma. It does

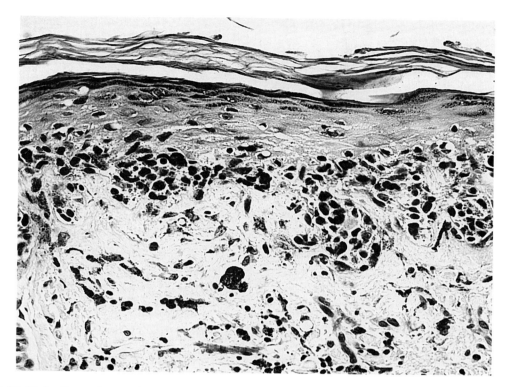

Figure 49–16. Lentigo maligna melanoma, radial growth phase, microinvasive. The atypical melanocytes are present at the dermoepidermal interface, with bare protrusion into the papillary dermis. The nests extend down into the papillary dermis. The cells tend to be small, pleomorphic, and show diminished cohesiveness. Invasion is usually inconspicuous in the radial growth phase of lentigo maligna melanoma.

not occur along a broad front but is seen in inconspicuous small areas frequently widely separate from each other. Here a few cells traverse the basement membrane zone to lie in the immediately subjacent dermis. The response of lymphocytes and macrophages is rather sparse and patchy, being related to the small invasive zones in most instances. It is not copious as in superficial spreading melanoma. The dermis almost always shows moderate to advanced solar

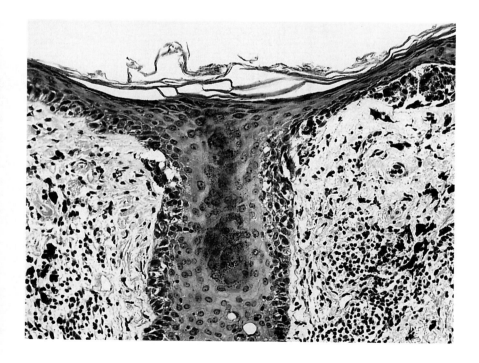

Figure 49–17. Lentigo maligna. There is no invasion here, and the proper designation of the lesion is lentigo maligna. Invasion was present immediately adjacent to this area. The micrograph illustrates a typical nest (upper right) and pilar involvement (center), a common feature of lentigo maligna and lentigo maligna melanoma.

degeneration. The histology of regression, to be described as a separate phenomenon, is commonly present.

Vertical Growth Phase. The histologic features required for the recognition of the vertical growth phase are similar to those delineated for superficial spreading melanoma. There is, however, greater variability in the kinds of cells that may make up the vertical growth phase of lentigo maligna melanoma. The cells may be large, epithelioid, and pigmented, but not infrequently are small or may be purely spindled in form. Desmoplastic and neurotropic melanoma may constitute the entire vertical growth phase. The histology of this kind of vertical growth phase will be described in detail under rare and unusual forms of melanoma.

MELANOMA OF THE ACRAL LENTIGINOUS TYPE AND THE MUCOSAL LENTIGINOUS TYPE

Clinical Features
Melanoma of the acral lentiginous type is a disease of the palms, soles, and subungual regions. Mucosal lentiginous melanoma is similar to, if not identical with, acral lentigi-nous melanoma but usually is named differently because of its anatomic site. The clinical and histologic descriptions given here apply to both the mucosal and acral lesions. The radial growth phase is richly colored with deep shades of tan, brown, and black; black may be the dominant color. Large areas may be covered. Lesions 3 to 4 cm in width are not uncommon, and they are flat. The margins are not palpable. Irregular involvement of the skin of the posterior nail fold with tan-brown pigmentation (Hutchinson's sign) is essentially diagnostic of subungual melanoma. The radial growth phase may be partially or completely amelanotic. Consequently, one may see histologic involvement of excision margins when the plane of excision was well beyond recognizable clinical lesion. The blue and blue-white hallmarks of regression are not uncommon clinical features. The vertical growth phase is often a pink or black spheroid nodule.

Histologic Features
Radial Growth Phase. The cells tend to be in the basilar epidermal region and are associated with a highly characteristic and commonly brisk lymphocytic response (Fig. 49–18). Such a response is usually lichenoid, and it may be so dense as to obscure the dermoepidermal interface. Individual cells are more common than nests. When nests do occur, their cells tend to be spindle shaped. The individual

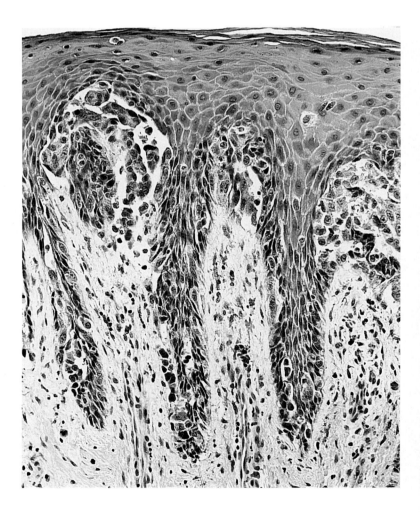

Figure 49–18. Acral lentiginous melanoma, radial growth phase. The rete are characteristically elongated and pointed. The melanoma cells tend to be at the dermoepidermal interface, as in lentigo maligna melanoma, but they are larger. Nests of melanoma cells are between rete, and individually disposed melanoma cells tend to grow along rete. Upward invasion is not as prominent as in superficial spreading melanoma, but it may be seen especially near areas of invasion where the vertical growth phase is formed.

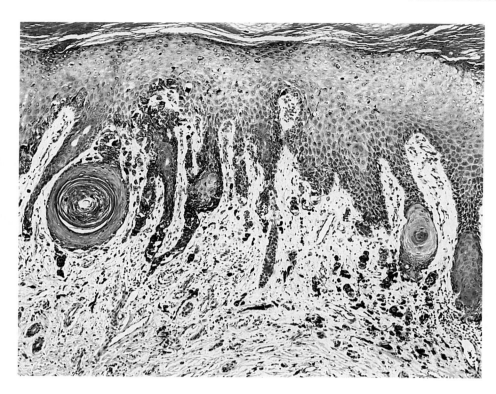

Figure 49–19. Acral lentiginous melanoma, radial growth phase. Much of the tumor is intraepidermal, but there are small clusters of tumor cells in the dermis. No nest has a growth preference over others; the vertical growth phase has not been established.

cells may show well-preserved dendrites (Figs. 49–19 and 49–20). These may be more prominent than in any kind of melanocytic pathology. Such dendrites may traverse the width of three to five keratinocytes. Epithelioid melanocytes are also seen and, especially near areas of invasion, may grow upward and be similar in appearance to superficial spreading melanoma. Both superficial spreading melanoma and nodular melanoma occasionally occur in acral sites. The site, therefore, is not the only determinant of the biologic form of the melanoma. The histology of regression, when present, is not different from that in other forms of melanoma.

Vertical Growth Phase. The cells of the acral vertical growth phase may form the classic spheroid nodule. However, other cell types and patterns are relatively common. An ill-defined collection of spindled melanocytes infiltrating the dermis is one such pattern. The acral and mucosal melanomas (especially those of the lower lip) are biologic forms of the disease, in addition to lentigo maligna melanoma, in which the vertical growth phase may be desmoplastic and neurotropic. Neurotropism may be such a dominant histologic feature that the entire primary tumor may be properly designated neurotropic melanoma.

MALIGNANT MELANOMA OF THE NODULAR TYPE

Clinical Features

Nodular melanomas do not resemble the other forms of the disease, but present as smooth spheroid nodules. In color, the lesion may be a uniform dark, thundercloud gray or bright pink. The tumors generally arise more rapidly than other forms of melanoma. They may develop on any cutaneous or mucosal surface but are usually seen on the trunk.

Histologic Features

Vertical Growth Phase. By definition, all nodular melanomas are in the vertical growth phase. The tumorigenic, pure vertical growth phase nodules are similar to tumorigenic nodules in other biologic forms of melanoma (Figs. 49–21 and 49–22). The criterion for classification as a nodular melanoma is the absence of a radial growth phase peripheral to the dermal tumor. The tumors arise from epidermal melanocytes and may or may not have a demonstrable precursor nevus. The precursors, when present, are melanocytic nevi, with or without dysplasia. The tumors do not reveal convincing evidence of extensive intraepidermal growth or extension of individual cells and small clusters of cells into the papillary dermis—that is, a radial growth phase is not recognizable. The smallest lesions that have been observed show dermal invasion and simultaneously a tendency for the cells to form a distinct nodule in the dermis. This melanoma apparently has competence for metastasis concomitant with its extension across the basement membrane zone. The cells are usually large and epithelioid, but may be small. Invasion well into the reticular dermis may be noted when such melanomas are no more than 7 to 8 mm wide. When there is no precursor lesion, nodular melanomas are the prototype of direct tumor progression—that is, the appearance of a neoplasm with competence for metastasis, without evidence of prior stepwise evolution.

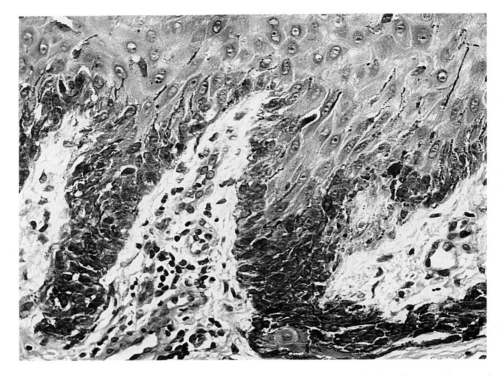

Figure 49–20. Acral lentiginous melanoma, radial growth phase. The melanocytic dendrites are long and unusually prominent, a common feature of the intraepidermal component of this form of melanoma.

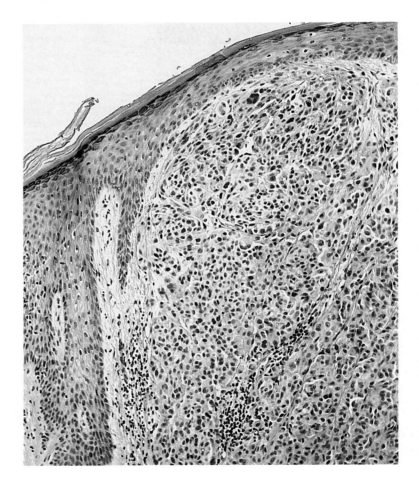

Figure 49–21. Nodular melanoma, edge of lesion. There is no radial growth phase. Its absence defines the lesion as nodular melanoma.

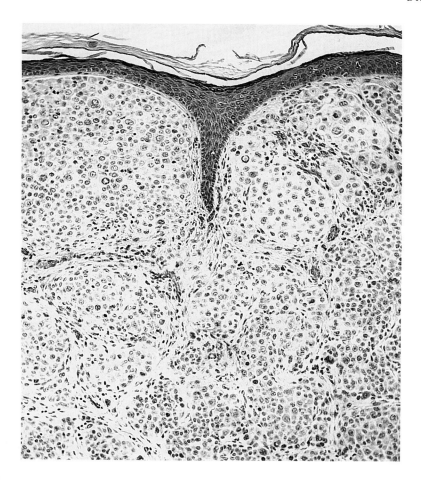

Figure 49–22. Nodular melanoma, center of lesion. An intraepidermal component is not illustrated. Multiple sections will demonstrate such a component, but it is rarely prominent.

FINE STRUCTURE OF MELANOMAS

Electron microscope studies of melanomas have had diverse goals: (1) to examine melanin synthesis, especially in relationship to melanosomes; (2) to compare fine structure of the different biologic forms of melanoma; (3) to examine changes in melanoma cells reflecting the steps of tumor progression; and (4) in diagnostic surgical pathology, to determine whether or not a given neoplasm is or is not malignant melanoma.

Most fine structural studies have used an approach emphasizing melanosomal morphology. These studies have classified normal and abnormal melanosomes variously. The abnormal forms are generally referred to as variant or aberrant (organelles with a single melanofilament having a periodic structure or concentric membranous lamellae without periodicity); finely and coarsely granular without recognizable melanofilaments; and ring or hollow forms (peripheral deposition of melanin). In general, melanogenesis is usually quite abnormal, and it obviously follows that melanoma cells are not particularly suitable for the investigation of normal melanin synthesis. There is great variation in cellular and melanosomal morphology in all forms of melanoma and in all stages of tumor progression. This variation may be overcome by adequate sampling of the lesions to be studied, the adequacy of the sample being somewhat dependent on the objectives of the study. One must select the site within the melanoma to be studied (for example, radial growth phase, vertical growth phase, and metastasis) and one must have multiple blocks. With appropriate sampling, one may distinguish between the radial growth phase of superficial spreading, lentigo maligna, and acral lentiginous melanoma; the latter form of melanoma has been the least studied by electron microscopy, but fits between lentigo maligna and superficial spreading melanoma with regard to cellular and organelle disarray. In general, the radial growth phase of lentigo maligna melanoma shows many melanosomes with an internal structure that approaches normal, and the same growth phase of superficial spreading melanoma shows a dominance of abnormal melanosomal forms, especially aberrant and granular forms. Vertical growth phase and metastatic melanoma show even greater disarray. Even studying the vertical growth phase (the invasive nodule), Hunter and associates found the fine structure of lentigo maligna melanoma to be quite characteristic.[68] The cells tended to be dendritic and presented large numbers of ellipsoid and normal-looking melanosomes. Except for this study, the cells of the vertical growth phase of the various forms of melanoma tend to be similar in their state of disorganization and resemble metastatic melanoma.

Electron microscopy is now used to identify the nature of the poorly differentiated and amelanotic neoplasm. Mazur and colleagues carefully addressed this present use of fine structure in the study of melanoma.[69] They studied 26 metastatic melanomas, 13 pigmented and 13 amelanotic, and properly emphasized the entire form of the melanoma and its cells, commenting on 12 characteristics in addition to the ubiquitous melanosomal aberrations. Briefly, they made the following observations. The tumors tended to grow in small, compact clusters of three to six cells with tightly apposed plasma membranes. Some of the clusters manifested an ensheathing arrangement of their processes, reminding one of the basic behavior of schwannian tissue. Dendritic cell processes were usually present. Microvilli or filopodia were present focally on the cell surfaces of every case studied. Nuclei were heterogeneous with mutilobate forms. Nucleoli were prominent, as were cytoplasmic nuclear invaginations. Rare cells showed the cytoplasmic organization of a fibroblast (see the section on desmoplastic melanoma). About half of the cases had mitochondria with tubular cristae. Other features reminiscent of schwannian tissue were noted, including formation of fragments of a basement membrane zone, complex cell membrane interdigitations, and prominent cytoplasmic processes. Various abnormal filaments and inclusions were observed. The melanosomes were quite abnormal, but present even in the amelanotic cases. Some of the granular forms, however, overlap with lysosomes in structure and are not, as a result, specific in configuration. In most instances, diligent search reveals a melanosome with one or more typical melanofilaments.

PHENOMENON OF REGRESSION

Clinical Features

Regression may occur in a portion of the radial growth phase of any of the melanomas. It is recognized as a blue-white or white area within the confines of the primary lesion. The skin markings are usually effaced, and the area resembles parchment. Patients may give a clear history of regression, stating that "the tumor began to break up and go away." Regression may be complete and may presumably occur in tumors that have entered the vertical growth phase. In such instances, patients may present with lymph node metastases, though the true incidence of this phenomenon is difficult to establish in totally regressed melanomas, many of which may evade clinical detection. Examination of the skin within the lymphatic drainage areas of the affected node group with a Wood's light reveals an irregular, stark white, flat area. Histologic examination after excision of such an area reveals the classic histology of regression to be presently described. Multiple sections though the regressed lesion occasionally pick up the odd tumor cell or two. We have documented complete regression of a primary (based on strongly suggestive histologic and convincing clinical evidence) without concurrent or subsequent metastases. Regression of the vertical growth phase and nodular melanomas is more difficult to establish directly and probably is quite uncommon, but from time to time one does see the histology of regression deep in the dermis, further presumptive evidence that vertical growth phase disease may also regress.

Histologic Features

Regression is easily recognized in the gross specimen, and appropriate sections should be taken through such areas for histologic examination. Microscopically, regression is an area where there is no melanoma, intraepidermal or dermal, and in many instances is flanked on either side by melanoma (Fig. 49–23). The area devoid of melanoma presents a thickened papillary dermis as a result of an increased amount of collagen disposed as delicate fibrils without organization into a bundle pattern. There is increased vascularity of this newly formed collagen. The papillary dermis, thus altered, is interspersed with a few scattered lymphocytes and moderate numbers of melanophages. The presence of regression should be recorded in pathology reports, as it is an adverse prognostic attribute.

Biologic Significance

Regression, as just described, is best conceptualized as the result of a host immune response that is at least partially successful. We have documented a few examples of putatively completely regressed melanomas that have not recurred or metastasized after complete excision of the site of the regressed tumor. More commonly, a patient presents with metastatic melanoma without an obvious primary lesion, and careful search locates a completely regressed primary site. Such cases may constitute an important caveat to the concept that radial growth phase (nontumorigenic) melanoma lacks competence for metastasis and is curable in 100% of cases. It is not knowable, faced with a completely regressed primary tumor, whether or not such a tumor was entirely within the radial growth phase. Radial growth phase (nontumorigenic) primaries with extensive regression (perhaps 75% or more of the surface area) may have some potential for metastasis, and a note should be entered into the pathology report to this effect. Ronan and associates have shown that thin melanomas with regression may metastasize.[70] At least one of their cases was clearly in the vertical growth phase, but others may have been regressed radial growth phase cases, again unknowable. When regression is only focal within the primary, one may note an area of vertical growth emerging at its margin or, occasionally, as an island within the pale regressed zone. The explanation of these curious phenomena and the prognostic adversity of regression must be speculative. It could be that the immune response to the radial growth phase is, in some instances, an immunoselective phenomenon permitting cells with a biologic potential for metastasis to grow preferentially, form a vertical growth phase, and metastasize.

PROGNOSTIC ATTRIBUTES

The maximum thickness of a melanoma has been the most valuable single prognostic attribute. The thickness method developed by the late Alexander Breslow involves measurement of tumor thickness from the outermost granular layer of the epidermis or from the base of an ulcer at the surface of a primary to the greatest depth of the tumor.[62] As useful as the method is, there is no thickness group (e.g., < 0.76 mm) that is not associated with a small percentage of metas-

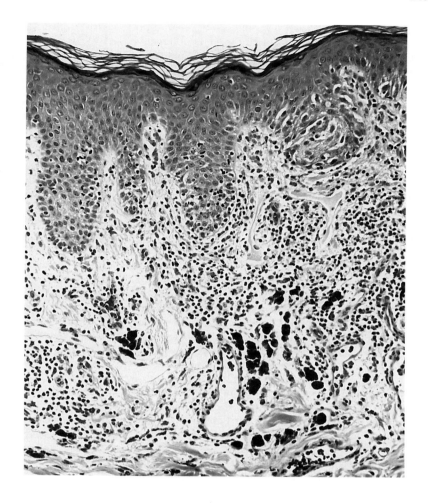

Figure 49–23. Regressive phenomenon, malignant melanoma, superficial spreading type, radial growth phase. Represented in the upper right is a bit of the radial growth phase of the melanoma. Below and to the left of this one notes a widened papillary dermis in which are lymphocytes, macrophages, and prominent blood vessels. The lymphocytes extend into the epidermis, a common feature of areas of regression.

tases and no group so thick (e.g., > 3.60 mm) that there are no long-term survivors. Although survival is related to thickness in an approximately linear way, other factors also influence survival. These factors may be integrated into a probability formula that is more valuable than thickness alone in predicting survival.[5,11] The following is a discussion of these factors.

Radial Growth Phase

The histologic features of the radial growth phase have been described and illustrated (see Figs. 49–10, 49–11, and 49–12). In most instances, the radial growth phase is easily identified. If there is any evidence, even equivocal, of the presence of the vertical growth phase, the pathology report should indicate that the early vertical growth phase is present.

When a melanoma has been designated as "radial growth phase present, vertical growth phase absent" (nontumorigenic melanoma), no other attribute is required to determine prognosis as the survival is essentially 100%. Such pure radial growth phase cases constitute about 30% of our data base, at present. As a matter of practice, we usually report thickness and levels and the presence or absence of a precursor lesion in these cases. (See the following section on the form of pathology reports on primary malignant melanomas.)

Vertical Growth Phase

We have investigated 23 attributes that, based on the literature or on theoretical grounds, could influence prognosis. Six attributes have been found, through multivariable analysis, to give some prognostic information not given by the other attributes (independent predictor variables). This statistical result does not mean that the other attributes may not be of prognostic importance. A larger data base, for example, may result in a prognostic model using more attributes than those to be presently discussed and illustrated. Angioneogenesis, satellitosis, ulceration, a brisk plasma cell infiltrate, and level IV–V invasion all are adverse prognostic attributes when tested separately, but in our present data set do not give prognostic information that is additive to the attributes of the present model. The attributes to be discussed apply *only* to those primaries that have entered the vertical growth phase in clinical stage I patients.[11]

The Mitotic Count per Square Millimeter. The earliest attempts to determine prognosis in melanoma on the basis of the pathology of the primary have shown a high mitotic rate to be an adverse prognostic attribute. Alistair Cochran developed a prognostic score in 1968, and mitotic count was an important attribute in that study, a forerunner to many subsequent studies on prognosis.[71,72] Schmoeckel and associates developed a prognostic index based on the product of mitotic rate and thickness.[73] We have found the number of mitotic figures per square millimeter, when used as a single attribute, to be related to prognosis as a continuous variable, but when integrated into our probability model, three ranges of mitotic counts are used: $0/mm^2$, 0.1 to $6.0/mm^2$, and $>6.1/mm^2$. These ranges of mitotic rate are statistically signficant and are wide enough to be consistently reproducible between observers. The microscope should be carefully calibrated before doing mitotic counts. The combined use of an ocular micrometer and a mounted calibrated scale (in divisions of 0.01mm) for the microscope stage permits one to determine the size of a given microscopic field in square millimeters. One should then count, at a magnification of 400 times, more than 1 mm^2, reporting the results as mitoses per square millimeter. Occasionally the vertical growth phase is < 1 mm^2. In such instances, one should report the number of mitoses observed and extrapolate to x/mm^2, reporting the results as extrapolated. The vertical growth phase should be carefully surveyed before starting the mitotic count. The mitotic count varies from area to area, and the count should be done where it is apparently the highest, so-called hot spots. Counts that are near one of the divisions of mitotic rates (e.g., about $6/mm^2$) should be done with unusual care: The search for hot spots should be quite careful, and when possible, 2 mm^2 should be counted.

Cellular Immune Response (Tumor Infiltrating Lympho-cytes). A number of studies of the lymphocytic response to primary melanomas have been reported with conflicting results. These studies have been reviewed by Kornstein and Guerry.[74] The lymphocytic response to the cells of the vertical growth phase has a powerful influence on prognosis if evaluated both quantitatively and qualitatively.[11] The qualitative evaluation was based on the presence or absence of infiltration of the lymphocytic response to the tumor. In an infiltrative host response, the lymphocytes disrupt and surround tumor cells (Fig. 49–24). One may actually observe rosette formation around tumor cells in routine histologic preparations (Figs. 49–25 and 49–26). If such a response is focal at the base of or within the vertical growth phase, it is reported as sparse or moderate depending on the denisty of the lymphocytes. If, on the other hand, the infiltrate is present across the entire base of the vertical growth phase or present throughout its substance as occasionally happens, the response is said to be brisk. Thus, the cellular immune response is reported as (1) noninfiltrative or absent, (2) sparse or moderate (nonbrisk) and infiltrative, or (3) brisk and infiltrative. One may get some idea about the importance of this attribute by comparing 8-year survival in those patients with a brisk infiltrative host response compared with those with a noninfiltrative or absent host response. If all other prognostic attributes are held statistically constant, patients whose tumors exhibited a brisk response were 11 times more likely to survive than those with an absent or noninfiltrative response. It is interesting to note that the presence of lymphocytes that do not infiltrate among tumor cells, even when they are present

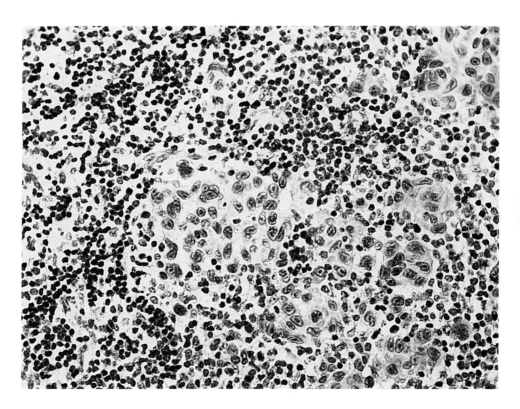

Figure 49–24. Tumor-infiltrating lymphocytes: the histology of the lymphocytic response that is an independent prognostic attribute when present in the vertical growth phase. The tumor cells of the vertical growth phase are actually disrupted by the infiltrating lymphocytes. Tumor cell nests and individual tumor cells are separated by lymphocytes.

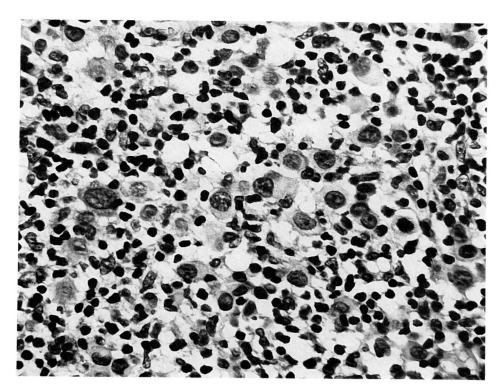

Figure 49–25. Tumor-infiltrating lymphocytes. Individual cells are separated and surrounded by lymphocytes. Rosette formation may be seen in routine histologic preparations.

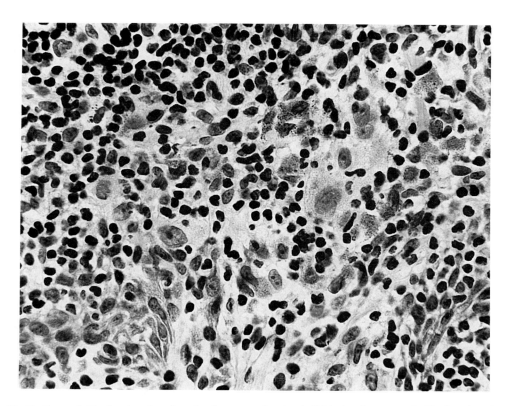

Figure 49–26. Tumor-infiltrating lymphocytes. Another area showing individual cells surrounded by lymphocytes. If such an infiltrate is present throughout the vertical growth phase or entirely across the base of the vertical growth phase, it is said to be brisk. All other patterns of tumor-infiltrating lymphocytes are classified as nonbrisk for the purpose of attribute assignment.

in abundance, has a similar significance to the complete absence of lymphocytes. Similarly, the presence or absence of lymphocytes in the nontumorigenic compartment (radial growth phase) of melanomas has no relevance to survival.

Maximum Tumor Thickness. When tumor thickness is used as a single prognostic attribute to evaluate outcome at 8 years, survival is related to thickness in a linear fashion. When used in a probability model, however, two thickness ranges are significant: ≤1.70 mm and >1.70 mm. Reports should always give the exact thickness, but the foregoing ranges are the important ones in using our model to calculate a probability of survival.

Anatomic Site. In quite large data bases, it is likely that more than two anatomic sites will modulate survival. For example, our present data indicate that volar-subungual tumors have the worst prognosis, followed by head, neck, and trunk (treated as a single site, termed axial) and extremities (the best prognosis). The difference in survival between volar subungual and axial is not great, and the model in current use combines these two sites as axial. Although we believe that site of the primary should be reported as precisely as possible, two sites (axial and extremity) as defined here are sufficient for statistical analysis of prognosis.

Sex. Sex is a categorical attribute needing no explanation. Females do better than males when all other attributes are held constant, including site.

Regression
The presence of regression in the radial growth phase is an adverse prognostic attribute *when* the vertical growth phase is present. This is not statistically demonstrable when regression is present and the vertical growth phase is absent (radial growth phase present). A detailed comment about the work of Ronan and associates is in order here.[70] They studied 103 patients with tumors ≤0.76 mm. Thirty of these tumors showed histologic evidence of partial regression, and six of these patients died of metastatic melanoma. All six of these patients had regression of >77%. Of the 24 patients who did not die, only 1 had regression >77%. However, one of their illustrated cases clearly shows that the tumor was in the vertical growth phase. At least four of the six fatal cases were likely to be in the vertical growth phase as judged by tumor area. Consequently, it seems probable that regression is an adverse attribute only in tumors in the vertical growth phase. However, if regression is extensive and no vertical growth phase is demonstrated, it should be reported. In such rare instances, one should not assume that survival will be 100%, as has been our experience in radial growth phase cases.

Probability Formula and Probability Tables Using Multiple Prognostic Attributes
The probability tables we currently use are shown as Tables 49–7 and 49–8. A shorter table is less accurate but useful when all prognostic attributes are not available (Table 49–9). This table uses four thickness groups, site, and sex—attributes that are available in virtually every primary melanoma. The value of using all of the prognostic attributes may be appreciated from studying Table 49–7. Tumors ≤1.70 mm, using thickness as a single attribute, have an expected survival at 8 years of about 84% (95% confidence interval: 75 to 92%). Using all six prognostic attributes for tumors ≤1.70 mm, one notes that survival probability varies

TABLE 49–7. PROBABILITIES OF 8-YEAR SURVIVAL—POINT ESTIMATE AND 95% CONFIDENCE INTERVAL THICKNESS ≤ 1.70 MM

Mitotic Rate per mm^2	Tumor-Infiltrating Lymphocytes	Regression	Female		Male	
			Extremities	Axial*/Subvol†	Extremities	Axial/Subvol
0.0	Brisk and infiltrative	Absent	1.0 .99–1.0	1.0 .96–1.0	1.0 .97–1.0	.99 .91–1.0
		Present	1.0 .97–1.0	.99 .92–1.0	.99 .93–1.0	.96 .81–.99
	Nonbrisk and infiltrative	Absent	1.0 .97–1.0	.98 .92–1.0	.99 .93–1.0	.96 .81–.99
		Present	.99 .93–1.0	.96 .80–.99	.97 .83–.99	.89 .60–.98
	Absent or noninfiltrative	Absent	.99 .93–1.0	.95 .78–.99	.96 .82–.99	.86 .57–.97
		Present	.96 .81–.99	.87 .54–.97	.89 .59–.98	.69 .30–.92
0.1 to 6.0	**Brisk and infiltrative**	Absent	1.0 .98–1.0	.98 .94–1.0	.99 .94–1.0	**.95 .85–.99‡**
		Present	.99 .95–1.0	.96 .86–.99	.97 .87–.99	.88 .70–.96
	Nonbrisk and infiltrative	Absent	.99 .96–1.0	.95 .87–.98	.96 .88–.99	.87 .71–.94
		Present	.96 .89–.99	.87 .71–.95	.90 .72–.97	.70 .47–.86
	Absent or noninfiltrative	Absent	.95 .88–.98	.84 .68–.93	.87 .70–.95	.65 .43–.82
		Present	.88 .69–.96	.66 .40–.85	.71 .42–.90	.40 .19–.65
	Brisk and infiltrative	Absent	.99 .93–1.0	.95 .79–.99	.96 .82–.99	.86 .58–.96
		Present	.96 .84–.99	.86 .61–.96	.89 .64–.97	.68 .37–.88
>6.1	Nonbrisk and infiltrative	Absent	.95 .85–.99	.84 .62–.95	.88 .66–.96	.65 .37–.85
		Present	.88 .68–.96	.66 .38–.86	.72 .41–.90	.40 .18–.66
	Absent or noninfiltrative	Absent	.85 .66–.95	.61 .35–.81	.67 .38–.86	.34 .16–.59
		Present	.68 .38–.88	.35 .15–.63	.42 .17–.72	.16 .06–.37

* Axial includes head, neck, and trunk.
† Subvol includes subungual and volar locations.
‡ The highlighted cells illustrate a case with a thickness of 1.45 mm, a mitotic count of 3/mm^2 with brisk tumor-infiltrating lymphocytes, absent regression, on the trunk of a male patient.

TABLE 49–8. PROBABILITIES OF 8-YEAR SURVIVAL—POINT ESTIMATE AND 95% CONFIDENCE INTERVAL THICKNESS > 1.70 MM

Mitotic Rate per mm^2	Tumor-Infiltrating Lymphocytes	Regression	Female		Male	
			Extremities	Axial[*]/Subvol[†]	Extremities	Axial/Subvol
0.0	Brisk and infiltrative	Absent	.99 .95–1.0	.98 .86–1.0	.98 .88–1.0	.95 .69–.99
		Present	.99 .89–1.0	.95 .70–.99	.96 .74–.99	.86 .47–.98
	Nonbrisk and infiltrative	Absent	.98 .90–1.0	.94 .71–.99	.95 .76–.99	.84 .47–.97
		Present	.95 .75–.99	.85 .46–.97	.88 .52–.98	.66 .24–.92
	Absent or noninfiltrative	Absent	.94 .73–.99	.82 .43–.96	.85 .49–.97	.60 .21–.90
		Present	.86 .47–.98	.61 .19–.91	.67 .23–.93	.35 .08–.77
0.1 to 6.0	Brisk and infiltrative	Absent	.98 .93–1.0	.94 .80–.98	.95 .82–.99	.84 .60–.95
		Present	.95 .84–.99	.84 .62–.95	.87 .65–.96	.65 .38–.84
	Nonbrisk and infiltrative	Absent	.95 .87–.98	.82 .65–.92	.86 .69–.94	.61 .42–.78
		Present	.86 .69–.95	.62 .40–.81	.68 .43–.86	.36 .20–.57
	Absent or noninfiltrative	Absent	.83 .66–.93	.57 .36–.76	.63 .39–.82	.31 .17–.51
		Present	.64 .37–.85	.32 .14–.57	.38 .16–.67	.14 .06–.31
>6.1	Brisk and infiltrative	Absent	.94 .78–.99	.81 .51–.95	.85 .56–.96	.60 .28–.85
		Present	.85 .60–.96	.60 .31–.84	.67 .34–.88	.35 .14–.63
	Nonbrisk and infiltative	**Absent**	.84 .65–.93	.57 .33–.78	.63 .38–.83	.31 .16–.53
		Present	**.64 .39–.84**[‡]	.32 .15–.56	.38 .17–.65	.14 .06–.29
	Absent or noninfiltrative	Absent	.59 .36–.78	.28 .13–.49	.33 .15–.57	.12 .05–.24
		Present	.34 .15–.61	.12 .05–.28	.15 .05–.36	.04 .02–.12

[*] Axial includes head, neck, and trunk.
[†] Subvol includes subungual and volar locations.
[‡] The highlighted cells illustate a case with a thickness of 2.20 mm, a mitotic count of 8/mm^2 with sparse tumor-infiltrating lymphocytes, present regression, on the extremity of a female patient.

TABLE 49–9. CLINICAL STAGE I VERTICAL GROWTH PHASE PROGNOSIS— THICKNESS, SEX, AND SITE

Thickness	Female		Male	
	Extremities	Axial/Subvol	Extremities	Axial/Subvol
≤ 1.70 mm	.97 .92–.99	.88 .79–.94	.92 .83–.97	.76 .64–.85
> 1.70–3.60 mm	.85 .73–.92	.61 .45–.75	.70 .51–.84	.39 .27–.53
> 3.61 mm	.68 .45–.84	.36 .19–.58	.46 .25–.69	.19 .09–.34

from 0.16% (95% confidence interval 6 to 37%): mitotic count ≥6.1/mm^2, absent or noninfiltrative host response, regression present, axial lesion in a male patient; to 100% (95% confidence interval: 99 to 100%): mitotic count 0/mm2; brisk, infiltrative host response, absent regression, extremity site in a female patient. Obviously, the significance of thickness as a guide to prognosis in vertical growth phase disease is greatly modulated by other attributes.

Form of Pathology Reports for Primary Malignant Melanomas

Our pathology reports currently use the following format, using a hypothetical case as an example.

Diagnosis:	Malignant melanoma
Type:	Superficial spreading type
Growth phase:	Radial growth phase present, vertical growth phase present (tumorigenic)
Mitotic Count*:	4.2/mm^2
Tumor infiltrating lymphocytes*:	Present, brisk
Thickness:	1.95 mm
Level of invasion:	Level IV
Site*:	Back (axial lesion)
Sex*:	Male
Regression*:	Present
Precursor lesion:	Compound nevus with melanocytic dysplasia of the type seen in the dysplastic nevus syndrome
Risk factors:	The tumor has entered the vertical growth phase and has potential for metastasis. The probability of survival at 8 years is 65%, with a 95% confidence interval of 38 to 84%

The italicized attributes are the independent predictors of prognosis for tumors in the vertical growth phase. The characteristics indicated by an asterisk are those reported solely for tumors with vertical growth phase present. For pure radial growth phase lesions, we state, "Survival approaches 100%. Only a theoretical potential for metastasis exists."

METASTATIC MELANOMA AND THE BIOLOGY OF METASTASIS

The essence of the concept of the vertical growth phase is the acquisition of competence for metastasis by a primary melanoma. However, metastases are manifest in only about 30% of vertical growth phase cases in our data base. Does the failure to *express* the capacity for metastasis reflect a modulation of metastatic potential by the prognostic attributes listed (and others, doubtless, not listed)? Or, is the nonexpression of metastasis a failure of some of the vertical growth phase cases (tumorigenic melanomas) to produce cells capable of completing the entire metastatic cascade? Such questions may not be answered with certitude at the present stage of study, but speculative answers may be rooted in enough detail to give them substance. In order to speculate from details of knowledge, brief mention must be made of the metastatic cascade. A review of the biology of metastasis by Liotta and associates, with particular reference to melanoma, is helpful in considering mechanisms of metastasis from vertical growth phase melanomas.[34]

Metastatic Cascade

The metastatic cascade constitutes that series of mechanistic steps that a cell or group of cells must complete in order to extend from its primary site to a site anatomically separate from the primary. For the purpose of this limited discussion, two anatomic sites will serve as prototypes for metastasis. The sites, lung (or other viscera) and regional lymph nodes, illustrate the possibility that at least partially disparate mechanisms may be involved in the biology of metastasis. The rubric under which the cascade exists is autonomous growth (at least partial); without this, metastasis does not occur.

The challenge to survival of a melanoma cell from its origin in the epidermis to proliferation in the lung is formidable. Consider this brief list of tasks as minimal requirements for the formation of a pulmonary metastatic nodule: (1) growth in the epidermis; (2) motility to traverse the basement membrane zone; (3) attachment to the lamina lucida mediated by elaboration of laminin/fibronectin (attachment glycoproteins) plasma membrane receptors; (4) production of hydrolytic enzymes to degrade the attachment glycoproteins; (5) traversal of the lamina densa related to synthesis of type IV collagenase; (6) migration into the papillary dermis (motility again); (7) selection of a population of cells capable of tumorigenic growth—vertical growth phase; (8) detachment of cells from the vertical growth phase; (9) induction of angioneogenesis; (10) chemotactically directed motility toward a blood vascular bed associated with synthesis of autocrine motility factor; (11) blood vascular intravasation requiring the crossing of the lamina densa, lamina lucida, and endothelium, in part via enzymatic mechanisms; (12) survival in the blood vascular circulation; (13) formation of cohesive factors (disialogangliosides) promoting tumor cell aggregation to enhance lodgment in a capillary bed before extravasation; (14) extravasation, necessitating endothelial adhesion, endothelial cell retraction, and passage through the lamina lucida and lamina densa; (15) migration into the pulmonary matrix; and (16) replication and survival at that site.

The evidence that lymph vascular metastases may be qualitatively different from blood vascular metastases is, in essence, mortality. Some 25% of patients with lymph node metastases survive; survival after nonregional metastases is exquisitely rare. Both forms of metastasis are discontinuous spread of cancer. Yet, in the one, survival likelihood is significant and, in the other, essentially nonexistent. Further, one must infer that lymph-borne metastases and blood-borne metastases traverse the same first eight steps listed in the previous paragraph. At this point, a qualitative dichotomy in the biology of metastasis could occur. On the one hand, the selection process at step 7 could select cells capable of completing only a lymph vascular cascade. On the other hand, the selection process could select a cell population capable of blood vascular *and* lymph vascular metastasis. The technique of lymph vascular intravasation and blood vascular intravasation should be quite different. Lymphatics do not have a basement membrane zone, no lamina lucida, no lamina densa.[75] Therefore, lymphatic entry should not require attachment glycoprotein receptors, hydrolytic enzymes to degrade these, nor type IV collagenase to permeate a lamina densa. Cells could complete the lymphatic metastatic cascade and yet fail to express some of the properties required for completion of the blood vascular metastatic cascade.

Failure of Melanoma Cells of the Radial Growth Phase to Metastasize

The melanoma cells of the microinvasive but nontumorigenic radial growth phase have acquired, at least, the properties of autonomous growth, motility, and may or may not have elaborated those surface receptors and proteolytic enzymes necessary for passage through the basement membrane zone. The cells enter the papillary dermis but, in our experience, do not metastasize. An inference from the manifest ability to negotiate a basement membrane zone is that such cells could complete either the lymphatic or blood vascular cascade. The cells may, however, traverse the basement membrane zone similar to the nevic cell mechanism. The cells have not acquired the ability to replicate in the dermis: to become tumorigenic and form the vertical growth phase. Growth in the radial growth phase is intraepidermal. A few cells extend into the papillary dermis, where they encounter a brisk and usually infiltrative host response. Mitotic figures in melanoma cells in the papillary dermis are rarely seen. Most of these cells do not survive and are replaced from the dividing epidermal population of melanoma cells. The essence of radial growth phase biology is intraepidermal growth with desultory extension into the papillary dermis without growth in the dermis. Until a new genetic event produces a subclone capable of replicating and becoming tumorigenic in the dermis, metastasis does not occur.

Possible Modulation of the Traverse of the Metastatic Cascade by Some Prognostic Attributes

This section posits that there are vertical growth phase cases that have acquired competence for metastasis and that competence may not be realized because of the influence of one or more of the prognostic attributes discussed in this chapter. The following paragraphs discuss the possibility of tumorigenic dermal growth of cells incompetent for metastasis.

The inference that vertical growth phase cases metastasize is an actuality, for some 30% of such cases persons die of metastatic disease. That this metastatic potential is modulated is inferred from the wide variation in survival probability with tumors of a given thickness. For tumors ≤1.70 mm in thickness, the survival probability varies from 16% to 100%; for tumors >1.70 mm, the survival probability varies from 4 to 99%. Here, we shall consider the three most powerful of the prognostic attributes.

A patient bearing a vertical growth phase melanoma with a mitotic count of $0/mm^2$ has an 11.7 times greater chance of survival than a patient with a vertical growth phase melanoma having mitotic count of $>6/mm^2$, all other attributes being held statistically constant. A high mitotic rate could reflect a cell population having a number of properties required for metastasis such as independence from exogenous growth factors. In the present context, the evidence suggests that mitotic rate has control over the number of cells accomplishing the afferent limb (intravasation) of the metastatic cascade. If mitotic rate is treated as a single prognostic attribute, it is related to survival in a linear fashion, indicating that the greater the mitotic rate the greater is the likelihood of metastasis. One may thus speculate that mitotic rate is one factor controlling the number of cells available for intravasation. Obviously, mitotic rate is also influenced by time. A mitotic rate of $8/mm^2$ in effect for 1 year will produce a dosage of intravasated tumor cells greater than the same mitotic rate will during 3 months, other attributes being constant.

Tumor-infiltrating lymphocytes that are brisk confer an 11.3 times greater chance of survival when compared with melanomas without tumor-infiltrating lymphocytes (all other attributes being held statistically constant). These lymphocytes could indicate such a rate of killing of melanoma cells at the primary site that few cells are available for intravasation (immunologic decrease of melanoma cell dosage). Tumor-infiltrating lymphocytes could also inhibit melanoma cell motility. More obviously, the attribute could mirror the presence of circulating tumor-specific lymphocytes capable of killing melanoma cells in the blood stream or, possibly, inhibiting extravasation of tumor cells.

A tumor thickness of ≤1.70 mm confers a survival advantage when, compared with tumors >1.70 mm in thickness, of 4.0 times. This could also be a reflection of tumor cell dosage available for intravasation. For example, treat the vertical growth phase as a sphere of tumor cells. A sphere 1.0 mm in diameter has a surface area of 3.1 mm^2, whereas a sphere 4.0 mm in diameter has a surface area of 50.3 mm^2. Not only does the larger sphere have a 16 times greater surface area but, given a constant mitotic rate, has existed for a much longer time. The larger tumor would be expected to produce many more tumor cells available for intravasation.

Tumorigenic Melanoma Cells Lacking Properties for Completion of the Full Metastatic Cascade

Melanomas that have evolved to the vertical growth phase are, doubtless, a heterogeneous population of tumors. As a matter of fact, Reed's concept of the minimal deviation melanomas is, in part, an attempt to classify the tumorigenic nodules (vertical growth phase) of melanoma according to their biologic potential.[65] Some vertical growth phase

melanomas predicted to give rise to metastases on the basis of the prognostic attributes herein discussed do not do so. Other attributes probably explain this. Surely, one such explanation lies in the cell properties of some of the vertical growth phase cases. To evolve to the vertical growth phase, it would seem that tumor cells need only to be able to survive in the dermis and grow in a tumorigenic manner. The properties required for metastasis may require further selection during dermal growth or may not be acquired at all. Such tumors, though in the vertical growth phase, may not have competence for metastasis.

STATISTICAL DATA COMPARING THE BIOLOGIC FORMS OF MELANOMA

Superficial spreading melanoma forms 67.5% of our data base, followed by nodular melanoma, lentigo maligna melanoma, and acral lentiginous melanoma, in order of frequency. Six percent of the cases had a radial growth phase that could not be classified because of histologic nonspecificity, whereas 4.4% of the cases were unusual biologic forms of melanoma or could not be classified by type for technical reasons (Table 49–10). This table is based on 501 cases reviewed by two different pathologists on three separate occasions.

IN VITRO CHARACTERISTICS OF MELANOMA CELLS

The in vitro and antigenic characteristics of the cells of the distal lesions of distal tumor progression reflect the biologic potential of the different lesional classes. These characteristics have recently been reviewed. Presented here are a few points that reflect the biologic behavior of these lesions, the central theme of this chapter. First, it is extremely difficult to establish long-term cell lines from radial growth phase primary melanomas. Second, when cultured, these cells are not tumorigenic in nude mice and have nonrandom chromosomal abnormalities only at chromosome 6. Third, the antigen profile of radial growth phase tumors is more similar to dysplastic nevi than to vertical growth phase and metastatic melanoma. Permanent cell lines can be readily established from vertical growth phase melano-

TABLE 49–10. BIOLOGICAL FORMS OF MALIGNANT MELANOMA

Biologic Type	Frequency	Percent
Superficial spreading melanoma	337	67.2
Nodular melanoma	54	10.8
Lentigo maligna melanoma	38	7.6
Acral lentiginous melanoma	19	3.8
Mucosal lentiginous melanoma	1	.2
Unclassified radial growth phase	30	6.0
Other and unknown	22	4.4
Total	501	100.0%

mas. These cell lines are tumorigenic in nude mice and have chromosomal abnormalities at chromosomes 1, 6, and 7. Metastatic cell lines usually have the same nonrandom chromosomal abnormalities, but may have multiple additional abnormalities. They are also tumorigenic and react with the same monoclonal antibody panels that are reactive with vertical growth phase cells (see Tables 49–3, 49–4, and 49–5).

RARE AND UNUSUAL FORMS OF MELANOMA

DESMOPLASTIC MELANOMA

Desmoplastic melanoma is an uncommon form of differentiation of the cells of the vertical growth phase.[76] It is most commonly seen in lentigo maligna melanoma but may be seen as all or part of the vertical growth phase of other forms of melanoma. Rarely, a melanoma may be entirely desmoplastic, with nothing but a row of atypical melanocytes in the basal layer of the epidermis to serve as a clue to the epidermal histogenesis of the lesion. Desmoplastic melanoma is a manifestation of the capacity of neural crest-derived cells to synthesize collagen.

Clinical Features

The lesion presents as a firm nodule or plaque covered with a tan or brown epidermis that may lack the distinctive colors of other forms of melanoma. The melanoma that is entirely desmoplastic may be so unusual in substance and appearance (e.g., a hard pink, dermal mass) that the possibility of melanoma may not be considered by the clinician. In spite of a histologic appearance simulating but distinguishable from mature fibrous tissue, the lesions may grow quite rapidly; a nodule several centimeters in diameter may form in a few months.

Histologic Features

The neoplasm is composed of spindle-shaped cells embedded in an abundant matrix of collagen, which widely separates the nuclei (Fig. 49–27). On casual inspection, the tumor may be mistaken for scar tissue but is distinguished by the lack of organization of its fibrous tissue. The fibroblasts of a surgical scar tend to have their long axes parallel to each other and to the overlying epidermis, and the newly formed blood vessels tend to be perpendicular to the fibroblastic polarity. In contrast, the cells of desmoplastic melanoma are disposed in poorly organized fascicles having a haphazard array (Figs. 49–27 and 49–28). With study of multiple sections, nuclear atypia is observed and may be quite striking (Fig. 49–29). The fibroblast-like areas of des-

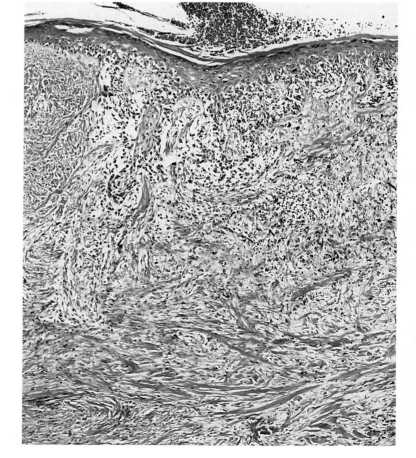

Figure 49–27. Malignant melanoma, lentigo maligna type with a desmoplastic vertical growth phase. The basilar region of the epidermis presents a row of atypical melanocytes with scattered foci of nest formation. From these nests there is a suggestion of streaming into the subjacent dermis. The remainder of the picture shows fascicles of collagen that do not resemble reticular dermis at all. Except for their somewhat haphazard array, the histology of the collagen is not terribly worrisome at this magnification. The histology depicted in this picture may be the only initial clue that the process is desmoplastic melanoma.

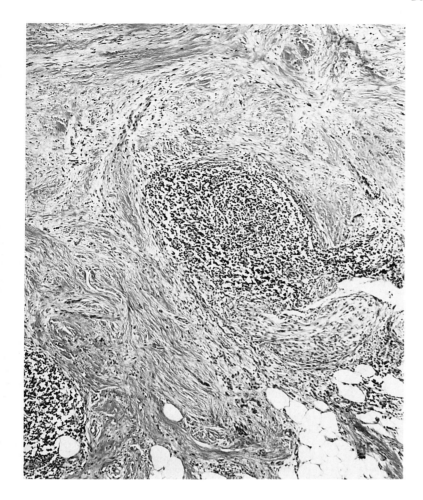

Figure 49–28. Malignant melanoma, lentigo maligna type with a desmoplastic vertical growth phase. Deeper in the dermis, approaching the subcutaneous tissue, the collagen bundle pattern is even more atypical. There is a suggestion of cytological atypia in the fibroblasts, even at this magnification. A patchy lymphocytic infiltrate is well shown. This feature is a hallmark of desmoplastic melanoma. Adjacent to the lymphocytic infiltrate there is neurotropism (shown at higher magnification in Figure 49–30).

moplastic melanoma are not, however, fibroblasts, nor is the fibroplasia comparable to the stromal response induced by most malignant neoplasms. The spindle cells are positive with antibodies of S-100 protein. Such positivity is variable, involving only a few cells or much of the neoplasm. Fine structural studies are especially informative. A given spindle cell shows a prominent endoplasmic reticulum filled with flocculent material and occasional collagen fibrils, the appearance of the cytoplasm of a fibroblast. The same cell may present nonmembrane-bound melanin granules and premelanosomes.[48] Scattered about the periphery of the tumor small patches of lymphocytes are frequently seen (see Fig. 49–28). This is a characteristic feature of desmoplastic melanoma. Neurotropism is of great importance and is a subtle histologic finding. At the periphery and within the substance of the lesion, one may see the fibroblast-like tumor cells around small nerves; they may instead be within the endoneurium (Fig. 49–30). In some tumors, neurotropism is extensive and much of the lesion may simulate a tangled collection of small nerves. The neoplasm may extend along nerves for several centimeters beyond the clinical extent of the lesion. Such extension, if not recognized and appropriately excised, may be responsible for local recurrence. Desmoplastic melanoma may not be correctly diagnosed by the pathologist, and neurotropism involving

excision margins may be overlooked. In such instances, local recurrences may be numerous before the true situation is recognized. Desmoplasia may be only a part of the vertical growth phase of a melanoma, and here it is diagnosed with greater ease. However, one may still fail to diagnose neurotropism, with unfortunate consequences. Reexcision specimens, after a biopsy has established that a melanoma exhibits neurotropism, should be examined carefully with multiple sections and inking of the margins. Close attention should be paid to small nerve fibers in searching for neurotropism.

NEUROTROPIC MELANOMA

Clinical Features

Melanomas that are predominantly neurotropic include those whose growth pattern simulates small peripheral nerves. The tumors may not have a distinctive surface coloration. Tan, brown, or black may be present, but the tumors may also present as rapidly growing amelanotic nodules. Nothing about the appearance or history of such nodules may suggest that the lesion is malignant melanoma, unless one is aware of such a clinical presentation of some forms of neurotropic melanoma. Additionally, neurotropism may

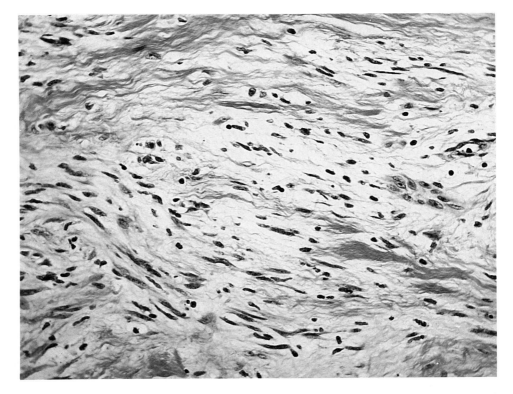

Figure 49–29. Malignant melanoma, lentigo maligna type with a desmoplastic vertical growth phase: atypia of the fibroblast-like cells that are a unique trait of the lesion. Search of these lesions will reveal fibroblasts with variable atypia. The depiction is prototypical of the fibroblastic atypia.

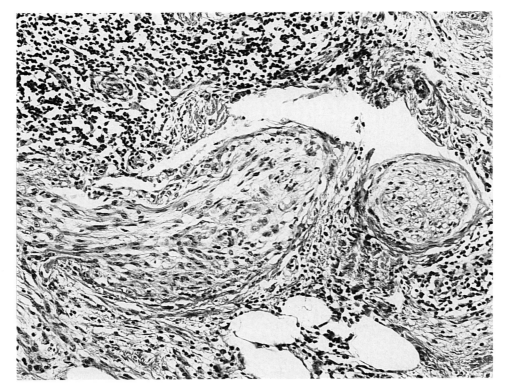

Figure 49–30. Malignant melanoma, lentigo maligna type with a desmoplastic vertical growth phase: neurotropism. A distended nerve is infiltrated by the elongate cells of the tumor. An area of lymphocytic infiltrate is also shown.

be a microscopic finding in a portion of the vertical growth phase of any form of melanoma, especially lentigo maligna melanoma and acral lentiginous melanoma. The clinical appearance of these melanomas is similar to those without neurotropism.

The tumors usually occur on the head and neck; only 4 of 22 of Reed and Leonard's cases occurred away from this anatomic site.[77] We have seen cases on the hands and feet, and the tumors are uncommonly seen at other sites. The lip, as a site, should be noted. Of the 18 head and neck cases reported by Reed and Leonard, 4 were on the lip. The lip tumors may present as rapidly evolving pink nodules. There may be no discoloration of the surface.

Histologic Features

Portions of neurotropic melanomas may appear as solid collections of spindle-shaped cells, and such areas have no histologic characteristics that distinguish them from other malignant dermal neoplasms composed of spindle cells. This group of tumors generally presents formidable problems in proper classification. At the periphery of the closely packed aggregates of spindle cells one may see a few nerves surrounded by the spindle cells, or these cells may actually be within the nerves, the latter finding being required for the diagnosis of true neurotropic melanoma. Other neurotropic melanomas are composed of numerous small tubules of cells that simulate peripheral nerves. (Figs. 49–31, 49–32, 49–33, and 49–34). Some of these tubular growths may entrap preexisting nerves or grow within them. The neurotropism may extend well beyond the main body of the tumor. More commonly, the characteristic form of neurotropic melanoma is composed of fascicles of spindle cells with pale cytoplasm and oval nuclei (see Reed and Leonard[77]). As in desmoplastic melanoma, histogenetic origin from epidermal melanocytes may not be obvious. A

row of large melanocytes may be seen in the epidermis. Even this minimal manifestation of abnormality of epidermal melanocytes may require multiple sections of several blocks of tissue. In other instances, the epidermal melanocytic pathology is that of obvious lentigo maligna and, much less commonly, the radial growth phase of some other form of melanoma.

GENERAL CONCEPT OF MINIMAL DEVIATION MELANOMA

Minimal deviation melanoma may be defined as the histologic variants of dermal tumorigenic melanoma of unknown biologic potential, but with *some* potential for metastasis. In Reed's terms, the category is a histologic hodge-podge, but a useful one in the language of the everyday practice of pathology: "A section presenting a nodule of unusual melanocytes in the dermis that defies ready classification into the schema of melanoma is likely to be a minimal deviation melanoma." Six forms of minimal deviation melanoma have been described.[65] Some of these have been treated in this and other sections of the chapter in various degrees of detail. The kinds of minimal deviation melanoma are as follows:

1. A small nodule of melanocytes that show moderate to moderately severe atypism and impinge on the reticular dermis (see Fig. 49–14). The nodules are <0.76 mm thick, as a rule. Metastases are uncommon but occur, and thus they may be justifiably designated as minimal deviation melanomas by Reed's concepts. We have called such lesions as early (but definite) vertical growth phase (tumorigenic melanoma). In our experience, about 10% of such melanomas metastasize. These have been discussed elsewhere in this chapter.

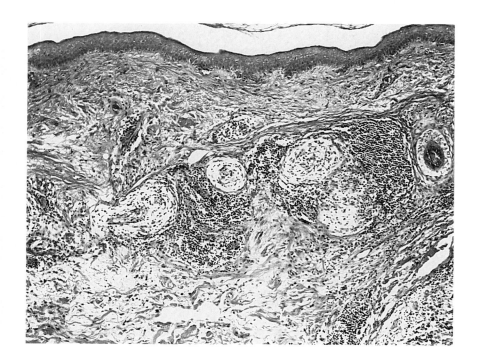

Figure 49–31. Neurotropic melanoma. The epidermis is virtually normal in this picture, but in other areas there was basilar melanocytic hyperplasia with atypia. The epidermal component of the lesion may be inconspicuous and is not diagnostic. Well below the epidermis there are circular areas of tumor cell proliferation resembling hypertrophied nerves in cross section. Some of the cells in the lower right are clearly atypical. The virtually ubiquitous lymphocytic infiltrate tends to surround each nest of nervelike or neurotropic tumor.

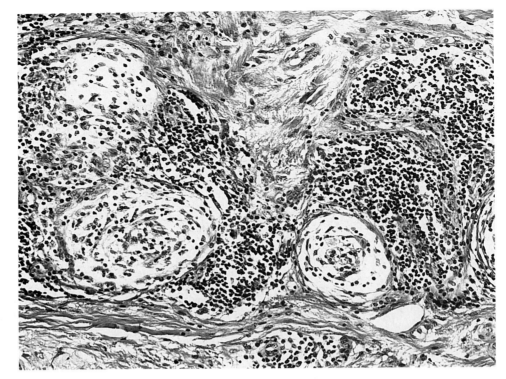

Figure 49–32. Neurotropic melanoma. At higher magnification, the nests of tumor show elongate cells in concentric array. The cells are small and, doubtless, differentiated along schwannian lines. They are malignant. The central portions of some of these distinctive structures are remnants of small nerves. Again note the lymphocytes. These can be a helpful reminder that unusual lesions may be neurotropic or desmoplastic melanoma.

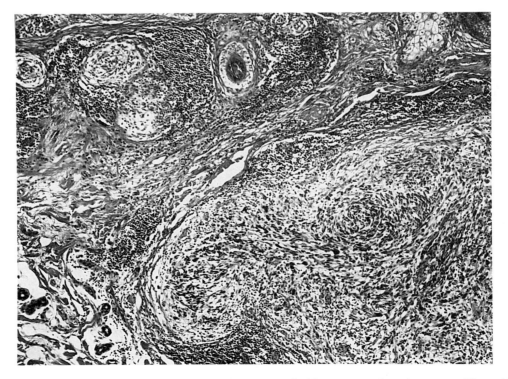

Figure 49–33. Neurotropic melanoma. A large area of tumor, atypical in pattern and cytology, resembling a bizarre, giant nerve.

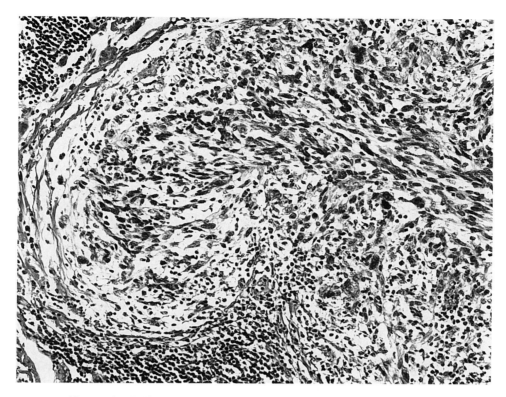

Figure 49–34. Neurotropic melanoma. Higher magnification of Figure 49–33.

2. Minimal deviation melanomas that share some histologic features with a Spitz tumor (see below).

3. Halo nevus variant of minimal deviation melanoma. These small globoid (or plaquelike) tumors are composed of closely aggregated nests of cells with moderate atypia. They are suffused with lymphocytes. Pigment may or may not be present, and the cells are usually smaller than the classic epithelioid melanoma cells (Figs. 49–35 and 49–36). They lack the deep component of an orderly dermal nevus admixed with lymphocytes so characteristic of the paradigmatic halo nevus. The term *halo nevus form of minimal deviation melanoma* does not imply that a halo will be present, nor does it implicate a sequential relationship with a benign halo nevus.

4. The various melanocytic proliferations occurring in congenital melanocytic nevi. (See the section devoted to this topic.)

5. Melanoma occurring in the dermal component of a nevus. (See the section devoted to this topic.)

6. Pigmented spindle cell lesions. This category of minimal deviation melanoma could well be a topic unto itself. The disparate forms of spindle cell melanomas are covered in several areas: pure spindle cell dermal tumors (the problem of the malignant blue nevus), some examples of desmoplastic melanoma, some neurotropic melanomas, and atypical nevi with dermal schwannian differentiation.

It is difficult to draw generalizations about minimal deviation melanoma because inherent in the concept is an attempt to codify *all* of the histologic diversity and address the biologic potential of the cellular variants of the vertical growth phase (tumorigenic melanoma). It is of value to practicing pathologists to know that these variants exist and something of a balm to know that others have been confused in recognition and understanding of them (a major understatement). Metastases are more surprising than common in the group. However, we have seen metastases with some frequency in those minimal deviation melanomas arising in the dermal component of a nevus. Desmoplastic and neurotropic melanomas that are not promptly diagnosed and properly treated early in their course commonly give rise to metastases.

MALIGNANT MELANOMA OF THE MINIMAL DEVIATION TYPE THAT IS SIMILAR TO A SPITZ TUMOR

These are tumors that uncommonly metastasize to lymph nodes, but they have not been associated with dissemination to distant organs or tissues and do not, consequently, cause death due to metastatic disease. It is important that this disorder be recognized by the pathologist. Otherwise, the patient, the patient's family, and the clinician may be justifiably alarmed by two things. First, the pathology of the primary lesion may be diagnosed as a malignant melanoma. Second, with or without an initial diagnosis of malignant melanoma, the development of positive lymph nodes may be regarded as an unduly grave sign.

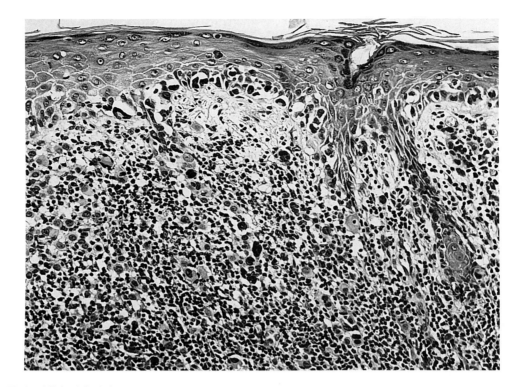

Figure 49–35. Minimal deviation melanoma, halo type. The intraepidermal melanocytes are quite atypical. Similarly atypical tumor cells are in the dermis admixed with a brisk infiltrate of lymphocytes. In this regard, the process has a similarity with a halo nevus. However, these lesions do not have a histological nevic component and do not present a clinical halo.

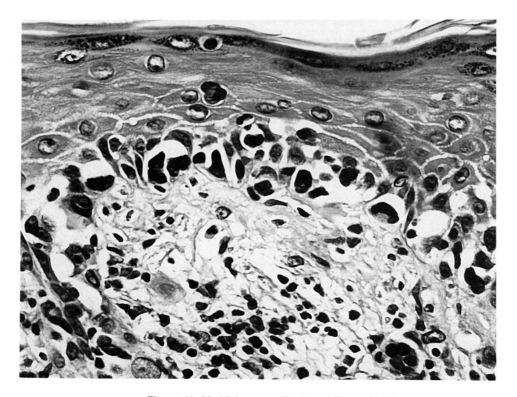

Figure 49–36. Higher magnification of Figure 49–35.

Clinical Features

These tumors are uncommon, and generalities about their appearance are unwarranted. They have been seen as extremity and as axial lesions. In our experience and in Reed's cases, the thigh and face are the more common sites. A history of rapid growth to an elevated pink nodule may be given but does not distinguish these lesions from ordinary Spitz tumors. In some instances, however, growth may be quite rapid, the neoplasms reaching a size greater than that of most Spitz tumors in a matter of 6 to 8 weeks. The tumors occur in childhood, but not exclusively so.

Histologic Features

Portions of the lesions have the appearance of Spitz tumors and, as such, are described elsewhere in this chapter and in this text. They differ from ordinary Spitz tumors in size, symmetry, and cytologic features. They are usually larger and present an area in the dermis that clearly has a growth preference over the remainder of the lesion and is responsible for asymmetry when examining the lesion at low-power microscopic magnification (Fig. 49–37). This area may be an irregular spheroid nodule or may present as one or more peninsula-like extensions from the base of the tumor. Such extensions may protrude into the subcutis. The cells

of the areas of asymmetric growth may be bizarre indeed, and some of this startling atypia may be present throughout the lesion (Figs. 49–38 and 49–39). The cells are larger than the rest and clearly pleomorphic; the nuclei are quite prominent and hyperchromatic; and mitotic figures may be numerous and abnormal.

Metastases and Biologic Significance

Reed has estimated that about 25% of minimal deviation melanomas of the spitzian type are associated with metastases to a single lymph node, rarely two nodes.[78] None of Reed's cases or ours has been associated with metastasis beyond the lymph nodes. This brings up the intriguing possibility that these particular minimal deviation melanomas are malignancies of a phenotype that is only partially transformed: The cells are capable of traversing a metastatic cascade involving lymphatics and lymph nodes, but not venules and distant organs. Certainly this is theoretically possible. A cutaneous lymphatic does not have a lamina densa, and one can envision lymphatic intravasation by tumor cells that have not acquired, for example, the ability to synthesize type IV collagenase. The postulated absence of this enzyme and, perhaps, the absence of a laminin receptor should not preclude lymphatic metastasis but

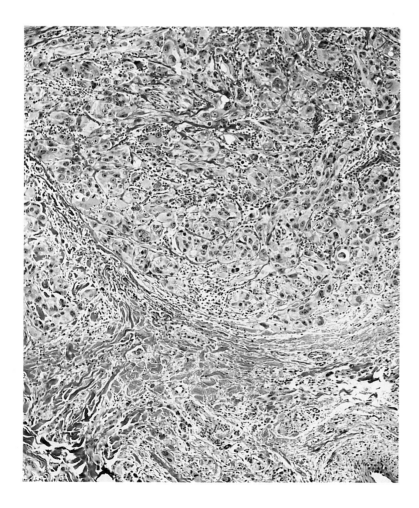

Figure 49–37. Minimal deviation melanoma, spitzian type. On the right there is an asymmetric nodule of large, epithelioid melanocytes. This nodule is deep in the reticular dermis, approaching the subcutis. The lesion was from a child with concurrent lymph node metastases. There has been no dissemination of the disease after long-term follow-up.

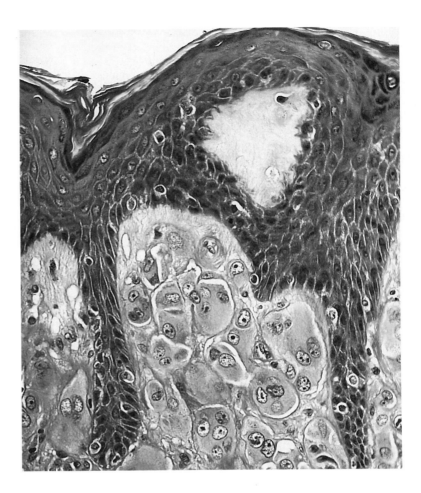

Figure 49–38. Minimal deviation melanoma, spitzian type. The bizarre cytology of the epithelioid melanocytes is shown.

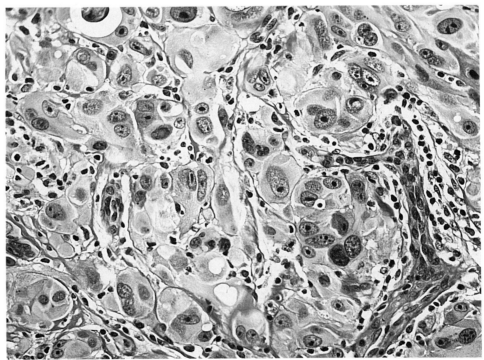

Figure 49–39. Minimal deviation melanoma, spitzian type: the cytology deep within the tumor.

would not permit metastasis via venular intravasation—that is, the afferent limb of the blood vascular metastatic cascade.

VARIOUS OVERGROWTHS, NEOPLASIAS, AND MALIGNANT MELANOMAS ARISING IN CONGENITAL MALFORMATIONS OF NEURAL CREST-DERIVED TISSUES (CONGENITAL MELANOCYTIC NEVI)

Congenital nevi may be so large and so grotesque that they emotionally devastate the family of an infant and seriously diminish the quality of the entire life of the affected individual. To pathologists, the lesions also present major problems in interpretation.

Problems with Terminology and Concepts

Those pigmented lesions present at birth and composed of *nests* of melanocytes in the epidermis and (usually) in the dermis are called congenital melanocytic nevi or congenital nevomelanocytic nevi. Such terms do not adequately describe these lesions. The lesions are usually composed of diverse tissues in addition to melanocytes. It is unlikely, in contrast to acquired melanocytic nevi, that these congenital lesions are derived from an initial growth of epidermal melanocytes. Nevertheless, the introduction of terms deemed to be more descriptive and accurate is likely to meet resistance of cherished semantic fetishes and cause confusion. We will therefore continue with the term *congenital melanocytic nevus*.

Differentiation Potential of Neural Crest Derivatives
The intraepidermal melanocyte of putatively normal skin in children and adults has limited potential for expression of the almost ineffable array of diverse cells and tissues originating from the neural crest. In postfetal life, melanocytes and cells seemingly derived from intraepidermal or dermal melanocytes restrict their manifestation of origin from the neural crest to three lines of differentiation: (1) continued existence as a melanocyte; (2) formation of neurosustentacular tissue, largely schwannian tissue, during differentiation of the dermal component of a nevus; and (3) differentiation into a collagen-synthesizing cell, demonstrated for example in the formation of the fibrotic matrix of a blue nevus. In contrast, no such apparent restrictions on expression of the embryologic potential of the neural crest apply to overgrowths and malformations developing in early fetal life from several adjacent neurocristic somites. Such lesions are commonly composed of melanocytes and neurosustentacular tissue exclusively, but the constituent cells usually involve the deeper tissues of the skin when compared with lesions developing in later fetal life, in infancy, in childhood, and in older individuals. Some large congenital nevi developing in early fetal life may express much of the phenotypical potential of the neural crest. These lesions present as irregular, large nodular overgrowths within the congenital melanocytic nevus. The nodules may be quite large in a neonate and may grow at such an alarming

rate that extensive areas of ulceration occur. When faced with such a clinical presentation, it is hard to dispute malignancy. Except in rare cases, however, subsequent events, histology, and in vitro studies mitigate against explication of the masses as melanoma. The growths may express the full neural crest potential for the formation of diverse cells and tissues. This potential includes, in addition to melanocytes and neurosustentacular tissue, one third of the cephalad mesenchyme of the body. This mesenchyme has been shown to originate from the cephalad neural crest and to give rise to the cranial skin, the dermis of the head and neck, the cranial skeleton, the muscle of some cranial blood vessels, the thymic stroma, the tracheal cartilages, and even odontoblasts. If one studies the neural crest in birds, the list of tissue potential must be extended to include striated muscle and fat. We have seen each of these tissue varieties in the nodular, bumpy masses presenting at birth. This includes, for example, small segments of cartilage, evenly separated one from the other, as one would expect tracheal cartilage to be separated.

Melanoma
Large, rapidly growing lesions present at birth are frequently called malignant melanoma, but with rare exceptions the lesions should not be so designated. The problem has been explained in the excellent report by Hendrickson and Ross[79]: "We do not believe the designation 'melanoma' captures the rich variety of differentiated features encountered in many of the neoplasms. In these complex cases we prefer the diagnosis 'malignant neoplasm arising in congenital giant nevus' and then further specify in the microscopic description the components encountered." One must even be quite cautious in the use of the term *malignant* in spite of seemingly compelling clinical and some histologic indications that a tumor is indeed malignant. As will be clarified in the discussion of these difficult and complex problems, most of the tumors presenting in congenital melanocytic nevi at birth or immediately thereafter, regardless of clinical appearance or histology, do not behave as malignant tumors by causing death due to metastasis. It is also true that convincing histologic examples of melanoma (simulating rather precisely malignant melanoma of the superficial spreading type) appearing in congenital melanocytic nevi at birth or shortly thereafter do not behave as biologic melanoma.

Melanocytic Nevi of the Congenital Type
Further problems are presented by the phrase *congenital type*. Some acquired melanocytic nevi as well as congenital melanocytic nevi present at birth, as defined by history, show involvement of the lower reticular dermis by nevic tissue, a feature that has been considered to some extent diagnostic of a congenital nevus. Such involvement is much deeper and more extensive in the truly congenital lesions than it is in the acquired lesions, but both may or may not show involvement of the reticular dermis. Such histology has been used to determine whether or not a given lesion is congenital when no history is available. It is a good but imperfect criterion for true "congenitalness." We have photographically documented the emergence of nevi in the later years of childhood that microscopically showed

involvement of the deep reticular dermis. This feature may also be encountered in nevi of the face and head that were not congenital by history. Consequently, the designation of a lesion of this group as congenital cannot be done with certitude on histological grounds alone. We use the phrase *of the congenital type* to indicate involvement of the deep reticular dermis by nevic tissue in small lesions likely to be acquired and reserve *congenital melanocytic nevus* for those actually present at birth, as judged by the extent of involvement of the reticular dermis and subcutis or, preferably, by a dependable clinical history.

Histology of the Congenital Melanocytic Nevus

This description is of those nevi that are relatively flat but have substance on palpation and are tan to brown and rather uniformly colored. The tissue composing such lesions forms the bulk of congenital melanocytic nevi. The melanocytes of the epidermis are variable in distribution. They may be disposed, individually, along elongated rete or as orderly nests at the tips of rete. The characteristic histology is in the dermis. Small, pigment-free cells, about 6 μm in diameter, permeate through the entire dermis and extend into the subcutis, involving the fibrous trabeculae and tending to spare the fat. The nevic cells seem to use the connective tissue of the dermis and subcutis as their stroma, differing from common acquired nevi, which form their own stroma as they differentiate in their dermal component. The dermal appearance of congenital melanocytic nevi is one of small cell monotony. It is on this background that the various neurocristic neoplasias and overgrowths are superimposed. Rhodes and colleagues have discussed the histology of these congenital nevi in considerable detail.[80] In addition to the finding of nevus cells in the lower third of the reticular dermis, they have shown that the finding of nevus cells "around" and "within" skin appendages and structures such as hair follicles, sebaceous glands, nerves, and lymphatics adds specificity to the histologic diagnosis. It is likely, however, that none of these findings is completely pathognomonic in small nevi. The best single criterion, in fact, is size greater than 1.5 cm.

Lesions Arising in Congenital Melanocytic Nevi

At Birth or in the Neonatal Period

Simulants of Superficial Spreading Melanoma. The epidermis may present an increased number of large epithelioid melanocytes disposed as individual cells and in nests at all levels of the epidermis. A similar cellular pattern may also be present in the immediately subjacent dermis (Fig. 49–40). Such histology is, of course, suggestive of malignant melanoma of the superficial spreading type. Cytologically, the cells are somewhat different from melanoma. The nuclei are relatively uniform, circular, uniformly chromatic, and lack prominent macronucleoli. The cytoplasm is uniformly pigmented, but the pigment is coarsely rather than finely granular. This dermoepidermal pathology may be seen in association with large nodular neurocristic hamartomas, but is also common in black areas of congenital melanocytic nevi that are relatively flat and without any tumorous overgrowths. We usually report the changes just described as "atypical melanocytic proliferation in a congenital melanocytic nevus." This is followed by a note stating that lesions with this histology have not behaved as malignant melanoma in our experience.

Simulants of Nodular Melanoma

MULTIPLE BLACK NODULES <5 MM IN DIAMETER. The lesions are globoid, smooth, uniformly black nodules. One may see several such lesions. Progressive growth does not occur, and the lesions become lighter and less conspicuous during the next several months. These small nodules are composed of epithelioid melanocytes significantly larger than the surrounding nevic tissue. The contrast between the cells of the nodules and the nevus may be striking, but the two

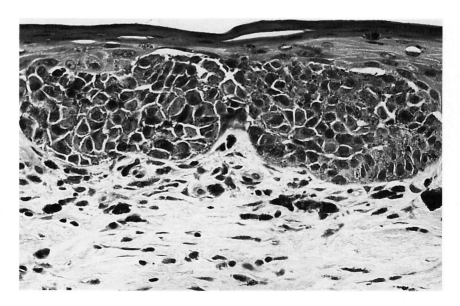

Figure 49–40. Congenital melanocytic nevus with an area that is a simulant of superficial spreading melanoma. The nests of large, atypical melanocytes bulge downward from the dermoepidermal interface. In other areas there was intraepidermal pagetoid growth of melanocytic, further simulating melanoma.

cell types often seem to blend at the periphery of the nodule. A few mitotic figures may be observed. No necrosis is present. The changes suggest a small nodular melanoma, but there is no evidence that such lesions presenting in the perinatal period behave as biologic melanoma. We usually diagnose these lesions as "atypical dermal melanocytic proliferation in a congenital melanocytic nevus." An appended note indicates the lack of biologic malignancy. Similar lesions developing in older children and adults should be given a more guarded prognosis, but the biologic melanomas occurring in childhood are distinguishable from these small nodules of proliferative melanocytes. (See the section on melanoma developing in congenital melanocytic nevi.)

SINGLE BLACK NODULES >5 MM IN DIAMETER. These lesions are uncommon and have occurred in smaller congenital melanocytic nevi, some 3 to 8 cm wide, as well as in the large lesions. They are present at birth and grow rapidly. Ulceration and bleeding may occur but are not notable or disturbing. Metastases have not been observed, but the natural history of these lesions is not known for their clinical presentation has been an imperative for their removal. Microscopically, the constituent cells are large, epithelioid, and have an abundance of amply pigmented cytoplasm (Fig. 49–41). Nuclei are uniform and nucleoli inconspicuous.

There is no lymphocytic response. The lesions and the cells composing them are much larger than the multiple small black nodules just described. These lesions, seen in neonates, are also signed out as atypical dermal melanocytic proliferation, with a detailed descriptive note.

Large, Multinodular, Rapidly Growing Overgrowths: Congenital, Proliferative Neurocristic Hamartomas

CLINICAL APPEARANCE. These malformations usually occur in the large truncal congenital melanocytic nevi. More than 50% of the trunk may be involved by a saddlelike lesion that tends to wrap around the body dorsoventrally. The nevus is multicolored, hairy, and thick on palpation. Irregular black areas are common. The superimposed proliferative hamartomas are large and may involve a significant portion of the underlying lesion. They may present as a glistening, partially ulcerated excrescence that is pink, gray, and black. Such lesions are polypoid and have a broad attachment at the base rather than a narrow stalk. An alternative appearance is that of multiple irregular nodular masses, firm on palpation and ill defined at the margins. Ulceration is less prominent than in the polypoid masses but is usually seen. The hamartomas are present at birth and may grow rapidly during the first few weeks of life. Apparently, some of

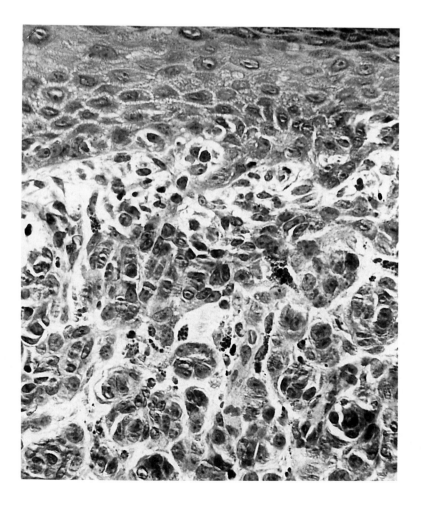

Figure 49–41. Congenital melanocytic nevus with an area that is a simulant of nodular melanoma. The histology is that of a black nodule >5 mm in diameter present at the time of birth and growing rapidly immediately thereafter.

these may appear after birth, in the neonatal period or in the early months of life.

PATHOLOGY. The pathology is as dramatic as the clinical picture is alarming. The bulk of the tissue forming these large masses is a nondescript mesenchyme, doubtless a neuromesenchyme akin to schwannian tissue. Within this one may see a variety of tissue forms reflecting their neural crest ancestry. Cartilage may be orderly and disorderly (Fig. 49–42); differentiated schwannian tissue attempts to ensheathe nonexistent nerve twigs and simulate them in the process (Fig. 49–43); skeletal muscle and even small foci of extramedullary hematopoieses are a part of the hamartoma. Melanocytes or their obvious derivatives are invariably present. Immediately deep to the epidermis they are seen as small epithelioid cells with some coarsely granular pigment arrayed singly or in small nests (Fig. 49–44). These areas are similar to the outer portion of the dermal component of acquired nevi. Other melanocytic components include areas similar to the single black nodules described in a previous section. These areas present as ill-defined islands of epithelioid melanocytes. The cells are pigmented with coarse, granular melanin. Their nuclei are rather small and uniform. Mitoses are rare. If one should see aggregates of small, relatively pigment-free pleomorphic melanocytes with a high mitotic rate, malignant melanoma is to be feared. Such histology is rare in the congenital, proliferative hamartomas.

Malignant Melanoma. The terminology applied to congenital neurocristic hamartomas as just described is imprecise. Many such lesions are called malignant melanoma, but it is difficult to state with clarity the histology of melanomas that are biologically malignant. As far as we can determine from the literature and from our experience, those lesions that have given rise to metastases are composed of small "blastic" pleomorphic cells. These unquestioned melanomas are described more fully in the next section.

Proliferations in Childhood and in Adult Life

Intraepidermal Melanocytic Growth Simulating a Dysplastic Nevus. Most congenital melanocytic nevi, regardless of size, show continuing intraepidermal melanocytic growth throughout life; the purely dermal congenital nevus does not occur or is rare. The intraepidermal melanocytic growth is commonly along narrow, elongated rete. The melanocytes may be large, and casual inspection may result in some worry and even diagnoses of dysplasia or in situ melanoma; overdiagnosis is common in these lesions. These large melanocytes lack the hyperchromatism, the folded nuclear envelope, the prominent nucleolus, and the occasional mitotic figure seen in various degrees in melanoma in situ and to a lesser extent in dysplastic nevi. The congenital melanocytic nevus is not, however, spared from developing either dysplasia or melanoma. The histologic criteria required for the diagnosis of either of these entities should be compelling

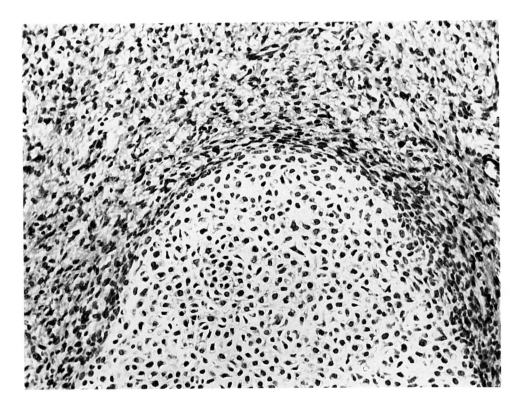

Figure 49–42. Congenital, proliferative neurocristic hamartoma arising in a large, congenital melanocytic nevus. An island of cartilage is depicted in a background of neuromesenchymal tissue, the latter forming the bulk of a massive tumor.

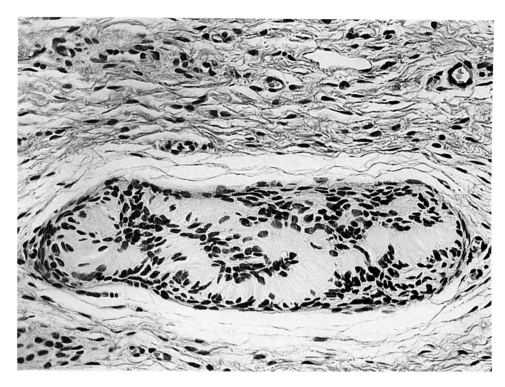

Figure 49–43. Congenital, proliferative neurocristic hamartoma arising in a large, congenital melanocytic nevus. A structure is shown that simulates a giant Wagner-Meissner corpuscle.

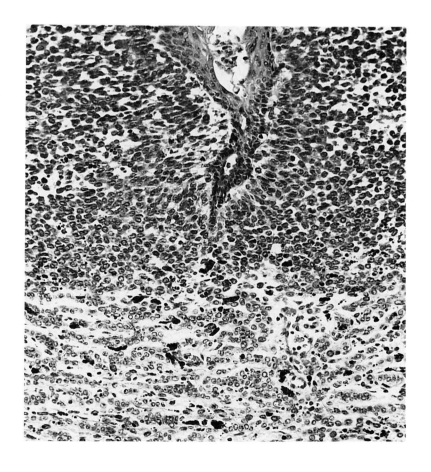

Figure 49–44. Congenital, proliferative neurocristic hamartoma arising in a large congenital melanocytic nevus. A subepidermal area that resembles the kinds of true melanoma occasionally arising in congenital melanocytic nevi. The cells are small and blastlike but not as disturbing as those in Figures 49–45 and 49–46. Further, they tend to blend with the subjacent smaller cells of orderly nevic tissue.

and classic before one can be certain that dysplasia or melanoma has developed within a congenital melanocytic nevus.

Deep Spindle Cell Neoplasms. Nodular tumors that are 1 cm or less in width when first detected may develop within congenital nevi of children or adults. Search for these relatively deep nodules should be a part of the routine follow-up of patients with congenital melanocytic nevi, and patients should be advised to search for them during self-examination. Histologically, these tumors are composed of tightly packed spindle cells that are essentially pigment free. There is no unanimity in terminology or concepts of biologic potential with regard to these lesions. We have heard them called malignant blue nevi, malignant melanomas, and malignant spindle cell neoplasms. We are not sure that these lesions are malignant in spite of their histology. A spindle cell morphology has not been the histology of the malignant melanomas we have seen in congenital melanocytic nevi. We sign out these tumors descriptively, "atypical spindle cell neoplasm of unknown biologic potential, arising in a congenital melanocytic nevus." This is followed by a note suggesting moderate excision margins and careful monitoring of the patients. We have not encountered dissemination of disease from this sort of tumor, but the cases are so uncommon as to preclude any generalizations concering their biology.

Malignant Melanoma. Some firm conclusions may be drawn about what is malignant melanoma in these lesions. The difficulty arises in determining what is *not* malignant melanoma. First we address the melanomas. The lesions usually arise beyond the neonatal period and may be inconspicuous. A small nodule appears, with a history of a short time of growth. This as a rule occurs in a congenital melanocytic nevus without a congenital neurocristic hamartoma. The lesion is sharply circumscribed and composed of partially confluent nests of small, pleomorphic, epithelioid melanocytes (Figs. 49–45 and 49–46). The cells of the melanoma do not blend or fuse with the surrounding nevic tissue, as is common in the superficial melanoma simulants. Pigment is sparse or absent and mitoses common (may be > 6/mm^2). Nuclear chromatin is condensed irregularly at the nuclear envelope, macronucleoli are prominent, and the intervening nucleoplasm relatively clear. Such nuclear characteristics are common in malignancy, especially melanoma. A lymphocytic response to these small nodules of melanoma cells is lacking. There is clear evidence that such cells are growing in an expansile form with growth preference over the surrounding tissues. The latter are pushed aside and replaced by the focus of malignancy. In the congenital neurocristic hamartoma, clusters of small pigment-synthesizing epithelioid melanocytes occurring deep to an epidermis showing pagetoid intraepidermal melanocytic growth must

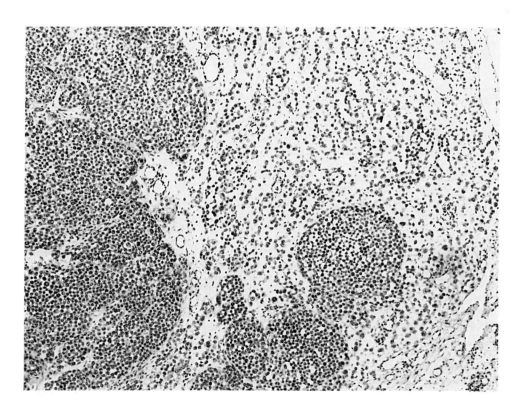

Figure 49–45. Malignant melanoma arising in a large congenital melanocytic nevus in a 2.5-year-old child. The tumor presented as a new small red papule. The cells are blastic but large compared with those of Figure 49–44. The cells are sharply delineated from the surrounding nevus; blending does not occur. The nodule was immediately deep to the epidermis without a demonstrable epidermal component.

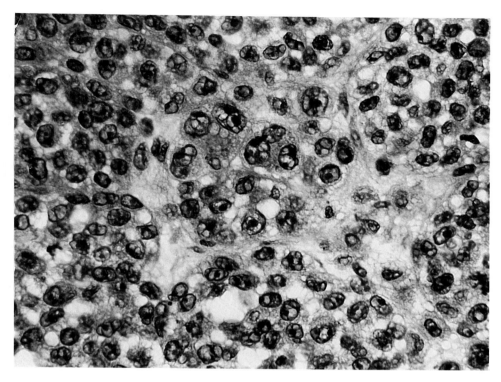

Figure 49–46. Malignant melanoma arising in a large congenital melanocytic nevus in a 2.5-year-old child. The cellular detail of the melanoma cells is illustrated. The child died of metastatic disease 5 months after definitive therapy.

be distinguished from the true melanomas. These areas simulate malignant melanoma of the superficial spreading type and are not melanoma. In the presence of the disorderly growth of neural crest-derived tissue in congenital proliferative neurocristic hamartomas, it is difficult to state that some other cell and tissue types will not behave as malignancies. When in doubt, it is best to follow the advice of Ross and Henderson and carefully describe the lesions, suggesting that malignant behavior may occur.

MELANOMAS ARISING IN THE DERMAL COMPONENT OF A NEVUS

One occasionally sees a lesion at scanning magnification that is similar to a large dermal nevus and that proves to be quite the contrary on examination at higher magnification. Much of the lesion (the amount is quite variable) has the histology of a dermal nevus, but foci of the nevus are replaced by relatively large epithelioid melanocytes with variable amounts of pigment. These cells grow contiguously and replace a portion of the background nevus. If one actually sees the epithelioid melanocytes and considers the diagnosis, recognition of these lesion as melanoma is not difficult. The cells are large, pleomorphic, and clearly different from the surrounding nevic tissue. Mitotic figures are present almost invariably. They may not be numerous, and painstaking search at 400 magnification may be required. When found, they strongly suggest the diagnosis of melanoma. An intraepidermal component may be inconspicuous

or absent. From this and the association of these lesions with the dermal component of a large dermal nevus, the inference of histogenesis from the dermal component of a nevus is generated.

ATYPICAL DERMAL MELANOCYTIC TUMORS SIMILAR TO SPONTANEOUS AND INDUCED MELANOMAS IN ANIMALS

These rare tumors present as slowly evolving black nodules. The surface is rough and the border irregular while tending to be circular. The first reaction to the histology of the tumor is surprise, in that it seems to be entirely composed of melanophages (Fig. 49–47). It is a nodular collection of cells so burdened with pigment that nuclei are obscured. Careful study reveals that many cells are distinguishable from melanophages. Some nuclear detail is discernible: nucleoli are prominent, chromatin condensed peripherally, and nucleoplasm generally clear. The melanin produces an opaque brown cytoplasm lacking most of the resolvable coarse granules of the melanophage. The melanin-rich melanocytes aggregate and, apparently with growth, become less melanized and then may be more easily distinguished from the melanophages. An occasional mitotic figure may be identified, and bleached sections may be quite helpful in revealing these and other nuclear characteristics. In experimental systems, the less pigmented cells will, in time, form distinctive clusters and after this will metastasize.[3] Precisely analogous events have not been encountered in

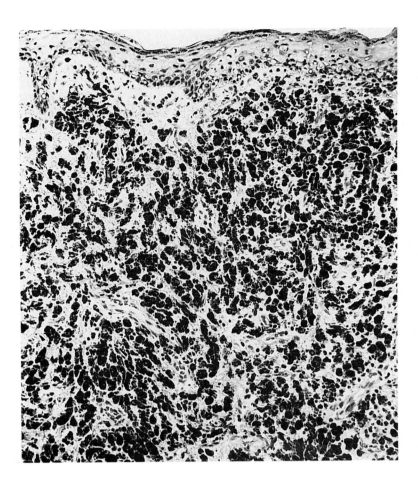

Figure 49–47. Atypical dermal melanocytic tumor, ? malignant melanoma. The lesion is composed almost entirely of melanophages. Multiple sections showed some large epithelioid melanocytes. The neoplasm is similar to some induced and spontaneous melanomas in animals. The biologic potential is unknown. Metastasis to regional nodes has been observed, but not dissemination. Usually there are no metastases of any kind.

the similar human tumors we have seen. The biologic potential of these tumors consequently remains unknown. A single example metastasized to a regional lymph node, but dissemination did not follow. These lesions are signed out descriptively and cautiously, indicating the possibility of malignancy and the similarity to induced and spontaneous animal tumors. Excision with moderate margins and careful monitoring of the patients are required. Unequivocal designation as melanoma is not appropriate.

DERMAL MELANOMAS THAT ARE OF A PURE POPULATION OF SPINDLE CELLS

Is there such a thing as a malignant blue nevus? One occasionally encounters spindle cell dermal neoplasms, closely applied to the epidermis, of such form that a diagnosis of malignancy is required. These lesions are commonly located on the face and, less commonly, on the foot. In the former location, the differential diagnosis includes atypical fibroxanthoma (superficial malignant fibrous histiocytoma) and spindle cell squamous cell carcinoma, along with such uncommon possibilities as fibrosarcoma in a radiation scar. The actual melanomas in this group may have an inconspicuous increase in atypical intraepidermal melanocytes and some pigment. Antibodies to S-100 protein and low-molecular-weight keratins are valuable in the proper classification of these lesions. In routine histological preparations, the cells of spindle cell melanomas tend to be closely apposed and do not blend with the connective tissue of the dermis as is characteristic of atypical fibroxanthomas and spindle cell squamous cell carcinomas. Further, the melanomas tend to be less pleomorphic than the other two common, confounding, spindle cell neoplasms.

Malignant blue nevus is also a diagnostic problem. Many pathologists call a malignant dermal spindle cell malignancy of melanocytic origin a malignant blue nevus for want of any other diagnosis. Such shoehorning of difficult lesions into existing categories is a serious error diffused throughout pathology and medicine and is discussed in the last section of this chapter. True malignant blue nevi must be preciously rare. The criteria for the appropriate use of this diagnostic category include the presence of some remnant of a blue nevus with classical histologic features. One notes a compact, cellular spindle cell neoplasm superimposed on this. Almost without exception, some pigment is seen in these cells. Mitotic figures are present, and areas of necrosis are seen. If mitotic figures are inconspicuous and necrosis absent, the diagnosis of melanoma should not be made. However, worrisome cases should be reported with a good descriptive note indicating that attributes of malignancy such as local recurrence or even metastasis are possible. Complete excision should be carried out. All of the problematic spindle cell neoplasms should be carefully searched for neurotropism.

MALIGNANT MELANOMA OF SOFT PARTS

A deep-seated soft tissue tumor bound to tendon, aponeurosis, or fascia was described by Enzinger in 1965.[81] The glycogen-filled clear cells in routine hematoxylin and eosin preparations led to the designation clear cell sarcoma. Since that time, many examples of the tumor have been shown to contain melanin. Chung and Enzinger have reviewed the literature and reported 141 cases of the neoplasm.[82] Melanin was demonstrated in 72% of 92 tumors examined by the Warthin-Starry and Fontana methods. Thirteen of 19 tumors reacted with S-100 protein. They concluded that "(1) clear cell sarcoma represents a malignant neuroectodermal tumor derived from potentially melanogenic cells that have migrated from the neural crest during embryonal life and (2) that the tumor is in many aspects akin to malignant melanoma and malignant blue nevus." The tumors occur at a median age of 27 years and may be seen in both children and the elderly. They are somewhat more common in females than in males. Some 12% of soft part melanomas occur in blacks and 5% in patients of Asiatic origin, racial predilections that are quite different from other forms of melanoma. For example, superficial spreading melanoma does not occur in blacks and is uncommon in Asiatics, whereas blacks and Asiatics form a significantly higher percentage of acral lentiginous melanomas (in this country) than they do of soft part melanomas. The tumors present as slowly growing masses, frequently of long duration, of the foot, ankle, and knee region or, less commonly, of the upper extremities. Examples on the trunk, head, and neck are rare. The prognosis is poor. The natural history of the disease is marked by chronicity with multiple recurrences over a period of years, and 43.5% of patients died of metastases in the series reported by Chung and Enzinger.

Grossly, the lesions are similar to sarcomas, and one fourth of them have brown or black areas. Microscopically, the cells are disposed in compact nests and short fascicles (Figs. 49–48 and 49–49); the cytoplasm is clear or granular and eosinophilic (Fig. 49–50); multinucleated cells are observed (Fig. 49–51); and mitotic figures are not numerous. Pigment is obvious or may be demonstrated in about two thirds of the cases.

DIFFERENTIAL DIAGNOSIS, ESPECIALLY HISTOLOGIC DIFFERENTIAL DIAGNOSIS

The distinctive features of the early stages of the radial growth phase of malignant melanoma of the superficial spreading type have been discussed and tabulated while discussing dysplastic nevi. The reader should review these characteristics before studying other aspects of the differential diagnosis.

EPITHELIOID CELL NEVUS: SPITZ TUMOR

Clinical Features
Spitz tumors appear and grow rapidly over a period of 6 weeks to several months, reaching a size of about 4 to 6 mm. At this size, growth usually ceases. The prototypical lesion is an elevated globoid pink lesion. A small percentage

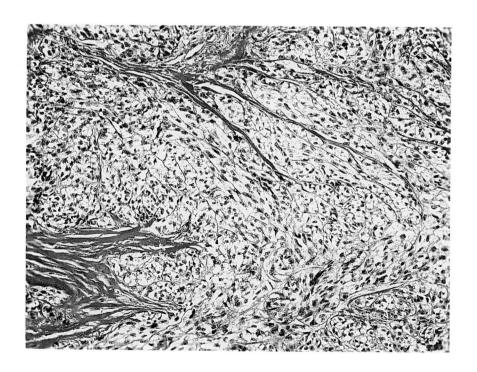

Figure 49–48. Soft tissue melanoma (clear cell sarcoma). The fasciculated pattern of clear cells, separated by fibrous septa, is illustrated. A characteristic histologic picture (*Courtesy of Sharon Weiss. AFIP Photograph 1203352*).

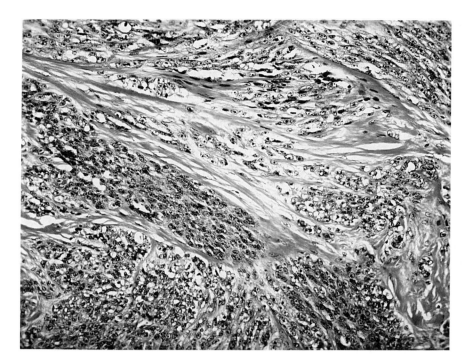

Figure 49–49. Soft tissue melanoma (clear cell sarcoma). The cytoplasm of the cells is less clear than those of Figure 49–48, but the fasciculated pattern is still obvious (*Courtesy of Sharon Weiss. AFIP Photograph 1650739*).

of the lesions are pigmented. The subsequent life history of the tumor includes the options of persistence with stability, fibroplasia, or differentiation along lines resembling a common acquired nevus. The tumors are common over the lower extremities, face, and buttocks but may be seen almost anywhere on the skin. The age incidence is skewed toward the early decades of life, but the elderly may develop classic Spitz tumors. When the diagnosis is made after the fourth decade of life, the clinical and histologic features should be compellingly classic. There are malignant melano-

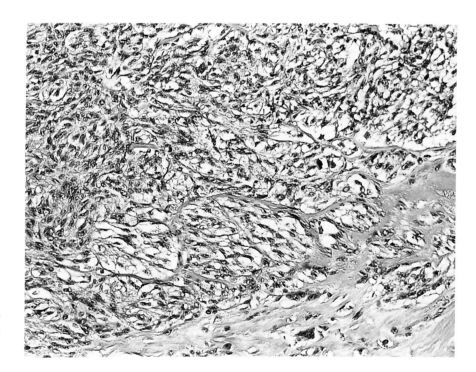

Figure 49–50. Soft tissue melanoma (clear cell sarcoma). The clear cells and delicate septa are pictured (*Courtesy of Richard J. Reed*).

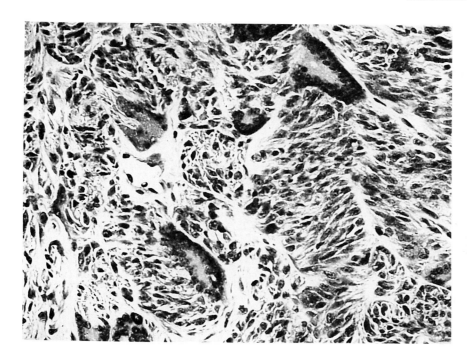

Figure 49–51. Soft tissue melanoma (clear cell sarcoma). Large giant cells, seen with some frequency in these lesions, are represented. Similar cells are seen, interestingly enough, in a variety of cutaneous melanocytic lesions (*Courtesy of Sharon Weiss*).

mas that somewhat resemble Spitz tumors (and here we are not referring to minimal deviation melanomas of the spitzian type). Such melanomas are usually at a stage having a high risk for metastasis. The differential diagnosis, in relationship to a Spitz tumor, is therefore between a high-risk melanoma and the benign epithelioid cell nevus.

Histologic Features

This description applies primarily to those epithelioid cell nevi that are pigment free or oligomelanotic, about 80 to 90% of the cases. The microscopic pathology of the lesions may be conveniently divided into the following areas: the intraepidermal component, the superficial dermal component, the deep dermal component and the manner of infiltration of the reticular dermis, the cytology of the individual cells, the stroma and the host cellular immune response, and the architecture of the lesions.

The Intraepidermal Component. The cells are usually disposed in nests. Such nests may be quite large and may bridge the entire thickness of the epidermis. They are more commonly in the lower half of the epidermis and at the dermoepidermal interface, bulging into the papillary dermis. Individual cells are not as prominent as the nests and are in the basal layer of the epidermis or in the lower spinous layers. The occasional presence of a few individual cells in the upper layers of the epidermis, in and of itself, is not an imperative for the diagnosis of melanoma. Occasionally a Spitz tumor may be entirely or largely intraepidermal. Such lesions may be difficult to distinguish from malignant melanoma of the superficial spreading type. They can be differentiated, as a rule on the basis of cytology (to be presently addressed), by the tendency to dominance of nests over single cells and by the presence of eosinophilic globular bodies in the epidermis and at the dermoepidermal inter-

face. These bodies, described by Kamino and co-workers, are similar to the fibrillary bodies seen in lichenoid reactions.[83] Such bodies are frequently about the size of one of the large epithelioid melanocytes and are roughly circular and somewhat irregular in outline. The pink bodies are usually dispersed individually but may be seen in small clusters. They may occur in other entities, including malignant melanoma, but are numerous enough in Spitz tumors to be of diagnostic help in conjunction with other histologic features. There are examples of Spitz tumors without an intraepidermal component.

The Superficial Dermal Component. Immediately deep to the epidermis the cells are disposed in large nests, frequently larger than the intraepidermal nests. In some instances, such nests may be within the dermal papillae, one nest to a papilla, and the undulating appearance of the dermoepidermal interface is preserved. When present, this finding is helpful in distinguishing Spitz tumors from malignant melanoma. When melanoma cells grow contiguously at the dermoepidermal interface or in nests in the papillary dermis, the rete-papillae pattern is usually effaced and appears as a relatively straight line. Infrequently, the superficial dermal component of a Spitz tumor appears as a solid collection of cells; nesting is inapparent.

The Deep Dermal Component and the Manner of Infiltration of the Reticular Dermis. Below the nested or solid pattern of growth, just described, the cells may permeate as individual cells between the collagen bundles of the reticular dermis. The cells, usually retaining their large epithelioid form, appear well into the reticular dermis, where they may be seen alone, as it were, without host response or other tumor cells. This pattern of extension into the reticular dermis is one of the most helpful histologic features for distinguishing the lesions from malignant melanoma. Melanoma cells do not permeate the reticular dermis in this manner; the malignant cells appear as columns or strands. Maturation of the large cells of epithelioid cell nevi into cells similar to those of an ordinary dermal nevus occurs but is uncommon. There is evidence, however, that some Spitz tumors may mature, in their entirety, to an ordinary melanocytic nevus. We have seen convincing examples of this kind of maturation occur in multiple eruptive Spitz tumors appearing within giant hairy nevi.

The Cytology of the Individual Cells. The epithelioid cell that is the prototype of this tumor is large, commonly 15 to 25 μm wide. The cytoplasm is a dull pink, having taken a bit of hematoxylin in routine preparations. The cytoplasm may have a fine fibrillary quality. Nuclei are large, and macronucleoli are routinely observed. Mitotic figures, even abnormal ones, may occasionally be numerous. One more often sees only a few typical mitoses, which are more common superficially than deep. Many Spitz nevi have no mitoses at all, a negative finding that may be quite reassuring in a difficult case. The cytology of the cells may be very disturbing. If one observes but a single microscopic field, at 250 to 400 magnification, one is tempted to call the lesion malignant. There is, however, in contrast to melanoma, a monotony to the disturbing cytology: As one moves from field to field, the cells look the same except for some tendency to mature (become smaller) as they descend into the dermis, a feature by no means present in every case. Melanomas are much more heterogeneous, the cells varying from small to large, from bizarre to a normal appearance, and from copious amounts of dusty tan pigment to none. At the fine structural level, most melanosomes in epithelioid cell nevi show many melanofilaments, frequently with the distinctive striated appearance. The melanosomes may be much larger than normal, but the granular melanosomes and melanosomes with only a suggestion of a melanofilament or two, so characteristic of melanoma, are uncommon in epithelioid cell nevi. The essential absence of evidence of pigment synthesis on melanosomes of Spitz tumors distinguishes them from all but the rare primary melanoma.

Stroma and the Host Cellular Immune Response. The stroma is frequently very vascular, contributing to the pink color of many of these lesions. In some instances, there may be no epidermal component, and the dermis may be so sclerotic as to widely separate the tumor cells. Such fibrotic variants have been called desmoplastic nevi by Barr and associates.[84] The response of host cells of the cellular immune system is variable. There may at times be a relatively dense infiltrate of lymphocytes. More frequently the response is patchy and sparse. Macrophages are occasionally common, and when admixed with the large cells of the tumor, the lesion has something of a granulomatous appearance.

Architecture of the Lesions. The tumors that are dominated by a dermal component are usually symmetrical in cross section, appearing as a coronal hemisection of a hot-air balloon. Such symmetry obviously does not apply to the lesions that are largely intraepidermal.

Lesions Demonstrating Pigment Synthesis. Pigment synthesis, when present, may be exuberant and is usually present throughout the lesion. Intraepidermal Spitz nevi commonly show pigment synthesis, and some of the cells in such lesions may have prominent pigment-containing dendrites. The pigment may be coarsely granular and rarely has the dusty quality of the cells of malignant melanoma of the superficial spreading type.

PIGMENTED SPINDLE CELL NEVUS

Some observers tend to incorporate the pigmented spindle cell nevi with classic Spitz tumors, as attested to by the names *epithelioid* and *spindle cell nevus*. There is overlap between the two lesions, but we classify them as separate entities because the clinical presentation and the histology are distinctive for each of the lesions in their most common forms.[85] Furthermore, codification as disparate entities emphasizes the difference between the two lesions in relationship to the reticular dermis. Pigmented spindle cell nevi do not involve the reticular dermis. A distinguishing feature of Spitz tumors is the permeation of individual large epithelioid cells into the reticular dermis.

Clinical Features

Pigmented spindle cell nevi appear, grow rapidly, and become stable at a size of 4 to 6 mm and in these respects are similar to the classic epithelioid cell nevus. In contrast to that lesion, however, these tumors are invariably pigmented and deeply so, being dark brown or deep black. In addition, they appear with some frequency as a circular plaque or disk rather than a globoid lesion, though the latter form is also seen. The lesions occur at an older median age and are more frequent on the lower extremity of female patients than are Spitz tumors. A common presentation is that of black lesion on the thigh of a female between 20 and 40 years of age; it appeared suddenly, grew rapidly, and was then stable. In contrast to Spitz nevi, in which the clinical diagnosis is often benign (angioma or nevus), pigmented spindle cell nevi may be submitted to pathologists with a clinical diagnosis of melanoma. This may be partly responsible for overdiagnosis by some pathologists.

Histologic Features

The lesion presents nests of spindle-shaped melanocytes at the dermoepidermal interface. The long axis of the nests and the cells composing the nests tends to be perpendicular to the epidermal surface (Fig. 49–52). The nests tend to be rather regularly spaced, in contrast to melanoma, in which nests are haphazardly spaced and are variable in size and form. Mitotic figures may be numerous in these nests, and cellular pleomorphism may be alarming in a few lesions. This feature, alone, in the nests of the dermoepidermal interface is insufficient evidence for a diagnosis of melanoma. The cells are deeply pigmented, and the pigment is coarsely granular. The lesion involves the papillary dermis in virtually all cases. Here the cells are also nested, spindle shaped, and pigmented. The nests have a more haphazard array than those of the dermoepidermal interface. A host response of lymphocytes is routine, as are many melano-

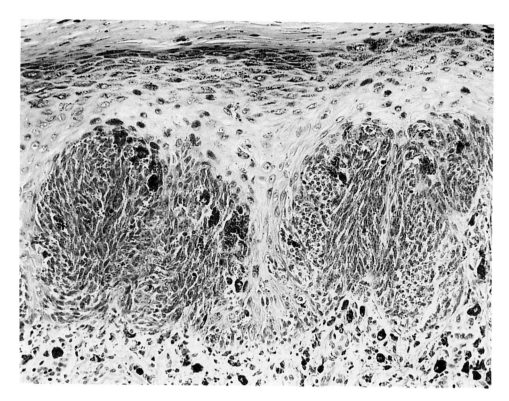

Figure 49–52. Compound pigmented spindle cell tumor (nevus) of Reed. The melanocytes are spindled in form and, as a rule, nested. The long axis of the nests and the cells tend to be perpendicular to the epidermis. The lesions are distinguishable from true epithelioid cell nevi (Spitz tumors).

phages. If there is significant involvement of the reticular dermis, one should not make a diagnosis of a pigmented spindle cell nevus, because the lesion could be a melanoma or some other spindle cell melanocytic neoplasm.

CELLULAR BLUE NEVUS

The diagnosis of cellular blue nevus is used rather permissively by pathologists, being applied somewhat casually to various blue nevi with areas of closely packed spindle cells. If the term is appropriately applied, it defines a distinct clinicopathologic entity that presents as an elevated nodular blue lesion, usually on the buttocks. A somewhat less well-defined lesion that occurs on the scalp may also be called a cellular blue nevus. These two forms of cellular blue nevi are somehwat different in clinical presentation, pathology, and biologic significance.

Histologic Features
The cellular blue nevus of the buttocks is usually greater than 1 cm wide and is somewhat larger than most ordinary blue nevi. It is firm, blue, and has an ill-defined margin. The lesion of the scalp is a firm blue plaque, irregular in outline, and commonly greater than 1.5 cm wide.

Pathology
The cellular blue nevus of the buttocks presents a unique histology. There is a background lesion similar to an ordinary fibrotic blue nevus. Bipolar, elongate pigment-containing cells are separated from each other by a rather acellular collagenous matrix. Superimposed on this are islands and peninsula-like collections of plump, closely packed, large spindle cells that are deeply pigmented (Figs. 49–53 and 49–54). The peninsulas of these cellular areas may project downward into the subcutaneous tissue. At first glance, the overall form of the lesion may be somewhat startling, and the compact cellularity in the islands and peninsulas may also be worrisome if one is not familiar with these lesions. One may occasionally see a suggestion of neurotropism and a rare mitotic figure without necrosis. We have not seen one of these lesions behave in a malignant fashion. There is, therefore, no evidence that these distinctive lesions undergo tumor progression to malignant melanoma (malignant blue nevus). True malignant blue nevi are exquisitely rare and are discussed as a separate category.

The cellular blue nevi of the scalp are a somewhat different matter. There may or may not be an ordinary blue nevus as a background lesion. The cellular component is not as sharply circumscribed as in the buttock lesions. It is composed of tightly packed spindle cells that may not contain much melanin. Pleomorphism is not usually striking, the worrisome histologic feature being hypercellularity. Such a histologic picture may dominate the entire lesion. These lesions, in contrast to the buttock lesions, may show progressive local growth requiring removal of the entire lesion. The tumors that are likely to be locally aggressive usually show mitotic activity and occasionally

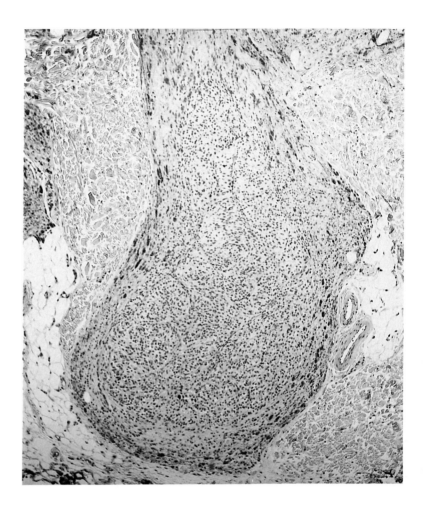

Figure 49–53. Cellular blue nevus. The peninsula-like base of the lesion is shown. At the periphery, the cells are elongate and bipolar, similar to the cells of an ordinary blue nevus. Centrally, the lesion is more cellular. The cells are rounded and contain less pigment.

foci of neurotropism. We have not seen such lesions metastasize nor behave as truly neurotropic melanomas. Necrosis, hardly ever seen in cellular blue nevi, is a finding that should strongly suggest frank malignancy.

ATYPICAL MELANOCYTIC NEVI OF THE GENITAL (VULVAR) TYPE

Clinical Features

The lesions are characteristically seen during the reproductive years but occasionally are encountered in children and in postmenopausal women. They have a monotonously uniform history: Discovery occurs during routine pregnancy examination, at delivery, or during self-examination. The lesions are black or dark brown with a hazy border and usually present a papular component. They generally do not clinically suggest melanoma of the mucosal lentiginous type. They are rarely larger than 5 mm in diameter and may be smaller.

Histologic Features

With only the rarest of exceptions, these lesions have a dermal component, which is an orderly dermal nevus. Over this is a broad and uniformly atypical area of melanocytic proliferation (Fig. 49–55).[86] It usually extends beyond the lateral margins of the underlying dermal nevus. This extension tends to be uniform, not ectopic as in melanocytic dysplasia. As a consequence, a given section of one of these genital atypical melanocytic nevi presents a dermal component capped by a broad T of melanocytic atypia. The melanocytes form an ill-defined band (a plate in three dimensions) that separates the keratinocytes above from the dermal nevus and dermis below. There may be considerable atypia of melanocytes and some extension into the dermis. Upward growth of the melanocytes is not seen to any extent, but the lesions may be suggestive of melanoma. The lesions may be seen in children and in postmenopausal women but are uncommon in these age-groups. Rarely, similar lesions have been seen on the male genitalia.

LENTIGO MALIGNA

The histology of lentigo maligna is unique when fully developed.[87] The epidermis is atrophic and overlies a dermis with advanced solar degeneration. The melanocytes are increased in number and dispersed as a row of large pigmented cells in the basilar region. The melanocytes are not usually contiguous, being separated from each other

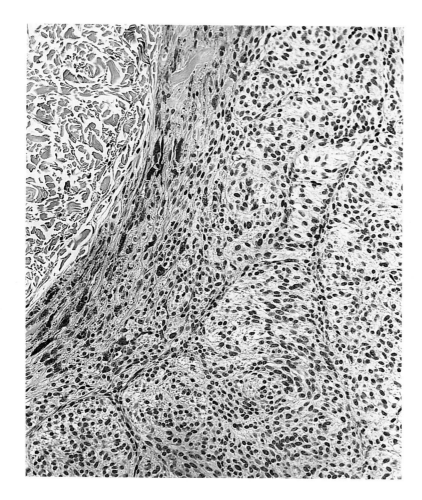

Figure 49–54. Cellular blue nevus. Higher magnification of Figure 49–53.

by one or more basilar keratinocytes. At irregular intervals a nest of melanocytes is noted at the dermoepidermal interface. The long axis of the nest tends to parallel the basal layer. The cells of the nest show dyshesion, being somewhat separate from each other. Such nested cells tend to be small, but a few moderately large and hyperchromatic nuclei are noted, giving evidence of some pleomorphism. Involvement of the external root sheath of pilar units is a common histologic feature. In some areas of lentigo maligna, the histology only shows elongated, narrow rete with an increased number of large melanocytes. Such areas may overlap some changes seen in dysplastic nevi. Additional biopsies or careful clinicopathologic correlation may be required to solve the problem. Lentigo maligna melanoma is distinguished from lentigo maligna by the presence of invasion. Invasion is not an obligate event in lentigo maligna. Though it has been stated to occur in one third to one half of the lesions of lentigo maligna, epidemiologic studies addressed to this point indicate that the actual progression to melanoma from lentigo maligna is less than 5%. This uncommon progression from lentigo maligna to lentigo maligna melanoma militates against classifying lentigo maligna as a form of melanoma in situ. For a lesion to be called melanoma in situ, progression to the invasive state should be the rule rather than the exception.

ACRAL MELANOCYTIC NEVI

Some melanocytic nevi removed from volar skin may show features that suggest the possibility of melanoma. Intraepidermal melanocytic growth often persists well into adult life. When most nevi on other parts of the skin have an inconspicuous intraepidermal component, volar nevi may present large intraepidermal nests of melanocytes that tend to bridge the entire thickness of the epidermis. Between the nests are an increased number of basilar melanocytes. These may be large but not atypical. The dermal component of such lesions is usually orderly, but some of the more superficial cells may be more prominent than those of most dermal nevi. A host lymphocytic response is absent, in contrast with the radial growth phase of acral lentiginous melanoma, which of course is typically much larger and more cellular.

CONJUNCTIVAL MELANOCYTIC NEVI

Conjunctival melanocytic nevi may show varying degrees of atypia histologically, and cursory inspection may suggest melanoma (Figs. 49–56, 49–57, and 49–58). Do not examine them cursorily. They are difficult. Folberg has provided

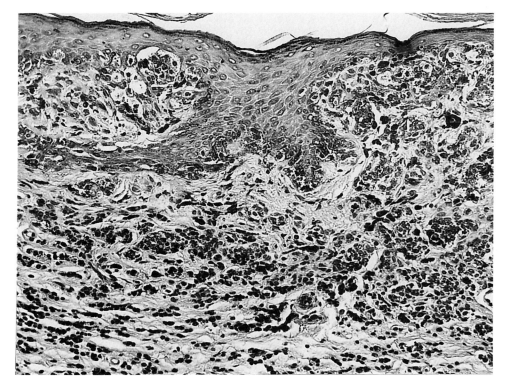

Figure 49–55. Atypical melanocytic hyperplasia of the genital (vulvar) type. The worrisome cells appear at the dermoepidermal interface, almost as a plaque of disturbing melanocytes, separating epidermis above from orderly nevic tissue below. Similar lesions occasionally appear on the male genitalia.

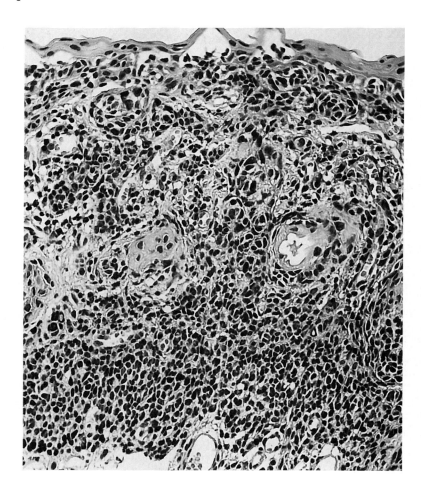

Figure 49–56. Compound nevus of the conjunctiva. The epithelium is almost replaced by small melanocytes, arrayed in a disorganized pattern (*Courtesy of Robert M. Folberg*).

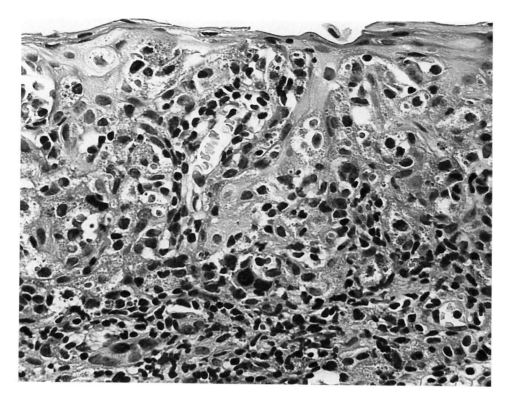

Figure 49–57. Compound nevus of the conjunctiva. The intraepithelial growth of melanocytes simulates a melanoma, but the cells are smaller. Lesion occurring in a prepubertal child (*Courtesy of Robert M. Folberg*).

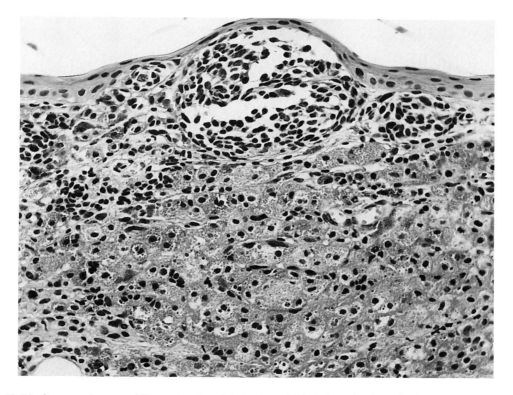

Figure 49–58. Compound nevus of the conjunctiva. A lesion in a child at about the time of puberty. The cells just below the epithelium have an abundance of finely pigmented cytoplasm. The changes are similar to dermal melanocytic hyperplasia (see Fig. 49–68) (*Courtesy of Robert M. Folberg*).

the following guidelines for the examination of histologically borderline melanocytic conjunctival lesions. Conjunctival melanomas are rare in childhood and adolescence. Conjunctival nevi that are entirely juctional are rare, even in childhood. One should be exceedingly cautious before making a diagnosis of a pure junctional nevus, especially in an adult. Such pure lesions, even when accompanied by nesting of melanocytes, are likely to be precursors of melanoma in an adult (known clinically to ophthalmologists as *primary acquired melanosis*). Most conjunctival nevi occur in the bulbar conjunctiva in the interpalpebral fissure (a light-exposed surface). Ordinary nevi are uncommon on the palpebral conjunctiva (the conjunctiva lining the inner surface of the eyelid). The intraepithelial component of a benign compound nevus terminates usually near the edge of the subepithelial component. Extension of intraepithelial melanocytes beyond the peripheral limits of the subepithelial component should raise the suspicion of a lesion more ominous than a compound nevus. It should be kept in mind that there are no firm rules separating the atypical nevus from melanoma. For example, it is frequently stated that epithelial cysts occur in benign lesions. However, melanomas may arise in nevi containing epithelial cysts. Dense lymphocytic infiltrates are said to be a disturbing feature, but benign nevi with very dense lymphocytic plasma cell infiltrates are common at the time of puberty (Fig. 49–59). Mitotic

figures suggest malignancy, but a few mitoses are not compellingly diagnostic of melanoma without other features. Finally, classic examples of Spitz tumors are seen on the conjunctiva.

CUTANEOUS METASTATIC MALIGNANT MELANOMA

A small epidermotropic metastasis may show extensive epidermal involvement and may precisely simulate a primary nodular melanoma (Figs. 49–60 and 49–61). The clue to its recognition as a metastasis is size, the invariable absence of a radial growth, and the routine paucity of a lymphocytic response. Most such lesions, when no more than about 3 to 4 mm in width, show extension well into the reticular dermis, and tumor cell groups are occasionally noted in dermal lymphatics. Such a combination of size and deep invasion is unusual—not unheard of—in a primary melanoma. Tumor cells may be found in a dermal lymphatic at the lesional edge. However, we have noted this finding in lesions judged to be benign (Spitz nevi, for example). Final determination of the nature of such lesions frequently requires detailed clinical information. We have encountered lesions with histology suggestive of an epidermotropic metastasis that proved to be primary melanomas, and the

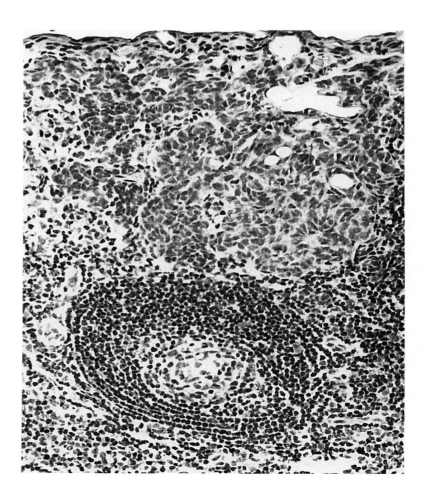

Figure 49–59. Compound nevus of the conjunctiva. A lymphocytic infiltrate with a germinal center associated with the nevus is portrayed, a feature at times seen in these lesions (*Courtesy of Robert M. Folberg*).

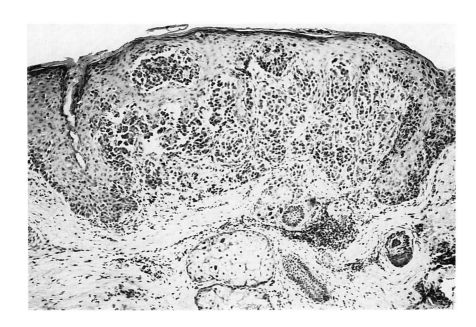

Figure 49–60. Metastatic, epidermotropic melanoma. The lesions may precisely mimic a primary melanoma. It is unusual, however, for a primary melanoma to show this much dermal invasion in a lesion this small.

converse error is also common in our referral practices. At times, the cutaneous metastasis may be composed of very orderly and small melanocytes, and in such instances the differential diagnosis is between a benign nevus and melanoma. Cursory examination at low-power magnification may overlook the features indicating malignancy: the presence of mitotic figures in the dermal component and involvement of the epidermis by individual melanocytes above the basal layer.

HALO NEVI

The usual halo nevus shows a dense lymphocytic infiltrate into the dermal component of the lesion associated with some intraepidermal melanocytic hyperplasia (Fig. 49–62). In some instances, however, the hyperplasia of melanocytes at the dermoepidermal interface and in the upper dermis may be extensive, with cytologic atypia. The absence of upward growth of melanocytes in the epidermis and the

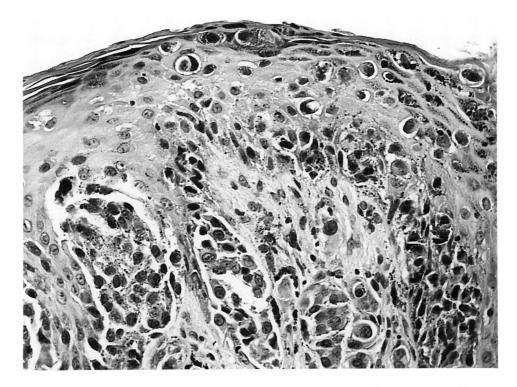

Figure 49–61. Metastatic, epidermotropic melanoma. Higher magnification of Figure 49–60.

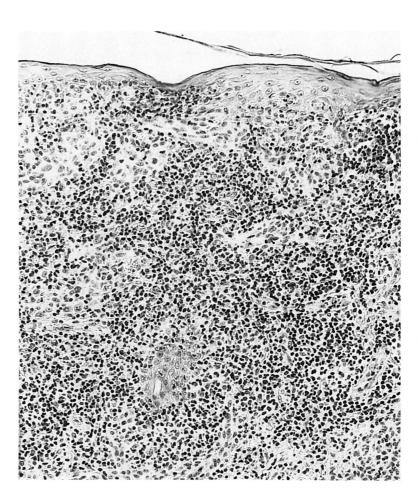

Figure 49–62. Halo nevus. The depths of the lesion are composed of orderly nevic tissue. Above this there is a brisk lymphocytic infiltrate. Superficially, the melanocytes are disorderly. Atypia may be quite striking in some lesions at the dermoepidermal interface. Numerous halo nevi may appear in patients affected by the dysplastic nevus syndrome.

presence, deeper, of lymphocytes admixed with mature dermal nevic cells serve to distinguish the halo nevus from melanoma. When there is atypia of the nevus cells in the upper dermis, it is important to demonstrate continuity with mature nevus cells at the base of the lesion. If there are two distinct populations, and especially if the deep cells are not involved by inflammation, the upper part of the lesion could be melanoma. Patients with dysplastic nevi occasionally develop multiple halos about some of their lesions. Consequently, if the pattern and cytology of dermoepidermal melanocytes simulates that of a dysplastic nevus and the dermal component has the features of a halo nevus, one should consider the possibility of the halo phenomenon occurring in a patient with dysplastic nevi.

ATYPICAL DERMAL MELANOCYTIC LESIONS

Those Characterized by Apparent Differentiation Along Schwannian Lines
The dermal component of some melanocytic lesions may present as small tubular structures permeating both papillary and reticular dermis (Figs. 49–63, 49–64, and 49–65). Such a pattern of growth may compose the entire dermal component of the lesion or may be a part of a conventional

dermal nevus. The cells of these unusual lesions are plump spindle cells and simulate small peripheral nerves (Fig. 49–66). Such lesions have been recently described under the term deep penetrating nevus.[91] An occasional focus of neurotropism may be noted, but the lesions do not behave as neurotropic melanomas. We have seen lesions with occasional mitoses, and some of these have recurred locally but have not shown further progression after complete removal. The epidermis of these lesions shows an increased number of melanocytes, presenting as a row of large cells with or without an occasional nest of melanocytes. There is no consistency in the terminology applied by pathologists to these lesions, and we are not aware of good descriptions of them in the literature. Until they are precisely defined by appropriate clinicopathologic studies, we sign them out descriptively: "compound melanocytic lesion with dermal differentiation along schwannian lines." If mitotic figures are present, reports should indicate the possibility of behavior as a malignant lesion with some potential for local recurrence, at least. As in other difficult dermal melanocytic lesions, necrosis is suggestive of overt malignancy.

Foci of Melanocytic Hyperplasia in the Dermal Component of a Nevus
A rather common histologic problem is caused by melanocytic hyperplasia in the dermal component of an otherwise straightforward compound or dermal nevus. As a matter

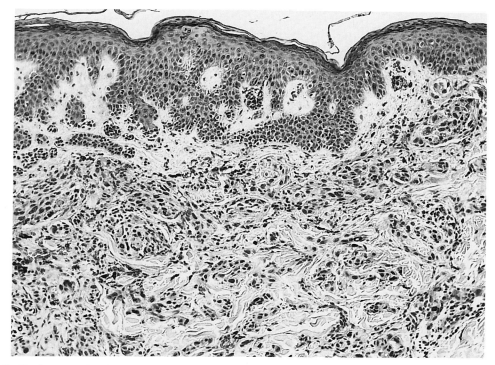

Figure 49–63. Compound melanocytic neoplasm with dermal differentiation along schwannian lines. The epidermis shows basilar melanocytic hyperplasia, with the formation of an occasional small melanocytic nest. The dermal component of the lesion dominates and may be admixed, in some lesions, with normal nevic tissue. The cells are in a haphazard array that tends to be in small fascicles or tubules. The growth is reminiscent of small nerves. Most cells show some pigment synthesis.

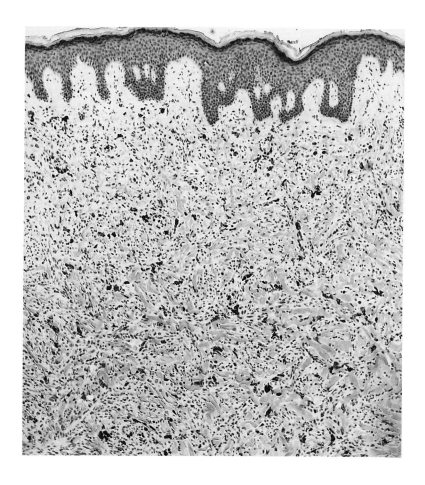

Figure 49–64. Compound melanocytic neoplasm with dermal differentiation along schwannian lines. Much of the dermis is replaced by the small schwannian cells of the tumor.

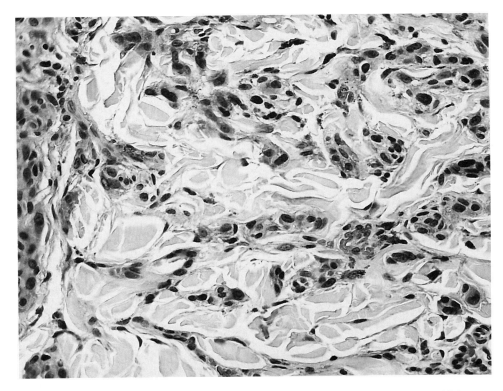

Figure 49–65. Compound melanocytic neoplasm with dermal differentiation along schwannian lines. Higher magnification of the cells in the dermis, arrayed in small clusters or solid tubes.

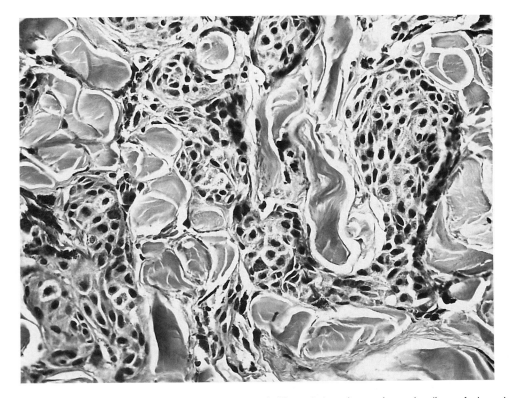

Figure 49–66. Compound melanocytic neoplasm with dermal differentiation along schwannian lines. A dermal pattern imitating the growth of small nerves.

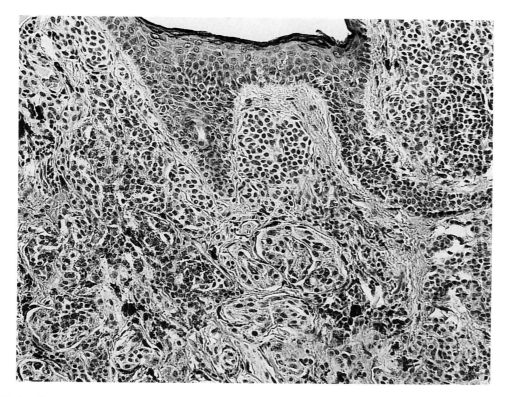

Figure 49–67. Compound nevus with dermal melanocytic hyperplasia. Just below the center of the micrograph there are larger cells, readily distinguishable from the dermal nevi cells. They contain finely divided pigment. Such lesions are seen on the face (especially of children) and are sometimes called combined nevi, a term that is imprecise and loosely used by various observers.

of fact, the clinical history ("a black spot has developed in this mole") may suggest the possibility of such a hyperplasia. Microscopically, a circumscribed aggregate of epithelioid melanocytes with dusty tan cytoplasm is responsible for the black spot (Figs. 49–67 and 49–68). Even though the nuclei are uniform in size, shape, and staining, the dusty cytoplasm in dermal melanocytes is a worry to those who have not previously seen such lesions. As is the case with other unusual dermal melanocytic lesions, one should always search for necrosis and mitotic figures as helpful indicators of malignancy. The dermal melanocytic proliferations are frequently signed out as combined nevi, of one sort or another (e.g., compound and blue nevus), but we prefer to record them descriptively, indicating clearly the nature of the various melanocytic elements. Melanocytic nevi with dermal melanocytic hyperplasia tend to occur in the young, and on the face, but there are numerous exceptions to this statement.

DISPARATE PROBLEMS PRESENTED BY SUPERFICIAL AND DEEP LESIONS THAT MAY BE CONFUSED WITH MELANOMA

It is helpful to separate the difficult histological problems of atypical melanocytic lesions into superficial and deep categories, as Sagebiel has done.[88,89] If one eliminates early vertical growth phase melanoma from the superficial atypical melanocytic lesions, the remainder pose no threat to the patient after complete excision with margins of only a few millimeters depending on the nature of the lesion. In one sense, after elimination of the cases of thin vertical growth phase, the name assigned to the superficial atypical lesions is inconsequential insofar as the physical welfare of the patient is concerned. It obviously is of great concern when one makes a diagnosis of melanoma in relationship to the psychological well-being of the patient (see the following section). The proper classification of the superficial lesions is also of biologic importance if their nature is to be understood and if patients are to be appropriately managed (Table 49–11).

PHILOSOPHICAL, HUMANISTIC, AND MORAL CONSIDERATIONS ATTENDANT ON THE DIAGNOSIS OF MALIGNANT MELANOMA AND RELATED LESIONS

Philosophical Considerations

"The world contains far more objects than we have concepts—so we make mistakes all the time." The foregoing quotation is paraphrased from Stephen Jay Gould and could well serve as a central theme for this chapter.[90] The objects

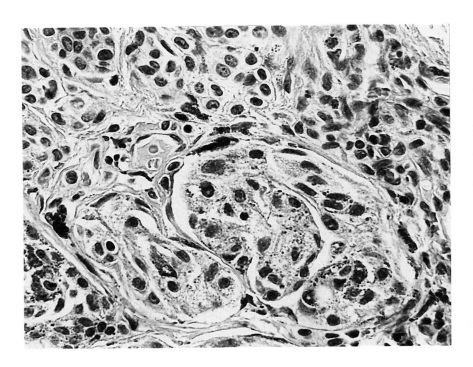

Figure 49–68. Compound nevus with dermal melanocytic hyperplasia. Higher magnification of Figure 49–67.

in the study of melanoma and its development are those changing aggregates of cells that reflect the saltatory progression of events of abnormal cellular evolutionary biology forming the neoplastic system affecting human cutaneous melanocytes. The concepts are mirrored by the words used to formulate a diagnosis of the changing aggregates of cells. Words are packages of information. Thus, a diagnosis couched in thoughtfully selected words reflects a concept. Our concepts and the windows exposing them to view (our words) are terribly flawed: So much information is missing. We have attempted to present the pathology of the disease melanoma in such a way that it suggests the history of a given tumor and in a way that will forecast, with some precision, its future impact or lack of impact

TABLE 49–11. THE SUPERFICIAL AND DEEP ATYPICAL MELANOCYTIC LESIONS

Superficial	Deep
Radial growth phase melanoma of any type	Vertical growth phase melanoma > 1.70 mm
Vertical growth phase melanoma ≤ 1.70 mm (some thin cases)	Spitz tumor
Lentigo maligna	Malignant melanoma arising in a dermal nevus
Dysplastic nevi of the type seen in the dysplastic nevus syndrome	Atypical dermal melanocytic hyperplasia in a congential melanocytic nevus
Atypical melanocytic hyperplasia in the epidermal component of a congenital melanocytic nevus in the neonatal period	Malignant melanoma arising the dermal component of a congenital melanocytic nevus
A largely intraepidermal Spitz tumor	Compound melanocytic lesion with dermal differentiation along schwannian lines
Compound pigmented spindle cell tumor	Atypical dermal melanocytes in acquired and congenital nevi
Halo nevus	Cellular blue nevus
Acral and conjunctival melanocytic nevi	Metastatic malignant melanoma
Atypical melanocytic hyperplasia of the genital (vulvar) type	

(cure) on an individual patient. We do not have enough concepts nor precisely defined diagnostic terms to properly and consistently classify all of the objects (entities, steps, states, lesions, events) of melanocytic neoplasia. It follows that one will not find a readily circumscribed niche for all of the melanocytic tumors encountered. If one attempts to force the odd and difficult lesions into existing categories, the fit is likely to be poor. Do not force the problem case into a category to assuage the diagnostic compulsiveness inherent in all but a few pathologists. A properly worded diagnosis transmits predefined information. If that diagnosis has been coerced from microscopic observations, incorrect information will be transmitted. The liberal use of descriptive diagnoses avoids the errors inherent in our flawed and numerically deficient concepts—concepts that fail to encompass all of the neoplastic objects we confront.

Humanistic and Moral Considerations

A pathology specimen and its derived histologic preparations are small preserved bits of a fellow human being; the specimen, though detached, is and will be bonded to its human and living source. *A pathologist should never forget nor underestimate that bond.* The diagnosis of the specimen will in many instances, especially cases of melanoma, travel along the ties of the bond and profoundly influence the life of that patient. The life will be influenced for its duration: For any one person that is *forever.* Do not ever make the diagnosis of melanoma quickly, casually, and without vigilant forethought about its consequences. We are especially cautious in making the diagnosis of melanoma in situ. These lesions, in and of themselves, are of no biologic consequence to a patient after excision. This does not preclude a frequent state of alarm in patients who are told that they are affected by melanoma. Furthermore, there is still egregious overtreatment, from time to time, when a diagnosis of melanoma is made, even an in situ one. We rarely use in situ melanoma as a formal diagnosis in a pathology report. If the histology is that of florid pagetoid growth of extremely atypical melanocytes throughout the epidermis, the diagnosis may be reluctantly rendered. More commonly the process is described and a footnote indicates that the features could be termed melanoma in situ. In due course and after extensive professional education, we will probably arrive at Reed's position: use the term cancer (in this context, melanoma) only for those tumors with known and proven potential for metastasis.[65] This does not solve the dilemma of the cancer biologist, "What is the proper term for the lesions we have termed radial growth phase (nontumorigenic) melanoma?" The lesions do show persistently autonomous growth; they are composed of abnormal cells; and one may occasionally culture these abnormal cells and the cultured cells show nonrandom chromosomal abnormalities. Of greater importance than these traits is the strong tendency to progress to the vertical growth phase (tumorigenic melanoma). All of the lesional steps of tumor progression preceding the radial growth phase (nontumorigenic melanoma) are indolent, stationary, or regressing; progression is the rare exception. The opposite is true of radial growth phase. For this reason and its cellular characteristics, we still desig-

nate radial growth phase (nontumorigenic melanoma) as cancer. It seems reasonable to regard this step as the biologic beginning of cancer. However, we are not comfortable with the name cancer for this pivotal, bridging lesion in neoplasia. The step of *human* import is the next one: vertical growth phase (tumorigenic melanoma).

Considerations, similar in principle, apply to the diagnosis of a dysplastic nevus and the dysplastic nevus syndrome. It needs to be emphasized again (indeed, over and over) that the words of a properly rendered diagnosis transmit a package of information. The information package may be extensive and include such aspects as therapy. The diagnosis "melanocytic dysplasia of the type that may be seen in the dysplastic nevus syndrome," in a defined clinical setting, conveys specific information concerning relative risk of melanoma development and provides guidelines for patient management. If a diagnosis of a dysplastic nevus is made without all of the required histologic characteristics, the diagnostic term will connote information that is incorrect for that patient.[32] As a specific example, consider the melanocytic nevus that shows an abnormal pattern of intraepidermal melanocytic growth in which this growth extends beyond the peripheral limits of the dermal component of a nevus: an abnormal architecture of epidermal melanocytes. The nature of lesions with such histologic characteristics is not known. They have not yet been subjected to epidemiologic study. They are not dysplastic nevi. If they are erroneously called dysplastic nevi, the information transmitted by the term may be, and usually is, wrong. Such nosologic and judgmental errors incorrectly transmit *this* information to a patient: "You are at risk for the development of malignant melanoma (a form of skin cancer that may spread to other parts of your body and may be fatal), and because of that risk you must be seen at regular intervals by a physician for the rest of your life." The proper histologic criteria for the diagnosis of a dysplastic nevus have been set forth here, and they should be used with care or a patient will be subjected to needless and costly anguish. The criteria may be consistently used by any trained pathologist after a period of thoughtful study.

In any life setting, humanistic and moral considerations are inextricably enmeshed with each other and should be deeply entwined in the deliberations of the pathologist challenged by the mysteries of melanocytic neoplasia.

ACKNOWLEDGMENTS

The invaluable and patient production of photomicrographs by Mr. William Witmer is gratefully acknowledged.

Doreen Gallo and Carol Blumenthal devoted generous hours and ideas to the manuscript. Patricia Clark provided patience and meticulous proofreading.

Richard J. Reed, MD spent painstaking and indulgent hours leading us through minimal deviation melanoma and other concepts of melanoma biology. He also furnished material on soft tissue melanomas.

Robert Folberg led us through the difficult melanocytic lesions of the conjunctiva and furnished excellent examples for photography.

Sharon Weiss, MD was of generous help with cases and thought concerning soft tissue melanomas.

John Brooks, MD also loaned an excellent case of soft tissue melanoma for study.

The work was supported by NCI Grants Ca-25298, Ca-25874, and Ca-16520.

BIBLIOGRAPHY

Balch CM, Milton GW, Shaw HM, et al. *Cutaneous Melanoma. Clinical Management and Treatment Results Worldwide.* Philadelphia, Pa: JB Lippincott; 1985.

Clark WH Jr, Goldman LI, Mastrangelo MJ, eds. *Human Malignant Melanoma.* Grune & Stratton; New York, NY: 1979.

Elder DE, ed. *Pathobiology of Malignant Melanoma,* New York, NY: Karger; 1987.

Elwood JM, ed. *Melanoma and Nevi. Incidence, Interrelationships and Implications.* New York, NY: Karger, 1988.

Mihm MC Jr, Murphy GF. *Pathobiology and Recognition of Malignant Melanoma.* Baltimore, Md: Williams & Wilkins, 1988.

Rhodes AR. Neoplasms: benign neoplasias, hyperplasias, and dysplasias of melanocytes. In: Fitzpatrick TB, Eisen AZ, Wolff K, et al, eds. *Dermatology in General Medicine.* 3rd ed. New York, McGraw-Hill International Book Co; 1987.

REFERENCES

1. Palowski A, Haberman HF, Menon IA. Junctional and compound pigmented nevi induced by 9,10-dimethyl-1,2-benzanthracene in the skin of albino guinea pigs. *Cancer Res.* 1976; 36:2813–2821.
2. Palowski A, Haberman HF, Menon IA. Skin melanoma induced by 7,12 dimethylbenzanthracene in albino guinea pigs and its similarities to skin melanomas of humans. *Cancer Res.* 1980; 40:3652–3660.
3. Clark WH Jr, Min BH, Kligman LHL. The developmental biology of induced malignant melanoma in guinea pigs and a comparison with other neoplastic systems. *Cancer Res.* 1976; 36:4079–4091.
4. Clark WH Jr, Elder DE, Guerry D IV, et al. A study of tumor progression: the precursor lesions of superficial spreading and nodular melanoma. *Hum Pathol.* 1984; 15:1147–1165.
5. Clark WH Jr, Elder DE, van Horn, M. The biologic forms of malignant melanoma. *Hum Pathol.* 1986; 17:443–450.
6. Elder DE, Clark WH Jr. Tumor progression and prognosis in malignant melanoma. In: Elder DE, ed. *Pathobiology of Malignant Melanoma.* London, England: S Karger AG; 1987:51–81.
7. Farber E, Cameron R. The sequential analysis of cancer development. In: Klein G, Weinhouse S, eds. *Advances in Cancer Research.* New York, NY: Academic Press Inc, 1980:125–226.
8. Farber E, Sarma DSR. Biology of disease: hepatocarcinogenesis: a dynamic cellular perspective. *Lab Invest.* 1987; 56:4–22.
9. Foulds L. *Neoplastic Development.* Vol 1, London, England: Academic Press Inc; 1969:439.
10. Pardee AB. Principles of cancer biology: biochemistry and cell biology. In: Devita VT Jr, Hellman S, Rosenberg SA, ed. *Cancer. Principles and Practice of Oncology.* 2nd ed. Philadelphia, Pa: JB Lippincott; 1985:4.
11. Clark WH, Elder DE, Guerry DG, et al. A model predicting survival in stage I melanoma based upon tumor progression. *J Nat Cancer Inst.* 1989; 81:1893–1904.
12. Foulds L. *Neoplastic Development.* Vol 1. London, England: Academic Press Inc; 1969:79.
13. Anders A, Dess G, Nishimura S, et al. A molecular approach

to the study of malignancy and benignancy in melanoma of *Xiphophorus.* In: Bagnara J, Klaus SN, Paul E, et al, eds. *Biological, Molecular, and Clinical Aspects of Pigmentation.* Tokyo, Japan: University of Tokyo Press; 1985:315–324.
14. Ley R. Personal communication, March 1, 1988.
15. Holman CDJ, Armstrong BK, Heenan PJ. Relationship of cutaneous malignant melanoma to individual sunlight-exposure habits. *J Nat Cancer Inst.* 1986; 76:403–414.
16. Kopf AW, Kripke ML, Stern RS. Sun and malignant melanoma. *J Am Acad Dermatol.* 1984; 11:674–684.
17. Østerlind A, Tucker MA, Hou-Jensen K, et al. The Danish case control study of cutaneous malignant melanoma. I: importance of host factors. *Int J Cancer.* In Press, 1988; 48:200–206.
18. Østerlind A, Tucker MA, Stone BJ, et al. The Danish case control study of cutaneous malignant melanoma. II: importance of UV-light exposure. *Int J Cancer.* 1988; 42:319–324.
19. Green A, Bain C, McLennan R, et al. Risk factors for cutaneous melanoma in Queensland. *Recent Results Cancer Res.* 1986; 102:76–97.
20. Rhodes AR, Weinstock MA, Fitzpatrick TB, et al. Risk factors for cutaneous melanoma. A practical method for recognizing predisposed individuals. *JAMA.* 1987; 258:3147–3154.
21. Green A, Siskind V, Bain C, et al. Sunburn and malignant melanoma. *Br J Cancer.* 1985; 51:393–397.
22. Green A. Sun exposure and the risk of melanoma. *Aust J Dermatol.* 1984; 25:99–102.
23. Holman CJ, Armstrong BK: Pigmentary traits, ethnic origin, benign naevi, and family history as risk factors for cutaneous malignant melanoma. *J Nat Cancer Inst.* 1984; 72:257–266.
24. Elwood JM, Gallagher RP, Davison J, et al. Sunburn, suntan, and the risk of cutaneous malignant melanoma: the Western Canada Melanoma Study. *B J Cancer.* 1985; 51:543–549.
25. Holman CDJ, Armstrong BK: Cutaneous malignant melanoma and indicators of total accumulated exposure to the sun: an analysis separating histogenetic types. *J Nat Cancer Inst.* 1984; 73:75–82.
26. Holly EA, Kelly JW, Schpall SN, et al. Number of melanocytic nevi as a major risk factor for malignant melanoma. *J Am Acad Dermatol.* 1987; 17:459–468.
27. Rampen FHJ, Fleuren BAM, de Boo ThM, et al. Prevalence of common "acquired" nevocytic nevi and dysplastic nevi is not related to ultraviolet exposure. *J Am Acad Dermatol.* 1988; 18:679–683.
28. Schreiber MM, Bozzo PD, Moon TE. Malignant melanoma in southern Arizona. *Arch Dermatol.* 1981; 117:6–11.
29. Jensen OM, Bolander AM. Trends in malignant melanoma of the skin. *World Health Stat Q.* 1980; 33:2–26.
30. Roush GC, Schymura MJ, Holford TR. Risk for cutaneous melanoma in recent Connecticut birth cohorts. *Am J Public Health.* 1985; 75:679–682.
31. MacKie RM, Doherty VR. Educational activities aimed at earlier detection and treatment of malignant melanoma in a moderate risk area. In: Elwood JM. *Melanoma and Nevi. Incidence, Interrelationships and Implications.* London, England, S Karger AG; 1988:140–153.
32. Clark WH Jr: The dysplastic nevus syndrome. *Arch Dermatol.* 1988; 124:1207–1210.
33. Yaar M, Woodley DT, Gilchrist BA: Human nevocellular nevus cells are surrounded by basement membrane components. Immunohistochemical studies of human nevus cells and melanocytes in vivo and in vitro. *Lab Invest.* 1988; 58:157–162.
34. Liotta LA, Guirguis R, Stracke M. Biology of melanoma invasion and metastasis. *Pigm Cell.* 1987; 1:5–15.
35. MacKie RM. Personal communication, February, 1988.
36. Greene MH. Dysplastic nevus syndrome. *Hosp Pract.* 1984; 19:91–108.
37. Greene MH, Clark WH Jr, Tucker MA, et al. Acquired precur-

sors of cutaneous malignant melanoma: the familial dysplastic nevus syndrome. *N Engl J Med.* 1985; 312:91–97.

38. Frichot BC III, Lynch HT, Guirgis HA, et al. A new cutaneous phenotype in familial malignant melanoma. *Lancet.* 1977; 1:864–865.

39. Clark WH Jr, Reimer RR, Greene MH, et al. Origin of familial malignant melanoma from heritable melanocytic lesions. "The B-K mole syndrome." *Arch Dermatol.* 1978; 114:732–738.

40. Bale SJ, Dracopolli NC, Tucker MA, et al. Mapping the gene for cutaneous malignant melanoma-dysplastic nevus to chromosome *N Engl J Med* 1989; 320:1367–1372.

41. Howell JN, Greene MH, Corner RC, et al. Fibroblasts from patients with hereditary cutaneous malignant melanoma are abnormally sensitive to the mutagenic effect of simulated sunlight and 4-nitroquinoline 1-oxide. *Proc Natl Acad Sci USA.* 1984; 81:1179–1183.

42. Smith PJ, Greene MH, Devlin DA, et al. Abnormal sensitivity to UV-radiation in cultured skin fibroblasts from patients with hereditary cutaneous malignant melanoma and dysplastic nevus syndrome. *Int J Cancer.* 1982; 30:39–45.

43. Sanford K, Parshad R, Greene MH, et al. Hypersensitivity to G_2 chromatid radiation damage in familial dysplastic naevus syndrome. *Lancet.* 1987; 2:1111–1116.

44. Elder DE. The dysplastic nevus. *Pathology.* 1985; 17:291–297.

45. Aronson PJ, Kaoru I, Fukaya T, et al. Monoclonal antibody (AFH1) immunoreactive on morphologically abnormal basal melanocytes within dysplastic nevi, nevocellular nevus nests, and melanoma. *J Invest Dermatol.* 1988; 90:452–458.

46. Rhodes AR, Seki Y, Fitzpatrick TB, et al. Melanosomal alterations in dysplastic nevi: a quantitative ultrastructural investigation. *Cancer.* 1988; 61:358–369.

47. From L, Wedad H, Kahn H, et al. Origin of desmoplasia in desmoplastic malignant melanoma. *Hum Pathol.* 1983; 14:1072–1080.

48. Jampel RM, Friedman KF, Hood AF, et al. Atypical melanocytic lesions of the vulva. *J Cutan Pathol.* 1988; 15:316.

49. Christensen WN, Friedman KF, Woodruff JD, et al. Histologic characteristics of vulvar nevocellular nevi. *J Cutan Pathol.* 1987; 14:87–91.

50. Guerry D IV, Elder DE, Clark WH Jr, et al. Dysplastic nevi are precursors and risk markers of sporadic melanoma. *Proc Am Assoc Cancer Res.* 1987; 28:1006.

51. Cooke KR, Spears GFS, Skegg DCG. Frequency of moles in a defined population. *J Epidemiol Community Health.* 1985; 39:48–52.

52. Kraemer KH, Tucker M, Tarone R, et al. Risk of cutaneous melanoma in dysplastic nevus syndrome types A and B. *N Engl J Med.* 1986; 315:1615–1616.

53. Bale SJ, Chakravarti A. Evidence for autosomal dominance and pleiotropy of the cutaneous malignant melanoma (CMM)/dysplastic nevus (DN) gene. *Am J Hum Genet.* 1987; 40:466–467.

54. Greene MH, Clark WH Jr, Tucker MA, et al. High risk malignant melanoma in melanoma-prone families with dysplastic nevi. *Ann Intern Med.* 1985; 102:458–465.

55. Nakanishi T, Hashimoto K. The differential reactivity of benign and malignant nevomelanocytic lesions with mouse monoclonal antibody TNKH1. *Cancer.* 1987; 59:1340–1344.

56. Imam A, Mitchell MS, Modlin RL, et al. Human monoclonal antibodies that distinguish cutaneous malignant melanoma from benign nevi in fixed tissue sections. *J Invest Dermatol.* 1986; 86:145–148.

57. Elder DE, Rodeck U, Thurin J, et al. Antigenic profile of tumor progression stages in human melanocytic nevi and melanomas. *Cancer Research.* 1989; 49:5091–5096.

58. Herlyn M, Clark WH, Rodeck U, et al. Biology of tumor progression in human melanocytes. *Lab Invest.* 1987; 56:461–474.

59. Takahashi H, Takashi H, Jimbow K. Fine structural characterization of melanosomes and dysplastic nevi. *Cancer.* 1985; 56:111–123.

60. Rhodes AR, Seki Y, Fitzpatrick TB, et al. Melanosomal alterations in dysplastic melanocytic nevi: a quantitative, ultrastructural investigation. *Cancer.* 1988; 61:358–369.

61. Elder DE, Guerry D IV, Epstein MN, et al. Invasive malignant melanomas lacking competence for metastasis. *Am J Dermatopathol* 1984; 6 (suppl 1): 55–61.

62. Breslow A. Thickness, cross-sectional areas and depth of invasion in the prognosis of cutaneous melanoma. *Ann Surg.* 1970; 172:902–908.

63. Kheir SM, Bines SD, Vonroenn JH, et al. Prognostic significance of DNA aneuploidy in Stage I cutaneous melanoma. *Ann Surg.* 1988; 207:455–461.

64. Reed RJ. The histologic variance of malignant melanoma: the interrelationship of histological subtype, neoplastic progression, and biological behavior. *Pathology.* 1985; 17:301–312.

65. Reed RJ. Minimal deviation melanoma. In Mihm MC Jr, Murphy GF, eds. *Pathobiology and Recognition of Malignant Melanoma.* Baltimore, Md: Williams & Wilkins; 1988:110–152.

66. Arrington JH III, Reed RJ, Ichinose H, et al. Plantar lentiginous melanoma: a distinctive variant of human cutaneous malignant melanoma. *Am J Surg Pathol.* 1977; 1:131–143.

67. Ackerman AB: Unifying concept of malignant melanoma. *Hum Pathol.* 1980; 11:591–595.

68. Hunter JAA, Zaynoun S, Paterson WD, et al. Cellular fine structure in the invasive nodules of the different histogenetic types of malignant melanoma. *Br J Dermatol.* 1978; 98:255–272.

69. Mazur MT, Katzenstein ALA. Metastatic melanoma: the spectrum of ultrastructural morphology. *Ultrastruct Pathol.* 1980; 1:337–356.

70. Ronan SG, Eng AM, Briele HA, et al. Thin malignant melanomas with regression and metastases. *Arch Dermatol.* 1987; 123:1326–1330.

71. Cochran AJ. Malignant melanoma: review of 10 year's experience in Glasgow, Scotland. *Cancer.* 1969; 23:1190–1199.

72. Cochran AJ. Method of assessing prognosis in patients with malignant melanoma. *Lancet.* 1968; 2:1062–1064.

73. Schmoekel C, Braun-Falco O: Prognostic index in malignant melanoma. *Arch Dermatol.* 1978; 114:871–873.

74. Kornstein MJ, Guerry D IV: The immunopathology of the mononuclear cell infiltrate in malignant melanoma. In: Elder DE, ed. *Pathobiology of Malignant Melanoma,* Basel: AG Karger, 1987:147–165.

75. Fawcett DW: *Bloom and Fawcett. A Textbook of Histology.* Philadelphia, Pa: WB Saunders Co, 1986:401.

76. Conley J, Lattes R, Orr W: Desmoplastic malignant melanoma (a rare variant of spindle cell melanoma). *Cancer.* 1971; 28:914–936.

77. Reed RJ, Leonard DD. Neurotropic melanoma: a variant of desmoplastic melanoma. *Am J Surg Pathol.* 1979; 3:301–311.

78. Reed RJ: Personal communication concerning clinical appearance of minimal deviation melanomas and the incidence of lymph node metastases. December 28, 1987.

79. Hendrickson MR, Ross JC: Neoplasms arising in congenital giant nevi: morphologic study of seven cases and a review of the literature. *Am J Surg Pathol.* 1981; 5:109–135.

80. Rhodes AR, Silverman RA, Harrist TJ, et al. A histologic comparison of congenital and acquired nevomelanocytic nevi. *Arch Dermatol.* 1985; 121:1266–1273.

81. Enzinger FM: Clear cell sarcoma of tendons and aponeuroses: an analysis of 21 cases. *Cancer.* 1965; 18:1163–1174.

82. Chung EB, Enzinger FM: Malignant melanoma of soft parts. A reassessment of clear cell sarcoma. *Am J Surg Pathol.* 1983; 7:405–413.

83. Kamino H, Misheloff E, Ackerman AB, et al. Eosinophilic glo-

bules in Spitz's nevi: new findings and a diagnostic sign. *Am J Dermatopathol* 1979; 1:319–324.

84. Barr RJ, Morales V, Graham JH. Desmoplastic nevus: a distinct variant of mixed spindle and epithelioid cell nevus. *Cancer.* 1980; 46:557–564.

85. Reed RJ, Ichinose H, Clark WH Jr, et al. Common and uncommon melanocytic nevi and borderline melanomas. *Semin Oncol.* 1975; 2:119–147.

86. Friedman RJ, Ackerman AB. Difficulties in the histologic diagnosis of melanocytic nevi on the vulvae of premenopausal women. In: Ackerman AB, ed. *Pathology of Malignant Melanoma.* New York, NY: Masson Publishing USA, Inc; 1981:119–128.

87. Clark WH Jr, Mihm MC. Lentigo maligna and lentigo-maligna melanoma. *Am J Pathol.* 1969; 53:39–67.

88. Sagebiel RW. Histopathology of borderline and early malignant melanomas. *Am J Surg Pathol.* 1979; 3:543–552.

89. Sagebiel RW. Problems in microstaging of melanoma vertical growth. In: Mihm MC Jr, Murphy GF, eds. *Pathobiology and Recognition of Malignant Melanoma.* Baltimore, Md: Williams & Wilkins; 1988:94–109.

90. Gould SJ: *An Urchin in the Storm.* New York, NY: WW Norton & Company; 1987:222.

91. Seab JA, Graham JH, Helwig EB. Deep penetrating nevus *Am J Surg Path.* 1989; 13:39–44.

CHAPTER 50
Tumors of Fibrous Tissue

Kenneth J. Friedman

In this chapter, an attempt is made to review tumors of the fibroblastic type that may present as a skin mass either from origin within the skin itself or from involvement of deeper structures with secondary skin manifestations. This large, heterogeneous group of lesions form a spectrum of entities ranging from localized benign reactive processes to poorly circumscribed infiltrative lesions with a tendency toward recurrence and, finally, to frankly malignant neoplastic tumors. Precise categorization of lesions such as the fibromatoses as reactive versus neoplastic, tumor or tumorlike, benign versus malignant, is difficult because of the lack of universal agreement.

NODULAR FASCIITIS

Nodular fasciitis has been generally considered to be a benign, pseudoneoplastic, reactive fibroblastic growth. The first cases were reported in 1955,[1] and, since that time, many names including infiltrative fasciitis, pseudosarcomatous fasciitis, and subcutaneous pseudosarcomatous fibromatosis have been applied to this lesion. Several large series have helped to more clearly define the clinical and pathologic findings of this rather common fibroblastic tumor, which is often mistaken for a malignancy because of its rapid growth, hypercellularity, cellular pleomorphism, and prominent mitotic activity.[2–9] Unusual subtypes worthy of special designation include proliferative fasciitis,[10] proliferative myositis,[11,12] cranial fasciitis,[13] parosteal fasciitis,[14] and intravascular fasciitis.[15]

Clinical Features
Although nodular fasciitis can occur at any age, it is most common in young adults, with a peak incidence in the fourth decade. The vast majority of cases occur between 10 and 50 years of age. There is no sex predilection. It may occur anywhere on the body but the most common site is the upper extremity and, in particular, the forearm, with other common sites of involvement including the shoulder, chest wall, back, and thigh. Multiple lesions are very rare.

More than 75% of patients have a history of a rapidly growing lesion that has been present for less than 4 weeks. A duration greater than 3 months is uncommon. Tenderness or pain may be present and a history of trauma is given in a minority of cases. Most lesions are located in the subcutis with adhesion to underlying fascia, and are round to oval nonencapsulated masses that may or may not be well circumscribed. The overwhelming majority of lesions measure less than 3 cm in greatest diameter. Tumors 4 cm or greater should be treated with suspicion, and the possibility of fibromatosis or sarcoma must be considered.

Simple excision is curative. Even in cases of incomplete excision, no recurrence is expected. Although a recurrence rate of 1% to 2% has been reported,[6] recurrence of a lesion originally classified as nodular fasciitis should lead to review and reappraisal of the diagnosis.[7] Spontaneous regression has been observed.

Histologic Features
The subcutaneous lesions, which are the most common type, tend to be well circumscribed; the lesions that grow along the fascia are irregular in contour (Fig. 50–1). The histologic pattern can be quite variable within the same lesion. Spindle, plump, or stellate fibroblasts with vesicular nuclei and prominent nucleoli are arranged either in short irregular bundles, in a vaguely storiform pattern, or haphazardly within a myxomatous stroma rich in hyaluronidase-sensitive acid mucopolysaccharides. This characteristic loosely textured or "feathery" pattern is an important diagnostic feature (Fig. 50–2).

Small vessel proliferation, often with prominent endothelial cells, microhemorrhages, and inflammatory cells are intermixed with the fibroblasts. A small hematoma or fibrin may be present within the central portion of the lesion surrounded by radially arranged small vessels and loose fibroblasts. Zones of higher cellularity with decreased ground substance may be present. The fibroblasts in these zones tend to be larger, crowded, and more plump (Fig.

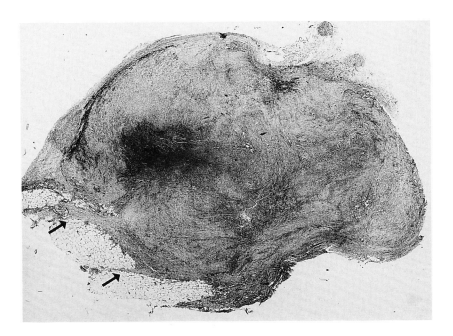

Figure 50–1. Nodular fasciitis. Moderately circumscribed fibrous nodule in subcutis with focal irregular infiltration into fat (arrows) and central hemorrhage. (H&E, ×10.)

50–3). Other zones may demonstrate decreased cellularity and increased collagen deposition with hyalinization. These three patterns, namely, loosely myxoid, cellular, and fibrous, may coexist in a single lesion or one growth pattern may predominate, although the combination of myxoid and fibrous patterns rarely occurs within the same lesion. Nodular fasciitis may progress in time from the myxoid to the cellular and finally to the collagen type as the lesion ages.[8]

Mitotic activity is easily noted and is greatest within the cellular areas of the myxoid zones where the mitotic rate is generally not significantly greater than one to two mitoses per high-power field. Abnormal mitoses are generally not observed. Varying numbers of large ganglion-like cells or osteoclast-like giant cells may be present (Fig. 50–3).

Differential Diagnosis

Myxoma is notably hypocellular and poorly vascularized. Fibrous histiocytoma displays a more prominent storiform growth pattern and is largely present within the dermis (dermatofibroma). Nodular fasciitis does not extend into the dermis. Clusters of foamy macrophages, touton-type giant cells, and hemosiderin deposition favor fibrous histiocytoma. Fibromatosis is a larger, more bulky tumor that displays a more infiltrative growth pattern. It is characterized by fascicles of uniform splender spindle cells embedded in a richly collagenous stroma. Mitotic activity is less than in nodular fasciitis.

Malignant fibrous histiocytoma is generally a disease of older patients and usually achieves a size greater than 3 cm at presentation. In addition, significant cellular pleomorphism and numerous mitoses, including atypical ones, are present. Inflammation and myxoid features can be present in both nodular fasciitis and malignant fibrous histiocytoma and do not serve as discriminating features; however, the infiltrate in inflammatory fibrous histiocytoma is most often dominated by neutrophils and foamy histiocytes as opposed to lymphocytes in nodular fasciitis. Fibrosarcoma is larger, deeper, and of longer duration than nodular fasciitis. Fibrosarcoma is composed of tightly interwoven fascicles in a herringbone pattern with cellular pleomorphism and prominent mitotic activity, including atypical mitoses.

Variants

Proliferative Fasciitis. Proliferative fasciitis demonstrates clinical features similar to those of nodular fasciitis, namely, smalll size, rapid growth, frequent history of trauma, preferential occurrence on the extremities, and subcutaneous location. For that reason, its distinction from nodular fasciitis

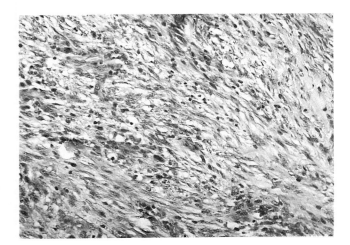

Figure 50–2. Nodular fasciitis. Spindle and plump fibroblasts embedded in a loosely textured "feathery" stroma with scattered lymphocytes. (H&E, ×235.)

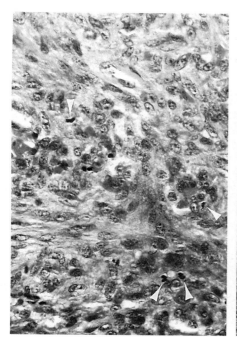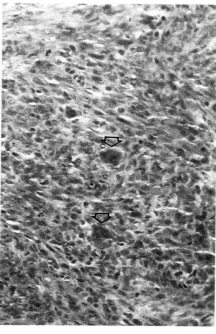

Figure 50–3. Nodular fasciitis. Left: Cellular zone containing larger, plumper, and more crowded fibroblasts with notable mitotic activity (arrowheads). Right: Multinucleated giant cells within a cellular zone (arrows). (Left: H&E, ×330; right: H&E, ×265.)

is not great. It occurs in adult life with a peak incidence between ages 40 and 70.[10] The lesion tends to grow along the fascial planes in an irregular stellate fashion. The histology is quite similar to that of nodular fasciitis, with the exception of numerous basophilic to pink-staining giant cells, with large nuclei and prominent nucleoli (Fig. 50–4). These cells resemble ganglion cells or immature muscle cells. Mitoses may be present within these giant cells. These cells have ultrastructural features of fibroblasts.[10,16] The lesion is benign and self-limited; simple excision is curative.

Proliferative Myositis. Proliferative myositis is the intramuscular analog of proliferative fasciitis with preference for the trunk and shoulder of adults in the fifth and sixth decade.[11] In its rapid onset and small size it is comparable to proliferative and nodular fasciitis. Proliferating spindle cells separate striated muscle bundles without degeneration, replacement, or regeneration of muscle tissue. The cellularity, including the presence of giant ganglion-like or myoid cells within the most rapidly proliferating foci, is identical to that of nodular fasciitis. Cartilaginous meta-

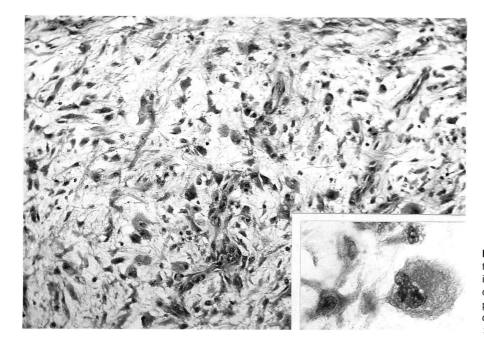

Figure 50–4. Proliferative fasciitis. Loosely textured "feathery" myxoid stroma containing plump fibroblasts and large ganglion-like or myoid cells. Inset: Large cells showing prominent nuclei, large nucleoli, and abundant cytoplasm. (H&E, ×130; inset: H&E, ×625.)

plasia and ossification may be present. Lesions in which bone formation is prominent and diffuse have been termed *myositis ossificans*.[17]

Cranial Fasciitis. A proliferative, rapidly growing fibroblastic lesion, cranial fasciitis involves the calvernium and overlying subcutaneous tissues of infants and children and closely resembles nodular fasciitis on histologic grounds. This lesion may originate from deep fascial layers of the scalp. Recurrence after complete excision has not been reported.[13]

Parosteal Fasciitis. Parosteal fasciitis, also histologically indistinguishable from nodular fasciitis, takes origin from the periosteum of long bones. Adjacent reactive cortical bone formation is seen. Like nodular fasciitis, this lesion is rapidly growing and of short duration. No progression of disease or metastasis has been reported.[14]

Intravascular Fasciitis. Intravascular fasciitis presents as a slowly growing mass present from 2 to several months, most often on the extremities or head and neck. It is characterized by histologic features of nodular fasciitis but with intraluminal, intramural, and extramural involvement of small to medium-sized veins and arteries and multinodular or serpential growth along the course of the affected vessels. Rarely, local recurrence has been reported.[15]

FIBROMATOSIS

The fibromatoses are a poorly understood spectrum of nonencapsulated, poorly circumscribed fibroblastic lesions that are biologically intermediate between benign and malignant tumors. They have an infiltrative growth pattern with a tendency toward recurrence; however, they do not metastasize. The recurrence rate varies significantly and depends on the patient's age, the location of the lesion, and the mode of therapy. Histologic findings do not appear to govern recurrence potential. These lesions can occur at any age, and frequently affect infants and children. Certain forms have a particular affinity for certain anatomic sites and age groups. Histologically, nearly all lesions are composed of varying numbers of well-differentiated uniform fibroblasts embedded in a mature collagenous stroma.

PALMAR (DUPUYTREN'S CONTRACTURE) AND PLANTAR (LEDDERHOSE'S DISEASE) FIBROMATOSIS

Clinical Features

A firm, subcutaneous, slowly growing, long-standing nodule is present adherent to the fascia in the palm or sole.[18-22] Bilaterality is common. Contracture of one or more digits is common with palmar involvement, but is rare in the plantar form. Palmar fibromatosis is seldom seen in patients younger than 30 years; its incidence increases rapidly with advancing age. Plantar fibromatosis, on the other hand, is found more commonly in young adults and children. Both forms are more common in men. Coexistence of palmar fibromatosis with plantar fibromatosis and other forms of fibromatosis (penile, knuckle pads) is well recognized, as is an association with epilepsy, diabetes, alcoholism, and liver cirrhosis.[23] Surgical removal is the treatment of choice.

Histologic Features

A single nodule or an aggregate of several multinodular masses is associated with the aponeurosis and subcutaneous fat. The nodules are small, usually measuring less than 1 cm. The nodules are composed of a moderately cellular proliferation of uniform slender fibroblasts associated with small to moderate amounts of mature collagen arranged in parallel or intersecting fascicles (Fig. 50–5). The collagen fibers are often wavy. Both palmar and plantar fibromatoses can be highly cellular. Scattered mitoses can be present. Older lesions tend to be less cellular and highly collagenous.

Differential Diagnosis

Fibrosarcomas exhibit higher cellularity, greater atypia with both nuclear and cellular pleomorphism, and a higher mitotic rate.

APONEUROTIC FIBROMATOSIS (CALCIFYING APONEUROTIC FIBROMATOSIS)

Clinical Features

This uncommon tumorlike proliferation most commonly affects the palms, fingers, and soles of children and young adults with a male predominance.[24] It is slow growing, and usually causes no discomfort or limitation of movement. Its relationship to palmar/plantar fibromatosis is unclear.

Histologic Features

A fibrous growth of variable cellularity is present, irregularly extending into surrounding tissues. Plump fibroblasts embedded in a densely collagenous stroma associated with foci of calcification and cartilaginous metaplasia are seen (Fig. 50–6). Palisading of fibroblasts around the zones of calcification is common.

Differential Diagnosis

Palmar/plantar fibromatosis does not display calcification or cartilage formation and tends to have less irregular extension into surrounding fat and muscle.

KNUCKLE PADS

Clinical Features

Knuckle pads are hyperkeratotic firm papules present over the dorsal aspects of the interphalangeal joints.[25] They are inherited as an autosomal dominant trait and appear during young adulthood. An association with palmar or plantar fibromatoses has been observed.

Histologic Features

Microscopically, knuckle pads resemble palmar and plantar fibromatosis.

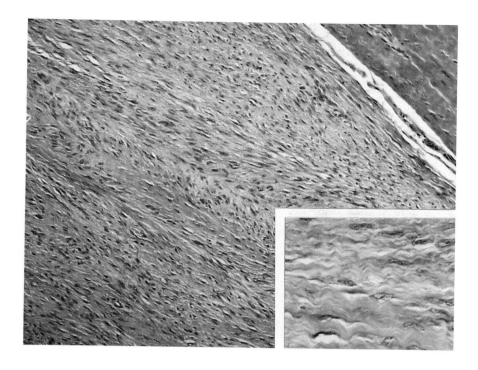

Figure 50–5. Palmar fibromatosis. Moderately cellular interlacing fascicles comprising elongated fibroblasts. Tendon is present at upper right. Inset: Uniform slender fibroblasts embedded in a richly collagenous wavy stroma (H&E, ×115; inset: H&E, ×360.)

INFANTILE DIGITAL FIBROMATOSIS

Clinical Features

Infantile digital fibromatosis occurs during infancy and early childhood on the dorsal and lateral surfaces of the distal fingers and toes. It often occurs in multiple locations.[26] Rare reports of sites of involvement other than the digits exist.[27] The lesion presents in the first year of life in 75% of cases; approximately one third are present at birth.[28] They are small, rarely exceeding 2 cm. The lesions appear as well-circumscribed waxy nodules, often red in color, bound to overlying skin. Recurrence after surgical removal is high, approximately 65%.[28] Functional impairment or joint deformities may occur, even in those cases associated with spontaneous remission.

Histologic Features

A poorly circumscribed proliferation of numerous intersecting bundles of uniform spindled fibroblasts embedded in a densely collagenous stroma is seen replacing the dermis

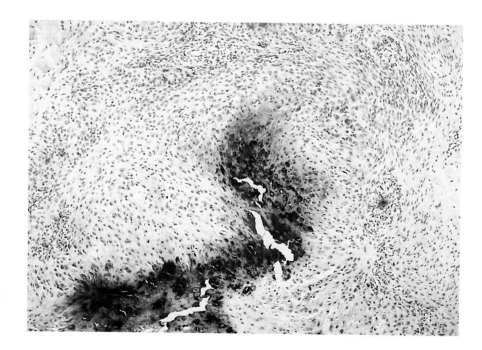

Figure 50–6. Aponeurotic fibromatosis. Central zone of calcification with cartilaginous metaplasia surrounded by uniform, somewhat palisaded, plump fibroblasts embedded in a collagenous stroma. (H&E, ×65.)

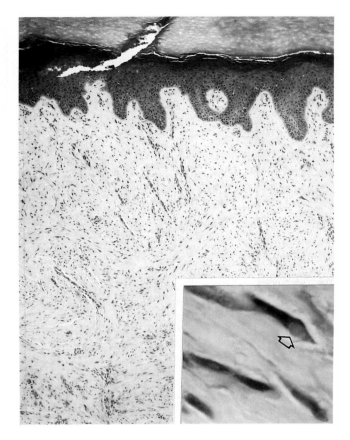

Figure 50–7. Infantile digital fibromatosis. Uniform spindled fibro-blasts embedded in a densely collagenous stroma. Note needle tract artifact within epidermis. Inset: Round, paranuclear inclusion within a fibroblast (arrow). (H&E, ×65; inset: H&E, ×800.)

extending into the fat (Fig. 50–7). Mitotic figures are rare. The characteristic histologic finding is the presence of vari-able numbers of small round, intracytoplasmic, paranuclear inclusions within the fibroblasts ranging in size from 1.5 to 15 μm. They are visible with hematoxylin and eosin staining but are highlighted with trichrome and phospho-tungstic acid and hematoxylin (PTAH) staining.[29] Ultra-structural studies show the inclusions to consist of densely packed microfilaments. Bundles of myofilaments have been demonstrated extending from the spherical inclusions run-ning along the bodies of the cells associated with dense bodies similar to those seen in smooth muscle and myofibroblasts.[30] Actin has been demonstrated in the tumor cells by immunohistochemistry.[31] These findings suggest that infantile digital fibromatosis may represent a neoplasm of myofibroblasts.

PENILE FIBROMATOSIS (PEYRONIE'S DISEASE)

Clinical Features
In penile fibromatosis, a long-standing, slowly growing mass on the dorsum of the penis is present that may involve the ventral or lateral surfaces.[32] Most patients are middle-aged and older males. Painful erections and deformities

result. An increased association with palmar and plantar fibromatosis, epilepsy, and diabetes has been reported.[33]

Histologic Features
The histology may vary considerably, depending largely on the age of the lesion. The initial phase consists of a perivascular chronic inflammatory infiltrate and endothelial cell hyperplasia followed by proliferation of fibroconnective tissue with ossification and destruction of muscle fibers within the corpus cavernosum.

FIBROUS HAMARTOMA OF INFANCY (SUBDERMAL FIBROMATOUS TUMOR OF INFANCY)

Clinical Features
Fibrous hamartoma of infancy most often occurs in infants within the first year of life, with a male predominance.[34] It appears most commonly in the region of the shoulder, axilla, and upper arm as a rapidly growing, 3- to 5-cm-deep dermal or subcutaneous nodule. Local excision is nearly always curative.

Histologic Features
The lesion is poorly circumscribed and comprises three components.[34] Interlacing trabeculae of cellular fibrous tis-sue containing uniform well-oriented spindled fibroblasts and abundant mature collagen are admixed in an organoid fashion with zones of loose fibrous tissue containing abun-dant hyaluronic acid and small rounded immature cells, resembling primitive neural tissue (Figs. 50–8, 50–9). The third component consists of variable amounts of mature fat cells interspersed among the two other components. Boundaries between tumor fat cells and normal subcutane-ous fat are often indistinct.

JUVENILE HYALINE FIBROMATOSIS

Clinical Features
Juvenile hyaline fibromatosis is a rare autosomal recessive disease presenting with multiple, slowly growing subcuta-neous nodules, gingival hyperplasia, flexural contractures, and radiolucent bone destructions.[35] The disease starts ap-pearing between 2 months and 4 years of age. The skin lesions consist of small fleshy papules over the face, neck, and nose and behind the ear and widely distributed subcuta-neous nodules or large tumors, with a predilection for the scalp, neck, and trunk.

Histologic Features
The cutaneous tumors consist of interlacing cords or strands of spindle cells with granular, pale-staining cytoplasm within the dermis and subcutis embedded in a dense, hya-line-like, eosinophilic ground substance that stains posi-tively with PAS and alcian blue.[35] Occasionally, the spindle cells form vascular channels.[36] Younger lesions are more cellular; older lesions are less cellular and tend to contain more ground substance.[37] Ultrastructurally, cystic Golgi vesicles contain a fine fibrillar material that is also found in the ground substance. Type I and III collagen have been

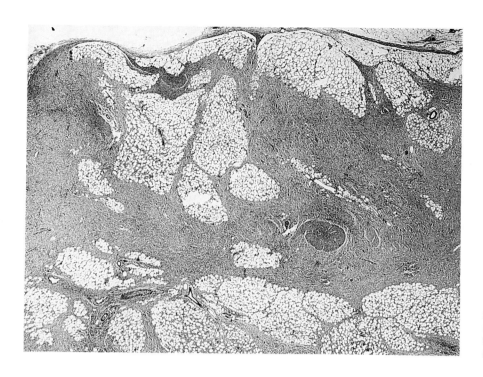

Figure 50–8. Fibrous hamartoma of infancy. Interlacing bundles of fibrous tissue admixed with mature fat and loose fibrous tissue in an organoid fashion. (H&E, ×12.)

identified in the hyaline material through immunohistochemical examination.

CONGENITAL FIBROMATOSIS (INFANTILE MYOFIBROMATOSIS)

Clinical Features
Congenital fibromatosis is used to designate a group of fibroblastic tumors that present at birth or manifest within the first few months of life. They are subdivided into a solitary type; a multiple type, in which numerous tumors involve the subcutis, muscle, and bone; and a generalized type, in which visceral involvement is noted as well. The solitary form is most common with a predilection for the head, arms, and upper torso.[32] The dermal and subcutaneous nodules tend to be small, measuring an average of 0.5 to 1.5 cm in greatest diameter.[38] The most common sites of visceral involvement in the generalized type are the lung, myocardium, and gastrointestinal tract.[39]

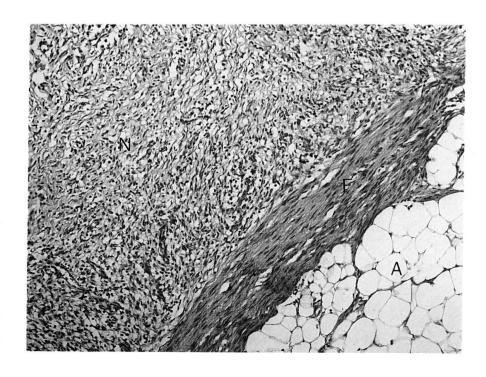

Figure 50–9. Fibrous hamartoma of infancy. Bundle of fibrous tissue (F) comprising slender fibroblasts, separate zones of mature adipose tissue (A), and loose fibrous tissue resembling primitive neural tissue (N). (H&E, ×110.)

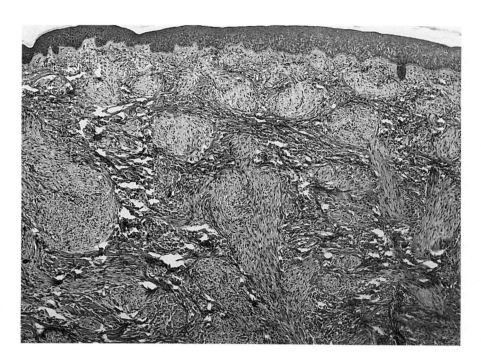

Figure 50–10. Congenital fibromatosis. Proliferation of short bundles and fascicles of plump and elongate spindle cells associated with abundant collagen deposition. (H&E, ×55.)

The prognosis of the types confined to soft tissue and bone is generally good. Recurrence may occur but reexcision is generally curative. Spontaneous regression may occur in the solitary and multiple types. Visceral involvement, and lung involvement in particular, afford a poor prognosis with a frequently fatal outcome.[39] There is some evidence to suggest that congenital fibromatosis is a heritable condition.[40]

Histologic Features

A fairly well circumscribed proliferation of short bundles and fascicles of plump or elongated spindle cells is present, resembling smooth muscle tissue (Figs. 50–10, 50–11).[38–40] Occasional PTAH-positive intracytoplasmic fibers can be detected, as in smooth muscle cells. Abundant collagen is associated with these zones. There may be a more cellular central zone in which rounded cells grow in solid sheets

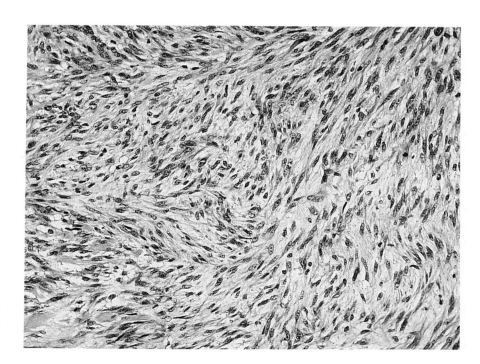

Figure 50–11. Congenital fibromatosis. Short interfacing fascicles of plump spindle cells with some features of smooth muscle (blunt-ended nuclei). (H&E, ×220.)

or in a hemangiopericytoma-like fashion. Foci of necrosis and calcification are frequent. Intravascular extension may occur but does not influence behavior.[38] Ultrastructural features of myofibroblasts have been described. The histologic and ultrastructural features of myofibroblasts have prompted the use of the term *infantile myofibromatosis*.[38]

DESMOID TUMOR

Clinical Features

The desmoid tumor is a poorly circumscribed, deeply seated, infiltrative growth of well-differentiated fibroblasts arising in either fascia or musculoaponeurotic structures. Desmoid tumors of the abdominal wall predominate in females of childbearing age during or after pregnancy. Extraabdominal desmoid tumors may occur at any age, including children, but are most common between puberty and 50 years, with a male predominance. The shoulder, back, chest wall, neck, and lower extremity are the most common sites of involvement. Intraabdominal forms also exist and can be associated with Gardner's syndrome, an autosomal dominant trait characterized by intestinal polyposis often leading to adenocarcinoma, cutaneous cysts, osteomata, and fibromatosis.[41] The tumor is generally solitary and slow growing but multiple tumors can occur rarely.[42,43] The average size ranges from 5 to 10 cm. An episode of trauma may precede the formation of the mass in a small percentage of cases.[44] Classification of the *desmoid* is controversial, with some authors regarding it as a form of fibromatosis[42] and others regarding it as a low-grade fibrosarcoma.[45] It is clear that this tumor can display a marked potential for invasive local growth along with a very strong tendency to recur, even after radical excision; however, it is regarded herein as a form of fibromatosis because of its lack of potential for metastasis and its histologic resemblance to other forms of fibromatosis.

Histologic Features

The tumor is generally restricted to the muscle and overlying aponeurosis or fascia, but it occasionally may involve the subcutis (Fig. 50–12). It is poorly circumscribed with an infiltrative border. Large sweeping fascicles are present, comprising uniform plump fibroblasts with elongated vesicular nuclei embedded in a heavily collagenous stroma (Fig. 50–13). The degree of cellularity varies in different areas and in different tumors. Zones of the stroma may be myxomatous or hypocellular.[45] Cystic degeneration or necrosis is very rare. Keloidlike, thickened hyalinized collagen may be present.[41] Mitotic activity is scant or absent. Where the tumor infiltrates muscle, atrophic multinucleated striated muscle giant cells may be present. Ultrastructurally, features of fibroblasts and myofibroblasts are seen.[41]

Differential Diagnosis

Solitary or multiple congenital fibromatosis tends to be better circumscribed and more superficially located and has myofibroblastic cytologic features. Fibrosarcoma displays greater cellularity, cytologic atypia, and frequent mitoses, including atypical mitoses. (See Fibrosarcoma.)

CONNECTIVE TISSUE NEVUS: COLLAGEN TYPE

Connective tissue nevi in this discussion refer to a group of cutaneous hamartomas characterized by stable, but variable deposition of collagen or elastic fibers, usually within

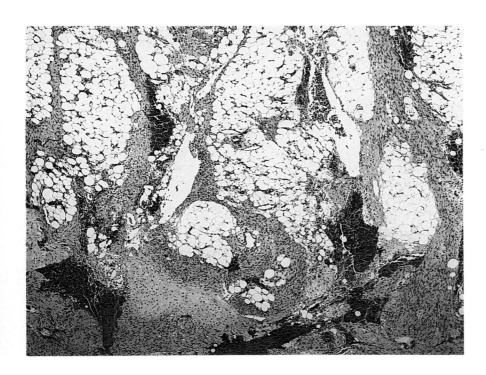

Figure 50–12. Desmoid tumor. Fascicles of uniform fibroblasts growing in an infiltrative pattern within subcutaneous fat and deeper soft tissue. (H&E, ×45.)

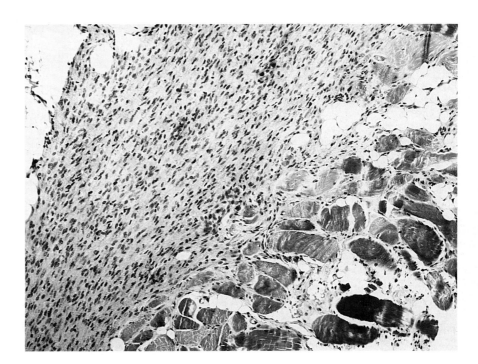

Figure 50–13. Desmoid tumor. Fascicle of slender uniform fibroblasts embedded in a collagenous stroma with infiltration between skeletal muscle bundles (lower right). (H&E, ×110.)

the deeper dermis, unassociated with inflammation. Connective tissue nevi can be subclassified as collagen or elastic tissue type, although a great amount of overlap can exist between patients and even within different lesions in the same patient.

FAMILIAL CUTANEOUS COLLAGENOMA

Clinical Features

Patients have an onset in the teenage years of multiple symmetric indurated nodules, particularly on the trunk and proximal arms. Lesions vary in size from a few millimeters to several centimeters. Accentuation of skin markings (orange peel appearance) may be present. There is no tendency toward grouping or coalescence into plaques. Nodules may increase in number during pregnancy. Inheritance is consistent with an autosomal dominant pattern. Hallmarks of tuberous sclerosis are absent as are skeletal abnormalities. Spontaneous resolution has not been reported. An association with cardiac pathology has been suggested.[46,47]

Histologic Features

There is a dermal thickening with an excessive accumulation of dense coarse variably oriented collagen, giving the dermis an acellular appearance.[46,47] Periadnexal adventitial dermis is replaced by a dense collagen network. The epidermis is normal. Elastic fibers are diminished, possibly representing a dilution effect of the collagen deposition. Focally, elastic fibers may be thin and fragmented.[47]

SHAGREEN PATCH IN TUBEROUS SCLEROSIS

Clinical Features

Tuberous sclerosis is an autosomal dominant condition with variable expressivity; however, up to 50% of cases have been estimated to represent new mutations. It is associated with mental retardation, epilepsy, visceral hamartomatous lesions, and skin lesions, which classically include adenoma sebaceum, soft fibromas of the face and scalp, periungual and subungual fibromas, shagreen patches, and hypopigmented leaf-shaped macules. The shagreen patch is a large, irregularly raised, thickened tumor or plaque, usually found in the lumbosacral region.

Histologic Features

Two patterns can be seen within the shagreen patch.[50] In one type, dense homogeneous collagen bundles are present within the deeper dermal levels, mimicking the appearance of morphea. The other type shows a uniform proliferation of tightly interwoven normal-appearing collagen bundles. At the periphery of the collagen bundles, elastic tissue may be broken or fragmented.[50]

Adenoma sebaceum histologically represents an angiofibroma. A downward displacement of adnexal structures by cellular fibrous connective tissue containing dilated capillary-like vessels is seen. Occasionally, large, stellate, glial-like stromal cells with large nuclei are present. Elastic fibers are absent.[48] Concentric perivascular and perifollicular accumulations of collagen can be seen; this pattern is characteristic of the larger facial fibromas. The ungual fibromas have an appearance similar to that of the facial angiofibromas.

Histologically, the shagreen patch is indistinguishable from connective tissue nevi of the collagen type unassociated with tuberous sclerosis. The facial angiofibromas are indistinguishable from fibrous papule of the nose or perifollicular fibroma.

NONFAMILIAL CUTANEOUS COLLAGENOMA

Clinical Features
Hamartomas of the collagen type unassociated with a family history have been reported.[48,51,52] Several patients with multiple lesions both clinically and histologically similar to familial collagenoma but without a family history have been described as eruptive collagenoma.[48] Connective tissue nevi in a zosteriform pattern have been described.[53,54] Connective tissue nevi of the collagen type have been reported in association with Becker's nevus[55] and multiple fibrofolliculomas.[56] In all cases, tuberous sclerosis must be excluded.

Histologic Features
All of these cases demonstrate dermal accumulation of altered collagen with or without accompanying elastic tissue abnormalities.

CONNECTIVE TISSUE NEVUS: ELASTIC TISSUE TYPE

DERMATOFIBROSIS LENTICULARIS DISSEMINATA IN THE BUSCHKE-OLLENDORFF SYNDROME

Clinical Features
Buschke-Ollendorff syndrome is an autosomal dominant condition that may present in both children and adults. It is characterized by multiple small radiographic densities in the bone, referred to as osteopoikilosis, and cutaneous connective tissue nevi, referred to as dermatofibrosis lenticularis disseminata.[57] The skin lesions are variable, comprising large dermal plaques, shagreen patches, or small, disseminated papules with a cobblestone appearance.[58]

Histologic Features
Microscopic findings differ somewhat from patient to patient, even within affected families.[57–59] In most cases there is alteration of dermal elastic tissue. Marked hyperplasia, clumping, and distortion of broad bands of interlacing elastic fibers is the predominant alteration. In other cases, hyperplasia of morphologically abnormal collagen is present with or without deficiency or fragmentation of elastic fibers, as in a connective tissue nevus of the collagen type.

ELASTOFIBROMA

Clinical Features
Elastofibroma is a slow-growing, deeply seated mass occurring almost exclusively in elderly persons, within the connective tissue between the lower portion of the scapula and the chest wall. Mechanical friction between the scapula and chest wall is the principal cause.[60]

Histologic Features
Overlap features exist between connective tissue nevus of the collagen and elastic tissue types. Within the deep dermis a mixture of swollen eosinophilic collagen and elastic fibers is seen in association with occasional fibroblasts and mature fat cells (Fig. 50–14). The elastic fibers have a degenerated beaded appearance or are fragmented into small globules or droplets having a linear appearance.[60] A flowerlike appearance is seen in elastic tissue cross section. Elastic tissue stains reveal branched and unbranched fibers with irregular serrated margins and a central dense core.

ISOLATED ELASTOMA

Isolated cases of connective tissue nevi of the elastic tissue type have been reported.[48] Juvenile elastoma demonstrates dermal nodules containing marked accumulation of normal-appearing elastic fibers.[61] Similar cases have been reported as nevus elasticus.[62] The grouped perifollicular papules of the pectoral region described as the Lewandowsky type of connective tissue nevus were mislabeled nevus elasticus because they are characterized by an absence or marked reduction in elastic fibers and normal collagen.[63]

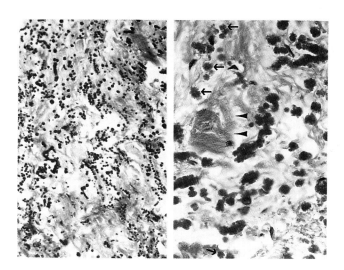

Figure 50–14. Elastofibroma. Left: Fragmented, globular aggregates of elastic tissue within swollen eosinophilic collagen bundles. Right: Beaded or globular appearance of altered elastic fibers with focal flowerlike arrangements seen in cross section (arrows) with swollen collagen bundles (arrowheads). (Left: H&E, ×145; right: H&E, ×385.)

BENIGN TUMORS OF FIBROUS TISSUE

DERMATOFIBROMA (CUTANEOUS BENIGN FIBROUS HISTIOCYTOMA)

Clinical Features

Dermatofibroma is a common tumor of the skin that can be found at any age, with an increased frequency between the third and fifth decades.[64,65] There is a female predominance and the most frequent sites of involvement are the lower extremities, but the tumors can occur at any site. The lesion is usually solitary or few in number. Multiple forms have been described.[66] Multiple dermatofibromas have been reported in association with systemic lupus erythematosus and myasthenia gravis,[67,68] and a familial variant has been described.[69]

The lesion presents as a slowly-growing, firm dermal nodule ranging in size from 3 mm to 2cm and in color from brown to red-brown to yellow or ivory. Lateral compression will dimple the central portion of the lesion, a clinical finding considered as an aid in differentiation from other tumors including melanoma.[70] Recurrence after local excision is uncommon.[71]

Histologic Features

A poorly circumscribed proliferation of varying cellularity containing fibroblasts, histiocytes, and mature collagen occupies the dermis (Fig. 50–15).[72] Focal superficial extension into the subcutis can be seen; however, massive infiltration of the fat is not a feature. Margins are not sharply defined and the degree of cellularity often dissipates at the tumor edges. The cellular proliferation may abut on the epidermis or leave a grenz zone. The epidermis characteristically demonstrates basilar hyperpigmentation and notable irregular acanthosis, with lengthening, widening, and distortion of the rete. Irregular downward basaloid proliferations of the epidermis may be seen, in some cases showing differentiation into primitive hair follicle tissue (Fig. 50–15).[73] Superficial and invasive basal cell carcinoma has been reported in association with dermatofibroma.[74–76]

The tumor is usually predominantly fibrous with dense collagen arranged in a vague storiform or whorled pattern containing a scanty number of slender fibroblastic cells; however, some lesions may demonstrate a high degree of cellularity while maintaining a predominantly spindle cell morphology (Fig. 50–16). Mitoses are rare without atypical forms. Rounded histiocytic cells can participate as a minor component. Lesions in which large histiocytic cells predominate are rare and have been referred to as histiocytomas. In these cases, the collagen stroma is delicate with prominent vasculature, and Touton cells, xanthoma cells, and multinucleated cells are common (Fig. 50–17). When hemosiderin deposition within the large cells is prominent, the term *hemosiderotic histiocytoma* is employed.[77]

In all variants of dermatofibroma a prominent capillary network can be seen. Secondary elements, including foam cells, multinucleated cells, hemosiderin-laden cells, and lymphocytes, are characteristic. Lymphoid nodules may rarely be present at the periphery.[78] Cystic areas of hemor-

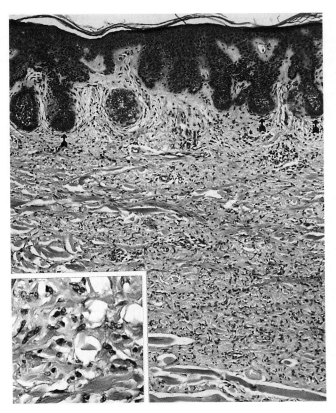

Figure 50–15. Dermatofibroma. Mildly cellular lesion with sparse spindle and stellate cells embedded in fibrous stroma. Note the overlying epidermal hyperplasia, in this case showing notable basaloid hyperplasia and hair follicle differentiation with miniature hair bulbs (arrows). Inset: Oval, elongated, and stellate cells percolating between collagen bundles. (H&E, ×65; inset: H&E, ×165.)

rhage can be present. In a small number of cases, prominent stromal and vascular hyalinization is present. These lesions were, in the past, referred to as sclerosing hemangioma (Fig. 50–18).

Aneurysmal (angiomatoid) fibrous histiocytoma demonstrates large blood-filled spaces lacking endothelial lining and surrounded by histiocytes that show xanthomatization and hemosiderin deposition.[79] More solid zones of spindled fibroblasts and red cell extravasation are present as well. The lesion may arise within an aneurysmal blood vessel.[80] Zones of marked focal cellular atypia have been reported.

Lesions described as "atypical cutaneous fibrous histiocytoma" demonstrate large, atypical, often multinucleated cells with nuclear pleomorphism, hyperchromatism, and prominent nucleoli.[81–83] Mitotic figures are scarce or absent. These lesions tend to be rich in histiocytes, which are often xanthomatized.

Immunohistochemistry demonstrates cytoplasmic α_1-antitrypsin and/or lysozyme in 13% to 63% of cases.[84,85] Positive staining is higher in cellular variants. Between 30% and 70% of the constituent cells label with factor XIIIa, suggesting a large population of dermal dendritic cells.[86] Electron microscopy demonstrates a spectrum of cell types including fibroblasts, myofibroblasts, and histiocytes.[87]

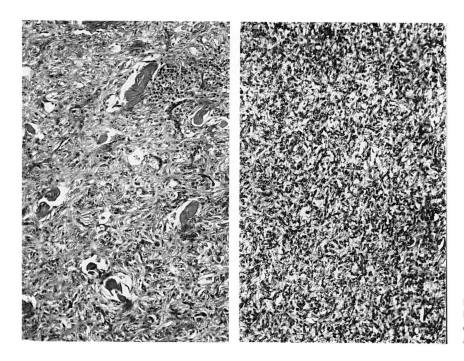

Figure 50–16. Dermatofibroma. Left: Hypocellular, predominantly fibrous type. Right: Hypercellular variant with little collagen stroma. (Left and right: H&E, ×100.)

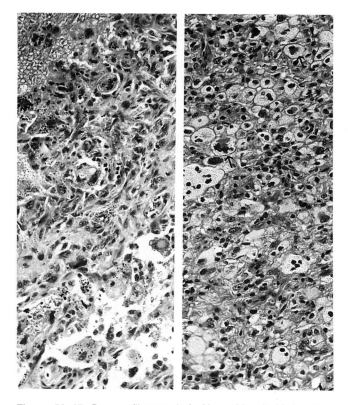

Figure 50–17. Dermatofibroma. Left: Hemosiderotic histiocytoma variant containing mono- and multinucleated foamy cells with abundant hemosiderin deposition and red cell extravasation (upper left corner). Right: Histiocytoma variant containing numerous mononucleated foamy cells with occasional multinucleated cells, some Tounton-like (arrows). (Left: H&E, ×120; right: H&E, ×165.)

Differential Diagnosis

Neurofibroma displays a more loose edematous stroma, wavy nuclei, and absent storiform or cartwheel growth pattern. Leiomyoma displays a more prominent fascicular growth pattern with characteristic blunt-ended nuclei. Dermatofibrosarcoma protuberans displays a more uniform cellular population with absence of secondary elements (foam cells, multinucleated cells, inflammatory cells) and shows a more prominent, monotonous storiform growth pattern with involvement of the subcutis and absence of the proliferative epidermal changes characteristic of dermatofibroma. Malignant fibrous histiocytoma is pleomorphic and deeply seated, with numerous typical and atypical mitoses. Xanthoma can be difficult to exclude in dermatofibroma rich in foam cells, but fibrous zones with storiform growth pattern and epidermal hyperplasia favor dermatofibroma.

FIBROEPITHELIAL POLYP (ACROCHORDON, SKIN TAGS) AND FIBROMA

Clinical Features

These extremely common lesions appear as multiple, skin-colored to light brown soft fleshy tags occurring most commonly about the neck, upper chest, and axillae.[88,89] They are more frequent in women and have their onset in middle adult life. Most lesions are small, measuring 1 to 5 mm in maximum diameter. Lesions larger than 1 cm may ocur; these are often pedunculated, occur on the lower trunk, and are sometimes referred to as soft fibromas. Twisting with subsequent infarction as well as repeated minor trauma is common. Multiple fibromas have been described in asso-

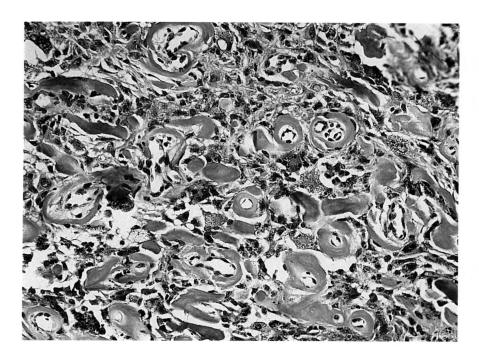

Figure 50–18. Dermatofibroma, sclerosing hemangioma type. Prominent sclerotic thick-walled proliferating vessels within the tumor. (H&E, ×175.)

ciation with Cowden's disease,[90,91] in addition to the multiple facial hair follicle tumors. Multiple soft fibromas on the face and scalp, as well as subungual and periungual fibromas, are a cutaneous manifestation of tuberous sclerosis.[92]

Histologic Features and Differential Diagnosis

The lesion is polypoid with a loose edematous stroma rich in dilated thin-walled vessels. Distinction from hemangioma can be difficult in some cases. Adnexal structures are not present. The epidermis displays varying degrees of hyperkeratosis, irregular acanthosis, and papillomatosis. These changes, along with occasional pseudoinclusion horn cyst formation, can make distinction from seborrheic keratosis difficult and arbitrary in some cases. Mature fat cells may occupy a large portion of the center of the polyp. If extensive fatty replacement, including fat tissue herniating into the papillary dermis, is present, a diagnosis of nevus lipomatosus superficialis can be considered. Older, involuting nevi may display similar gross morphology; therefore nevus cells can be found in numerous fibroepithelial polyp–like lesions. Soft fibromas display a loose edematous stroma without significant epidermal changes. If the stroma is composed of dense collagen, the term *fibroma* can be used.

The fibromas associated with Cowden's disease are well-circumscribed, nonencapsulated tumors of the mid- and upper dermis comprising an organized pattern of interwoven fascicles of coarse, widely spaced, hyalinized collagen bundles separated by broad mucin-rich spaces.[90,91] A moderate increase in fibroblasts is seen. Fibromas of the soft fibroma type, as well as multiple skin tags, can be seen as well.

The face and scalp fibromas associated with tuberous sclerosis demonstrate thickened sclerotic collagen bundles arranged concentrically around atrophic pilosebaceous

units.[92] The peri- and subungual fibromas demonstrate fibrosis and proliferation of gliallike, large, stellate fibroblasts.[92]

TUMORS OF PERIFOLLICULAR CONNECTIVE TISSUE

Clinical Features

The three tumors of perifollicular connective tissue, namely, trichodiscoma, perifollicular fibroma, and fibrofolliculoma, look quite similar clinically, presenting as small, skin-colored, flat or dome-shaped papules that are generally multiple and localized symmetrically on the face, ears, trunk, and extremities.[93–99]

Trichodiscomas have been reported (1) as nonfamilial generalized and multiple forms,[93] (2) as a dominantly inherited pure form,[94] and (3) as a dominantly inherited form associated with multiple fibrofolliculomas and acrochordons.[95,96] Perifollicular fibromas have been described in nonfamilial, limited forms,[97] as well as a generalized, familial form.[98] Fibrofolliculomas have been reported in pure and mixed forms.[95,96,99] Fibrofolliculoma is discussed in greater detail in Chapter 45.

Histologic Features

Trichodiscomas are fibrovascular tumors of the hair disk, which is a touch receptor consisting of well-vascularized dermal connective tissue and thick myelinated nerves in contact with Merkel cells adjacent to the hair follicle in the papillary dermis.[93] The trichodiscoma is an elliptical parafollicular lesion comprising interwoven fascicles of fine fibrillar collagen embedded in abundant alcian blue–positive ground substance with a moderate increase in fibroblasts (Fig. 50–19).[93] An increased density of telangiectatic blood

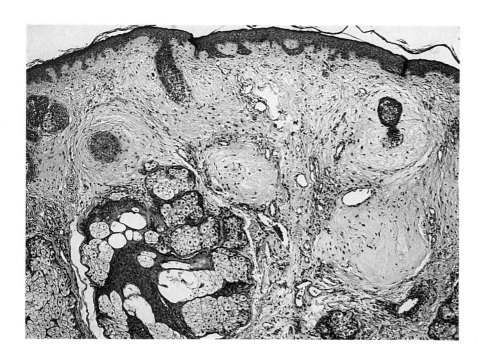

Figure 50–19. Trichodiscoma. Parafollicular, sparsely cellular proliferation of fibroblasts and fine fibrillar collagen within a myxoid stroma with telangiectases. (H&E, ×120.)

vessels is seen. Endothelial cell proliferation including endothelial cell aggregates can be present.[94] There is flattening of the overlying epidermis and bent rete ridges at the periphery.

Perifollicular fibroma is characterized by marked connective tissue proliferation of the fibrous root sheath with young hypercellular collagen surrounding hair follicles in a concentric fashion. The follicles are small, vellus type, and may be dilated and keratin filled.[97,98]

Fibrofolliculoma shows a cystically dilated, keratin-filled follicle surrounded by proliferative fibrous connective tissue. Numerous thin, anastomosing bands of outer root sheath epithelium extend from the infundibulum into the surrounding expanded fibrous root sheath.[95,96]

FIBROUS PAPULE OF THE NOSE (FACE)

Clinical Features

Fibrous papule is a very common lesion that appears as a small, solitary dome-shaped papule generally on the nose of adults.[100] Its clinical appearance may suggest a nevus or basal cell carcinoma. It may rarely occur elsewhere on the head and neck.

Histologic Features

The dermis is fibrous, containing variable numbers of fibroblasts which can be spindled, plump, oval, multinucleate, or stellate, resembling ganglion cells.[100] There is an increase in dilated blood vessels. Coarse collagen fibers wrap around vellus hair follicles in a concentric pattern, as is seen in perifollicular fibroma (see preceding section) (Fig. 50–20). Perivascular fibrosis may be present. Ultrastructural analysis of the cellular component supports a fibrohistiocytic origin.[62,101]

These features are quite similar to those seen in angiofibromas associated with tuberous sclerosis, and, for this reason, fibrous papule is regarded by some authors as a form of solitary angiofibroma.[103]

ANGIOFIBROMA (TUBEROUS SCLEROSIS, PEARLY PENILE PAPULES)

Clinical Features

Multiple angiofibromas form an essential component of tuberous sclerosis, a dominantly inherited disorder, which includes mental deficiency, epilepsy, fibromas of the face and scalp, subungual and periungual fibromas, shagreen patches (a form of connective tissue nevus), and white macules.[104,105] Systemic involvement includes gliomas of the central nervous system and retina, cardiac rhabdomyomas, renal angiomyolipomas, and cystic lesions of bone, kidney, and lung.[106]

The facial angiofibromas of tuberous sclerosis are variably sized, firm, red or light-brown papules in a symmetric centrofacial distribution about the chin, nasolabial folds, and cheeks. These develop in childhood and most often appear as the presenting sign of the disease.[105] They were, in the past, referred to as adenoma sebaceum.

Pearly penile papules, a form of acral angiofibroma, consist of one to five rows of discrete 1- to 4-mm papules distributed circumferentially around the coronal sulcus.[107]

Histologic Features

Angiofibroma demonstrates similar histology regardless of its clinical association. There is dermal fibrosis with a proliferation of fibroblasts displaying either a spindled, plump oval, or stellate (glial) appearance (Fig. 50–21). Multinucleated cells may be seen. There is vascular proliferation

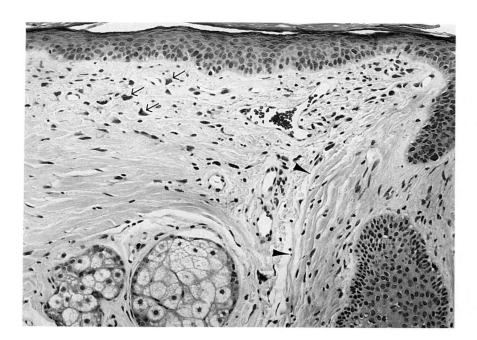

Figure 50–20. Fibrous papule. Fibrous dermis containing plump, oval, spindled, and stellate fibroblasts (arrows) with proliferation of dilated blood vessels and perifollicular fibrosis (arrowheads). (H&E, ×175.)

and dilatation. Perivascular and concentric perifollicular fibrosis can be seen.[104]

These histologic features can be indistinguishable from fibrous papule of the face. For differentiation from tumors of perifollicular connective tissue see that section.

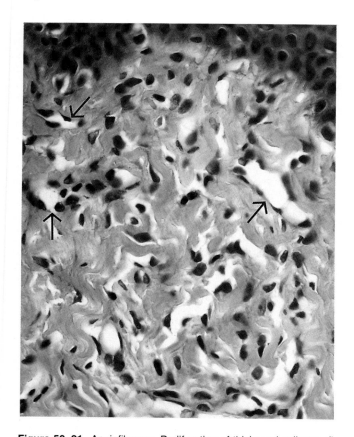

Figure 50–21. Angiofibroma. Proliferation of thickened collagen, fibroblasts, and blood channels (arrows). (H&E, ×500.)

ACQUIRED (DIGITAL) FIBROKERATOMA

Clinical Features

Acquired fibrokeratoma consists of a solitary, firm, hyperkeratotic protrusion that tends to occur around interphalangeal joints, but may occur on the palms, soles, dorsal hands, feet, and legs.[108–110] They are generally less than 1.5 cm, but larger lesions can occur.[111] The lesions may be pointed or dome-shaped, sessile, or pedunculated. Acquired fibrokeratoma occurs in adults.

Histologic Features

The tumor is composed of thickened collagen bundles that may have a parallel or interwoven growth pattern. Cellularity is generally sparse; however, in some cases, increased fibroblast density is notable.[109] Elastic tissue is generally reduced or absent. Foci of increased deposition of hyaluronic acid may be seen.[108–110] Nerves are small and sparse, in contrast to supernumerary digit. Adnexal structures are few to absent. Vascular proliferation has been noted in some cases.[109,110] The epidermis demonstrates hyperorthokeratosis and a variable degree of acanthosis (Fig. 50–22).

FIBROMA OF TENDON SHEATH

Clinical Features

Fibroma of tendon sheath presents as a solitary, slowly growing, occasionally painful nodule usually arising from, or near, a tendon sheath on the fingers, hands, wrists, and feet.[112,113] This fibroma occurs in adults of any age with a predominance in middle-aged males. It is rarely larger than 3 to 4 cm in maximum diameter.[113] Local recurrence has been reported in 25% of cases.[112]

Histologic Features

There is a sharply demarcated deposition of hyalinized, whorled fibrous tissue of variable cellularity located within

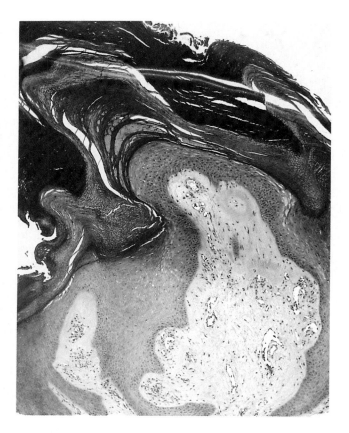

Figure 50–22. Acquired fibrokeratoma. Orthohyperkeratosis, irregular acanthosis, and dermal fibrosis with sparse cellularity. (H&E, ×170.)

the dermis or superficial subcutis (Fig. 50–23).[112,113] Hypocellular zones predominate. Zones of notably increased cellularity can be seen in which scattered, normal-appearing mitoses may be present.[112] Vascular channels, many slitlike,

are a prominent feature.[112,113] Focal myxoid generation can be seen.[113]

GIANT CELL TUMOR OF TENDON SHEATH (PIGMENTED VILLONODULAR SYNOVITIS AND TENOSYNOVITIS)

Clinical Features

Giant cell tumor of tendon sheath is a common tumor of the fingers and hands. It can occur at any age, with a predominance between the ages of 30 and 50.[114] It typically appears as a painless, 0.5- to 4-cm, slowly growing nodule arising predominantly on the fingers and less commonly on the knee, hand, wrist, foot, and hip.[114–117] On the finger, it is typically located adjacent to the interphalangeal joint. The tumors are not fixed to skin unless they are located in the distal finger. Pressure erosion of the adjacent bone without bone invasion can be seen on x-ray in a small portion of patients.[114] Although benign, giant cell tumors of tendon sheath may recur in 10% to 44% of cases.[116,117] A diffuse form of this tumor has been reported in which notable, poorly confined soft tissue extension is present with or without adjacent joint involvement.[118]

Histologic Features

The tumor is circumscribed and lobulated with attachment to a tendon sheath. A dense collagenous capsule surrounds and penetrates the tumor, dividing it into poorly formed nodules. There are variable numbers of mononuclear cells, xanthoma cells, and giant cells associated with variable amounts of collagen (Fig. 50–24). Typically, moderately cellular sheets of mononuclear cells blend with less cellular, collagenized zones in which the cells may display spindle morphology. Multinucleated giant cells are scattered about the tumor; these display hypereosinophilic cytoplasms containing anywhere from 4 to 60 nuclei. Hemosiderin-laden cells are common. Mitotic figures can be present.[117,118]

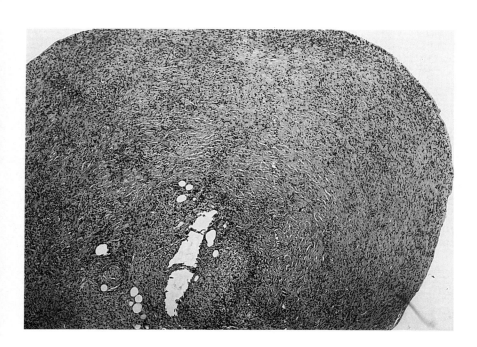

Figure 50–23. Fibroma of tendon sheath. Well-circumscribed tumor showing alternating cellular and hypocellular zones. (H&E, ×45.)

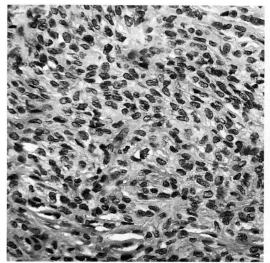
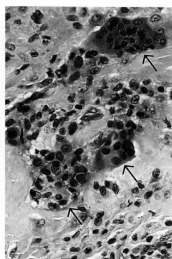

Figure 50–24. Giant cell tumor of tendon sheath. Left: Moderately cellular sheets of oval mononuclear and plump spindle cells. Right: Scattered multinucleated giant cells containing numerous nuclei (arrows). (Left: H&E, ×250; right: H&E, ×260.)

FIBRO-OSSEOUS PSEUDOTUMOR OF THE DIGITS

Clinical Features

Fibro-osseous pseudotumor of the digits presents as a fusiform swelling or mass, most often in the region of the proximal phalanx of the index or middle finger.[119] It predominates in adults between 20 and 30 years of age. The lesion appears suddenly in most cases. Overlying erythema of the skin is common. The lesion occurs in children and adults. Recurrence is rare and complete local excision is curative.

Histologic Features

The lesion is a poorly defined multinodular tumor involving the subcutis and adjacent fibrous structures without muscle involvement. A mixture of typical and atypical fibroblasts, osteoblasts, and bony trabeculae of variable maturity is seen. Zones of loosely arranged fibroblasts in a myxoid stroma are intermixed with more cellular fibrous zones. The fibroblasts can display nuclear pleomorphism and mitotic activity. The osteoblasts are without cellular atypism. Osteoclasts are rare.

GIANT CELL FIBROBLASTOMA

Clinical Features

A rare tumor, giant cell fibroblastoma occurs mainly in males under the age of 10; the majority of patients are under 5 years of age.[120–122] Young and middle-aged adults can be affected.[122] The tumors are superficial, measuring from 1 to 6 cm in maximum diameter, and are slowly growing and usually painless. Predominant locations are the trunk, inguinal or scrotal regions, thigh, and neck. Recurrence is present in roughly 50% of cases[120,122] in most cases, recurrence may be the result of involvement of the margins of excision.[120] No metastasis has been reported. None of the tumors have been multiple or familial. Some authors believe that this tumor should be grouped with the juvenile fibromatoses.[121]

Histologic Features

There may be involvement of the dermis, subcutis, and deeper soft tissue. This tumor consists of variable proportions of solid and angiectoid zones (Fig. 50–25). Scattered randomly throughout both zones are multinucleated giant

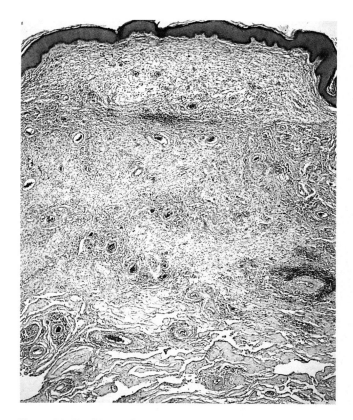

Figure 50–25. Giant cell fibroblastoma. Solid spindle cell zones of moderate cellularity within the superficial dermis and middermis. Superficial portion shows myxoid stroma; middermis demonstrates more densely collagenous stroma. Angiectoid zone with pseudosinusoids is present in deep dermis. Vascular proliferation is present throughout. (H&E, ×35.)

cells containing 5 to 15 nuclei, usually arranged circumferentially around the periphery of the cell in a wreath- or floret-like pattern (Fig. 50–26). The cytoplasm is pink, without foamy features. The solid areas vary in cellularity from hypocellular, with only scattered fibroblasts and floret-type giant cells embedded in dense hyalinized collagen, to moderately cellular, with plump fibroblasts, wavy collagen, and myxoid stroma. The angiectoid zones are formed by pseudosinusoids separated by loose connective tissue containing abundant ground substance. The pseudosinusoids vary from huge gaping sinuses as seen in cavernous hemangioma to small compressed slitlike spaces. Red cells are commonly present within these spaces as a result of the surgical procedure. These spaces are lined in part by floret cells, in part by similar, smaller mononucleated cells, and in part by collagen fibers. Mitoses are rare in all cell types. Small aggregates of entrapped degenerating fat are seen in some tumors.

Immunohistochemical staining for factor VIII antigen is negative in the floret and mononucleated cells lining the angiectoid spaces, as well as in the spindle and floret cells in the solid areas.[120,121] Electron microscopy demonstrates fibroblastic features in both the mononuclear and multinucleate cells, as well as in the spindle cells. Long, thin cytoplasmic processes are present.[120,121]

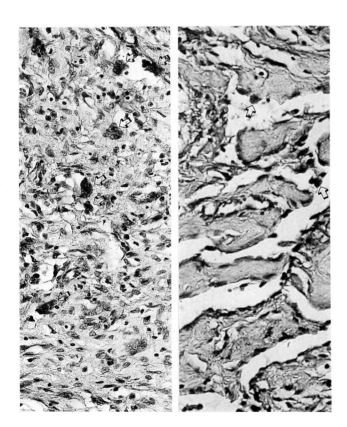

Figure 50–26. Giant cell fibroblastoma. Left: Moderately cellular zone containing plump fibroblasts, abundant collagen, and numerous floret-type giant cells (arrows). Right: Angiectoid zone with pseudosinusoids lined by mononuclear cells, some flattened, and rare multinucleated cells (arrows). (Left and right: H&E, ×225.)

MALIGNANT TUMORS OF FIBROUS TISSUE

ATYPICAL FIBROXANTHOMA

Clinical Features

Atypical fibroxanthoma (AFX) is an uncommon solitary tumor of the skin that has been reported as paradoxical fibrosarcoma,[123] pseudosarcoma,[124–126] pseudosarcomatous dermatofibroma,[127] and pseudosarcomatous reticulohistiocytoma.[128]

It occurs most on sun- or irradiation-damaged skin of the head and neck of elderly people, the median age being approximately 69 years. Less commonly, it may occur on the limbs and trunk of young and middle-aged persons, with the median age of such patients being approximately 40 years.[129,130] The ears, cheek, and nose are the most commonly affected sites. An approximate 3:2 male predominance is seen.[131]

The tumor presents as a firm, solitary, often ulcerated nodule, usually measuring less than 2 cm in diameter, although large tumors have been reported.[129] The lesion generally appears as a rapidly growing tumor of a few months' duration; only rarely, its growth may extend 10 years or longer, and these lesions are usually associated with previous radiation therapy.[131,132] Lesions on the trunk and limbs are slower growing and of longer duration than those on the head and neck.

The common occurence of this tumor on actinically damaged skin and its frequent association with other actinic-related lesions suggests solar radiation as a predisposing factor.[129] The relationship of prior irradiation and trauma is less clear, although many cases of AFX developing after exposure to therapeutic radiation have been reported with latent periods in excess of 10 years. This time interval is compatible with a radiation-induced tumor.[132] Many of these tumors reported as AFX may have actually represented spindle cell squamous carcinomas, as immunohistochemistry for cytokeratin was not applied in these cases.

The biologic nature of AFX has been controversial. In the majority of studies of this tumor, growth has been self-contained and curable by local excision, arguing in favor of a benign process despite its malignant histologic appearance.[129,131] Even in some cases in which primary excision was considered incomplete, recurrence was not observed.[133] Arguing against a benign process is a well-recognized potential for local recurrence[129,132] and five well-documented cases of metastasis.[129,130,134–136] These cases of metastasis were not histologically distinguishable from other cases of AFX, with the exception of vascular invasion and subcutaneous involvement in one case.[129]

Although AFX has an excellent prognosis after conservative, but complete, excision, it should best be regarded as a low-grade sarcoma because of its potential, albeit small, for metastasis. Its lack of aggressive biologic behavior may, in large part, result from its superficial location.

Histologic Features

These tumors are moderately well-circumscribed dermal nodules, although minor extension into the subcutis can be seen. Invasion of deeper soft tissues is not present.[137] Ulceration is common. The nonulcerated epidermis is effaced and atrophic. The epidermis at the edges of the tumor nodule may be hyperplastic and form a collarette. Adnexal structures are sparse and may be entrapped or distorted. The tumor is highly cellular with a disorganized haphazard arrangement. Most tumors display zones of interlacing bundles of plump spindle cells in a vague fascicular pattern alternating with haphazardly arranged large polyhedral cells, although either growth pattern may predominate (Figs. 50–27 to 50–29).[129,132,137] A well-developed storiform or broad fascicular growth pattern is generally not observed.

The cell constituents are polymorphous with cellular and nuclear pleomorphism.[129,131,132,137] These include plump spindle cells with vesicular to hyperchromatic nuclei, pleomorphic polyhedral histiocytoid cells with prominent nucleoli and abundant vacuolated cytoplasm, and bizarre mono- and multinucleated giant cells with giant, irregular hyperchromatic nuclei and enlarged nucleoli. Xanthoma cells are uncommon. Both typical and atypical mitototic figures are numerous, averaging one per high power field.[132,137] Occasional inflammatory cells may be present. Reactive vascular proliferation is present commonly both within and surrounding the tumor. Only small amounts of collagen are seen. Necrosis is rare and, if prominent, argues against the diagnosis of AFX.[138] Osteoid production as been described in a single case.[139]

Ultrastructural studies have shown cells possessing fea-

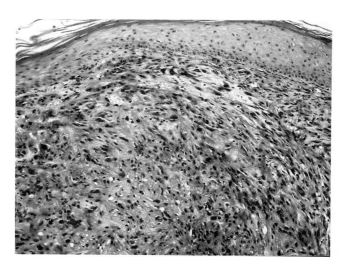

Figure 50–28. Vague interlacing bundles of atypical spindle cells with epidermal flattening and atrophy. (H&E, ×165.)

tures of fibroblasts, myofibroblasts, and histiocytes, including intermediate forms with overlapping features.[140,141] Langerhans granules, characteristic of Langerhans cells, have been described in two cases.[140,142] This finding, albeit

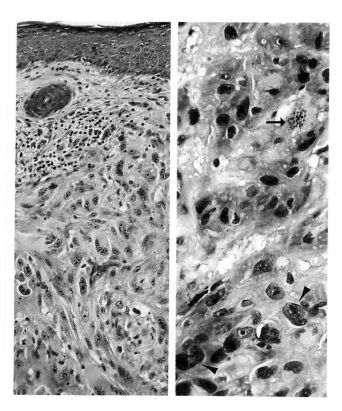

Figure 50–27. Atypical fibroxanthoma. Left: Predominantly large polyhedral histiocytoid cells, suggestive of carcinoma, fill the dermis. Right: Striking cytologic atypia with numerous mitoses (arrow) and scattered multinucleated cells (arrowheads). (Left: H&E, ×165; Right: H&E, ×340.)

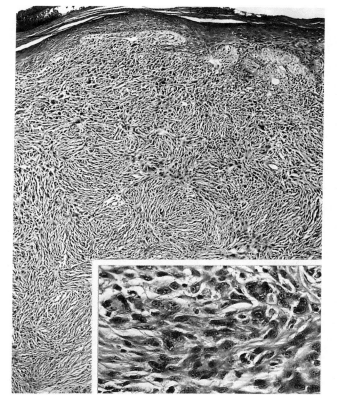

Figure 50–29. Atypical fibroxanthoma. Prominent spindle cell morphology with vague fascicles and more abundant collagen than is usual. Inset: Marked cytologic atypia of both mono- and multinucleated cells. (H&E, ×115; inset: H&E, ×285.)

rare, may suggest tumor heterogenicity among AFXs. Ultrastructural features of melanocytic or epithelial differentiation are absent.

Differential Diagnosis

The differential diagnosis includes spindle cell squamous cell carcinoma, spindle cell melanoma, malignant fibrous histiocytoma, leiomyosarcoma, and dermatofibrosarcoma protuberans. In the absence of features specific for either melanoma or carcinoma (i.e., junctional melanocytic nests, intracytoplasmic melanin, invasive islands of discernible epithelium), differentiation from melanoma and squamous cell carcinoma can be extremely difficult, even after thorough sampling of the lesion. The basement membrane in AFX often becomes indistinct without clear separation of tumor cells from overlying basilar epidermal cells. This fact and the frequent presence of ulceration further hamper separation from squamous carcinoma or melanoma.[131] In this application, immunohistochemistry can be extremely useful.[137,143–145] Squamous cell carcinoma is positive for cytokeratin and usually positive for epithelial membrane antigen; AFX is negative for these determinates. Vimentin is present as an intermediate filament in both AFX and melanoma, but is absent in squamous carcinoma.[145] The majority of AFXs demonstrate positivity for α_1-antitrypsin and α_1-antichymotrypsin; however, squamous carcinoma and melanoma may be positive for these enzymes, making their usefulness somewhat limited. Positivity for S100 protein, a consistent feature of melanoma, is absent in the vast majority of AFXs;[137,145] however, minimally positive S100 protein staining has been reported in AFX.[144] In these cases, the S100-positive cells were dendritic in nature and were observed in greatest concentration at the periphery of the lesion associated with inflammatory cells, suggesting that they represented dermal dendritic cells and not true tumor cells. Ultrastructural studies can also be utilized to exclude melanoma and squamous carcinomas.

Malignant fibrous histiocytoma generally displays a more prominent storiform or myxoid growth pattern and is situated more deeply, extensively involving the subcutis with extension into fascia or muscle. Dermatofibrosarcoma protuberans is a proliferation of relatively uniform spindle cells in a prominent storiform pattern. Giant cells and the degree of pleomorphism seen in AFX are absent. Leiomyosarcoma displays a well-organized fascicular growth pattern with interlacing fascicles of relatively uniform plump spindle cells with blunt-ended nuclei and longitudinal cytoplasmic filaments apparent with trichrome stains.

DERMATOFIBROSARCOMA PROTUBERANS

Clinical Features

Dermatofibrosarcoma protuberans (DFSP) is a slowly growing, locally aggressive, rarely metastasizing, malignant neoplasm which frequently recurs after attempts at excision.[146–152] It occurs at any age but generally affects adolescents, young adults and middle-aged adults principally, with a male preference. The tumor most often presents on the trunk and extremities, but may occur at any site.

It begins as a firm, sclerodermoid plaquelike thickening of the skin inducing a red-blue discoloration of the overlying skin. The plaque eventually gives rise to one or more nodules, resulting in the protuberant appearance that its name suggests. The tumor may appear initially in a nodular configuration.[146] Although DFSP is generally stationary or slow growing over months to years, the appearance of a nodular character heralds a phase of accelerated growth. Ulceration may occur. In rare cases, despite advanced stage of tumor growth, no protrusion of the tumor is noted clinically.[150] These tumors clinically resemble morphea or morpheaform basal cell carcinoma.[150] The overall size is variable, averaging 5 cm.

The recurrence rate is high, ranging from 20% to 60%;[146–152] tumors recur generally within 1 to 3 years of surgery, although a small group can recur very late. Metastasis to lymph nodes and viscera has been reported. The overall frequency of metastasis varies considerably between series; however, it is generally considered to be less than 1%.[153,154] Appropriate therapy consists of wide local excision at the earliest detectable phase of the tumor.

Histologic Features

The tumor diffusely infiltrates the dermis and subcutis and may appose the epidermis or leave a grenz zone of papillary dermal sparing.[146–152] The epidermis, as a rule, does not display the type of hyperplasia associated with dermatofibroma (cutaneous fibrous histiocytoma). Epidermal atrophy or ulceration may occur. DFSP exhibits a uniform cellular proliferation of fibroblasts in a prominent storiform (matlike), whorled or cartwheel pattern, whereby the fibroblasts arrange themselves in whorls or bundles around central acellular zones (Figs. 50–30, 50–31).[146–152] In a minority of cases, this storiform growth pattern is inapparent or focal, requiring study of multiple tissue blocks. The cells intermingle with collagen bundles of varying thickness. The tumor is cellular centrally, becoming less so peripherally. Although the collagen stains with trichrome, it is not usually polarizable in DFSP and this absence of polarizable collagen as been suggested as a useful differentiating feature between DFSP and dermatofibroma.[155] The superficial portion of the tumor may be deceptively hypocellular, making diagnosis on the basis of superficial biopsy very difficult.

The tumor cells are monomorphic, plump spindle cells with elongated nuclei. Nuclear hyperchromatism or pleomorphism is not prominent. There is scanty, ill-defined eosinophilic cytoplasm. Cells within more cellular zones may be more rounded or histiocytic in appearance. Foam cells and giant cells are not features of DFSP. Mitotic activity is generally present, but usually does not exceed 5 mitoses/10 high-power fields.[146–152] A low mitotic rate does not preclude aggressive behavior.

Thin-walled capillaries are randomly distributed throughout, occasionally occupying the center of individual cartwheel zones. Perivascular and peripheral accumulations of lymphocytes are commonly seen. Tumor necrosis is rare. Myxoid zones with sparse cellularity are not uncommon. Totally myxoid variants of DFSP have been described, demonstrating a monotonous pattern of sparse, uniform cellularity and pale myxoid stroma with rare foci of storiform growth.[156] Metastases may consist predominantly of large

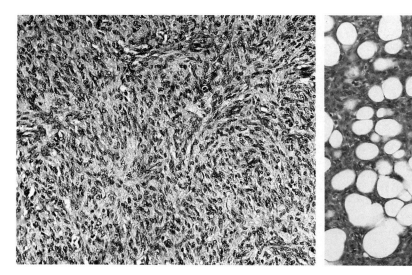

Figure 50–30. Dermatofibrosarcoma protuberans. Left: Uniform cellular proliferation of fibroblasts in a storiform pattern. Right: Characteristic massive diffuse infiltration between fat cells of the subcutis. (Left: H&E, ×190; Right: H&E, ×165.)

histiocytic cells or may demonstrate the same spindled growth pattern of the primary tumor.[148,149,153,154,157]

The pigmented DFSP or Bednar tumor contains, in addition to areas characteristic of DFSP, a population of deeply pigmented bipolar or multiple dendritic cells scattered randomly throughout the tumor (Fig. 50–32).[158] The pigment is Fontana-Masson positive, iron negative. These cells fail to demonstrate immunoreactivity for S100 protein.

Immunohistochemistry of DFSP demonstrates focal lysozyme and antichymotrypsin staining in only a small minority of cases.[146,159] Ultrastructural studies have provided conflicting evidence of either fibroblastic, histiocytic, or schwannian differentiation.[160–162]

Differential Diagnosis

Benign cutaneous fibrous histiocytoma (dermatofibroma) differs from DFSP in its characteristic hyperplastic epidermal changes, confinement to the dermis, smaller size, and uninodularity. Microscopically, dermatofibroma has more cellular polymorphism, including large histiocytic cells, foamy and hemosiderin-laden macrophages, and multinucleated cells. If only a superficial biopsy of DFSP is obtained, however, differentiation from dermatofibroma can be difficult. Thorough sampling of DFSP is crucial for accurate diagnosis. Malignant fibrous histiocytoma is characterized by far more pleomorphism, mitotic activity, and necrosis than is seen in DFSP, and, in addition, its deeper location and more rapid growth differ from the more superficial, slow-growing nature of DFSP. If histologic features of both DFSP and malignant fibrous histiocytoma are present within the same tumor, the lesion should be regarded as a high-grade sarcoma.[163]

Neurofibromas, particularly the diffuse type, may invade the subcutis and mimic DFSP; however, the lack of a prominent storiform pattern, and the presence of corpuscles or other features of neuroid differentiation, numerous mast cells, and S100 protein immunoreactivity help to distinguish neurofibroma from DFSP. Fibrosarcomas are deep-seated tumors that rarely occur in the skin and are composed of interlacing fascicles of uniformly atypical cells with numerous mitoses growing in a herringbone, rather than storiform, pattern. Atypical fibroxanthoma displays marked cellular polymorphism and pleomorphism with numerous mitoses and a poorly organized growth pattern. Myxoid DFSP must be distinguished from myxoid malignant fibrous histiocytoma, myxoid liposarcoma, and nodular fasciitis. The superficial location and complete absence of lipoblasts differentiates DFSP from liposarcoma. Nodular fasciitis is characterized by its small size, rapid growth, and absence of recurrence as well as its variable growth pattern when compared with DFSP.

MALIGNANT FIBROUS HISTIOCYTOMA

Clinical Features

Although malignant fibrous histiocytoma (MFH) is the most common sarcoma of soft tissues in middle to late adult

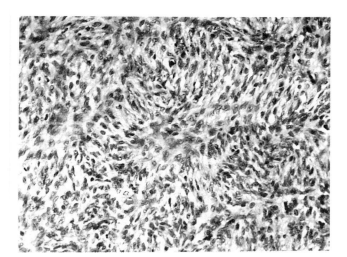

Figure 50–31. Dermatofibrosarcoma protuberans. Uniform proliferation of fibroblasts with prominent storiform growth pattern seen centrally. (H&E, ×270.)

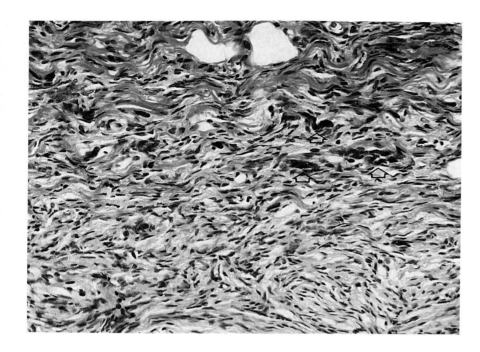

Figure 50–32. Pigmented dermatofibrosarcoma protuberans (Bednar tumor). Uniform proliferation of fibroblasts with scattered deeply pigmented dendritic cells (arrows). (H&E, ×290.)

life, its presentation as a primary skin tumor is rare because only a small proportion are confined exclusively to the subcutis.[164] Approximately two thirds are located within skeletal muscle, spreading along the fascial planes or between muscle fibers. MFH is quite rare in children. The majority of cases arise between the ages of 50 and 70, more frequently in men. The most common locations are the lower extremity, the thigh and buttock in particular, the upper extremity, and the retroperitoneum.[164,165] The tumor generally presents as a painless enlarging mass of several months' duration.[164] The tumors are solitary, measuring 5 to 10 cm in diameter; superficially positioned tumors are smaller that their more deeply seated counterparts.[164–166] MFH has been reported as developing in association with radiation treatment,[167,168] burn scar,[169] chronic ulceration,[170] and previous surgical sites.[171]

The angiomatoid MFH deserves special mention because, unlike the other histologic subtypes of MFH, it occurs most often in children and young adults and it occupies the dermis and subcutis, rather than the deeper muscle layers.[172] Systemic symptoms, such as anemia and weight loss, may be associated with even rather small lesions.

Overall recurrence with MFH is in the range 24% to 34%.[164,166] The overall rate of metastasis ranges from 10% to 55%,[164–166] depending on the series examined. Metastases generally occur within 2 years of diagnosis and most frequently involve the lung, lymph nodes, liver, and bone.[164] Histologic features correlate poorly with the prediction of recurrence or metastasis. Depth of tumor invasion is the single most important predictive parameter. Less than 10% of tumors confined to the subcutis metastasize, and 4-year survival is 65%, whereas tumors involving skeletal muscle metastasize in 43% of cases with a 40% 4-year survival.[164,165] Smaller tumor size, location on the lower extremity, and presence of a marked lymphocytic host response are also

favorable prognostic indicators.[164,165] Treatment of choice is wide local excision.

Histologic Features

MFH has been divided into several histologic variants.[164,165,173] The most common variant, the *storiform-pleomorphic* type, displays short, highly cellular fascicles in a storiform or cartwheel pattern comprising elongated to plump fibroblastic cells (Figs. 50–33, 50–34). A delicate, elaborate vascular pattern is present throughout. Other zones may display larger, pleomorphic, rounded histiocytic cells in a less organized, often haphazard, growth pattern. Numerous typical and atypical mitoses can be found. Large atypical tumor giant cells, as well as xanthoma cells and modest numbers of chronic inflammatory cells, are commonly present. Tumors containing numerous large atypical xanthoma giant cells have been referred to as fibroxanthosarcoma.[174] The stroma can vary considerably from sparsely to heavily collagenous, but the majority of the stroma consists of delicate collagen bundles.

Focal myxoid change is common; however, the *myxoid type* of MFH demonstrates a myxoid appearance in greater than 50% of the tumor (Fig. 50–35). In these hypocellular areas, spindled and stellate fibroblasts lie in a stroma rich in hyaluronic acid. The vascular pattern is quite prominent. The myxoid zones may blend smoothly with cellular areas or may appose cellular zones sharply. The cytology varies from well-differentiated fibroblasts to highly pleomorphic forms with multinucleation and prominent mitotic activity.

The *inflammatory type* of MFH displays numerous xanthoma cells in sheets admixed with predominantly neutrophils, although chronic inflammatory cells can predominate in a minority of cases (Fig. 50–35).[175] Atypia, multinucleation, and mitoses are prominent, although large zones of

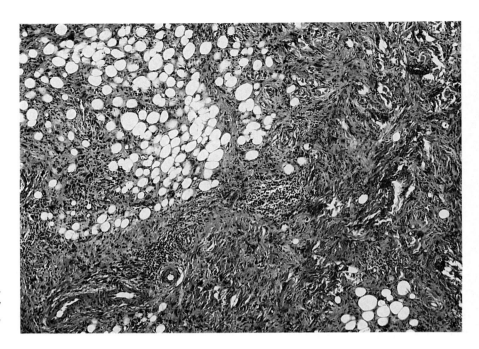

Figure 50–33. Malignant fibrous histiocytoma. Atypical pleomorphic cells massively invading subcutis and deeper tissues. (H&E, ×65.)

mature-appearing xanthoma cells can be seen. The stroma is hyaline-like with sparse collagen.

The *giant cell type* of MFH, also referred to as malignant giant cell tumor of soft parts,[176] displays varying amounts of histiocytes, fibroblasts, and osteoclast-type giant cells with abundant eosinophilic cytoplasm arranged in a multinodular pattern separated by thick fibrous bundles. Cellular pleomorphism and mitotic activity are present. Osteoid formation can be seen.

The *angiomatoid type* of MFH involves the deep dermis and subcutis as a circumscribed nodular or cystic mass.

Atypical fibroblastic and histiocytic cells form solid masses associated with extensive, multifocal hemorrhages, irregular dilated blood vessels, and inflammatory cells (Fig. 50–36). The hemorrhagic spaces are often lined by histiocytic tumor cells. A thick fibrous pseudocapsule as well as germinal center formation can be seen and may lead to an erroneous interpretation of lymph node metastasis.

Although there are no ultrastructural features specific for MFH,[177,178] ultrastructural studies have defined cells with features of fibroblasts, myofibroblasts, and histiocytes. Immunohistochemistry has demonstrated α_1-antitrypsin,

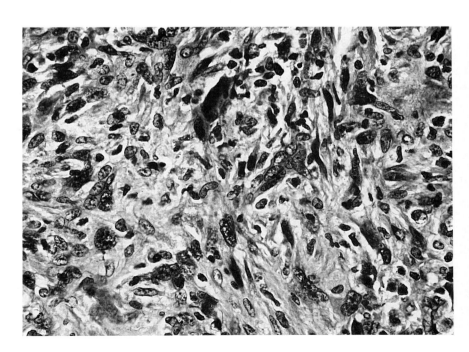

Figure 50–34. Malignant fibrous histiocytoma, storiform-pleomorphic type. Large pleomorphic spindled and rounded mono- and multinucleated cells with marked atypia. (H&E, ×340.)

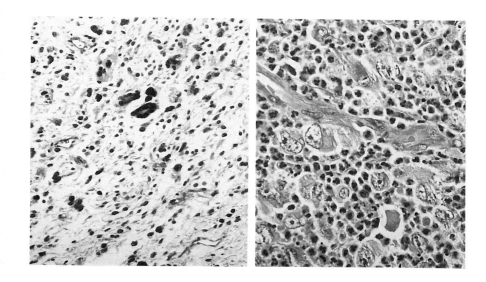

Figure 50–35. Malignant fibrous histiocytoma. Left: Myxoid type. Right: Inflammatory type. (Left: H&E, ×150; right: H&E, ×345.)

α_1-antichymotrypsin, ferritin, and lysozyme in 12% to 37% of MFHs.[179,180]

Differential Diagnosis

The differential diagnosis of MFH and its histologic variants is broad and is beyond the scope of this discussion. Many of these lesions are discussed in detail elsewhere in this text. The pleomorphic variant must be differentiated from other pleomorphic sarcomas including liposarcoma, leiomyosarcoma, malignant schwannoma, and rhabdomyosarcoma. Differentiation from atypical fibroxanthoma can be made based on the smaller size and superficial location of atypical fibroxanthoma. Dermatofibroma and dermatofibrosarcoma protuberans have a prominent storiform growth pattern and lack the marked pleomorphism and atypical

mitoses seen in MFH. The myxoid variant must be distinguished from myxoma, nodular fasciitis, and myxoid liposarcoma.

FIBROSARCOMA

Clinical Features

In the adult form, fibrosarcoma arises most commonly between the ages of 30 and 55 with a predilection for the thigh, knee, trunk, and distal extremities.[181–184] A large, slowly growing, deeply seated mass is typical. Deep structures including muscle, fascia, aponeuroses, and tendons are involved, but subcutaneous tissue can be involved, particularly in those cases associated with scarring, radiation,

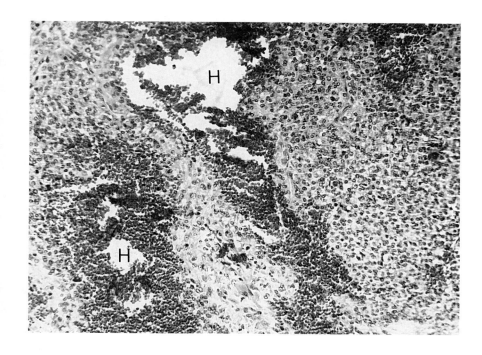

Figure 50–36. Malignant fibrous histiocytoma, angiomatoid type. Solid sheets of uniform large atypical rounded cells surround irregular cystic hemorrhagic zones (H). (H&E, ×100.)

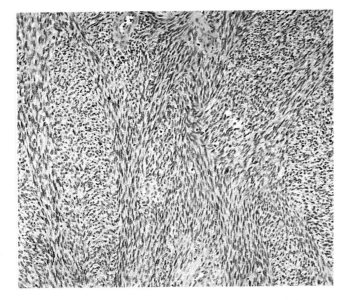

Figure 50–37. Fibrosarcoma. Broad interlacing hypercellular fascicles of uniformly atypical spindle cells in a prominent herringbone pattern. (H&E, ×100.)

or thermal injury. The behavior of this tumor is largely dependent on the histologic grade and degree of differentiation. Data on recurrence, metastasis, and survival of fibrosarcoma are difficult to evaluate because many authors include desmoid tumors as low-grade or grade 1 fibrosarcoma in their series. Others include high-grade pleomorphic lesions, which may represent malignant fibrous histiocytoma rather than fibrosarcoma. Prognosis is least favorable in tumors that display high cellularity, little interstitial collagen, and frequent mitoses (greater than two per high-power field).[184] A 35% 5-year survival is reported in high-grade tumors.[182] Recurrence occurs in approximately 50% of cases. Metastases are bloodborne, and occur most commonly in the lungs.[184] Patients treated by radical excision have a significantly higher 5-year survival than patients treated with local excision (70% versus 30%).[183] Tumor size or location appears to have little effect on survival.[181]

The congenital and infantile forms of fibrosarcoma present from birth through early childhood, with the majority of cases present either at birth or within the first year of life.[185,186] The tumor presents as a nontender mass involving principally the extremities. The 5-year survival is approximately 84%, which is significantly better than that of the adult form.[181] Histologic parameters are not predictive of the clinical course in the congenital and infantile forms.

Histologic Features

Adult and infantile forms share similar histologic features. Small tumors are moderately circumscribed; larger tumors are not and invade surrounding structures. Well-differentiated fibrosarcoma displays well-defined broad fascicles that interlace, forming a prominent herringbone pattern (Fig. 50–37). A dense network of reticulin is present around the tumor cells. The cells are uniform spindle cells with scanty cytoplasm. Mitotic activity is present but variable (Fig. 50–38). Some cases may show large amounts of collagen, which may be hyalinized, separating tumor cells. Poorly differentiated tumors are more cellular, with more densely packed, less well organized tumor cells that may be more oval or round than spindled. A distinct, well-defined fascicular growth pattern is not seen. More cellular pleomorphism and mitotic activity are present than in the well-differentiated forms; however, marked cellular pleomorphism, multinucleated cells, and atypical giant cells are not features of fibrosarcoma. Rarely, there may be foci of myxoid change or zones of osseous or chondroid metaplasia.

Differential Diagnosis

Nodular fasciitis is a smaller, more rapidly growing tumor with a more irregular growth pattern, prominent myxoid matrix, and notable lymphocytic infiltrate. Fibrous histiocytoma, benign and malignant, exhibits prominent storiform

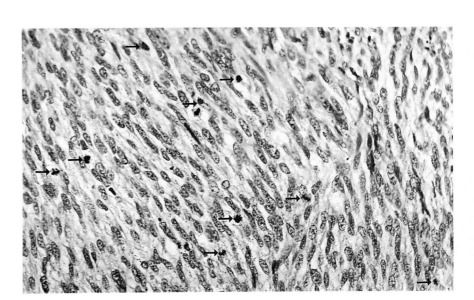

Figure 50–38. Fibrosarcoma. Uniformly atypical plump spindle cells in well-defined fascicles with numerous mitoses (arrows). (H&E, ×330.)

architecture with cellular pleomorphism and polymorphism. Fibromatosis is less cellular than fibrosarcoma, with few to absent mitoses and more interstitial collagen. Malignant schwannoma displays more prominent whorling or palisading, as well as more prominent myxoid features. The epithelial component of synovial sarcoma is lacking in fibrosarcoma.

EPITHELIOID SARCOMA

Clinical Features
Epithelioid sarcoma is a soft tissue sarcoma of uncertain histogenesis. It usually occurs in young adults, with approximately three quarters of cases presenting between the ages of 10 and 39.[187-189] The predominant sites of involvement are the distal upper extremities, particularly the hands and forearms, followed by the lower extremities. Unusual sites of involvement include the penis[190] and vulva.[191] Epithelioid sarcoma generally presents as an asymptomatic, firm mass in the deep soft tissues but may infrequently involve the dermis or subcutis primarily. Ulceration may occur in the more superficial forms. The duration before diagnosis is most often 1 to 3 years.[187,189] A history of trauma is present in a minority of cases.[187] Recurrence is common, occurring in approximately 75% of cases.[187,188] Metastasis develops in approximately 30% to 50%, with lymph nodes and lungs being the most frequent initial sites of metastatic involvement.[187,188] Unfavorable prognostic factors include proximal location, male sex, diagnosis at a later age, large tumor size (greater than 2.5 cm), high mitotic activity, tumor necrosis, and vascular invasion. Aggressive early surgery is the treatment of choice; the extent of the tumor is usually greater than clinically appreciated.[187,188]

Histologic Features
The lesion is nodular, with infiltrating margins. The most common growth pattern is multinodular and pseudopalisading, comprising polygonal epithelioid cells with abundant eosinophilic cytoplasm and spindle cells forming irregular cohesive collars around central, acellular, necrotic zones (Figs. 50–39, 50–40). This growth pattern simulates palisading granulomatous processes such as granuloma annulare and rheumatoid nodule. The central necrotic zones may contain degenerated or hyalinized collagen, necrotic tumor cells, amorphous debris, or glycosaminoglycans. Tumors showing little or no necrosis display a more diffuse pattern of growth of plump epithelioid cells blending with spindle cells, with subtle transition between the two cell types; a distinct biphasic pattern or formation of glandular structures, as seen in synovial sarcoma, is absent.

These cells infiltrate diffusely between mature collagen bundles. Avascular cleftlike spaces can be seen lined by tumor cells. Although typical histologic growth patterns of epithelioid sarcoma can be seen in all cases through careful examination of all tissue available, unusual features include multinucleated giant cells, zones of prominent storiform growth, and cartilaginous or osseous metaplasia. Cytologic atypia, with regard to large, irregular hyperchromatic nuclei with prominent nuclei and notable mitotic activity, can be seen in at least some zones of the tumor, although large zones of the lesion may be devoid of significant cellular atypia and mitotic activity (Fig. 50–41). Intracytoplasmic vacuolization may be present.

Immunohistochemical studies have demonstrated cytokeratin in the vast majority of cases.[157,192-194] In addition, carcinoembryonic antigen, epithelial membrane antigen, neuron-specific enolase, S100 protein, lysozyme, α_1-antitrysin, and α_1-antichymotrypsin have been identi-

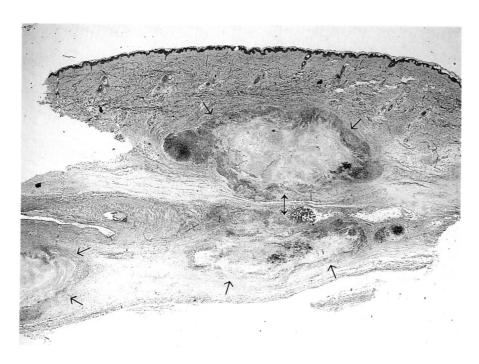

Figure 50–39. Epithelioid sarcoma. Multinodular growth in a pseudopalisading pattern (arrows). (H&E, ×11.)

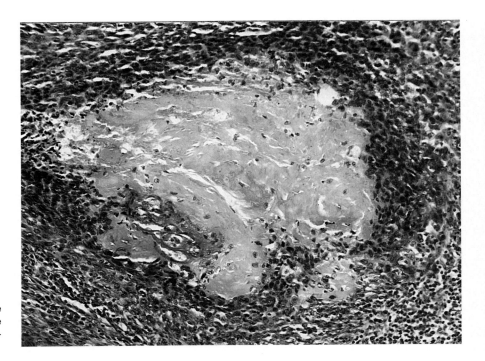

Figure 50–40. Epithelioid sarcoma. Spindle cells and epithelioid cells forming a cohesive collar around a central acellular zone of degenerated collagen. (H&E, ×145.)

fied.[187,192–194] Leukocyte common antigen (LCA) is negative in the large epithelioid cells of epithelioid sarcoma, but may be positive in reactive peritumoral cells.[192] The keratin-positive, LCA-negative profile of the epithelioid cells in epithelioid sarcoma helps to distinguish it from the necrobi-

otic granulomas, in which the epithelioid cell component would exhibit keratin-negative, LCA-positive staining.

Electron microscopy demonstrates cytoplasmic filaments and occasional junctional specializations. Lysozymes are not present.[189]

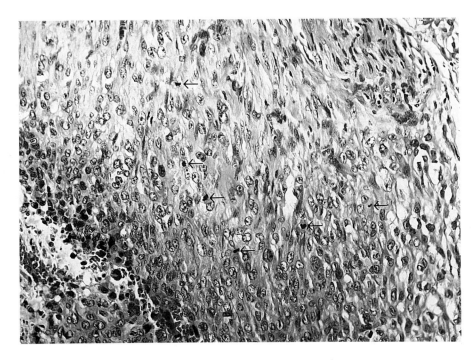

Figure 50–41. Epithelioid sarcoma. Plump spindle and epithelioid cells with notable cytologic atypia and mitoses (arrows). Central necrotic zone is present at lower left. (H&E, ×220.)

Differential Diagnosis

Necrobiotic granulomas contain smaller epithelioid cells, more diverse inflammatory elements, less cellular pleomorphism, and lower mitotic activity. The keratin-positive, LCA-negative profile of epithelioid sarcoma helps to distinguish it from necrobiotic granulomas (see Histologic Features). Malignant fibrous histiocytoma displays more cellular pleomorphism with bizarre tumor giant cells and a more prominent, consistent storiform growth pattern, without the multinodular pattern present in most cases of epithelioid sarcoma. Squamous cell carcinoma displays more cohesive sheets of cells with intercellular bridging and participation of the overlying epidermis. Keratin pearls are not seen in epithelioid sarcoma.

Melanoma may contain melanin pigment and will display melanosomes ultrastructurally; epithelioid sarcoma does not. Atypical melanocytic proliferation of the overlying epidermis is expected in a primary melanoma. The multinodular, pseudopalisading growth pattern of epithelioid sarcoma is uncommon in metastatic melanoma. The distinct biphasic pattern, with or without glandular structures, seen in synovial sarcoma, is absent in epithelioid sarcoma. Epithelioid hemangioendothelioma does not display the multinodular growth pattern with central necrosis as seen in epithelioid sarcoma.[195] The polygonal cells in epithelioid hemangioendothelioma are factor VIII antigen positive, keratin negative, a staining pattern opposite that of epithelioid sarcoma.

SYNOVIAL SARCOMA

Clinical Features

Synovial sarcoma may occur at any age, with a peak incidence in the third and fourth decades.[196–198] Preferred sites of involvement are the thigh, foot, knee, shoulder, and forearm. The tumor is felt to arise from synovial lining cells. The tumor presents as a slowly enlarging painless mass in the deep soft tissue. Recurrence occurs in more than one half of patients. The average 5-year survival is approximately 50%. Small tumors (5 cm or less) have a far better prognosis (75%, 5-year survival) than large tumors (more than 5 cm) of the same locations (26%, 5-year survival).[197] Tumors located on the distal extremities have a more favorable prognosis.[197]

Histologic Features

Although the lesion may appear grossly circumscribed, infiltration into adjacent tissues is common. A biphasic histologic pattern is seen (Fig. 50–42).[196–198] An epithelium-like element appears either as solid nests of polygomal cells with clear cytoplasm or as cuboidal to columnar cells enclosing slitlike spaces or surrounding apparent tubules or ducts. Small papillary excrescences may be seen projecting into the enclosed spaces. The spaces often contain mucicarmine-positive material. Surrounding and encasing the epithelial component is a uniform spindle cell proliferation in an irregular nodular arrangement. Transition between spindle and epithelial forms can be seen. Monophasic synovial sarcoma composed solely of either the epithelial or spindle cell component has been described. Focal calcifications are common and are a useful diagnostic aid, particularly in the monophasic variants. Ultrastructural studies demonstrate features of epithelial cells, fibroblast-like cells, and transitional forms.

Differential Diagnosis

Distinction of monophasic fibrous synovial sarcoma from fibrosarcoma can be impossible on histologic grounds; however, fibrosarcoma displays a more prominent herringbone

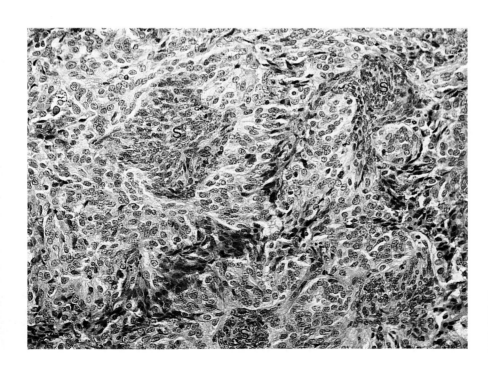

Figure 50–42. Synovial sarcoma. Biphasic pattern including an epithelial component, here without glandular structures and a plump spindle cell component (S). (H&E, ×225.)

fascicular growth pattern and generally a higher mitotic rate.

CLEAR CELL SARCOMA (MALIGNANT MELANOMA OF SOFT PARTS)

Clinical Features

A rare tumor, clear cell sarcoma occurs predominantly in young patients between 15 and 35 years of age. It originates from tendons, aponeuroses, and fascial structures with a predilection for the feet and ankles.[199–201] Recurrence and metastases are common, with lung, lymph nodes, and bone being the most common sites for metastatic disease.[199–201] Death from metastatic tumor occurs in up to 43% of patients.[199] Radical local excision is the treatment of choice.[199] The exact histogenesis of this tumor remains unclear, but the presence of intracellular melanin and S100 protein in the majority of cases suggests that clear cell sarcoma is of neuroectodermal derivation from potentially melanogenic cells of neural crest origin. Malignant melanoma of soft parts has thereby been suggested as an appropriate designation for this neoplasm.[199] It is included in this chapter because of its uncertain histogenesis and its relationship microscopically to synovial sarcoma.

Histologic Features

The tumor ranges in diameter from 1 to 5 cm, with a median of 3 cm. It is lobulated, consisting of nests and short fascicles of fusiform or polygonal cells with indistinct clear to granular eosinophilic cytoplasm, vesicular nuclei, and prominent nucleoli (Fig. 50–43).[199–202] No acinar or glandular structures are seen. Multinucleated giant cells containing 10 to 15 nuclei are present in the majority of cases. Mitotic activity is generally scarce, but may range from absent to extremely high. The tumor is separated and surrounded by fibrous septa of varying thickness. Intracellular glycogen is present in roughly two thirds of cases.[199]

Intracellular melanin is demonstrable in approximately 75% of cases; intra- and extracellular iron pigment can be present as well.[199] Immunohistochemistry demonstrates S100 protein positivity in the majority of tumors.[199] Ultrastructural studies show overlapping features with synovial sarcoma; however, unlike synovial sarcoma, clear cell sarcoma is monomorphous and displays melanin, melanosomes, and premelanosomes in approximately two thirds of cases.[199,202,203]

Differential Diagnosis

Clear cell sarcoma can be distinguished from synovial sarcoma by its lack of an epithelial component, glandular structures, and calcification, and presence of intracellular melanin. Fibrosarcoma demonstrates a more densely cellular growth with prominent herringbone architecture and dense reticulin meshwork. The absence of origin from a large nerve and prominent palisading help to differentiate clear cell sarcoma from malignant schwannoma.

Metastasis from melanoma, and, in particular, from acral lentiginous melanoma and melanoma of the ocular choroid, may simulate clear cell sarcoma although metastatic melanoma generally displays a more pleomorphic histology. Both of these tumors may display intercellular melanin, glycogen, and S100 protein.

Acknowledgment

I thank Dr. Jonathan Epstein, who graciously provided valuable slide material.

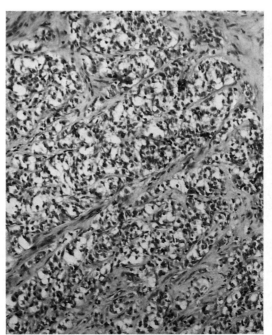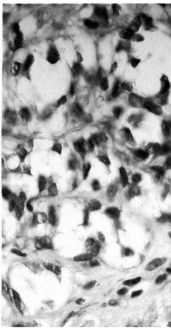

Figure 50–43. Clear cell sarcoma. Left: Lobulated proliferation of nests of clear cells. Right: Polygonal cells with indistinct clear cytoplasm. (Left: H&E, ×125; right: H&E, ×425.)

REFERENCES

1. Kornwaler BE, Keasbey L, Kaplan L: Subcutaneous pseudosarcomatous fibromatosis (fasciitis). *Am J Clin Pathol* 1955;25:241–252.

2. Stout AP: Pseudosarcomatous fasciitis in children. *Cancer* 1961;14:1216–1222.

3. Price EB Jr, Silliphant WM, Shuman R: Nodular fasciitis. A clinicopathologic analysis of 65 cases. *Am J Clin Pathol* 1961;35:122–136.

4. Hutter RVP, Stewart FW, Foote FW Jr: Fasciitis. A report of 70 cases with follow-up proving the benignity of the lesion. *Cancer* 1962;15:992–1003.

5. Soule EH: Proliferative (nodular) fasciitis. *Arch Pathol* 1962;73:437–444.

6. Meister P, Buckmann FW, Konrad EA: Nodular fasciitis: Analysis of 100 cases and review of the literature. *Pathol Res Pract* 1978;162:133–165.

7. Enzinger FM, Weiss SW: *Soft Tissue Tumors.* St. Louis, Mo, CV Mosby, 1983, pp 15–31.

8. Bernstein KE, Lattes R: Nodular (pseudosarcomatous) fasciitis, a nonrecurrent lesion: Clinicopathologic study of 134 cases. *Cancer* 1982;49:1668–1678.

9. Shimizu S, Hashimoto H, Enjoji M: Nodular fasciitis: An analysis of 250 patients. *Pathology* 1984;16:161–166.

10. Chung EB, Enzinger FM: Proliferative fasciitis. *Cancer* 1975;36:1450–1458.

11. Enzinger FM, Dulcey F: Proliferative myositis: Report of 33 cases. *Cancer* 1967;20:2213–2223.

12. Meister P, Konrad EA, Buckmann PW: Nodular fasciitis and proliferative myositis as variants of one disease entity. *Invest Cell Pathol* 1979;2:277–281.

13. Lauer DH, Enzinger FM: Cranial fasciitis of childhood. *Cancer* 1980;45:401–406.

14. Hutter RV, Foote FW, Francis KC, et al.: Parosteal fasciitis. A self-limited benign process that simulates a malignant neoplasm. *Am J Surg* 1962;104:800–807.

15. Patchefsky AS, Enzinger FM: Intravascular fasciitis. *Am J Surg Pathol* 1981;5:29–36.

16. Rose AG: An electron microscopic study of the giant cells in proliferative myositis. *Cancer* 1974;33:1543–1546.

17. Ackerman LV: Extraosseous localized non-neoplastic bone and cartilage formation (so-called myositis ossificans). *J Bone Joint Surg* 1958;40A(2):279–298.

18. Conway H: Dupuytren's contracture. *Am J Surg* 1954;87:101–119.

19. Larsen D, Posche L: Dupuytren' contracture: With special reference to pathology. *J Bone Joint Surg* 1958;40A:773–792.

20. Mikkelson OA: Dupuytren's disease—Initial symptoms, age of onset and spontaneous course. *Hand* 1977;9:11–15.

21. Allen RA, Woolner LB, Ghormley RD: Soft tissue tumors of the sole. With special reference to plantar fibromatosis. *J Bone Joint Surg* 1955;37A:14–26.

22. Aviles E, Arlen M, Miller T: Plantar fibromatosis. *Surgery* 1971;69:117–120.

23. Enzinger FM, Weiss SW: *Soft Tissue Tumors.* St. Louis, Mo. CV Mosby Company, 1983, p 46.

24. Allen PW, Enzinger FM: Juvenile aponeurotic fibroma. *Cancer* 1970;26:857–867.

25. Allison JR Jr, Allison JR Sr: Knuckle pads. *Arch Dermatol* 1966;93:311–316.

26. Shapiro L: Infantile digital fibromatosis and aponeurotic fibroma. *Arch Dermatol* 1969;99:37–42.

27. Miyamoto T, Mihara M, Hagan, et al.: Posttraumatic occurrence of infantile digital fibromatosis. *Arch Dermatol* 1986;122:915–918.

28. Dabney KW, MacEwen GD, David NE: Recurring digital fibrous tumor of childhood. Case report with long-term follow-up and review of the literature. *J Pediatr Orthop* 1986;6:612–617.

29. Mehregan AH, Nabai H, Matthews JE: Recurring digital fibrous tumor of childhood. *Arch Dermatol* 1972;106:375–378.

30. Mehregan AH: Superficial fibrous tumors in childhood. *J Cutan Pathol* 1981;8:321–334.

31. Zina AM, Rampini E, Fulcheri S, et al.: Recurrent digital fibromatosis of childhood. An ultrastructural and immunohistochemical study of two cases. *Am J Dermatopathol* 1986;8:22–26.

32. Smith BH: Peyronie's disease. *Am J Clin Pathol* 1966;45:670–681.

33. Lund M: Dupuytren's contracture and epilepsy. Clinical connection between Dupuytren's contracture, fibroma plantae, periathrosis humeri, helodermia, induratio penis plastica and epilepsy with attempt at pathogenetic evaluation. *Acta Psychiatr Neurol* 1971;16:465–471.

34. Enzinger FM: Fibrous hamartoma of infancy. *Cancer* 1965;18:241–248.

35. Fayad MN, Tacoub A, Salman S, et al.: Juvenile hyalin fibromatosis: Two new patients and review of the literature. *Am J Med Genet* 1987;26:123–131.

36. Ramberger K, Krieg T, Kunze D, et al.: Fibromatosis hyalinica multiplex (juvenile hyalin fibromatosis). *Cancer* 1985;56:614–624.

37. Kitano Y: Juvenile fibromatosis. *Arch Dermatol* 1976;112:86–88.

38. Chung EB, Enzinger FM: Infantile myofibromatosis. *Cancer* 1981;48:1807–1818.

39. Spraker MK, Stack C, Esterly N: Congenital generalized fibromatosis: A review of the literature and report of a case associated with porencephaly, hemiatrophy and cutis marmorata telangiectatica congenita. *J Am Acad Dermatol* 1984;10:365–371.

40. Brill PW, Yandow DR, Langer LO, et al.: Congenital generalized fibromatosis. Case report and literature review. *Pediatr Radiol* 1982;12:269–278.

41. Gardner EJ: Follow-up study of a family group exhibiting dominant inheritance for a syndrome including intestinal polyps, osteomas, fibromas and epidermal cysts. *Am J Hum Genet* 1982;14:376–390.

42. Enzinger FM, Weiss SW: *Soft Tissue Tumors.* St. Louis, Mo, CV Mosby, 1983, pp 52–66.

43. Reitamo JJ, Hayry P, NyKyn E, et al.: The desmoid tumor. Incidence, sex, age and anatomical distribution in the Finnish population. *Am J Clin Pathol* 1982;77:665–673.

44. Rock MG, Pritchard DJ, Reiman HM, et al.: Extraabdominal desmoid tumors. *J Bone Joint Surg* 1984;66:1359–1374.

45. Hajdu SI: *Pathology of Soft Tissue Tumors.* Philadelphia, Lea and Febiger, 1979, pp 122–125.

46. Uitto J, Santa-Cruz DJ, Eisen AZ: Familial cutaneous collagenoma: Genetic studies on a family. *Br J Dermatol* 1979;101:185–195.

47. Henderson RR, Wheeler CE Jr, Abele DC: Familial cutaneous collagenoma. Report of cases. *Arch Dermatol* 1968;98:23–27.

48. Uitto J, Santa-Cruz DJ, Eisen AZ: Connective tissue nevi of the skin. *J Am Acad Dermatol* 1980;3:441–461.

49. Pierard GE, Lapiere CM: Nevi of connective tissue. A reappraisal of their classification. *Am J Dermatopathol* 1985;7:325–333.

50. Nickel WR, Reed WB: Tuberous sclerosis. Special reference to the microscopic alterations in the cutaneous hamaromas. *Arch Dermatol* 1962;85:209–226.

51. Sosis AC, Johnson WC: Connective tissue nevus. *Dermatologica* 1972;144:57–62.

52. Rocha G, Winkelmann RK: Connective tissue nevus. *Arch Dermatol* 1962;85:722–729.

53. Steiner K: Connective tissue nevus. *Arch Dermatol Syphilol* 1944;50:183–190.

54. Kozminsky ME, Bronson DM, Barsky S: Zosteriform connective tissue nevus. *Cutis* 1985;36:77–80.

55. Fenske NA, Donelan PA: Becker's nevus coexistent with connective tissue nevus. *Arch Dermatol* 1984;102:1347–1351.

56. Weintraub R, Pinkus H: Multiple fibrofolliculomas associated with a large connective tissue nevus. *J Cutan Pathol* 1977;4:289–299.

57. Schorr WF, Optiz JM, Reyes CN: The connective tissue nevus—Osteopoikilosis syndrome. *Arch Dermatol* 1972;106:208–214.

58. Morrison JG, Jones EW, MacDonald DM: Juvenile elastoma and osteopoikilosis (the Buschke Ollendorff syndrome). *Br J Dermatol* 1977;97:417–422.

59. Cole GW, Barr RJ: An elastic tissue defect in dermatofibrosis lenticularis disseminata. Buschke Ollendorff syndrome. *Arch Dermatol* 1982;118:44–46.

60. Enzinger FM, Weiss SW: *Soft Tissue Tumors.* St. Louis, Mo, CV Mosby, 1983, pp 33–36.

61. Weidman FD, Anderson NP, Ayres S: Juvenile elastoma. *Arch Dermatol Syphilol* 1933;28:182–189.

62. Starricco R, Mehregan AH: Nevus elasticus and nevus elasticus vascularis. *Arch Dermatol* 1961;84:943–947.

63. Lewandowsky F: Naevus elasticus regionis mammariae. *Arch Klin Exp Dermatol* 1921;90:131.

64. Gonzalez S, Duarte I: Benign fibrous histiocytoma of the skin. A morphologic study of 290 cases. *Pathol Res Pract* 1982;174:379–391.

65. Niemi KM: The benign fibrohistiocytic tumors of the skin. (Review) *Acta Dermatol Venereol* 1970;50(suppl)63:1–66.

66. Baraf CS, Shapiro L: Multiple histiocytomas. *Arch Dermatol* 1970;101:588–590.

67. Lin RY, Landsman L, Krey PR, et al.: Multiple dermatofibromas and systemic lupus erythematosus. *Cutis* 1986;37:45–49.

68. Bargmen HB, Fefferman I: Multiple dermatofibromas in a patient with myasthenia gravis treated with prednisone and cyclophosphamide. *J Am Acad Dermatol* 1986;14:351–352.

69. Roberts JT, Byrne EH, Rosenthal D: Familial variant of dermatofibroma with malignancy in the proband. *Arch Dermatol* 1981;117:12–15.

70. Fitzpatrick TB, Gilchrist BA: Dimple sign to differentiate benign from malignant cutaneous lesions. *N Engl J Med* 1977;296:1518.

71. Enzinger FM, Weiss SW: *Soft Tissue Tumors.* St. Louis, Mo. CV Mosby, 1983, pp 135.

72. Shoenfeld RJ: Epidermal proliferations overlying histiocytomas. *Arch Dermatol* 1964;90:266–270.

73. Dalziel K, Marks R: Hair follicle–like changes over histiocytomas. *J Am Dermatopathol* 1986;8:461–466.

74. Halpryn HJ, Allen AC: Epidermal changes associated with sclerosing hemangiomas. *Arch Dermatol* 1959;80:160–166.

75. Goette DK, Helwig EB: Basal cell carcinomas and basal-cell carcinoma–like changes overlying dermatofibromas. *Arch Dermatol* 1975;111:589–592.

76. Buselmeier TJ, Ueker JH: Invasive basal cell carcinoma with metaplastic bone formation associated with a longstanding dermatofibroma. *J Cutan Pathol* 1979;6:496–500.

77. Bernstein JC: Hemosiderin histiocytoma of the skin. *Arch Dermatol* 1939;40:390–396.

78. Barker SM, Winkelmann RK: Inflammatory lymphadenoid reactions with dermatofibroma/histiocytoma. *J Cutan Pathol* 1986;13:222–226.

79. Santa Cruz DJ, Kyriakos M: Aneurysmal (angiomatoid) fibrous histiocytoma of the skin. *Cancer* 1981;47:2053–2061.

80. Sood U, Mehregan AH: Aneurysmal (angiomatoid) fibrous histiocytoma. *J Cutan Pathol* 1985;12:157–167.

81. Leyva WH, Santa Cruz DJ: Atypical cutaneous fibrous histiocytoma. *Am J Dermatopathol* 1986;8:467–471.

82. Fukamizu H, Oku T, Inoue K, et al.: Atypical (pseudosarcomatous) cutaneous histiocytoma. *J Cutan Pathol* 1983;10:327–333.

83. Tamada S, Ackerman AB: Dermatofibroma with monster cells. *Am J Dermatopathol* 1987;9:380–387.

84. Gonzalez B: Benign fibrous histiocytomas of the skin. An immunohistochemical analysis of 30 cases. *Pathol Res Pract* 1985;180:486–489.

85. Letini M, Grosso M, Carrozza G, et al.: Fibrohistiocytic tumors of soft tissues. An immunohistochemical study of 183 cases. *Pathol Res Pract* 1986;181:713–717.

86. Cerio R, Spaull J, Jones EW: Dermatofibroma: A tumor of dermal dendrocytes? (Abstract) *J Cutan Pathol* 1987;14:351.

87. Fine G, Morales MD, Pardo V: Ultrastructure of histiocytomas. *Am J Clin Pathol* 1977;67:214.

88. Waisman M: Cutaneous papillomas of the neck: Papillomatous seborrheic keratoses. *South Med J* 1957;50:725–731.

89. Templeton HJ: Cutaneous tags of the neck. *Arch Dermatol* 1936;33:495–505.

90. Starink TM, Meijer CJ, Braunstein MH: The cutaneous pathology of Cowden's disease: New findings. *J Cutan Pathol* 1985;12:83–93.

91. Starink TM, Van Der Veen JP, De Waal LP, et al.: The Cowden syndrome: A clinical and genetic study in 21 patients. *Clin Genet* 1986;29:222–233.

92. Nickel WR, Weed WB: Tuberous sclerosis (review of cutaneous lesions). *Arch Dermatol* 1962;85:209–226.

93. Pinkus H, Coskey R, Burgess GH: Trichodiscoma: A benign tumor related to the haarscheibe (hair disk). *J Invest Dermatol* 1974;63:212–218.

94. Starink TM, Kisch LS, Meijer CJ: Familial multiple trichodiscomas. *Arch Dermatol* 1985;121:888–891.

95. Birt AR, Hogg GR, Dube WJ: Hereditary multiple fibrofolliculomas with trichodiscomas and acrochordons. *Arch Dermatol* 1977;113:1674–1677.

96. Fujita WH, Barr RJ, Headley JL: Multiple fibrofolliculomas with trichodiscomas and acrochordons. *Arch Dermatol* 1981;117:32–35.

97. Zackheim HS, Pinkus H: Perifollicular fibroma. *Arch Dermatol* 1960;82:913–917.

98. Hornstein OP, Knickenberg M: Perifollicular fibromatosis cutis with polyps of the colon. *Arch Dermatol Res* 1975;253:161–175.

99. Foucar K, Rosen T, Foucar E, et al.: Fibrofolliculoma: A clinicopathologic study. *Cutis* 1981;28:429–432.

100. Graham JH, Sanders JB, Johnson WC, et al.: Fibrous papule of the nose. *J Invest Dermatol* 1965;45:194–203.

101. Santa Cruz DJ, Prioleau PG: Fibrous papule of the face. An electron microscopic study of two cases. *Am J Dermatopathol* 1979;1:349–352.

102. Ragaz A, Berezowsky V: Fibrous papule of the face. A study of five cases by electron microscopy. *Am J Dermatopathol* 1979;1:353–355.

103. Ackerman AB, Kornberg R: Pearly penile papules. Acral angiofibromas. *Arch Dermatol* 1973;108:673–675.

104. Nickel WR, Reed, WB: Tuberous sclerosis (review of cutaneous lesions). *Arch Dermatol* 1962;85:209–226.

105. Fitzpatrick TB, Szabo G, Hori Y, et al.: White leaf-shaped macules. *Arch Dermatol* 1968;98:1–6.

106. Reed WB, Nickel WR, Campion G: Internal manifestations of tuberous sclerosis. (Review) *Arch Dermatol* 1963;87:715–718.

107. Ackerman AB, Kornberg R: Pearly penile papules. Acral angiofibromas. *Arch Dermatol* 1973;108:673–675.

108. Bart RS, Andrade R, Kopf AW, et al.: Acquired digital fibrokeratoma. *Arch Dermatol* 1968;97:120–128.

109. Kint A, Baran R, De Keyser H: Acquired (digital) fibrokeratomas. *J Am Acad Dermatol* 1985;12:816–821.

110. Verallo WM: Acquired digital fibrokeratomas. *Br J Dermatol* 1968;80:730–736.

111. Cooper PH, Mackel SE: Acquired fibrokeratoma of the heel. *Arch Dermatol* 1985;121:386–388.

112. Chung EB, Enzinger FM: Fibroma of tendon sheath. *Cancer* 1979;44:1945–1954.

113. Humphreys S, McKee PH, Fletcher CD: Fibroma of tendon sheath: A clinicopathologic study. *J Cutan Pathol* 1986;13:331–338.

114. Jones FE, Soule EH, Coventry MB: Fibrous histiocytoma of synovium (giant cell tumor of tendon sheath, pigmented nodular synovitis): A study of 118 cases. *J Bone Joint Surg Am* 1969;51(pt A):76–86.

115. Phalen GS, McCormack LJ, Gazale WJ: Giant cell tumor of tendon sheath (benign synovioma) in the hand. Evaluation of 56 cases. *Clin Orthop* 1959;15:140–151.

116. King DT, Millman AJ, Gurevitch AW, et al.: Giant cell tumor of the tendon sheath involving skin. *Arch Dermatol* 1978;114:944–946.

117. Wright CJE: Benign giant cell synovioma: An investigation of 85 cases. *Br J Surg* 1951;38:257–271.

118. Enzinger FM, Weiss SW: *Soft Tissue Tumors.* St. Louis, Mo, CV Mosby, 1983, pp 502–517.

119. Dupree WB, Enzinger FM: Fibro-osseous pseudotumor of the digits. *Cancer* 1986;58:2103–2109.

120. Abdul-Karim FW, Evans HL, Silva EG: Giant cell fibroblastoma: A report of three cases. *Am J Clin Pathol* 1985;83:165–170.

121. Dymock RB, Allen PW, Stirling JW, et al.: Giant cell fibroblastoma. A distinctive, recurrent tumor of childhood. *Am J Surg Pathol* 1987;11:263–272.

122. Shmookler BM, Enzinger FM: Giant cell fibroblastoma: A peculiar childhood tumor. (Abstract) *Lab Invest* 1983;46:7A.

123. Bourne RG: Paradoxical fibrosarcoma of the skin (pseudosarcoma): A review of 13 cases. *Med J Aust* 1963;50:504–510.

124. Finlay-Jones LR, Nicoll P, Ten Seldam REJ: Pseudosarcoma of the skin. *Pathology* 1971;3:215–222.

125. Samitz MH: Pseudosarcoma. Pseudomalignant neoplasia as a consequence of radiodermatitis. *Arch Dermatol* 1967;96:283–285.

126. Woyke S, Domagala W, Olszewski W, et al.: Pseudosarcoma of the skin. An electron microscopic study and comparison with the fine structure of the spindle-cell variant of squamous carcinoma. *Cancer* 1974;33:970–980.

127. Levan NE, Hirsch P, Kwong MQ: Pseudosarcomatous dermatofibroma. *Arch Dermatol* 1963;88:908–912.

128. Gordon HW: Pseudosarcomatous reticulohistiocytoma. A report of four cases. *Arch Dermatol* 1964;90:319–324.

129. Fretzin DF, Helwig EB: Atypical fibroxanthoma of the skin. A clinicopathologic study of 140 cases. *Cancer* 1973;31:1541–1552.

130. Dahl L: Atypical fibroxanthoma of the skin. A clinicopathologic study of 57 cases. *Acta Pathol Microbiol Scand* 1976;84:183–197.

131. Starink TM, Hausman R, VanDelden L, et al.: Atypical fibroxanthoma of the skin. Presentation of 5 cases and a review of the literature. *Br J Dermatol* 1977;97:167–177.

132. Hudson AW, Winkelmann RK: Atypical fibroxanthoma of the skin: A reappraisal of 19 cases in which the original diagnosis was spindle-cell squamous carcinoma. *Cancer* 1972;29:413–422.

133. Kroe OJ, Pitcock JA: Atypical fibroxanthoma of the skin. Report of ten cases. *Am J Clin Pathol* 1969;51:487–492.

134. Jacobs DS, Edwards WD, Ye RC: Metastatic atypical fibroxanthoma of skin. *Cancer* 1975;35:457–463.

135. Kemp JP, Stenn KS, Arons M, et al.: Metastasizing atypical fibroxanthoma. Coexistence with chronic lymphocytic leukemia. *Arch Dermatol* 1978;1144:1533–1535.

136. Glavin FL, Cornwell ML: Atypical fibroxanthoma of the skin metastatic to a lung. *Am J Dermatopathol* 1985;7:57–63.

137. Kuwano H, Hashimoto H, Enjoji M: Atypical fibroxanthoma distinguishable from spindle cell carcinoma in sarcoma-like skin lesions. A clinicopathologic and immunohistochemical study of 21 cases. *Cancer* 1955;40:172–180.

138. Enzinger FM, Weiss SW: *Soft Tissue Tumors.* St. Louis, Mo, CV Mosby, 1983, p 167.

139. Chen KTK: Atypical fibroxanthoma of the skin with osteoid production. *Arch Dermatol* 1980;116:113–114.

140. Alguacil-Garcia AA, Unni KK, Goellner JR, et al.: Atypical fibroxanthoma of the skin. An ultrastructural study of two cases. *Cancer* 1977;40:1471–1480.

141. Barr RJ, Wuerker RB, Graham GH: Ultrastructure of atypical fibroxanthoma. *Cancer* 1977;40:736–743.

142. Carson JW, Schwartz RA, McCandless CM, et al.: Atypical fibroxanthoma of the skin. Report of a case with Langerhans-like granules. *Arch Dermatol* 1984;120:234–239.

143. Lentini M, Grosso M, Carrozza G: Fibrohistiocytic tumors of soft tissues. An immunohistochemical study of 183 cases. *Pathol Res Pract* 1986;181:713–717.

144. Winkelmann RK, Peters MS: Atypical fibroxanthoma. A study with antibody to S-100 protein. *Arch Dermatol* 1985;121:753–755.

145. Silvis NG, Swanson PE, Manivel JC, et al.: Spindle-cell and pleomorphic neoplasms of the skin. A clinicopathologic and immunohistochemical study of 30 cases, with emphasis on "atypical fibroxanthomas." *Am J Dermatopathol* 1988;10:9–19.

146. Fletcher CDM, Evans BJ, Macartney JC, et al.: Dermatofibrosarcoma protuberans: A clinicopathological and immunohistochemical study with a review of the literature. *Histopathology* 1985;9:921–938.

147. Bendix-Hansen K, Myhre-Jensen O, Kaae S: Dermatofibrosarcoma protuberans. A clinicopathological study of nineteen cases and review of world literature. *Scand J Plast Reconstruct Surg* 1983;17:247–252.

148. Taylor HB, Helwig EB: Dermatofibrosarcoma protuberans: A study of 115 cases. *Cancer* 1962;15:717–725.

149. McPeak CJ, Cruz T, Nicastri AD: Dermatofibrosarcoma protuberans: An analysis of 86 cases—5 with metastases. *Ann Surg* 1967;166(suppl 2):803–816.

150. Burkhardt BR, Soule EH, Winkelman RK, et al.: Dermatofibrosarcoma protuberans. Study of 58 cases. *Am J Surg* 1986;111:638–644.

151. Pack GT, Tabah EJ: Dermatofibrosarcoma protuberans. A report of 39 cases. *Arch Surg* 1951;62:391–411.

152. Lambert WC, Abramovits W, Gonzalez-Sevra A, et al.: Dermatofibrosarcoma non-protuberans: Description and report of five cases of a morpheaform variant of dermatofibrosarcoma. *J Surg Oncol* 1958;28:7–11.

153. Volpe R, Carbone A: Dermatofibrosarcoma protuberans metastatic to lymph nodes and showing a dominant histiocytic component. *Am J Dermatopathol* 1983;5:327–334.

154. Brennar W, Schaefler K, Chhabra R, et al.: Dermatofibrosarcoma protuberans metastatic to a regional lymph node. Report of a case and review. *Cancer* 1975;36:1897–1902.

155. Barr RJ, Young EM, King DF: Non-polarizable collagen in dermatofibrosarcoma protuberans: A useful diagnostic aid. *J Cutan Pathol* 1986;13:339–346.

156. Frierson HF, Cooper PH: Myxoid variant of dermatofibrosarcoma protuberans. *Am J Surg Pathol* 1983;7:445–450.

157. Hajdu SI: *Pathology of Soft Tissue Tumors.* Philadelphia, Lea and Febiger, 1979, p 90.

158. Dupree WB, Langloss JM, Weiss SW: Pigmented dermatofibrosarcoma protuberans (Bednar tumor). A pathologic, ultra-

structural and immunohistochemical study. *Am J Surg Pathol* 1985;9:630–639.

159. Lentini M, Grosso M, Carozza G, et al.: Fibrohistiocytic tumors of soft tissues. An immunohistochemical study of 183 cases. *Pathol Res Pract* 1986;181:713–717.

160. Escalona-Zaptu JE, Fernandez EA, Escuin FL: The fibroblastic nature of dermatofibrosarcoma protuberans. *Virchow's Arch (Pathol Anat)* 1981;391:165–175.

161. Ozzello L, Hamels J: The histiocytic nature of dermatofibrosarcoma protuberans: Tissue culture and electron microscopic study. *Am J Clin Pathol* 1976;65:136–148.

162. Hashimoto K, Brownstein MH, Jakobiec FA: Dermatofibrosarcoma protuberans. *Arch Dermatol* 1974;110:874–885.

163. Enzinger FM, Weiss SW: *Soft Tissue Tumors.* St. Louis, Mo, CV Mosby, 1983, p 161.

164. Weiss SW, Enzinger FM: Malignant fibrous histiocytoma. An analysis of 200 cases. *Cancer* 1978;41:2250–2266.

165. Kearney MM, Soule EH, Ivins JC: Malignant fibrous histiocytoma. A retrospective study of 167 cases. *Cancer* 1980;45:167–178.

166. Hajdu SI: *Pathology of Soft Tissue Tumors.* Philadelphia, Lea and Febiger, 1979, pp 110–121.

167. Goette DK, Deffer TA: Post-irradiation malignant fibrous histiocytoma. *Arch Dermatol* 1985;121:535–538.

168. Yamamoto Y, Arata J, Yonezawa S: Angiomatoid malignant fibrous histiocytoma associated with marked bleeding arising in chronic radiodermatitis. *Arch Dermatol* 1985;121:275–276.

169. Yamamura T, Aozasa K, Honda T, et al.: Malignant fibrous histiocytoma developing in a burn scar. *Br J Dermatol* 1984;110:725–730.

170. Routh A, Hickman BT, Johnson WW: Malignant fibrous histiocytoma arising from chronic ulcer. *Arch Dermatol* 1985;121:529–531.

171. Inoshita T, Youngberg GA: Malignant fibrous histiocytoma arising in previous surgical sites. *Cancer* 1984;53:176–183.

172. Enzinger FM: Angiomatoid malignant fibrous histiocytoma: A distinct fibrohistiocytic tumor of children and young adults simulating a vascular neoplasm. *Cancer* 1979;44:2147–2157.

173. Enzinger FM, Weiss FM: *Soft Tissue Tumors.* St. Louis, Mo, CV Mosby, 1983, pp 170–196.

174. Kempson RI, Kyriakos M: Fibroxanthosarcoma of the soft tissues. A type of malignant fibrous histiocytoma. *Cancer* 1972;29:961–976.

175. Kyriakos M, Kempson RL: Inflammatory fibrous histiocytoma. An aggressive and lethal lesion. *Cancer* 1976;37:1584–1606.

176. Guccion JG, Enzinger FM: Malignant giant cell tumor of soft parts. An analysis of 32 cases. *Cancer* 1972;29:1518–1529.

177. Alguacil-Garcia A, Unni KK, Goellner JR: Malignant fibrous histiocytoma: An ultrastructural study of six cases. *Am J Clin Pathol* 1978;69:121–129.

178. Churg AM, Kahn LB: Myofibroblasts and related cells in malignant fibrous and fibrohistiocytic tumors. *Hum Pathol* 1977;8:205–218.

179. Lentini M, Grosso M, Carozza G, et al.: Fibrohistiocytic tumors of soft tissues. An immunohistochemical study of 183 cases. *Pathol Res Pract* 1986;181:713–717.

180. duBoulay CE: Demonstration of alpha-1-antitrypsin and alpha-1-antichymotrypsin in fibrous histiocytomas using the immunoperoxidase technique. *Am J Surg Pathol* 1982;559–564.

181. Pritchard DJ, Soule EH, Taylor WF, et al.: Fibrosarcoma, a clinicopathologic and statistical study of 199 tumors of the soft tissues of the extremities and trunk. *Cancer* 1974;33:888–897.

182. MacKenzie DH: Fibrosarcoma: A dangerous diagnosis. A review of 205 cases of fibrosarcoma of soft tissues. *Br J Surg* 1964;51:607–613.

183. Bizer LJ: Fibrosarcoma: Report of 64 cases. *Am J Surg* 1971;121:586–587.

184. Enzinger FM, Weiss SW: *Soft Tissue Tumors.* St. Louis, Mo, CV Mosby, 1983, p 113.

185. Chung EB, Enzinger FM: Infantile fibrosarcoma. *Cancer* 1976;38:729–739.

186. Soule EH, Pritchard DJ: Fibrosarcoma in infants and children. A review of 110 cases. *Cancer* 1977;40:1711–1721.

187. Chase DR, Enzinger FM: Epithelioid sarcoma. Diagnosis, prognostic indicators, and treatment. *Am J Surg Pathol* 1985;9:241–263.

188. Part J, Woodruff JM, Marcove RC: Epithelioid sarcoma: An analysis of 22 cases indicating the prognostic significance of vascular invasion and regional lymph node metastasis. *Cancer* 1978;41:1472–1487.

189. Heenan PJ, Quirk CJ, Papadimitriou JM: Epithelioid sarcoma. A diagnostic problem. *Am J Dermatopathol* 1986;8:95–104.

190. Iossifides I, Ayala AG, Johnson DE: Epithelioid sarcoma of the penis. *Urology* 1979;14:190–191.

191. Ulbright TM, Brokaw SA, Stehman FB, et al.: Epithelioid sarcoma of the vulva. Evidence supporting a more aggressive behavior than extra-genital epithelioid sarcoma. *Cancer* 1983;52:1462–1469.

192. Wick MR, Manivel JC: Epithelioid sarcoma and isolated necrobiotic granuloma: A comparative immunocytochemical study. *J Cutan Pathol* 1986;13:253–260.

193. Daimaru Y, Hashimoto H, Tsuneyoshi M, et al.: Epithelial profile of epithelioid sarcoma. *Cancer* 1987;59:134–141.

194. Schmidt D, Harms D: Epithelioid sarcoma in children and adolescents. An immunohistochemical study. *Virchow's Arch* 1987;410:423–431.

195. Weiss SW, Enzinger FM: Epithelioid hemangioendothelioma. A vascular tumor often mistaken for carcinoma. *Cancer* 1982;50:970–981.

196. Evans HL: Synovial sarcoma: A study of 123 biphasic and 17 probable monophasic examples. *Pathol Annu* 1980;15:309–331.

197. Hadju SI, Shiu MH, Fortner JG: Tendosynovial sarcoma. A clinicopathological study of 116 cases. *Cancer* 1977;39:1201–1217.

198. Krall RA, Kostiarovsky M, Patchefsky AS: Synovial sarcoma: A clinical, pathological, and ultrastructural study of 26 cases supporting the recognition of a monophasic variant. *Am J Surg Pathol* 1981;5:137–151.

199. Chung EB, Enzinger FM: Malignant melanoma of soft parts. A reassessment of clear cell sarcoma. *Am J Surg Pathol* 1983;7:405–413.

200. Pavlidis NA, Fisher C, Wiltshaw E: Clear cell sarcoma of tendons and aponeuroses: A clinicopathologic study. *Cancer* 1984;54:1412–1417.

201. Amr SS, Farah GR, Muhtaseb HH, et al.: Clear cell sarcoma: Report of two cases with ultrastructural observations and review of the literature. *Clin Oncol* 1984;10:59–65.

202. Lombardi L, Rilke F: Ultrastructural similarities and differences of synovial sarcoma, epithelioid sarcoma, and clear cell sarcoma of the tendons and aponeuroses. *Ultrastruct Pathol* 1984;6:209–219.

203. Warner TF, Hafez GR, Padmalatha C, et al.: Acral lentiginous melanoma simulating "clear cell sarcoma of tendon and aponeuroses." *J Cutan Pathol* 1983;10:193–200.

CHAPTER 51
Tumors of Neural Differentiation

Jerome B. Taxy

Primary cutaneous tumors expressing neural differentiation occur infrequently[1] and constitute a heterogeneous group of lesions, not all of which represent true neoplasms. Despite the appearance of *neural and neuroma* in the terminology, neurons are not a histopathologic feature of these tumors, which are composed of sustentacular or peripheral nerve sheath cells.

Cutaneous nerves consist of single or groups of axons, associated Schwann, cells and fibroblasts. The unmyelinated nerves are enveloped by crudely overlapping Schwann cell processes; the myelinated fibers are enveloped by complex laminations of these processes, which form the nodes of Ranvier (Fig. 51–1). External to the Schwann cells are the perineural fibroblasts.[1,2] In cutaneous neural tumors, therefore, axons, Schwann cells, fibroblasts, and the peculiar but distinctive granular cells, which probably represent variants of Schwann cells, are the common proliferating constituents. Some would prefer the generic designation *nerve sheath tumors* for this group of lesions.[3]

Electron microscopy has been of great assistance in identifying the cellular constituents of a given tumor.[2] Schwann cells are characterized by long, overlapping cytoplasmic processes outlined by a discrete, often multilayered, basal lamina. Associated Luse bodies, or long-spaced (1500–2000 Å) collagen fibers, are common.[4,5] Fibroblasts have less complicated cytoplasmic extensions, only segments of which have a parallel basal lamina. Subplasmalemmal pinocytosis and intracytoplasmic filaments are also common. Granular cells are distinguished by the polymorphic intracytoplasmic granules resembling lysosomes that pack the cytoplasm almost to the exclusion of other organelles.

Immunohistochemically, the most commonly used antibody in the evaluation of neural tumors is S-100 protein. This acidic, calcium-binding protein (molecular weight [MW] 21,000), completely soluble in ammonium sulfate and originally isolated from bovine brain, consists of two polypeptide chains that exhibit dimeric association of unknown functional significance.[5–7] The distribution of this antigen is widespread and includes glia, neurons, Schwann cells, Langerhans cells, meningothelium, melanocytes, and hyaline cartilage[6,7] (Fig. 51–2). Benign tumors composed of these cell types, including granular cell tumors,[8,9] also express this antigen; malignant tumors are less reproducibly positive.[5,6]

Myelin basic protein (MBP) is a basic polypeptide of about 170 amino acid residues, constituting about 30% of normal myelin, and is synthesized by Schwann cells. An antibody to MBP has been used in conjunction with S-100 protein to study Schwann cell lesions.[10,11] Less extensively studied antigens are Leu-7 (MW 110,000), expressed primarily by T-killer lymphocytes but shared by neurons, glia, Schwann cells, and certain neuroendocrine cells,[12] and type IV collagen, quantitatively plentiful in association with Schwann cells.[13] Antibodies to vimentin, an intermediate filament expressed primarily by mesenchymal cells, may also be positive in cutaneous neural tumors.[11]

The effective diagnostic use of immunohistochemistry is tempered by the increasing number of antigens that have been purified for antibody preparation, the many commercial sources whose preparation methods may vary, the polyclonal or monoclonal nature of the antibody, and the tendency to let traditional light microscopic morphology assume secondary importance.

PALISADED ENCAPSULATED NEUROMA

Clinical Features
In 1972, Reed et al.[14] described 44 cases of a solitary, painless, nonpigmented facial tumor often present for several years to which the designation *palisaded encapsulated neuroma* was applied. A similar group of 63 cases has been presented recently.[15] The male:female ratio was about equal in both studies and the patients were middle-aged.

Histologic Features
Histologically, these are well-delineated dermal masses composed of compact fascicles of spindle cells. There is often a grenz zone between the tumor and the lower border of the occasionally attenuated epidermis (Fig. 51–3). Al-

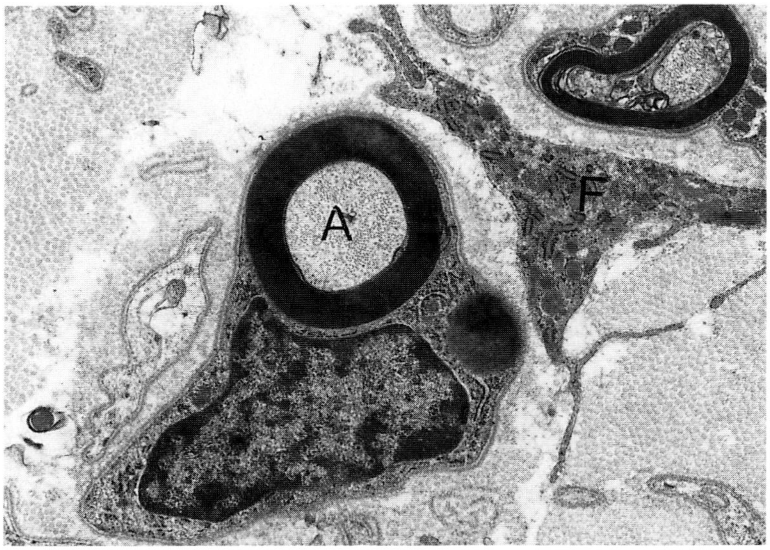

Figure 51–1. From a neurofibroma, a Schwann cell and adjacent cytoplasmic processes are each enveloped by a discrete but single-layered basal lamina. An axon in the center (A) and a similar structure (upper right) are surrounded by a myelin sheath. Between the two is a portion of a perineural fibroblast (F). The background consists of cross-sectioned collagen fibers. (×4000.)

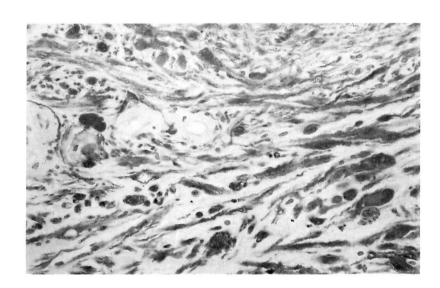

Figure 51–2. From a schwannoma, positive cytoplasmic staining for S100 protein. (Immunoperoxidase-ABC, ×200.)

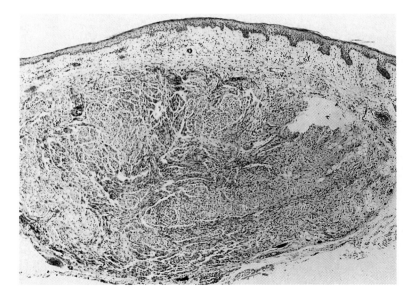

Figure 51–3. Palisaded encapsulated neuroma. Well-defined dermal nodule of compactly arranged interlacing fascicles, overlying grenz zone and attenuated epidermis. (H&E, ×20.)

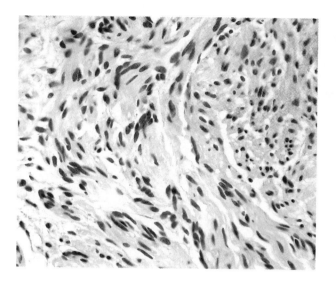

Figure 51–4. Palisaded encapsulated neuroma. Interlacing fascicles of benign fusiform cells with suggestion of palisading. (H&E, ×400.)

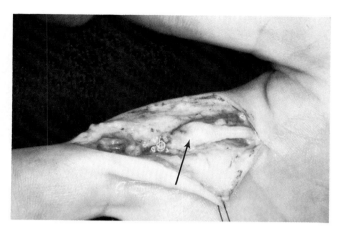

Figure 51–5. Clinical exposure of digital nerve at the base of the right index finger several weeks after injury, demonstrating a small fusiform mass (arrow) representing a traumatic neuroma. (*Photograph courtesy of Ho Min Lim, M.D.*)

though the cells resemble Schwann cells, palisading of the nuclei is inconstant (Fig. 51–4). Axon content, as determined by a Bodian stain, is variable; occasional nonmyelinated nerve fibers partially enveloped by Schwann cells may be seen ultrastructurally.[15] The histologic features are similar to those encountered in mucosal neuromas, but in contrast, no associated clinical syndrome is recognized. The behavior is benign after simple excision.

TRAUMATIC NEUROMA

Clinical Features

The severing of a peripheral nerve results in degeneration and eventual atrophy in the distal segment and, after an initial degenerative reaction in the proximal portion, a proliferative attempt to repair the damage. This process involves growth of axons and proliferation of Schwann cells. Unfortunately, the reparative attempt often results in a localized but random tangle of nerve fascicles that is functionless and often painful. The designation *traumatic neuroma* implies an accidental exogenous event; however, any cutaneous breach, including incision of the skin during surgery, can result in nerve damage and neuroma formation. In the foot, such iatrogenic neuromas may follow elective foot surgery, with patients complaining of pain, paresthesia, dysesthesia, anesthesia, or combinations thereof.[16] Amputation sites are common locations for traumatic neuromas where they may, in part, be responsible for the phantom pain the patient experiences. Less commonly, the lesion may be clinically represented as a mass (Fig. 51–5), usually less than 1 cm.

Histologic Features

Histologically, in relatively early stages, the nerve stump will demonstrate an edematous background containing a

poorly organized proliferation of Schwann cells (Fig. 51–6). In a more established lesion, a focally edematous, disorganized array of small discrete nerve fascicles is present (Fig. 51–7), each surrounded by bands of fibrous tissue (Fig. 51–8). The ratio of axons to Schwann cells is high.[1]

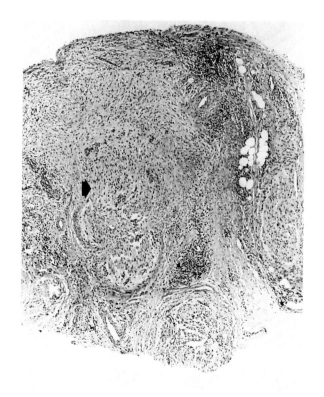

Figure 51–6. Relatively early traumatic neuroma showing an abrupt disruption of the nerve fiber (arrow) with a distal diffuse cellular proliferation. (H&E, ×40.)

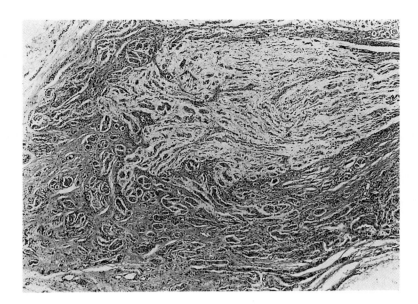

Figure 51–7. More established traumatic neuroma. Partially edematous nerve fascicle is surrounded by numerous disorganized nerve twigs. (H&E, ×40.)

NEUROFIBROMA

Clinical Features

Neurofibroma is probably the most common neural tumor, and its various morphologic forms take on added significance because the question of the clinical presence of neurofibromatosis is often raised. Von Recklinghausen's disease, or neurofibromatosis, is inherited as an autosomal dominant trait, occurring with variable expression but 100% penetrance in about 1 of 3,000 births. Approximately 80,000 Americans are affected by this condition, 50% of whom probably represent new mutations. This disease exhibits no racial or ethnic bias.[17] Although its potential severity cannot be predicted in initially mildly affected patients, it is progressive in all cases, with neurofibromas beginning to appear at the end of the first decade or during puberty. The long-term risk of malignancy may have been overemphasized, but remains substantial particularly in affected female relatives of proband cases.[18]

There are three major clinical defining features[17]: (1) café-au-lait spots, present in almost all patients, possibly present at birth and increasing in size over time; (2) Lisch nodules, lesions of the iris present in about 94% of cases over 6 years of age, not symptom producing and of diagnostic significance only; (3) neurofibromas. Virtually all patients with neurofibromatosis will have the soft, pendunculated, small lesions that eventually cover the cutaneous surfaces in severely affected cases; however, not all patients with an isolated occurrence of this variety of neurofibroma are afflicted with the syndrome. Whether these patients represent a forme fruste of the disease or whether there are just sporadic tumors is debatable. All neurofibromas represent an expansion and destruction of a given peripheral nerve, which in the skin usually implies a small nerve twig.

Histologic Features

The pedunculated neurofibroma may occur on any cutaneous area and is primarily dermal in position (Fig. 51–9). This is not an encapsulated lesion and consists of spindled cells with bland, slightly wavy nuclei and slender elongated cytoplasmic processes in a myxoid background, in which mast cells and collagen bands are often apparent (Fig. 51–10). Degrees of nuclear pleomorphism are occasionally encountered in otherwise routine neurofibromas (Fig. 51–10, inset) and should not lead to an interpretation of malignancy. Axons can be seen on a Bodian stain (Fig. 51–11) or can be visualized ultrastructurally[2] (Fig. 51–1). The nature of the spindled tumor cells is probably a mixture. Some are Schwann cells, although some of these are probably preexistent, being apposed to the axons. Most others exhibit long cell processes without the usual Schwann cell complexity, and with segments of variable length outlined by basal

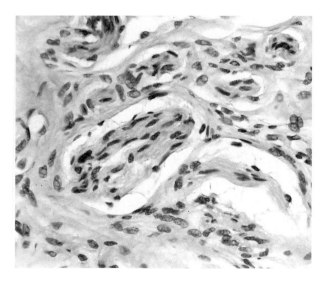

Figure 51–8. Traumatic neuroma. Small nerve twigs each surrounded by a fibrous band. (H&E, ×250.)

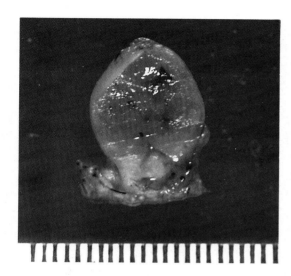

Figure 51–9. An excised, hemisected, pedunculated neurofibroma. Tumor is small and extends to the rim of skin at the base. Line markings are in millimeters.

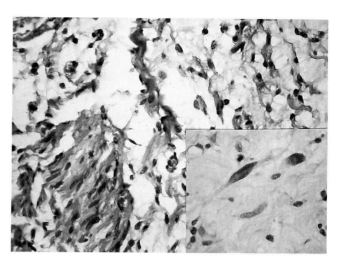

Figure 51–10. Neurofibroma. Bland spindled cells, slightly wavy nuclei, and a myxoid background. Inset: Atypical cells in an otherwise typical pedunculated neurofibroma. (H&E, ×160; inset: H&E, ×400.)

lamina (Fig. 51–12). Long-spaced collagen is occasionally seen.[2] Irrespective of their ultrastructural features, these cells exhibit positive staining for S100 protein.[6,7,10,11]

All patients with plexiform neurofibromas do have von Recklinghausen's disease, and the histologic diagnosis may occasionally establish the clinical diagnosis of the syndrome. These bulky lesions are usually deep, but may have an overlying, café-au-lait spot and will produce obvious cutaneous distortions. This tumor is represented by hypertrophic nerve fascicles that produce a ropelike mass in which each fascicle is individually accentuated (Fig. 51–13). The cellular composition of these fascicles is similar to that of the pedunculated variety of neurofibroma. Surgically, removal of this mass is a much more complicated issue.

Still a third variety is the diffuse neurofibroma, on which the literature is scant.[19] This neurofibroma commonly affects the skin, extending to the deeper soft tissues and results in obvious disfigurement (Fig. 51–14). It may occur in about 10% of neurofibromatosis patients.[19] In addition to the usual histologic features of neurofibroma, these poorly circumscribed tumors exhibit the formation of tactoid (Meissner) bodies, which are aggregates of tumor cells without any axonal association. The palisaded nuclear arrays define intervening fibrillary cell processes (Fig. 51–15). Two cases have been examined ultrastructurally by the author, one from the breast region of a 13-year-old boy with several café-au-lait spots, and the other, the illustrated buttock lesion from a 36-year-old man without any stigmata of neurofibromatosis (Fig. 51–14). The cells in both were Schwann cells; long-spaced collagen was found in one case.

All three variants of neurofibroma are benign. As an isolated phenomenon, the pedunculated variety is innocuous. As a component of neurofibromatosis, the myriad of

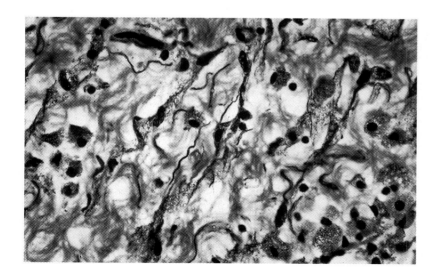

Figure 51–11. Neurofibroma with elongated or spiral axonal processes. (Bodian stain, ×400.)

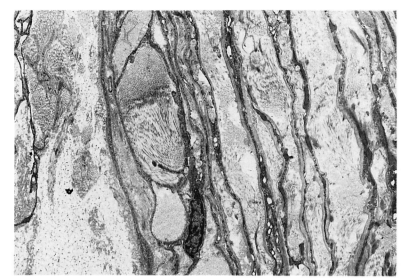

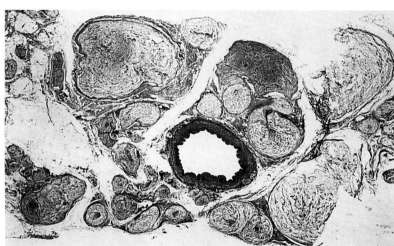

Figure 51–12. Neurofibroma. Tumor cells with elongated cell processes, most of which are outlined by a single layer of basal lamina. (×2500.)

Figure 51–13. Cross section of a plexiform neurofibroma with varying sized hypertrophied nerves. (Masson trichrome, ×10.)

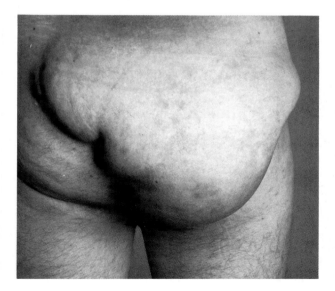

Figure 51–14. A 36-year-old man with a diffuse neurofibroma affecting the right buttock. (*Photograph courtesy of J. Ralph Seaton, M.D.*)

these lesions can be disfiguring. Plexiform and diffuse neurofibromas may present greater surgical challenges; because of anatomic bulk and/or location, they are not easily nor completely removed. Neurofibromas, especially of deep soft tissues and body cavities, are associated with malignant changes.

SCHWANNOMA

Clinical Features
Neurofibromas arise within a given nerve fascicle and produce a mass by expanding within and thereby obliterating the nerve. Schwannomas, theoretically, merely push the nerve fascicle aside while remaining attached to it.[20] Therefore, axons are found within neurofibromas but not within schwannomas. The latter are probably true neoplasms, being well circumscribed and composed of a homogeneous population of cells. A schwannoma of the eighth cranial nerve is generically referred to as an acoustic neuroma.

These tumors are usually sporadic occurrences and

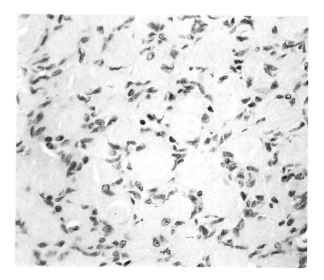

Figure 51–15. Diffuse neurofibroma. Palisaded nuclear arrays and intervening fibrillary material. (H&E, ×250.)

carry no sinister connotations specifically with regard to von Recklinghausen's disease, although patients with that condition obviously can harbor a schwannoma as well as a neurofibroma. Rarely, a schwannoma may assume a multinodular or plexiform appearance, making the distinction from a plexiform neurofibroma difficult and clouding the clinical implications.[21] An association between schwannoma and prior childhood head and neck irradiation has been reported, but a cause-and-effect relationship was not statistically significant.[22]

Histologic Features

The histologic features of this tumor are highly characteristic. The vessels are typically grouped and thick walled or hyalinized. There are two growth patterns, often seen side by side: One consists of dense fascicles of spindled cells in which nuclei are lined up in the same plane and are separated by pink, fibrillar cytoplasmic processes (Antoni A). This palisaded nuclear arrangement and fibrillar material are termed a Verocay body (Fig. 51–16). The second is a more haphazard arrangement of the same bland spindled cells in a loose, myxoid background (Antoni B) (Fig. 51–17). Occasionally, there are groups of xanthoma cells between the dense cellular areas. The nature of these foamy cells is not clear, although histiocytes, probably marrow derived, are often seen in degenerating nerves.[23]

Electron microscopically, the tumor cells are well-developed Schwann cells with complex arrays of overlapping and interdigitating slender cytoplasmic processes. Each process is outlined by a well-defined basal lamina, sometimes layered, and occasional bundles of long-spaced collagen, i.e., Luse bodies (Fig. 51–18).[2,4]

Variants

As the cellular density in a schwannoma is seldom worrisome and the individual cytologic features are usually benign, a correct diagnosis virtually ensures benign behavior. Although malignant change is not thought to occur, rare histologic variants have caused concern. **Cellular schwannoma,** described by Woodruff et al.,[24] is an encapsulated, usually deep lesion with occasional cystic change and focal hemorrhage. One tumor occurred in a patient with neurofibromatosis. The dense cellularity seen histologically is without Verocay bodies. Ultrastructurally, the cells were Schwann cells[2,24]; Luse bodies were also seen. Nuclear pleomorphism and mitotic activity, albeit of low frequency, may be present even though the behavior is benign. One of their 14 cases recurred, although the initial removal had been incomplete. The distinction between this tumor and a malignant schwannoma may be difficult.

Pigmented schwannomas are also usually more deeply seated tumors and contain melanin.[24–27] In addition to a spindle cell element, there may be cells with a more polygonal component.[25] This, plus the occasional mitosis and pleomorphism, raises the issue of malignant melanoma. Ultrastructurally, the cells are Schwann cells, which are

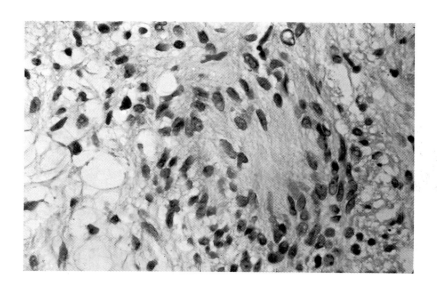

Figure 51–16. Schwannoma. A Verocay body consisting of two areas of nuclear palisading separated by fibrillary material. Portion of myxoid Antoni B area to left. (H&E, ×400.)

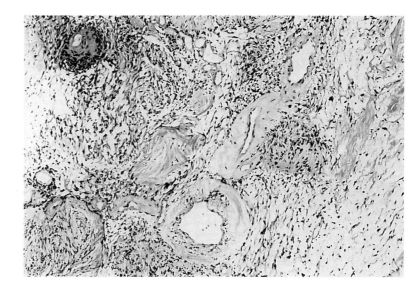

Figure 51–17. Schwannoma. Denser cellular areas (Antoni A) centrally, adjacent to looser areas (Antoni B). Focally hyalinized stromal vessels are also present. (H&E, ×160.)

presumed to be the sources of the melanin.[27] Recurrences are uncommon.

Epithelioid schwannoma is another unusual variant.[28] The tumors are grossly circumscribed but may, on histologic examination, exhibit local invasiveness. Groups of active, but bland, polygonal cells are separated by a myxoid matrix. Defined cell borders and elongated cytoplasmic processes can be discerned (Fig. 51–19). Electron microscopically, the overlapping complex of cytoplasmic processes outlined by basal lamina is easily apparent (Fig. 51–20). S100 staining is strongly positive. Despite some nuclear pleomorphism and occasional mitotic activity, clinical behavior is benign.

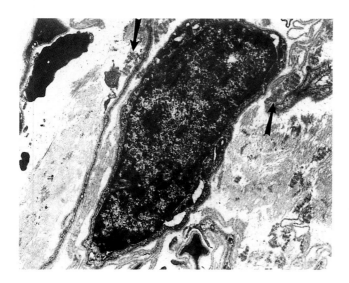

Figure 51–18. Schwannoma. Schwann cell nucleus surrounded by a thin cytoplasmic rim. In the background are thin cytoplasmic processes, all enveloped by several layers of basal lamina. Note long-spaced collagen, i.e., Luse bodies (arrows). (×6000.)

Differential Diagnosis

In the preceding histologic variants of schwannoma, the differential diagnosis may include malignant schwannoma, melanoma, or possibly a metastatic epithelial malignancy. Judicious use of immunohistochemistry for keratin and S100 would resolve the last possibility, but not the first two, as both are potentially positive for S-100 protein. The ultra-structural features of Schwann cells are not observed in melanoma, nor are they typically well developed in malignant schwannoma[29]; however, the interpretation of a Schwann cell tumor can be made by electron microscopy if the Schwann cell features are well developed. In this context, electron microscopic observation of well-differentiated Schwann cells in a histologically difficult lesion may indicate a benign process.

GRANULAR CELL TUMOR

Clinical Features

The granular cell tumor is a histologically and electron microscopically distinctive tumor occurring in the skin and subcutaneous tissues; mucosal surfaces, especially of the head and neck; and deep soft tissues. In a series of 118 tumors, 38 were in the oral cavity or tongue and 48 were cutaneous in location.[30] The tumors are usually small (under 2.0 cm) and solitary, although multiple synchronous tumors are occasionally encountered.[30,31] Grossly, they appear deceptively well demarcated (Fig. 51–21) and have smooth, firm, yellow-tan and gritty sectioned surfaces simulating a carcinoma.

Histologic Features

Histologically, the tumor is locally invasive, composed of nests and cords of polygonal cells with bland nuclei and ample granular cytoplasm. Multinucleation, mild nuclear pleomorphism, and an occasional mitosis may be seen, but are not common[30] (Fig. 51–22). Often, in the skin and

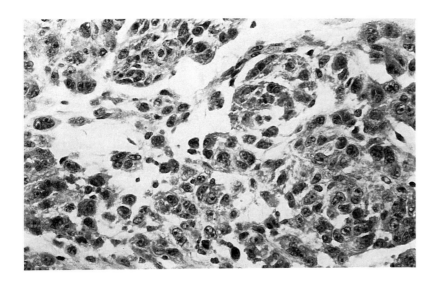

Figure 51–19. Epithelioid schwannoma. Groups of polygonal cells with active but uniform nuclei and prominent nucleoli. Cell borders are relatively defined and processes in the background are discernible. (H&E, ×400.)

mucosal sites, proliferation of the overlying epithelium results in elongation of the rete pegs, hyperkeratosis and acanthosis. The designation *pseudoepitheliomatous hyperplasia* for this phenomenon denotes a reactive process, although rare instances of true in situ carcinoma have been reported[30] (Fig. 51–23).

The cytoplasmic granules characteristic of this tumor are periodic acid-Schiff positive, diastase resistant. Histochemistry for acid phosphatase is positive, thus supporting the notion that these are lysosomal granules. This impression is reinforced by their ultrastructural appearance, a polymorphous population of dark granules with heterogeneous

electron density and occasional residual bodies (Fig. 51–24). Frequent observations of cytoplasmic processes, some outlined by basal lamina, and positive S100 immunostaining[8,9,30,31] have supported the idea that the granular cell tumor is formed by variants of a Schwann cell.

Neither cellular pleomorphism nor mitotic activity nor clear margins are reliable indicators of tumor recurrence. In the study by Lack et al.,[30] five tumors recurred in which the initial margins had been negative; conversely, 19 cases with positive margins did not recur. Truly malignant granular cell tumors are indistinguishable histologically and ultrastructurally from the benign tumors,[32–34] so that the only reliable parameter of malignancy is clinical behavior.[35] In one report, the metastases of one lesion were floridly malignant histologically despite a lack of such features in the initial lesion. The metastases demonstrated strong immunopositivity for carcinoembryonic antigen.[35]

A clinicopathologic variant of the granular cell tumor

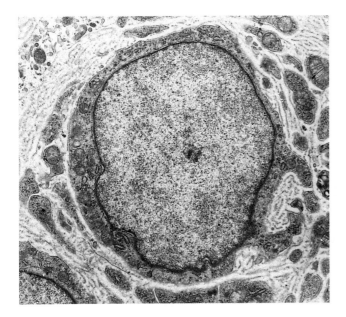

Figure 51–20. Epithelioid schwannoma. Tumor cell is surrounded by numerous cytoplasmic processes, each outlined by several layers of basal lamina. (×6000).

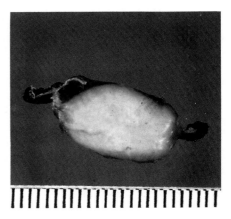

Figure 51–21. Granular cell tumor. Excision of a small cutaneous lesion (skin blackened by india ink) demonstrating apparent gross demarcation and uniform cut surface. Line markings are in millimeters.

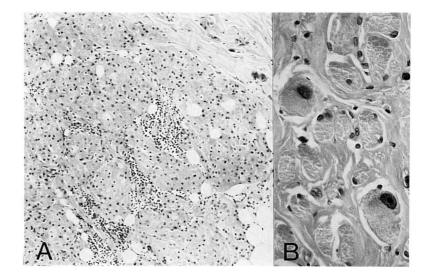

Figure 51–22. A. Typical granular cell tumor infiltrating fat. Confluent nests of histologically bland cells. **B.** Cytologically atypical cells in an otherwise conventional granular cell tumor. (A: H&E, ×160; B: H&E, ×400.)

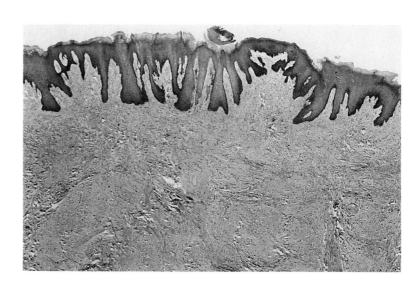

Figure 51–23. Pseudoepitheliomatous hyperplasia overlying a benign granular cell tumor. (H&E, ×20.)

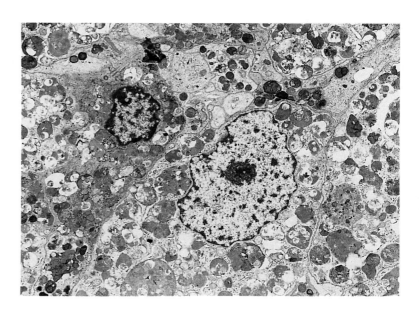

Figure 51–24. Granular cell tumor. An electron micrograph demonstrating the typical polymorphous lysosomal granules packing the cytoplasm of the tumor cells. (×4000.)

is the congenital epulis. This rare condition is apparent at birth and is represented by a pedunculated mass attached to the maxillary or mandibular alveolar ridge.[36,37] The size of the tumor may range from under 1 cm to several centimeters in diameter. The patients are almost all females. In a literature review and report of new cases totaling 81 patients, only 7 males were noted.[36] Morphologically, the lesions are identical to conventional granular cell tumors, except that the overlying epithelium is smooth and attenuated. The clinical behavior is benign, even if resection is incomplete.[36] Spontaneous involution has been documented.[37]

NEUROTHEKEOMA (NERVE SHEATH MYXOMA)

Clinical Features

In 1980, Gallager and Helwig[38] reported 53 cases of a benign tumor of the dermis and subcutaneous tissue histologically suggestive of a Schwann cell tumor that they termed *neurothekeoma*. They suggested a resemblance to nerve sheath myxoma, but felt the two tumors were different. Subsequent authors have disagreed, concluding that the two represent the same tumor.[39–41] In the report by Gallager and Helwig, the lesion was rare over the age of 25, had a 4:1 female: male occurrence, historically was present for years, and appeared primarily on the face, shoulder, or arm. Subsequent reports confirm these clinical features.

Histologic Features

The lesions are small, averaging about 1.0 cm in diameter. Histologically, the tumors are not well circumscribed and frequently extend into surrounding soft tissue. They have an overall lobulated architecture, the lobules being composed of epithelioid cells with ample cytoplasm and small spindled cells with thin cytoplasmic prolongations (Fig. 51–25). Multinucleated giant cells, cytologic atypia, and mitoses

(as many as 5 per 10 high-power fields) are common. The lobules of cells are separated by a mucinous or myxoid background (Fig. 51–26).

Although the histologic features surely suggest a Schwann cell lesion, especially the epithelioid variant, ultrastructural and immunohistochemical confirmation has not been apparent. Electron microscopy in a few cases has demonstrated long cell processes with absent or only scant basal lamina[38,41]; one report indicated well-developed, occasionally multilayered basal lamina.[39] That report, as well as one other, also indicated strong positive staining for S100 protein.[39,40] This experience has not been uniform,[6,41] although one case yielded a positive reaction to AHMY-1, a monoclonal antibody similar to myelin basic protein, thus suggesting Schwann cell composition. Most reports have indicated that axons or nerves are not associated with this tumor.[38–40] The two cases the author has studied have also been S100 negative and one has shown entrapped small nerve fibers.

MALIGNANT SCHWANNOMA

Clinical Features

The designation commonly given to a malignant peripheral nerve tumor is malignant schwannoma or malignant peripheral nerve sheath tumor. For convenience, the former is employed here. These tumors are deep lesions, affecting the skin only secondarily by bulk or by ulceration. Primary presentation in the skin is exceptional. Malignant schwannoma is a diagnosis established in any of the following situations: a sarcoma arising in a patient with neurofibromatosis; a sarcoma arising in or inseparable from a nerve; a sarcoma arising in a preexistent neurofibroma. A sarcoma without any of the preceding associations can be interpreted as a malignant schwannoma if the histologic characteristics of the tumor are similar to those of tumors arising in an accepted setting.[29]

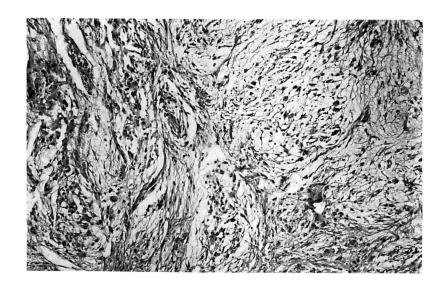

Figure 51–25. Neurothekeoma. Lobulated low-power growth of spindled and polygonal cells with slender cytoplasmic processes. (H&E, ×160.)

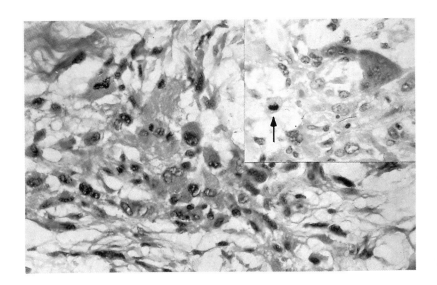

Figure 51–26. Neurothekeoma. Cytologically atypical epithelial-like cells with cytoplasmic processes in a myxoid background. Inset: Neurothekeoma with a multinucleated giant cell and a mitotic figure (arrow). (H&E, ×400.)

Histologic Features

Grossly, these are bulky, poorly circumscribed fleshy tumors, similar to other types of sarcoma. Histologically, there are alterations in cellular density, with some areas more loosely textured than others. The cells are fusiform, with wavy nuclear contours and poor cell demarcation. Palisading nuclei are uncommon. Heterologous differentiation, e.g., cartilage, osteoid, skeletal muscle, and mucin-producing glands, may be encountered.

Ultrastructural examination should be concerned with the better differentiated regions by light microscopy. These areas present long, overlapping processes and incomplete basal lamina formation, and are not the features of well-developed Schwann cells. They can be used to support a light microscopic diagnosis only. S100 staining is positive in only about half the cases interpreted light microscopically as malignant schwannoma.[6]

REFERENCES

1. Reed ML, Jacoby RA: Cutaneous neuroanatomy and neuropathology: Normal nerves, neural-crest derivatives and benign neural neoplasms in the skin. *Am J Dermatopathol* 1983;5:335–362.
2. Erlandson RA, Woodruff JM: Peripheral nerve sheath tumors: An electron microscopic study of 43 cases. *Cancer* 1982;49:273–287.
3. Feigin I: Skin tumors of neural origin. *Am J Dermatopathol* 1983;5:397–399.
4. Sian CS, Ryan SF: The ultrastructure of neurilemoma with emphasis on Antoni B tissue. *Hum Pathol* 1981;12:145–160.
5. Erlandson RA: Diagnostic immunohistochemistry of human tumors: An interim evaluation. *Am J Surg Pathol* 1984;8:615–624.
6. Weiss SW, Langloss JM, Enzinger FM: Value of S-100 protein in the diagnosis of soft tissue tumors with particular reference to benign and malignant Schwann cell tumors. *Lab Invest* 1983;49:299–308.
7. Kahn HJ, Marks A, Thom H, et al: Role of antibody to S-100 protein in diagnostic pathology. *Am J Clin Pathol* 1983;79:341–347.
8. Nakazato Y, Ishizek J, Takahashi K, et al.: Immunohistochemical localization of S-100 protein in granular cell myoblastoma. *Cancer* 1982;49:1624–1628.
9. Armin A, Connelly EM, Rowden G: An immunoperoxidase investigation of S-100 protein in granular cell myoblastomas: Evidence for Schwann cell derivation. *Am J Clin Pathol* 1983;79:37–44.
10. Penneys NS, Mogollon R, Kowalczyk A, et al.: A survey of cutaneous neural lesions for the presence of myelin basic protein: An immunohistochemical study. *Arch Dermatol* 1984; 120:210–213.
11. Roholls PJM, DeJong ASH, Ramaekers FCS: Application of markers in the diagnosis of soft tissue tumors. *Histopathology* 1985;9:1019–1035.
12. Smolle J, Walter GF, Kerl H: Myelin-associated glycoprotein in neurogenic tumours of the skin: An immunohistological study using Leu-7 monoclonal antibody. *Arch Dermatol Res* 1985;277:141–142.
13. Gay RE, Gay S, Jones RE Jr: Histological and immunohistological identification of collagens in basement membranes of Schwann cells of neurofibromas. *Am J Dermatopathol* 1983;5:317–325.
14. Reed RJ, Fine RM, Meltzer HD: Palisaded encapsulated neuromas of the skin. *Arch Dermatol* 1972;106:865–870.
15. Dover JS, From L, Lewis A: Clinicopathologic findings in palisaded encapsulated neuromas. *J Cutan Pathol* 1986;13:77.
16. Kenzora JE: Sensory nerve neuromas—Leading to failed foot surgery. *Foot Ankle* 1986;7:110–117.
17. Riccardi VM: Von Recklinghausen neurofibromatosis. *N Engl J Med* 1981;305:1617–1627.
18. Sorensen SA, Mulvihill JJ, Nielsen A: Long term follow-up of von Recklinghausen neurofibromatosis: Survival and malignant neoplasms. *N Engl J Med* 1986;314:1010–1015.
19. Enzinger FM, Weiss SW: *Soft Tissue Tumors.* St. Louis, Mo, CV Mosby, 1983, pp 610–615.
20. Harkin JC, Reed RJ: Tumors of the peripheral nerve system, in *Atlas of Tumor Pathology,* 2nd series. Washington, DC, American Pathologists, 1969, p 71.
21. Woodruff JM, Marshall ML, Godwin TA, et al.: Plexiform (mul-

tinodular) schwannoma: A tumor simulating the plexiform neurofibroma. *Am J Surg Pathol* 1983;7:691–697.

22. Shore-Freedman E, Abrahams C, Recant W, et al.: Neurilemoma and salivary gland tumors of the head and neck following childhood irradiation. *Cancer* 1983;51:2159–2163.

23. Liu HM: Schwann cell properties: II. The identity of phagocytes in the degenerating nerve. *Am J Pathol* 1974;75:395–416.

24. Woodruff JM, Godwin TA, Erlandson RA, et al.: Cellular schwannoma: A variety of schwannoma sometimes mistaken for a malignant tumor. *Am J Surg Pathol* 1981;5:733–744.

25. Font RL, Truoug LD: Melanotic schwannoma of soft tissues: Electron-microscopic observations and review of literature. *Am J Surg Pathol* 1984;8:129–138.

26. Mennemeyer RP, Hammer SP, Tytus JS, et al.: Melanotic schwannoma: Clinical and ultrastructural studies of three cases with evidence of intracellular melanin synthesis. *Am J Surg Pathol* 1971;3:3–10.

27. Burns DK, Silva FG, Forde KA, et al.: Primary melanocytic schwannoma of the stomach: Evidence of a dual melanocytic and schwannian differentiation in an extra-axial site in a patient without neurofibromatosis. *Cancer* 1983;52:1432–1441.

28. Taxy JB, Battifora H: Epithelioid schwannoma: Diagnosis by electron microscopy. *Ultrastruct Pathol* 1981;2:19–24.

29. Taxy JB, Battifora H, Trujillo Y, et al.: Electron microscopy in the diagnosis of malignant schwannoma. *Cancer* 1981;48:1381–1391.

30. Lack EE, Worsham GF, Callihan MD, et al.: Granular cell tumor: A clinicopathologic study of 110 patients. *J Surg Oncol* 1980;13:301–316.

31. Seo IS, Azzarelli B, Warner TF, et al.: Multiple visceral and cutaneous granular cell tumors: Ultrastructural and immuno-cytochemical evidence of Schwann cell origin. *Cancer* 1984;53:2104–2110.

32. Cadotte M: Malignant granular-cell myoblastoma. *Cancer* 1974;33:1417–1422.

33. Steffelaar JW, Nap M, v. Haelst UJGM: Malignant granular cell tumor: Report of a case with special reference to carcinoembryonic antigen. *Am J Surg Pathol* 1982;6:665–672.

34. Usui M, Ishii S, Yamawaki S, et al.; Malignant granular cell tumor of the radial nerve: An autopsy observation with electron microscopic and tissue culture studies. *Cancer* 1977;39:1547–1555.

35. Robertson AJ, McIntosh W, Lamont P, et al.: Malignant granular cell tumour (myoblastoma) of the vulva: Report of a case and review of the literature. *Histopathology* 1981;5:69–79.

36. Lack EE, Worshem GF, Callihan MD, et al.: Gingival granular cell tumors of the newborn (congenital "epulis"): A clinical and pathologic study of 21 patients. *Am J Surg Pathol* 1981;5:37–46.

37. O'Brien FV, Pielow WD: Congenital epulis: Its natural history. *Arch Dis Child* 1971;46:559–560.

38. Gallager RL, Helwig EB: Neurothekeoma: A benign cutaneous tumor of neural origin. *Am J Clin Pathol* 1980;74:759–764.

39. Angervall L, Kindbloom LG, Haglid K: Dermal nerve sheath myxoma: A light and electron microscopic, histochemical and immunohistochemical study. *Cancer* 1984;53:1752–1759.

40. Fletcher CDM, Chan JKC, McKee PH: Dermal nerve sheath myxoma: A study of 3 cases. *Histopathology* 1986;10:135–145.

41. Aronson PJ, Fretzin DF, Potter BS: Neurothekeoma of Gallager and Helwig (dermal nerve sheath myxoma variant): Report of a case with electron microscopic and immunohistochemical studies. *J Cutan Pathol* 1985;12:506–519.

CHAPTER 52

Vascular Tumors

Philip H. Cooper

A discussion of vascular tumors of the skin encompasses a diverse group of lesions. Only a few qualify as true neoplasms, defined as a new growth that exhibits loss of responsiveness to normal growth controls. Moreover, if one views Kaposi's sarcoma as a multicentric disease, angiosarcomas are the only cutaneous vascular tumors clearly capable of producing embolic-type metastases. Most vascular tumors of the skin represent malformations, self-limited proliferations, or acquired vascular dilations.

HEMANGIOMAS

Infantile Capillary Hemangioma

Clinical Features
Infantile capillary hemangioma, also called *strawberry nevus, benign infantile hemangioendothelioma,* and *cellular angioma of infancy,* is a distinctive clinicopathologic entity.[1-3] Cutaneous abnormalities are first noted a few days after birth.[2,4] The lesion then enlarges, assuming its characteristic, slightly nodular crimson appearance. The tumor usually continues to grow for several months or as long as a year, resulting in lesions that range in size from several millimeters to 6 cm or more. After a static phase, spontaneous involution commences, leading to an excellent cosmetic outcome in 50% of patients by the age of 5 years and in 75 to 90% after 7 years.[1,3] Most individuals have just a single lesion, but in 15 to 20% of cases, the tumor is multiple.[2,3] Females are affected twice as often as males. In referral populations, the head is the most common site,[2,3] but in a group of unselected patients, lesions were distributed in approximate proportion to the surface area of the affected part.[2] The parotid gland is an additional recognized location for infantile capillary hemangioma.[5,6]

Histologic Features
The microscopic appearance depends on the age of the lesion. Young tumors are quite cellular and consist of closely set nodules that create a mosaic or crude jigsaw puzzle pattern at low power. Depending on the size and depth of the lesion, cutaneous adnexa, adipose tissue, skeletal muscle, and remnants of parotid gland are buried within the nodules and trapped in fibrous septa between them. At high power, the vascular character of the tumor can be overlooked. There are large fields of uniform cells with modest amounts of light eosinophilic cytoplasm (Fig. 52–1). Nuclei are ovoid, vesicular, and contain one to three small nucleoli. Mitotic figures are numerous; several can often be found in a single high-power field. On further search, however, it is possible to locate foci where the cells form nests or cords, separated from one another by delicate collagenous stroma. Moreover, small lumina surrounded by tumor cells can be discerned, and some contain red blood cells. Reticulin stains are helpful in highlighting the cord and nestlike pattern and in identifying the vascular nature of the tumor in its cellular phase.

In older lesions, lumina are more widespread and, because of their increased caliber, more obvious. Individual capillaries are clearly separated by stroma. It may be possible to recognize an investing layer of fusiform pericytes. Increasing age of the lesion is signified by almost complete canalization (although cellular foci may persist), further increase of intercapillary stroma, and loss of definition of the nodular architecture (Fig. 52–2). Senescent lesions consist of poorly defined aggregates of greatly dilated capillaries, some of which show hyalinization of their walls.[7]

Electron Microscopy
Ultrastructurally, the capillaries are lined by a single continuous layer of endothelial cells and are bounded by a basement membrane.[6,8–10] One or several layers of pericytes surround the endothelium-lined tubes and are, themselves, invested in basement membrane. Crystalloid inclusions of uncertain nature have been observed in the endothelial cells.[10] Weibel-Palade bodies are either poorly formed or apparently absent, at least in the earlier stages of evolution of the lesion.[8–10]

Acquired Capillary Hemangiomas

Capillary hemangiomas that appear during later childhood or adult life are generally small lesions, often excised for

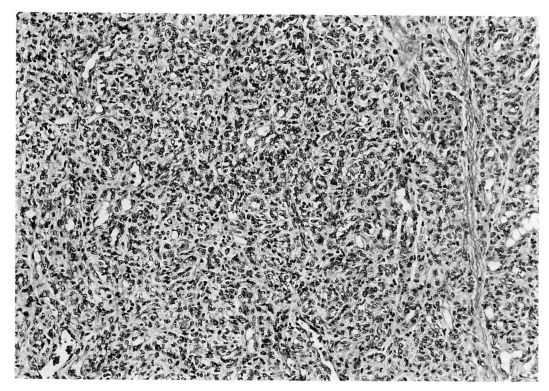

Figure 52–1. Infantile capillary hemangioma from a 4-month-old infant. Cellular nodules are separated from one another by a delicate fibrous band (right). A subtle pattern of cords and nests can be discerned, and tumor cells surround lumens, focally (H&E, ×175).

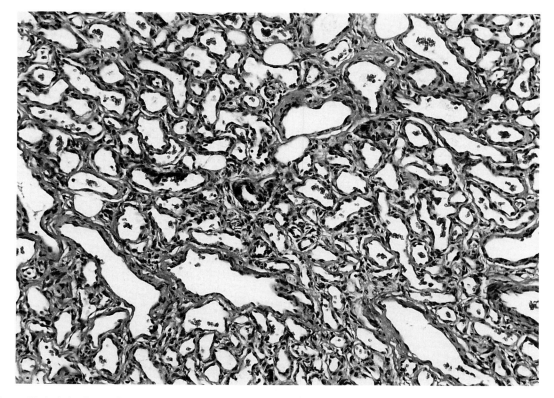

Figure 52–2. Infantile capillary hemangioma from a 2-year-old child. The lesion is extensively canalized, and lumina are lined by flattened endothelial cells. Individual capillaries are separated by fibrous stroma (H&E, ×160).

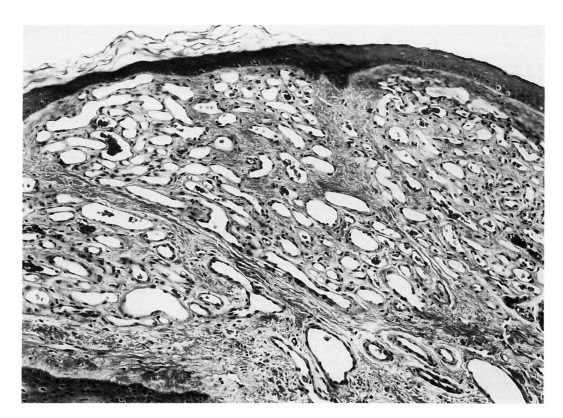

Figure 52–3. Cherry hemangioma. Aggregates of dilated capillaries are located in the superficial dermis (H&E, ×160).

cosmetic reasons or microscopic confirmation. They consist of aggregates of capillaries at various levels of the dermis or subcutis. *Cherry hemangiomas* are first seen in adolescents or young adults, increase in size and number later in life, and are present in most individuals older than 70 years. The lesions consist of ruby or cherry red papules, 1 to 5 mm in diameter, elevated 1 to 3 mm above adjacent skin. Microscopically, aggregates of dilated capillaries, with variably thickened walls, are located in the superficial dermis (Fig. 52–3).

Cavernous Hemangioma

Clinical Features
In the usual case, one or more circumscribed, soft, compressible or cystic, blue or skin-colored tumors become apparent in infancy, childhood, or early adulthood and persist thereafter. The lesions usually range in size from one to several centimeters but can be much larger, with involvement of an entire anatomic region (*angiomatosis*). Large cavernous hemangiomas (and a variety of other vascular tumors) may be complicated by consumptive coagulopathy (*Kasabach-Merritt syndrome*) and microangiopathic hemolytic anemia.[11–13] The consumption of clotting factors apparently takes place primarily within the hemangioma.[11,12]

The *blue rubber bleb nevus syndrome*[14–17] consists of the sporadic or familial occurrence of multiple cavernous hemangiomas of the skin, mucous membranes, gastrointestinal tract, and other viscera; gastrointestinal blood loss;

and iron deficiency anemia. The cutaneous lesions consist of pedunculated, sessile, intradermal, and subcutaneous tumors that range in size from a few millimeters to 3 cm or larger. The most superficial tumors are soft, somewhat lobulated, deep blue or black, and easily compressible. Some reports of blue rubber bleb nevus syndrome probably describe patients with multiple glomus tumors.[18] *Maffucci's syndrome*[16,19,20] consists of the nonfamilial occurrence of multiple cutaneous vascular tumors in association with enchondromatosis. The cutaneous lesions are usually cavernous hemangiomas, but capillary hemangiomas, phlebectasias, and lymphangiomas have also been observed.[19,20] The enchondromas most often involve the hands, feet, and long bones and result in gross deformities, bony shortening, and susceptibility to fracture. Affected patients are at risk for transformation of their enchondromas into chondrosarcomas.

Histologic Features
The microscopic diagnosis of cavernous hemangioma is, at times, arbitrary. Perhaps the most reproducible picture is of a circumscribed, subcutaneous nodule consisting of multiple large, blood-filled vascular channels lined by flat endothelial cells (Fig. 52–4). The walls of the vascular structures are thick, fibrous, variably hyalinized, and contain only sparse spindle cells consistent with adventitial fibroblasts. In some cases, a proportion of the vessels have thin, delicate walls. In the dermis, the diagnosis of cavernous hemangioma depends primarily on the presence of aggre-

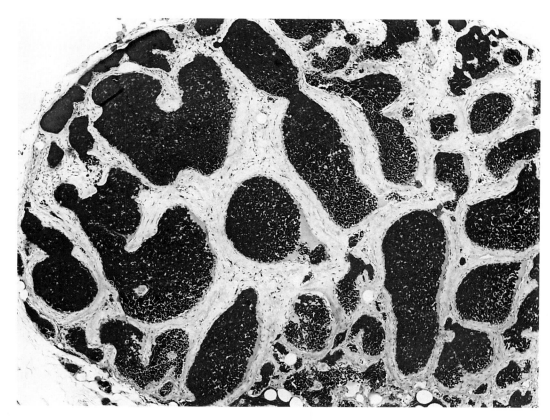

Figure 52–4. Cavernous hemangioma. A circumscribed, subcutaneous nodule consists of multiple large, blood-filled channels lined by flat endothelial cells. The thick walls consist of pale, hyalinized connective tissue containing sparse spindle cells (H&E, ×65).

gated or dispersed, large vascular spaces judged by the observer to be cavernous. Thick, fibrous walls are usually absent, and aside from their large caliber, the vessels resemble capillaries, venules, or small veins.[4] In other cases, the walls consist of thin, hyalinized bands. The microscopic spectrum just described can be found in individual patients with blue rubber bleb nevus syndrome (and, presumably, Maffucci's syndrome) if enough lesions are studied.[14,15] Cavernous hemangiomas are subject to thrombosis, papillary endothelial hyperplasia, and the formation of phleboliths. There may be epidermal hyperplasia similar to that observed in verrucous hemangiomas and angiokeratomas.[15]

Verrucous Hemangioma

Verrucous hemangiomas are either present at birth or appear within the first two decades of life.[21,22] The lower extremity is the most common site, followed by the trunk and upper extremity. The tumor first appears as one or more groups of red papules that lack epidermal abnormalities. With time, the lesions gradually expand, often become confluent, and result in red to purple verrucous plaques or linear streaks and bands, several centimeters or more in maximal dimension. Many cases reported as *angiokeratoma circumscriptum*[23] fall within the definition of verrucous hemangioma.

Microscopically, the underlying hemangioma is either of the capillary type, cavernous, or mixed.[21] It involves the entire dermis and extends into the subcutis. The overlying epidermis exhibits undulating or filiform papillomatosis, hyperkeratosis, and parakeratosis (Fig. 52–5). Rete ridges extend downward between dilated capillaries, partially or completely encompassing them in a manner similar to that observed in angiokeratomas. Dilated lymphatics may be found in small numbers mixed with the ectatic blood vessels.[21] Verrucous hemangiomas are fundamentally different from angiokeratomas, as they represent vascular tumors with extensive dermal involvement, rather than acquired telangiectasias, essentially limited to dermal papillae.

Lobular Capillary Hemangioma (Pyogenic Granuloma)

Clinical Features

Lobular capillary hemangioma is a specific clinicopathologic entity[24] that should not be confused with granulation tissue. It typically presents as a firm red polyp or papule, subject to ulceration and hemorrhage, that achieves its maximal size within a few weeks or months. Sites of predilection include the hands and face and the mucous membranes of the mouth and nose.[24,25] The lesion occasionally develops within a nevus flammeus.[26,27] The gingival tumor of preg-

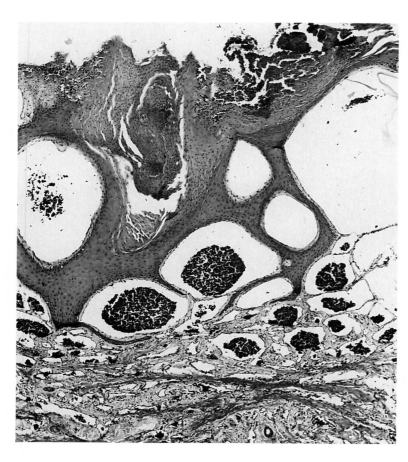

Figure 52–5. Verrucous hemangioma. Markedly dilated, capillary-type blood vessels involve the papillary and reticular dermis. The epidermis exhibits papillomatosis, hyperkeratosis, and parakeratosis. Rete ridges extend between individual capillaries, seeming to partially or completely surround them (H&E, ×60).

nant women (*pregnancy epulis*) is identical, clinically and pathologically, to lobular capillary hemangioma.[24,25]

Lobular capillary hemangiomas can recur after excision. Moreover, multiple *satellites* rarely develop adjacent to the site of a recently treated lesion.[26,28] Affected patients are nearly always less than 20 years of age, and their tumors are typically located on the upper trunk or shoulder. Rare patients develop multiple lobular capillary hemangiomas in a localized area[29] or widespread "disseminated" lesions.[30] Lobular capillary hemangiomas occasionally present as clinically nonspecific *dermal, subcutaneous,* or *intravenous* nodules.[31–33]

Histologic Features

The microscopic picture[24–26,31,32,34] is characteristic and almost always allows distinction from other vascular tumors. The lesion is composed of an aggregate of angiomatous lobules. In the typical polypoid tumor, individual lobules are most obvious in the deeper portions, where they are relatively discrete (Fig. 52–6). When superficially located, the aggregates of capillaries may lose their definition and assume a patchy or confluent pattern. The cellularity of the lobules probably depends, in part, on the age of the tumor. In lesions of short duration, the lobules are often quite cellular and exhibit few if any discernible capillary lumens. Nuclei are vesicular, but cytologically bland. Mitotic figures can be numerous.[24] In the usual case, however, most of the lobules contain angular, slightly branching,

open capillary lumina (Fig. 52–7). In older lesions, particularly in their superficial portions, the lobules are often considerably enlarged, primarily because of the appearance of additional lumina and dilation of others. Endothelial cells are flattened, and mitotic figures are few. Some lesions, particularly nasal[24] and intravenous examples,[32] contain large areas where the capillaries form a meshwork, and the lobular arrangement is only focally present.

In tumors uncomplicated by ulceration, the stroma is fibromyxoid or collagenous (Fig. 52–7). There may be stromal edema, superficially, but inflammatory cells are sparse. When the surface is ulcerated, the stroma becomes markedly infiltrated by inflammatory cells, including large numbers of neutrophils. Fibrin, hemorrhage, and necrosis may also be present. These secondary changes tend to obscure the lobular architecture, but it can usually be appreciated in deeper portions of the lesion. The stroma also contains arterioles and venules that connect with the larger capillaries of individual lobules,[24,31,32] suggesting that the latter have both an arterial supply and a venous drainage. The stromal venules occasionally contain foci of papillary endothelial hyperplasia.[24,32,35] In ideal sections, a small muscular artery and one or more veins can be observed extending perpendicularly within the dermis and entering the lesion. An epidermal collarette is seen in some exophytic tumors but is a nonspecific finding.[24] Intradermal and subcutaneous lesions consist of circumscribed groups of angiomatous lobules (Fig. 52–8).[31] Intravenous examples are polypoid, with a stalk providing attachment to the vein wall (Fig. 52–9).[32]

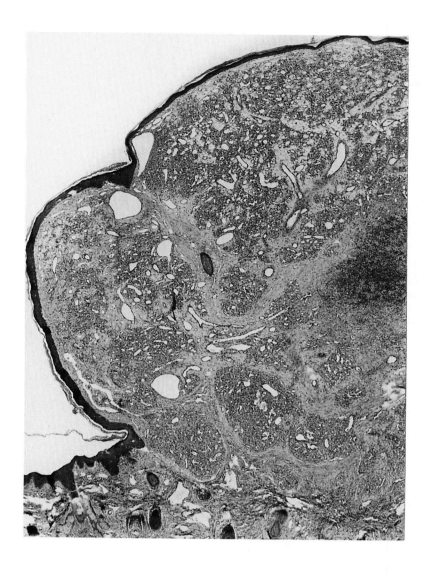

Figure 52–6. Lobular capillary hemangioma. The tumor consists of an aggregate of angiomatous lobules. The lobules are well outlined and relatively discrete in the deeper portions but partially lose their definition, superficially. In the absence of ulceration, the stroma shows only superficial edema and rare inflammatory cells (H&E, ×30).

Electron Microscopy

Ultrastructural observations document the essential capillary nature of lobular capillary hemangioma.[33,36,37] Factor VIII-related antigen is present in endothelial cells lining larger stromal vessels but is sparse or absent in proliferative, cellular foci.[38] *Ulex europaeus* lectin binds to endothelial cells in both larger vessels and cellular lobules.[39]

Differential Diagnosis

The microscopic diagnosis is usually straightforward. A differential diagnosis, when necessary, often centers on one or more of the other vascular lesions described elsewhere in this chapter. Particularly cellular examples, with numerous mitotic figures, can be cause for alarm, but familiarity with this microscopic aspect, appreciation of the lobular architecture, and knowledge of the clinical findings should be helpful. Occasional lobular capillary hemangiomas consist of just one large cellular lobule and may resemble a nonvascular lesion such as a histiocytic proliferation or even an epithelial tumor. Evidence of capillary differentiation can usually be found, however, and reticulin stains are helpful in outlining additional capillaries. The histologic picture of intravenous lobular capillary hemangioma is es-

sentially identical to that observed in more typical sites and should be distinguished from intravascular papillary endothelial hyperplasia and intravascular angiolymphoid hyperplasia.

As noted earlier, there has been confusion between lobular capillary hemangioma and ordinary *granulation tissue*. Granulation tissue develops as part of the injury-repair sequence. Capillary proliferation is fundamental to granulation tissue. Initially, the capillaries appear as cords of primitive-appearing spindle cells with frequent mitotic figures (Fig. 52–10). The stroma is edematous and contains acute and chronic inflammatory cells. As granulation tissue matures, the capillaries become canalized. Stromal collagenization signifies the emergence of scar. Granulation tissue occurs at sites of persistent injury such as chronic ulcers, ostomies, sites of intubation, and vaginal cuffs that result from hysterectomy. In these settings, granulation tissue often forms an elevated or polypoid nodule, with a characteristic pattern of capillaries that radiate toward the surface (Fig. 52–10).[40] Although such lesions are often submitted by clinicians as "pyogenic granuloma" or "granuloma," they are not granulomatous and bear no relation to lobular capillary hemangioma. Exuberant granulation tissue also

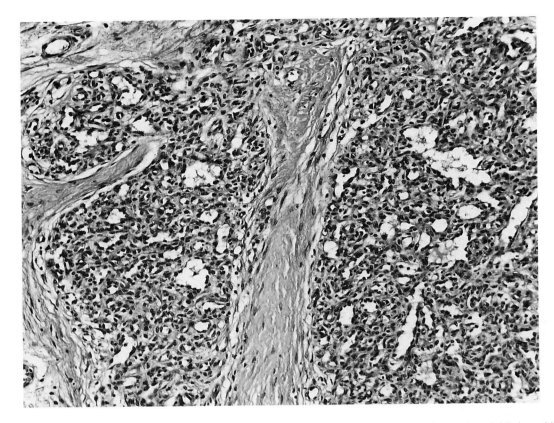

Figure 52–7. Lobular capillary hemangioma. Typical lobules are moderately cellular and contain angular, slightly branching, capillary-type vessels. The lobules are sharply circumscribed, and the intervening stroma lacks inflammatory infiltrate (H&E, ×160).

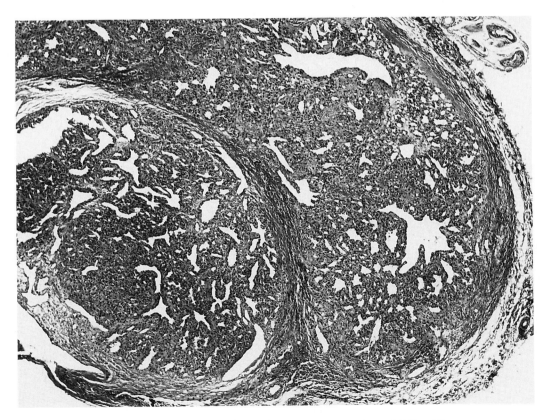

Figure 52–8. Subcutaneous lobular capillary hemangioma (H&E, ×65).

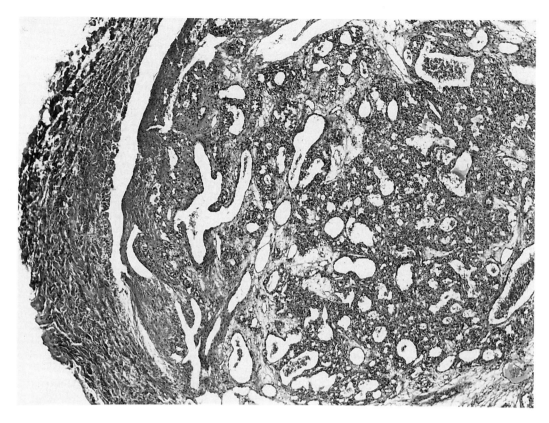

Figure 52–9. Intravenous lobular capillary hemangioma. The tumor forms an intraluminal polyp attached to the vein wall (left) by a fibrovascular stalk (lower left) (H&E, ×65).

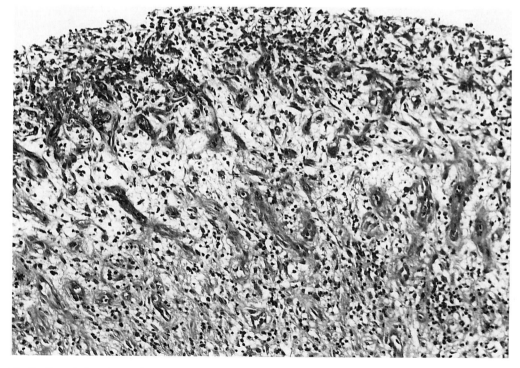

Figure 52–10. Granulation tissue. Capillaries are present in the form of cords of primitive-appearing spindle cells, some of which are canalized. Note the radiating pattern toward the surface (H&E, ×160).

occurs in patients receiving *retinoid therapy* for cystic acne or psoriasis.[41]

Acral Arteriovenous Hemangioma

Acral arteriovenous hemangioma appears as an asymptomatic red, purple, or flesh-colored papule with a predilection for the skin of the face.[42–44] A minority are situated on an extremity; the trunk is an occasional site. The tumor is nearly always solitary; when multiple, the lesions are grouped.

Microscopically, one observes a circumscribed aggregate of prominent blood vessels located within the superficial one half or two thirds of the dermis (Fig. 52–11). Many have thick walls with fibromyxoid ground substance and loosely arranged, circumferentially oriented spindle cells, some of which have histochemical characteristics of smooth muscle. The thick-walled vessels thus resemble arteries, but elastic fibers are delicate and discontinuous, and well-formed internal elastic membranes are absent. The remaining vessels within the tumor resemble ectatic venules or dilated capillaries. In fortuitous sections, connections between the thick- and thin-walled vascular elements can be observed.[42] A small muscular artery and one or more veins may be present in the dermis deep to the lesion and can be traced into it with serial sections. The precise nature of acral arteriovenous hemangioma is uncertain, but it seems possible, based on microscopic findings and the anatomic sites of predilection, that the lesion is centered on one or more preexisting arteriovenous anastomoses. The thick-walled vessels have microscopic features that render equivocal their designation as either arteries or veins. Their lack of a well-formed internal elastic membrane suggests that they are more closely related to veins, perhaps altered by local hemodynamic factors.

Acquired Tufted Angioma

Acquired tufted angioma is a rare form of benign, locally progressive capillary angiomatosis observed in both children and adults.[45–47] Some of the tumors reported as *angioblastomas*[48] may represent tufted angiomas; others are probably juvenile capillary hemangiomas. The lesions consist of slowly enlarging erythematous macules and plaques, several centimeters in size, with a predilection for the upper trunk and neck. Microscopically, there are numerous cellular lobules dispersed throughout the dermis (Fig. 52–12). The individual cells are ovoid or spindled and lack atypia. Cleftlike lumina are present within the lobules. The cellular masses themselves protrude into and greatly distort thin-walled, venule-like channels about their peripheries. This feature and the dispersed distribution of the angiomatous masses within the dermis allow distinction from intradermal lobular capillary hemangioma. The latter consists of a cir-

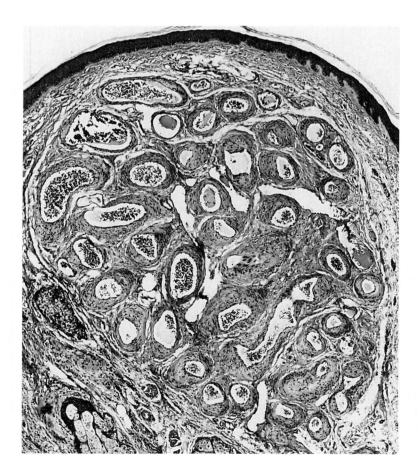

Figure 52–11. Acral arteriovenous hemangioma. The tumor consists of a circumscribed aggregate of blood vessels. Many have thick walls with fibromyxoid ground substance and loosely arranged, circumferentially oriented spindle cells. A scattering of thin-walled vessels is also present. (H&E, ×60).

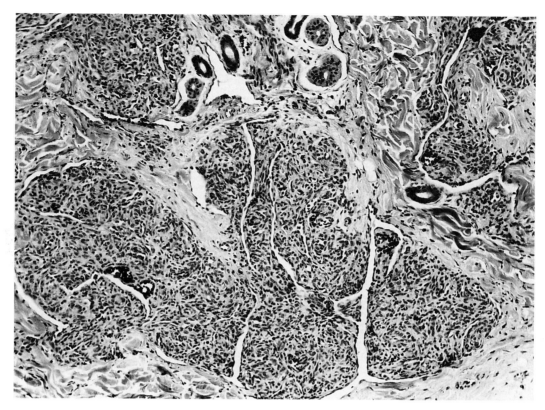

Figure 52–12. Acquired tufted angioma. Lobules of spindle cells contain cleftlike lumens. The lobules appear to protrude into and greatly distort venulelike channels about their peripheries. Compare these images with those of lobular capillary hemangioma (Figs. 52–6 and 52–7) (H&E, ×125).

cumscribed group of capillary lobules and clinically presents as a nodule.

LYMPHANGIOMA

In considering the classification of lymphangiomas, one is faced with a plethora of terms that lack clear definitions or universal usage. This is partly because of the fact that lymphangiomas represent a clinical and pathologic continuum. Individual patients often exhibit findings consistent with two or more of the subtypes to be outlined below.[49–51]

Most lymphangiomas are either apparent at birth or become evident within the first few years of life. They are believed to result from progressive dilation of primitive lymphatic anlage that lacks connections with the rest of the lymphatic system.[50,52] The head and neck are the most common sites, followed by the upper limb girdle, proximal extremities, and trunk. When the tumor presents as a multilocular cyst, typically in the neck or axilla, the term *cystic hygroma* is commonly employed. *Cavernous lymphangiomas* consist of swellings or thickenings of the skin, soft tissues, and mucous membranes (particularly of the mouth) that are either localized, multifocal within an anatomic region, or extensive, with involvement of adjacent anatomic areas or an entire extremity (*lymphangiomatosis*). As noted previously, large lesions can be cavernous in one area and cystic

in another.[50] It has been suggested that the areolar, fibrofatty tissue of the neck and axilla accommodates the enlargement of a lymphangioma to "cystic" proportions, whereas the more compact dermis, subcutis, and submucosa, with its interlacing skeletal muscle, confines the channels to merely "cavernous" size.[50]

The term *lymphangioma circumscriptum* has been applied with some latitude. In one study,[51] superficial lymph-filled vesicles, some of which were blood tinged or accompanied by verrucous changes, constituted an important part of the definition. The underlying lesions, however, ranged from small superficial dermal tumors (called *localized* lymphangioma circumscriptum) to larger contiguous or multifocal tumors with dermal and subcutaneous involvement (designated *classic* lymphangioma circumscriptum). Aside from the superficial vesicles, most of these latter lesions were otherwise identical to cavernous lymphangiomas as defined earlier. Some were also cystic. In another study,[53] lymphangioma circumscriptum was more strictly defined as a lesion confined to the upper part of the dermis. Tumors with deeper involvement were classified as cavernous. *Acquired lymphangiectasias*, closely resembling localized lymphangioma circumscriptum, can occur in sites of chronic lymphedema of either the congenital type or that secondary to surgery and/or radiation.[54,55]

Microscopically, the subepidermal vesicles consist of greatly dilated lymph capillaries (Fig. 52–13). These expand

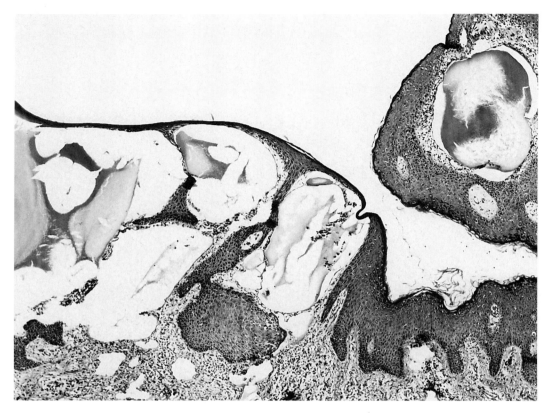

Figure 52–13. Lymphangioma. Greatly dilated lymph capillaries expand dermal papillae and are associated with epidermal hyperplasia and papillomatosis. Similar channels were present throughout the dermis and superficial subcutaneous tissue, and the lesion was classified as a cavernous lymphangioma. Tumors with similar features have also been called classic lymphangioma circumscriptum. Lesions with identical appearances, but limited to the superficial dermis, have been designated localized lymphangioma circumscriptum. (H&E, ×75).

dermal papillae and, depending on the plane of section, can appear to be entirely surrounded by epidermis. There may be associated epidermal hyperplasia and hyperkeratosis. In most lymphangiomas, additional thin-walled channels are numerous within the dermis and often the subcutis. Some of the vessels may have fibrous walls (Fig. 52–14), and in deeper locations, it is not uncommon to observe bundles of smooth muscle within the walls of the greatly ectatic lymphatics. Lumina are either empty or contain light eosinophilic coagulum admixed, in some cases, with lymphocytes, red blood cells, macrophages, and neutrophils. The interstitium of lymphangiomas, particularly the deeper examples, often contains lymphoid cells and exhibits fibroplasia. Some cases also have numerous blood-filled channels, and the designation *hemolymphangioma* seems appropriate.

For diagnostic purposes, the term *lymphangioma* should usually be sufficient. If a pathologist wishes to include additional descriptive terminology, it should be understood that the terms employed lack precision and often add little diagnostic or prognostic information. There is value in commenting on the extent and depth of the lymphangioma within the specimen. If the tumor is confined to the superficial dermis and appears encompassed by the surgical procedure,

the likelihood of recurrence is quite small.[51,52] For larger lymphangiomas, the prospect of obtaining a cure with just a single operation depends on the anatomic location, extent and depth of the tumor, and the skill of the surgeon.

ACQUIRED PROGRESSIVE LYMPHANGIOMA

Only a few cases of acquired progressive lymphangioma have been reported.[45,56–58a] Clinically, there is a slowly enlarging, red-brown or dusky macule or plaque, usually on an extremity, that ranges in size from 1 to several centimeters. Affected patients have ranged in age from 5 to 57 years. Microscopically, there is an anastomosing network of generally bloodless vascular spaces throughout the dermis, at times accompanied by patchy lymphoid infiltrates (Fig. 52–15). Most of the endothelial cells are flattened, but a minority may be enlarged and hyperchromatic. Clinical findings and absence of proliferative foci, prominent atypia, and mitotic activity should allow distinction from angiosarcoma. The pattern of vascular structures closely resembles that seen in patch stage Kaposi's sarcoma, and clinical findings may be necessary for an accurate diagnosis.

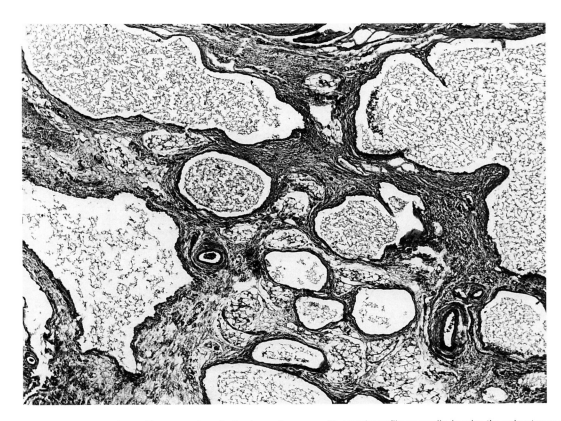

Figure 52–14. Lymphangioma. Cavernous lymphatic channels, some with prominent fibrous walls, involve the subcutaneous tissue. This lesion also had superficial changes identical to those observed in Fig. 52–13 and, in addition, a prominent "cystic" component (H&E, ×65).

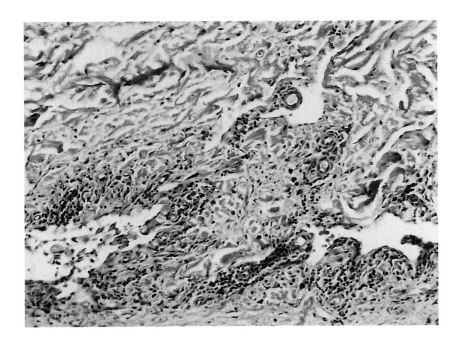

Figure 52–15. Acquired progressive lymphangioma. An anastomosing network of generally bloodless vascular spaces dissects through the dermis. A few of the endothelial cells are enlarged and have hyperchromatic nuclei (H&E, ×150).

ANGIOMATOSIS

The term *angiomatosis* has been applied to unusually extensive tumors composed of benign appearing, generally thin-walled blood vessels or lymphatics that affect large segments of skin and contiguous soft tissue.[59] The process is often accompanied by bony and visceral involvement. The distinction between angiomatosis and extensive, but otherwise ordinary, hemangiomas or lymphangiomas can be arbitrary. At times, one encounters a *localized* cutaneous vascular proliferation with either an infiltrative or multicentric pattern of growth within the dermis. Lobular capillary hemangioma with satellites, tufted angioma, acquired progressive lymphangioma, and acral angiomatosis (see below) are specific examples. When a vascular proliferation with the characteristics just mentioned defies specific classification, it can be designated as a *localized angiomatosis*. Such lesions have not been described in detail. They are capable of local recurrence but lack metastatic potential.

ACRAL CAPILLARY ANGIOMATOSIS (PSEUDO-KAPOSI'S SARCOMA, ACROANGIODERMATITIS)

Acral capillary angiomatosis is often associated with an arteriovenous malformation of the leg or foot.[60–62] Patients are typically in their early 20s at the time of diagnosis, but the first clinical abnormalities can appear during childhood. Lesions consist of unilateral red or purple nodules and plaques on the toes or foot. Patients may suffer persistent pain and troublesome ulceration. Additional findings include stasis dermatitis, varicosities, bruits, and bounding pulses. The affected extremity may be enlarged and exhibit increased temperature, hyperhidrosis, and hypertrichosis. Similar cutaneous lesions can develop adjacent to surgically constructed arteriovenous shunts[63] or in individuals with venous insufficiency unassociated with a vascular malformation.[64]

The microscopic picture is generally similar to that of marked stasis dermatitis.[64] A proliferation of well-formed, thin- to thick-walled capillaries often forms discrete groups or larger nodules (Fig. 52–16). Changes are most marked in the superficial dermis, but the deep dermis and subcutis may be involved. There is associated fibroplasia, accompanied by red blood cell extravasations, hemosiderin deposits, and sparse lymphoid infiltrate. An erroneous diagnosis of Kaposi's sarcoma was initially rendered in many of the reported cases,[60–62] but the microscopic features of that entity are lacking in acral angiomatosis.

TELANGIECTASIAS

Nevus Flammeus

Nevus flammeus is present at birth as a pink macule on the face or neck and occasionally at other sites.[65] Most small lesions (*salmon patch*) disappear during infancy or childhood, but large facial nevi (*port-wine stain*) persist. During adult-

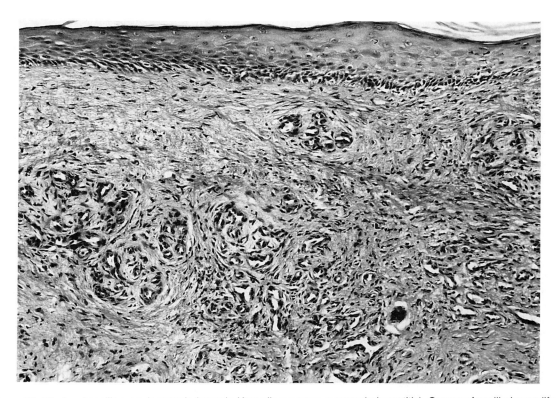

Figure 52–16. Acral capillary angiomatosis (pseudo-Kaposi's sarcoma, acroangiodermatitis). Groups of capillaries proliferate in the superficial dermis and are accompanied by interstitial fibroplasia, hemosiderin deposits, and a sparse lymphoid infiltrate (H&E, ×160).

hood, port-wine stains often thicken, become purple, and may develop nodular, warty, or cobblestone-like elevations. The *Sturge-Weber syndrome* consists of a large nevus flammeus in the distribution of the ophthalmic branch of the trigeminal nerve, accompanied by ipsilateral meningeal angiomatosis, "tram line" meningeal calcifications, mental retardation, seizures, ipsilateral glaucoma, and contralateral hemiparesis. The *Klippel-Trenaunay syndrome* consists of a nevus flammeus of one or more extremities, accompanied by soft tissue and bony hypertrophy and venous varicosities.[66] The presence, in addition, of an underlying arteriovenous malformation (*racemose, circoid aneurysm*) defines the *Parkes Weber syndrome*.[66]

The primary abnormality in nevus flammeus is an increased number of ectatic, thin-walled dermal blood vessels. Vascular profiles are most numerous just beneath the epidermis (Fig. 52–17), and their number rapidly decreases at deeper levels.[65] The number of abnormal vessels remains little changed over time, but their caliber progressively increases (Fig. 52–18), resulting in an increase in total vascular cross-sectional area. This latter parameter correlates with thickening and darkening of the lesion.[65] The superficial nodules seen in some cases are due to the presence of foci variously designated as cavernous hemangiomas, arteriovenous hemangiomas, and localized exaggerations of the ectatic process.[67] Lobular capillary hemangiomas (pyogenic granulomas) also rarely develop within port-wine stains.[26,27]

Hereditary Hemorrhagic Telangiectasia (Osler's Disease)

Hereditary hemorrhagic telangiectasia is an autosomal dominant condition that presents with nosebleeds in childhood. Lesions appear during the second or third decade as punctiform or linear telangiectatic mats involving the mucous membranes of the upper aerodigestive tract and the skin of the face, ears, nail beds, palms, and less commonly the extremities and trunk. Similar lesions are found in viscera, and arteriovenous malformations of the brain and lungs, major arterial aneurysms, and hepatic fibrosis may also be present.

The mucocutaneous lesions consist of aggregates of greatly dilated, thin-walled vessels, some of which are closely apposed to overlying epidermis or mucous membrane.[68] Ultrastructurally, the vessels resemble post capillary venules.[68] Gaps between endothelial cells result from loss of normal connections between their cell processes. Fibrin-platelet thrombi fill these gaps and rest directly against the basal lamina. Perivascular connective tissue may also be defective, as it consists primarily of amorphous and finely filamentous material.[68] Although isolated observations suggest defects in the clotting system, perhaps the anatomic abnormalities result in fragile, ectatic venules that are liable to rupture, either spontaneously or as a result of trauma or inflammation.

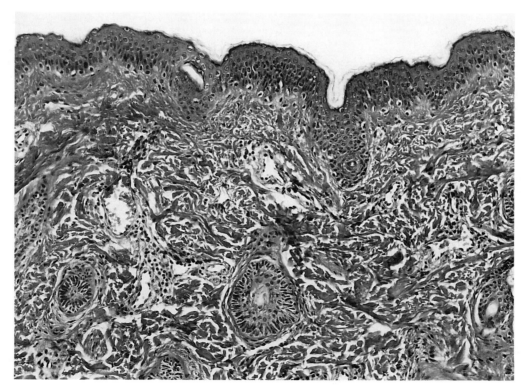

Figure 52–17. Nevus flammeus from a 2-year-old child. Dilated vessels in the superficial dermis are relatively inconspicuous (H&E, ×160).

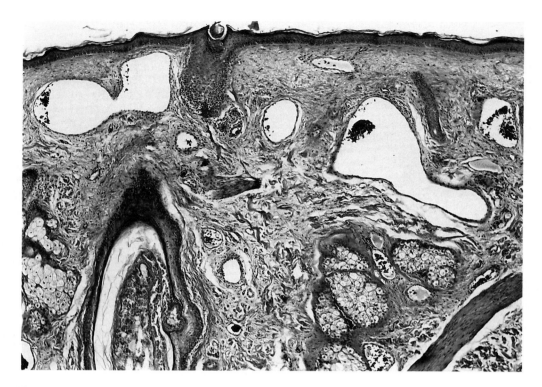

Figure 52–18. Nevus flammeus from a 61-year-old man. The number of abnormal vessels remains little changed over time, but their caliber progressively increases (H&E, ×65).

Unilateral Nevoid Telangiectasia and Generalized Essential Telangiectasia

Most patients with unilateral nevoid telangiectasia are females whose lesions appear at puberty or during pregnancy.[69] A minority of cases are congenital or associated with alcoholic cirrhosis. The lesions often have a predilection for the C3, C4, and trigeminal dermatomes.[69] Generalized essential telangiectasia is seen primarily in middle-aged women.[70] The lesions vary considerably in extent, distribution, and configuration. In both syndromes, ectatic, thin-walled blood vessels are seen microscopically, most notably in the superficial dermis. It is uncertain whether these telangiectasias are based on increased end-organ progesterone or estrogen receptors.[71]

Angioma Serpiginosum

Angioma serpiginosum usually affects females and typically becomes apparent within the first two decades of life.[72–74] The extremities are the most common site. Lesions consist of red or purple puncta, usually no larger than a pinhead, that bleed when traumatized. New puncta continue to develop, and the process thus expands slowly but progressively. Ultimately, the lesions are arranged in various patterns and groupings that may include serpiginous, gyrate, and linear arrays.

Microscopically, dilated capillary-type blood vessels, some with thickened walls, are seen individually or in clusters in dermal papillae and the subpapillary dermis. Lymphocytic infiltrates are slight or nonexistent. Purpura and hemosiderin deposits are absent. Ultrastructurally, more than one capillary may be invested by a single connective tissue sheath, suggesting either marked tortuosity or a microangiomatous alteration at the capillary level.[74] Thickening of the walls is due either to a nonspecific increase in basement membrane that contains embedded collagenous fibers[74] or to the presence of numerous concentrically arranged pericytes.[75]

Angiokeratoma

Angiokeratomas represent acquired telangiectasias, perhaps due to trauma or chronic irritation.[76] Epidermal hyperplasia is secondary. Clinical lesions consist of verrucoid red or purple papules several millimeters in size. In the *Mibelli* type, multiple lesions are present on the dorsa and sides of the fingers and toes, most commonly in adolescent girls with a history of cold intolerance. In the *Fordyce* variant, solitary or more commonly multiple lesions affect the scrotal skin, with onset usually in the third decade or later.[77] When multiple, the process can spread onto contiguous nonscrotal skin, and there may be evidence of increased venous pressure such as varicocele.[77] Analogous lesions occur on the vulva.[78] Isolated or multiple angiokeratomas can occur at

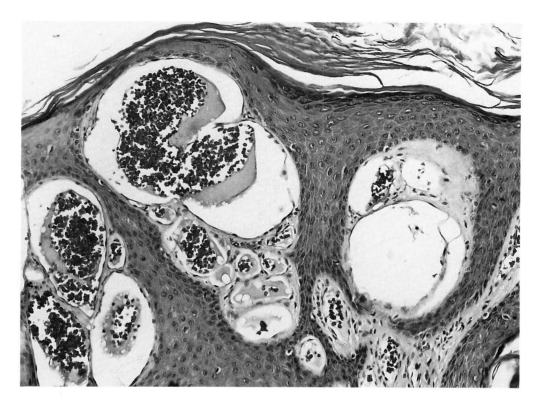

Figure 52–19. Angiokeratoma. Dermal papillae are expanded by greatly dilated capillaries. Hyperplastic rete ridges extend between groups of capillaries, appearing to partially or completely surround them. The vascular channels are lined by flat endothelium, and a thin layer of connective tissue separates them from the epidermis (H&E, ×165).

essentially any other anatomic site, but in particular the lower extremity.[76] Such cases are designated as *solitary, multiple,* or *papular* angiokeratoma. Angiokeratoma-like changes occasionally develop over conventional capillary or cavernous hemangiomas, in association with a nevus flammeus, in the *hemangiectatic hypertrophy (Klippel-Trenaunay) syndrome,* and in *Cobb's syndrome* (cutaneous hemangioma with a dermatomal distribution closely related to an associated angioma of the spinal cord).[79] *Angiokeratoma circumscriptum* is improperly classified with the angiokeratomas, as defined previously, and is discussed with *verrucous hemangioma.*

Histologic Features

The microscopic appearance of the various clinical forms of angiokeratoma is similar. A group of dermal papillae is expanded and distorted by enormously dilated capillaries (Fig. 52–19). The lumina are either empty or contain proteinaceous material mixed with blood. Thrombosis may be present. Hyperkeratosis and acanthosis are more prominent in older lesions and at acral sites.[76] Rete ridges extend between the dilated capillaries, partially or completely encompassing them. The plane of section may create the impression of intraepidermal blood cysts, but it is usually possible to appreciate that such structures are lined by a layer of flattened endothelium and separated from closely applied epidermis by a thin layer of eosinophilic connective tissue. A small number of additional ectatic vessels may be present in the superficial or mid-dermis, beneath the lesion, and

dilated veins are often prominent in the deep dermis in angiokeratomas of the scrotum and vulva.[77,78]

Venous Lake, Capillary Aneurysm, Thrombosed Vessel

Venous lakes are static or slowly enlarging, slightly loculated papules, one to several millimeters in size, usually observed in elderly men with long-term actinic exposure.[80] Often multiple, the lesions occur on the ears, face, lips, neck, and occasionally at other sites. Venous lakes are usually compressible and not likely to be confused with malignant melanoma. In comparison with venous lakes, capillary aneurysms are usually solitary.[81,82] The age range of patients is broader, the anatomic distribution is more diverse, and the sexes are affected equally. Capillary aneurysms often evolve rapidly and consist of firm black papules, easily mistaken for malignant melanoma. Similar lesions occur in the oral mucous membranes.[83]

Histologic Features

Microscopically, venous lakes consist of one or multiple interconnecting, greatly dilated, blood-filled vascular channels situated in actinically damaged dermis. The walls of the vessels consist of fibrous membranes that rarely contain a few smooth muscle cells.[80] There may be connections with small veins in the mid-dermis. Capillary aneurysms are quite similar to venous lakes. Typically, just a single greatly dilated vessel (Fig. 52–20) is observed beneath the

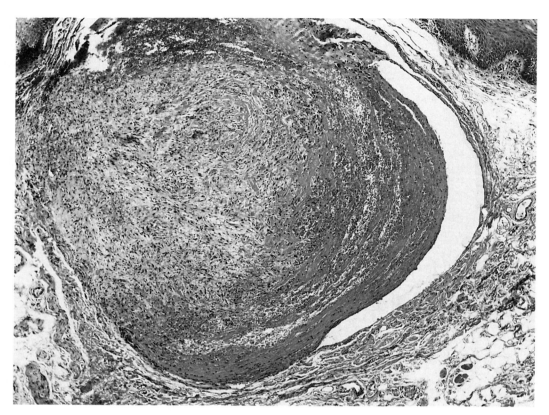

Figure 52–20. Thrombosed capillary aneurysm. An enormously dilated vessel consistent with a capillary contains partially organized, laminated thrombus (H&E, ×65).

epidermis.[81] It either lacks a discernible wall or is surrounded by a delicate fibrous layer. Thrombus, with or without organization, is present in some but not all lesions (Fig. 52–20). In the oral cavity, the dilated vessel has a more prominent wall consistent with a small vein.[83]

Distinction between the foregoing lesions is not always clear cut. The venous lake appears to be a specific clinical entity and most likely represents a superficial venous varicosity.[80] It is uncertain whether aneurysmal dilation of a capillary precedes or is caused by thrombosis, but the lesion typically occurs in previously normal-appearing skin. Failure to find thrombus in lesions with histories consistent with thrombosed capillary aneurysm can be explained by lysis of the thrombus before excision. Thrombosis can also occur in venous lakes, in which case the distinction from thrombosed capillary aneurysm may be impossible. Venous lakes and capillary aneurysms may be the sites of papillary endothelial hyperplasia.

INTRAVASCULAR PAPILLARY ENDOTHELIAL HYPERPLASIA

Clinical Features
Intravascular papillary endothelial hyperplasia is a benign lesion, usually situated within the lumen of a dermal or subcutaneous vein or within one or more lumina of a hemangioma or vascular malformation.[35,84–86] The process can also occur in venous lakes,[87] multiple superficial phlebectasias,[88] capillary aneurysms,[89] and lymphangiomas.[85,90]

When located in a vein, papillary endothelial hyperplasia produces a flesh-colored, red, or blue nodule that ranges in size from a few millimeters to 2 or 3 cm. Most are located on the extremities, with a predilection for the fingers, or on the head, where, in addition to the face and scalp, the oral mucous membranes can be involved.[91,92] When the lesion occurs in a preexisting vascular tumor, the findings are usually those of the latter.

Histologic Features
Microscopically, proliferation of endothelial cells is confined to one or more vascular lumina (Figs. 52–21 and 52–22). In the fully developed form, numerous delicate or more bulbous papillae extend from the wall of the affected structure. They may appear to float freely within its lumen or to form a spongelike meshwork, partially or completely filling the lumen. The papillae are lined by endothelial cells and have cores that consist either of fibrin and trapped red blood cells or of hyalinized connective tissue, which, itself, may contain capillaries (Fig. 52–23). The endothelial cells have mildly enlarged, oval, hyperchromatic nuclei with small distinct nucleoli. They occasionally form several layers, tufts, or strands that lack stromal support. Mitotic figures are either rare or absent, and necrosis is not found. In most cases, the affected lumen also contains laminated or fragmented thrombus in varying stages of organization (see Figs. 52–21 and 52–22), and a continuum from unorganized thrombus to well-developed papillary structures may be noted. Hemosiderin deposits are not unusual.

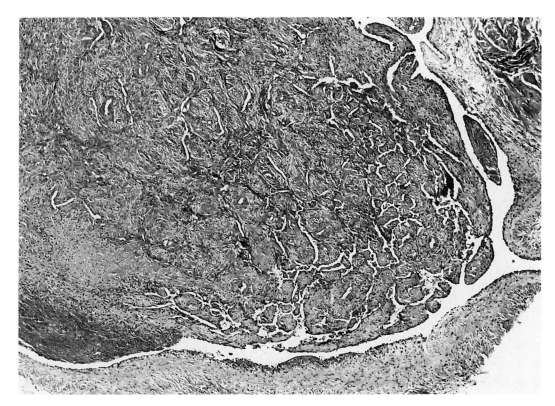

Figure 52–21. Intravascular papillary endothelial hyperplasia. The lesion is situated within the lumen of a superficial digital vein and consists of generally coarse papillae that are lined by endothelial cells and have cores consisting of fibrous tissue. Portions of the vein wall can be seen surrounding the lesion, and partially organized thrombus is present (lower left) (H&E, ×65).

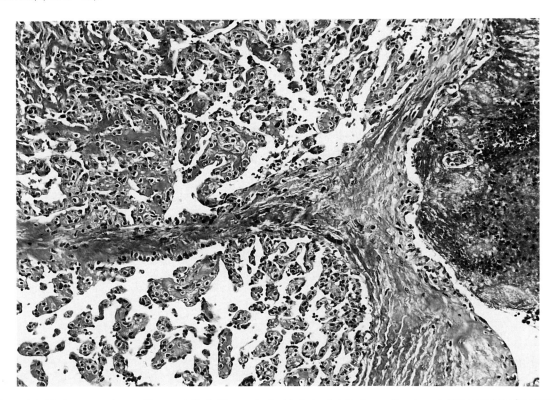

Figure 52–22. Intravascular papillary endothelial hyperplasia. Myriads of delicate papillae occupy three lumina of a cavernous hemangioma. The papillae are lined by endothelial cells and have cores that consist either of fibrin and red blood cells or of hyalinized connective tissue. One of the lumina (right) contains thrombus. The entire cavernous hemangioma showed similar changes (H&E, ×160).

821

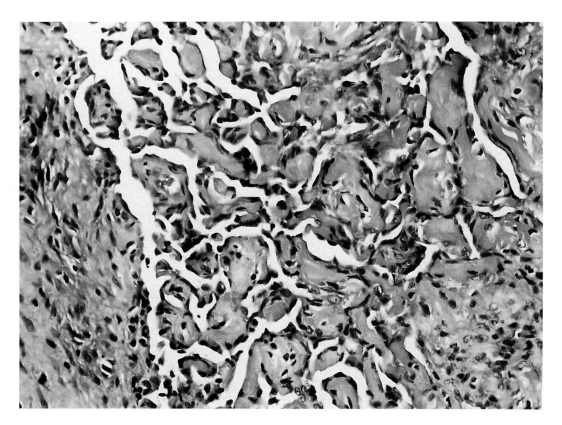

Figure 52–23. Intravascular papillary endothelial hyperplasia. High-power view of papillae reveals cores of hyalinized connective tissue. The papillae are lined by endothelial cells with mildly enlarged, hyperchromatic nuclei. Pleomorphism and mitotic figures are absent (H&E, ×300).

When intravascular papillary endothelial hyperplasia is superimposed on a preexisting vascular tumor, involvement is only partial and recognition of the underlying lesion is straightforward (see Fig. 52–22). When the process distends just a single vein (see Fig. 52–21), its intravascular location can be more difficult to appreciate, as hyalinization of the vein wall may partially or completely obliterate recognizable smooth muscle cells and elastic fibers.[35,84] Small segments of vein can often be identified, however, either surrounding the lesion or in adjacent tissue. There can also be discontinuities of the vein wall and focal extension of the papillary proliferation into perivascular connective tissue.[84]

Papillary endothelial hyperplasia has been viewed by most observers as an unusual pattern of organization of a thrombus. Indeed, the process has been well documented in organizing arterial thromboemboli and venous thrombi.[93] The possibility, however, that endothelial proliferation is the primary event in some cases is not completely excluded. Ultrastructurally, the lesion resembles granulation tissue.[94]

Differential Diagnosis

High-power fields of papillary endothelial hyperplasia can be indistinguishable from well-differentiated angiosarcoma, but the intravascular location, lack of mitotic activity and pleomorphism, and absence of an infiltrative, dissecting pattern of vascular spaces within adjacent tissue exclude a malignant diagnosis. The microscopic appearance differs markedly from that of lobular capillary hemangioma (pyo-

genic granuloma) or angiolymphoid hyperplasia with eosinophilia, both of which can be intravascular.

ANGIOLYMPHOID HYPERPLASIA WITH EOSINOPHILIA

A number of terms have been applied to this relatively common entity including *atypical* or *pseudopyogenic granuloma*,[95,96] *inflammatory angiomatous nodule*,[96] *angiolymphoid hyperplasia with eosinophilia*,[97–101] *papular angioplasia*,[102] *inflammatory arteriovenous hemangioma*,[42] *intravenous atypical vascular proliferation*,[103] and *epithelioid hemangioma*.[59] Tumors with similar, but not necessarily identical, microscopic findings also occur in deeper soft tissues, viscera, and bones. The term *histiocytoid hemangioma*[104,105] has been suggested to encompass this entire clinicopathologic spectrum, although some authors designate the more cellular, potentially malignant, deep-seated examples as *epithelioid hemangioendotheliomas*.[106–108] The discussion to follow will confine itself primarily to the benign dermal and subcutaneous tumors most likely to be encountered by dermatopathologists. *Kimura's disease* (*eosinophilic hyperplastic lymphogranuloma, eosinophilic lymphofolliculosis*) probably represents a separate entity[109,109A] and will be commented on at the close of this section.

Clinical Features

The usual clinical presentation is of one or multiple pink,

dull red, or red-brown cutaneous papules and small nodules that have been present for either several months or more than a year.[96,98,101] When multiple, the lesions tend to be grouped or confluent. Some patients have larger dermal or subcutaneous masses.[97,98,101] Sites of predilection include the skin in and about the ears, the forehead, the scalp, other facial sites, and the neck. Lesions can also develop on the trunk or extremities[98,99,101] and, rarely, in the mouth.[110] Most patients with angiolymphoid hyperplasia are betwen the ages of 20 and 50 years, and approximately two thirds are female. Only a few have peripheral eosinophilia.

Histologic Features

Microscopically, angiolymphoid hyperplasia consists of one or several nodules within the dermis, subcutis, or both; they are either well circumscribed or blend with adjacent tissue. Inflammatory infiltrate and abnormal vessels lined by unusual endothelial cells are usually apparent at low power (see Fig. 52–24). The characteristic endothelial cells, required for the diagnosis, are grossly enlarged and assume fusiform, polygonal, ovoid, cuboid, and hobnail shapes (Figs. 52–25 and 52–26). Their enlargement is due to an increase in both cytoplasmic and nuclear volume. The cytoplasm is dense, faintly granular, and either eosinophilic or amphophilic. Cytoplasmic vacuoles may be observed and can be large enough to distend the cell and distort the nucleus. The vesicular nuclei are oval or irregularly indented or grooved and often contain a prominent eosinophilic nucleolus. Mitotic figures are usually rare or absent, but in occasional cases they are more plentiful.

The diagnostic endothelial cells line well-formed vascular spaces in most lesions, at least focally. The abnormal vessels may be outlined by a cuff of loosely arranged spindle cells embedded in myxoid ground substance (see Fig. 52–26). The angiomatous nature of the lesion may be less apparent when the endothelial cells are disposed in sheets or nodules (Fig. 52–27). A pattern of nests and cords can usually be discerned in such cases, however, and this arrangement is highlighted with a reticulin stain. Moreover, careful inspection indicates that small lumina are indeed present within the nests and cords and that they seem to form by fusion of cytoplasmic vacuoles of adjacent cells (Fig. 52–28). Red blood cells may be present within such incipient lumina.

The stroma consists of fibrovascular tissue that invariably contains lymphocytes and eosinophils. Mast cells are common, and macrophages, at times containing hemosiderin, and plasma cells are not unusual. In a minority of cases, most notably subcutaneous tumors, lymphoid follicles with germinal centers are also present, particularly around the periphery of the lesion. Thrombosis and hemorrhage are not rare and may be associated with foci of papillary endothelial hyperplasia in which the endothelial cells retain their epithelioid appearance.

Angiolymphoid hyperplasia can involve medium-sized

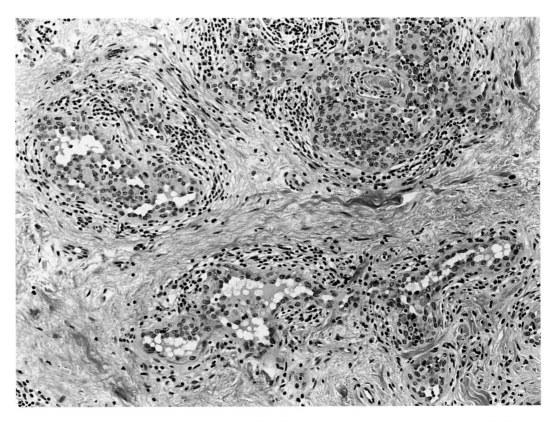

Figure 52–24. Angiolymphoid hyperplasia with eosinophilia. Characteristic abnormal vessels are situated in fibrous stroma that contains lymphocytes and eosinophils. The endothelial cells are epithelioid and exhibit a spectrum of arrangements from nearly solid cords to well canalized vascular structures (H&E, ×160).

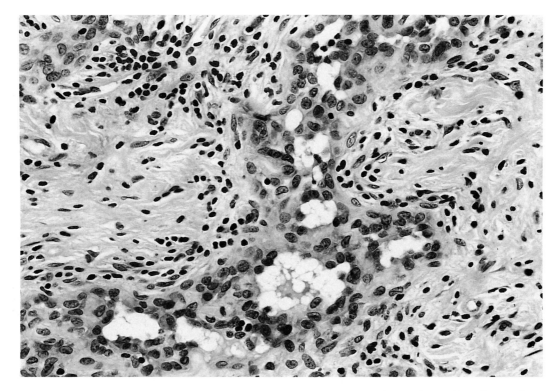

Figure 52–25. Angiolymphoid hyperplasia with eosinophilia. High-power view of an abnormal vessel from the case illustrated in Figure 52–24. The channel is lined by enlarged epithelioid endothelial cells. Lumina seem to form by aggregation of cytoplasmic vacuoles and lysis of membranes between them (H&E, ×300).

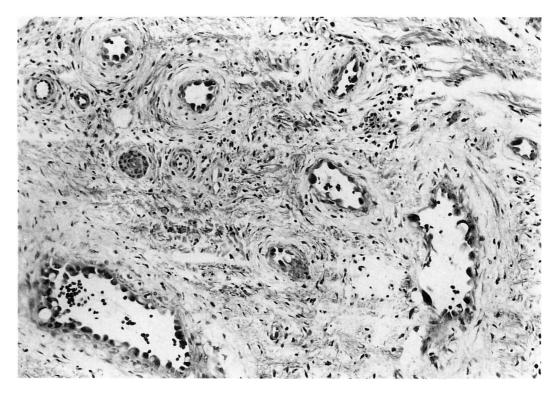

Figure 52–26. Angiolymphoid hyperplasia with eosinophilia. Several diagnostically important abnormal blood vessels are present in this field. They are lined by enormously enlarged endothelial cells that protrude into the lumina. Cytoplasmic vacuoles distend the cells and distort the nuclei. Several of the vessels are cuffed by a layer of loosely arranged spindle cells (H&E, ×160).

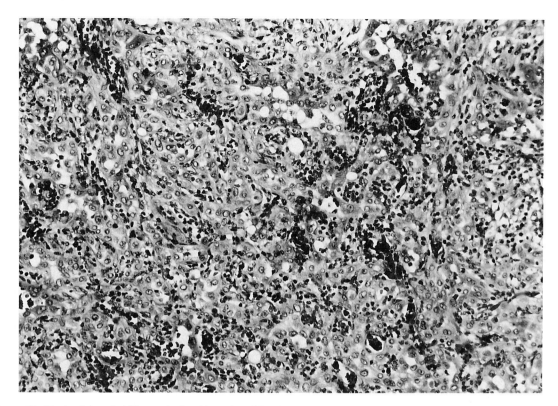

Figure 52–27. Angiolymphoid hyperplasia with eosinophilia. The vascular nature of the lesion is not immediately obvious. The cells are arranged in cords and nests separated by sparse stroma that contains lymphocytes and eosinophils. Many of the endothelial cells are vacuolated, and careful inspection indicates that the vacuoles coalesce to form lumina (H&E, ×175).

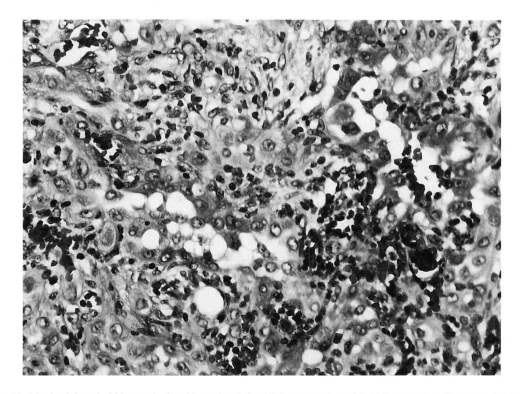

Figure 52–28. Angiolymphoid hyperplasia with eosinophilia. High-power view of field illustrated in Figure 52–27. Lumina appear to form by aggregation of cytoplasmic vacuoles and lysis of membranes between them. Sparse red blood cells can be identified within the lumina (H&E, ×300).

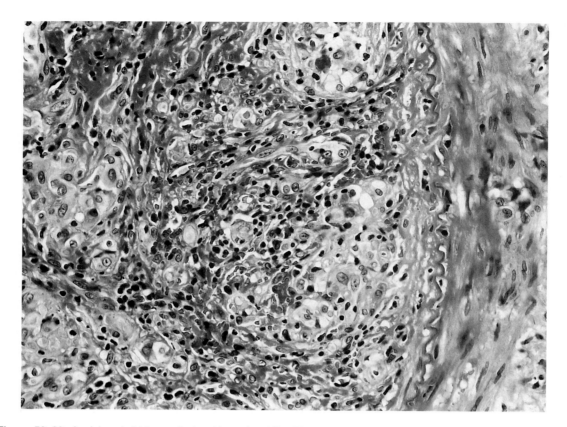

Figure 52–29. Angiolymphoid hyperplasia with eosinophilia. The lesion fills the lumen of a temporal artery. Nests of epithelioid endothelial cells are associated with sparse fibrous stroma that contains lymphocytes and eosinophils. Cytoplasmic vacuoles aggregate to form incipient lumina. The internal elastic membrane of the affected artery and a portion of its media can be recognized (right) (H&E, ×300).

arteries and veins,[59,99,101,103,111,112] particularly when the lesion is subcutaneous. The presence of such large vessels is sometimes obvious microscopically (Fig. 52–29), but in most instances, only short segments of artery or vein wall can be identified in and around the lesion. The remainder of the involved vessels and their lumina are partially or completely replaced by the tumor. Stains for elastic fibers are helpful in such cases.

Electron Microscopy

Ultrastructurally,[100,110,112–117] the characteristic endothelial cells have straight or folded cell membranes connected by specialized attachments. The cytoplasm contains diverse, nonspecific organelles and, in addition, Weibel-Palade bodies, pinocytotic vesicles, and intermediate filaments indicative of endothelial differentiation. Thin filaments, with focal condensations (dense bodies), lipid droplets, and lysosomes may also be observed. Large membrane-bound cytoplasmic vacuoles correlate with vacuoles observed light microscopically. The altered endothelial cells either abut the stroma directly or are surrounded by one or several layers of smooth muscle cells and pericytes. Some of the abnormal vessels thus resemble venules.[114] A basal lamina may be situated between the endothelial and perithelial cells but is often discontinuous or fragmented. Extracellular material consistent with elastin is occasionally seen in the vessel walls, but well-formed membranes are lacking. The enlarged endothelial cells exhibit strong activity for both respiratory and hydrolytic enzymes and a weak or absent reaction for alkaline phosphatase.[100,114] Factor VIII-related antigen is consistently present,[101,110,112,115–117] but the number of positive cells varies. The endothelial cells also bind *U. europaeus* lectin.[112,117] Both vimentin and actin have been documented within the endothelial cells.[112] Lysozyme and α_1-antitrypsin are absent[112,115,116] as are cytokeratin and epithelial membrane antigen.[112] The lymphoid infiltrate consists primarily of polytypic B cells.[115]

Differential Diagnosis

The question of whether angiolymphoid hyperplasia is related to *Kimura's disease* is still debated, but for the present it seems wise to draw a distinction between the two. Patients with the latter condition are usually male, manifest large subcutaneous nodules and plaques, and regularly exhibit peripheral eosinophilia. In addition to the cervicofacial area, many other body sites can be involved in Kimura's disease, and there is a predilection for subcutaneous tissue overlying lymph node-bearing areas. Microscopically, Kimura's disease seems best classified as a form of lymphoid hyperplasia.[109,109a] Germinal centers are numerous. Tissue eosinophilia is typically extensive, with the formation of microabscesses and diffuse sheets. Vascular changes are just a minor finding, consisting of that degree of increased vascularity and endothelial swelling to be expected in a chronic reactive process. The grossly enlarged endothelial cells characteristic of angiolymphoid hyperplasia are lacking.

The distinction between angiolymphoid hyperplasia and *epithelioid hemangioendothelioma* needs further study, particularly because both can affect large blood vessels and the latter occasionally metastasizes.[106] Initial observations suggest that the absence of well-formed vessels and inflammatory infiltrate and the presence of distinctive mucoid-hyaline stroma support the diagnosis of epithelioid hemangioendothelioma.[106] The relation between the recently described *epithelioid angiomatosis*[117a] observed in patients with acquired immunodeficiency syndrome (AIDS) and typical cases of angiolymphoid hyperplasia is also uncertain. According to available information, the former exhibits a range of appearances from pyogenic granuloma-like lesions to tumors resembling angiosarcoma. Neutrophilic microabscesses are also present, and clusters of organisms, possibly representing the cat-scratch disease bacillus, have been identified in lesional tissue.

SPINDLE CELL HEMANGIOENDOTHELIOMA

Spindle cell hemangioendothelioma is a recently described clinicopathologic entity[117b,117c] that is characterized by the gradual development of one or multiple dermal-subcutaneous nodules with a predilection for the extremities, particularly the hands and feet. In some patients, several separate sites are involved. Microscopically, a characteristic combination of cytologically uniform spindle cells is seen, with variable numbers of intervening cavernous vascular spaces. Clusters and cords of vacuolated, epithelioid endothelial cells are also present. Mitotic figures are rare or absent. Local recurrences are common.

GLOMUS TUMOR

Glomus tumors were first described in 1924,[118] and detailed discussions were published by 1935.[119,120] *Solitary* lesions have a marked predilection for the extremities, particularly the upper extremity, where most are located subungually.[59,120–122] They also occur on the trunk, head and neck, and genitalia. When *multiple,* the number of lesions ranges from a few to several hundred.[18,123–130] They often appear in early childhood or even at birth[126] and are either confined to a localized area or scattered randomly about the body. Subungual tumors are rare. Families affected by multiple glomus tumors have been reported.[18,129]

Clinical Features

Clinically, most glomus tumors are small, firm, deep red or blue papules or nodules, a few millimeters or a centimeter in size. Larger tumors, at times exceeding 3 cm, tend to occur at sites other than the hands and feet, are generally softer and somewhat compressible, and exhibit either lighter shades of red or blue or no distinctive color. Glomus tumors are usually painful and tender. The classic symptoms, characteristic of the smaller, acral lesions, consist of paroxysms of excruciating, radiating pain, often elicited by minor pressure or exposure to cold. Glomus tumors rarely recur after excision.[121,122] Subungual lesions can erode the distal phalanx.[120,121]

Histologic Features

Microscopically, the typical case appears as one or several circumscribed nodules in the dermis or subcutis. Each nodule consists of a tangle of convoluted vascular channels, the walls of which contain glomus cells (Fig. 52–30). In many cases, the channels have obvious lumina lined by flattened endothelial cells, but in some instances the lumina are greatly compressed and easily overlooked (Fig. 52–31). The glomus cells are disposed in multiple layers, patches, or nests, situated either immediately adjacent to the endothelium or separated from it by a layer of connective tissue that may be hyalinized. Glomus cells are cytologically monotonous, although there is some variation from tumor to tumor. In most instances, they are of medium size and possess modest amounts of lightly or densely eosinophilic cytoplasm. Partial cytoplasmic clearing, when present, reveals delicate, eosinophilic cell borders and rounded or polygonal cell shapes. The nuclei of glomus cells are ovoid or round and centrally placed. Chromatin is either finely stippled or vesicular. There may be small nucleoli. Mitotic figures are exceptional or completely lacking. In some cases, the glomus cells merge with spindle cells that resemble or are indistinguishable from smooth muscle (see Fig. 52–30).

Most glomus tumors are surrounded by a capsulelike rim of compressed fibrous tissue. Small pseudopods of tumor can extend through defects in the fibrous rim, and vessels in the immediate vicinity of the tumor may also be cuffed by several layers of glomus cells. It is usually possible to identify small nerves around the tumor, and they can occasionally be traced into the substance of the lesion. Except for the presence of mast cells, the stroma is characteristically devoid of inflammatory infiltrate and is either collagenous, hyalinized, or myxoid (see Fig. 52–30). The stroma also contains normal-appearing arterioles and venules, and connections may be seen between these and vessels cuffed by glomus cells.

Some glomus tumors are partially or completely dominated by cavernous spaces lined by just one or a few layers of glomus cells (Fig. 52–32). Such tumors are less well-circumscribed and may be multifocal within the dermis or subcutis. This variant, called *glomangioma,* has been emphasized as the type observed in patients with multiple glomus tumors.[18] The separation of glomangioma, however, from ordinary glomus tumors seems artificial. Indeed, the microscopic distinction is arbitrary when the tumor contains both cavernous and cellular foci. Moreover, solitary lesions, when located elsewhere than the digits, are more likely to have the cavernous appearance of glomangioma.[120,122] The fact that this pattern is often observed in patients with multiple tumors may be explained by the anatomic distribution of their lesions rather than any intrinsic difference between solitary and multiple glomus tumors. The term *glomangiomyoma* has been used to identify glomus tumors with a prominent component of smooth muscle.[59] Such lesions can be viewed as minor variants. It has also been suggested that the *vascular leiomyoma (angiomyoma)* is a form of glomus tumor,[131] but these lesions are perhaps better classified with the cutaneous leiomyomas.

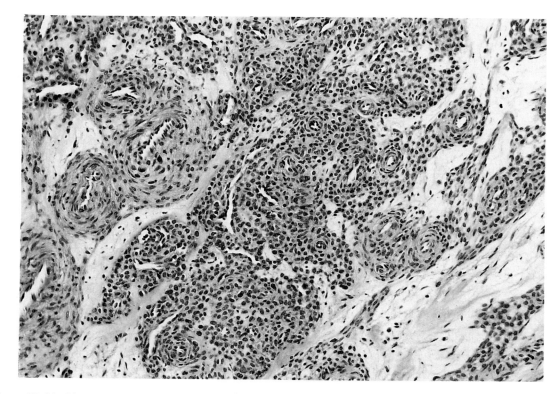

Figure 52–30. Glomus tumor. The lesion consists of a tangle of convoluted vascular structures. Each is lined by a layer of flattened endothelial cells and cuffed by layers or nests of rounded or polygonal glomus tumor cells. Note that some vessels are surrounded by layers of fusiform cells exhibiting transitional features between those of glomus tumor cells and smooth muscle. The stroma is both hyalinized and myxoid (H&E, ×160).

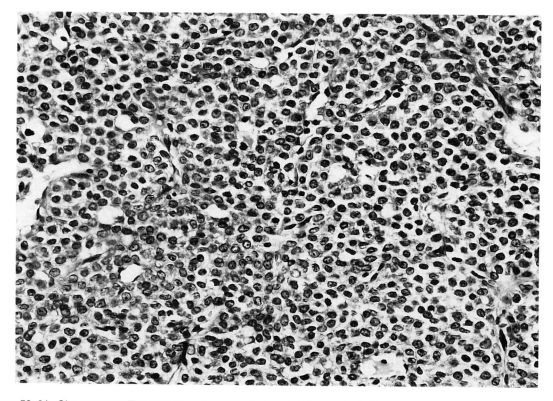

Figure 52–31. Glomus tumor. The vascular nature of the lesion might be overlooked in this cellular field. Nestlike aggregates of rounded or polygonal glomus tumor cells compress slitlike vessels. The vessels are lined by flattened endothelial cells. The glomus tumor cells contain sparse to modest amounts of eosinophilic or partially cleared cytoplasm and uniform rounded or ovoid nuclei with vesicular or stippled chromatin. Small nucleoli can be appreciated (H&E, ×300).

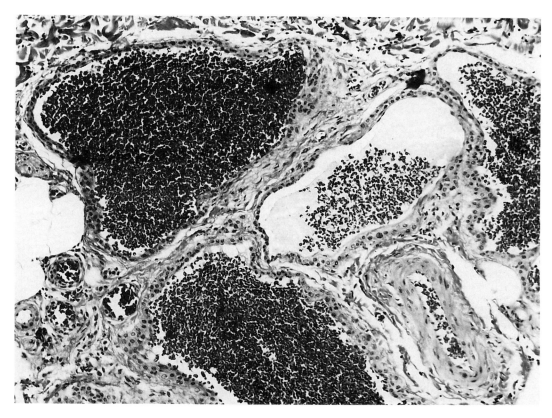

Figure 52–32. Glomangioma. The lesion closely resembles a cavernous hemangioma, but one or two layers of cuboidal glomus tumor cells are present within the walls of the greatly ectatic vessels (H&E, ×160).

The glomus tumor mimics the normal glomus microscopically. Normal glomera, most prevalent on the tips of the digits and in the nail beds, are microscopically distinctive, dermally situated arteriovenous anastomoses with thermoregulatory function.[59,118–120] The preglomic arteriole gives rise to several branches, some of which transform into convoluted vascular structures known as Sucquet-Hoyer canals. These are lined by flattened endothelium and surrounded by several layers of glomus cells. They lack an internal elastic membrane. The canals drain into collecting veins. Additional normal arterioles nourish the glomus and connect directly with draining venules. Thin, nonmyelinated nerves are intimately associated with the vascular tangle. The diagnostic vessels of glomus tumors closely mimic the Sucquet-Hoyer canal. Ultrastructurally,[18,59,122,124,125,127,129,130,132–134] glomus tumor cells are essentially identical to normal glomus cells.[135] Aside from their shape, they have the characteristics of smooth muscle including abundant thin filaments with condensations (dense bodies) and plasmalemmal insertions, intermediate filaments, pinocytotic vesicles, and an investing basement membrane. One dissimilarity between glomus tumor cells and normal smooth muscle is the presence of abundant vimentin in the former.[134] A similar distribution of intermediate filament types is seen, however, in vascular smooth muscle in certain sites.[134] Moreover, desmin, a marker of smooth muscle, has recently been identified in glomus tumor cells.[136] Delicate nonmyelinated nerves can often be

identified in the capsule or stroma of glomus tumors, thus completing the analogy with the normal glomus.

Differential Diagnosis

Diagnostic confusion is unlikely once experience has been gained with a few cases. The glomangioma variant can be mistaken for a cavernous hemangioma. Spiradenomas with extreme stromal edema or marked dilation of stromal vessels may be confused with glomangiomas, and spiradenomas lacking stromal changes can resemble ordinary glomus tumors. The cells of spiradenomas are generally smaller, however, with more hyperchromatic nuclei, and lack the well-developed eosinophilic cytoplasm of glomus cells. Neither a "two-cell" pattern nor ductal differentiation is present in glomus tumors. Glomus tumors with abundant myxoid and hyaline stroma might conceivably be confused with chondroid syringoma, and those with partially cleared cytoplasm, with acrospiroma. In problem cases, the reticulin stain highlights the vascular pattern of glomus tumor, the characteristic relation of glomus cells to vessels, and the fact that individual glomus cells are surrounded by a delicate layer of reticulin.

HEMANGIOPERICYTOMA

Hemangiopericytomas are neoplasms of somatic soft tissues. They rarely arise in the subcutis, but to the author's knowledge, no convincing examples have been documented

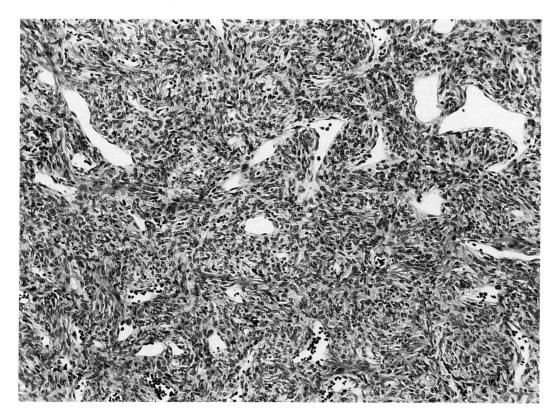

Figure 52–33. Hemangiopericytoma. Monotonous spindle cells are disposed about blood vessels that branch in a distinctive staghorn or antlerlike pattern (H&E, ×160).

as primary dermal neoplasms. Hemangiopericytomas do not, therefore, fall easily within the domain of dermatopathology, and only a brief summary can be given here. The reader is referred to several excellent discussions published elsewhere.[59,137,138]

Hemangiopericytomas are slowly growing tumors that often attain large size before surgical intervention. The age range of affected individuals is wide, as is the anatomic distribution of the tumors. The most common sites are the lower extremity, pelvic fossa and retroperitoneum, and the head and neck. The tumor typically involves skeletal muscle, deep fascia, and periosteum. Microscopically, monotonous spindle cells are disposed around blood vessels that branch in a distinctive staghorn or antlerlike pattern (Fig. 52–33). The cells are separated from one another by a meshwork of reticulin. The potential for metastatic behavior is suggested by the presence of marked cellularity, more than four mitotic figures per 10 high-power fields, and necrosis.

KAPOSI'S SARCOMA

Clinical Features

In the *classic* form, Kaposi's sarcoma occurs in middle-aged or elderly individuals, most of whom are white males.[139,140] The disease is usually indolent or only slowly progressive and clinically consists of red-brown or violaceous macules (patches), plaques, and nodules that initially appear on the lower extremities. Most patients die of unrelated causes, although at autopsy, clinically silent visceral lesions may be found.

Kaposi's sarcoma accounts for as many as 9% of all malignancies in blacks of certain parts of equatorial Africa.[141] The *nodular* form resembles the classic type, clinically and biologically, although the patients are somewhat younger. Moreover, some of them develop a "florid" or "aggressive" variant, consisting of both exophytic and deeply infiltrative tumors that often involve bone. A frequently fatal *lymphadenopathic* form occurs in black African children and consists of widespread involvement of lymph nodes. Cutaneous and visceral lesions are minor or absent.

Kaposi's sarcoma is the most common tumor associated with AIDS.[142,143] Initial lesions have a predilection for the skin of the trunk, upper extremities, head, and oral mucous membranes. They are often small, subtle, pink or red macules and papules with round, polygonal, and fusiform shapes. The latter tend to be oriented along lines of skin cleavage. The cutaneous disease is progressive, and autopsy studies[144–146] have documented a high frequency of visceral involvement, most notably of lymph nodes, lungs, and gastrointestinal tract. Kaposi's sarcoma is also a complication of immunosuppressive therapy administered to renal transplant patients[147] or to individuals with various other conditions. Moreover, the tumor may develop as a second malignancy in patients with hematologic disorders, many of whom are receiving immunosuppressive therapy.[140,148]

Histologic Features

Microscopically, well-developed lesions of Kaposi's sarcoma are distinctive.[139–142,149,150] Proliferations of monotonous spindle cells produce one or more circumscribed nodules in the upper half of the dermis. The cells are arranged in fascicles that intersect at various angles and are, therefore, observed in transverse, oblique, and longitudinal planes of section (Figs. 52–34 and 52–35). Their cytoplasm is light eosinophilic, and cell borders are usually indistinct. The nuclei are ovoid or fusiform and have tapered or rounded ends. Nuclear contours are generally smooth, and chromatin rims are thin and delicate. The remaining chromatin is finely dispersed or focally condensed. In many cases, there are small nucleoli. Mitotic figures can almost always be found, and it is not unusual to observe three or four in a single high-power field.

Of great diagnostic importance is the presence of vascular slits. These are recognized by observing one or a few red blood cells wedged between individual spindle cells (see Fig. 52–34). Larger columns or lakes of erythrocytes may distend the slits (Fig. 52–35), and when further dilated, they can appear sinusoidal. If sectioned transversely, the slits appear as rounded holes of various sizes, situated both between and seemingly within individual cells. This pattern suggests that the slits are actually tubular. When many closely spaced slits are observed in transverse section, the tissue assumes a distinctive spongy or sievelike appearance (see Figs. 52–34 and 52–35). The finding of even small intact fields that demonstrate the spindle cells and slits in both longitudinal and transverse section is of particular help in arriving at a firm diagnosis in small specimens or in those complicated by marked edema, inflammation, or hemorrhage.

The dermis between individual nodules of tumor contains normal arterioles, capillaries, venules, and ectatic lymphatics. Perivascular lymphocytic infiltrates, at times accompanied by plasma cells, are frequently present, and similar cells are usually scattered within the tumor nodules. In most cases, hemosiderin can be found within tumor cells and macrophages and free within the stroma. Clusters of light eosinophilic, hyaline bodies of uncertain nature, ranging in size from 1 to 10 μm, are identifiable in the large majority of specimens, both between and within the spindle cells.[149] Although these bodies may represent phagocytized red blood cells, their tinctorial qualities and highly variable size usually allow distinction from intact red blood cells.

With the advent of AIDS, pathologists are frequently required to recognize Kaposi's sarcoma in its patch or plaque stage.[142,150,151] Strictly defined, the *patch* contains few, if any, of the spindle cells that typify the nodule. Instead, one observes dilated, jagged, irregularly branching, fre-

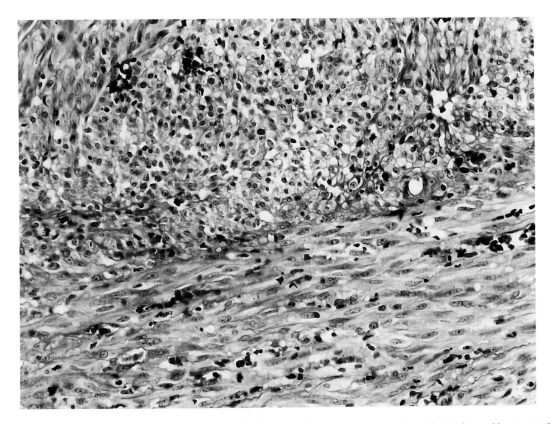

Figure 52–34. Kaposi's sarcoma. In the typical nodule, fascicles of medium-sized spindle cells interlace with one another. In this field, they are sectioned both longitudinally (bottom) and transversely (top). Nuclei have generally smooth contours, delicate chromatin rims, finely dispersed chromatin, and small nucleoli. Vascular slits are discerned by observing the presence of one or a few red blood cells wedged between individual tumor cells (H&E, ×300).

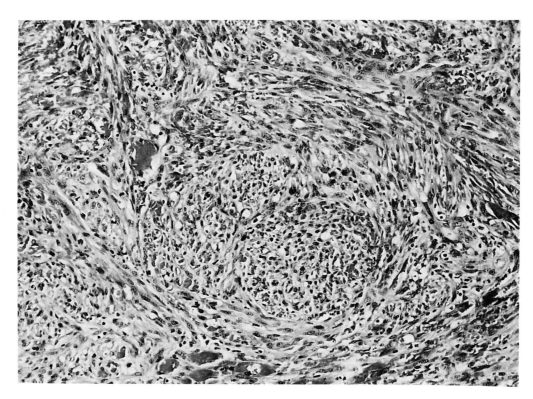

Figure 52–35. Kaposi's sarcoma. The microscopic features are generally similar to those illustrated in Figure 52–34, but there is somewhat more cytological atypia, and vascular slits are more prominent (H&E, ×175).

quently empty vascular spaces, most notably in the superficial dermis (Fig. 52–36). These surround normal-appearing vessels and dissect between fibers of the reticular dermis. The endothelial cells lining these vessels are small, flat, widely spaced, and essentially indistinguishable from normal endothelial cells. A perivascular lymphocytic infiltrate, often accompanied by plasma cells, is usually present. Extravasations of erythrocytes and hemosiderin deposits may or may not be seen. Careful study of such specimens with multiple sections often discloses at least rare foci containing small numbers of spindle cells characteristic of Kaposi's sarcoma, frequently immediately adjacent to the ectatic vessels (see Fig. 52–36). It may be possible to identify incipient slits in such fields. The *plaque* stage is typified by the further development of the spindle cell component at multiple foci within the dermis (Fig. 52–37).

The microscopic appearance of Kaposi's sarcoma in lymph nodes and viscera is usually similar to that seen in cutaneous nodules, but the full microscopic spectrum has been observed. Moreover, postmortem studies[144–146] and a review of open-lung biopsy specimens[152] have disclosed deviant microscopic appearances, thought to represent polymorphous, inflammatory, or sclerotic variants of Kaposi's sarcoma. In such lesions, dense infiltrates of lymphocytes and plasma cells, diffuse interstitial sclerosis, and prominent hemosiderin deposits greatly obscure the underlying vasoformative proliferation of spindle cells. Whether these changes represent a type of incipient Kaposi's sarcoma or, more likely, the effects of spontaneous involution and/or therapy has not been determined, but the interpretation

that such lesions are, indeed, Kaposi's sarcoma is supported both by their distinctive distribution within lymph nodes and viscera and the presence of adjacent, more typical Kaposi's sarcoma. In one postmortem study, lesions with similar appearances were also observed in the skin.[144] An additional microscopic variant, documented in both skin and lymph nodes, consists of an extensive, anastomosing pattern of vascular spaces lined by flattened endothelial cells[145,153] that appears to be a florid expression of the ectatic vessels that characterize the patch stage. The microscopic findings mimic those of lymphangioma and well-differentiated angiosarcoma. Several reports have briefly described and illustrated an anaplastic variant of Kaposi's sarcoma or a transition to fully developed angiosarcoma.[139,141,149] Individual cases have not been documented in great detail, and the evolution of Kaposi's sarcoma to fully developed angiosarcoma needs further study.

Histogenesis

The histogenesis of Kaposi's sarcoma is still uncertain. A comprehensive ultrastructural study, with careful light microscopic correlation, has not been published. Available observations indicate that the ectatic vessels seen in patches are lined by endothelial cells, but that basal lamina is often absent and pericytes are greatly reduced in number in comparison with normal capillaries.[154] The less well-differentiated spindle cells that characterize plaques and nodules have been variably interpreted,[155–162] but their tendency to form aggregates around slitlike lumina suggests their vasoformative nature. The presence of erythrocytes, lyso-

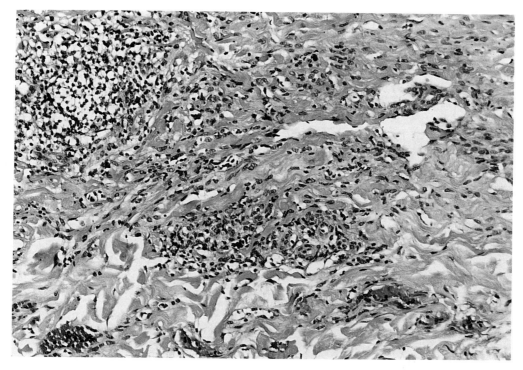

Figure 52–36. Kaposi's sarcoma, patch stage. Jagged, branching, ectatic, vascular channels dissect between fibers of the reticular dermis and partially surround normal blood vessels (upper right). They are lined by widely spaced, flat endothelial cells. Lymphoplasmacytic infiltrates, sparse red blood cell extravasations, and hemosiderin deposits are also present. A small number of spindle cells characteristic of better-developed lesions of Kaposi's sarcoma can be discerned (left center) (H&E, ×175).

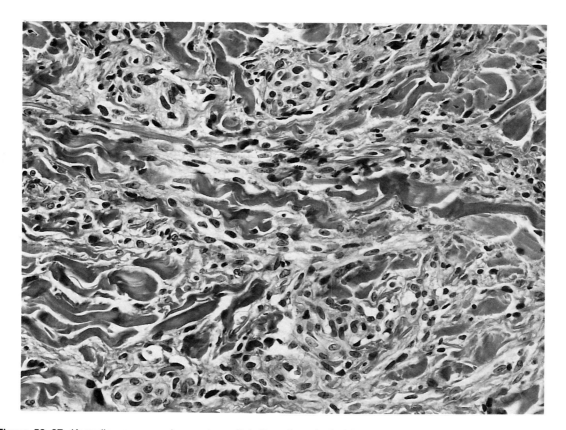

Figure 52–37. Kaposi's sarcoma, plaque stage. Spindle cells typical of Kaposi's sarcoma form an interlacing pattern within the dermis. Compare the cytological details of these cells with those illustrated in Figure 52–34 (H&E, ×300).

somes, and ferritin within the spindle cells indicates phago-cytic capabilities.[155–158]

Immunohistochemistry

The results of immunohistochemical studies are conflicting and, to some degree, confusing.[160–170] Well-formed vessels in lesions of Kaposi's sarcoma are lined by cells that contain factor VIII-related antigen and have the capacity to bind *U. europaeus* lectin, features consistent with endothelial cells and, more specifically, with those of blood vessels rather than lymph capillaries. Some of these structures may be part of the nonneoplastic vasculature ordinarily observed in and around foci of Kaposi's sarcoma. *U. europaeus* binding has consistently been noted in the spindle cells, but the results for factor VIII-related antigen have been variable or essentially negative. More recent studies, using newly developed antibodies and additional enzyme histochemical procedures, have provided further evidence that the spindle cells are, indeed, endothelial, but opinions differ regarding their lymphatic[167,169] versus blood vascular nature.[168,170] The same can be said of the ectatic vessels in patch lesions. Further confusing the issue is the presence of abundant laminin and type IV collagen surrounding many individual spindle cells[161,168] despite the sparseness of ultrastructurally recognizable basal lamina in such foci.[161] These findings further support the endothelial nature of the spindle cells and have been interpreted as evidence favoring their blood vascular rather than lymphatic origin.[161,168]

From the foregoing, it can be tentatively concluded that the underlying lesion in Kaposi's sarcoma is a proliferation of poorly differentiated endothelial cells. It remains to be determined whether they are derived from the endothelium that lines the ectatic vessels of the patch stage or from primitive perivascular mesenchyme adjacent to such vessels.

ANGIOSARCOMA

Angiosarcomas of the skin occur almost exclusively in three specific settings: (1) the scalp and face, usually in elderly patients[45,171–177]; (2) lymphedematous extremities[175,176,178–185]; and (3) skin that has been irradiated.[175,186] The diagnosis should be entertained with caution under any other circumstances.

Clinical Features

Patients with angiosarcoma of the head are usually in their seventh or eighth decade at the time of diagnosis. The scalp is more commonly affected. On the face, the central and upper portions are favored. Most angiosarcomas of lymphedematous extremities develop on an upper extremity in women who have had an ipsilateral mastectomy and axillary lymphadenectomy, from 1 to 30 or more years previously (median of 10 years). Moderate or severe chronic lymphedema is nearly always present. Angiosarcomas also

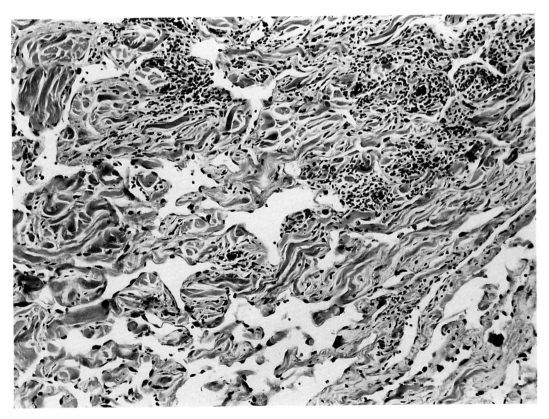

Figure 52–38. Angiosarcoma. A freely anastomosing network of generally bloodless vascular channels dissects throughout the reticular dermis, seeming to use the latter as a supporting structure. Endothelial cells are widely spaced. Their nuclei are generally enlarged and hyperchromatic, and there are scattered bizarre forms. Nodular lymphoid infiltrates are also present (H&E, ×160).

occur on extremities (more often the lower) of individuals suffering from congenital lymphedema,[182,183] lymphedema praecox, and lymphedema due to a variety of other inflammatory, surgical, traumatic, and radiation-related mechanisms.[181] The disease has also been documented in filarial lymphedema.[185] Postirradiation angiosarcomas of the skin develop many years after therapeutic radiation administered for either superficial benign conditions or more deep-seated malignancies. The lower abdominal wall and suprapubic area are the most common sites.[186]

The lesions are generally similar regardless of the clinical setting. In some cases, only edema or patchy erythema is evident. In others, multiple bruiselike changes dominate the picture. In more advanced cases, there are also nodules and plaques that range in color from flesh tones to red or violaceous. Some angiosarcomas are surmounted by superficial vesicles containing clear or bloody fluid. The lesions are typically multifocal, and their clinical borders are indistinct. Cutaneous angiosarcomas recur locally and ultimately metastasize. The median survival is approximately 20 months, and the 5-year survival approximately 15%.

Histologic Features

Microscopically, angiosarcomas of the skin evolve within the dermis, but often infiltrate subcutaneous tissue or deeper structures. They characteristically exhibit a multifocal distribution within a biopsy specimen. Moreover, there is a broad but distinctive spectrum of architectural patterns,[45,171,173,175,176] and a substantial part of the spectrum

may be present within the biopsy specimen. Generally speaking, the tumors are composed of either spindle or epithelioid cells.[176]

The better-differentiated lesions are obviously vasoformative and display angular, jagged, or rounded endothelium-lined spaces that form freely anastomosing networks within the dermis (Figs. 52–38 through 52–41). The neoformed channels spread or "dissect" between fibers of the reticular dermis, using them as a supporting structure. They abut adnexa but do not destroy them. The cells lining the abnormal vessels can closely resemble normal endothelium or show only mild nuclear enlargement and hyperchromasia. In most cases, however, more markedly enlarged endothelial cells, with either densely hyperchromatic or vesicular nuclei, are also present. The neoplastic cells may form multiple layers or isolated tufts that lack supporting structures. They can also line intraluminal papillae that have collagenous cores consisting of dermal remnants. The lumina of the neoplastic vessels are often empty but may contain combinations of lymphlike material, desquamated neoplastic cells, lymphocytes, and red blood cells. Nodular lymphoid infiltrates can obscure the microscopic picture. Mitotic figures are often sparse.

Architecturally less well-differentiated angiosarcomas tend to retain a dissecting pattern between fibers of the reticular dermis. They exhibit more marked endothelial proliferation, however, often accompanied by increased cytologic pleomorphism and mitotic activity (Fig. 52–42). When the neoplastic cells are spindled, lumina often consist of

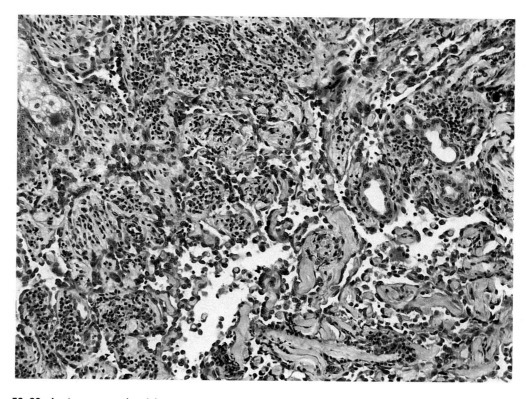

Figure 52–39. Angiosarcoma. An elaborate, anastomosing network of vascular spaces extensively dissects the dermis. Endothelial nuclei are enlarged and hyperchromatic. Note that intraluminal papillae have cores that consist of dermal remnants. Adnexal structures (left and right) are abutted by the tumor but not destroyed (H&E, ×175).

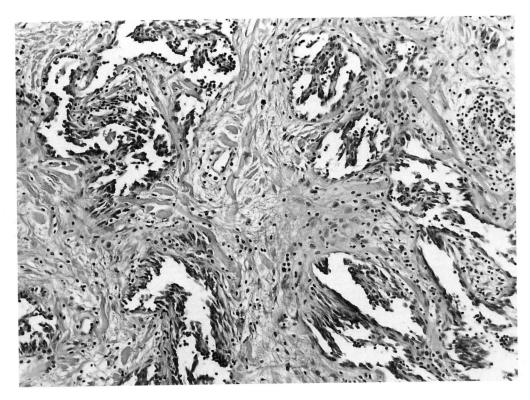

Figure 52–40. Angiosarcoma. This tumor is characterized by large jagged vascular spaces lined by one or several layers of moderately atypical spindled endothelial cells (H&E, ×175).

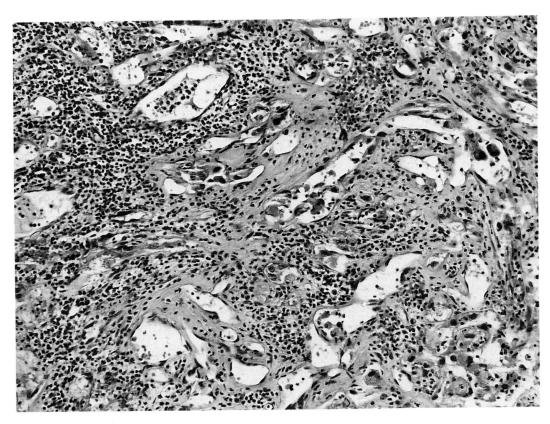

Figure 52–41. Angiosarcoma. Obvious vascular spaces are lined by pleomorphic, generally fusiform endothelial cells. There is a prominent interstitial inflammatory infiltrate (H&E, ×160).

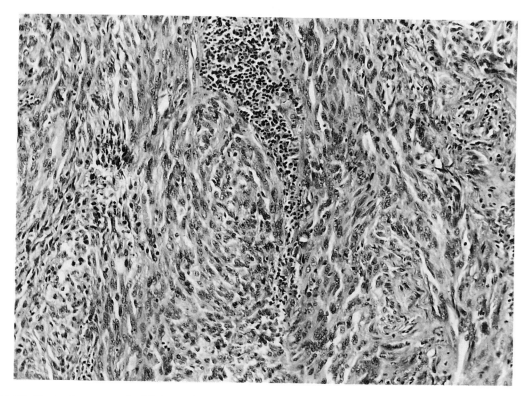

Figure 52–42. Angiosarcoma. In this less obviously vasoformative tumor, atypical, spindled endothelial cells form an interlacing syncytium that obliterates most of the dermis. Lumina are seen as cleftlike spaces (H&E, ×175).

narrow intercellular clefts or slits. When the cells are epithelioid, lumina appear as intracytoplasmic vacuoles or more obvious spaces lined by neoplastic cells.

In their least well-differentiated fields, angiosarcomas take the form of expansile cellular nodules or large sheets of cells (Figs. 52–43 and 52–44). Pleormorphism is prominent, and mitotic figures numerous. Such tumors may at first seem patternless, but it can often be appreciated that the cells tend to surround small lumina. There is often a meshwork, sievelike, or sinusoidal appearance. Blood elements or lymphlike material, if present, are localized within the lumina and sparse or absent between them. Inflammatory infiltrate is minimal. Adnexa are destroyed.

Electron Microscopy

Ultrastructurally, the neoplastic cells of angiosarcomas consistently exhibit one or more features of endothelial differentiation[173,176,182,187–189] including pinocytosis, intermediate filaments, specialized cell connections, cytoplasmic flaps, Weibel-Palade bodies, and basement membrane production. They typically form vascular structures, at times surrounded by pericytes.[173] In fact, the preponderance of ultrastructural evidence indicates that angiosarcomas often show differentiation toward blood vessels rather than lymph channels.

Immunohistochemistry

It is often possible to make an objective diagnosis of angiosarcoma based on hematoxylin and eosin-stained sections of an adequate biopsy specimen. The regular presence of factor VIII-related antigen in the neoplastic endothelial cells, as demonstrated by immunohistochemical techniques,[176,189–191] can be of considerable diagnostic aid in difficult cases. *U. europaeus* lectin can also be quite helpful,[188,191,192] as it binds avidly to endothelial cells of all classes, including those of angiosarcomas. Vimentin is present in angiosarcomas, whereas cytokeratin is absent.[188]

Differential Diagnosis

The differential diagnosis of angiosarcoma can include one or more of the benign vascular proliferations described elsewhere in this chapter. The architecture of angiosarcoma may resemble that of Kaposi's sarcoma, but pleomorphism is more marked in the former. Angiosarcomas of epithelioid cells (see Fig. 52–44) can be mistaken for malignant melanoma, but they rarely interact with the epidermis in a way that simulates junctional change. Epithelioid endothelial cells occasionally contain finely divided hemosiderin resembling melanin, but appropriate stains should be helpful. Epithelioid angiosarcomas with a nesting pattern, tubulelike lumina, and intracytoplasmic vacuoles may also resemble primary or metastatic adenocarcinoma. Epithelial mucin is lacking, however, and adenocarcinomas regularly contain cytokeratin and epithelial membrane antigen. Angiosarcomas of spindle cells raise the differential diagnosis of a broad array of other spindle cell tumors of the dermis. Knowledge of the clinical findings of angiosarcomas, familiarity with their distinctive architectural patterns, directed search for vasoformative features, and a high index of suspicion can usually solve these diagnostic dilemmas.

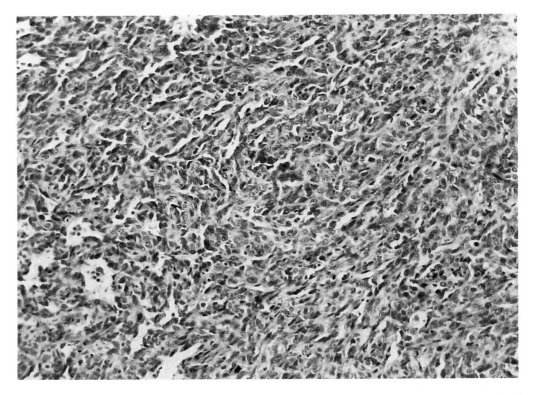

Figure 52–43. Angiosarcoma. This poorly differentiated tumor is composed of pleomorphic spindle cells. Cleftlike and sinusoidal spaces between tumor cells suggest the vasoformative nature of the neoplasm. Inflammatory infiltrate is absent (H&E, ×160).

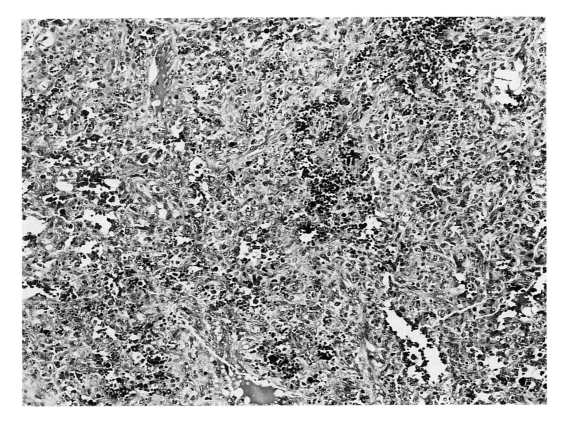

Figure 52–44. Angiosarcoma. This poorly differentiated tumor is composed of nodules and sheets of large pleomorphic epithelioid endothelial cells. Isolated lumina help to identify the tumor as vascular. This field resembles some cases of angiolymphoid hyperplasia with eosinophilia (see Fig. 52–27), but the cytologic picture indicates malignancy (H&E, ×160).

ENDOVASCULAR PAPILLARY ANGIOENDOTHELIOMA OF CHILDHOOD

Reports of endovascular papillary angioendothelioma (*Dabska tumor*) are few,[193–196] and its nature remains uncertain. With one exception,[194] the patients have been children, and in several instances, the lesion was present at birth. Clinically, one observes either a diffuse swelling or a nodule. Microscopically, dilated vessels in the dermis and subcutis are lined by enlarged cuboidal or columnar endothelial cells that form ramifying, intraluminal papillae with hyalinized, globular cores (Fig. 52–45). Nuclei are hyperchromatic, but overt pleomorphism is lacking and mitotic figures are sparse. Lymphocytes may also be observed within the lumina, adherent to the endothelial cells.[196] The stroma contains additional dilated vessels that are lined by flat endothelium and contain proteinaceous material. Resected lymph nodes in two cases contained foci of endothelial proliferation.[193] All patients thus far reported remained well after surgical therapy.

Much remains to be learned about endovascular papillary angioendothelioma. Certain clinical and pathologic findings suggest that, in some cases, the lesion may be superimposed on a preexisting lymphangioma or hemangioma. In fact, the tumor has certain microscopic features in common with intravascular papillary endothelial hyperplasia, an alteration well known to be superimposed on preexisting vascular tumors. Lymph nodal foci may represent multifocality rather than true embolic-type metastases.[196] The affinity of lymphocytes for the enlarged endothelial cells suggests that the latter may be related to "high" endothelial cells present in postcapillary venules of lymph nodes.[196] High endothelial cells selectively interact with lymphocytes based on the presence of a surface receptor system.

INTRAVASCULAR LYMPHOMATOSIS (MALIGNANT ANGIOENDOTHELIOMATOSIS) AND REACTIVE (BENIGN) ANGIOENDOTHELIOMATOSIS

Since first being described,[197,198] angioendotheliomatosis has remained an enigmatic entity. In most patients, the process appears cytologically malignant and is often rapidly fatal.[198–209] Recent evidence indicates that, with few exceptions, the cells in this form of the disease have a *lymphoid* nature.[202,204–209] On the other hand, reactive (benign) angioendotheliomatosis is a true endothelial proliferation, apparently related to subacute bacterial endocarditis in some cases.[197,209–213] The clinical appearances in both intravascu-

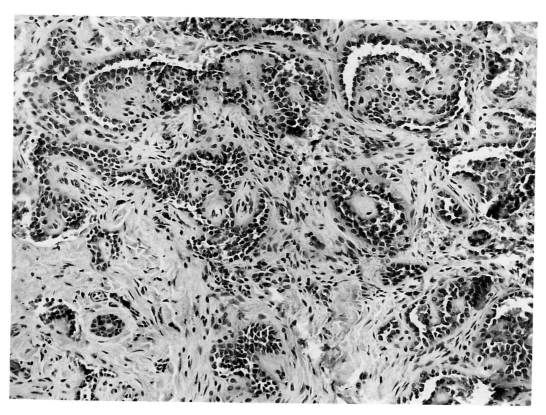

Figure 52–45. Endovascular papillary angioendothelioma (Dabska tumor). Vascular spaces are lined by cuboidal or columnar endothelial cells with enlarged, hyperchromatic nuclei. The endothelial cells line intraluminal papillae, some of which have hyalinized, globular cores (H&E, ×175).

lar lymphomatosis and reactive angioendotheliomatosis are approximately similar and consist of erythematous or violaceous cutaneous nodules and plaques. Individuals with intravascular lymphomatosis may lack cutaneous lesions and present, instead, with nonlocalizing neurologic signs or progressive dementia.

When patients with intravascular lymphomatosis come to autopsy, multiple infarcts of the central nervous system are often the most obvious gross findings, but infiltrates of the skin or viscera (notably the adrenal glands and, on occasion, the spleen or lymph nodes) may also be visible.[198,208] Microscopically, there is systemic involvement by a florid proliferation of malignant-appearing cells within the lumens of capillaries, venules, and arterioles (Fig. 52–46). The cells may be enmeshed in fibrin-platelet thrombi. Sometimes they form an eccentric subendothelial layer.[201] The cells are noncohesive, rounded, and have sparse amphophilic cytoplasm. The nuclei have either coarse clumped chromatin or appear vesicular and typically contain prominent nucleoli. Mitotic figures are usually obvious. Affected vessels may be distended by the malignant cells and can appear tortuous or coiled.[198,209] Extension of the infiltrate into vessel walls or perivascular connective tissue is not rare. In most cases, flattened, normal-appearing endothelial cells of affected vessels are easily distinguished from the cytologically atypical intravascular proliferation. Extravascular infiltrates closely resemble those of malignant

lymphoma.[198,208,214] Based on published descriptions and illustrations,[197,209–213] the proliferating cells of the reactive variant resemble endothelial cells. They have spindled, vesicular nuclei but lack cytological pleomorphism (Fig. 52–47). Extravascular spread is lacking.

As noted earlier, recent work has shed new light on the nature of malignant angioendotheliomatosis. Early observers remarked on a similarity between the proliferating cells and those of lymphomas and leukemias.[198] Scott and associates,[214] noting the microscopic appearance of extravascular infiltrates and a history of nasopharyngeal lymphoma in one of their patients, considered the possibility that malignant angioendotheliomatosis represented an "unusual form of reticuloendothelial sarcoma," and Ansell and colleagues,[215] in 1982, described a patient with diffuse large cell lymphoma who subsequently developed malignant angioendotheliomatosis. More recently, a substantial number of cases have been studied immunocytochemically,[202,204–208] and it has become apparent that, in nearly every instance, the cells in question have lymphoid features. They contain leukocyte common antigen, a sensitive and specific marker of lymphoid cells, and detailed marker studies on a handful of cases have demonstrated either a B-cell or T-cell phenotype.[202,207,208] Prior workers pointed to the presence of factor VIII-related antigen, an endothelial marker, as evidence for the endothelial nature of malignant angioendotheliomatosis.[201,203] Many cases are negative for

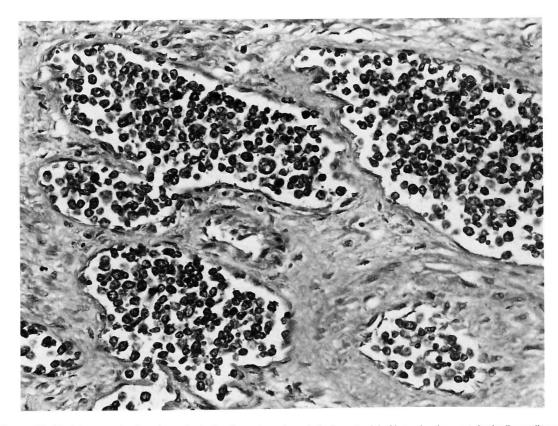

Figure 52–46. Intravascular lymphomatosis (malignant angioendotheliomatosis). Noncohesive, cytologically malignant-appearing, round cells distend the lumina of thin-walled vessels. Nuclei are hyperchromatic and vesicular. Cytoplasm is sparse. Note the presence of normal-appearing, flat endothelial cells (H&E, ×300).

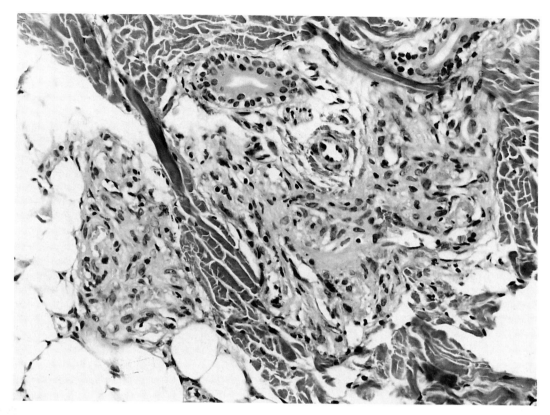

Figure 52–47. Reactive angioendotheliomatosis. A proliferation of enlarged endothelial cells with ovoid, vesicular nuclei obscures the lumina of several capillaries at the dermal-subcutaneous junction (H&E, ×300).

factor VIII-related antigen, however,[200–203,206,207] and the extravascular infiltrates are consistently negative.[205,208] Moreover, *U. europaeus* lectin, a highly sensitive endothelial marker, has consistently failed to bind to both intravascular and extravascular infiltrates.[205,206,208] It can be speculated that factor VIII-related antigen, present in serum and platelets, is coated upon or absorbed by the malignant intravascular cells, thus explaining their positive reactions.[204,205,208] Cytokeratin and epithelial membrane antigen have been consistently lacking,[208] thus excluding an epithelial origin.

Ultrastructural evidence supporting the endothelial nature of malignant angioendotheliomatosis has been critically reviewed,[202,205,208] and it seems likely that prior observers mistook reactive endothelial cells for the malignant cells in question.[199,200,203,214] It should be kept in mind that benign, albeit reactive, endothelium is often intimately intermingled with the malignant cells.[202] When illustrated at low power, in their entirety, the malignant cells closely resemble those of malignant lymphoma.[199,201,202,205,208]

Despite the foregoing evidence that malignant angioendotheliomatosis is actually a lymphoma, several questions remain. In the large majority of cases, there is no obvious nodal lymphoma at the time of autopsy. Moreover, hematopoietic organs are typically spared or show only minor involvement. Hence the origin of the malignancy and the reason for its angiotropism are unknown. Rare cases are negative for all pertinent markers,[208] and their nature requires explanation.

As noted above, the reactive form of angioendotheliomatosis is a true endothelial proliferation. The cells partially or completely fill affected vessels but, despite their enlargement, are readily recognizable as endothelial in character, both in routine sections and with the use of immunohistochemical markers.[213] The precise nature of reactive angioendotheliomatosis and its clinical associations need further study.

REFERENCES

1. Lister WA. The natural history of strawberry naevi. *Lancet.* 1938; 1:1429–1434.
2. Walsh TS Jr, Tompkins VN. Some observations on the strawberry nevus of infancy. *Cancer.* 1956; 9:869–904.
3. Bowers RE, Graham EA, Tomlinson KM. The natural history of the strawberry nevus. *Arch Dermatol.* 1960; 82:667–680.
4. Hidano A, Nakajima S. Earliest features of the strawberry mark in the newborn. *Br J Dermatol.* 1972; 87:138–144.
5. Campbell JS. Congenital capillary hemangiomas of the parotid gland: a lesion characteristic of infancy. *N Engl J Med.* 1956; 254:56–60.
6. Nagao K, Matsuzaki O, Shigematsu H, et al. Histopathologic studies of benign infantile hemangioendothelioma of the parotid gland. *Cancer.* 1980; 46:2250–2256.
7. Nakayama H. Clinical and histological studies of the classification and the natural course of the strawberry mark. *J Dermatol.* 1981; 8:277–291.

8. Taxy JB, Gray SR. Cellular angiomas of infancy: an ultrastructural study of two cases. *Cancer.* 1979; 43:2322–2331.

9. Tani M, Kaibuchi S, Murata Y, et al. Ultrastructure of hypertrophic hemangioma. *J Cutan Pathol.* 1983; 10:133–137.

10. Pasyk KA, Grabb WC, Cherry GW. Crystalloid inclusions in endothelial cells of cellular and capillary hemangiomas: a possible sign of cellular immaturity. *Arch Dermatol.* 1983; 119:134–137.

11. Inceman S, Tangün Y. Chronic defibrination syndrome due to a giant hemangioma associated with microangiopathic hemolytic anemia. *Am J Med.* 1969; 46:997–1002.

12. Straub PW, Kessler S, Schreiber A, et al. Chronic intravascular coagulation in Kasabach-Merritt syndrome: preferential accumulation of fibrinogen[131] I in a giant hemangioma. *Arch Intern Med.* 1972; 129:475–478.

13. Lang PG, Dubin HV. Hemangioma-thrombocytopenia syndrome: a disseminated intravascular coagulopathy. *Arch Dermatol.* 1975; 111:105–107.

14. Rice JS, Fischer DS. Blue rubber-bleb nevus syndrome. Generalized cavernous hemangiomatosis or venous hamartoma with medulloblastoma of the cerebellum: case report and review of the literature. *Arch Dermatol.* 1962; 86:503–511.

15. Fretzin DF, Potter B. Blue rubber bleb nevus. *Arch Intern Med.* 1965; 116:924–929.

16. Sakurane HF, Sugai T, Saito T. The association of blue rubber bleb nevus and Maffucci's syndrome. *Arch Dermatol.* 1967; 95:28–36.

17. Hagood MF, Gathright JB Jr. Hemangiomatosis of the skin and gastrointestinal tract: report of a case. *Dis Colon Rectum.* 1975; 18:141–146.

18. Rycroft RJG, Menter MA, Sharvill DE, et al. Hereditary multiple glomus tumours: report of four families and a review of the literature. *Trans St Johns Hosp Dermatol Soc.* 1975; 61:70–81.

19. Lewis RJ, Ketcham AS. Maffucci's syndrome: functional and neoplastic significance: case report and review of the literature. *J Bone Joint Surg.* 1973; 55:1465–1479.

20. Loewinger RJ, Lichtenstein JR, Dodson WE, et al. Maffucci's syndrome: a mesenchymal dysplasia and multiple tumour syndrome. *Br J Dermatol.* 1977; 96:317–322.

21. Imperial R, Helwig EB. Verrucous hemangioma: a clinicopathologic study of 21 cases. *Arch Dermatol.* 1967; 96:247–253.

22. Klein JA, Barr RJ. Verrucous hemangioma. *Pediatr Dermatol.* 1985; 2:191–193.

23. Lynch PJ, Kosanovich M. Angiokeratoma circumscriptum. *Arch Dermatol.* 1967; 96:665–668.

24. Mills SE, Cooper PH, Fechner RE. Lobular capillary hemangioma: the underlying lesion of pyogenic granuloma: a study of 73 cases from the oral and nasal mucous membranes. *Am J Surg Pathol.* 1980; 4:471–479.

25. Kerr DA. Granuloma pyogenicum. *Oral Surg Oral Med Oral Pathol.* 1950; 4:158–176.

26. Warner J, Wilson Jones E. Pyogenic granuloma recurring with multiple satellites: a report of 11 cases. *Br J Dermatol.* 1968; 80:218–227.

27. Swerlick RA, Cooper PH. Pyogenic granuloma (lobular capillary hemangioma) within port-wine stains. *J Am Acad Dermatol.* 1983; 8:627–630.

28. Zaynoun ST, Juljulian HH, Kurban AK. Pyogenic granuloma with multiple satellites. *Arch Dermatol.* 1974; 109:689–691.

29. Juhlin L, Hjertquist S-O, Pontén J, et al. Disseminated granuloma pyogenicum. *Acta Derm Venereol.* 1970; 50:134–136.

30. Nappi O, Wick MR. Disseminated lobular capillary hemangioma (pyogenic granuloma): a clinicopathologic study of two cases. *Am J Dermatopathol.* 1986; 8:379–385.

31. Cooper PH, Mills SE. Subcutaneous granuloma pyogenicum:

32. Cooper PH, McAllister HA, Helwig EB. Intravenous pyogenic granuloma: a study of 18 cases. *Am J Surg Pathol.* 1979; 3:221–228.

33. Ulbright TM, Santa Cruz DJ. Intravenous pyogenic granuloma: case report with ultrastructural findings. *Cancer.* 1980; 45:1646–1652.

34. Oehlschlaegel G, Müller E. Zum Granuloma pyogenicum sive teleangiectaticum als Sonderfall des capillaren Hamangioms und uber dessen Beziehung zu anderen Angiomen und gefassgebundenen Naevi. *Arch Klin Exp Dermatol.* 1964; 218:126–157.

35. Kuo T, Sayers CP, Rosai J. Masson's "vegetant intravascular hemangioendothelioma": a lesion often mistaken for angiosarcoma: study of seventeen cases located in the skin and soft tissues. *Cancer.* 1976; 38:1227–1236.

36. Davies MG, Barton SP, Atai F, et al. The abnormal dermis in pyogenic granuloma: histochemical and ultrastructural observations. *J Am Acad Dermatol.* 1980; 2:132–142.

37. Marsch WC. Zur Ultrastruktur des eruptiven kapillären Hämangioms ("Granuloma pyogenicum sive teleangiectaticum"). *Hautarzt.* 1984; 35:92–96.

38. Burgdorf WHC, Mukai K, Rosai J. Immunohistochemical identification of factor VIII-related antigen in endothelial cells of cutaneous lesions of alleged vascular nature. *Am J Clin Pathol.* 1981; 75:167–171.

39. Miettinen M, Holthofer H, Lehto V-P, et al. Ulex europaeus I lectin as a marker for tumors derived from endothelial cells. *Am J Clin Pathol.* 1983; 79:32–36.

40. Fechner RE, Cooper PH, Mills SE. Pyogenic granuloma of the larynx and trachea: a causal and pathologic misnomer for granulation tissue. *Arch Otolaryngol.* 1981; 107:30–32.

41. Campbell JP, Grekin RC, Ellis CN, et al. Retinoid therapy is associated with excess granulation tissue responses. *J Am Acad Dermatol.* 1983; 9:708–713.

42. Girard C, Graham JH, Johnson WC. Arteriovenous hemangioma (arteriovenous shunt): a clinicopathological and histochemical study. *J Cutan Pathol.* 1974; 1:73–87.

43. Carapeto FJ, Garcia-Perez A, Winkelmann RK. Acral arteriovenous tumor. *Acta Derm Venereol.* 1977; 57:155–158.

44. Connelly MG, Winkelmann RK. Acral arteriovenous tumor: a clinicopathologic review. *Am J Surg Pathol.* 1985; 9:15–21.

45. Wilson Jones E. Malignant vascular tumours. *Clin Exp Dermatol.* 1976; 1:287–312.

46. Alessi E, Bertani E, Sala F. Acquired tufted angioma. *Am J Dermatopathol.* 1986; 8:426–429.

47. Padilla SR, Orkin M, Rosai J. Acquired "tufted" angioma (progressive capillary hemangioma): a distinctive clinicopathologic entity related to lobular capillary hemangioma. *Am J Dermatopathol.* 1987; 9:292–300.

48. Kumakiri M, Muramoto F, Tsukinaga I, et al. Crystalline lamellae in the endothelial cells of a type of hemangioma characterized by the proliferation of immature endothelial cells and pericytes—angioblastoma (Nakagawa). *J Am Acad Dermatol.* 1983; 8:68–75.

49. Harkins GA, Sabiston DC Jr: Lymphangioma in infancy and childhood. *Surgery.* 1960; 47:811–822.

50. Bill AH Jr, Sumner DS. A unified concept of lymphangioma and cystic hygroma. *Surg Gynecol Obstet.* 1965; 120:79–86.

51. Peachey RDG, Lim C-C, Whimster IW. Lymphangioma of skin: a review of 65 cases. *Br J Dermatol.* 1970; 83:519–527.

52. Whimster IW. The pathology of lymphangioma circumscriptum. *Br J Dermatol.* 1976; 94:473–486.

53. Flanagan BF, Helwig EB. Cutaneous lymphangioma. *Arch Dermatol.* 1977; 113:24–30.

54. Prioleau PG, Santa Cruz DJ. Lymphangioma circumscriptum

following radical mastectomy and radiation therapy. *Cancer.* 1978; 42:1989–1991.

55. Leshin B, Whitaker DC, Foucar E. Lymphangioma circumscriptum following mastectomy and radiation therapy. *J Am Acad Dermatol.* 1986; 15:1117–1119.

56. Gold SC. Angioendothelioma (lymphatic type). *Br J Dermatol.* 1970; 82:92–93.

57. Watanabe M, Kishiyama K, Ohkawara A. Acquired progressive lymphangioma. *J Am Acad Dermatol.* 1983; 8:663–667.

58. Zachary CB, Wilson Jones E, Spaull J. Progressive lymphangioma: differential diagnosis and endothelial cell marker studies. *Arch Dermatol.* 1984; 120:1617. Abstract.

58a. Tadaki T, Aiba S, Masu S, et al. Acquired progressive lymphangioma as a flat erythematous patch on the abdominal wall of a child. *Arch Dermatol.* 1988; 124:699–701.

59. Enzinger FM, Weiss SW. *Soft Tissue Tumors.* St. Louis, Mo: CV Mosby; 1983.

60. Earhart RN, Aeling JA, Nuss DD, et al. Pseudo-Kaposi sarcoma: a patient with arteriovenous malformation and skin lesions simulating Kaposi sarcoma. *Arch Dermatol.* 1974; 110:907–910.

61. Rusin LJ, Harrell ER. Arteriovenous fistula: cutaneous manifestations. *Arch Dermatol.* 1976; 112:1135–1138.

62. Marshall ME, Hatfield ST, Hatfield DR. Arteriovenous malformation simulating Kaposi's sarcoma (pseudo-Kaposi's sarcoma). *Arch Dermatol.* 1985; 121:99–101.

63. Goldblum OM, Kraus E. Bronner AK. Pseudo-Kaposi's sarcoma of the hand associated with an acquired, iatrogenic arteriovenous fistula. *Arch Dermatol.* 1985; 121:1038–1040.

64. Mali JWH, Kuiper JP, Hamers AA. Acro-angiodermatitis of the foot. *Arch Dermatol.* 1965; 92:515–518.

65. Barsky SH, Rosen S, Geer DE, et al. The nature and evolution of port wine stains: a computer-assisted study. *J Invest Dermatol.* 1980; 74:154–157.

66. Lindenauer SM. The Klippel-Trenaunay syndrome: varicosity, hypertrophy and hemangioma with no arteriovenous fistula. *Ann Surg.* 1965; 162:303–314.

67. Finley JL, Noe JM, Arndt KA, et al. Port-wine stains: morphologic variations and developmental lesions. *Arch Dermatol.* 1984; 120:1453–1455.

68. Hashimoto K, Pritzker MS. Hereditary hemorrhagic telangiectasia: an electron microscopic study. *Oral Surg Oral Med Oral Pathol.* 1972; 34:751–768.

69. Wilkin JK, Smith JG Jr, Cullison DA, et al. Unilateral dermatomal superficial telangiectasia: nine new cases and a review of unilateral dermatomal superficial telangiectasia. *J Am Acad Dermatol.* 1983; 8:468–477.

70. McGrae JD Jr, Winkelmann RK. Generalized essential telangiectasia: report of a clinical and histochemical study of 13 patients with acquired cutaneous lesions. *JAMA.* 1963; 185:909–913.

71. Person JR, Longcope C. Estrogen and progesterone receptors are not increased in generalized essential telangiectasia. *Arch Dermatol.* 1985; 121:836–837.

72. Frain-Bell W. Angioma serpiginosum. *Br J Dermatol.* 1957; 69:251–268.

73. Stevenson JR, Lincoln CS Jr. Angioma serpiginosum. *Arch Dermatol.* 1967; 95:16–22.

74. Kumakiri M, Katoh N, Miura Y. Angioma serpiginosum. *J Cutan Pathol.* 1980; 7:410–421.

75. Chavaz P, Laugier P. Angiome serpigineux de Hutchinson: etude ultrastructurale. *Ann Dermatol Venereol.* 1981; 108:429–436.

76. Imperial R, Helwig EB. Angiokeratoma: a clinicopathological study. *Arch Dermatol.* 1967; 95:166–175.

77. Imperial R, Helwig EB. Angiokeratoma of the scrotum (Fordyce type). *J Urol.* 1967; 98:379–387.

78. Imperial R, Helwig EB. Angiokeratoma of the vulva. *Obstet Gynecol.* 1967; 29:307–312.

79. Jessen RT, Thompson S, Smith EB. Cobb syndrome. *Arch Dermatol.* 1977; 113:1587–1590.

80. Bean WB, Walsh JR. Venous lakes. *Arch Dermatol.* 1956; 74:459–463.

81. Epstein E, Novy FG Jr, Allington HV. Capillary aneurysms of the skin. *Arch Dermatol.* 1965; 91:335–340.

82. Weiner MA. Capillary aneurysms of the skin. *Arch Dermatol.* 1966; 93:670–673.

83. Weathers DR, Fine RM. Thombosed varix of oral cavity. *Arch Dermatol.* 1971; 104:427–430.

84. Clearkin KP, Enzinger FM. Intravascular papillary endothelial hyperplasia. *Arch Pathol Lab Med.* 1976; 100:441–444.

85. Amérigo J, Berry CL. Intravascular papillary endothelial hyperplasia in the skin and subcutaneous tissue. *Virchows Arch (A).* 1980; 387:81–90.

86. Hashimoto H, Daimaru Y, Enjoji M. Intravascular papillary endothelial hyperplasia: a clinicopathologic study of 91 cases. *Am J Dermatopathol.* 1983; 5:539–546.

87. Barr RJ, Graham JH, Sherwin LA. Intravascular papillary endothelial hyperplasia: a benign lesion mimicking angiosarcoma. *Arch Dermatol.* 1978; 114:723–726.

88. Reed CN, Cooper PH, Swerlick RA. Intravascular papillary endothelial hyperplasia: multiple lesions simulating Kaposi's sarcoma. *J Am Acad Dermatol.* 1984; 10:110–113.

89. Paslin DA. Localized primary cutaneous intravascular papillary endothelial hyperplasia. *J Am Acad Dermatol.* 1981; 4:316–318.

90. Kuo T, Gomez LG. Papillary endothelial proliferation in cystic lymphangiomas: a lymphatic vessel counterpart of Masson's vegetant intravascular hemangioendothelioma. *Arch Pathol Lab Med.* 1979; 103:306–308.

91. Heyden G, Dahl I, Angervall L. Intravascular papillary endothelial hyperplasia in the oral mucosa. *Oral Surg Oral Med Oral Pathol.* 1978; 45:83–87.

92. Escasany RT, Millet PU. Masson's pseudoangiosarcoma of the tongue: report of two cases. *J Cutan Pathol.* 1985; 12:66–71.

93. Salyer WR, Salyer DC. Intravascular angiomatosis: development and distinction from angiosarcoma. *Cancer.* 1975; 36:995–1001.

94. Kreutner A Jr, Smith RM, Trefny FA. Intravascular papillary endothelial hyperplasia: light and electron microscopic observations of a case. *Cancer.* 1978; 42:2304–2310.

95. Peterson WC Jr, Fusaro RM, Goltz RW. Atypical pyogenic granuloma: a case of benign hemangioendotheliosis. *Arch Dermatol.* 1964; 90:197–201.

96. Wilson Jones E, Bleehen SS. Inflammatory angiomatous nodules with abnormal blood vessels occurring about the ears and scalp (pseudo or atypical pyogenic granuloma). *Br J Dermatol.* 1969; 81:804–816.

97. Wells GC, Whimster IW. Subcutaneous angiolymphoid hyperplasia with eosinophilia. *Br J Dermatol.* 1969; 81:1–15.

98. Mehregan AH, Shapiro L. Angiolymphoid hyperplasia with eosinophilia. *Arch Dermatol.* 1971; 103:50–57.

99. Reed RJ, Terazakis N. Subcutaneous angioblastic lymphoid hyperplasia with eosinophilia (Kimura's disease). *Cancer.* 1972; 29:489–497.

100. Castro C, Winkelmann RK. Angiolymphoid hyperplasia with eosinophilia in the skin. *Cancer.* 1974; 34:1696–1705.

101. Olsen TG, Helwig EB. Angiolymphoid hyperplasia with eosinophilia: a clinicopathologic study of 116 patients. *J Am Acad Dermatol.* 1985; 12:781–796.

102. Wilson Jones E, Marks R. Papular angioplasia: vascular papules of the face and scalp simulating malignant vascular tumors. *Arch Dermatol.* 1970; 102:422–427.

103. Rosai J, Akerman LR. Intravenous atypical vascular proliferation: a cutaneous lesion simulating a malignant blood vessel tumor. *Arch Dermatol.* 1974; 109:714–717.

104. Rosai J, Gold J, Landy R. The histiocytoid hemangiomas: a unifying concept embracing several previously described entities of skin, soft tissue, large vessels, bone, and heart. *Hum Pathol.* 1979; 10:707–730.

105. Rosai J. Angiolymphoid hyperplasia with eosinophilia of the skin: its nosological position in the spectrum of histiocytoid hemangioma. *Am J Dermatopathol.* 1982; 4:175–184.

106. Weiss SW, Enzinger FM. Epithelioid hemangioendothelioma: a vascular tumor often mistaken for a carcinoma. *Cancer.* 1982; 50:970–981.

107. Ishak KG, Sesterhenn IA, Goodman ZD, et al. Epithelioid hemangioendothelioma of the liver: a clinicopathologic and follow-up study of 32 cases. *Hum Pathol.* 1984; 15:839–852.

108. Tsuneyoshi M, Dorfman HD, Bauer TW. Epithelioid hemangioendothelioma of bone: a clinicopathologic, ultrastructural, and immunohistochemical study. *Am J Surg Pathol.* 1986; 10:754–764.

109. Kung ITM, Gibson JB, Bannatyne PM. Kimura's disease: a clinico-pathological study of 21 cases and its distinction from angiolymphoid hyperplasia with eosinophilia. *Pathology.* 1984; 16:39–44.

109a. Urabe A, Tsuneyoshi M, Enjoji M. Epithelioid hemangioma versus Kimura's disease: a comparative clinicopathologic study. *Am J Surg Pathol.* 1987; 11:758–766.

110. Massa MC, Fretzin DF, Chowdhury L, et al. Angiolymphoid hyperplasia demonstrating extensive skin and mucosal lesions controlled with vinblastine therapy. *J Am Acad Dermatol.* 1984; 11:333–339.

111. Moesner J, Pallesen R, Sorensen B. Angiolymphoid hyperplasia with eosinophilia (Kimura's disease): a case with dermal lesions in the knee region and a popliteal arteriovenous fistula. *Arch Dermatol.* 1981; 117:650–653.

112. Angervall L, Kindblom L-G, Karlsson K, et al. Atypical hemangioendothelioma of venous origin: a clinicopathologic angiographic, immunohistochemical, and ultrastructural study of two endothelial tumors within the concept of histiocytoid hemangioma. *Am J Surg Pathol.* 1985; 9:504–516.

113. Daniels DG, Schrodt GR, Fliegelman MT, et al. Ultrastructural study of a case of angiolymphoid hyperplasia with eosinophilia. *Arch Dermatol.* 1974; 109:870–872.

114. Eady RAJ, Wilson Jones E. Pseudopyogenic granuloma: enzyme histochemical and ultrastructural study. *Hum Pathol.* 1977; 8:653–668.

115. Wright DH, Padley NR, Judd MA. Angiolymphoid hyperplasia with eosinophilia simulating lymphadenopathy. *Histopathology.* 1981; 5:127–140.

116. Ose D, Vollmer R, Shelburne J, et al. Histiocytoid hemangioma of the skin and scapula: a case report with electron microscopy and immunohistochemistry. *Cancer.* 1983; 51:1656–1662.

117. Srigley JR, Ayala AG, Ordóñez NG, et al. Epithelioid hemangioma of the penis. A rare and distinctive vascular lesion. *Arch Pathol Lab Med.* 1985; 109:51–54.

117a. Le Boit P, Berger T, Egbert B, et al. Atypical cutaneous vascular proliferations in patients with AIDS are associated with the cat scratch disease bacillus. Presented at the annual meeting of the United States and Canadian Academy of Pathology (abstract 314); March 1, 1988; Washington, DC.

117b. Weiss SW, Enzinger FM. Spindle cell hemangioendothelioma: a low-grade angiosarcoma resembling a cavernous hemangioma and Kaposi's sarcoma. *Am J Surg Pathol.* 1986; 10:521–530.

117c. Scott GA, Rosai J. Spindle cell hemangioendothelioma: report of seven additional cases of a recently described vascular neoplasm. *Am J Dermatopathol.* 1988; 10:281–288.

118. Masson P. Le glomus neuromyo-artériel des régions tactiles et ses tumeurs. *Lyon Chir.* 1924; 21:257–280.

119. Bailey OT. The cutaneous glomus and its tumors—glomangiomas. *Am J Pathol.* 1935; 11:915–935.

120. Stout AP. Tumors of the neuromyo-arterial glomus. *Am J Cancer.* 1935; 24:255–272.

121. Shugart RR, Soule EH, Johnson EW Jr. Glomus tumor. *Surg Gynecol Obstet.* 1963; 117:334–340.

122. Tsuneyoshi M, Enjoji M. Glomus tumor: a clinicopathologic and electron microscopic study. *Cancer.* 1982; 50:1601–1607.

123. Kohout E, Stout AP. The glomus tumor in children. *Cancer.* 1961; 14:555–566.

124. Tarnowski WM, Hashimoto K. Multiple glomus tumors: an ultrastructural study. *J Invest Dermatol.* 1969; 52:474–478.

125. Venkatachalam MA, Greally JG. Fine structure of glomus tumor: similarity of glomus cells to smooth muscle. *Cancer.* 1969; 23:1176–1184.

126. Conant MA, Wiesenfeld SL. Multiple glomus tumors of the skin. *Arch Dermatol.* 1971; 103:481–485.

127. Goodman TF, Abele DC. Multiple glomus tumors: a clinical and electron microscopic study. *Arch Dermatol.* 1971; 103:11–23.

128. McEvoy BF, Waldman PM, Tye MJ. Multiple hamartomatous glomus tumors of the skin. *Arch Dermatol.* 1971; 104:188–191.

129. Pepper MC, Laubenheimer R, Cripps DJ. Multiple glomus tumors. *J Cutan Pathol.* 1977; 4:244–257.

130. Murata Y, Tsuji M, Tani M. Ultrastructure of multiple glomus tumor. *J Cutan Pathol.* 1984; 11:53–58.

131. Wood JH. Vascular tumors of the skin. In: Helwig EB, Mostofi FK, eds. *The Skin.* Baltimore, Md: Williams & Wilkins; 1971.

132. Murad TM, von Haam E, Murthy MSN. Ultrastructure of a hemangiopericytoma and a glomus tumor. *Cancer.* 1968; 22:1239–1249.

133. Harris M. Ultrastructure of a glomus tumour. *J Clin Pathol.* 1971; 24:520–523.

134. Miettinen M, Lehto V-P, Virtanen I. Glomus tumor cells: evaluation of smooth muscle and endothelial cell properties. *Virchows Arch (B).* 1983; 43:139–149.

135. Goodman TF. Fine structure of the cells of the Suquet-Hoyer canal. *J Invest Dermatol.* 1972; 59:363–369.

136. Brooks JJ, Miettinen M, Virtanen I. Desmin immunoreactivity in glomus tumors. *Am J Clin Pathol.* 1987; 87:292.

137. McMaster MJ, Soule EH, Ivins JC. Hemangiopericytoma: a clinicopathologic study and long-term followup of 60 patients. *Cancer.* 1975; 36:2232–2244.

138. Enzinger FM, Smith BH. Hemangiopericytoma: an analysis of 106 cases. *Hum Pathol.* 1976; 7:61–82.

139. Cox FH, Helwig EB. Kaposi's sarcoma. *Cancer.* 1959; 12:289–298.

140. Reynolds WA, Winkelmann RK, Soule EH. Kaposi's sarcoma: a clinicopathologic study with particular reference to its relationship to the reticuloendothelial system. *Medicine.* 1965; 44:419–443.

141. Templeton AC. Kaposi's sarcoma. *Pathol Annu.* 1981; 16:315–336.

142. Gottlieb GJ, Ackerman AB. Kaposi's sarcoma: an extensively disseminated form in young homosexual men. *Hum Pathol.* 1982; 13:882–892.

143. Safai B, Johnson KG, Myskowski PL, et al. The natural history of Kaposi's sarcoma in the acquired immunodeficiency syndrome. *Ann Intern Med.* 1985; 103:744–750.

144. Moskowitz LB, Hensley GT, Gould EW, et al. Frequency and anatomic distribution of lymphadenopathic Kaposi's sarcoma in the acquired immunodeficiency syndrome: an autopsy series. *Hum Pathol.* 1985; 16:447–456.

145. Niedt GW, Schinella RA. Acquired immunodeficiency syn-

drome: clinicopathologic study of 56 autopsies. *Arch Pathol Lab Med.* 1985; 109:727–734.

146. Lemlich G, Schwam L, Lebwohl M. Kaposi's sarcoma and acquired immunodeficiency syndrome: postmortem findings in twenty-four cases. *J Am Acad Dermatol.* 1987; 16:319–325.

147. Penn I. Kaposi's sarcoma in organ transplant recipients: report of 20 cases. *Transplantation.* 1979; 27:8–11.

148. Ulbright TM, Santa Cruz DJ. Kaposi's sarcoma: relationship with hematologic, lymphoid, and thymic neoplasia. *Cancer.* 1981; 47:963–973.

149. O'Connell KM. Kaposi's sarcoma: histopathological study of 159 cases from Malawi. *J Clin Pathol.* 1977; 30:687–695.

150. Blumenfeld W, Egbert BM, Sagebiel RW. Differential diagnosis of Kaposi's sarcoma. *Arch Pathol Lab Med.* 1985; 109:123–127.

151. Francis ND, Parkin JM, Weber J, et al. Kaposi's sarcoma in acquired immune deficiency syndrome (AIDS). *J Clin Pathol.* 1986; 39:469–474.

152. Purdy LJ, Colby TV, Yousem SA, et al. Pulmonary Kaposi's sarcoma: premortem histologic diagnosis. *Am J Surg Pathol.* 1986; 10:301–311.

153. Gange RW, Wilson Jones E. Lymphangioma-like Kaposi's sarcoma: a report of three cases. *Br J Dermatol.* 1979; 100:327–334.

154. McNutt NS, Fletcher V, Conant MA. Early lesions of Kaposi's sarcoma in homosexual men: an ultrastructural comparison with other vascular proliferations in skin. *Am J Pathol.* 1983; 111:62–77.

155. Hashimoto K, Lever WF, Kaposi's sarcoma: histochemical and electron microscopic studies. *J Invest Dermatol.* 1964; 43:539–549.

156. Niemi M, Mustakallio KK. The fine structure of the spindle cell in Kaposi's sarcoma. *Acta Pathol Microbiol Scand.* 1965; 63:567–575.

157. Mottaz JH, Zelickson AS. Electron microscope observations of Kaposi's sarcoma. *Acta Derm Venereol* 1966; 46:195–200.

158. Braun-Falco O, Schmoeckel C, Hübner G. Zur Histogenese des Sarcoma idiopathicum multiplex haemorrhagicum (Morbus Kaposi): eine histochemische und elektronenmikroskopische Studie. *Virchows Arch (A).* 1976; 369:215–227.

159. Sterry W, Steigleder G-K, Bodeux E. Kaposi's sarcoma: venous capillary haemangioblastoma: a histochemical and ultrastructural study. *Arch Dermatol Res.* 1979; 266:253–267.

160. Akhtar M, Bunuan H, Ali MA, et al. Kaposi's sarcoma in renal transplant recipients: ultrastructural and immunoperoxidase study of four cases. *Cancer.* 184; 53:258–266.

161. Bendelac A, Kanitakis J, Chouvet B, et al. Basement membrane in Kaposi's sarcoma: an immunohistochemical and ultrastructural study. *Pathol Res Pract.* 1985; 180:626–632.

162. Leu HJ, Odermatt B. Multicentric angiosarcoma (Kaposi's sarcoma): light and electron microscopic and immunohistological findings of idiopathic cases in Europe and Africa and of cases associated with AIDS. *Virchows Arch (A).* 1985; 408:29–41.

163. Guarda LG, Silva EG, Ordóñez NG, et al. FActor VIII in Kaposi's sarcoma. *Am J Clin Pathol.* 1981; 76:197–200.

164. Nadji M, Morales AR, Ziegles-Weissman J, et al. Kaposi's sarcoma: immunohistologic evidence for an endothelial origin. *Arch Pathol Lab Med.* 1981; 105:274–275.

165. Modlin RL, Hofman FM, Kempf RA, et al. Kaposi's sarcoma in homosexual men: an immunohistochemical study. *J Am Acad Dermatol.* 1983; 8:620–627.

166. Flotte TJ, Hatcher VA, Friedman-Kien AE. Factor VIII-related antigen in Kaposi's sarcoma in young homosexual men. *Arch Dermatol.* 1984; 120:180–182.

167. Beckstead JH, Wood GS, Fletcher V. Evidence for the origin of Kaposi's sarcoma from lymphatic endothelium. *Am J Pathol.* 1985; 119:294–300.

168. Kramer RH, Fuh G-M, Hwang CBC, et al. Basement membrane and connective tissue proteins in early lesions of Kaposi's sarcoma associated with AIDS. *J Invest Dermatol.* 1985; 84:516–520.

169. Russell Jones R, Spaull J, Spry C, et al. Histogenesis of Kaposi's sarcoma in patients with and without acquired immune deficiency syndrome (AIDS). *J Clin Pathol.* 1986; 39:742–749.

170. Rutgers JL, Wieczorek R, Bonetti F, et al. The expression of endothelial cell surface antigens by AIDS-associated Kaposi's sarcoma: evidence for a vascular endothelial cell origin. *Am J Pathol.* 1986; 122:493–499.

171. Wilson Jones E. Malignant angioendothelioma of the skin. *Br J Dermatol.* 1964; 76:21–39.

172. Reed RJ, Palomeque FE, Hairston MA III, et al. Lymphangiosarcomas of the scalp. *Arch Dermatol.* 1966; 94:396–402.

173. Rosai J, Sumner HW, Kostianovsky M, et al. Angiosarcoma of the skin: a clinicopathologic and fine structural study. *Hum Pathol.* 1976; 7:83–109.

174. Hodgkinson DJ, Soule EH, Woods JE. Cutaneous angiosarcoma of the head and neck. *Cancer.* 1979; 44:1106–1113.

175. Maddox JC, Evans HL. Angiosarcoma of skin and soft tissue: a study of forty-four cases. *Cancer* 1981; 48:1907–1921.

176. Cooper PH. Angiosarcomas of the skin. *Semin Diagn Pathol.* 1987; 4:2–17.

177. Holden CA, Spittle MF, Wilson Jones E. Angiosarcoma of the face and scalp, prognosis and treatment. *Cancer.* 1987; 59:1046–1057.

178. Stewart FW, Treves N. Lymphangiosarcoma in postmastectomy lymphedema: a report of six cases in elephantiasis chirurgica. *Cancer.* 1948; 1:64–81.

179. Herrmann JB. Lumphangiosarcoma of the chronically edematous extremity. *Surg Gynecol Obstet.* 1965; 121:1107–1115.

180. Eby CS, Brennan MJ, Fine G. Lymphangiosarcoma: a lethal complication of chronic lymphedema: report of two cases and review of the literature. *Arch Surg.* 1967; 94:223–230.

181. Woodward AH, Ivins JC, Soule EH. Lymphangiosarcoma arising in chronic lymphedematous extremities. *Cancer.* 1972; 30:562–572.

182. Dubin HV, Creehan EP, Headington JT. Lymphangiosarcoma and congenital lymphedema of the extremity. *Arch Dermatol.* 1974; 110:608–614.

183. Laskas JJ Jr, Shelley WB, Wood MG. Lymphangiosarcoma arising in congenital lymphedema. *Arch Dermatol.* 1975; 111:86–89.

184. Sordillo PP, Chapman R, Hajdu SI, et al. Lymphangiosarcoma. *Cancer.* 1981; 48:1674–1679.

185. Muller R, Hajdu SI, Brennan MF. Lymphangiosarcoma associated with chronic filarial lymphedema. *Cancer.* 1987; 59:179–183.

186. Goette DK, Detlefs RL. Postirradiation angiosarcoma. *J Am Acad Dermatol.* 1985; 12:922–926.

187. Silverberg SG, Kay S, Koss LG. Postmastectomy lymphangiosarcoma: ultrastructural observations. *Cancer.* 1971; 27:100–108.

188. Miettinen M, Lehto V-P, Virtanen I. Postmastectomy angiosarcoma (Stewart-Treves syndrome): light-microscopic, immunohistological, and ultrastructural characteristics of two cases. *Am J Surg Pathol.* 1983; 7:329–339.

189. Capo V, Ozzello L, Fenoglio CM, et al. Angiosarcomas arising in edematous extremities: immunostaining for factor VIII-related antigen and ultrastructural features. *Hum Pathol.* 1985; 16:144–150.

190. Guarda LA, Ordonez NG, Smith JL Jr, et al. Immunoperoxidase localization of factor VIII in angiosarcomas. *Arch Pathol Lab Med.* 1982; 106:515–516.

191. Ordonez NG, Batsakis JG. Comparison of *Ulex europaeus* I lectin and factor VIII-related antigen in vascular lesions. *Arch Pathol Lab Med.* 1984; 108:129–132.

192. Holden CA, Spaull J, Das AK, et al. The histogenesis of angio-sarcoma of the face and scalp: an immunohistochemical and ultrastructural study. *Histopathology*. 1987; 11:37–51.

193. Dabska M. Malignant endovascular papillary angioendotheli-oma of the skin in childhood: clinicopathologic study of 6 cases. *Cancer*. 1969; 24:503–510.

194. de Dulanto F, Armijo-Moreno M. Malignant endovascular papillary hemangioendothelioma of the skin: the nosological situation. *Acta Derm Venereol*. 1973; 53:403–408.

195. Patterson K, Chandra RS. Malignant endovascular papillary angioendothelioma: cutaneous borderline tumor. *Arch Pathol Lab Med*. 1985; 109:671–673.

196. Manivel JC, Wick MR, Swanson PE, et al. Endovascular papil-lary angioendothelioma of childhood: a vascular lesion possi-bly characterized by "high" endothelial cell differentiation. *Hum Pathol*. 1986; 17:1240–1244.

197. Pfleger L, Tappeiner J, Zur Kenntnis der systemisierten En-dotheliomatose der cutanen Blutgefässe (Reticuloendothe-liose?). *Hautarzt*. 1959; 10:359–363.

198. Braverman IM, Lerner AB. Diffuse malignant proliferation of vascular endothelium: a possible new clinical and patholog-ical entity. *Arch Dermatol*. 1961; 84:72–80.

199. Petito CK, Gottlieb GJ, Dougherty JH, et al. Neoplastic an-gioendotheliosis: ultrastructural study and review of the litera-ture. *Ann Neurol*. 1978; 3:393–399.

200. Wick MR, Scheithauer BW, Okazaki H, et al. Cerebral angio-endotheliomatosis. *Arch Pathol Lab Med*. 1982; 106:342–346.

201. Fulling KH, Gersell DJ. Neoplastic angioendotheliomatosis: histologic, immunohistochemical, and ultrastructural findings in two cases. *Cancer*. 1983; 51:1107–1118.

202. Bhawan J, Wolff SM, Ucci AA, et al. Malignant lymphoma and malignant angioendotheliomatosis: one disease. *Cancer*. 1985; 55:570–576.

203. Kitagawa M, Matsubara O, Song S-Y, et al. Neoplastic an-gioendotheliosis: immunohistochemical and electron micro-scopic findings in three cases. *Cancer*. 1985; 56:1134–1143.

204. Mori S, Itoyama S, Mohri N, et al. Cellular characteristics of neoplastic angioendotheliosis: an immunohistochemical marker study of 6 cases. *Virchows Arch (A)*. 1985; 407:167–175.

205. Wrotnowski U, Mills SE, Cooper PH. Malignant angioendo-theliomatosis: an angiotropic lymphoma? *Am J Clin Pathol*. 1985; 83:244–248.

206. Carroll TJ Jr, Schelper RL, Goeken JA, et al. Neoplastic an-gioendotheliomatosis: immunopathologic and morphologic evidence for intravascular malignant lymphomatosis. *Am J Clin Pathol*. 1986; 85:169–175.

207. Sheibani K, Battifora H, Winberg CD, et al. Further evidence that "malignant angioendotheliomatosis" is an angiotropic large-cell lymphoma. *N Engl J Med*. 1986; 314:943–948.

208. Wick MR, Mills SE, Scheithauer BW, et al. Reassessment of malignant "angioendotheliomatosis": evidence in favor of its reclassification as "intravascular lymphomatosis." *Am J Surg Pathol*. 1986; 10:112–123.

209. Bhawan J. Angioendotheliomatosis proliferans systemisata: an angiotropic neoplasm of lymphoid origin. *Semin Diagn Pa-thol*. 1987; 4:18–27.

210. Ruiter M, Mandema E. New cutaneous syndrome in subacute bacterial endocarditis. *Arch Intern Med*. 1964; 113:283–290.

211. Pasyk K, Depowski M. Proliferating systemetized angioendo-theliomatosis of a 5-month-old infant. *Arch Dermatol*. 1978; 114:1512–1515.

212. Martin S, Pitcher D, Tschen J, et al. Reactive angioendothe-liomatosis. *J Am Acad Dermatol*. 1980; 2:117–123.

213. Wick MR, Rocamora A. Reactive and malignant "angioendo-theliomatosis": a discriminant clinicopathologic study. *J Cutan Pathol*. 1988; 15:260–271.

214. Scott PWB, Silvers DN, Helwig EB. Proliferating angioendo-theliomatosis. *Arch Pathol*. 1975; 99:323–326.

215. Ansell J, Bhawan J, Cohen S, et al. Histiocytic lymphoma and malignant angioendotheliomatosis: one disease or two? *Cancer*. 1982; 50:1506–1512.

CHAPTER 53

Tumors with Smooth Muscle Differentiation

Karen A. Sherwood and Marc D. Chalet

Tumors with smooth muscle differentiation may present in the dermis or subcutaneous tissue as hamartomas or benign or malignant neoplasms. The location of the lesion depends on the muscle in which it arises. The more superficial dermal neoplasms arise from the arrectores pilorum or genital smooth muscle, and are discernible from the surrounding stroma, but are less well circumscribed than the somewhat deeper neoplasms that arise in vascular smooth muscle.

SMOOTH MUSCLE HAMARTOMAS

Clinical Features
Smooth muscle hamartomas represent a hyperplasia of the arrectores pilorum. Although rarely reported, they may be more common than currently believed.[1] Clinically, these lesions have been noted at birth[2-9] except one.[10] They appear as large indurated macules or plaques (2–10 cm in diameter or larger).[5,10,11] Some may develop perifollicular papules,[3,4] hyperpigmentation,[4-6,9] or hypertrichosis.[3,4] The total number of hairs within the lesion is not actually increased, but the hairs do appear both thicker and longer.[3] On stroking, the lesions may become transiently elevated (pseudo-Darier's sign) or exhibit vermiform movement.[4-6,9] Smooth muscle hamartomas are located primarily on the trunk, especially the lumbosacral area, and also on the extremities. No treatment is necessary. With time, the hyperpigmentation, prominent hair, and induration all diminish.[8] Becker's nevi have been associated with smooth muscle hamartomas. They develop in the second decade of life, usually in the deltoid region. Initially, the area becomes hyperpigmented. This is followed by hypertrichosis. On histologic examination, acanthosis, elongation of the rete ridges, and hyperpigmentation of the basal cell layer are noted. Occasionally, smooth muscle hyperplasia is also found.[7]

Histologic Features
There is hyperplasia of the smooth muscle bundles in the dermis. The bundles are well circumscribed, oriented in varying directions, and exhibit a characteristic clear space (Fig. 53–1) separating them from the surrounding collagen.[2,3,8] In some areas, the bundles are arranged around a hair follicle. In cases with hyperpigmentation, increased epidermal melanin pigment is also noted.

In smooth muscle hamartoma the smooth muscle bundles are more sharply demarcated than those of the piloleiomyoma. The muscle bundles may be separated from one another by varying amounts of collagen, but the characteristic clear spaces seen in smooth muscle hamartoma are not present in the piloleiomyoma.

LEIOMYOMAS

Clinical Features
Leiomyomas are benign neoplasms of smooth muscle. The cutaneous leiomyomas may be subdivided into three groups depending on the site of origin, be it arrectores pilorum, genital, or vascular smooth muscle. Piloleiomyomas are the most common cutaneous smooth muscle tumors. They may be solitary, but usually are multiple. Multifocal familial piloleiomyomas have been reported in several generations,[12] twins,[13] and siblings.[14] The pattern of inheritance is believed to be autosomal dominant with incomplete penetrance.[15] These tumors arise in the second and third decades of life and are slow growing. Clinically, they appear as small intradermal nodules without overlying epidermal change. They are located on the trunk and the extremities, predominantly the extensor surfaces. Piloleiomyomas may attain a size of 2 cm in diameter. Pain, a common symptom, may be induced by pressure, change in temperature, or sexual excitation.[16] In larger lesions there is histologic evidence that the neoplasm compresses peripheral nerves[12,17] supporting the concept that pain is initiated by direct tumor compression of nerve fibers. Electron microscopy of painful lesions has demonstrated that the myelin sheath of associated peripheral nerves may be distorted, disrupted, or absent.[18] In a nonpainful tumor, the nerve was noted to be unaltered.[12]

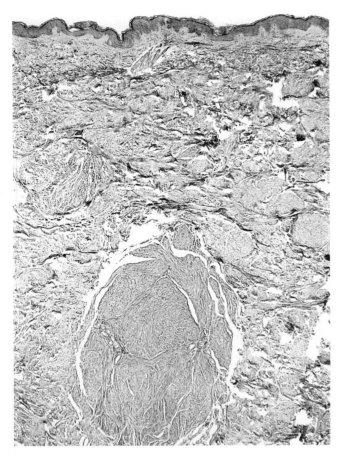

Figure 53–1. A smooth muscle hamartoma consisting of well-circumscribed muscle bundles arranged in varying directions and exhibiting a clear space separating the bundles from the surrounding collagen. (H&E, ×20.) (*Courtesy of J. Wollman, M.D., Pathology Service, Wadsworth VA Medical Center.*)

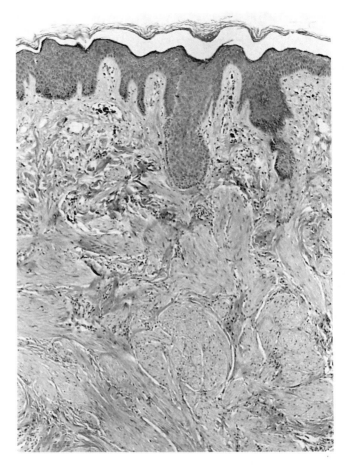

Figure 53–2. Piloleiomyoma composed of closely arranged muscle fascicles that are separated from each other by the surrounding collagen at the periphery of the lesion. (H&E, ×40.) (*Courtesy of J. Wollman, M.D., Pathology Service, Wadsworth VA Medical Center.*)

Association with uterine leiomyomas has been documented, but this is probably coincidental given the relatively frequent occurrence of uterine leiomyomas in the general population (1 of 10 women).[19] The neoplasms may be surgically removed if symptomatic. Numerous lesions or a large area of involvement, however, may preclude surgical intervention. Pain control has been achieved with oral administration of benoxybenzamide or nifedipine.[20]

Histologic Features

The neoplasm, composed primarily of spindle-shaped cells, is present in the dermis. The dermis contains individual fascicles of smooth muscle fibers that are closely arranged but not necessarily contiguous, especially at the periphery of the lesion where the fascicles may be separated by the surrounding collagen (Fig. 53–2). The neoplasm is therefore discrete, but is neither necessarily well circumscribed nor encapsulated. The muscle fibers are elongated, are more eosinophilic than the surrounding collagen, and have elongated nuclei, which are blunt tipped. These nuclei have been described as "eel-like"[21] or "cigar-shaped."

When fascicles are seen on end (in cross section), the nuclei are placed centrally within the muscle fibers and perinuclear vacuolization is noted (Figs. 53–3, 53–4). They can be further distinguished with special stains. Phosphotungstic acid–hematoxylin and Masson's trichrome stain muscle blue, purple and red, respectively.

Immunocytochemical staining with immunoperoxidase is more useful than immunofluorescent staining techniques. The purified rabbit anti-chicken gizzard myosin antibody (RAMA) identifies both benign and malignant smooth muscle tumors. Creatine phosphokinase (CPK) isoenzyme assays are used to differentiate skeletal muscle from smooth muscle. In all smooth muscle neoplasms the predominance of the smooth muscle component is demonstrated by a skeletal muscle:smooth muscle ratio of less than 0.05. This is both sensitive and specific.[22]

Electron microscopy reveals abundant, fine actin filaments in smooth muscle cells as well as in myoepithelial cells and myofibroblasts. Smooth muscle is characterized by abundant actin filaments which aggregate into dense bodies.[18,23] Numerous pinocytotic vesicles are located near

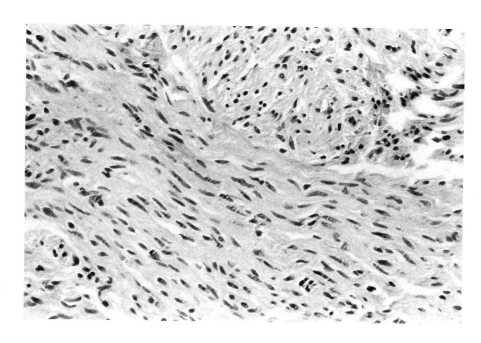

Figure 53–3. A piloleiomyoma with muscle fascicles arranged both longitudinally and in cross section (top right). The perinuclear vacuolization characteristic of smooth muscle when seen in cross section is prominent here. (H&E, ×200.) (*Courtesy of J. Wollman, M.D., Pathology Service, Wadsworth VA Medical Center.*)

the plasma membrane. The cell is surrounded by a continuous basal lamina. Rough endoplasmic reticulum (RER) is sparse or absent. The absence of rough endoplasmic reticulum distinguishes the smooth muscle cell from the myofibroblast.[23]

GENITAL LEIOMYOMAS

Genital leiomyomas occur on the scrotum, labia majora, and areola. They appear as small solitary intradermal nodules. Pain is not a clinical feature of these lesions. The site of origin is the dartoic muscle in the scrotum and labia and the mammary erectile muscle in the areola. Histopathologically the tumor is identical to the leiomyoma of the arrectores pilorum muscle.[24]

ANGIOLEIOMYOMAS

Clinical Features

Angioleiomyomas are small, solitary, slow-growing intradermal or subcutaneous nodules that usually arise on the

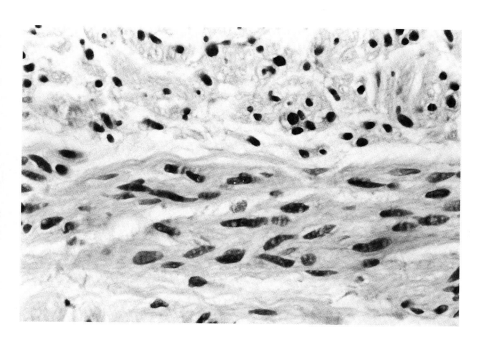

Figure 53–4. A high-power view of a muscle bundle showing the plump, elongated, blunt-tipped nuclei characteristic of smooth muscle. On cross section, the perinuclear vacuolization is again noted. (H&E, ×400.) (*Courtesy of J. Wollman, M.D., Pathology Service, Wadsworth VA Medical Center.*)

lower extremity.[25] Infrequently they occur on the upper extremity and trunk, and rarely they have been reported to occur in the oral cavity.[26,27] The peak incidence occurs between the fourth and sixth decades of life. Women are more frequently affected than men (female:male ratio of 2:1).[12] In half of the cases, pain is a presenting symptom.

Histologic Features

Angioleiomyomas are found in the subcutaneous tissue, but may be located in the deep dermis. They are sharply demarcated, solitary nodules that are separated from the surrounding dermis by a thin band of compressed connective tissue. The neoplasm contains numerous blood vessels. Originating from the muscular walls of the vessels are smooth muscle fibers arranged in orderly concentric layers. The vessel lumina are small and rounded, slitlike, or stellate[28] and they are lined by a single layer of endothelial cells. The muscle fibers extend tangentially from the vessels and merge with the surrounding muscular stroma (Fig. 53–5). Hyalinization, myxoid degeneration, and fat may rarely be present in the stroma.[24] The vessel of origin is thought to be a vein, as it lacks both an internal and an external elastic lamina.[29] Nerve fibers are not a prominent histologic feature, yet some authors think that it is the compression of nerves that causes the associated pain.[17] Ischemia produced by vessel constriction is another theory that has been postulated to account for the occurrence of pain in these lesions.[28]

Electron microscopy of angioleiomyomas demonstrates the same features seen in piloleiomyomas.

Differential Diagnosis

Dermatofibromas differ from leiomyomas in that the nodule present in the dermis is composed centrally of new amphophilic collagen. At the periphery, the fibrosing inflammatory process entraps more mature eosinophilic collagen bundles. Fibroblasts are present in the nodule as spindle-shaped cells, whose nuclei both are shorter than those of the leiomyomas and are tapered at their ends. The overlying epidermis is hyperplastic and often hyperpigmented. Neurofibromas may be differentiated from piloleiomyomas because the surrounding stroma in these lesions is loosely arranged and amphophilic. In addition, neurofibromas have spindle-shaped cells with nuclei that are curved, wavy, or S-shaped and have tapered ends. Scattered mast cells are present as well in the neurofibromas.[21]

LEIOMYOSARCOMAS

Clinical Features

Superficial leiomyosarcomas are extremely rare neoplasms. They may be subdivided into two types by location; **cutaneous leiomyosarcoma**, which arises from the arrectores pilorum or the dartoic muscle of genital skin,[30] and **subcutaneous leiomyosarcoma**, which arises from muscle of arterioles and veins of the subcutaneous tissue.[31] They are generally located on the extremities, usually the proximal lower extremity. Other areas of involvement include the head and neck,[32] torso,[33] and more rarely the scrotum,[34,35] labia majora,[36] areola,[37] and penis.[38] Superficial leiomyosarcomas present between the ages of 60 and 70[39]; however, they may occur in younger patients, even neonates.[32] A male:female ratio of 2:1 has been noted.[39] If multiple nodules exist, metastases from an abdominal or retroperitoneal primary neoplasm must be considered.[39] Trauma,[40] and ionizing radiation[41] have been cited as predisposing factors. One reported case arose in a chronic stasis ulcer.[42] Clinically, both appear as solitary, slow-growing nodules. The cutaneous tumors are smaller, attaining a size of up to 6 cm in diameter, whereas subcutaneous leiomyosarcomas may attain a size up to 13 cm in diameter. Discoloration has been noted more frequently in cutaneous neoplasms, whereas subcutaneous neoplasms tend to be painful. Both may ex-

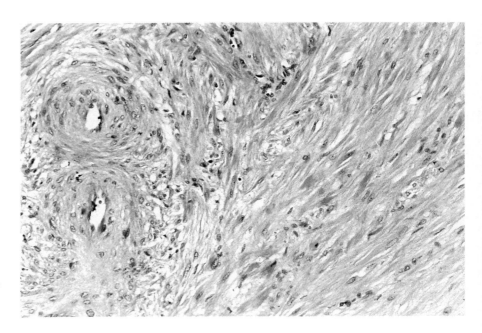

Figure 53–5. Within an angioleiomyoma small blood vessels with muscular walls merge with surrounding muscle fascicles of the neoplasm. (H&E, ×200.) *(Courtesy of J. Wollman, M.D., Pathology Service, Wadsworth VA Medical Center.)*

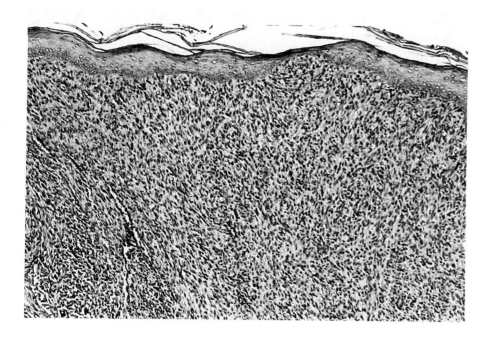

Figure 53–6. Highly cellular and irregular fascicles replace the reticular and papillary dermis in this section of a cutaneous leiomyosarcoma. (H&E, ×100.) (*Courtesy of the California Tumor Tissue Registry.*)

hibit epidermal changes such as ulceration, scaling, and crusting.[40] Superficial leiomyosarcomas have a good prognosis compared with leiomyosarcomas arising in deeper soft tissues, retroperitoneum, gastrointestinal tract, genitourinary tract and large blood vessels. There is potential for local recurrence (40% to 60%)[40,43] and metastasis. The frequency with which metastases occur is directly related to the depth of tumor extension. The reported metastatic rate for cutaneous leiomyosarcomas is 10%,[39] whereas that for subcutaneous leiomyosarcomas is 33% to 40%.[39,40] In one study, neoplasms confined to the dermis did not metastasize.[40] The most common site for metastasis is the lung (secondary to hematogenous spread) followed by the regional lymph nodes.[44,45]

The most important prognostic factor in one series[39] was the initial surgery where early wide local excision proved to be curative. If the neoplasms recur, they tend to be larger and to extend more deeply.[40]

Histologic Features

Cutaneous leiomyosarcomas are present in the dermis, and may penetrate the subcutaneous fat as well as occasionally ulcerate the overlying epidermis. Subcutaneous leiomyosarcomas are present in the superficial subcutaneous tissues with varying degrees of extension up into the lower reticular dermis. Both neoplasms are composed of highly cellular, poorly circumscribed fascicles of spindle-shaped cells (Fig. 53–6). The fascicles are arranged in irregular, interlacing bundles, often intersecting at right angles. The bundles are surrounded by a thin network of reticulin fibers, as are the cells.[39] The nuclei are elongated and blunt ended, and tend to align within the bundles in a palisaded fashion. The degree of differentiation may vary within one neoplasm. In the well-differentiated areas, the cells resemble the smooth muscle cells of leiomyomas. In poorly differentiated areas the nuclei appear more plump and have prominent nucleoli (Fig. 53–7).[40] The neoplasm contains bizarre

multinucleated giant cells in varying numbers scattered throughout the lesion, as well as numerous atypical mitoses. The neoplasm can be easily identified as differentiating toward muscle by staining with Masson's trichrome and hematoxylin-van Gieson, which stain muscle fibers red and yellow, respectively. Longitudinal intracytoplasmic myofibrils stain purple with phosphotungstic acid. In one study, subcutaneous leiomyosarcomas were found to be composed of atypical spindle cells arranged haphazardly throughout the neoplasm. Fascicular bundles tended to be absent. Endothelium-lined spaces surrounded by smooth muscle cells may be a feature that suggests differentiation toward vascular smooth muscle.[40]

In the past, the number of mitoses per high-power field (grading) was used as a criterion for determining biologic behavior or prognosis. It has been shown, however, that the number of mitoses present does not correlate well with the clinical prognosis.[40,46] Furthermore, scattered mitotic figures can be seen in benign leiomyomas.

Electron microscopy of leiomyosarcoma reveals fine actin filaments, dense bodies, and pinocytotic vesicles as seen in benign leiomyomas. The plasma membrane, however, is discontinuous and the nuclei are atypical.[47]

Differential Diagnosis

Atypical fibroxanthomas and malignant fibrous histiocytomas may be differentiated from cutaneous and subcutaneous leiomyosarcomas by the presence of polygonal cells, resembling histiocytes, admixed with spindle-shaped cells. The cytoplasm may be foamy or vacuolated. Bizarre multinucleated giant cells are present, and show more marked nuclear atypia than is seen in leiomyosarcomas. Occasionally, a storiform pattern is noted in malignant fibrous histiocytoma. Dermatofibrosarcoma protuberans is composed of cells with large spindle-shaped nuclei, arranged in "storiform" or "cartwheel" patterns. In spindle cell squamous cell carcinomas, continuity with the overlying epidermis

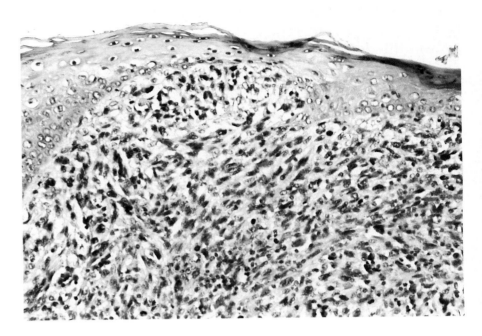

Figure 53–7. Marked nuclear pleomorphism and occasional multinucleated giant cells, in addition to the blunt-tipped elongated nuclei, characterize this leiomyosarcoma. The overlying epidermis is thinned in this section. Often, the overlying epidermis is ulcerated. (H&E, ×200.) (*Courtesy of the California Tumor Tissue Registry.*)

may be noted in addition to focal evidence of keratinization. Fibrosarcomas penetrate the subcutaneous tissues, muscle, and fascia. The cells are arranged in fascicles in a "herringbone" pattern. The nuclei are spindle-shaped and may appear thin in the well-differentiated lesions. In the more poorly differentiated lesions, the nuclei tend to be more plump and to demonstrate greater pleomorphism.[21]

REFERENCES

1. Metzker A, Merlob P: Congenital smooth muscle hamartoma. *J Am Acad Dermatol* 1986;14:691.
2. Berger TG, Levin MW: Congenital smooth muscle hamartoma. *J Am Acad Dermatol* 1984;11:709–712.
3. Tsambaos D, Orfanos CE: Cutaneous smooth muscle hamartoma. *J Cutan Pathol* 1982;9:33–42.
4. Stokes JH: Nevus pilaris with hyperplasia of nonstriated muscle. *Arch Dermatol Syphilol* 1923;7:479–481.
5. Kern F, Hambrick GW: Smooth muscle hamartoma. *Birth Defects* 1971;7:346–347.
6. Slifman NR, Harrist TJ, Rhodes AR: Congenital arrector pili hamartoma. *Arch Dermatol* 1985;121:1034–1037.
7. Urbanek WR, Johnson WC: Smooth muscle hamartoma associated with Becker's nevus. *Arch Dermatol* 1978;114:104–106.
8. Truhan AP, Esterly NB: Hypertrichotic skin-colored patches in an infant. *Arch Dermatol* 1985;121:1197.
9. Karo KR, Gange RW: Smooth-muscle hamartoma. *Arch Dermatol* 1981;117:678–679.
10. Wong RC, Solomon AR: Acquired dermal smooth-muscle hamartoma. *Cutis* 1985;35(4):369–370.
11. Metzker A, Amir J, Rotem A, et al.: Congenital smooth muscle hamartoma of the skin. *Pediatr Dermatol* 1984;2:45–48.
12. Chen-Chen JS, Zelman J, Toker C: Familial cutaneous leiomyomata: A case report with electron microscopic study. *Mt Sinai J Med* 1980;47(1):40–44.
13. Rudner JD, Schwartz OD, Grekin JH: Multiple cutaneous leiomyomas in identical twins. *Arch Dermatol* 1964;90:81–82.
14. Joliffe DS: Multiple cutaneous leiomyomata. *Clin Exp Dermatol* 1978;3(1):89–92.
15. Kloepfer HW, Krafchuk J, Derbes V, et al.: Hereditary multiple leiomyomas of the skin. *Am J Hum Genet* 1958;10:48.
16. Fox SR: Leiomyomatosis cutis. *N Engl J Med* 1960;263(24):1248–1250.
17. Montgomery H, Winklemann RK: Smooth-muscle tumors of the skin. *Arch Dermatol* 1959;79:32–39.
18. Mann PR: Leiomyoma cutis: An electron microscope study. *Br J Dermatol* 1970;82:463–469.
19. Robbins SL, Cotran RS: *Pathologic Basis of Disease*, ed 6. Philadelphia, Saunders, 1979.
20. Thompson JA: Therapy of painful cutaneous leiomyomas. *J Am Acad Dermatol* 1985;13:865–867.
21. Lever WF, Schaumburg-Lever G: *Histopathology of the Skin*, ed 6. Philadelphia, Lippincott, 1983.
22. Bures JC, Barnes L, Mercer D: A comparative study of smooth muscle tumors utilizing light and electron microscopy, immunocytochemical staining and enzymatic assay. *Cancer* 1981; 48:2420–2426.
23. Seymour AE, Henderson DW: Electron microscopy in surgical pathology: A selective review. Pathology 1981;13:111–135.
24. Enzinger EM, Weiss SW: *Soft Tissue Tumors*. St. Louis, Mo, Mosby, 1983.
25. Duhig JT, Ayer JP: Vascular leiomyoma. *Arch Pathol* 1959;68:424–430.
26. Mechlin DC, et al.: Leiomyoma of the maxilla—Report of a case. *Laryngoscope* 1980;90:1230–1233.
27. Reichart P, Reznik-Schuller H: The ultrastructure of an oral angiomyoma. *J Oral Pathol* 1977;6:25–34.
28. MacDonald DM, Sanderson KV: Angioleiomyoma of the skin. *Br J Dermatol* 1974;91:161–168.
29. Seifert HW: Ultrastructural investigation on cutaneous angioleiomyoma. *Arch Dermatol Res* 1981;271:91–99.
30. Flotte TJ, et al.: Leiomyosarcoma of the dartos muscle. *J Cutan Pathol* 1981;8:69–74.
31. Kilgour CS: Cutaneous leiomyosarcoma. *Br J Plast Surg* 1955; 8:144–146.
32. Heiech JJ, Organ CH: Leiomyosarcoma of the scalp in a newborn. *Arch Dermatol* 1970;102:213–215.
33. Chaves E, et al.: Leiomyosarcoma in the skin. *Acta Dermatol Venereol* 1972;52:288–290.
34. Johnson S, Rundell M, Platt W: Leiomyosarcoma of the scro-

tum, a case report with electron microscopy. *Cancer* 1978;41: 1830–1835.

35. Gaffney EF, Harte PJ, Browne HJ: Paratesticular leiomyosarcoma: An ultrastructural study. *J Urol* 1984;134:133–134.

36. Pandhi RK, Bedi TR, Dhawan IK: Leiomyosarcoma of the labium majus with extensive metastases. *Dermatologica* 1975;150:70–74.

37. Hernandez FJ: Leiomyosarcoma of male breast originating in the nipple. *Am J Surg Pathol* 1978;2(3):299–303.

38. Kathuria S, Jablokow VR, Molnar Z: Leiomyosarcoma of the penile prepuce with ultrastructural study. *Urology* 1986;27(6): 556–557.

39. Dahl I, Angervall L: Cutaneous and subcutaneous leiomyosarcoma: A clinicopathologic study of 47 patients. *Pathol Eur* 1974;9:307–315.

40. Fields JP, Helwig EB: Leiomyosarcoma of the skin and subcutaneous tissue. *Cancer* 1981;47:156–169.

41. Hietanen A, Sakai Y: Leiomyosarcoma in an old irradiated lupus lesion. *Acta Dermatol Venereol* 1960;40:167–172.

42. Nunnery EW, et al.: Leiomyosarcoma arising in a chronic stasis ulcer. *Hum Pathol* 1981;12(10):951–953.

43. Stout AP, Hill WT: Leiomyosarcoma of the superficial soft tissues. *Cancer* 1958;11(4):844–854.

44. Phelan JT, Sherer W, Mesa P: Malignant smooth-muscle tumors (leiomyosarcomas) of soft-tissue origin. *N Engl J Med* 1962; 266:1027–1030.

45. Levack J, Dick A: Cutaneous leiomyosarcoma with lymphatics spread: A report of two cases. *Glasgow Med J* 1955;36:337–342.

46. Headington JT, Beals TF, Niederhuber JE: Primary leiomyosarcoma of the shin: A report and critical appraisal. *J Cutan Pathol* 1977;4:308–317.

47. Harris M: Differential diagnosis of spindle cell tumors by electron microscopy—Personal experience and a review. *Histopathology* 1981;5:81–105.

CHAPTER 54
Tumors with Adipose and Cartilage Differentiation

Karl H. Anders and Marc D. Chalet

TUMORS WITH ADIPOSE DIFFERENTIATION

Subcutaneous adipose tissues provide an abundant energy reservoir, act as a protective barrier against trauma, and help conserve body heat. Tumors of the subcutaneous fat are frequently encountered clinical lesions. Benign neoplasms predominate, but malignant lesions and hamartomas also occur (Table 54–1). The distinction between some benign neoplasms and hamartomas is vague, as the etiology of these lesions is poorly understood. Generally, most tumors occurring in infancy are considered hamartomatous; those occurring in maturity are probably neoplastic.

NEVUS LIPOMATOSUS CUTANEOUS SUPERFICIALIS

Clinical Features

Nevus lipomatosus cutaneous superficialis (of Hoffman-Zurhelle) is a rare idiopathic lesion which often presents at birth, but which usually has developed by the third decade.[1–3] Soft, pale, yellow or flesh-colored papules, with smooth or wrinkled surfaces, characterize the entity. Growth is slow and usually confined to one side of the midline. Coalescence of these nodules can result in large, cosmetically deforming plaques measuring up to 30 cm in diameter.[4] Lesions are painless and linear in distribution, affecting predominantly the pelvic girdle, especially the buttocks. Involvement of trunk, legs, and other sites is reported.[5] Solitary nevus lipomatosus may be difficult to distinguish from an acrochordon.

Histologic Features

Groups of mature, nonencapsulated adipocytes permeate the dermal collagen. These fat cells may extend to the papillary dermis and are centered around blood vessels. The quantity of fat is variable, but may constitute up to 50%

of dermal tissues and can result in great irregularity of the dermal–subcutaneous interface. The surrounding tissues may show slightly disoriented collagen bundles, increased numbers of blood vessels, and spindle cells (identified by electron microscopy as immature fat cells[6]). The epidermis and skin appendages are minimally altered.

FOLDED SKIN WITH LIPOMATOUS NEVUS

Clinical Features

Folded skin with underlying lipomatous nevus ("Michelin tire baby") is an extremely rare disorder.[7–9] Patients present at birth with widespread convoluted skin folding. These soft fatty folds are cosmetically compromising but seem to diminish in size during childhood.

Histologic Features

The subcutaneous fat is thickened. Lobules of mature adipocytes extend into and thin the reticular dermis; adnexal structures are enveloped by fat. The papillary dermis and epidermis are not significantly affected.

CONGENITAL LIPOMATOSIS

Clinical Features

Congenital lipomatosis is a benign hamartomatous tumor usually diagnosed during the first few months of life.[10,11] Large, well-defined, subcutaneous masses of adipose tissue are found primarily in the thoracic region and are associated with fatty infiltration of underlying skeletal muscle. Recurrences after incomplete resection are common, but metastases do not occur.

Congenital lipomatosis has been described in the Proteus syndrome.[12,13] In addition to lipomas and fatty overgrowth, these infants have partial gigantism of the hands or feet, "pigmented nevi," hemihypertrophy, and other subcutaneous tumors (hemangiomas, lymphangiomas, mesenchymomas). The fatty tumors may grow quite rapidly.[13]

Histologic Features

The subcutaneous lesions of congenital lipomatosis are composed of benign, mature (partially encapsulated) adipose tissue, often infiltrating the deep skeletal muscle. There is no nuclear atypia.

ANGIOMYOLIPOMA

Clinical Features

The existence of angiomyolipomas originating in the skin has not been established, although a few cases arising in pericutaneous soft tissues have been reported.[14–16] These circumscribed, rubbery lesions have a benign clinical course; local excision is curative. Unlike renal angiomyolipomata, superficial tumors are not associated with tuberous sclerosis.[15,17]

Histologic Features

Histologic studies show a variable combination of mature adipose tissue, thick-walled blood vessels, and irregularly arranged bundles of benign smooth muscle cells. Hemorrhage is frequent. The varying proportions of these elements result in a diversity of macroscopic appearances, with color ranging from gray to red.

LIPOMA

Clinical Features

Lipomas are one of the most common mesenchymal neoplasms.[17–21] These benign tumors are solitary (occasion-

ally multiple), slowly growing lesions that often present during the fifth decade of life. Lipomas are round, "lozenge"- or disk-shaped, mobile masses with a soft doughy consistency. They are usually found in the back, shoulder, or neck, but may be encountered at any subcutaneous site. Although most lipomas are small and asymptomatic, some patients develop large masses (larger than 10 cm), which may cause pain secondary to nerve compression. These well-circumscribed fatty masses are easily "shelled out" by surgeons. Rarely there is local recurrence, especially with nonencapsulated, locally infiltrative tumors; such lesions necessitate a wide local excision.[22]

Histologic Features

Lipomas are usually defined by a thin fibrous capsule and have a sparse intralesional collagenous framework, producing a lobular pattern. These tumors are composed of sheets of mature, fairly uniform lipocytes (Fig. 54–1), indistinguishable from the white fat cells in the surrounding subcutaneous tissue. Lipocytes are spherical to polygonal and have a large, single, lipid vacuole compressing and causing eccentric localization of the cytoplasm and nucleus. Lipomas are easily and accurately diagnosed by fine-needle aspiration biopsy.[23]

Occasional lipomas may contain other mesenchymal elements. *Fibrolipomas* have abundant hyalinized connective tissue and perivascular spindle cells (containing ultrastructural cytoplasmic lipid droplets[21]). *Myxolipomas* contain plentiful myxoid ground substance.

Lipomas may rarely infarct secondary to trauma or ischemia, causing hemorrhage and cyst formation. *Infarcted lipomas* contain necrotic fat cells surrounded by lipophages, multinucleated giant cells, lymphocytes, and plasma cells (Fig. 54–2). Fibrosis and dystrophic calcification are commonly seen.

MULTIPLE LIPOMA SYNDROMES

Clinical Features

Some adults have multiple subcutaneous fatty tumors that, although histologically not distinctive, are of clinical interest.

Adiposis dolorosa (Dercum's disease)[24–27] usually occurs in middle-aged adults, often postmenopausal females. Patients characteristically are obese and have multiple, extremely tender lipomas involving primarily the arms, trunk, and periarticular soft tissues. Pain is cyclical with frequent periods of exacerbation. Chronic analgesic therapy is often necessary; rarely, intravenous lidocaine has been successfully used with long-lasting relief.[27] Although the etiology is unknown, patients frequently have associated emotional disturbances.[27]

Benign symmetric lipomatosis (Madelung's disease) is characterized by massive, bilateral, poorly circumscribed lipomas around the neck, suboccipital area, upper trunk, and proximal extremities.[17,28–31] Coalescence of lipomas results in the classic "horse-collar" appearance, which is disfiguring and may interfere with neck mobility and respiration. Although these tumors are not painful, surgery may be required. This idiopathic disease usually afflicts non-

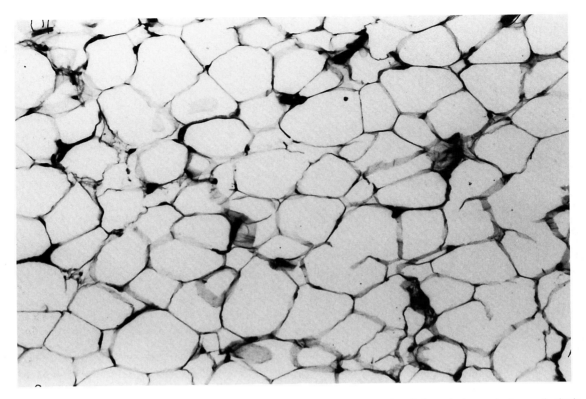

Figure 54–1. Section of lipoma consisting of mature adipocytes with minimal variation of size and shape. A single, large, cytoplasmic lipid vacuole, causing eccentric nuclear displacement, is characteristic of white fat. (H&E, ×100.)

obese, middle-aged males, often with a history of heavy alcohol consumption or liver disease.[17]

Familial multiple lipomatosis is transmitted in an autosomal dominant fashion and usually manifests by the third decade.[32–35] Patients may have from one to hundreds of slowly growing, asymptomatic, subcutaneous lipomas of varying size and widespread distribution. Lipomas may also occur in the gastrointestinal tract and other deep sites.

Histologic Features

Lesions in these syndromes are histologically indistinguishable from ordinary lipomas. Occasional tumors may be fibrolipomas or may show infarction. Malignant changes are not known to occur.

ANGIOLIPOMA

Clinical Features

Angiolipomas usually occur in young adults.[17,36–39] Although clinically resembling lipomas, they are less prevalent, are usually multiple, are often painful, and may be surprisingly mobile.[40] The forearm, trunk, and upper arm are the favored sites of origin. Angiolipomas are benign, usually small (less than 2 cm), encapsulated, subcutaneous nodules; rarely, they are larger masses having a poorly defined, infiltrative margin.[22] Muscular infiltration usually occurs in the lower extremity, but may be found elsewhere.[38,40–42] Infiltrating angiolipomas are solitary lesions that should be widely excised to prevent local recurrence.

Histologic Features

Angiolipomas are composed primarily of mature adipocytes, but have a much richer vascular pattern than ordinary lipomas (Fig. 54–3).[17,36] Vascular regions are most pronounced subcapsularly and result in a reddish coloration. The vessels are usually well-formed capillaries of variable number, ranging from few vascular foci to lesions composed primarily of blood vessels. Vascular channels are often filled with erythrocytes. Intraluminal fibrin thrombi are seen in most cases. Pericyte proliferation, mast cell infiltration, and stromal fibrosis may be present.

Lesions with a prominent vascular pattern may be hypercellular and can be confused with Kaposi's sarcoma or angiosarcoma, especially if they are infiltrative. Cells in angiolipomas, however, are small and typical. Mitoses are rare.

SPINDLE CELL LIPOMA

Clinical Features

Spindle cell lipomas are small (usually less than 5 cm), firm, solitary, subcutaneous tumors found predominantly in men 45 to 70 years of age; their presence in women or young adults is uncommon.[17,43–45] They are slow growing, painless nodules, found usually in the shoulder or posterior

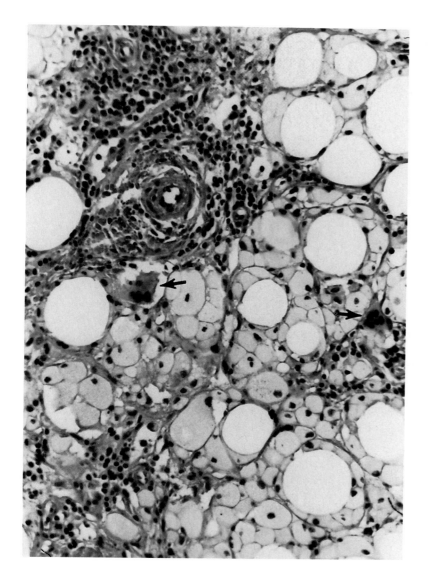

Figure 54–2. An infarcted lipoma with a prominent lymphoid infiltrate (top left). Numerous foamy histiocytes (lipophages) surround necrotic adipocytes (center, right). Arrows highlight multinucleated giant cells. (H&E, ×100.) (*Courtesy of the California Tumor Tissue Registry.*)

neck region. Spindle cell lipomas are adequately treated by simple excision. They neither recur nor metastasize. Grossly they resemble lipomas, but contain gray-white gelatinous foci.

Histologic Features

Spindle cell lipomas are usually well-circumscribed, nonencapsulated, round neoplasms; rarely, however, they have infiltrative borders.[44,45] They are composed of mature adipocytes, spindle cells, and a myxoid stroma (Fig. 54–4).

The spindle cells are small, well oriented, uniform, and typical. Rarely they exhibit multinucleation and pleomorphism analogous to "ancient neurilemmomas."[44] Ultrastructural studies favor a fibroblastic origin.[43,46] Within lesions, spindle cells are usually irregularly distributed. Some areas show only occasional spindle cells intermingled with lipocytes; elsewhere, large fascicles of spindle cells may conceal the lipomatous nature of the tumor. Mitoses are not commonly seen.

The stroma is usually myxoid and contains small collagen fibers. Mast cells may be numerous. Vessels tend to be inconspicuous, but may occasionally be prominent.[47]

The differential diagnosis includes sclerosing liposarcoma and fibrosarcoma. Spindle cell lipomas are distinguished by their uniform, nonpleomorphic nuclei and the absence of mitoses and lipoblasts.

PLEOMORPHIC LIPOMA

Clinical Features

Pleomorphic lipomas are rare subcutaneous neoplasms with clinical features similar to those of spindle cell lipomas.[48] They are solitary, painless tumors occurring primarily in the back or posterior neck, but rarely elsewhere.[49] As with spindle cell lipomas, elderly men are most commonly affected. Pleomorphic lipomas do not metastasize. If excision is inadequate, however, there may be recurrences.

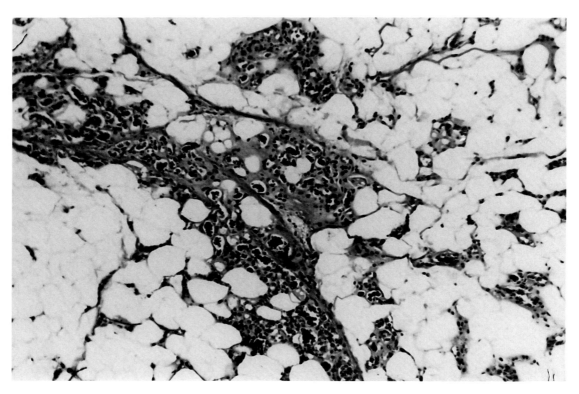

Figure 54–3. Angiolipomas contain a mixture of mature fat cells and blood vessels. The vascular channels are lined by small, typical, endothelial cells and contain numerous erythrocytes. (H&E, ×40.) (*Courtesy of the California Tumor Tissue Registry.*)

Histologic Features

Pleomorphic lipomas exhibit an extremely variable morphologic picture.[48,50] A key to the diagnosis is the presence of characteristic bizarre, multinucleated, "floret-type" giant cells (Fig. 54–5, 54–6). These cells contain multiple, hyper-chromatic, overlapping nuclei arranged in a circular pattern resembling a flower's petals. The cytoplasm is eosinophilic. Floret giant cells may be rare and focal or numerous and diffusely distributed.

Pleomorphic lipomas also contain mature adipocytes

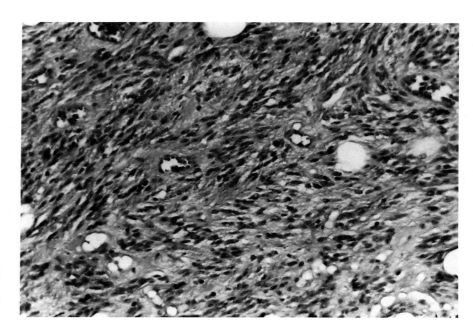

Figure 54–4. Spindle cell lipoma. The cellular region, composed of numerous, small, uniform, spindle cells, is admixed with mature adipocytes. Such lesions may be misinterpreted as sarcoma. (H&E, ×100.) (*Courtesy of the California Tumor Tissue Registry.*)

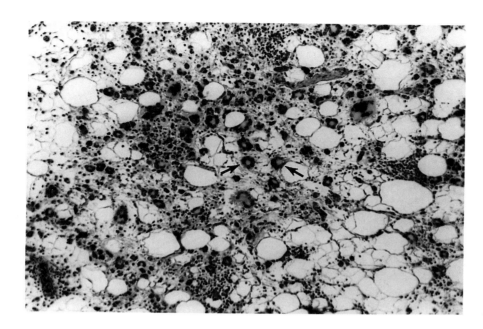

Figure 54–5. Pleomorphic lipomas are composed of mature fat cells, multinucleated, floretlike giant cells (arrows), rare spindle cells, and scattered lymphocytes. The stroma is myxoid. (H&E, ×40.) (*Courtesy of the California Tumor Tissue Registry.*)

of variable size, occasionally with atypical, enlarged nuclei. Occasional scattered lipoblast-like cells may be found, as may fibroblastic spindle cells resembling those seen in spindle cell lipoma. The stroma is myxoid or collagenous; blood vessels are not conspicuous. Scattered lymphocytes, plasma cells, and mast cells may also be seen.

Although clinically benign, pleomorphic lipomas are often histologically misinterpreted as liposarcomas. Unlike

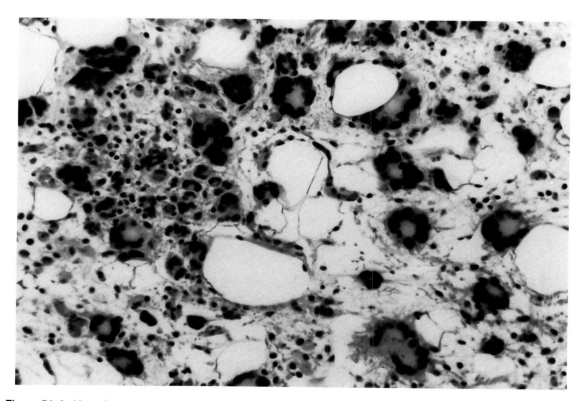

Figure 54–6. Many floretlike giant cells are seen in this pleomorphic lipoma. These cells have numerous hyperchromatic nuclei arranged in a circular pattern resembling the petals of a flower, hence the name. The cytoplasm is deeply eosinophilic. (H&E, ×100.) (*Courtesy of the California Tumor Tissue Registry.*)

liposarcomas, however, pleomorphic lipomas are superficial in location and do not infiltrate surrounding tissues. Less nuclear pleomorphism, no atypical mitoses, and only rare lipoblasts are seen in pleomorphic lipoma.

BENIGN LIPOBLASTOMA

Clinical Features
Benign lipoblastoma (lipoblastomatosis) is a rare entity occurring exclusively in infants and young children.[51-54] Patients have a solitary, subcutaneous mass that is usually asymptomatic. These tumors are most common in the extremities and, with slow growth, may reach considerable size (up to 15 cm). Lipoblastomas have a pale, myxomatous, lobulated appearance.

Two variants of lipoblastoma are recognized. *Benign lipoblastomas* are superficial and well circumscribed, and are the more common type seen in dermatologic practice. Recurrences are rare after conservative local excision. *Diffuse lipoblastomas* are deep, poorly defined neoplasms that infiltrate skeletal muscle. These tumors are less common, but may recur and can become progressively more well differentiated with each recurrence.[55]

Histologic Features
Lipoblastomas are composed of fetal fat cells in a myxoid stroma (Fig. 54–7), separated into small, irregular lobules by highly vascularized collagenous septae. Most cells present are lipoblasts with a single cytoplasmic fat vacuole that eccentrically displaces the nucleus and produces a "signet-ring" appearance. A few lipoblasts are multivacuolated, with a scalloped nuclear contour. The nuclei are slightly enlarged and hyperchromatic. Scattered mature adipocytes are often seen as well. Rarely, a lesion contains hibernoma-like fat cells. Occasional primitive stellate or spindle-shaped mesenchymal cells are present.

Lipoblastomas may be histologically confused with well-differentiated or myxoid liposarcoma. Lipoblastomas, however, occur only in children, whereas liposarcomas are exceedingly rare in this age group. In addition, mitoses, bizarre lipoblasts, giant cells, and atypical nuclei are not seen in lipoblastomas.

HIBERNOMA

Clinical Features
Hibernomas are rare, benign, solitary, subcutaneous tumors that are clinically indistinguishable from lipomas.[17,56-58] They usually arise in young adults and are most commonly found in the interscapular region. These tumors may measure up to 12 cm in diameter, are circumscribed, and are tan to reddish brown in color. Conservative excision is curative.

Histologic Features
Hibernomas are easily recognized, being composed of lobules of round to oval cells divided by well-vascularized fibrous tissue (Fig. 54–8). The characteristic cell type is the "mulberry" cell (Fig. 54–9), thought to be of brown fat origin.[59] These cells have prominent, round, central nuclei and granular, eosinophilic cytoplasm containing numerous, variably sized fat vacuoles. No atypia is seen and mitoses are absent. Univacuolar adipocytes may be present in these tumors, and some lesions resemble transitions between hibernomas and lipomas.

Electron microscopic studies reveal numerous, large mitochondria with abundant transverse cristae.[57-59] These account for the granular cytoplasm of "mulberry" cells and the brown macroscopic appearance of the tumor. A recent study reports endocrine-like activity in a hibernoma, identified by electron microscopy.[60]

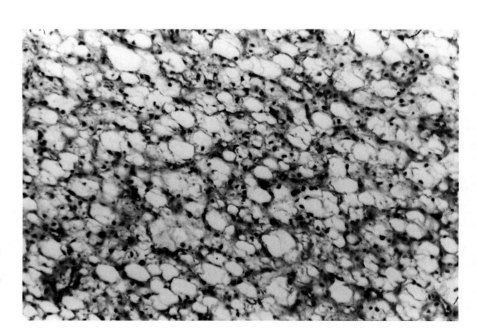

Figure 54–7. A tumor lobule from a benign lipoblastoma. Many small, atypical, univacuolar fat cells—analogous to embryonic fat—are seen in a myxoid stroma. (H&E, ×100.) (*Courtesy of the California Tumor Tissue Registry.*)

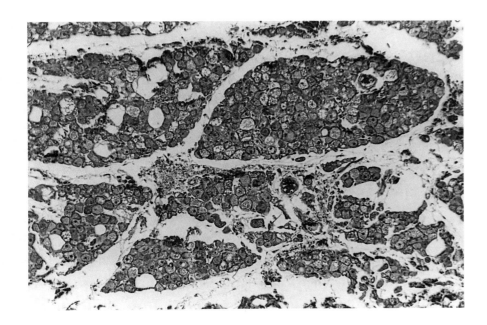

Figure 54–8. The characteristic lobular pattern of a hibernoma is readily apparent. (H&E, ×40.) (*Courtesy of the California Tumor Tissue Registry.*)

Liposarcoma

Clinical Features

Liposarcomas are among the most common sarcomas of adult life.[61] Despite the prevalence of lipomas in subcutaneous tissues, malignant neoplasms of fatty origin only rarely occur in the skin,[62,63] where they often have extended from deep fascial or intermuscular origin.[64,65] Liposarcomas are thought to arise de novo from primitive mesenchymal cells and, with rare exceptions,[66–68] not from preexisting lipomas.

Liposarcomas are most frequent in adults 40 to 60 years of age, and are extremely rare in children and young adults.

The skin overlying these tumors may be tense, red and inflamed, or ulcerated. Some liposarcomas are painful, but most present as rapidly enlarging masses. Therapy usually includes wide excision and radiation. Recurrences are common after incomplete resection, but only poorly differentiated lesions metastasize, usually to the lungs, but rarely to the skin.[69] Amputation may be necessary.

Frequently, liposarcomas are large lobulated masses (larger than 10 cm) that have a poorly defined margin. Grossly, their appearance is variable, reflecting histologic composition. Some are firm and yellow; others are soft, gray, and myxoid. Hemorrhage, necrosis, and fibrosis are frequent.

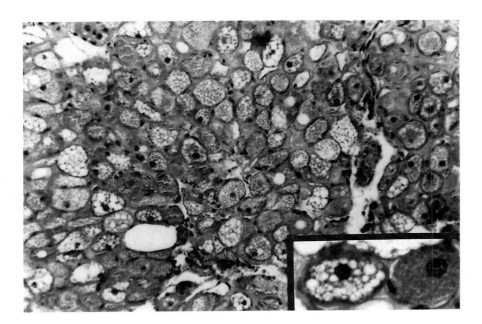

Figure 54–9. Hibernomas are composed of round, multivacuolated cells, characteristic of brown fat. These "mulberry" cells have prominent, round, central nuclei and granular, eosinophilic, or vacuolated cytoplasm (inset, lower right). (H&E, ×100; inset, ×200.) (*Courtesy of the California Tumor Tissue Registry.*)

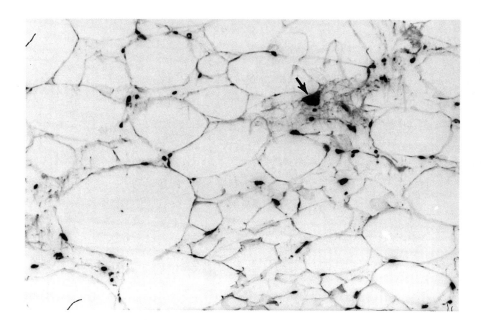

Figure 54–10. Well-differentiated liposarcoma may closely resemble lipoma; however, lipocytes display a greater size variation and more pronounced nuclear atypia. A single, large, pleomorphic, mesenchymal cell is seen in a thin band of collagenous stroma (arrow). (H&E, ×100.)

Histologic Features

Four categories of liposarcoma are recognized. These can occur in pure form or combined patterns[61]: (1) well-differentiated, (2) myxoid, (3) round cell, (4) pleomorphic. The latter two variants have the worst prognosis. Malignant lipoblasts are the cell type common to all of these neoplasms.[61,70]

Well-differentiated (lipoma-like) **liposarcoma** closely resembles a lipoma at scanning magnification (Fig. 54–10); however, the univacuolated fat cells are of more variable size and have slightly enlarged, hyperchromatic nuclei. Fibrous septae between lobules of tumor cells contain large, atypical, primitive, mesenchymal cells with pleomorphic nuclei and occasional lipoblasts. Rare mitotic figures are present. Such lesions must be extensively sampled to detect possible foci of poor differentiation, which herald a worse prognosis.

Myxoid liposarcoma is the most frequent variant. Tumors have an abundant myxoid stroma with a prominent, complex, capillary network (Fig. 54–11). These tumors contain malignant lipoblasts, signet-ring cells, and a variable number of more differentiated adipocytes. Some myxoid liposarcomas, with prominent nuclear atypia and low lipid content, may metastasize.

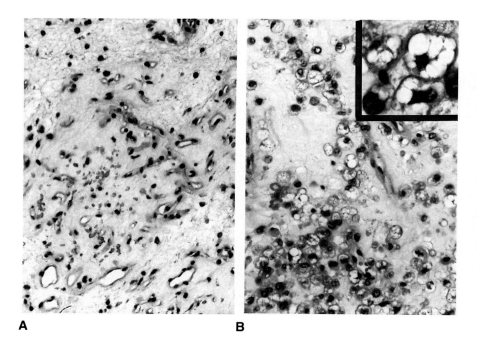

Figure 54–11. A. Myxoid liposarcoma with abundant myxoid stroma and complex vascular pattern, but few lipoblasts. **B.** Numerous lipoblasts are seen in this myxoid liposarcoma. Lipoblasts (inset, upper right) are characterized by scalloped, hyperchromatic nuclei and multiple, well-defined cytoplasmic lipid vacuoles. (H&E, ×100; inset, ×200.)

A   B

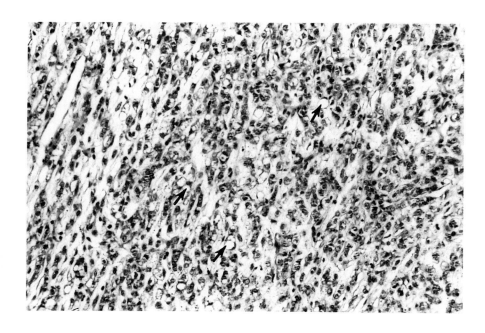

Figure 54–12. Cords of densely packed, small, round to oval cells in round cell liposarcoma. Most cells have a signet-ring shape (arrows). (H&E, ×100.) (*Courtesy of the California Tumor Tissue Registry.*)

Round cell liposarcomas are characterized by small, uniform, round to oval cells (Fig. 54–12), frequently with a single cytoplasmic lipid vacuole (signet-ring cells) and lipoblasts. The cells are closely packed and show large, atypical, hyperchromatic nuclei and fairly numerous mitoses. Although there are frequently areas resembling myxoid liposarcoma, these tumors are more cellular, show a less prominent vascular pattern, and less myxoid stroma. Round cell liposarcomas have an aggressive clinical course.

Pleomorphic (poorly differentiated) **liposarcomas** have bizarre, giant, uni- or multivacuolated lipoblasts (Fig. 54–13) with one or more large anaplastic nuclei. These malignant lipoblasts are admixed with smaller, pleomorphic, round to spindle-shaped cells; stroma is sparse. Pleomorphic liposarcomas are very aggressive tumors with frequent systemic dissemination. Electron microscopic examination may be necessary for a definitive diagnosis (to exclude pleomorphic malignant fibrous histiocytoma or pleomorphic rhabdomyosarcoma.[71,72]

TUMORS WITH CARTILAGE DIFFERENTIATION

Benign and malignant cutaneous tumors with cartilaginous differentiation are uncommon, and rarely described in the dermatologic literature. Such lesions are extraskeletal and

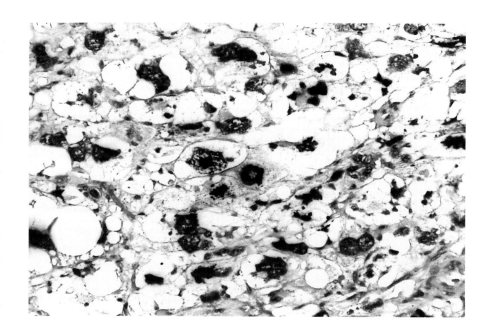

Figure 54–13. Bizarre, giant, multinucleated lipoblasts characterize this pleomorphic liposarcoma. (H&E, ×100.)

not attached to underlying bone. The etiology of these neoplasms is unknown.

CUTANEOUS CARTILAGE TUMOR

Clinical Features

Cutaneous cartilage tumors (extraskeletal chondromas) are slowly enlarging, nontender masses involving primarily the extremities, especially the fingers and toes.[73-76] Attachment to tendons and tendon sheaths is common, but some lesions are primarily dermal in location.[74] Adults 30 to 60 years of age are usually affected.

Cutaneous cartilage tumors are well demarcated, are easily enucleated by surgeons, and have a firm, gritty texture. Most measure less than 3 cm in diameter and none metastasize. Recurrences, however, after incomplete removal are common.

Histologic Features

These tumors are well circumscribed and have a lobular pattern. Areas of mature, hyaline cartilage are necessary for the diagnosis. Frequently, the cartilaginous stroma exhibits calcification, fibrosis, myxoid changes, and hemorrhage. Foci of immature-appearing chondroblastic cells with slightly pleomorphic nuclei may be found; the stroma surrounding these cells is myxoid and such regions are suggestive of chondrosarcoma. Granulomatous inflammation may be seen around the periphery of the cartilage lobules.[75,76]

Although the histologic features of cutaneous cartilage tumor may be suggestive of extraskeletal chondrosarcoma—especially if the chondrocytes appear immature—these tumors are always benign. Cutaneous cartilage tumor shows a lower cellularity, less pleomorphism, and no mitoses. Chondrosarcoma involves primarily the deep, proximal soft tissues, whereas cutaneous cartilage tumor affects the hands and feet.

EXTRASKELETAL CHONDROSARCOMA

Clinical Features

Extraskeletal chondrosarcomas are very rare tumors that infrequently involve the subcutaneous tissues.[76-78] A cutaneous metastasis from an osseous primary must be excluded in the diagnosis of this lesion. Although the greatest frequency of neoplasia occurs in no well-defined age group, many patients are young adults. Tumors are usually found in the extremities and may grow rapidly. The overlying skin is tense and may ulcerate. Radical local excision should be performed; nonetheless, recurrence and lung metastases are frequent. The probability of dissemination is directly related to the tumor's cellularity.

Histologic Features

Abundant myxoid stroma, bands and cords of chondroblastic cells, and a nodular architecture characterize **myxoid chondrosarcoma. Mesenchymal chondrosarcomas** are composed of sheets of primitive mesenchymal cells (with a prominent vascular pattern), containing islands of well-

differentiated cartilaginous tissue. An excellent, detailed review of these tumors is found elsewhere.[76]

REFERENCES

1. Girglia HS, Bhattacharya SK: Nevus lipomatosus cutaneous superficialis. *Int J Dermatol* 1975;14:273–276.
2. Wilson Jones E, Marks R, Pongsehirun D: Naevus superficialis lipomatosus. A clinicopathological report of twenty cases. *Br J Dermatol* 1975;93:121–133.
3. Dotz W, Prioleau PG: Nevus lipomatosus cutaneous superficialis. A light and electron microscopic study. *Arch Dermatol* 1984;120:376–379.
4. Kopf AW, Bart RS: Giant nevus lipomatosus. *J Dermatol Surg Oncol* 1983;9:279–281.
5. Weitzner S: Solitary nevus lipomatosus cutaneous superficialis of scalp. *Arch Dermatol* 1968;97:540–542.
6. Reymond JL, Stoebner P, Amblard P: Nevus lipomatosus cutaneus superficialis. An electron microscopic study of four cases. *J Cutan Pathol* 1980;7:295–301.
7. Ross CM: Generalized folded skin with an underlying lipomatous nevus. "The Michelin tire baby." *Arch Dermatol* 1969;100:320–323.
8. Ross CM: Generalized folded skin with underlying lipomatous nevus: The Michelin tyre baby. (Letter) *Arch Dermatol* 1972;106:766.
9. Gardner EW, Miller HM, Lowney ED: Folded skin associated with underlying nevus lipomatosus. *Arch Dermatol* 1979;115:978–979.
10. Nixon HH, Scobie WG: Congenital lipomatosis: A report of four cases. *J Pediatr Surg* 1971;6:742–745.
11. Lachman RS, Finklestein J, Mehringer CM, et al.: Congenital aggressive lipomatosis. *Skeletal Radiol* 1983;9:248–254.
12. Wiedemann HR, Burgio GR, Aldenhoff P, et al.: The Proteus syndrome. Partial gigantism of the hands and/or feet, nevi, hemihypertrophy, subcutaneous tumors, macrocephaly or other skull anomalies and possible accelerated growth and visceral affections. *Eur J Pediatr* 1983;140:5–12.
13. Mücke J, Willgerodt H, Künzel R, et al.: Variability in the Proteus syndrome: Report of an affected child with progressive lipomatosis. *Eur J Pediat* 1985;143:320–323.
14. Bures C, Barnes L: Benign mesenchymomas of the head and neck. *Arch Pathol Lab Med* 1978;102:237–241.
15. Chaitin BA, Goldman RL, Linker DG: Angiomyolipoma of penis. *Urology* 1984;23:305–306.
16. Chen KTK, Bauer V: Extrarenal angiomyolipoma. *J Surg Oncol* 1984;25:89–91.
17. Enzinger FM, Weiss SW: *Soft Tissue Tumors.* St. Louis, Mo, Mosby, 1983, pp 199–241.
18. Adair FE, Pack GT, Farrior JH: Lipomas. *Am J Cancer* 1932;16:1104–1120.
19. Osment LS: Cutaneous lipomas and lipomatosis. *Surg Gynecol Obstet* 1968;127:129–132.
20. Braisfield RD, Das Gupta TK: Soft tissue tumors: Benign tumors of adipose tissue. *CA* 1969;19:3–7.
21. Kim YH, Reiner L: Ultrastructure of lipoma. *Cancer* 1982;50:102–106.
22. Dionne GP, Seemayer TA: Infiltrating lipomas and angiolipomas revisited. *Cancer* 1974;33:732–738.
23. Layfield LJ, Anders KH, Glasgow BJ, et al.: Fine-needle aspiration of primary soft-tissue lesions. *Arch Pathol Lab Med* 1986;110:420–424.
24. Mella BA: Adiposis dolorosa. *Univ Mich Med Cent J* 1967;33:79–81.
25. Eisman J, Swezey RL: Juxta-articular adiposis dolorosa: What is it? Report of 2 cases. *Ann Rheum Dis* 1979;38:479–482.

26. Palmer ED: Dercum's disease: Adiposis dolorosa. *Am Fam Physician* 1981;24:155–157.

27. Atkinson RL: Intravenous lidocaine for the treatment of intractable pain of adiposis dolorosa. *Int J Obes* 1982;6:351–357.

28. Taylor LM, Beahrs OH, Fontana RS: Benign symmetric lipomatosis. *Mayo Clin Proc* 1961;36:96–100.

29. Kodish ME, Alsever RN, Block MB: Benign symmetric lipomatosis: Functional sympathetic denervation of adipose tissue and possible hypertrophy of brown fat. *Metabolism* 1974;23:937–945.

30. Schuler FA III, Graham JK, Horton CE: Benign symmetrical lipomatosis (Madelung's disease). *Plast Reconstruct Surg* 1976;57:662–665.

31. Uhlin SR: Benign symmetric lipomatosis. *Arch Dermatol* 1979;115:94–95.

32. Kurzweg FT, Spencer R: Familial multiple lipomatosis. *Am J Surg* 1951;82:762–765.

33. Shanks J, Paranchych AW, Tuba J: Familial multiple lipomatosis. *Can Med Assoc J* 1957;77:881–884.

34. Stephens FE, Isaacson A: Hereditary multiple lipomatosis. *J Hered* 1959;50:51–53.

35. Mohar N: Familial multiple lipomatosis. *Acta Dermatol Venereol (Stockh)* 1980;60:509–513.

36. Howard WR, Helwig EB: Angiolipoma. *Arch Dermatol* 1960;82:924–931.

37. Belcher RW, Czarnetzki BM, Carney JF, et al.: Multiple (subcutaneous) angiolipomas. Clinical, pathologic and pharmacologic studies. *Arch Dermatol* 1974;110:583–585.

38. Lin JJ, Lin F: Two entities in angiolipoma. A study of 459 cases of lipoma with review of literature on infiltrating angiolipoma. *Cancer* 1974;34:720–727.

39. Dixon AY, McGregor DH, Lee SH: Angiolipomas: An ultrastructural and clinicopathologic study. *Hum Pathol* 1981;12:739–747.

40. Sahl WJ Jr: Mobile encapsulated lipomas. *Arch Dermatol* 1978;114:1684–1686.

41. Walling AK, Companioni GR, Belsole RJ: Infiltrating angiolipoma of the hand and wrist. *J Hand Surg [Am]* 1985;10:288–291.

42. Puig L, Moreno A, de Moragas JM: Infiltrating angiolipoma: Report of two cases and review of the literature. *J Dermatol Surg Oncol* 1986;12:617–619.

43. Enzinger FM, Harvey DJ: Spindle cell lipoma. *Cancer* 1975;36:1852–1859.

44. Angervall L, Dahl T, Kindblom LG, et al.: Spindle cell lipoma. *Acta Pathol Microbiol Scand* 1976;84:477–487.

45. Brody HJ, Meltzer HD, Someren A: Spindle cell lipoma. *Arch Dermatol* 1978;114:1065–1066.

46. Bolen JW, Thorning D: Spindle-cell lipoma: A clinical, light- and electron-microscopic study. *Am J Surg Pathol* 1981;5:435–441.

47. Warkel RL, Rehme CG, Thompson WH: Vascular spindle cell lipoma. *J Cutan Pathol* 1982;9:113–118.

48. Shmookler BM, Enzinger FM: Pleomorphic lipoma: A benign tumor simulating liposarcoma. A clinicopathologic analysis of 48 cases. *Cancer* 1981;47:126–133.

49. Bryant J: A pleomorphic lipoma in the scalp. *J Dermatol Surg Oncol* 1981;7:323–325.

50. Evans HL, Soule EH, Winkelmann RK: Atypical lipoma, atypical intramuscular lipoma, and well differentiated retroperitoneal liposarcoma. *Cancer* 1979;43:574–584.

51. Vellios F, Baez J, Shumacker HB: Lipoblastomatosis: A tumor of fetal fat different from hibernoma. *Am J Pathol* 1958;34:1149–1159.

52. Chung EB, Enzinger FM: Benign lipoblastomatosis. An analysis of 35 cases. *Cancer* 1973;32:482–492.

53. Alba Greco M, Garcia RL, Vuletin JC: Benign lipoblastomatosis. Ultrastructure and histogenesis. *Cancer* 1980;45:511–515.

54. Chaudhuri B, Ronan SG, Ghosh L: Benign lipoblastomata. Report of a case. *Cancer* 1980;46:611–614.

55. Van Meurs DP: The transformation of an embryonic lipoma to a common lipoma. *Br J Surg* 1947;34:282–284.

56. Novy FG Jr, Wilson JW: Hibernomas, brown fat tumors. *Arch Dermatol* 1956;73:149–157.

57. Seemayer TA, Knaack J, Wang NS, et al.: On the ultrastructure of hibernoma. *Cancer* 1975;36:1785–1793.

58. Fleishman JS, Schwartz RA: Hibernoma: Ultrastructural observations. *J Surg Oncol* 1983;23:285–289.

59. Dardick I: Hibernoma: A possible model of brown fat histogenesis. *Hum Pathol* 1978;9:321–329.

60. Allegra SR, Gmuer C, O'Leary GP Jr: Endocrine activity in a large hibernoma. *Hum Pathol* 1983;14:1044–1052.

61. Enzinger FM, Weiss SW: *Soft Tissue Tumors.* St. Louis, Mo, Mosby, 1983, pp 242–296.

62. Sampson CC, Saunders EH, Green WE, et al.: Liposarcoma developing in a lipoma. *Arch Pathol* 1960;69:506–510.

63. Weitzner S, Kornblum S: Subcutaneous liposarcoma of forearm. *Am Surg* 1972;38:176–178.

64. Phelan JT, Perez-Mesa C: Liposarcoma of the superficial soft tissues. *Surg Gynecol Obstet* 1962;115:609–614.

65. Saunders JR, Jaques DA, Casterline FF, et al.: Liposarcomas of the head and neck. A review of the literature and addition of four cases. *Cancer* 1979;43:162–168.

66. Wright CJE: Liposarcoma arising in a simple lipoma. *J Pathol Bacteriol* 1948;60:483–487.

67. Sternberg SS: Liposarcoma arising within a subcutaneous lipoma. *Cancer* 1952;5:975–978.

68. Enterline HT, Culberson JD, Rochlin DB, et al.: Liposarcoma. A clinical and pathologic study of 53 cases. *Cancer* 1960;13:932–950.

69. Peison B, Benisch B, Williams MC: Retroperitoneal liposarcoma metastatic to scalp. *Arch Dermatol* 1978;114:1358–1359.

70. Rossouw DJ, Cinti S, Dickersin GR: Liposarcoma. An ultrastructural study of 15 cases. *Am J Clin Pathol* 1986;85:649–667.

71. Reddick RL, Michelitch H, Triche TJ: Malignant soft tissue tumors (malignant fibrous histiocytoma, pleomorphic liposarcoma, and pleomorphic rhabdomyosarcoma): An electron microscopic study. *Hum Pathol* 1979;10:327–343.

72. Weiss LM, Warhol MJ: Ultrastructural distinctions between adult pleomorphic rhabdomyosarcomas, pleomorphic liposarcomas, and pleomorphic malignant fibrous histiocytomas. *Hum Pathol* 1984;15:1025–1033.

73. Dahlin DC, Salvador AH: Cartilaginous tumors of the soft tissues of the hands and feet. *Mayo Clin Proc* 1974;49:721–726.

74. Holmes HS, Bovenmeyer DA: Cutaneous cartilaginous tumor. *Arch Dermatol* 1976;112:839–840.

75. Chung EB, Enzinger FM: Chondroma of soft parts. *Cancer* 1978;41:1414–1424.

76. Enzinger FM, Weiss SW: *Soft Tissue Tumors.* St. Louis, Mo, Mosby, 1983, pp 698–719.

77. Korns ME: Primary chondrosarcoma of extraskeletal soft tissue. A case report. *Arch Pathol* 1967;83:13–15.

78. Enzinger FM, Shiraki M: Extraskeletal myxoid chondrosarcoma. An analysis of 34 cases. *Hum Pathol* 1972;3:421–435.

CHAPTER 55
Metastatic Tumors

N. Scott McNutt and Patricia M. Fishman

GENERAL PATHOBIOLOGY OF TUMOR METASTASIS

The fundamental basis of metastasis to skin has not been investigated thoroughly. Probably it is very similar to metastasis to the parenchymal organs, particularly those that have blood vessels with a continuous endothelium separated from the parenchyma by basement membranes. Primary cancers of internal viscera do not seem to metastasize specifically or selectively to the skin. The incidence of metastasis to the skin from internal cancers is low.[1] This is surprising when one considers the size of the skin as an organ and realizes that it is one of the largest organs in the body. The rate of metastasis is not as low as to skeletal muscle and not as high as to brain, both of which also have continuous endothelium. The localization of metastases in the skin relates to patterns of blood and lymphatic flow in the skin as well as to sites of surgical procedures (Fig. 55–1).

Metastasis as a general process has been divided into several steps through which the tumor cells must pass (Table 55–1). Some of these steps require diverse and opposing properties in the cell population.[2] When metastasis occurs via a blood route, the first step requires that the tumor cells have the ability to invade through the walls of blood or lymphatic vessels. In order to do this, the tumor cells must have the ability to degrade basement membrane proteins by proteolysis. They also must have cell motility, which allows them to push into a vessel wall. In those instances in which medium-sized blood vessels are invaded, the cell motility must be capable of working against considerable local hydrostatic pressure. A second step requires that cell adhesion be defective enough to allow cells or clusters of cells to break off the main tumor mass and to be carried downstream in the veins (Fig. 55–2) or lymphatics via the thoracic duct to the general blood circulation. If the tumor induces rapid and complete thrombosis of the blood vessel during the invasive process, the tumor cells remain trapped at the local site and no metastasis occurs. Consequently, the tumor cells cannot be too thrombogenic. A third step is required to localize the tumor cells at a distant site. Either

the clusters of cells must be large enough to form an embolic plug of a small blood vessel, or the individual tumor cells must have cell adhesion properties that allow them to attach to the endothelial surface of the vessels at the distant site.[3] In a fourth step, the tumor cells must grow at the distant site and invade the tissues at the site of metastasis in order to establish a permanent colony of cells. In this sequence of steps, it is evident that opposing properties are involved in detachment from endothelium and then reattachment to endothelium. The cells in the population need diversity in the strength of adhesion of tumor cells to other tumor cells and also of tumor cells to endothelium in order to go through the sequence. The production and degradation of certain cell adhesion proteins produced by the tumor cells seems intimately involved in the metastatic process.[4–6] For example, tumors that produce the adhesion protein laminin, a normal basement membrane component, have an increased propensity to form metastases in experimental systems in which the cells are injected intravenously.[7] Also, antibodies to laminin and fragments of the laminin molecule can reduce the number of metastases following intravenous injection of the tumor cells. In addition, a different cell adhesion protein, fibronectin, can be degraded or can fail to attach to the tumor cell surface. Such events may facilitate the invasive process and facilitate the shedding of tumor cells into the bloodstream.

In the experimental laboratory setting, it is possible to demonstrate that some types of tumors have a selective ability to metastasize to certain anatomic sites. Nicolson et al.[8] found that, with the mouse B16 melanoma cell line, it is possible to obtain a strain of cells with a heightened propensity to metastasize to the brain. In their experiment, tumor cells were injected into mice, and metastases were widespread, particularly in lung, liver, and brain. If only cells from the brain metastases were removed for subsequent passage into mice, by the tenth such passage, the melanoma cells metastasized to brain very selectively and not much to lung and liver. In certain clinical settings, there are examples of selective metastatic propensity, for example, bronchogenic carcinomas that form metastases

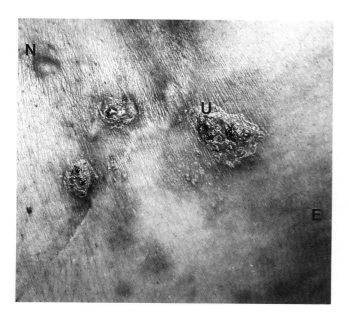

Figure 55–1. Gross photograph of metastatic adenocarcinoma of the breast. A diagonal surgical scar is present from the surgery that removed the primary tumor. Several appearances of metastases are demonstrated. At the upper left, a small nonulcerated nodule (N) is present. Near the center, several nodules have early ulceration (U). At the lower middle and right, there is diffuse erythema and induration (E).

in the adrenal glands bilaterally and gastric carcinomas that form metastases in the ovaries bilaterally. The skin has not been demonstrated to be such a site of selective metastasis, but it remains a theoretical possibility in isolated cases.

In the skin, and indeed in most metastases in general, the gross patterns of metastasis follow simple routes of

TABLE 55–1. STEPS IN THE METASTATIC PROCESS

Step	Requirements
1. Invasion into a blood or lymphatic vessel wall	1. a. Degradation of basement membrane proteins b. Cell motility
2. Detachment of cells or clusters of cells into blood or lymph	2. a. Defective cell to cell adhesion b. Lack of thrombosis
3. Attachment of cells or clusters of cells at a distant site	3. a. Embolic plugging of vessels b. Activation of the coagulation system c. Binding to endothelial or subendothelial surfaces
4. Growth at the new site	4. a. Mitosis b. Degradation of basement membrane proteins c. Cell motility d. Escape from immune destruction e. Stimulation of vascular ingrowth

blood and lymphatic flow. Embolism of clusters of tumor cells may account for metastasis to the skin without invoking any selective adhesive interactions between tumor cells and the vascular endothelium (Fig. 55–2). Likewise, simple embolism could account for the formation of liver metastases from primary gastrointestinal tumors and for lung metastases from renal tubular cell adenocarcinomas. After the establishment of small or large pulmonary metastases, tumor cells may be shed into the arterial circulation, with subsequent embolism to almost any organ, including the skin. However, the wider diameter and lower resistance of the pulmonary capillary bed compared to the systemic capillary bed may allow tumor cells to flow through the lungs and into the arterial circulation without establishment of a definite pulmonary metastasis.[9] Endothelial injury can increase the tendency to form metastases at a particular site, as has been demonstrated in the lung.[10] The size of the tumor cells themselves and their interaction with the blood coagulation system and platelets may be very important in determining the hydrodynamic radius of tumor cell clusters in the circulation and, consequently, in determining where the tumor cells will lodge to form metastases.[11] (Fig. 55–2). In experimental systems, pretreatment with warfarin [3-(alpha-acetonylbenzyl)-4-hydroxycoumarin] or heparin may reduce the number of metastases following injection of tumor cells[12,13] or following spontaneous metastasis.[14–18] Endothelial damage may enhance the ability of tumor cells to adhere at a site of injury. In experimental injury systems, tumor cells can be found associated with small platelet and fibrin thrombi at sites of denuded vascular basement membrane.[10]

After the tumor embolus has lodged in the blood or lymphatic vessels of the skin, it must have the ability to grow in the skin. There are several steps required in this process also. Mitosis and the formation of an expanding mass of tumor cells would produce a hydrostatic pressure, or growth pressure, which could account for the shape of most cutaneous metastases, that is, an expanding spherical nodule in the deep dermis and subcutis (Fig. 55–3). However, some metastases have a diffusely infiltrative pattern of growth that requires more than growth pressure to explain (Figs. 55–4, 55–5). Ameboid movement by tumor cells has been observed experimentally in cell culture and in skin window preparations. Also, some tumors have a loss of adhesive contacts between tumor cells, that is, loss of cohesion. Together these two factors, motility and decreased cohesion, may account for the phenomenon of diffuse infiltration by metastases (or even primary tumors).

The mass of tumor cells must survive any host immunologic response, which usually is associated with lymphocytic infiltration of the tumor (Fig. 55–6). The clinical observation that squamous cell carcinomas of the skin are more frequent in immunosuppressed renal transplant patients suggests that immunologic competence is important in suppressing tumor growth; that is, it suggests that so-called immune surveillance does occur.[19] Other evidence for immune surveillance derives from observations that Kaposi's sarcoma may appear in immunosuppressed renal transplant patients and may regress after immunosuppressive drugs are decreased or stopped.[20] The appearance of metastases many years after removal of the primary tumor implies that the

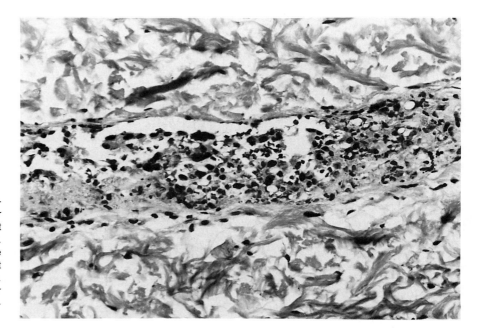

Figure 55–2. In this light micrograph at intermediate magnification, there is intravascular growth of adenocarcinoma of the breast at the edge of a metastatic nodule in the skin. Pleomorphic hyperchromatic tumor cells are entrapped in a loose fibrin meshwork. Most of the erythrocytes have been washed away. Such loose clusters of poorly adherent tumor cells may be dislodged easily to form metastases downstream. (H&E, ×300.)

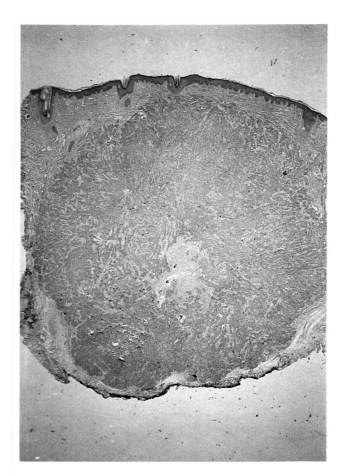

Figure 55–3. Low magnification light micrograph of metastatic carcinoma of the lung. This tumor forms a spherical nodule centered on the junction of the deep dermis and subcutis. It has a sunburst pattern with a central fibrotic region. (H&E, ×30.)

tumor cells have survived a period of equilibrium with the host immune response and have later escaped this suppression. Certainly, immune destruction of the tumor is desirable for the host, but there is some experimental evidence indicating that the effects of an immunologic response are not always purely beneficial.[2] Sharkey and Fogh[21] have reviewed the literature and studied a large series of tumors transplanted into nude mice (deficient in T cell immunity) and concur with previous authors that, when injected subcutaneously into nude mice, many tumors produce expanding spherical nodules that can achieve great size but usually do not kill the nude mouse by metastasis. North and Nicolson[22] have studied an experimental system in which breast adenocarcinoma cells are injected into nude rats. No metastases were present in the nude rats at a time when age-matched immunocompetent controls had lung and lymph node metastases. These studies indicate that a T cell immune response in some instances actually may enhance metastatic spread perhaps either by disseminating cells in the inflammatory response or by forming intravascular clusters with circulating tumor cells.[2,23] Prehn[24] has proposed that primary tumor growth has two phases in some instances: first, a lymphocyte-dependent phase and, second, a lymphocyte-independent phase. Primary tumors often have a prominent lymphocytic response, whereas metastases usually do not. Consequently, speculation has been made that metastasis involves the escape from a lymphocyte-dependent phase of growth as well as an escape from destruction of the tumor cells by lymphocytes. It is difficult to understand exactly what lymphocyte-dependent tumor growth means in cell biologic terms. Perhaps it relates to a need for an inflammatory response to disrupt cell to cell adhesions in order to achieve an infiltrative pattern of growth, but investigation of the mechanism is needed.

Finally, in order for a metastasis to form a tumor mass greater than approximately 1 to 2 mm in diameter, there

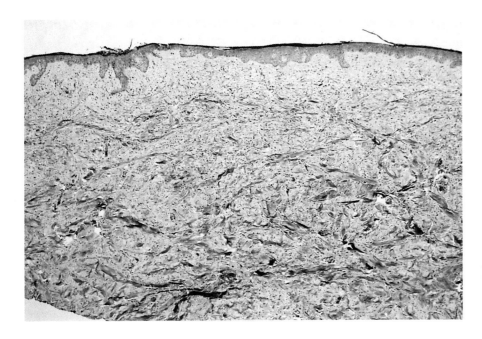

Figure 55–4. Low magnification light micrograph of a diffuse pattern of metastasis in the dermis. Between the collagen bundles, the interspaces are widened, and there is an increase in dotlike nuclei. Appendages are lost. (H&E, ×60.)

needs to be some type of vascular response, such as capillary ingrowth into the tumor[25,26] (Fig. 55–7). A number of tumor angiogenesis factors have been demonstrated in experimental models. Several have been fully purified and cloned. There are factors that act directly on endothelial cells and stimulate motility and mitosis. There are also factors that may stimulate other cells, such as macrophages, to release endothelial growth factors. Examples of direct endothelial growth factors are acidic and basic fibroblast growth factor (FGF) and endothelial cell growth factor (ECGF). An example of an indirect endothelial growth factor may be beta-transforming growth factor (TGF), which is very strongly chemotactic for macrophages. Heparin, as well as low molecular weight saccharides derived from the cleavage of heparin, and copper chelates, such as ceruloplasmin, also may be angiogenic.[26] Suppression of tumor angiogenesis has been demonstrated experimentally using a small fragment of heparin in conjunction with corticosteroids.

In summary, the acquisition by a tumor of the properties necessary to produce a metastasis is a complex and probably multistep phenomenon. The presence within a tumor of cells with different cell surface and other properties facilitates the ability of the colony of tumor cells to go through all the necessary steps to produce a successful

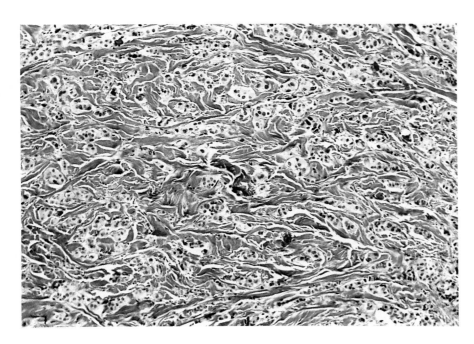

Figure 55–5. At higher magnification, the infiltrate of pale-staining tumor cells can be seen between the collagen bundles, in this metastatic carcinoma of the breast. (H&E, ×150.)

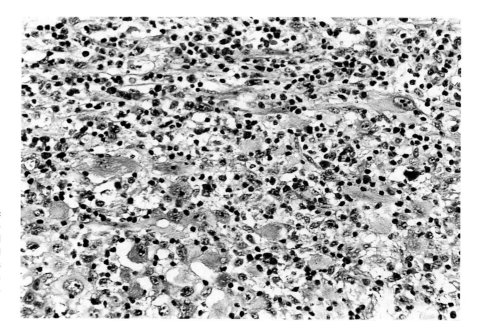

Figure 55–6. Light micrograph of metastatic renal cell adenocarcinoma in skin after treatment with interleukin 2 to enhance T cell immunity. In contrast to untreated renal cell carcinoma (e.g., Fig. 55–7), this metastasis has a diffuse infiltrate of lymphoid cells. Such a reaction may destroy tumor cells as indicated by cell vacuolation and shrinkage. (H&E, ×300.)

metastasis. Evolution on a cellular level would select for cell variants that have the capacity not only to grow but also to spread into new regions of nutrient supply and to stimulate the ingrowth of their own vascular supply.

CLINICAL FEATURES OF CUTANEOUS METASTASIS

Gross Appearance

Brownstein and Helwig[1,27,28] and McKee[29] have reviewed the clinical presentations and histologic appearances of metastatic tumors in the skin. The usual presentation of a cuta-

neous metastasis is as a nodule or group of nodules frequently near a surgical scar from the excision of the primary tumor (Fig. 55–1). The nodules are usually painless, freely mobile, and flesh colored. They often grow rapidly, then reach a maximum size, and tend to remain static. Certainly, there is some variation depending on the type of tumor and the degree of host response to the growth. Metastatic nodules generally do not ulcerate except after trauma or diagnostic biopsy.[1,29,30] Tumors that tend to metastasize by blood vascular routes also tend to have hemorrhage in their metastatic deposits. Renal cell carcinoma and choriocarcinoma are good examples of tumors with hemorrhagic metastases, but other tumors can do this as well, such as

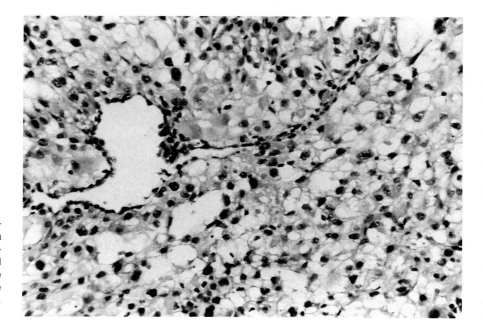

Figure 55–7. Light micrograph of an untreated metastatic renal cell adenocarcinoma in skin. This tumor lacks the prominent lymphoid infiltrate seen in Figure 55–6. A general characteristic of this tumor is the presence of large, thin-walled blood vessels that have been induced to form within the tumor mass. (H&E, ×300.)

thyroid carcinoma, adenocarcinoma of the lung, or even lymphomas and leukemic infiltrates. Metastases often are thought clinically to represent simple cysts or benign dermal tumors,[29] so that a high index of suspicion is needed on the part of the histopathologist to recognize the true nature of the disease process.

Diffuse induration also may be one of the types of gross appearances of metastatic cancer in the skin (Fig. 55–1). Occasionally, the diffuse induration is accompanied by signs of inflammation, such as warmth, tenderness, erythema, and swelling of the skin. This produces the pattern of so-called inflammatory carcinoma.[28] The appearance of erysipelas is mimicked. The term "carcinoma erysipelatoides" was coined by Rasch[31] for this entity. In contrast to true infectious cellulitis, usually there is an absence of fever, chills, and leukocytosis. Partial clinical response to antibiotics can be misleading, particularly in cases where ulceration is present. Skin biopsy is necessary to make the diagnosis. Inflammatory carcinoma is most commonly due to infiltration of the skin lymphatics by breast carcinoma[1,28] but has been reported to be due to carcinomas of the lung,[32,33] stomach,[28] pancreas,[34] rectum,[35] and pelvic organs.[32]

Diffuse induration at times may be less inflammatory than the carcinoma erysipeloides pattern and instead may mimic the appearance of a hard, white plaque produced by morphea, discoid lupus erythematosus,[36] or scleroderma. When this sclerodermoid presentation[28] is on the scalp, it may cause a scarring alopecia. A biopsy usually shows an adenocarcinoma, sometimes with a signet-ring appearance of the cells in a diffuse pattern of infiltration through a fibrotic stroma. Metastases from cancers of the breast, stomach, lung, or kidney have been reported to produce such lesions.[37, 38]

Su et al.[37] have reviewed several cases of unusual types of clinical presentations of metastatic cancer to the skin. They illustrate a case of metastasis from a squamous cell carcinoma of the penis that had a dermatomal or linear or zosteriform pattern of infiltration on the skin of the lower abdomen and thigh. In another case, they illustrate a presentation of skin metastases that resembled condylomata acuminata in the perianal region in a patient with mucinous adenocarcinoma of the rectum. Another patient had multiple small firm papules on the glans and on the shaft of the penis secondary to metastasis from a prostatic adenocarcinoma.

Special studies may be necessary to identify the type of metastatic cancer. Currently, immunoperoxidase methods to demonstrate specific antigens are definitive approaches and frequently can be used on formalin-fixed and paraffin-embedded tissue.[39] For example, Nadji et al.[40] have reported an immunohistochemical marker for prostatic neoplasms, called "prostate-specific antigen." When used in conjunction with antibody stains for prostatic acid phosphatase, a specific identification of a metastasis from a prostatic adenocarcinoma is possible. Electron microscopy also is a useful approach, but McKee[29] states that, in his experience, electron microscopic examination of tissue taken from paraffin-embedded blocks has very little to offer in comparison to a repeat biopsy of the patient and the fixation of fresh tissue for electron microscopy.

Incidence of Metastases

The most extensive and detailed study of tumors metastatic to the skin and subcutis was that of Brownstein and Helwig.[1,27,28] To understand the results of their study, one first must examine the structure of the study itself. Of 3500 patients with the diagnosis of cutaneous metastasis at the Armed Forces Institute of Pathology between 1948 and 1963, they studied 724 patients (21%) for whom there was adequate documentation of both the primary and the metastatic tumors. They excluded certain types of cases: (1) malignant melanomas whose primary lesion had been destroyed or never submitted for examination were excluded from study even though the pigmentation in the lesion revealed the nature of the process (approximately 30 cases), (2) patients in whom cutaneous metastases were noted only as part of the autopsy record, (3) dermatofibrosarcoma protuberans, (4) Kaposi's sarcoma, (5) lymphoma, (6) leukemia, (7) myeloma, (8) Paget's disease without dermal infiltration in the breast, and (9) patients with ulcerated metastases from squamous cell carcinoma of the oral cavity when the histologic study made it difficult to rule out a primary tumor of the skin (a few cases). Despite the usual bias of studies from the Armed Forces Institute of Pathology toward a male population, there were 242 women among the 724 patients, but the 482 males still give a 2:1 male predominance overall in the patient population studied. Another bias is that unusual and difficult diagnostic problems tend to be referred to the Armed Forces Institute, making it possible that their cases underrepresent the usual and routine types of cases, such as breast cancer metastatic to the skin near a mastectomy scar or malignant melanoma with satellite metastases in the skin. Despite these limitations, the study of Brownstein and Helwig is still the best so far in the literature.

Brownstein and Helwig[1] found that the incidence of the various tumors metastatic to the skin correlated well with the frequency of the primary malignant tumors in each sex (Table 55–2). the most common metastases to skin in men were from carcinomas of the lung and colon and in women from carcinomas of the breast.

In autopsy series, skin metastases are found in only 1 to 5% of autopsies of patients with metastatic cancer (Table 55–3). The incidence of tumors metastatic to the skin reflects the usual age distribution of cancer, with approximately

TABLE 55–2. METASTATIC TUMORS TO SKIN: INCIDENCE IN EACH SEX

Men		Women	
Site	%	Site	%
Lung	24	Breast	69
Colon	19	Colon	9
Melanoma	13	Melanoma	5
Squamous cell carcinoma of oral cavity	12	Ovary	4
		Lung	4
Kidney	6		

From ref. 1.

TABLE 55–3. INCIDENCE OF SKIN METASTASES IN AUTOPSY SERIES

Study	Incidence	%
Gates[44]	58/2298	2.5
Abrams et al.[106]	44/1000	4.4
Reingold[30]	32/2300	1.4
Leu[107]	34/1367	2.3
Willis[108]	3/ 430	0.7

80% of the cases being in patients over 40 years of age (82.6% for men and 79% for women).[1]

The risk of developing a skin metastasis must be related in part to the duration of disease. Consequently, since patients today live longer with their cancers despite metastases, we should expect to see a rise in the incidence of cutaneous metastases in autopsy series. However a dramatic increase seems unlikely, since Brady et al.[41] found approximately 100 patients with skin metastases among 10,675 patients appearing for radiotherapy (i.e., 0.9%), excluding breast cancer. With the rapid increase in the incidence of lung cancer in women and in the incidence of malignant melanoma in both sexes, future series can be expected to show a relative increase in the frequency of skin metastases from these types of tumors. In a review by Beerman in 1957,[42] stomach was listed as the site of origin for 15 to 31% of all cutaneous metastases. The decline in incidence of gastric adenocarcinoma in the general population should produce a decline in the incidence of skin metastases from this tumor.

Brownstein and Helwig[1] studied their incidence data with regard to whether or not the skin metastases were the presenting feature of the disease. Their data are somewhat astonishing in that 60% of the patients with skin metastases from carcinoma of the lung (squamous cell, adenocarcinoma, and oat cell) presented with those skin metastases. This clinical presentation also was true of 53% of patients with carcinoma of the kidney, 40% of patients with carcinoma of the ovary, 5% of patients with squamous cell carcinoma of the oral cavity, and 3% of the patients with breast cancer. Perhaps these percentages are so high because the Armed Forces Institute is a referral center for unusual cases. Less of this selective bias should have been present in the smaller series of 22 cases reported by Mehregan,[36] and still 45% of the patients had their skin metastasis at the same time or before the diagnosis of a known or unknown primary cancer. Concerning those patients who developed a skin metastasis after the recognition of a primary tumor, Brownstein and Helwig[1] state that one third of those patients developed a skin metastasis within 6 months, one half within 1 year, and more than 90% within 5 years. In the 10% who developed skin metastases more than 5 years after the primary, those patients had cancers of the breast, melanomas, or adenocarcinomas of the kidney or colon.

Sites of Metastasis

Brownstein and Helwig[1] have emphasized that metastasis to the skin is not a random phenomenon in many cases and that there are "patterns of metastases." In a review

of the available data, Caro and Bronstein[43] reaffirmed a general rule that cutaneous metastases often arise within the vicinity of the primary tumor. Beerman,[42] Gates,[44] and Rosenthal and Lever[45] observed the tendency of skin metastases to occur in the region of the primary growth and suggested that the internal tumor spread via the lymphatics to the skin in such cases. More distant spread was considered to be due to blood-borne metastases. Reingold[30] found that 15 of 17 patients with lung cancer with skin metastases had metastases to the skin of the chest (as well as elsewhere). Similarly, 7 of 8 patients with gastrointestinal cancer and skin metastases had metastases to the skin of the abdomen, and 6 of 10 patients with genitourinary cancers had metastases to the skin of the abdomen. Brownstein and Helwig[1] found that three fourths of the men in their series had metastases to the head, neck, anterior chest, and abdomen, which accounted for only one fourth of the total skin surface. In women, localization was more striking, since three fourths of the women had metastases to the anterior chest and abdomen, which corresponds to only one fifth of the body surface. Metastatic lesions also tended to be localized to one body region, since only 3% of the patients had involvement of multiple areas of the body at the time of initial biopsy or excision of a cutaneous metastasis.[1] In contrast, in the autopsy study of Reingold,[30] almost all of the patients had multiple anatomic regions involved. This multiplicity of sites may reflect the advanced state of disease in an autopsy series. Reingold[30] reported that only 4 of his 36 patients had solitary skin metastases (11%). Gates[44] is cited as having solitary metastases in only 19 of 231 patients (8.2%).

Consideration should be given to each of the body regions. The following discussion is based principally on data from Brownstein and Helwig[1] unless cited otherwise.

The scalp in men was the site of metastases from the lung and kidney,[1,46] and it was the presenting complaint in 50% of them, that is, 11 of 22 patients. Rosenthal and Lever[45] reviewed cases of renal cell carcinoma with cutaneous metastases and found that 28% had metastases to the head, especially the scalp. Breast cancer was responsible for most of the scalp metastases in women.[1]

The face was the site of metastases in 44 patients. Twelve of these were from squamous cell carcinoma of the oral cavity, 6 were from kidney, and 6 from lung.

The neck was the site of extension of tumor from underlying cervical lymph node involvement. The tumors that caused this usually were carcinomas of the oral cavity, lung, breast,[1] or thyroid.[47]

The upper extremity was an uncommon site of metastasis. Even though it is 18% of the body surface, only 6% of patients had metastases to the upper extremity. The most frequent causes were melanoma, or carcinomas of the breast, lung, or kidney.

The lower extremity was also an uncommon site, with only 4% of patients having metastases to this region, which is 36% of the body surface.

The anterior chest was the most frequent site of metastases in women, usually from cancer of the breast, lung, or kidney. In men, it was the site of metastases from cancers of the lung and from melanomas. Reingold[30] found that the anterior chest was the most frequent site of metastases in men. In contrast, the abdomen was found to be the most frequent site of metastases in men by Brownstein and Helwig.[1] For both sexes, the abdominal wall was the most common site for tumors with an initial presentation as a skin metastasis. The most common cancers were from the colon, lung, stomach, or ovary. Adenocarcinoma of the gallbladder also has been reported as a rare source of a hidden primary cancer that can occur as skin metastases.[48,49]

The umbilicus deserves separate consideration, since it has been taught for a long time that a metastasis to the umbilicus, that is, a Sister Mary Joseph's nodule, is an important diagnostic sign of internal malignancy.[50–58] Steck and Helwig[59] reviewed 112 tumors of the umbilicus collected at the Armed Forces Institute of Pathology. Of these, 48 were malignant and 64 were benign. Of the 48 malignant tumors, 40 were metastatic and 8 were primary. They stated that there were no gross features that were helpful in distinguishing the 40 metastatic cancers from the 8 primary malignancies. A hard nodular mass (in 37 of 40 patients) or an ill-defined induration (in 3 of 40 patients) was the usual appearance. Occasionally, they were ulcerated but rarely painful or tender. The value in clinical diagnosis was reaffirmed, since an umbilical tumor was the presenting symptom in 18 of the 40 patients (45%) and was present before the diagnosis of internal malignancy in 29 of the 40 patients (72%). The umbilical tumor appeared after surgery for internal cancer in 11 patients. Among the 40 cases of metastases, 36 were due to adenocarcinomas. Among the 40 metastatic tumors, there were primary tumors in the stomach (11 cases), pancreas (6 cases), sigmoid colon (4 cases), ovary (4 cases), and one case each for endometrium, cecum, transverse colon, penis, cervix, appendix, and liver. The 8 primary cancers of the umbilicus were malignant melanoma arising in a preexisting nevus (4 cases), basal cell carcinoma (2 cases), myosarcoma (1 case), and an adenocarcinoma in a cutaneous remnant of the omphalomesenteric duct in the presence of a Meckel's diverticulum. The benign tumors included melanocytic nevi (24 cases), endometriomas (28 cases), and skin tags (13 cases) as well as some other benign lesions. The routes of spread to the umbilicus were too inconstant in the cases of metastasis to be of any practical value.

The back and flank regions were uncommon sites of metastasis.[1] Only 8% of patients had metastases to this region, which corresponds to 20% of the body surface. The tumors were from lung or breast or were melanomas.

The pelvic region was a fairly common site of metastasis. Cancers of the colon and rectum were frequent causes. Cancers of the lower urinary tract and genitals would also be expected to involve this area.[60–73] Metastasis to the genitals is rare[74,75] but can mimic a syphilitic chancre.

In summary, Brownstein and Helwig[1] state that in men with cutaneous metastasis, the area of localization in the skin was of limited value in uncovering the primary tumor. In women, presentation on the skin of the chest was usually due to cancer of the breast and on the abdomen was usually due to cancer of the ovary.

Routes of Metastasis

True metastasis to the skin from a distant site usually occurs via hematogenous or lymphatic routes. However, in locations where the pleura or peritoneum is very close to the skin, a skin nodule may result by extension via subpleural or subperitoneal lymphatics from an underlying pleural or peritoneal metastasis.[76] An effusion fluid containing malignant cells may be present.

An important cause of skin metastasis is a prior surgical procedure on an internal or skin malignancy. Nodules in mastectomy scars or abdominal scars following removal of a breast or colon cancer are typical examples. These metastases may arise from direct implantation of tumor cells in the wound site at the time of surgery. An alternative explanation might be that circulating tumor cells are localized at the time of surgery to the region of acute injury to the vascular system. Injury to the blood vessels produces leakage of fluid into the tissue, which can be shown vividly after intravascular injection of tracers, such as trypan blue or colloidal carbon particles.[77]

There is no proof that biopsy of malignant skin tumors, such as malignant melanomas, affects the long-term prognosis of the disease.[78] However, biopsy through a growing dermal tumor nodule can be expected to increase the availability of lymphatic vessels and thin blood vessels to the tumor cells. Consequently, excisional biopsy of a suspected solitary malignant tumor nodule is recommended wherever possible.

Prognosis

The prognosis of patients is generally regarded as dismal at the time of detection of a cutaneous metastasis. Reingold[30] found in his series that the average duration of life after a skin metastasis was only 3 months. There is variation with different tumor types. For example, Gates[44] found 9 cases of breast cancer with an average duration of life of 16 months after skin metastasis. Taboada and Fred[79] studied 10 patients with cutaneous metastases and noted a 3-year survival of a patient with skin metastases to the scalp, arms, and thighs from a fibrosarcoma of the tibia. However, the other 9 patients survived only 1 to 4 months (mean 1.8 months). Steck and Helwig[59] reported an average duration of life of 11 months after detection of an umbilical metastasis, most of which were due to adenocarcinomas.

APPROACH TO THE DIAGNOSIS OF CUTANEOUS METASTASIS

Obtaining an Adequate Specimen

The clinical approach to the patient with a solitary tumor nodule varies with the anatomic location and the prior history of the patient. If the nodule is in a critical anatomic site, incisional biopsy and subsequent radiation therapy may be preferable to complete excision.

If there is a prior history of malignancy, the major clinical and pathologic question is whether the nodule is from the original tumor or is from a new primary site, such as a new primary tumor of the skin or even from a new primary internal malignancy. To answer such questions, one requires as much information as possible about the original tumor, including histologic slides and the pathology report on any previous tumor specimens. A paraffin block of the original tumor may be needed for further sectioning and for special staining procedures, immunostaining, or even electron microscopy.

At the time of incisional or excisional biopsy of a tumor nodule, all the available diagnostic procedures should be considered, since distinguishing a primary tumor from a metastatic one can be a difficult task. A portion of the nodule should be fixed in buffered 10% formalin (4% formaldehyde), a portion should be frozen, and a portion should be fixed in buffered glutaraldehyde–paraformaldehyde solution[80] in the event that the tissue will be submitted for electron microscopy.

Specimen Processing

Any portion of the tissue that is fresh should be frozen and stored at $-70°$ C, if possible, to preserve it for further study. The formalin-fixed tissue should be submitted for routine embedding in paraffin and sectioning. The sections should be stained with hematoxylin and eosin or other suitable stain and compared carefully to any sections available from previous tumors. Before resorting to more difficult methods, some standard special stains should be examined in order to formulate a differential diagnosis in difficult cases. The periodic acid-Schiff stain (PAS) before and after diastase digestion can aid in the recognition of glycogen, glycoprotein secretory droplets, and glycoprotein-rich brush border regions on epithelial cells in an adenocarcinoma. It is mainly neutral polysaccharides that stain with this technique. Mucicarmine stains may be useful also for detecting mucinous secretory material in the cytoplasm of cells. An alcian blue stain at pH 2.5 is also a good histochemical stain for acidic polysaccharide groups, such as hyaluronic acid, sialic acid, chondroitin sulfate, and heparin sulfate. Staining with alcian blue at more acid conditions, such as pH 0.5, will eliminate the staining of hyaluronic acid, but the staining of chondroitin sulfate and heparin sulfate will persist.[81] From these slides and stains, most cases of metastatic cancer to the skin can be classified, except for the anaplastic tumors.

Taylor and Sherrod[82] found that when difficult cases are selected, morphologic characteristics alone lead to incorrect classification of anaplastic tumors in almost 50% of cases. They published a proposed algorithm for the selection of antibody stains to use in the classification of anaplastic metastatic tumors from an unknown primary source. As a beginning panel of immunostains, they recommend staining for low molecular weight keratins (LK), high molecular weight keratins (HK), carcinoembryonic antigen (CEA), and vimentin (VIM). LKs tend to be found in simple epithelia, whereas the HKs tend to be found in growths derived from stratified squamous epithelia, as a general rule. CEA is found on the cell surface of some glandular epithelia. VIM is an intermediate filament protein that is found in many sarcomas, melanomas, and some lymphomas. Using these four antibody stains, Taylor and Sherrod[82] listed the several possible outcomes.

A group of tumors is keratin positive and VIM negative (Table 55–4). Almost all of these are epithelial tumors. If the LK is positive and HK is negative and CEA is also negative, these tumors usually are adenocarcinomas, such as from the endometrium, thyroid, kidney, and embryonal tumors. These can then be separated by staining for thyroglobulin, renal tubular antigen, and alpha-fetoprotein or human chorionic gonadotropin (HCG) in the thyroid, kidney, and embryonal tumors, respectively. Chordomas are usually LK positive, CEA negative, and S100 positive.

Those tumors that are LK positive, HK negative, and weakly CEA positive are usually adenocarcinomas of the prostate, liver, endometrium, salivary gland, or lung. As a second screening step, these tumors can be distinguished by staining for prostate-specific antigen and prostatic acid phosphatase obviously for prostatic tumors. Liver tumors often are positive for alpha-fetoprotein, or sometimes for alpha$_1$-antitrypsin. Lung bronchoalveolar adenocarcinomas may be positively stained for surfactant protein.

The tumors that are LK positive, HK negative, and CEA strongly positive, tend to be from the gastrointestinal tract, particularly from colon and stomach. However, medullary carcinoma of the thyroid gland has a similar pattern of staining but should be positive for calcitonin.

The tumors that are weakly LK positive, HK negative, and weakly CEA positive usually are adenocarcinomas derived from germ cell tumors, choriocarcinoma, carcinoids, oat cell carcinoma, or parathyroid carcinoma. Chordoma may be weakly positive for LK and CEA but is positive for S100.

Tumors that are positive for both LK and HK and weakly CEA positive are adenocarcinomas of sweat glands, breast, pancreas, bile ducts, or bladder. Tumors that are weakly positive for LK and HK and are CEA negative are follicular carcinoma of the thyroid, basal cell carcinoma, synovial sarcoma, and mesothelioma.

The group of tumors that is LK negative and strongly positive for HK usually have their origin from stratified squamous epithelia. CEA is negative to weakly or focally positive in some examples. This group includes the classic squamous cell carcinomas of the bronchi, skin, nasopharynx, esophagus, and cervix.

The weakly LK positive and VIM negative group also includes Merkel cell carcinomas and oat cell tumors. Merkel cell tumors are sometimes stained by neuron-specific enolase and Leu 7.

In contrast to these mostly epithelial tumors, there is the category of VIM-positive tumors (Table 55–5). Most of these are keratin negative and CEA negative. In this group are malignant melanomas and most of the sarcomas. They must be differentiated from each other by a second step that involves staining for common leukocyte antigen, S100 protein, desmin, glial fibrillary acidic protein, factor VIII-related antigen, neurofilament antigen, and neuron-specific enolase. The lymphomas are in this group of VIM-positive tumors that are common leukocyte positive. Further subdivision of the lymphomas is best done on frozen sections with monoclonal antibodies to T cell subsets and to kappa and lambda light chains. S100-positive members of the VIM-positive group include histiocytosis X, melanomas, schwannomas (neurilemmomas), neurofibromas, and granular cell tumors. Rhabdomyosarcomas and leiomyosarcomas are positive for desmin, myoglobin, and common muscle anti-

TABLE 55–4. KERATIN-POSITIVE, VIMENTIN-NEGATIVE TUMORS

LK	HK	CEA	VIM	Tumor Type	Other Tests
+	−	−	−	Adenocarcinomas	
				Thyroid	Thyroglobulin +
				Renal cell	Renal tubular Ag +
				Embryonal	Alpha-fetoprotein +
					HCG +
				Endometrium	
				Chordoma	S100 +
+	−	±	−	Adenocarcinomas	
				Prostate	Prostate-spec. Ag +
					Prostate acid phos +
				Liver	Alpha-fetoprotein +
					Alpha-$_1$-antitrypsin+
				Bronchoalveolar	Surfactant protein +
				Endometrium	
				Salivary gland	
+	−	+ +	−	Adenocarcinomas	
				Gastrointestinal tract	Calcitonin +
				Medullary	
				carcinoma	
				of thyroid	
±	−	±	−	Adenocarcinomas	
				Germ cell	Alpha-fetoprotein +
					and HCG +
				Choriocarcinomas	HCG +
				Carcinoids	Neuron-sp. enolase +
				Oat cell carcinoma	Neuron-sp. enolase +
				Parathyroid	
+	+	±	−	Adenocarcinomas	
				Sweat gland	
				Breast	Alpha-lactalbumin +
				Pancreas	
				Bile ducts	
				Bladder	
±	±	−	−	Follicular carcinoma	
				of thyroid	Thyroglobulin +
				Basal cell carcinoma	
				Synovial sarcoma	
				Mesothelioma	
−	+ +	±	−	Squamous cell carcinomas	
±	−	−	−	Neuroendocrine carcino-	
				mas	
				Merkel cell tumors	Neuron-specific enolase +
				Oat cell carcinoma	Neuron-specific enolase +

Adapted from ref. 82.

gen. Gliomas, astrocytomas, and ependymomas are positive for glial fibrillary acidic protein. Kaposi's sarcoma (particularly in frozen sections) and some angiosarcomas are positive for factor VIII-related antigen. The endothelial cell nature of these tumors is better shown by *Ulex europeaus* I lectin binding.

If keratin, VIM, and CEA are all positive, suspect a reason for nonspecific binding of the antibodies or for high endogenous peroxidase activity that has not been properly blocked. It is remarkable that granulocytic sarcoma gives a high endogenous peroxidase activity, which usually is blocked before the routine incubations.

HISTOLOGIC PATTERNS OF METASTASIS

Nodular Infiltrates

The most common histologic pattern, by far, is the expansile nodule centered in the deep dermis near the junction of deep dermis and subcutis, that is, centered near the deep vascular plexus (Fig. 55–3). This has been described as producing, at scanning magnification, a cannon ball or sunburst pattern of cells in the dermis. This sunburst pattern is formed by the radial growth of strands of tumor cells and stroma (Fig. 55–8), often emanating from a central area of

TABLE 55–5. VIMENTIN-POSITIVE KERATIN-NEGATIVE TUMORS

LK	HK	CEA	VIM	Tumor Type	Other Tests
—	—	—	+	Lymphomas	Common leukocyte Ag +
				Malignant melanomas	S100 +
				Histiocytosis X	S100 +
				Mesenchymal tumors and sarcomas	
				Schwannoma	S100 +
				Neurofibroma	S100 +
				Granular cell	S100 +
				Rhabdomyosarcoma	Desmin +
					Myoglobin +
					Common muscle Ag +
				Leiomyosarcoma	Desmin +
					Common muscle Ag +
				Gliomas	Glial fibrillary acidic protein +
					S100 +
				Kaposi's sarcoma	Factor VIII RA ±
					Ulex lectin +
				Angiosarcoma	Factor VIII RA ±
					Ulex lectin +

Adapted from ref. 82.

very dense fibrosis. Inflammatory reaction usually is minimal or absent, except in nodules with abundant necrosis. This pattern may be produced by any carcinoma (Fig. 55–9), any malignant melanoma, or any sarcoma.

The tumor nodule tends to flatten the overlying epidermis (Fig. 55–9) but rarely is attached to it. Often, there is a zone of papillary dermal tissue that is spared (Fig. 55–3), a so-called grenz zone. If the tumor nodule goes on to ulceration, these features are lost, of course. Epidermal appendages, such as sweat glands and hair follicles, tend to be destroyed by the tumor growth. Simple attachment of tumor cells to adnexal keratinocytes is not sufficient evidence of the origin of the tumor from the adnexal structure.

Metastatic tumor cells even may attach to normal cells. For example, it has been shown that metastatic cancer cells can attach by desmosomes to other cell types.[83] In Paget's disease, tumor cells may share desmosomes with normal keratinocytes of the epidermis.[84] Other evidence is needed to distinguish some metastases from primary adnexal tumors.

Evidence of histiotypic differentiation should be sought in different areas of the tumor. What may appear undifferentiated near the periphery or in a superficial biopsy actually can have glandular or squamous differentiation near the center of the nodule, which may be deep in the skin. In the most differentiated areas, certain features of the tumor

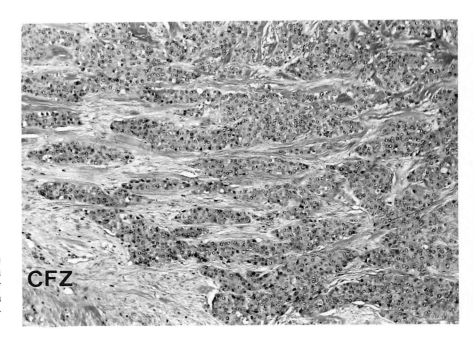

Figure 55–8. Intermediate magnification light micrograph of metastatic carcinoma from the lung. The radial growth of tumor cells from a central fibrotic zone (CFZ) is a common histologic feature in metastatic tumor nodules. (H&E, ×120.)

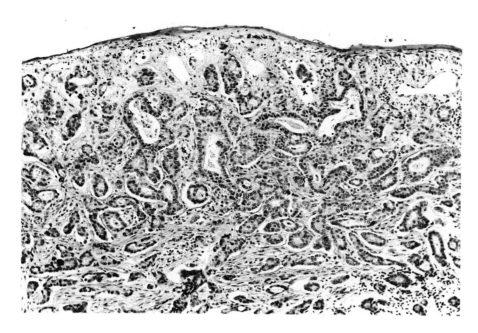

Figure 55–9. Metastatic adenocarcinoma from the breast to the skin. The well-formed glandular lumens indicate that this is a rather well differentiated adenocarcinoma. This lesion is not ulcerated; the epidermis is very flattened at the surface of the nodule. (H&E, ×150.)

cells can be clues to their cell type and, occasionally, to their organ of origin. For example, glandular lumens with PAS staining of the borders of the lumens after diastase digestion or with alcian blue staining suggest an adenocarcinoma. Hyaluronic acid production in the stroma may be abundant, so that stromal mucin in a variety of tumors must be distinguished from true epithelial mucin production. Pseudoglandular spaces may be formed by cell detachment in poorly differentiated squamous cell carcinomas. Zones of complete keratinization to form squamous pearls are indicative of squamous cell carcinoma. Mixed squamous and glandular differentiation may be in metastatic adeno-

squamous carcinoma or in teratocarcinoma. Transitional cell carcinoma of the urinary tract can have areas of squamous differentiation. Metastatic thyroid or ovarian carcinoma may have concentrically calcified bodies, called psammoma bodies (Fig. 55–10). Metastatic renal cell carcinoma often has a pattern of cells that are large and have abundant clear-staining cytoplasm containing glycogen and fat[46] (Fig. 55–11). There is also a tendency for hemorrhage into a highly vascular clear cell nodule of renal cell carcinoma. However, these features are not specific and may be seen in metastatic balloon-cell melanoma, anaplastic Kaposi's sarcoma, adrenal cell carcinoma, clear cell adenocarcinoma

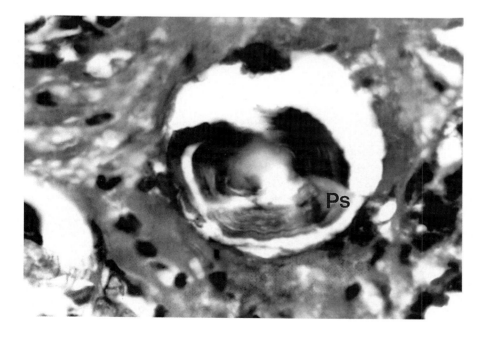

Figure 55–10. Primary papillary carcinoma of the thyroid gland photographed at high magnification to show psammoma bodies (Ps). These bodies are calcific masses with a concentrically laminated appearance. Sectioning tends to cause them to fracture or be pulled out of sections since they are so hard. (H&E, ×1200.)

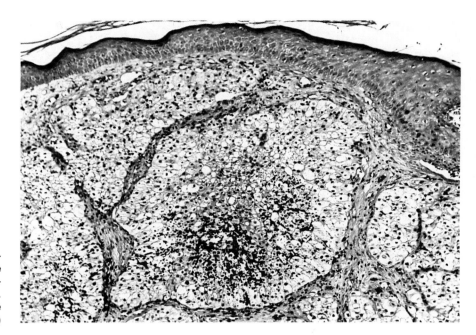

Figure 55–11. Metastatic renal cell carcinoma often has a pattern of clear cells due to abundant cytoplasm containing fat, glycogen, and hydropic swelling of organelles. Hemorrhage is present in the center of the nodules, a frequent finding. (H&E, ×150.)

of the lung, epithelioid sarcoma of the stomach, and even clear cell hidradenocarcinoma of the skin.[85]

Lymphatic Permeation

The histologic pattern of lymphatic permeation is found typically in so-called inflammatory carcinoma of the breast. It can be produced also by adenocarcinomas of the stomach, colon, and pancreas as well as carcinomas of the urinary bladder.

In the sections, at scanning magnification, small nests and ribbons of aggregated tumor cells appear scattered diffusely in the reticular dermis. At intermediate magnification, some of the nests of tumor cells may be seen to lie within a space lined by endothelial cells (Fig. 55–12). In many cases, this is difficult to demonstrate, since the tumor cells seem to have broken through the wall of the lymphatic or to have destroyed its endothelial lining. Superficial lymphatics of the papillary dermis may be dilated by the underlying lymphatic obstruction. The epidermis usually is spared, except for flattening of the rete ridge pattern. Appendages may be spared or destroyed. In the scalp, the hair follicles may be destroyed so that the metastasis has the appearance of a scarring alopecia.[37]

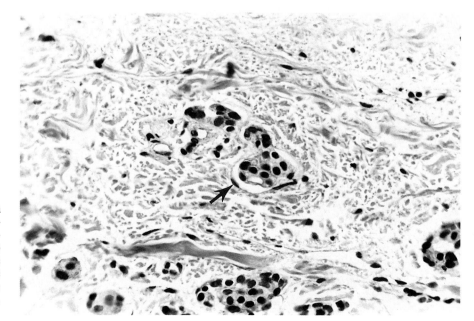

Figure 55–12. Metastatic adenocarcinoma of the breast having the pattern of an inflammatory carcinoma, since its gross appearance simulated erysipelas. Histologically, the infiltration of the tumor cells in lymphatics is characteristic. In the center, a lymphatic vessel retains some of its endothelial lining (arrow) and is nearly filled by tumor cells. (H&E, ×600.)

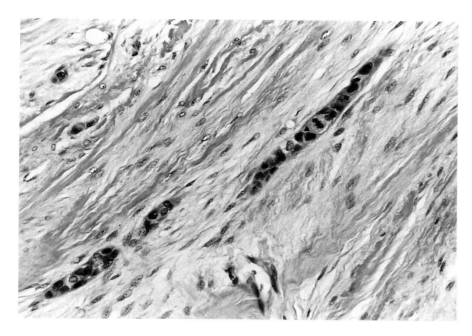

Figure 55–13. Metastatic adenocarcinoma of the breast having a densely fibrotic stroma. Thin cords of tumor cells are present and are one or two cell layers in thickness, called an "Indian file" array. (H&E, ×380.)

Diffuse Permeation

Metastatic carcinomas can infiltrate the dermis in a very subtle pattern produced by spindle-shaped cells and rounded cells that are widely scattered between the collagen bundles of the reticular dermis (Figs. 55–4, 55–5). At scanning magnification, a diffuse increase in cellularity of the dermis may be visible. Also the pattern of collagen bundles is altered frequently because of an increase in the number of small collagen bundles. Occasionally, the collagen bundles become so compact that a diffuse dense sclerosis is produced by the apparent fusion of collagen bundles. Within this collagen matrix, the tumor cells are dispersed as thin cords of cells, one or two cell layers in thickness (Fig. 55–13). The image of these individual tumor cells adjacent to each other in the cords has been referred to as the "Indian file" pattern. In some cases, the cells are even more dispersed in the matrix and do not form such arrays but instead are present as individual cells, widely separated in the stroma (Fig. 55–14). This very diffuse pattern is similar to the pattern of infiltration of the linitis plastica type of adenocarcinoma of the stomach, with its diffuse infiltrate

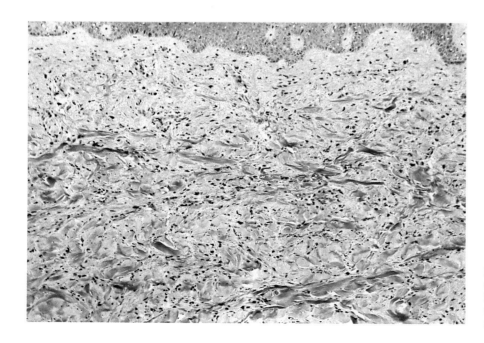

Figure 55–14. Metastatic adenocarcinoma of the breast having a widely dispersed population of tumor cells in the dermis. The atypical cells are so scattered in the dermis that recognition may be difficult. (H&E, ×150.)

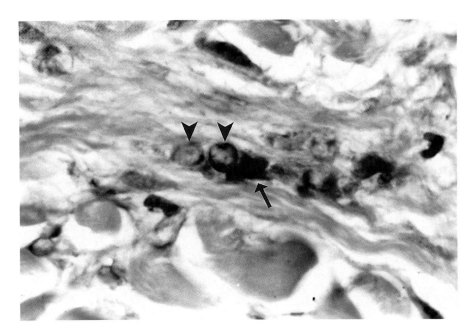

Figure 55–15. High magnification of the tumor in Figure 55–14. Here in a PAS stain after diastase digestion, the lumens of intracytoplasmic canaliculi can be seen as discrete vacuoles (arrowheads). The hyperchromatic nucleus of one of the tumor cells is just to the left of the pair of vacuoles (arrow) and is more homogeneously dark than the vacuoles. Such vacuoles containing mucin sometimes give the cell a so-called signet-ring appearance. (PASD, ×1200.)

of signet-ring cells. If the cytologic features, such as nuclear atypism and cytoplasmic mucin production, do not provide adequate clues to the underlying metastatic cancer, special techniques, such as special histologic stains, immunohistochemistry, or electron microscopy, may be required.

The pattern of diffuse infiltration usually is found in metastases from adenocarcinomas, particularly from breast, stomach, lung, and prostate cancers. Rarely, metastatic malignant melanoma (of the desmoplastic type) can have such a diffuse pattern. In most of the adenocarcinomas, a careful search for intracytoplasmic mucin usually is rewarding, with the help of such special stains as mucicarmine, alcian blue at pH 2.5, or PAS-D (Fig. 55–15). Occasionally, the alcian blue or PAS-D stain the brush border glycoproteins of intracytoplasmic canaliculi. This staining often appears as a positive rim around a moderate-sized cytoplasmic vesicle, 1 to 2 μm in diameter. Antibodies to LK should stain all of the adenocarcinomas but not the desmoplastic melanomas. Conversely, desmoplastic melanoma should stain for S100 protein and VIM but not for keratin.

In some cases, metastatic adenocarcinoma with a very subtle pattern of diffuse infiltration can be difficult to distinguish from some types of benign histiocytic infiltrates, such as nonpalisaded granuloma annulare or some types of fibroblastic tumors, such as dermatofibroma. A high index of suspicion is necessary in such instances even to know when to order special tests for making the distinction from metastasis. A clinical history of a prior cancer can be an important factor in arousing suspicion and stimulating further study. Stains for mucin, such as alcian blue at pH 2.5, should stain the extracellular space between collagen bundles and near macrophages (histiocytes) in granuloma annulare. This must be differentiated from intracellular mucin in a metastatic adenocarcinoma. Granuloma annulare should also be positive for histiocytic markers on immunoperoxidase stains. Dermatofibromas often have epidermal hyper-

plasia above the lesion, whereas metastases usually flatten the overlying epidermis. The battery of special immunoperoxidase stains previously discussed in the section, Specimen Processing, can be used to detect the difference between the adenocarcinoma cells and fibroblasts, since LK should be positive in the metastatic adenocarcinoma and VIM should be negative. This is in contrast to the fibroblasts of dermatofibroma, which are VIM positive and keratin negative. However, it is important to include antibodies to S100 protein and to CEA in the battery of stains.

PROBLEMS IN DETERMINING PRIMARY VERSUS METASTATIC TUMORS

MALIGNANT MELANOMA

Malignant melanoma may produce intracutaneous metastases near a primary skin lesion, and these are called satellites, or, if microscopic, they are called microsatellites (Fig. 55–16). Malignant melanomas also may form skin metastases when the primary is in an internal or hidden location, for example, rectal melanomas or ocular melanomas. If there is only a solitary metastasis from an unknown primary, distinguishing between a metastasis and a primary melanoma is a very real problem. The pattern of spread of the melanoma cells within the epidermis and dermis provides the best means to make such a distinction. Primary malignant melanoma usually has a phase of intraepidermal growth that precedes intradermal growth as a nodule.[86,87] In contrast, metastatic malignant melanoma often has no evidence of continuity with the overlying epidermis (Fig. 55–16). However, some metastatic nodules grow in the dermis until they abut on the epidermis and infiltrate into it. In such cases, the infiltration in the epidermis usually is

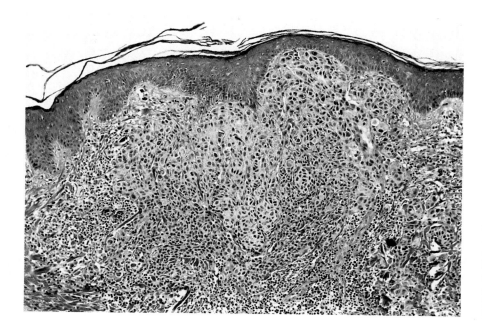

Figure 55–16. Metastatic malignant melanoma illustrating the occasional problem of differentiation from a new primary tumor. This metastasis was near a primary tumor and represented a satellite nodule. There is no infiltration of the epidermis. The lack of maturation with progressive depth in the dermis (see Fig. 55–17) and the resemblance to the primary tumor cells are important distinctive features. (H&E, ×120.)

confined to the epidermis just above the nodule in the dermis.[88] Infiltration in the epidermis for more than three to five rete ridges beyond the dermal portion should be considered strong evidence of a primary melanoma rather than a metastatic one. Maize and Ackerman[89] have summarized those microscopic features that have been helpful in their experience differentiating metastatic from primary malignant melanoma when both exhibit epidermotropism.[88] The features that to them favor the diagnosis of epidermotropic metastatic melanoma are (1) small size, sometimes 3 mm in diameter or less, (2) nests of melanocytes within the epidermis situated not primarily at the dermal–epidermal junction but above it, (3) thinning of the epidermis over a nodular aggregate of atypical melanocytes in the dermis, (4) dermal papillae that seem stretched wider by collections of atypical melanocytes, (5) elongation and inward turning of rete ridges or adnexal structures at the periphery of the lesion (probably an effect of rapid expansion of a nodule in the dermis or epidermis), (6) atypical melanocytes within vascular structures lined by endothelium, and (7) a zone of melanoma in the dermis that is equal to or broader than the zone of melanoma in the epidermis.

Despite these general rules, there remain a few cases in which it is difficult to make the distinction between primary nodular malignant melanoma and metastatic melanoma, or even a Spitz's nevus (spindle or epithelioid cell nevus), since infiltration into the epidermis may not be present. Consequently, it may be impossible to distinguish between these entities. If there is any evidence of a residual nevus, this would favor a diagnosis of primary nodular melanoma rather than metastatic melanoma. With regard to Spitz's nevus, a full discussion of diagnostic criteria is beyond the scope of this chapter and is included elsewhere in this book. Features of Spitz's nevus that are useful for distinguishing them from metastatic melanoma are that Spitz's nevi often are associated with epidermal hyperplasia

and almost always have a polarity to their organization in the dermis. That is, Spitz's nevi have the largest cells and almost all of the mitoses in the upper portion of the lesion.[90] In contrast, metastatic melanoma (Fig. 55–17) does not have the largest cells in the upper portion and does not have a restriction of mitoses to the upper portion. Metastatic melanoma at times also can mimic a blue nevus. The presence of mitoses and enlarged nuclei with prominent nucleoli usually allow recognition of a metastasis. However, there remain instances when all of these criteria fail to be helpful. In such rare instances, a judgment must be made based on whether the lesion in question is near a known primary melanoma or a site of resection of a melanoma and whether there are other lesions suggestive of metastasis. Following the patient's course may give the answer.

Rarely, a metastatic adenocarcinoma can produce a histologic pattern of cells in nests with extension into the epidermis that mimics nodular amelanotic melanoma. Immunoperoxidase stains for keratin and CEA are positive, and stains for S100 protein and VIM are negative in such adenocarcinomas. Malignant neuroendocrine or carcinoid tumors can produce this pattern of metastasis.[91,92]

SWEAT GLAND CARCINOMAS

At times, there may be a problem in differentiating between metastatic adenocarcinoma and a primary sweat gland carcinoma. For example, metastatic renal cell adenocarcinoma may mimic clear cell hidradenocarcinoma (malignant eccrine acrospiroma), since both tumors may contain numerous cells with a clear appearance to their cytoplasm. Metastatic adenocarcinoma with small glands may be very similar to a primary tubular adenocarcinoma of the sweat glands. A clue for making this distinction may be in the position of the tumor nodule in the dermis in some cases, but usually both the metastasis and the primary sweat gland tumor

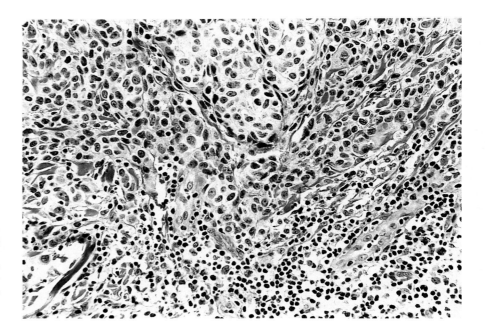

Figure 55–17. At the base of the cutaneous satellite metastasis (see Fig. 55–16), the lack of maturation of the cells and the resemblance to the primary tumor are diagnostic features. Also, mitoses near the base are important (not shown). A sparse lymphocytic infiltrate is present at the base of this tumor. (H&E, ×300.)

form a deep nodule near the junction of the reticular dermis and subcutis. However, if the tumor is in the upper portion of the dermis, a primary sweat gland tumor usually will have a region of continuity with the overlying epidermis and may even spread within the epidermis, whereas metastatic adenocarcinomas usually have no continuity with the epidermis. For example, the usual primary eccrine gland carcinoma in the upper dermis is the eccrine porocarcinoma. There usually is no difficulty in distinguishing it from a metastasis because of its attachment to and infiltration of the epidermis.

Immunohistochemical approaches are the most promising for distinguishing primary sweat gland tumors from metastatic adenocarcinomas when the lesions are deep in the dermis. For example, the milk protein alpha-lactalbumin may be detected in 67% of breast carcinomas and in 62% of their metastases.[93] There is a close correlation between the presence of this marker in the primary tumor and in the metastases. The current polyclonal antisera to alpha-lactalbumin also react with some skin appendage tumors and mesotheliomas.[93] If a monoclonal antibody against alpha-lactalbumin becomes available, it may be more useful, since the reported staining of breast carcinoma is blocked by prior incubation of the polyclonal antibody with excess purified alpha-lactalbumin, but the staining of primary sweat gland tumors is not blocked.[93]

Other antigens, such as CEA, are frequent both in sweat gland carcinomas and in internal adenocarcinomas of the gastrointestinal tract and, therefore, are not useful for this problem. Swanson et al.[94] studied 32 examples of sweat gland carcinomas using a panel of antibodies, that is, antiepithelial membrane antigen, anticytokeratin, anti-CEA, anti-S100 protein, anti-alpha-lactalbumin, antisalivary amylase, anti-beta-$_2$-microglobulin, anti-Leu M1, and anti-blood group antigens A,B,H. The authors conclude that these immunocytochemical markers appear unable to distinguish between primary malignant adnexal tumors and metastases to the skin.

Another approach, recently reported by Penneys and Matsuo,[95] may be useful. An antibody prepared against salivary gland mucin has been found to react with skin tumors of eccrine origin but not with tumors of apocrine origin. This or a similar antibody may provide a method for the positive identification of sweat gland carcinoma instead of metastasis, but this hypothesis needs to be tested.

NEUROENDOCRINE CARCINOMAS

Primary neuroendocrine carcinomas of the skin (trabecular carcinomas or Merkel cell carcinomas) must be distinguished from metastatic small cell melanomas and from metastatic small cell carcinomas (oat cell carcinomas), especially from the lung and gastrointestinal tract. At times, the distinction between Merkel cell tumor and a lymphoma of the Burkitt's type is a problem. The histology usually is only suggestive of the diagnosis, and special techniques, such as immunohistochemistry, are needed for confirmation of the diagnosis.

There are at least two types of distinctions that have to be made. One of them is easy, and the other is very difficult indeed. It is relatively easy to distinguish between primary neuroendocrine carcinoma cells and small cells of squamous carcinoma or adenocarcinoma using immunoperoxidase methods. Neuroendocrine carcinomas usually have positive staining in the cytoplasm for neuron-specific enolase and may also stain for neurofilament proteins.[96] Caution is needed in the interpretation of results. A battery of several antibody stains must be used, since no one antibody stain is specific. For example, neuroendocrine carcinomas stain often for LK or prekeratin, thereby making their distinction from metastatic adenocarcinomas difficult. Malignant melanomas may stain for neuron-specific enolase in almost 60% of reported cases.[97] However, malignant melanomas frequently are stained by antibodies against S100 protein, whereas neuroendocrine tumors are not. Consequently, testing a suspected case with stains for S100 protein, LK, HK, neuron-specific enolase, neurofilament protein, and VIM should provide for the proper distinction between neuroendocrine carcinomas and metastatic squamous carcinomas or adenocarcinomas.

A much more difficult problem is distinguishing between primary neuroendocrine carcinoma and metastatic neuroendocrine carcinoma. Wick et al.[96] have reported that, in 7 secondary metastatic neuroendocrine carcinomas, there was staining for the following neuropeptides: bombesin (4 of 7), leucine enkephalin (2 of 7), beta-endorphin (1 of 7). These substances have been demonstrated in neuroendocrine cells of the lung or foregut but not in Merkel cell carcinomas.[96] There is weak bombesin staining in Merkel cells of newborn skin but not in those of adult skin.[97]

SARCOMAS

The metastasis of sarcomas to the skin (Fig. 55–18) has received relatively little attention. In a series of 724 patients with skin metastases from known primary lesions, there were only 19 cases (2.6%) of sarcomas (27). These cases included leiomyosarcoma, rhabdomyosarcoma, fibrosarcoma, chondrosarcoma, Ewing's sarcoma, osteogenic sarcoma, and undifferentiated sarcomas. It is not clear how many of these sarcomas were true metastases and how many were cases of direct extension of a deep subcutaneous sarcoma to involve the overlying skin.

Perhaps the initial evaluation of a patient with a sarcomatous nodule in the skin should be guided by the principle that it is metastatic until proven otherwise, since primary sarcomas of the skin are very rare indeed. Metastasis of a primary internal sarcoma to the skin is not a common presentation but is more often an incidental finding late in the course of disease when the diagnosis is not a problem. We have observed two patients with metastatic leiomyosar-

coma, in which metastasis to the skin was the first sign of recurrence after removal and treatment of the primary tumor site. One patient had a leiomyosarcoma of the inguinal region and returned 4 years later with a metastasis to the scalp (Figs. 55–18, and 55–19). The other patient had a gastric leiomyosarcoma and developed metastases to the skin of the chest wall. Leiomyosarcoma metastatic to the umbilicus has been reported.[98]

There are few clues to the primary or secondary nature of cutaneous sarcomas. A multiplicity of such lesions is, of course, strong evidence of metastasis. Primary cutaneous sarcomas generally are rather indolent growths that do not appear very bizarre cytologically or have a high mitotic rate in the initial tumor. Very bizarre cytology and frequent mitoses in a sarcomatous nodule are more typical of a metastasis from an internal primary sarcoma or a recurrence of a partially excised primary sarcoma or a malignant fibrous histiocytoma or a rare lesion called an "atypical fibroxanthoma." Metastatic renal cell carcinoma can have a sarcomatous pattern of spindle cells, either with or without a clear appearance to the cytoplasm. Metastatic malignant melanoma also can have a spindle cell morphology, suggesting a sarcoma. Rarely, spindle cells can be so abundant in a primary eccrine acrospiroma (nodular hidradenoma or clear cell hidradenoma) that a careful search for eccrine glandular differentiation or immunoperoxidase stains are necessary to distinguish this tumor from a sarcoma.

ENDOMETRIOSIS AND ENDOSALPINGIOSIS

The occurrence of benign endometrial cysts (i.e., endometriosis) and cysts of the fallopian tubal epithelium (i.e., endosalpingiosis) have been reported in the skin. These benign ectopic structures must be distinguished from metastatic adenocarcinoma (Table 55–6). In the case of cutaneous

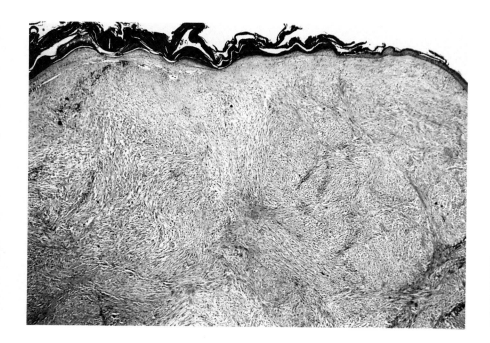

Figure 55–18. Low magnification light micrograph of a metastatic leiomyosarcoma to the scalp. The epidermis is very thin over this nodule. A relatively uniform proliferation of spindle-shaped tumor cells forms the nodule. (H&E, ×38.)

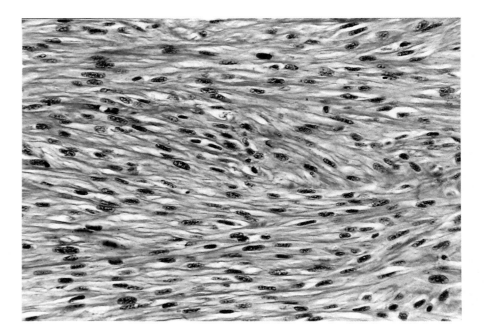

Figure 55–19. Intermediate magnification of metastatic leiomyosarcoma. The tumor cells are spindle-shaped, with atypical nuclei and moderately abundant eosinophilic cytoplasm. Immunocytochemistry may be necessary for the identification of this tumor. (H&E, ×300.)

endometriosis, the women affected are usually 35 to 55 years of age. They usually have lesions in or near the umbilicus or abdominal surgical scars from gynecologic operations.[99] The lesions are red, brown, or blue-black tumors that often noticeably enlarge and are painful and tender about the time of the menses. They usually are less than 3 cm in diameter.[100,101] They may discharge bloody fluid to the skin surface. It is curious that the reported cases often are not associated with widespread pelvic endometriosis. Chatterjee[102] reported 17 cases of endometriosis in surgical scars and stated that only 4 (24%) had pelvic endometriosis. Although theories of coelomic metaplasia have been invoked to explain some cases,[101] it seems more likely that implantation of epithelial fragments explains the association with surgical scars and uterine curettage.

With regard to cutaneous endosalpingiosis, the lesions have been reported only very rarely. Almost all cases of endosalpingiosis in general have been in females with tubal disease, that is, tubal pregnancy, chronic salpingitis, or a history of tubal lavage. Cases have been reported in women in their 30s with lesions near the umbilicus.[103] In contrast to endometrial cysts, endosalpingiosis does not enlarge or hemorrhage with the menses. The lesions of cutaneous endosalpingiosis reported by Doré et al.[103] had a brown color but only had mild pruritus associated with the menses, and they did not discharge fluid. Endosalpingiosis is more common in the omentum and as cysts near the tubes than in the skin. Zinsser and Wheeler[104] reported that 9 of 35 prospectively studied omenta contained endosalpingiotic cysts, all of which were associated with tubal disease. The relationship to the cutaneous ciliated cysts reported by Farmer and Helwig[105] is not known. However the 11 cases reported were single cysts generally on the lower extremity in female patients without any stated gynecologic disease.

Histologically, endometriosis and endosalpingiosis are easy to distinguish from each other. Endometriosis has many tubular glands and cysts in a fibrotic connective tissue (Fig. 55–20). The endometrial glands are lined by a columnar nonciliated epithelium without histologic evidence of se-

TABLE 55–6. DIFFERENTIAL HISTOLOGIC FEATURES OF ENDOMETRIOSIS, ENDOSALPINGIOSIS, AND ADENOCARCINOMA

Feature	Endometriosis	Endosalpingiosis	Adenocarcinoma
Epithelium	Columnar nonciliated	Three columnar cell types: ciliated, nonciliated, and peg cells	One columnar cell type, may be ciliated
Connective tissue	Endometrial stroma	Loose	Loose or fibrotic
Inflammation	Neutrophils	None	Lymphoid
Pigment	Hemosiderin abundant	None	None to small amount of hemosiderin
Cytology	Dispersed, fine chromatin; regular nuclei	Dispersed, fine chromatin; regular nuclei	Coarse, clumped chromatin; nuclear pleomorphism

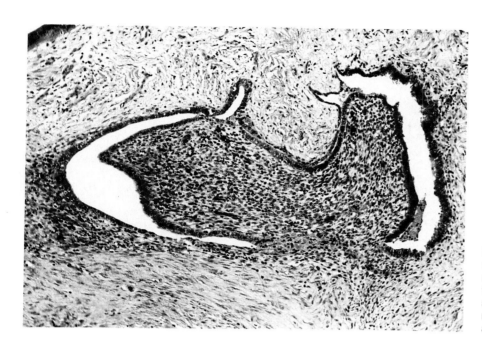

Figure 55–20. Intermediate magnification of cutaneous endometriosis. Note the presence of distinctive cellular endometrial stroma with the endometrial glandular epithelium. The stroma is important in distinguishing endometriosis from metastatic, well-differentiated adenocarcinoma. (H&E, ×148.)

cretion. The epithelium may undergo all of the cyclic changes of regular endometrium, including decidual change with pregnancy.[102] These glands are associated with a densely cellular stroma (Fig. 55–20), which can be found easily, although it may not be evident in all sections. This stroma resembles the distinctive stroma of the normal endometrium and usually is composed of rather closely packed basophilic cells, with a high nucleus/cytoplasm ratio, clustered near the basement membrane of the glands. The stroma may contain collections of neutrophils as well as hemorrhage and hemosiderin. The lumen of the glands often contains cellular debris from the breakdown of neutrophils, red blood cells, and epithelial cells. Hemosiderosis and dense fibrosis may be prominent features of the surrounding connective tissue. These lesions may be present in the dermis, subcutis, or underlying muscle. The glands themselves may have a rather distorted shape in the fibrosis, but cytologically the nuclei appear uniform and regular. Consequently, the benign cytologic characteristics and the endometrial stroma are the most helpful features distinguishing endometriosis from metastatic adenocarcinoma.

Endosalpingiosis is distinctive histologically in that the cysts are lined by an epithelium composed of three cell types: columnar ciliated cells, columnar secretory nonciliated cells, and rather dark, condensed, rod-shaped cells called "peg cells."[104] Each of these cell types has a benign cytology. There is no associated endometrial stroma or hemorrhage. There may be papillary projections into the lumen of the cysts, producing, along with the distinctive epithelium, a resemblance to the fallopian tube. Adenocarcinomas, such as those serous cystadenocarcinomas of the ovary which are low-grade or borderline tumors, can present a problem in the differential diagnosis of endosalpingiosis. Both types of lesions can be associated with stromal calcification and psammoma bodies. Zinsser and Wheeler[104] reported psammoma bodies in 75% of cases of omental endo-

salpingiosis. However, the benign cytology and the fact that the epithelium of endosalpingiosis contains three cell types serve to distinguish endosalpingiosis from metastatic adenocarcinoma, which would be composed of a single epithelial cell type. Adenocarcinoma may produce papillary projections also but shows more evidence of piling up of cells or stratification of the epithelium compared to endosalpingiosis. The nuclear morphology of borderline cystadenocarcinomas of the ovary can be remarkably uniform from cell to cell, including finely dispersed chromatin. This makes it important to rely on the cellular composition of the epithelium in distinguishing these borderline carcinomas from endosalpingiosis.

REFERENCES

1. Brownstein MH, Helwig EB. Patterns of cutaneous metastasis. *Arch Dermatol.* 1972;105:862–868.
2. Fidler IJ, Gersten DM, Hart IR. The biology of cancer invasion and metastasis. *Adv Cancer Res.* 1978;28:149–250.
3. Poste G, Nicolson GL. Arrest and metastasis of blood-borne tumor cells are modified by fusion of plasma membrane vesicles from highly metastatic cells. *Proc Natl Acad Sci USA.* 1980;77:399–403.
4. Liotta LA. Tumor invasion and metastases: role of the basement membrane. *Am J Pathol.* 1984;117:339–348.
5. Liotta LA. Tumor invasion and metastasis. Role of the extracellular matrix. *Cancer Res.* 1986;46:1–7.
6. Terranova VP, Williams JE, Liotta LA, Martin GR. Modulation of the metastatic activity of melanoma cells by laminin and fibronectin. *Science.* 1984;226:982–985.
7. Liotta LA, Rao CN, Wewer UM. Biochemical interactions of tumor cells with the basement membrane. *Annu Rev Biochem.* 1986;55:1037–1057.
8. Nicolson GL, Brunson KW, Fidler IJ. Specificity of arrest, survival, and growth of selected metastatic variant cell lines. *Cancer Res.* 1978;38:4105–4111.

9. Zeidman I, Buss JM. Transpulmonary passage of tumor cell emboli. *Cancer Res.* 1952;12:731–733.

10. Adamson IYR, Young L, Orr FW. Tumor metastasis after hyperoxic injury and repair of the pulmonary endothelium. *Lab Invest.* 1987;57:71–77.

11. Chew EC, Wallace AC. Demonstration of fibrin in early stages of experimental metastasis. *Cancer Res.* 1976;36:1904–1909.

12. Donati MB, Poggi A, Mussoni L, et al. Hemostasis and experimental cancer dissemination. In: Day SB, et al., eds. *Cancer Invasion and Metastasis: Biological Mechanisms and Therapy.* New York: Raven Press; 1977:151–160.

13. Fisher B, Fisher ER. Experimental studies of factors influencing hepatic metastases. VIII. Effect of anticoagulants. *Surgery.* 1961;50:240–247.

14. Dvorak HF. Thrombosis and cancer. *Hum Pathol.* 1987;18:275–284.

15. Dvorak HF, Senger DR, Dvorak AM. Fibrin as a component of the tumor stroma: origins and biological significance. *Cancer Metab Rev.* 1983;2:41–73.

16. Kohanna FH, Sweeney J, Hussey S, et al. Effect of perioperative low-dose heparin administration on the course of colon cancer. *Surgery.* 1983;93:433–438.

17. Zacharski LR, Henderson WG, Rickles FR, et al. Rationale and experimental design for the VA cooperative study of anticoagulants (warfarin) in the treatment of cancer. *Cancer.* 1979;44:732–741.

18. Zacharski LR, Henderson WG, Rickles FR, et al. Effect of warfarin on survival in small cell carcinoma of the lung. *JAMA.* 1981;245:831–835.

19. Penn I, Starzl TE. Malignant tumours arising de novo in immunosuppressed organ transplant recipients. *Transplantation.* 1972;14:407–417.

20. Gange RW, Wilson Jones E. Kaposi's sarcoma and immunosuppressive therapy: an appraisal. *Clin Exp Dermatol.* 1978;3:135–146.

21. Sharkey FE, Fogh J. Metastasis of human tumors in atymhic nude mice. *Int J Cancer.* 1979;24:733–738.

22. North SM, Nicolson GL. Effect of host immune status on the spontaneous metastasis of cloned cell lines of the 13762NF rat mammary adenocarcinoma. *Br J Cancer.* 1985;52:747–755.

23. Ishibashi T, Yamada H, Harada S, et al. Distant metastasis facilitated by BCG: spread of tumor cells injected in the BCG primed site. *Br J Cancer.* 1980;41:553–561.

24. Prehn RT. The immune system as a stimulator of tumor growth. *Science.* 1972;176:170–171.

25. Folkman J. Tumor angiogenesis. *Adv Cancer Res.* 1985;43:175–203.

26. Folkman J, Klagsbrun M. Angiogenic factors. *Science.* 1987;235:442–447.

27. Brownstein MH, Helwig EB. Metastatic tumors of the skin. *Cancer.* 1972;29:1298–1307.

28. Brownstein MH, Helwig EB. Spread of tumors to the skin. *Arch Dermatol.* 1973;107:80–86.

29. McKee PH. Cutaneous metastases. *J Cutan Pathol.* 1985;12:239–250.

30. Reingold IM. Cutaneous metastases from internal carcinoma. *Cancer.* 1966;19:162–168.

31. Rasch C. Carcinoma erysipelatoides. *Br J Dermatol Syph.* 1931;43:351–354.

32. Ingram JT. Carcinoma erysipelatoides and carcinoma telangiectaticum. *Arch Dermatol.* 1958;77:227–231.

33. Hazelrigg DE, Rudolph AH. Inflammatory metastatic carcinoma. Carcinoma erysipelatoides. *Arch Dermatol.* 1977;113:69–70.

34. Edelstein JM. Pancreatic carcinoma with unusual metastasis to the skin and subcutaneous tissue simulating cellulitis. *N Engl J Med.* 1950;242:779–781.

35. Reuter MJ, Nomland R. Inflammatory cutaneous metastatic carcinoma. *Wis Med J* 1941;40:196–201.

36. Mehregan AH. Metastatic carcinoma to the skin. *Dermatologica.* 1961;123:311–325.

37. Su WPD, Powell FC, Goellner JR. Malignant tumors metastatic to the skin. Unusual illustrative cases. In: Wick MR, ed. *Pathology of Unusual Malignant Cutaneous Tumors.* New York: Marcel Dekker; 1985:357–397.

38. Jaqueti G, Rodriguez P, Perez M. Cancer erisipelatoso: metastasis cutaneas de un carcinoma de mama. *Actas Dermosif.* 1962;53:211–217.

39. Borowitz MJ, Stein RB. Diagnostic applications of monoclonal antibodies to human cancer. *Arch Pathol Lab Med.* 1984;108:101–105.

40. Nadji M, Tabei SZ, Castro A, et al. Prostate-specific antigen: an immunohistologic marker for prostate neoplasms. *Cancer.* 1981;48:1229–1232.

41. Brady LW, O'Neill EA, Farber SH. Unusual sites of metastases. *Semin Oncol.* 1977;4:59–64.

42. Beerman H. Some aspects of cutaneous malignancy. *Am J Med Sci.* 1957;233:456–472.

43. Caro WA, Bronstein BR. Tumors of the skin. In: Moschella SL, Hurley HJ, eds. *Dermatology.* 2nd ed. Philadelphia: WB Saunders Co; 1985:1533–1638.

44. Gates O. Cutaneous metastases of malignant disease. *Am J Cancer.* 1937;30:718–730.

45. Rosenthal AL, Lever WF. Involvement of the skin in renal carcinoma. *Arch Dermatol.* 1957;76:96–102.

46. Connor DH, Taylor HB, Helwig EB. Cutaneous metastasis of renal cell carcinoma. *Arch Pathol.* 1963;76:339–346.

47. Horiguchi Y, Takahashi C, Imamura S. Cutaneous metastasis from papillary carcinoma of the thyroid gland. *J Am Acad Dermatol.* 1984;10:988–992.

48. Izuo M. A case of carcinoma of the gallbladder associated with skin metastases as the first sign. *Jpn J Cancer Clin.* 1965;11:213–218.

49. Tongco RC. Unusual skin metastases from carcinoma of the gallbladder. *Am J Surg.* 1961;102:90–93.

50. Powell FC, Cooper AJ, Massa MC, et al. Sister Mary Joseph's nodule: a clinical and histologic study. *J Am Acad Dermatol.* 1984;10:610–615.

51. Barrow MV. Metastatic tumors of the umbilicus. *J Chronic Dis.* 1966;19:1113–1117.

52. Chakraborty AK, Reddy AN, Grosberg SJ, Wapnick S. Pancreatic carcinoma with dissemination to umbilicus and skin. *Arch Dermatol.* 1977;113:838–839.

53. Charoenkul V, delCampo A, Derby A, et al. Tumors of the umbilicus. *Mt Sinai J Med (New York).* 1977;44:257–262.

54. Chatterjee SN, Bauer HM. Umbilical metastasis from carcinoma of the pancreas. *Arch Dermatol.* 1980;116:954–955.

55. Gilmore RA, Sharman JM. Small bowel tumour presenting as Sister Joseph's nodule. *NZ Med J.* 1980;91:176–177.

56. Horn JJ, Fred HL, Lane M, Hudgins PJ. Umbilical metastases. *Arch Intern Med.* 1964;114:799–802.

57. Samitz MH. Umbilical metastasis from carcinoma of the stomach: Sister Joseph's nodule. *Arch Dermatol.* 1975;111:1478–1479.

58. Zeligman I, Schwilm A. Umbilical metastasis from carcinoma of the colon. *Arch Dermatol.* 1974;110:911–912.

59. Steck WD, Helwig EB. Tumors of the umbilicus. *Cancer.* 1965;18:907–915.

60. Beautyman EJ, Garcia CJ, Sibulkin D, Snyder PB. Transitional cell bladder carcinoma metastatic to the skin. *Arch Dermatol.* 1983;119:705–707.

61. Bischoff AJ, Fishkin BG. Carcinoma of the urinary bladder with cutaneous metastasis—report of 4 cases. *J Urol.* 1956; 79:701–710.

62. Hollander A, Grots IA. Oculocutaneous metastases from carci-

noma of the urinary bladder: case report and review of the literature. *Arch Dermatol.* 1968;97:678–684.

63. Hsu CT, Sai YS. Skin metastases from genital cancer: report of two cases. *Obstet Gynecol.* 1962;19:69–75.

64. Ichikawa T, Kumamoto Y, Asano M. A case of prostatic carcinoma with metastases to the skin and both testes. *J Urol.* 1962;87:941–950.

65. Katske FA, Waisman J, Lupu AN. Cutaneous and subcutaneous metastases from carcinoma of prostate. *Urology.* 1982;19:373–376.

66. Landow RK, Rhodes DW, Bauer M. Cutaneous metastases: report of two cases of prostate cancer. *Cutis.* 1980;26:399–401.

67. Marquis W, Benson R. Long-term survival with skin metastases from carcinoma of the prostate. *Urology.* 1980;16:407–408.

68. McDonald JH, Heckel NJ, Kretchmer HL. Cutaneous metastases secondary to carcinoma of the urinary bladder: report of two cases and review of the literature. *Arch Dematol Syph.* 1950;61:276–284.

69. Safer LF, Pirozzi DJ. Extensive cutaneous metastases from urinary bladder carcinoma. *Cutis.* 1980;26:485–486.

70. Schiff BL. Tumors of testis with cutaneous metastases to scalp. *Arch Dermatol Syph.* 1955;71:465–467.

71. Schwartz RA, Fleishman JS. Transitional cell carcinoma of the urinary tract presenting with cutaneous metastasis. *Arch Dermatol.* 1981;117:513–515.

72. Scott LS, Head MA, Mack WS. Cutaneous metastases from tumors of the bladder, urethra, and penis. *Br J Urol.* 1954;26:387–400.

73. Venable DD, Hastings D, Misra RP. Unusual metastatic patterns of prostate adenocarcinoma. *J Urol* 1983;130:980–985.

74. Oka M, Nakashima K. Carcinoma of the prostate with metastases to the skin and glans penis. *Br J Urol.* 1982;54:61–63.

75. Powell FC, Venencie PY, Winkelmann RK. Metastatic prostate carcinoma manifesting as penile nodules. *Arch Dermatol.* 1984;120:1604–1606.

76. Lehman JA Jr, Smith GV, Cross FS. Lymphatic extension of carcinoma of the lung to the anterior chest wall. *Am J Surg.* 1965;110:944–947.

77. Cuenod HF, Joris I, Langer RS, Majno G. Focal arteriolar insudation. A response of arterioles to chronic nonspecific irritation. *Am J Pathol.* 1987;127:592–604.

78. Weedon D. Melanoma and other melanocytic skin lesions. In: Berry CL, ed. *Dermatopathology.* New York: Springer-Verlag; 1985:1–55.

79. Taboada CF, Fred HL. Cutaneous metastases. *Arch Intern Med.* 1966;117:516–519.

80. Karnovsky MJ. A formaldehyde–glutaraldehyde fixative of high osmolality for use in electron microscopy. *J Cell Biol.* 1965;27:137a–138a. Abstract.

81. Johnson WC. Histochemistry of the skin. In: Graham JH, Johnson WC, Helwig EB, eds. *Dermal Pathology.* New York: Harper and Row; 1972:75–117.

82. Taylor CR, Sherrod AE. Approach to the unknown primary anaplastic tumors. In: Taylor CR, ed. *Immunomicroscopy: A Diagnostic Tool for the Surgical Pathologist.* Philadelphia: Saunders; 1986:303–326.

83. Ghadially FN. *Diagnostic Electron Microscopy of Tumours.* London: Butterworths; 1980:51–67.

84. Sagebiel RW. Ultrastructural observations on epidermal cells in Paget's disease of the breast. *Am J Pathol.* 1969;57:49–64.

85. Keasbey LE, Hadley GG. Clear cell hidradenoma. Report of three cases with widespread metastases. *Cancer.* 1954;7:934–952.

86. Clark WH Jr, From L, Bernadino EA, Mihm MC Jr. The histogenesis and biologic behavior of primary human malignant melanomas of the skin. *Cancer Res.* 1969;29:705–715.

87. Ackerman AB. Malignant melanoma: a unifying concept. *Hum Pathol.* 1980;11:591–595.

88. Kornberg R, Harris M, Ackerman AB. Epidermotropically metastatic malignant melanoma. *Arch Dermatol.* 1978;114:67–70.

89. Maize JC, Ackerman AB. *Pigmented Lesions of the Skin. Clinicopathologic Correlations.* Philadelphia: Lea & Febiger; 1987.

90. LeBoit PE, Fletcher HV. A comparative study of Spitz nevus and nodular malignant melanoma using image analysis cytometry. *J Invest Dermatol.* 1987;88:753–757.

91. Norman JL, Cunningham PJ, Cleveland BR. Skin and subcutaneous metastases from gastrointestinal carcinoid tumors. *Arch Surg.* 1971;103:767–769.

92. Reingold IM, Escovitz WE. Metastatic cutaneous carcinoid. *Arch Dermatol.* 1960;82:971–975.

93. Lee AK, DeLellis RA, Rosen PP, et al. Alpha-lactalbumin as an immunohistochemical marker for metastatic breast carcinomas. *Am J Surg Pathol.* 1984;8:93–100.

94. Swanson PE, Cherwitz DL, Neumann MP, Wick MR. Eccrine sweat gland carcinoma: an histologic and immunohistochemical study of 32 cases. *J Cutan Pathol.* 1987;14:65–86.

95. Penneys NS, Matsuo S. A monoclonal antibody to salivary mucin identifies an epitope in eccrine ducts. *J Cutan Pathol.* 1986;13:458. Abstract.

96. Wick MR, Millns JL, Sibley RK, et al. Secondary neuroendocrine carcinoma of the skin. An immunohistochemical comparison with primary neuroendocrine carcinoma of the skin. *J Am Acad Dermatol.* 1985;13:134–142.

97. Gould VE, Moll R, Moll I, et al. Neuroendocrine (Merkel) cells of the skin: hyperplasias, dysplasias, and neoplasms. *Lab Invest.* 1985;52:334–353.

98. Powell FC, Cooper AJ, Massa MC, et al. Leiomyosarcoma of the small intestine metastatic to the umbilicus. *Arch Dermatol.* 1984;120:1604–1606.

99. Steck WD, Helwig EB. Cutaneous endometriosis. *JAMA.* 1965;191:167–170.

100. Williams HE, Barsky S, Storino W. Umbilical endometrioma (silent type). *Arch Dermatol.* 1976;112:1435–1436.

101. Popoff L, Raitchev R, Andreev VCh. Endometriosis of the skin. *Arch Dermatol.* 1962;85:66–69.

102. Chatterjee SK. Scar endometriosis: a clinicopathologic study of 17 cases. *Obstet Gynecol.* 1980;56:81–84.

103. Dore N, Landry M, Cadotte M, Schurch W. Cutaneous endosalpingiosis. *Arch Dermatol.* 1980;116:909–912.

104. Zinsser KR, Wheeler JE. Endosalpingiosis in the omentum. A study of autopsy and surgical material. *Am J Surg Pathol.* 1982;6:109–117.

105. Farmer ER, Helwig EB. Cutaneous ciliated cysts. *Arch Dermatol.* 1978;114:70–73.

106. Abrams HL, Spiro N, Goldstein N. Metastases in carcinoma. *Cancer.* 1950;3:76–85.

107. Leu F. Les metastases cutanees des cancers viscereaux. These. Universite de Lausanne, Lausanne, 1964.

108. Willis RA. *The Pathology of Tumors.* London: Butterworth and Co; 1960:179.

CHAPTER 56
Cutaneous Lymphoma

George F. Murphy

Recently we have begun to appreciate skin as a lymphoid organ. Closely allied with draining lymph nodes, it provides a microenvironment for a variety of immunologically competent, constantly trafficking mononuclear cells. It is not surprising, therefore, that the skin is often both primarily and secondarily affected by dysplastic and malignant lymphoid infiltrates.

In order to understand the pathogenesis and classification of lymphomas affecting the skin, it is necessary to first illustrate these processes as they arise in lymph nodes.

LYMPH NODAL LYMPHOMA

Morphology and Classification

The non-Hodgkin's lymphomas, excluding mycosis fungoides, are heterogeneous, both clinically and pathologically. A helpful feature in understanding their biology and classification, however, is that they often appear to represent clonal outgrowths of normal lymphoid cells at varying stages of their intranodal functional development. The most common systems of morphologic classification[1-3] rely on the cytologic and functional similarities between malignant cells and their benign counterparts. Unfortunately, each system has its own nomenclature, and categories are easily superimposed only by experienced hematopathologists. Fortunately, these systems have been evaluated by the non-Hodgkin's Lymphoma Pathologic Classification Project,[4] sponsored by the National Cancer Institute. The findings of this study indicate the reproducibility and clinical relevance of all three systems, and they proposed a clinically relevant nomenclature (Table 56–1). The architectural and cytologic features of each descriptive type are schematically depicted in Figure 56–1. Although this system was formulated for classifying primary lymph nodal lymphomas, it is conceptually helpful to view cutaneous involvement by B cell malignancies in a similar manner.

The architecture of nodal lymphoma, whether nodular (follicle-like) or diffuse, characteristically effaces the involved node, partially or fully obliterating preexisting structure. This observation is useful in initial recognition of lymphoma at low power magnification and can be applied to atypical and malignant lymphoid infiltration of the skin as well.

The cytology of nodal lymphoma varies from small lymphocytelike cells to larger cells with clefted nuclei to still larger cells resembling histiocytes. Both architecture and cytologic detail are used to assign predictions of biologic behavior (Fig. 56–1).

The immunomorphology of nodal lymphoma recently has been recognized as an important diagnostic adjunct. Normal lymph nodes are composed of a heterogeneous population of cells[5-10] (various subsets of lymphocytes, macrophages, dendritic cells) arranged in discrete anatomic sites, permitting efficient cell–antigen and cell–cell interactions. B cells are primarily localized in follicular regions, whereas T cells predominate in the paracortical and interfollicular regions. In lymphomas, this normal immune architecture generally is effaced, and the proliferating neoplastic cells are immunologically monomorphic. For example, in B cell lymphomas, there is often immunoglobulin light chain restriction, as detected by routine immunohistochemistry for lambda and kappa light chains.[11] This contrasts sharply with normal and hyperplastic nodes, which contain follicles with an admixture of cells expressing both light chain classes. In T cell malignancies, there is generally a marked preponderance of one functional subclass of T lymphocyte (e.g., helper-inducer cells in mycosis fungoides), although this feature is not in itself diagnostic.[12] More specific diagnostic methods relying on immunoglobulin and T cell receptor gene rearrangements[13,14] are now being applied to the routine diagnosis of B and T cell malignancies at some centers.

TABLE 56–1. NOMENCLATURE PROPOSED BY THE NON-HODGKIN'S PATHOLOGIC CLASSIFICATION PROJECT: THE WORKING FORMULATION

Clinical Type	Descriptive Type
Low-grade lymphomas	Small lymphocytic (consistent with chronic lymphocytic leukemia, plasmacytoid)
	Follicular
	Small cleaved cell
	Mixed (small cleaved and large cells)
Intermediate-grade lymphomas	Follicular
	Large cell
	Diffuse
	Small cleaved cell
	Mixed small and large cell
	Large cell (cleaved or non-cleaved)
High-grade lymphomas	Large cell immunoblastic
	Lymphoblastic
	Small noncleaved cell (Burkitt's)

CUTANEOUS LYMPHOMA

B CELL TYPE

Clinical Features

Cutaneous involvement occurs in less than 5% of patients with malignant nodal lymphoma of the B cell type[15,16] (Fig. 56–2), and its appearance often is late in the course of the disease. Although only a small percentage of patients primarily have skin involvement, when lesions occur, they are often the sole manifestation of disease.[17–19] Clinically, nodules are characteristically single or grouped and red to violaceous in color. In contrast to T cell malignancy, overlying epidermal alterations, such as scaling, are uncommon. Lesions show a predilection for the head, neck, or trunk.

Histologic Features

Histologically, infiltrates usually form sharply demarcated perivascular and periappendageal cellular aggregates within the mid- and deep dermis (B cell pattern), with frequent

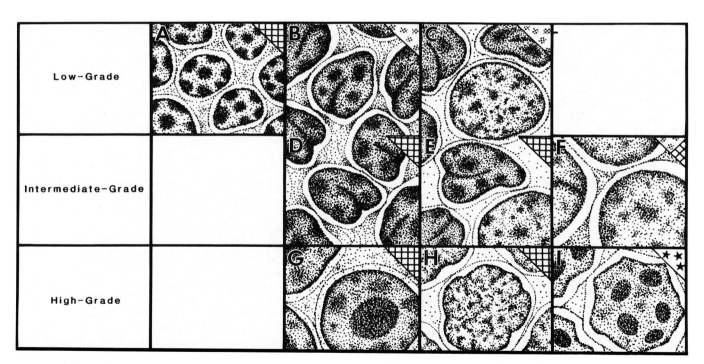

Figure 56–1. Schematic diagram of cytologic and architectural features of non-Hodgkin's lymphomas. **A.** Small lymphocytic lymphoma has a diffuse architecture (cross-hatched, upper right) and nuclei about the diameter of a benign lymphocyte. Small cleaved lymphomas have nuclei smaller in diameter than a reactive histiocyte, exhibit prominent clefts or nuclear membrane folds, and show either a nodular (**B,** clustered dots, upper right) or diffuse (**D**) architecture. Mixed lymphomas may be either nodular (**C**) or diffuse (**E**) and contain cells similar to B/D admixed, with large atypical cells with nuclear diameters approximating those of reactive histiocytes. Large cell lymphomas (**F**) may show either a nodular or diffuse architecture and contain preponderantly cells similar to the large lymphoid cell mentioned for C/E; hence the misnomer "histiocytic lymphoma." Large cells also predominate in the diffuse infiltrates of immunoblastic lymphomas (**G**), but these cells have prominent (blastlike) central nucleoli and often show plasmacytoid chromatin clumping. Lymphoblastic lymphoma (**H**) is diffuse and has a stippled chromatin pattern and frequently shows complex nuclear infoldings. Burkitt's lymphoma (**I**) has a diffuse architecture disrupted by numerous interspersed reactive histiocytes (stars, upper right) and contains cells with angulated nuclei and multiple (2 to 5) small nucleoli.

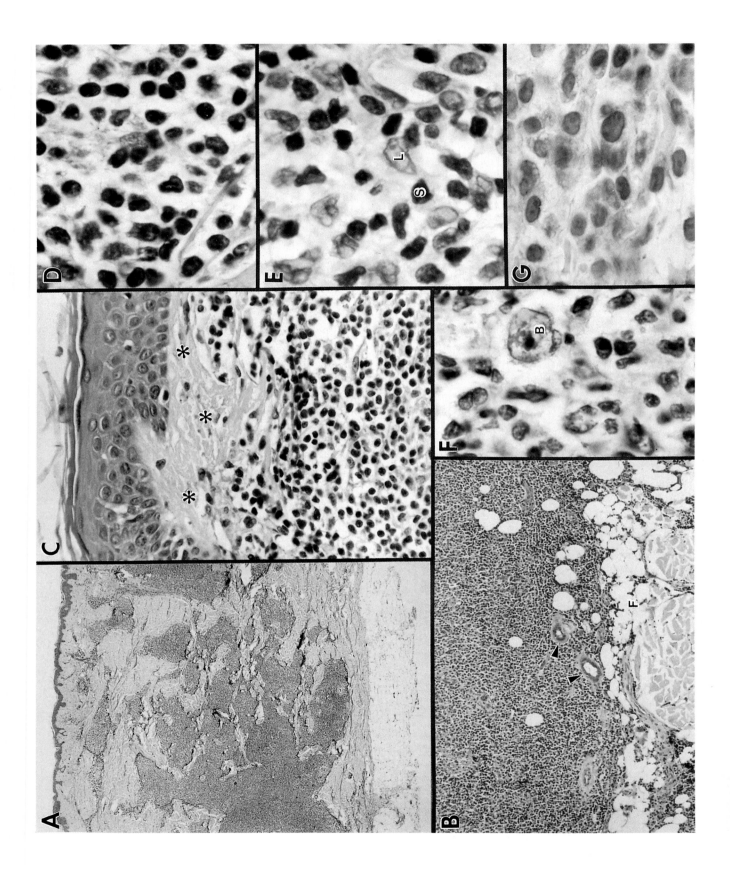

sparing of the subepidermal zone of collagen (so-called grenz zone). The B cell pattern alone, however, is not diagnostic of malignancy and may be seen in cutaneous pseudolymphoma. Cytologically, the nodular aggregates are composed of monomorphous populations of neoplastic cells showing one of the patterns depicted in Figure 56–1. Definitive cytologic classification of B cell lymphoma type on the basis of skin biopsy alone usually is not possible and requires sampling of involved lymph nodes. Even definitive diagnosis of malignancy may be difficult by routine morphology alone when skin infiltrates are composed of neoplastic cells that are small to intermediate in size, thus resembling reactive processes, or when they are composed of anaplastic large lymphoid cells that mimic carcinoma or melanoma. Thus, ancillary techniques, such as immunohistologic evaluation for surface immunoglobulin light chain type, may be required for diagnosis.

Differential Diagnosis

The differential diagnosis of cutaneous involvement by B cell lymphoma includes T cell lymphoma (nonepidermotropic variant or stage), reactive lymphoid hyperplasia (or pseudolymphoma), and leukemic infiltrates. The last, when of myelocytic derivation, characteristically contain cytoplasmic chloracetate esterase activity detectable cytochemically,[20] and cells of both myeloid and monocyte derivation contain cytoplasmic lysozyme, detectable by immunoperoxidase studies of paraffin sections.[21] These enzymes cannot be demonstrated in lymphoid neoplasms, although lymphoid cells characteristically react more strongly in paraffin sections than do myelomonocytic cells for leukocyte common antigen.[22] Thus, cutaneous involvement by acute myeloid and monocytic leukemias (granulocytic sarcoma) can usually be separated from lymphoma using these special diagnostic studies.

Although B cell lymphomas involving the skin may show plasmacytoid features, true plasma cell tumors of the skin are encountered infrequently. When they occur, they are divisable into the categories of (1) benign cutaneous plasmacytoma, (2) primary malignant cutaneous plasmacytoma, and (3) secondary malignant cutaneous plasmacytoma.[23] Whereas the last category most often occurs late in the course of multiple myeloma or plasma cell leukemia,[24,25] primary tumors are rare and require painstaking clinical testing to establish a diagnosis. Infiltrating cells form nodular dermal aggregates and are variably pleomorphic, although they generally retain a considerable degree of plasma cell differentiation and express monoclonal cytoplasmic immunoglobulin.

T CELL TYPE

Cutaneous T cell lymphoma (CTCL) represents a spectrum of related T cell proliferative lesions with variable clinical and histopathologic manifestations (Fig. 56–3). Included in this designation[26] are epidermotropic variants (mycosis fungoides) and nonepidermotropic variants, types with peripheral blood involvement (Sezary's syndrome), and presumed precursor lesions (e.g., parapsoriasis en plaques and poikiloderma vasculare atrophicans). In many instances, these seemingly disparate entities may simply represent different stages of disease evolution. Immunologically, CTCL is a neoplasm of the helper–inducer lymphocyte subset. Although the cause of CTCL is unknown, some authors have suggested a role for retroviruses and chronic antigen stimulation in its genesis.[27] It is thus of interest that Langerhans cells[28] appear to be intimately associated with the proliferating neoplastic cells in CTCL.

Clinical Features

Clinically, CTCL classically evolves from patches to plaques to nodules, although exceptions occur, and nodules may occur de novo. Plaques vary from pale pink to red-brown and usually exhibit scaling. Follicular involvement may result in alopecia. In early stages, lesions may be diagnosed as eczema or psoriasis, but they do not respond to traditional therapy for these entities. Ethrodermic variants may be confused with other causes of this clinical appearance, which correlates with an increased incidence of circulating malignant cells. When multiple lesions exist, biopsy of the center of the most established or advanced lesions will be most diagnostically instructive.

The histopathology of CTCL is as variable as its clinical appearance. Definitive evaluation of early lesions is difficult and may result in confusion with spongiotic dermatoses, benign (small plaque) forms of parapsoriasis, or nonspecific dermatitis. Epidermotropic variants of CTCL show a band-like infiltrate (T cell pattern) of atypical mononuclear cells in the upper dermis, no zone of subbasal lamina sparing (grenz zone) as in many B cell lesions, and variable migration of atypical mononuclear cells into the overlying epidermis (epidermotropism). Although the epidermis so affected may be hyperplastic and often shows abnormal scale formation, it is relatively devoid of spongiosis.[29] This is an important differential feature between epidermotropic CTCL and eczematous dermatitis. Small collections of atypical mononuclear cells in the epidermis form so-called Pautrier's microabscesses. In nonepidermotropic lesions, the mid- and deep dermis may be diffusely or focally infiltrated by atypical

---

Figure 56–2. Cutaneous B cell lymphoma. Architecturally **(A)**, malignant lymphoid cells tend to form nodules about dermal vessels and appendages. Infiltrates frequently involve the deep dermis **(B)**, destroying preexisting adnexal structures, such as eccrine glands (arrowheads), and may even expand into subcutaneous fat (F). The epidermis **(C)** is generally spared, separated from the malignant infiltrate by an uninvolved zone of papillary dermal collagen (*; grenz zone). Cytologically, a spectrum of cell size and morphology is seen ranging from well-differentiated lymphocytes to small hyperchromatic cleaved cells **(D)** to mixtures of large (L) and small (s) cells **(E)** to more pleomorphic large cell forms **(F)** in which immunoblastic cells (B) are frequently encountered. Care must be taken to differentiate these infiltrates from myelogenous leukemia **(G)**, which may occur primarily in the skin.

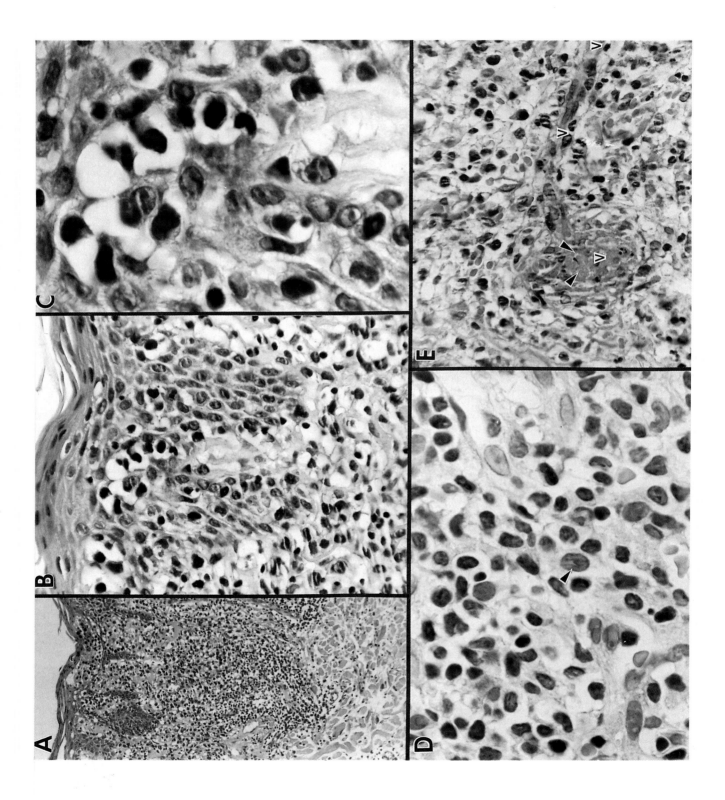

TABLE 56–2. DIFFERENCES BETWEEN ADULT T-CELL LEUKEMIA/LYMPHOMA (ATL) AND CLASSIC CTCL (MYCOSIS FUNGOIDES/SEZARY'S SYNDROME)

Characteristics	ATL	Classic CTCL
Clinical		
Highest incidence	Japan, Carribean	USA, Europe
Clustered outbreaks	Yes	No
Age	Younger	Older
Race	Asian/black	Caucasian
Visceral involvement	More frequent	Less frequent
Course	More fulminant	Often prolonged survival
Laboratory		
Hypercalcemia	Approximately 25%	No
Lytic bone lesion	May occur	Unusual
Antibodies to HTLV-I	Yes	No
Lymphocyte function	Suppressor	Helper
Tac (IL-2 receptor) expression	Yes	No
Morphology		
Gross appearance	Papules/nodules	Patches, plaques, nodules
Microscopic appearance	More lobulated nuclei	Cerebriform nuclei

mononuclear cells. These lesions often lack cytodifferentiation such that the differential diagnosis includes B cell malignancy or even poorly differentiated carcinoma and metastatic melanoma.

Histologic Features

The characteristic cytologic appearance of CTCL is a lymphoid cell with a hyperchromatic nucleus exhibiting a complex, infolded nuclear contour (convoluted or cerebriform nucleus). Similar cells are found in the peripheral blood in Sezary's syndrome. Although these Sezary-Lutzner cells are characteristic, they may be difficult to recognize in routine (6 μm-thick) sections, and plastic-embedded, 1-μm thick sections may be required to appreciate the degree of nuclear complexity. In addition, similar cells may occur in benign dermatoses or after exposure to certain cytokines, although in these latter situations, true Pautrier microabscesses do not occur, and cells with this morphology do not predominate among other mononuclear cells, as is characteristically seen in lesions of CTCL. Further, the degree of nuclear complexity of cerebriform cells in inflammatory dermatoses is not as profound as that of true Sezary-Lutzner cells, as judged by image analysis of transmission electron micrographs.[30]

Because of the diagnostic subtleties of early lesions of CTCL, attempts have been made to use immunohistochemistry in the diagnostic evaluation of this condition. Some investigators have found that cells of CTCL tend to lose pan-T antigens (e.g., those defined by anti-Leu 1,4,5, and 9 antibodies).[31] In addition, CTCL cells are unreactive with the antibody 3A1, which reacts with 70% of benign helper–inducer cells (Leu 3a+) and 95% of cytotoxic suppressor cells (Leu 2a+).[12] Although not entirely specific for CTCL, the monoclonal antibodies BE1 and BE2 appear to be useful in distinguishing CTCL cells from normally unreactive resting or activated T cells. Finally, Vonderheid et al.[32] have demonstrated the usefulness of the Leu 3a/Leu 2a ratio (≥ 6:1) in separating CTCL from reactive infiltrates characterized by a predominance (but often ≤ 6:1) of helper–inducer (Leu 3a+) cells. It is also of interest that CTCL cells generally lack markers of cellular activation (e.g., those defined by anti-HLA-DR and anti-Tac antibodies) that are expressed by benign, activated T lymphocytes.[30]

An interesting variant of CTCL has been discovered.[27,34–40] Although rare, it holds promise for promoting our understanding of lymphoid neoplasia in general. Called "adult T cell leukemia/lymphoma" (ATL), this disorder differs from classic CTCL in a number of respects (Table 56–2), although routine skin biopsy and immunophenotyping alone do not permit definitive diagnostic separation of these two entities. ATL is the first human malignancy shown to be of retroviral etiology. As such, it represents an important model of viral oncogenesis as well as a new disease entity which must be reckoned with both diagnostically and therapeutically. Careful consideration of clinical and laboratory parameters is necessary to exclude this possibility when a skin biopsy suggesting CTCL is evaluated; this is particularly true when disease progression is more rapid or fulminant than is usually expected for classic CTCL.

Differential Diagnosis

The establishment of a diagnosis of malignancy when faced with a clinically atypical lymphoid infiltrate frequently presents a significant challenge to the histopathologist. Pitfalls

Figure 56–3. Cutaneous T cell lymphoma. Architecturally, unlike B cell lymphoma, the infiltrate is closely associated with the epidermis **(A),** particularly in early lesions. The papillary dermis and epidermis are infiltrated by atypical hyperchromatic lymphoid cells **(B),** which aggregate to form Pautrier microabscesses **(C).** In the dermis **(D),** the complex nuclear infoldings (*arrowhead*) may be appreciated even in routinely prepared sections, particularly under 100× oil immersion via varying focal planes. CTCL shows a remarkable tendency to infiltrate and destroy preexisting structures, often resulting in follicular mucinosis as well as lymphomatous vasculitis. **E.** A dermal vessel (v) is infiltrated and destroyed by malignant T cells, resulting in focal fibrin thrombus formation (arrowheads).

of overdiagnosis and underdiagnosis can be overcome by use of adjunctive special diagnostic techniques, awareness of the plethora of disorders that may mimic cutaneous lymphoma, and appreciation of relevant clinical parameters. When lymphoma is suspected, it is advantageous to coordinate planning for specimen triage with a dermatopathologist or hematopathologist before the biopsy is performed. Fixation in formalin and subsequent embedding in paraffin is adequate for routine hematoxylin and eosin evaluation and for certain immunohistologic stains (e.g., S100 protein, cytoplasmic immunoglobulin, leukocyte common antigen) and histochemical reactions (e.g., chloroacetate esterase activity), but special fixatives may be required for optimal nuclear morphology (B-5 solution, a formalin–mercury mixture) or evaluation by 1-μm plastic-embedded sections (glutaraldehyde). Additionally, a rapidly frozen portion of the biopsy is required if most immunohistologic stains are required (e.g., surface immunoglobulins and B and T cell antigens).

There are a number of reactive, dysplastic, and malignant mononuclear cell infiltrates that may simulate cutaneous lymphoma. Although detailed discussion of each of these disorders is beyond the scope of this chapter, a number are listed in Table 56–3 along with differential diagnostic considerations.

SUMMARY

This chapter emphasizes general diagnostic features of malignant cutaneous lymphoid infiltrates. A complete discussion of relevant specific issues is available in volumes addressing this subject exclusively.[41,42] The spectrum of cutaneous lymphoma includes the diverse architectural patterns and cytologic features seen in the subtypes of B and T cell malignancy described. Because of this diversity, lymphomas can variously mimic conditions as different as insect bite reactions and metastatic carcinoma. Many lymphomas are exquisitely sensitive to treatment, and the skin is a highly accessible site for many therapeutic modalities. Thus, accurate recognition and classification of cutaneous lymphomas is essential. Accordingly, the dermatopathologist must approach these diagnostically subtle and problematic infiltrates with awareness of the morphologic diversity routinely expressed by these neoplastic proliferations as well as be

TABLE 56–3. REACTIVE, DYSPLASTIC, AND MALIGNANT MONONUCLEAR CELL INFILTRATES POTENTIALLY SIMULATING CUTANEOUS LYMPHOMA

Disorder	Lymphoma Simulated	Helpful Differential Feature(s)
Reactive		
Arthropod bite reaction	B cell or nonepidermotropic T cell	Lymphoid follicles; polyclonal immunoglobulin (Ig)
Pseudolymphomatous folliculitis	T cell or B cell	Disrupted pilosebaceous units; granulomatous response
Angiolymphoid hyperplasia with eosinophilia	T cell or B cell	Vascular proliferation; germinal centers
Lymphocytoma cutis	B cell or nonepidermotropic T cell	Lymphoid follicles; perivascular infiltrate without follicular or epidermal involvement
Actinic reticuloid	T cell	Primarily in actinically damaged skin; acanthosis of epidermis without significant epidermotropism
Collagen vascular disease	B cell or T cell	Clinical evaluation; direct immunofluorescence (e.g., positive lupus band test); benign cytology
Dysplastic (? premalignant; close follow-up required)		
Lymphomatoid papulosis	T cell	Clinical features (crops of papules and nodules); *caution:* may exhibit T cell receptor gene rearrangements
Lymphomatoid granulomatosis	B cell or nonepidermotropic T cell	Pulmonary and/or CNS involvement; angiocentricity with vessel injury
Angioimmunoblastic lymphadenopathy	B cell	Clinical features; spectrum including immunoblasts and plasma cells
Histiocytosis X[a]	B cell or T cell	Pale cell with reniform nuclei, S100 protein; T6 reactivity; Birbeck granules
Malignant histiocytosis	B cell or T cell	Clinical features; immunohistochemistry for histiocytic markers (e.g. lysozyme or α-I-antichymotrypsin).
Regressing atypical histiocytosis[b]	B cell or T cell	Clinical pattern of regression
Leukemic infiltrates	B cell or nonepidermotropic T cell	Peripheral blood (may be negative); myeloid and monocytic markers

[a] Clinical course variable from benign to malignant behavior.
[b] Biologic behavior controversial; some progress to malignancy.

equipped with a battery of special studies necessary for enhanced sensitivity in their detection.

REFERENCES

1. Rappaport H. Tumors of the hematopoietic system. In: *Atlas of Tumor Pathology*, Section 3, Fascicle 8. Washington, DC: US Armed Forces Institute of Pathology, 1966.
2. Lukes RJ, Collins RD. Immunological characterization of human malignant lymphomas. *Cancer.* 1974;34:1488–1503.
3. Lennert K, Mori N, Stein H, Kaiserling E. The histopathology of malignant lymphoma. *Br J Haematol.* 1975;31(suppl):193–203.
4. The Non-Hodgkin's Lymphoma Pathologic Classification Project. National Cancer Institute sponsored study of classifications of non-Hodgkin's lymphomas: summary and description of a working formulation for clinical usage. *Cancer.* 1982;49:2112–2135.
5. McCluskey RT, Bhan AK. Cell-mediated reaction in vivo. In: Gree I, Cohen S, McCluskey RT, eds. *Mechanisms of Tumor Immunity.* New York: Wiley; 1977:1.
6. Parrot DMV, de Sousa M. Thymus-dependent and thymus-independent populations: origin, migratory pattern and life span. *Clin Exp Immunol.* 1971;8:663.
7. Howard JC, Hunt SV, Gowans JL. Identification of marrow-derived and thymus-derived small lymphocytes in the lymphoid tissues and thoracic duct lymph of normal rats. *J Exp Med.* 1972;135:200.
8. Sprent J. Circulating T and B lymphocytes of the mouse, I: migratory properties. *Cell Immunol.* 1973;7:10.
9. Bhan AK, Reinisch CL, Levey RH, et al. T cell migration into allografts. *J Exp Med.* 1975;141:1210.
10. Gutman GA, Weissman IL. Lymphoid tissue architecture: experimental analysis of the origin and distribution of T-cells and B-cells. *Immunology,* 1972;23:465.
11. Aisenberg AC, Bloch KJ. Immunoglobulins on the surface of neoplastic lymphocytes. *N Engl J Med.* 1972;287:272.
12. Haynes BF, Metzgar RS, Menna JD, Bunna PA. Phenotypic characterization of cutaneous T-cell lymphoma. Use of monoclonal antibodies to compare with other malignant T cells. *N Engl J Med.* 1981;304:1319–1323.
13. Cleary ML, Chao J, Warnke R, Sklar J. Immunoglobulin gene rearrangement as a diagnostic criterion of B-cell lymphoma. *Proc Natl Acad Sci USA.* 1984;81:593.
14. Weiss LM, Hu E, Wood GS, et al. Clonal rearrangements of T-cell receptor genes in mycosis fungoides and dermatopathic lymphadenopathy. *N Engl J Med.* 1985;313:539.
15. Risdall R, Hoppe RT, Warnke R. Non-Hodgkin's lymphoma. A study of the evolution of the disease based upon 92 autopsied cases. *Cancer.* 1979;44:529.
16. Fisher ER, Park EJ, Wechsler HL. Histologic identification of malignant lymphoma cutis. *Am J Clin Pathol.* 1976;65:149.
17. Kim H, Dorfman RF. Morphological studies of 84 untreated patients subjected to laparotomy for the staging of non-Hodgkin's lymphoma. *Cancer.* 1974;33:657.
18. Wood GS, Burke JS, Horning S, et al. The immunologic and clinicopathologic heterogeneity of cutaneous lymphomas other than mycosis fungoides. *Blood.* 1983;62:464.
19. Evans HL, Winkelmann RK, Banks PM. Differential diagnosis of malignant and benign cutaneous lymphoid infiltrates. A study of 57 cases in which malignant lymphoma had been diagnosed or suspected in the skin. *Cancer.* 1979;44:699.
20. Yam LT, Li CY, Crosby WH. Cytochemical identification of monocytes and granulocytes. *Am J Clin Pathol.* 1971;55:283.
21. Pinkers GS, Said JW. Profile of intracytoplasmic lysozyme in normal tissues, myeloproliferative disorders, hairy cell leukemia, and other pathologic processes: an immunoperoxidase study of paraffin sections and smears. *Am J Pathol.* 1977;89:351.
22. Kurtin PJ, Pinken GS. Leucocyte common antigen, a diagnostic discriminant between hematopoietic and non-hematopoietic neoplasms in paraffin sections using monoclonal antibodies, correlation with immunologic studies and ultrastructural localization. *Hum Pathol.* 1985;16:353.
23. Headington JT. Plasma cell tumors of the skin. In: Murphy GF, Mihm MC, eds. *Lymphoproliferative Disorders of the Skin.* London: Butterworths; 1986:160.
24. River GL, Schorr WL. Malignant skin tumors in multiple myeloma. *Arch Dermatol.* 1966;93:432–438.
25. Alberts DS, Lynch P. Cutaneous plasmacytomas in myeloma. *Arch Dermatol.* 1978;114:1784–1787.
26. Edelson RL. Cutaneous T-cell lymphomas—perspective. *Ann Intern Med.* 1975;83:548–552.
27. Yoshida OL, Miyashi I, Hunuma Y. Isolation and characterization of retrovirus from cell lines of human adult T-cell leukemia and its implication in the disease. *Proc Natl Acad Sci USA.* 1982;79:2031–2035.
28. Chu A, Berger CL, Kung PC, Edelson RL. In situ identification of Langerhans cells in the dermal infiltrate of cutaneous T-cell lymphoma. *J Am Acad Dermatol.* 1982;6:350–359.
29. Sanchez JL, Ackerman AB. The patch stage of mycosis fungoides: criteria for histologic diagnosis. *Am J Dermatopathol.* 1979;1:5.
30. McNutt NS, Crain WR. Quantitative electron microscopic comparison of lymphocyte nuclear contours in mycosis fungoides and in benign infiltrates in skin. *Cancer.* 1981;47:698.
31. Picker LJ, Weiss LM, Medeires LJ, Wood GS, Warnke RA. Immunophenotypic criteria for the diagnosis of non-Hodgkin's lymphoma. *Am J Pathol.* 1987;128:181.
32. Vonderheid EC, Tan E, Sobel EL, Schwab E, Micaily B, Jegasothy BV. Clinical implications of immunologic phenotyping in cutaneous T cell lymphoma. *J Am Acad Dermatol.* 1987;17:40.
33. Hattor T, Uchiyama T, Toibana T, et al. Surface phenotype of Japanese adult T-cell leukemia cells characterized by monoclonal antibodies. *Blood.* 1979;58:145.
34. Uchiyama T, Yadoi J, Sagawa K, et al. Adult T-cell leukemia: clinical and hematologic features of 16 cases. *Blood.* 1977;50:481–492.
35. Broder S, Bunn PA, Jaffe E, et al. T-cell lymphoproliferative syndrome associated with human T-cell leukemia/lymphoma virus. *Ann Intern Med.* 1984;100:543–557.
36. Hinuma Y, Nagata K, Misoka M, et al. Adult T-cell leukemia antigen in an ATL cell line and detection of antibodies to the antigen in human sera. *Proc Natl Acad Sci USA.* 1981;78:6476–6480.
37. Gallo RC, Reitz MS. Human retroviruses and adult T-cell leukemia. *J Natl Cancer Inst.* 1982;69:1209–1214.
38. Blattner WA, Kalyanaraman VS, Robert-Guroff M, et al. The human type-C retrovirus, HTLV, in blacks from the Caribbean region, and relationship to adult T-cell leukemia/lymphoma. *Int J Cancer.* 1982;30:257–264.
39. Shimoyama M, Minato K, Saito H, et al. Comparison of clinical, morphologic, and immunologic characteristics of adult T-cell leukemia-lymphoma and cutaneous T-cell leukemia: a clinopathological study of five cases. *Blood.* 1983;62:758–766.
40. Jaffe E, Blattner W, Blayney D, et al. The pathologic spectrum of adult T-cell leukemia/lymphoma in the United States. *Am J Surg Pathol.* 1984;8:263–275.
41. Burg G, Braun-Falco O, eds. *Cutaneous Lymphomas, Pseudolymphomas, and Related Disorders.* Berlin: Springer-Verlag; 1983.
42. Murphy GF, Mihm MC, eds. *Lymphoproliferative Disorders of the Skin.* Boston: Butterworths; 1986.

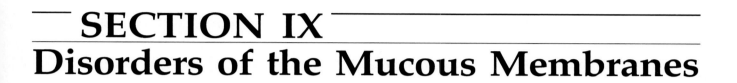

SECTION IX
Disorders of the Mucous Membranes

CHAPTER 57
Disorders of the Mucous Membranes

L. Stefan Levin

Many lesions affect oral mucous membranes. It is therefore not possible to describe them all in a book whose subject is primarily dermatopathology. Many textbooks deal exclusively with clinical and microscopic oral pathology; these sources cover the discipline in detail. The purpose of this section is to delineate the clinical and microscopic characteristics of a select group of oral mucous membrane lesions. Disorders were selected because they are common, they are peculiar to oral mucous membranes, they are important in the differential diagnosis of other more common lesions, or they may be premalignant.

REACTIVE MEMBRANE LESIONS

NECROTIZING SIALOMETAPLASIA

Clinical Features
This condition is a benign, self-limiting disorder of minor salivary glands and most commonly is found on the posterior portion of the hard palate, lateral to the midline.[1] It is characterized by a large, deep ulcer that is sharply delineated from the surrounding mucosa and can measure up to 3 cm in greatest dimension. In rare instances, the lesion may initially be non-ulcerated or begin as a localized enlargement.[1,2] While the overwhelming majority of cases are unilateral, bilateral occurrence has been reported.[3] The soft palate, retromolar trigone, lower lip, tongue, and buccal mucosa are other, although rare, intraoral sites of occurrence. The lesion occurs most commonly in the fifth and sixth decades of life, and has been reported more frequently in men than in women. Pain is a complaint in about one third of patients.

Most investigators attribute the etiology of necrotizing sialometaplasia to infarction and subsequent tissue necrosis[3]; the cause for infarction is unknown. Incisional biopsy is necessary to confirm the diagnosis. Neither complete excision nor further treatment is necessary after initial biopsy, because the condition resolves spontaneously. Long

term follow-up is not available for most patients; however, the lesion usually resolves within weeks to several months. Malignant change has not been described. Although recurrence at the site of the original lesion has not been reported, Rossie et al[4] described a patient in whom necrotizing sialometaplasia occurred on one side of the hard palate; five years later, the patient developed a similar lesion on the opposite side.

Histologic Features
On microscopic examination, the epithelium is ulcerated. Islands of well-differentiated squamous epithelium are found within the deep connective tissue; these islands are likely minor salivary gland ducts and acini that have undergone squamous metaplasia[3] (Fig. 57–1). Pseudoepitheliomatous hyperplasia is also seen. Necrotic minor salivary gland acini, mucous pooling, and an inflammatory infiltrate consisting of neutrophils, histiocytes, plasma cells, and lymphocytes are characteristic features. Outlines of necrotic minor salivary gland acini are also found.[2,3]

Differential Diagnosis
Because of the irregular shape of the lesion, as well as deep ulceration, necrotizing sialometaplasia may be misinterpreted as squamous cell carcinoma or as a minor salivary gland neoplasm. However, necrotizing sialometaplasia can be distinguished from squamous cell carcinoma by its rapid onset and sharp delineation from the surrounding mucosa. In addition, squamous cell carcinoma is rare on the hard palate. Although the hard palate is a common site for intraoral minor salivary gland tumors, they usually grow slowly, are of long duration, and usually present as a firm nodule that may be ulcerated, rather then only as a large ulcer.

On microscopic examination of necrotizing sialometaplasia, pseudoepitheliomatous hyperplasia, squamous metaplasia, and remnants of mucous glands may lead to the erroneous diagnosis of squamous cell carcinoma or mucoepidermoid carcinoma. However, there is no epithelial atypia, and the lobular architecture of the minor salivary glands is maintained. A syphilitic gumma, a tuberculous

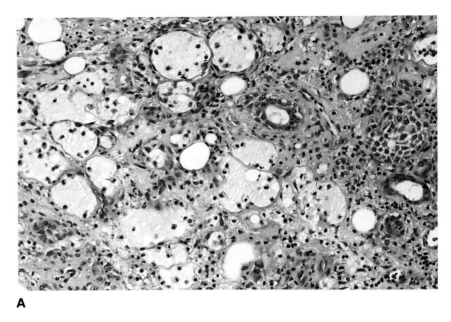

A

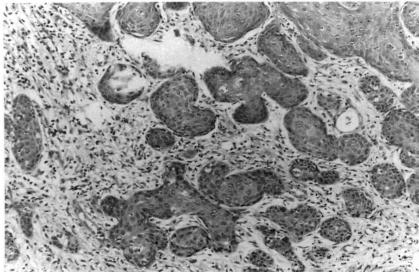

B

Figure 57–1. A. Necrotizing sialometaplasia. Necrotic salivary gland acini, ductal remnants, and an inflammatory cell infiltrate are seen. (H&E, ×170.) **B.** Necrotizing sialometaplasia. Pseudoepitheliomatous hyperplasia in the underlying connective tissue is seen. (H&E, ×40.)

ulcer, and midline lethal reticulosis may also be considered in the clinical differential diagnosis. Careful microscopic examination of a biopsy specimen of sufficient size to include all characteristics of the lesion, as well as correlation with clinical findings, are essential to establish the correct diagnosis.

MIGRATORY STOMATITIS (GEOGRAPHIC STOMATITIS)

Clinical Features

This disorder of oral mucous membranes is characterized by multiple, well-circumscribed, macular, circinate, erythematous lesions, each with a slightly raised, white periphery.

Lesions may be of different sizes in the same patient; some may be only a few millimeters in greatest dimension, while others may reach 1 cm or more in size. The most common sites are the dorsal surface and lateral borders of the tongue (where the condition is known as geographic tongue). On the tongue, the erythematous central portions of the lesions lack filiform papillae, although fungiform papillae remain. However, the condition may occur on any intraoral site.[5]

The lesions are usually asymptomatic and are only noted on routine examination.[5–7] However, burning, itching, or sensitivity to spicy foods is sometimes a complaint.[5–8] Lesions tend to disappear; when they recurr, they may do so at sites different from those found initially.[7] Migratory stomatitis heals without scarring. The condition is found associated with fissured tongue in about 30% of cases.[8]

No treatment is necessary. Because the clinical features of migratory stomatitis are usually diagnostic on clinical examination, biopsy is necessary only if presentation is atypical, or if the patient is concerned about malignant disease.

Histologic Features

On microscopic examination, the white peripheral portion of the lesion is hyperparakeratotic[6] (Fig. 57–2). Epithelium that corresponds clinically to the erythematous central portion of the lesion is spongiotic, and covered by a layer of parakeratotic and acanthotic stratified squamous epithelium that may exhibit intracellular and extracellular edema.[6] Filiform papillae are absent. An inflammatory cell infiltrate consisting of lymphocytes and polymorphonuclear neutrophils may be seen scattered throughout the entire epithelial thickness; microabscesses are found in the superficial epithelial layers. Connective tissue papillae extend almost to

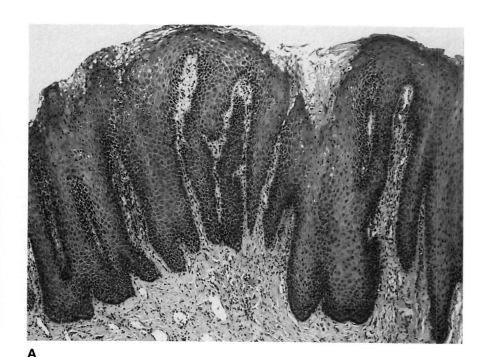

A

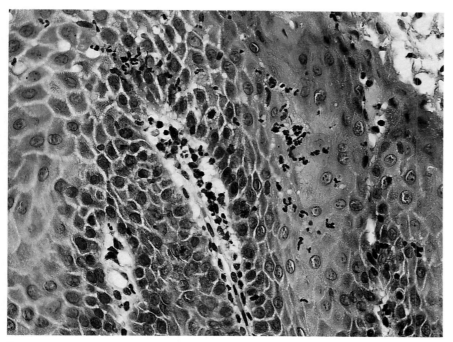

B

Figure 57–2. A. Migratory stomatitis. Hyperparakeratosis, acanthosis, and a chronic inflammatory cell infiltrate in the connective tissue are present. (H&E, ×75.) **B.** Migratory stomatitis. Clusters of polymorphonuclear neutrophils are found within the overlying epithelium. (H&E, ×200.)

the surface, producing suprapapillary thinning of the surface epithelium. An inflammatory cell infiltrate of lymphocytes, plasma cells, histiocytes, and polymorphonuclear neutrophils is found in the underlying connective tissue.

Differential Diagnosis

Clinical lesions of geographic stomatitis are similar to those of lichen planus, candidiasis, and lupus erythematosus. Although the intraoral lesions of lichen planus may be erosive and erythematous, they are not circinate and do not have a white periphery; in addition, lichen planus, when erosive, is frequently painful. The white pseudomembrane of candidiasis is easily removed with a tongue blade leaving a bleeding surface. The oral lesions of lupus erythematosus may also be erythematous, with radiating white striae at the periphery. Microscopic examination (as well as serologic studies in lupus erythematosus) should also serve to distinguish these disorders from migratory stomatitis.

The intraoral lesions of Reiter's syndrome are similar clinically and microscopically to those of migratory stomatitis. Oral lesions described in most patients with this syndrome are erosive and erythematous, although some reports describe intraoral ulcers as well as vesicles.[9–12] Associated features of arthritis, conjunctivitis, urethritis, and skin lesions should assist in distinguishing between these two conditions.

Oral lesions, similar on clinical and microscopic examination to those of migratory stomatitis, have been reported in many patients with psoriasis.[12] However, controversy exists over the frequency of these oral manifestations.[13–15]

INFLAMMATORY PAPILLARY HYPERPLASIA

Clinical Features

Inflammatory papillary hyperplasia is characterized by a cobblestone pattern of many erythematous, small, papillary projections of soft tissue on the hard palate, lingual surface of the maxillary alveolar ridge, and occasionally on the buccal surface of the ridge.[16] It is rare in the mandible.[17] The condition is found most commonly beneath ill-fitting maxillary dentures. In rare instances, the lesion has been reported in patients who do not wear dentures.[16–18] The condition is asymptomatic and the patient is usually unaware of its presence. Although removal of the denture usually results in remission of the inflammatory component of the lesion, complete regression usually does not occur.[18] Surgical removal is necessary, followed by fabrication of a new denture. Malignant change has not been reported.

Histologic Features

On microscopy, the surface of the lesion consists of many low papillary elevations. These projections are covered by parakeratotic and acanthotic stratified squamous epithelium[16,18] (Fig. 57–3). The surface is rarely ulcerated. Pseudoepitheliomatous hyperplasia is a frequent finding. The supporting connective tissue is loose and infiltrated densely with lymphocytes and plasma cells; rarely are polymorphonuclear leukocytes found. The inflammation is found in the connective tissue immediately subjacent to the basal cell layer. When mucous glands are found, they are usually inflamed and may exhibit squamous metaplasia and mucous pooling.

Differential Diagnosis

Clinical features of inflammatory papillary hyperplasia are characteristic and diagnostic. The presence of pseudo-epitheliomatous hyperplasia may lead to the erroneous diagnosis of squamous cell carcinoma. However, there is no evidence of dysplasia of the surface epithelium, and the islands of epithelium in the connective tissue show no atypia. Where ductal metaplasia is prominent and where there is mucous pooling, the lesion may be confused with mucoepidermoid carcinoma.

EPULIS FISSURATUM

Clinical Features

An epulis fissuratum is a mass of soft tissue in the labial or lingual vestibule at the periphery of an ill-fitting denture.[19] The condition is more common in the anterior regions of the jaws than in the posterior.[19,20] Lesions are asymptomatic in about half of affected patients.[20] An epulis fissuratum may be the color of normal oral mucous membrane or may be erythematous and bleed easily.[21] The epithelium may be clinically ulcerated. Although removal of the denture may result in partial resolution because of reduction in inflammation, total remission by this method is unusual.[19] Treatment is by surgical excision. Malignant change has not been documented.

Histologic Features

On microscopic examination, the surface epithelium is hyper-parakeratotic and acanthotic.[21] An ulcer is present in 25% of cases.[21] Deposits of eosinophilic homogeneous material may be found in the superficial epithelial layers[21,22] (Fig. 57–4). These deposits may be confined to the cytoplasm of individual cells, or they may become large, the result of rupture of adjacent epithelial cell membranes and coalescence.[22] Pyknotic nuclei may be found within these deposits. Electron microscopic studies indicate that this material is plasma, derived from the inflamed connective tissue below.[23] The underlying connective tissue is dense and contains variable numbers of neutrophils, lymphocytes, and plasma cells. Nodular aggregates of lymphoid tissue may also be seen.[21] Where muscle is involved, considerable numbers of eosinophils may be found. Adjacent minor salivary glands may exhibit ductal ectasia, squamous metaplasia, and fibrosis as well as a lymphocytic and plasma cell infiltrate. There is no evidence of epithelial dysplasia.

Differential Diagnosis

The clinical features distinguish epulis fissuratum from other oral lesions. Microscopic examination is necessary, however, to rule out a malignant neoplasm that has developed by chance at the denture edge.

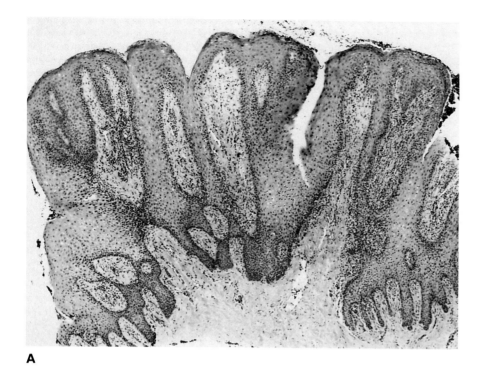

A

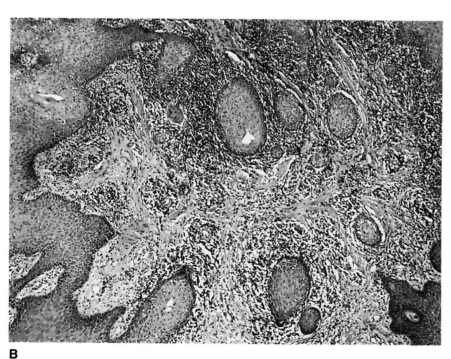

B

Figure 57–3. A. Inflammatory papillary hyperplasia. Surface papillary projections and a chronic inflammatory cell infiltrate are seen. (H&E, ×55.) **B.** Inflammatory papillary hyperplasia. Pseudoepitheliomatous hyperplasia and chronic inflammation are noted. (H&E, ×70.)

PERIPHERAL GIANT CELL GRANULOMA

Clinical Features

The peripheral giant cell granuloma is a sessile or pedunculated, localized, red or red-purple enlargement that occurs only on the gingiva or alveolar ridge. In some instances,

adjacent teeth may be displaced.[24] When the lesion occurs on the edentulous alveolar ridge, it may produce a cup-shaped depression in the underlying bone.[24] The peripheral giant cell granuloma occurs more commonly in the anterior regions of the jaws than in the posterior. The mandible is affected twice as often as the maxilla and females are more

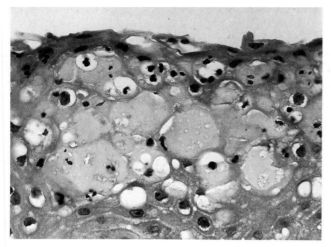

Figure 57–4. Epulis fissuratum. Eosinophilic deposits in the superficial epithelium are found. (H&E, ×400.)

frequently affected than males.[25] The average age of occurrence is in the fourth and fifth decades.[25,26] If the lesion is incompletely removed, or local factors such as calculus remain on the root surface, the lesion may recur. The recurrence rate is between 5 and 10%.

Histologic Features
The surface stratified squamous epithelium is usually intact but may be ulcerated.[26] A dense connective tissue zone usually separates the epithelium from the giant cell lesion beneath.[25] The lesion is characterized by variable numbers of multinucleated giant cells of the foreign body type, some of which are closely associated with blood vessel walls (Fig. 57–5). The number of nuclei in each giant cell may vary from few to many, and phagocytized red blood cells and hemosiderin may be found within the cytoplasm. The giant

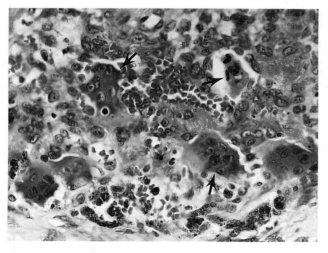

Figure 57–5. Peripheral giant cell granuloma. Multinucleated giant cells (arrows) in an active mesenchymal stroma with hemosiderin pigment are evident. (H&E, ×440.)

cells are separated from each other by a fibrovascular stroma containing oval or polyhedral nuclei that can show considerable mitotic activity. Osteoid, amorphous calcification, and extravasated red blood cells are often found in the stroma. Hemosiderin is frequently present, usually at the periphery of the lesion. A lymphocytic and plasma cell infiltrate is frequently found, either diffusely throughout the lesion or at the periphery.

Differential Diagnosis
Several other lesions occur on the gingiva that clinically resemble the peripheral giant cell granuloma. These include the peripheral ossifying fibroma, pyogenic granuloma, and fibroma. Although odontogenic neoplasms usually occur centrally within bone, they may rarely present as localized gingival enlargements that do not involve bone. Microscopic features distinguish these lesions from one another and from the peripheral giant cell granuloma.

The central giant cell granuloma is identical to the peripheral giant cell granuloma on microscopic examination. The central giant cell granuloma occurs in the body of the maxilla or mandible and usually does not communicate with the oral mucous membrane. Rarely, the central lesion may burst through the cortex and present as a gingival enlargement; thus, a dental radiograph is necessary prior to surgical removal of a peripheral giant cell granuloma to ensure that it has not originated centrally. The central giant cell granuloma on rare occasions has been associated with hyperparathyroidism, but no such association with the peripheral lesion has been documented.[27]

PERIPHERAL OSSIFYING FIBROMA

Clinical Features
Like the peripheral giant cell granuloma, the peripheral ossifying fibroma is a localized enlargement that occurs only on the gingiva.[28,29] The lesion is slightly more common in the incisor-canine region than in the premolar-molar region.[28,29] Two-thirds occur in the maxilla, while the remainder occur in the mandible.[28] The peripheral ossifying fibroma is either pedunculated or sessile, may be ulcerated, and is pink or red. It may move teeth[28] and produce superficial erosion of the alveolar bone.[30] The average size is between 0.1 and 1.0 cm, although lesions as large as 3.0 cm have been described.[29] The mean age of occurrence is the third decade. Complete removal is necessary. A recurrence rate of 15%–20% has been reported.[28,29]

Histologic Features
On microscopic examination, the oral epithelium may be intact and of normal thickness, but is usually ulcerated.[29] When ulcerated, the ulcer is covered by fibrin containing polymorphonuclear leukocytes. The connective tissue subjacent to the ulcer is distinctive and is composed of many fibroblasts with large round or oval nuclei (Fig. 57–6). Vascularity is not a prominent feature, and collagen is scant. Scattered throughout the connective tissue are deposits of calcified material that may be in the form of small grains, larger droplets, osteoid, or trabecular bone. A chronic inflammatory cell infiltrate, composed of lymphocytes and

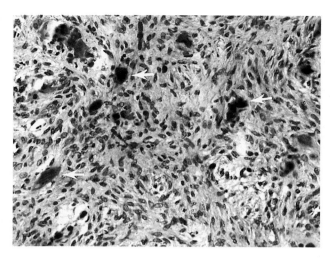

Figure 57-6. Peripheral ossifying fibroma. Droplet calcification (arrows) and an active mesenchymal stroma are seen. (H&E, ×270.)

plasma cells is seen; this infiltrate is usually more pronounced in the superficial portions of the lesion than in deeper portions.[29] In approximately 15% of lesions, multinucleated giant cells similar to those seen in the central giant cell granuloma are found.[29]

Differential Diagnosis
The peripheral giant cell granuloma is similar in clinical appearance to the peripheral ossifying fibroma. Multinucleated giant cells are present in both lesions; however, they are found singly and in small clusters in the peripheral ossifying fibroma, and many more are present in the peripheral giant cell granuloma. In addition, the rather distinctive connective tissue stroma, as well as lack of extravascular red blood cells and hemosiderin in the peripheral ossifying fibroma, should allow differentiation between these two lesions.

The pyogenic granuloma and fibroma also occur on gingiva and are similar clinically to the peripheral ossifying fibroma. However, both lack the characteristic connective tissue stroma of the peripheral ossifying fibroma, and neither demonstrate giant cells or calcified material.

Rarely, odontogenic neoplasms such as the ameloblastoma, adenomatoid odontogenic tumor, and the calcifying epithelial odontogenic tumor (Pindborg tumor), as well as the calcifying and keratinizing odontogenic cyst (Gorlin cyst), occur on the gingiva. The microscopic features of these lesions should distinguish them from the peripheral ossifying fibroma.

APHTHOUS STOMATITIS

Clinical Features
Aphthous stomatitis is a chronic disease characterized by one or more ulcers of oral mucous membranes.[31] Although most investigators conclude that there is no preceding vesicular stage, vesicles have been occasionally documented.[32] The ulcers each have a white necrotic center and an erythe-matous periphery, and are found on sites not bound tightly to bone by periosteum. Thus, the lips inside the wet line, buccal mucosa, mucolabial and mucobuccal folds, tongue, floor of mouth, soft palate, and faucies are affected sites, while the hard palate and gingiva are spared. The peak age of onset is the second decade of life.[33] More than 50% of individuals evaluated may be affected, depending on the population studied.[34]

Aphthous ulcers occur in at least two clinical forms. In one, called minor aphthous stomatitis, one or at most a few ulcers are present at the same time. They are small and range in size from 1 mm to 10 mm;[33] they remain for 7 to 14 days, and heal spontaneously without scarring. The recurrence rate is in terms of months or years.[34] The other form, called major aphthous stomatitis (periadenitis mucosa necrotica recurrens, Sutton's disease), is characterized by one or more large, deep ulcers that measure between 10 mm and 30 mm, last for up to 6 weeks, and heal with scarring.[31] New ulcers may form before older ones resolve, so that some patients are rarely free of lesions.[35] It is unknown whether minor aphthous stomatitis can transform into major aphthous stomatitis with time; however, patients may have both forms.[35]

The etiology of aphthous stomatitis is unknown. It is generally believed that virus is not the cause. However, many precipitating factors have been implicated, including trauma, hormonal changes during menses and pregnancy, psychogenic factors, and allergy.[36] A genetic component has been suggested.[37] It is likely that this condition is, in reality, a heterogeneous group of disorders, with the extent of this heterogeneity yet to be determined.

Histologic Features
Microscopic findings are non-specific. The ulcer is covered by a layer of fibrin, necrotic epithelial cells and polymorphonuclear neutrophils.[35] Bacteria may be present. The connective tissue underlying the ulcer bed is loose and supports an inflammatory cell infiltrate composed of lymphocytes, plasma cells, eosinophils, polymorphonuclear neutrophils, and histiocytes. Capillaries are prominent. Salivary gland, if present, demonstrate chronic sialadenitis with fibrosis.[36]

Differential Diagnosis
Oral ulcers, which are similar in clinical appearance to aphthous ulcers, occur in several other oral conditions, including Behçet's syndrome, Reiter's syndrome, neutropenia and disorders of neutrophil chemotaxis, coeliac disease, acquired immunodeficiency disease (AIDS), and Crohn's disease. They may also result from trauma and chemotherapy. In addition to oral ulcers, patients with Behçet's syndrome have genital ulcers and ocular lesions. Oral ulcers have also been described, although rarely, in Reiter's syndrome; conjunctivitis, arthritis, and skin lesions are also characteristic. The ulcers in neutropenia are associated with hematologic abnormalities, and ulcers in patients with defects in neutrophil chemotaxis are found in patients with chronic granulomatous disease, Chediak Higashi syndrome, and hyperimmunoglobulin E-recurrent infection (Job syndrome). Individuals with celiac disease have gastrointestinal abnormalities. Severe aphthous ulcers are among the many

manifestations of AIDS. The ulcers in all of these conditions are non-specific on microscopic examination.

Oral ulcers may occur in Crohn's disease, and fissures, a cobblestone appearance, and nodular masses have also been described. A history of gastrointestinal disease, as well as the microscopic finding of granulomatous inflammation in the oral lesions in most cases, will aid in making the diagnosis. Traumatically induced ulcers will regress upon removal of the injurious agent; a history of trauma may also be helpful in making the diagnosis. A drug history is helpful in determining the cause of some intraoral ulcers.

Aphthous ulcers are commonly confused with herpetic ulcers. However, herpetic ulcers are preceded by vesicles, which frequently occur in clusters. They are found on mucosa that is bound tightly to bone by periosteum, such as attached gingiva and hard palate. On microscopic examination, viral changes may be found.

VERRUCIFORM XANTHOMA

Clinical Features

The verruciform xanthoma is an asymptomatic, solitary lesion of the oral mucous membranes.[38] It is well delineated from the surrounding normal tissue and usually has a warty surface that is white, grey, or red. While the most common sites are the gingiva and hard palate, any other intraoral soft tissue sites may be affected. The average age of diagnosis is in the late fifth and early sixth decades of life.[39] Size usually ranges from 0.2 cm to 2.0 cm, although a lesion as large as 4.0 cm in greatest dimension has been noted.[40] No association with systemic disease has been reported. Recurrences have not been described following conservative surgical removal.

Histologic Features

On microscopic examination, the epithelial surface is verrucous (Fig. 57–7). It is covered by a layer of parakeratin, which varies in thickness and extends deeply into epithelial crevices.[39,41] Rete ridges are elongated and extend to the same relative depth into the connective tissue. Exocytosis of neutrophils into the epithelium has been described.[39,40,42] The pathognomonic features of the verruciform xanthoma are large foam cells that fill the connective tissue papillae. These cells contain numerous large and small vacuoles that contain lipid.[42] Slightly positive PAS granularity has been noted in the one specimen evaluated using this stain.[42] In most cases, foam cells do not extend more deeply into the connective tissue than the bases of the rete ridges. Connective tissue papilla may extend close to the epithelial surface. A chronic inflammatory cell infiltrate, consisting primarily of lymphocytes, may also be noted in the underlying connective tissue.[42]

Differential Diagnosis

The differential diagnosis includes papilloma. However, the microscopic features of the papilloma do not include foam cells. While foam cells may be found in individuals with abnormalities of lipid metabolism, normal blood lipid and glucose levels have been described in the few patients

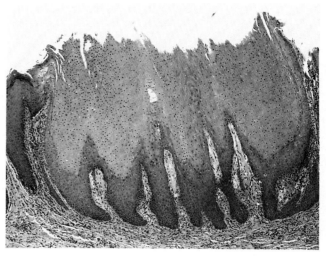

A

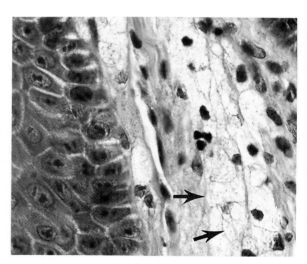

B

Figure 57–7. A. Verruciform xanthoma. A markedly thick layer of parakeratotic epithelium covers the surface. (H&E, ×60.) **B.** Verruciform xanthoma. Foamy histiocytes (arrows) are present in the connective tissue papillae. (H&E, ×550.) (Courtesy of Dr. Todd Beckerman, Baltimore, MD.)

with verruciform xanthoma studied, and no other systemic abnormalities have been noted.

REACTIVE LYMPHOID HYPERPLASIA (LYMPHOEPITHELIAL CYST, BENIGN CYSTIC LYMPHOID AGGREGATE)

Clinical Features

Lymphoid aggregates on the oral mucous membranes are common and are sometimes called oral tonsils.[43] They are pink, well-circumscribed, sessile, exophytic, round, smooth surfaced masses measuring 1 to 3 mm in diameter.[43] These aggregates are asymptomatic and found on routine examination. Sites of predilection are the posterior soft palate, floor of mouth, and ventral and posterior lateral surfaces of the tongue. As many as 25 have been reported in one patient.[43]

Lymphoid aggregates may become enlarged, presumably because of irritation. When they enlarge, they usually maintain their normal color and surface contours, although they may be more red or yellow than the surrounding tissues.[44] Lesions up to 1.5 cm in diameter have been reported.[44,45] They are usually asymptomatic and are detected on routine examination.[46]

Histologic Features

On microscopic examination, oral tonsils are characterized by a crypt lined most commonly by stratified squamous epithelium, which is continuous with the surface epithelium.[43] Pseudostratified columnar epithelium may also be present in the crypt lining.[43] Surrounding the crypt are aggregates of lymphoid tissue in a diffuse or nodular pattern.

When oral tonsils enlarge because of irritation, lymphoid tissue surrounding the crypt epithelium proliferates, resulting in development of many enlarged lymphoid follicles.[44] The epithelial-lined crypt may dilate to form a cystic cavity (Fig. 57–8). This cavity is lined by a thin layer of parakeratinized or orthokeratinized stratified squamous epithelium without rete ridges.[45] Occasionally, the lining is composed of pseudostratified columnar epithelium containing goblet cells or ciliated columnar epithelium.[45,46] Squamous cells with nuclei, keratin debris, lymphocytes, and polymorphonuclear leukocytes may be found in this cavity. Lymphoid tissue is found adjacent to the epithelial lining, most commonly in association with germinal centers; in some cases, there is a dense lymphocytic infiltrate only. Accessory salivary gland tissue may also be found near the lymphoid tissue.[45]

Differential Diagnosis

Neither normal lymphoid aggregates, nor those that have enlarged, should be confused with the normal opening of a minor salivary gland duct, or with a mucocele, fibroma, salivary gland tumor, or lipoma. These lesions may be distinguished from each other by clinical and microscopic examination.

AMALGAM TATTOO

Clinical Features

An amalgam tattoo is an asymptomatic, blue-grey or black, macular or (rarely) papular lesion of oral mucous membranes.[47] It results from introduction of amalgam into the oral soft tissues during dental restorative procedures or during tooth extraction. While this lesion may be found anywhere in the oral cavity, approximately half occur on the gingiva or alveolar mucosa, and almost 25% occur on the buccal mucosa. Many are located near the site of a large amalgam restoration; in some instances the lesion is located near a site from which a tooth with an amalgam restoration had been extracted some time before. Amalgam tattoos range in size from 0.1 cm to 2.0 cm in greatest dimension. In most patients only one amalgam tattoo is present, although several may be found in one individual. On radiologic examination, some are radiopaque.[47]

Histologic Features

On microscopic examination, the surface epithelium is normal (Fig. 57–9). Amalgam is present in the connective tissue either as fine black-brown granules, or as large masses. Fine, brown granules may also be found along connective tissue fibers, in multinucleated giant cells and macrophages, in nerve sheaths, in the walls of blood vessels, in the base-

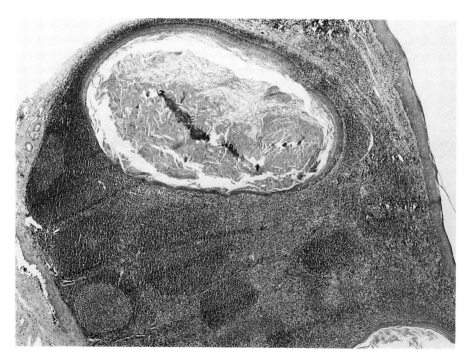

Figure 57–8. Benign cystic lymphoid aggregate. Epithelial-lined cyst, filled with keratin, and germinal centers at periphery are noted. (H&E, ×35.)

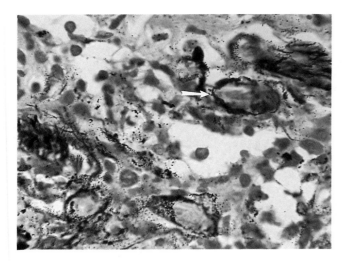

Figure 57–9. Amalgam tattoo. Granular pigment deposited in connective tissue and in wall of blood vessel (arrow) is seen. (H&E, ×500.)

ment membrane zone, and in skeletal muscle. However, selective binding to these structures may not be found in recently implanted amalgam.[48] In some cases, the granules are so fine that they cannot be seen under low-power magnification.[47] About half of all cases do not show a significant inflammatory reaction, while the remainder evoke a mild to moderate chronic inflammation response consisting of lymphocytes and macrophages.[48] A foreign body reaction may also be found.

Differential Diagnosis

Biopsy is required for definitive diagnosis. Because of the small size of most amalgam tattoos, excisional biopsy is recommended. Large lesions need not be completely removed once incisional biopsy confirms the diagnosis. The differential diagnosis includes graphite implantation (for example, from pencil lead), and implantation of other foreign materials. Graphite may be distinguished from amalgam since graphite does not bind to blood vessels, nerves, connective tissue fibers, and basement membrane. In addition, graphite and amalgam exhibit yellow birefringence under polarized light; however, while graphite maintains a yellow birefringence, after treatment with ammonium sulfide amalgam particles will develop a strong orange birefringence.[48] In addition, ammonium sulfide will change the dark particles of amalgam to granular semitranslucent structures, whereas graphite remains unchanged by this procedure.[48] Energy dispersive x-ray microanalysis can distinguish amalgam pigmentation from other foreign materials.[49]

The amalgam tattoo should be distinguished from hemosiderin and melanin pigment, varix, pigmented nevus, melanotic macule, and melanoma. Prussian blue and fontana stains will distinguish amalgam from hemosiderin and melanin, since amalgam will remain black-brown. Varices, nevi, and melanoma may be distinguished from an amalgam tattoo by their histologic characteristics.

Pigmentation of the oral mucous membranes may result from use of minocycline, chloroquine, and oral contracep-

tives. It also occurs in Peutz-Jegher syndrome, Albright's syndrome, hemochromatosis, and in malignant or suppurative lung disease. A history of drug ingestion, or signs of systemic disease will aid in arriving at the correct diagnosis.

The amalgam tattoo should also be differentiated from normal racial pigmentation.

MUCOCELE

Clinical Features

The mucocele is a painless, smooth-surfaced, soft, fluctuant lesion that originates in salivary glands.[50] Although rare in major salivary glands, mucoceles are common in the minor glands. Their color depends on location. If deep, the surface is the color of normal mucous membrane; if superficial, they are blue and translucent.[50] When close to the surface of the mucous membrane, they may appear vesicular and drain a clear fluid, either spontaneously or when traumatized.[50]

Two types of mucoceles have been described. The more common, the mucous extravasation phenomenon, results from trauma to minor gland ducts and subsequent escape of mucus into surrounding soft tissues.[50] The most frequent site for the mucous extravasation phenomenon is the lower lip. However, any oral mucous membrane site may be affected.[50,51] Almost half of all cases occur in individuals in the first and second decades.[50,51] The other type of mucocele, the mucous retention phenomenon, occurs most commonly on buccal mucosa and floor of mouth adjacent to, but not in continuity with, the major salivary gland ducts.[52] It is found most commonly in the fifth, sixth and seventh decades.[51,52] Treatment of both types of mucoceles consists of removal of the lesion along with adjacent minor salivary gland acini and ducts.

Histologic Features

On microscopic examination, the overlying oral epithelium is thin and intact (Fig. 57–10). The mucous extravasation phenomenon consists of a pool of eosinophilic mucus containing foamy histiocytes and polymorphonuclear leukocytes, surrounded by a wall of granulation tissue.[51] No epithelial-lined cyst wall is present. In some instances, a well-circumscribed space is not seen; rather, mucus is found within the connective tissue itself.[50] Salivary glands in the walls of some mucous extravasation phenomena may be chronically inflamed; acinar degeneration, ductal dilatation, and fibrosis may also be found.[50] On the other hand, the wall of the mucous retention phenomenon is composed of cuboidal, columnar or flattened epithelium;[51] this wall is likely an expanded minor salivary gland duct,[52] and may contain mucous cells.[53]

Two other types of minor salivary gland retention cysts have been described.[53] The first is characterized by oncocytic columnar cells in the epithelial lining; most are unicystic, while 30% are multicystic. Small papillary projections of the cyst lining may be noted. The second, termed mucopapillary cysts, are large and tortuous, and are lined by cuboidal, columnar, and stratified squamous epithelium with mucous metaplasia. Papillary projections extend into the cyst lumina.

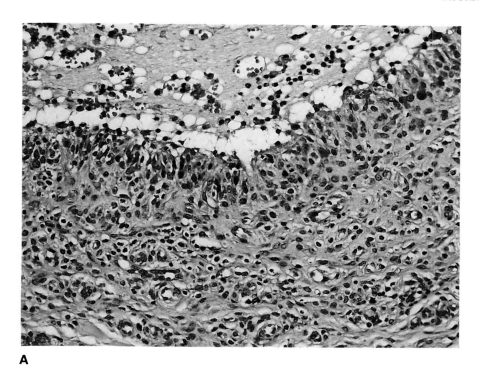

A

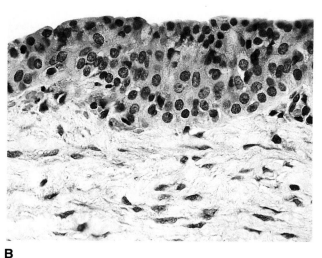

B

Figure 57–10. A. Mucous extravasation phenomenon. A wall of compressed granulation tissue surrounds a pool of mucus. (H&E, ×360.) **B.** Mucous retention phenomenon. A wall of metaplastic ductal epithelium is noted. (H&E, ×400.)

Differential Diagosis

On clinical examination, mucoceles may resemble minor salivary gland neoplasms. Although rare on the lower lip, these neoplasms can occur on many other intraoral sites, as do mucoceles. Thus, microscopic examination is necessary to distinguish these reactive lesions from more serious disease.

Mucoceles should also be differentiated from lymphangiomas of the alveolar ridges in neonates and eruption cysts. This type of lymphangioma and the eruption cyst occur on the alveolar ridges, and site where mucoceles do not develop. Furthermore, eruption cysts occur over the crowns of erupting teeth, while mucoceles do not. In addition, their microscopic features should also differentiate them from mucoceles.

Other lesions that should be included in the differential diagnosis of mucocele are hemangioma, neural neoplasm, and traumatic neuroma, especially if the lesion is deep-seated. These lesions should be easily distinguishable on microscopic examination.

MINOR SALIVARY GLAND CALCULI

Clinical Features

A minor salivary gland calculus presents as a firm, single, elevated mass that can freely move beneath the surface of the mucous membrane.[54] Most are between 3 mm and 5 mm in greatest dimension. The most common site affected is the upper lip; the buccal mucosa may also be affected, but somewhat less frequently. Rarer sites are the lower lip, mucobuccal fold, tongue, soft palate, and alveolar mucosa. The color of the mucous membrane over the lesion has not been described in most cases; however, some are yellow, and others are white or blue.[54] Rarely, purulent discharge from the lesion may occur.[54,55] The sialolith may project from a small punctum on the surface of the overlying soft tissue.[55] Soft tissue radiographs of the lesion may demonstrate a radiopaque mass.

Histologic Features

On gross examination, a yellow or brown calculus is usually found. Some are calcified enough to require demineralization prior to sectioning, and others are non-mineralized.[54] On microscopic examination, the central portions of the calculi are homogeneous (Fig. 57–11). The peripheral portions are composed of concentric layers that are pronounced in most calculi but absent in others. Surrounding the calculus is a dilated extralobular salivary gland duct composed of flattened simple squamous epithelium or simple cuboidal epithelium.[54] The duct may exhibit squamous metaplasia, mucous glands, respiratory epithelium, and oncocytic change.[54] Inflammation of varying severity, usually consisting of lymphocytes and plasma cells but sometimes of polymorphonuclear neutrophils, is usually seen in the connective tissues surrounding the dilated duct. The surrounding minor salivary gland acini exhibit a chronic inflammatory cell infiltrate and may also be atrophic or sclerotic.

Differential Diagnosis

The differential diagnosis includes mucocele and phlebolith. Unlike a sialolith, the most common site for the mucocele is the lower, rather than the upper, lip. In addition, the median age of occurrence of the sialolith of minor salivary glands is the sixth decade, and the most common age for the mucous extravasation type of mucocele is the first and

second decades. On microscopic examination of a mucocele, no sialolith is seen; rather, a pool of mucus is surrounded by a layer of granulation tissue (mucous extravasation phenomenon), or by a layer of epithelium (mucous retention phenomenon). The phlebolith may be distinguished from the sialolith on microscopic examination by phlebolith's surrounding blood vessel wall.

HAIRY LEUKOPLAKIA

Clinical Features

A recently described condition, hairy leukoplakia occurs primarily in male homosexuals who either have developed, or will develop, AIDS.[56] It is an asymptomatic, frequently corrugated ("hairy"), slightly raised, poorly circumscribed white lesion that does not rub off when scraped with a tongue blade. The size of the lesion ranges from a few millimeters to over 3 cm in greatest dimension.[57] Other individuals infected with the human immunodeficiency virus (HIV), may also develop the condition, including intravenous drug abusers,[58] non-homosexual hemophiliacs and other individuals whose only risk factor has been receipt of blood transfusions,[59,60] and women who have been partners of HIV-infected men.[59]

The most common site for hairy leukoplakia is the lateral border of the tongue, where the lesion is frequently bilateral.[56] Hairy leukoplakia also occurs with less frequency on the ventral surface of the tongue, buccal mucosa, floor of mouth, and tongue dorsum.[61]

Some studies report that 20% to 25% of all individuals with this condition develop AIDS in a mean time of less than 1 year following diagnosis of hairy leukoplakia.[61,62] Another study indicated that the probability of AIDS developing in patients with hairy leukoplakia is 48% by 16 months and 83% by 31 months.[63]

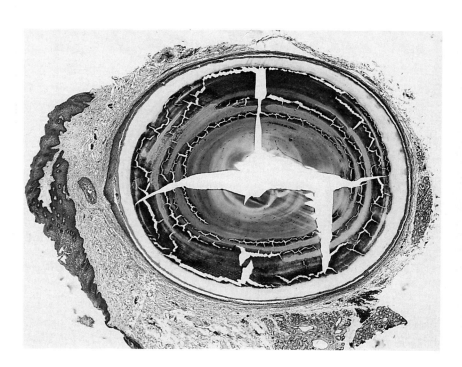

Figure 57–11. Minor salivary gland calculus. The calculus is present in a dilated minor salivary gland duct. (H&E, ×20.)

Histologic Features

On microscopic examination, the surface epithelium is hyperparakeratotic (Fig. 57–12).[56] Superficial colonies of *Candida* are found in 43% to 88% of cases,[56,61] and bacteria are present on the surface in about 50%.[56] Hair-like projections of parakeratin extend from the surface in 80% of cases.[56] A prominent zone of enlarged epithelial cells, each with a pyknotic nucleus and a perinuclear halo, may be found in the superficial spinous cell layer; sometimes, these cells are seen in the suprabasal region.[56,61] In some lesions, only a few such cells are found.[61] Chromatin clumping at the nuclear membrane of these enlarged cells have been described.[64] While some reports have described these enlarged cells as "koilocytoid"[64] or koilocytes,[61] other investigators[65] contend that they lack the extensive clear cytoplasm and nuclear atypia reported in typical koilocytes of flat condylomatous lesions of the cervix. Neutrophils are rarely found in the parakeratin layer of hairy leukoplakia,[61] and in most cases there is no inflammatory cell infiltrate in the underlying connective tissue.[56,61]

Papilloma virus in the epithelial cells of hairy leukoplakia has been noted by one group of investigators,[66] although these findings have not been substantiated by others.[64,65,67] Intranuclear herpesvirus (Epstein-Barr virus) has been found more consistently.[64,65,67]

Eversole and colleagues[61] concluded that parakeratosis and koilocytosis are not specific for hairy leukoplakia; these features may also be found in biopsies from patients with candidiasis unassociated with AIDS, and in idiopathic leukoplakia with parakeratosis, although they are not as striking. Kanas et al[65] also concluded that a definitive diagnosis cannot be made without demonstration of Epstein-Barr virus, either biochemically or by electron microscopic examination. Thus, clinical-pathological correlation is necessary when making the diagnosis of hairy leukoplakia.

Differential Diagnosis

The differential diagnosis of hairy leukoplakia includes idiopathic leukoplakia and snuff dippers' leukoplakia, lichen planus, galvanic lesions, hairy tongue, tongue chewing, and chronic hyperplastic candidiasis. Also included are white sponge nevus, dyskeratosis congenita, pachyonychia congenita, and hereditary benign intraepithelial dyskeratosis.

The most common sites for idiopathic leukoplakia are the buccal mucosa and commissure, and for snuff dippers' leukoplakia, areas where the smokeless tobacco is held, namely, the mucobuccal fold; none of these sites is common for hairy leukoplakia. In addition, the lesion of smokeless tobacco can be fissured. The microscopic features of idiopathic leukoplakia and snuff dippers' leukoplakia range from hyperkeratosis, dysplasia, and carcinoma in situ to squamous cell carcinoma. While hyperkeratosis is also a feature of hairy leukoplakia, the epithelium of hairy leukoplakia is not dysplastic.

Lichen planus may also be white; however, when white, it is usually reticulated or plaque-like. On microscopic examination, a band-like inflammatory response is present in the region immediately subjacent to the surface epithelium; in contrast, little if any inflammation is seen in hairy leukoplakia. The white lesions produced by galvanism frequently regress after removal of the offending restorations.

White sponge nevus, dyskeratosis congenita, pachyonychia congenita, and hereditary benign intraepithelial dyskeratosis may be difficult to differentiate from hairy leukoplakia. However, these genetic diseases are usually multifocal; a family history may also be helpful. With the exception of white sponge nevus, all have findings in other organ systems.

Hairy tongue usually occurs on the tongue dorsum rather than on the lateral borders. Microscopic features in-

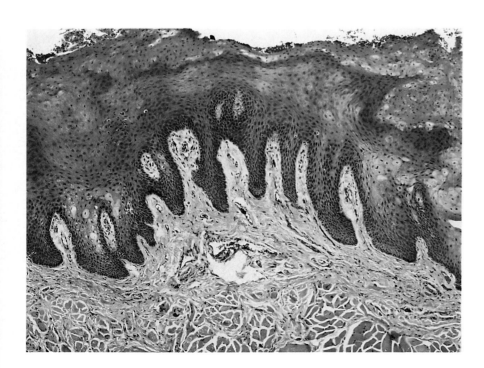

Figure 57–12. Hairy leukoplakia. Hyperparakeratosis and a few epithelial cells, each with a pyknotic nucleus and a perinuclear halo are seen. (H&E, ×75.) (Courtesy Dr. E. James Cundiff, II, Dallas, TX.)

clude elongated and sharply pointed filiform papillae vertically oriented to the surface of the specimen. In contrast, "hairy" projections on the surface of hairy leukoplakia are more ragged and oriented more parallel to the epithelial surface. The lesions of tongue and cheek biting are difficult to microscopically differentiate from hairy leukoplakia. However, the clinical lesions of tongue chewing and cheek biting are more diffuse than hairy leukoplakia and have a more ragged surface. Chronic hyperplastic candidiasis is characterized by a chronic inflammatory cell infiltrate in the underlying connective tissue as well as microabscesses in the epithelium.

CHEEK AND LIP CHEWING (CHEEK BITING)

Clinical Features

This factitial injury results from habitual chewing of oral mucosa.[68–70] Regions involved are those accessible to the patient's teeth. The buccal mucosa is the site most frequently affected, and lesions are usually bilateral.[70] The mucous membranes of the lips are less frequently affected; the lower lip is more commonly affected than the upper.[69] The lesion is diffuse. Affected regions are white, rough, and covered by macerated small flakes of epithelium that remain attached to the mucosa. Areas of erythema may be found between the flakes.[70] Malignant degeneration has not been reported.

Histologic Features

On microscopic examination, the epithelial surface is rough and flaky, reflecting the clinical appearance of the lesion[68,70] (Fig. 57–13). A layer of hematoxyphilic bacteria covers the surface, and no fungi are demonstrable on PAS-staining.[68] The superficial layer of epithelium is characterized by large cells with darkly staining, pyknotic nuclei, and clear cytoplasm.[68,70] Beneath this zone is a region of normal epithelial maturation. The cytoplasm of these cells may be clear. This characteristic is found in normal buccal and labial mucosae. No significant inflammatory cell infiltrate is present in the supporting connective tissue.[68]

Differential Diagnosis

The differential diagnosis includes chemical burn, leukoplakia, hairy leukoplakia, candidiasis, lichen planus, leukoedema, white sponge nevus, hereditary benign intraepithelial dyskeratosis, pachyonychia congenita, and dyskeratosis congenita. Any oral mucous membrane site may be affected by a chemical burn; however, the white, necrotic pseudomembrane is dissimilar from the lesion in cheek or tongue chewing. On microscopic examination, significant numbers of bacteria are not found on the epithelial surface of a chemical burn, nor is the rough epithelial surface characteristic of cheek or lip chewing seen. The microscopic findings in leukoplakia range from hyperkeratosis to squamous cell carcinoma; bacterial colonies are not usually found on the surface of these lesions. The lesions of cheek and tongue chewing are more ragged than those of hairy leukoplakia, although it may be difficult to distinguish one from the other on microscopic examination.

Candidiasis on microscopic examination is characterized by fungal forms in the epithelium, as well as an acute and chronic inflammatory cell infiltrate; intraepithelial microabscesses are also found. The clinical lesions of lichen planus are reticular or erythematous, and a bandlike inflammatory infiltrate immediately adjacent to the epithelium consisting chiefly of lymphocytes is characteristic. Superficial necrosis is not seen in the lesions of leukoedema or of white sponge nevus. Individuals with white sponge nevus, hereditary benign intraepithelial dyskeratosis, pachyonychia congenita, and dyskeratosis congenita may have a

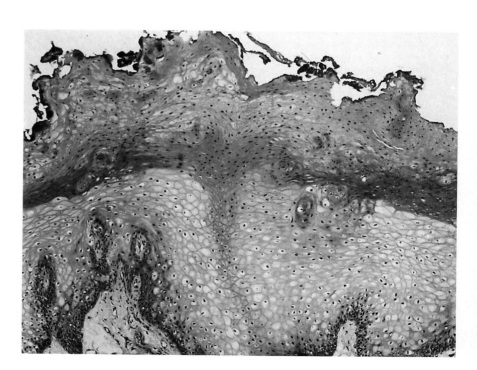

Figure 57–13. Cheek and lip chewing. A thick, ragged layer of parakeratin is covered by a layer of bacteria. (H&E, ×85.)

family history of the disorders. In addition, these conditions may be identified by their associated systemic findings.

IRRITATION FIBROMA (FIBROMA, FIBROUS HYPERPLASIA)

Clinical Features

This common oral lesion is an asymptomatic, well-circumscribed, soft, usually sessile enlargement, most commonly found on the buccal mucosa.[71] It is usually similar in color to the surrounding soft tissues, although the lesion may be white. More than half occur in the fourth, fifth, and sixth decades.[72] Although controversy exists over whether this lesion is a neoplasm, the lesion is likely reactive in etiology.

Histologic Features

On microscopic examination the specimen is covered by a layer of normally maturing, stratified squamous epithelium that may be thinner than normal and that may exhibit flattening and shortening of the rete ridges[73] (Fig. 57–14). The epithelial surface may be hyperorthokeratotic or hyperparakeratotic, and occasionally is ulcerated. The subjacent connective tissue is composed of dense, intertwining bundles of collagen fibers. Only a few spindle-shaped fibroblastic nuclei and few vascular channels are found; vessels are usually small. Aggregates of adipose tissue occasionally are seen. Although the lesions are not microscopically encapsulated, they are usually well-circumscribed. Few if any inflammatory cells are noted.

Differential Diagnosis

The differential diagnosis includes lipoma, minor salivary gland neoplasm, neuroma, neural neoplasm, and granular cell tumor. Microscopic examination should distinguish between these conditions.

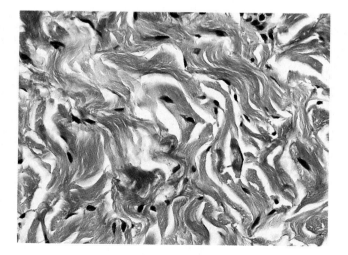

Figure 57–14. Irritation fibroma. Spindle-shaped fibroblasts are scattered throughout the dense connective tissue. (H&E, ×360.)

GIANT CELL FIBROMA

Clinical Features

The giant cell fibroma, unlike the irritation fibroma, is found most commonly on the gingiva.[74,75] Most are less than one cm in greatest dimension, and frequently they are less than 0.5 cm in size. The surface is often nodular. Unlike the irritation fibroma, the majority of giant cell fibromas occur in the first three decades.[74,75]

Histologic Features

Microscopic examination demonstrates a mass of soft tissue, covered by a layer of epithelium that in some areas is thin and in other regions is acanthotic.[74,75] The underlying connective tissue is myxomatous or dense, and has many small vessels. Distributed throughout are large, spindle-shaped or angular fibroblasts, with dendritic-like cytoplasmic processes extending from the periphery[74,75] (Fig. 57–15). These cells may be multinucleated and nucleoli are prominent. The cytoplasm is basophilic and sometimes vacuolization is present. Intracellular melanin granules are found. There is no inflammatory component.

Differential Diagnosis

When on the gingiva, the giant cell fibroma is similar clinically to the peripheral ossifying fibroma, giant cell granuloma, pyogenic granuloma, and peripheral odontogenic tumors. Microscopic examination will assist in delineating these conditions from each other. When on other sites, the lipoma, minor salivary gland neoplasm, neuroma, neural neoplasm, and granular cell tumor should be considered.

PAPILLOMA

Clinical Features

This common lesion is a sessile or pedunculated, white, pink or red exophytic growth, with a cauliflower-shaped surface.[76] Although the most common oral site according to some investigators is the complex of the hard palate, soft palate, and uvula,[76] others contend that the tongue is the most frequent location.[77] The majority of cases occur in the third, fourth, and fifth decades of life.[76,77] Most papillomas are less than 1 cm in greatest dimension, although lesions 2 to 3 cm have been described.[76] The overwhelming number of patients have one papilloma only; in a rare instance, several have been described in one patient.[76] Recurrence is rare once the lesion has been removed.[76] There is no evidence that papillomas are premalignant disorders.

Histologic Features

On microscopic examination, the external surface of a papilloma is composed of many fingerlike projections of epithelium, each supported by a vascular connective tissue core[77] (Fig. 57–16). Most papillomas are covered by a thickened layer of parakeratin, although hyperorthokeratosis may also be present.[76] The epithelium in approximately 20% of all papillomas demonstrates individual cell keratinization, atypical mitotic figures, increased nuclear-cytoplasmic ratio,

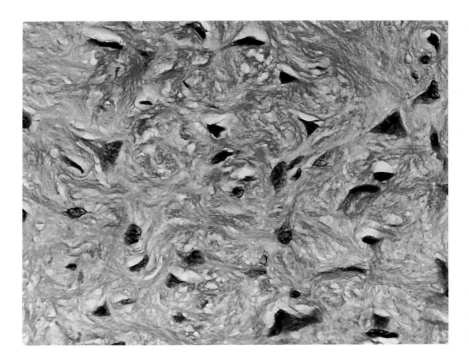

Figure 57–15. Giant cell fibroma. The connective tissue is dense. Distributed throughout are angular shaped fibroblasts. (H&E, ×440.) (Courtesy Dr. Dean K. White, Lexington, KY.)

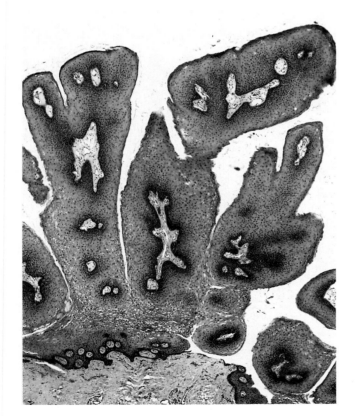

Figure 57–16. Papilloma. Fingerlike projections with fibrovascular connective tissue cores are present. (H&E, ×45.)

or basal cell hyperplasia.[76] An inflammatory cell infiltrate in the connective tissue is a frequent finding.[76,77]

Differential Diagnosis

The differential diagnosis includes other unifocal oral papillary lesions, including verruciform xanthoma, verruca vulgaris, and condyloma acuminatum. Although the papilloma and verruciform xanthoma each have a warty surface, the papilloma lacks foam cells characteristic of verruciform xanthoma. Some investigators have indicated that it is not possible to differentiate between the oral lesions of verruca vulgaris, condyloma acuminatum, and papilloma using routine staining methods for light microscopic examination.[76,78] However, lesions in which microscopic characteristics are consistent with verruca vulgaris of the skin[79] and anogenital condyloma acuminatum[80] have been found in the oral cavity. Human papilloma virus has been detected in both of these oral lesions,[79–81] as well as in some oral papillomas.[82]

NICOTINE STOMATITIS

Clinical Features

This condition is characterized by macular, round, well-circumscribed, asymptomatic white lesions on the posterior portion of the hard palate and anterior soft palate, each with a depressed, erythematous center. The anterior hard palate may also rarely be affected.[83] The palatal mucosa between the macules may be diffusely white and fissured.[84] Nicotine stomatitis is more common in pipe-smokers, but it has also been reported in cigarette smokers.[83,84] The lesion

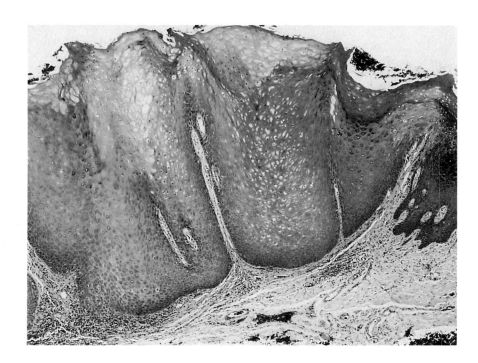

Figure 57–17. Nicotine stomatitis. The epithelium is hyperparakeratotic and acanthotic, and the rete ridges are broad. Chronic inflammatory cells are present in the connective tissue. (H&E, ×50.)

is the result of direct, local action of smoke on the soft tissues. Patients who wear dentures while smoking do not develop nicotine stomatitis under their dentures, but the mucosa posterior to the denture edge develops the characteristic lesions.[84,85] Upon cessation of smoking, nicotine stomatitis has been reported to disappear.[84,85]

There is no evidence that nicotine stomatitis is premalignant when it results from placement of the unlit end of the cigarette or pipe into the mouth when smoking. However, nicotine stomatitis also develops in reverse smokers (individuals who smoke with the lit end of a homemade cigar in their mouths). Nicotine stomatitis produced by this process is believed to predispose to development of squamous cell carcinoma of the palate.[86]

Histologic Features

On microscopic examination, the surface of the epithelium is hyperkeratotic (Fig. 57–17). Acanthosis with broadening of the rete ridges is also noted.[84] The subjacent connective tissue is infiltrated with a predominantly lymphocytic infiltrate which also involves the mucous glands. Minor salivary gland ducts may be occluded by desquamated keratin,[84] and squamous metaplasia of the ducts (3) and duct enlargement may also be found.[84,85]

Differential Diagnosis

The lesions of nicotine stomatitis are characteristic on clinical examination. The microscopic features are distinctive if sections through the center of the lesion are taken. However, examination of sections taken from the periphery may be suggestive of, but not diagnostic of, nicotine stomatitis. In such instances, clinical-pathologic correlation is necessary.

MEDIAN RHOMBOID GLOSSITIS

Clinical Features

Median rhomboid glossitis is an oval, erythematous, depapillated, sometimes nodular lesion on the dorsum of the tongue at the midline, anterior to the foramen cecum and circumvallate papillae. It is usually well-demarcated from the surrounding normal tongue, and its size may range from less than 0.5 cm to greater than 2.0 cm in greatest dimension.[87] Although the condition is usually asymptomatic, some patients have slight pain, "irritation," or itching.[88]

Controversy exists concerning the etiology of median rhomboid glossitis. Some investigators have proposed that the lesion is developmental in origin,[89] and others conclude that infection by *Candida* is the cause.[90] The lesion is rare in children: No cases of median rhomboid glossitis were found in a prevalence study of 10,010 schoolchildren by Baughman,[91] although a few cases have been reported in children under age 10.[92] The lesion is most common in the fifth decade of life.[90] There is no evidence that malignant change occurs.

Histologic Features

On microscopic examination, tongue papillae are absent[90] (Fig. 57–18). The lesion is covered by a layer of parakeratin that is of normal thickness, or by a hyperparakeratotic layer of stratified squamous epithelium. *Candida* hyphae are found in the superficial epithelial layers in many cases. Rete ridges are elongated and sometimes anastomose with one another. The underlying connective tissue is infiltrated with lymphocytes and plasma cells, and an increased number of blood vessels is also noted. Polymorphonuclear neu-

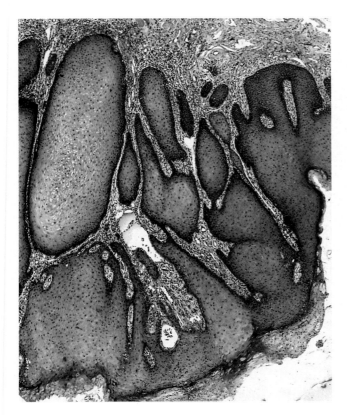

Figure 57–18. Median rhomboid glossitis. The surface is hyper-parakeratotic, rete ridges are elongated, and there is a chronic inflammatory cell infiltrate in the underlying connective tissue. PAS-D stain of this specimen was positive for *Candida*. (H&E, ×45.)

trophils are frequently found in the parakeratin layer. Degeneration of skeletal muscle is found deeper within the connective tissue.

Differential Diagnosis

The clinical and microscopic features taken together are characteristic of this condition.

LICHEN PLANUS

Clinical Features

Lichen planus is a relatively common disorder of oral mucous membranes that is usually diagnosed after age 40. Intraoral lesions may assume several clinical forms: reticulated, papular, plaque-like, atrophic, hypertrophic, erosive, ulcerative, and bullous.[93] The cause of this clinical heterogeneity is unknown. Radiating striae, a predominant feature of the reticulated form, may be seen in the other types as well. The reticulated and papular patterns are white, usually asymptomatic, and first found on routine examination.[94] The erosive and bullous forms are frequently painful.

The most common sites for all types of oral lichen planus are the buccal mucosa and lateral border of the tongue, although any intraoral site, including the gingiva, may be affected. When on the gingiva, the condition is

clinically a desquamative gingivitis. More than one intraoral site is usually affected and the condition is frequently bilateral. Over 50% of individuals with oral mucous membrane lichen planus have the condition on their skin.[93] However, it is difficult to determine the exact frequency of this association, because most patients with oral disease do not receive complete dermatologic examinations, and follow-up may not be adequate.

Controversy exists over whether oral lichen planus is a premalignant disorder. Many patients have been reported in whom squamous cell carcinoma presumably developed in oral lichen planus. However, because both lichen planus and oral squamous cell carcinoma are relatively common disorders, both would be expected to occur together by chance alone in some patients. In addition, some cases of lichenoid dysplasia may have been erroneously diagnosed as lichen planus.[95] Silverman et al.[96] prospectively studied 570 patients with lichen planus for an average of 3.4 years, and were unable to support the hypothesis that disorder was a premalignant condition. However, it appears that patients with lichen planus who develop oral squamous cell carcinoma are more likely to have the erosive form.

Histologic Features

On microscopic examination, the surface is covered by normally maturing, hyperparakeratotic or hyperorthokeratotic stratified squamous epithelium[93,97] (Fig. 57–19). The epithelium may be atrophic and lack rete ridge formation, the rete ridges may be saw-toothed, or the epithelium may be acanthotic. Individually keratinizing squamous cells, so-called cytoid bodies or Civatte bodies, are found primarily in the lower spinous cell layer. Degeneration of basal cells is characteristic. These cells are replaced by an acellular eosinophilic band. Immediately subjacent to the epithelium is a dense band of lymphocytes; histiocytes and plasma cells may rarely be present. The inflammatory infiltrate may obscure the epithelial-connective tissue junction. Few inflammatory cells are seen in the deeper connective tissues. Microscopic ulceration as well as vesicle formation may be seen.

Minimal criteria have not been established for the microscopic diagnosis of lichen planus. However, Krutchkoff and Eisenberg[95] have suggested that the presence of epithelial dysplasia precludes the diagnosis of lichen planus, even if the other microscopic features characteristic of lichen planus are present.

Differential Diagnosis

The differential diagnosis of lichen planus includes lichenoid drug eruption, lupus erythematosus, leukoplakia and lichenoid dysplasia, pemphigus, pemphigoid, epidermolysis bullosa, erythema multiforme, and graft-versus-host disease. Drug reactions in oral mucous membranes can resemble lichen planus both clinically and histologically; thus, a drug history is essential. The inflammatory cell infiltrate in lupus erythematosus is more diffuse than in lichen planus and is perivascular. Serologic studies should also aid in distinguishing between the two disorders. Leukoplakia, as well as a lichenoid dysplasia, are conditions that histologically and clinically may resemble lichen planus. A feature shared by all three lesions may be a subepithelial bandlike

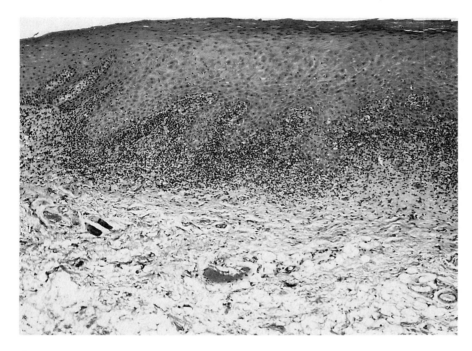

A

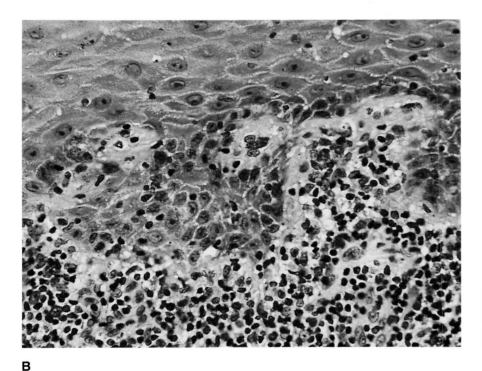

B

Figure 57–19. A. Lichen planus. There is a dense, band-like infiltrate immediately subjacent to the epithelium. (H&E, ×60.) **B.** Lichen planus. The basal cell layer is absent and the infiltrate is primarily lymphocytic. (H&E, ×400.)

inflammatory infiltrate. However, dysplastic epithelium precludes the diagnosis of lichen planus, regardless of the character of this infiltrate. In both leukoplakia and lichenoid dysplasia, the basal cell layer is usually intact.

Pemphigus may be distinguished from lichen planus by the site of vesicle formation. In both lichen planus and pemphigoid, the vesicle forms between the epithelium and connective tissue. However, in lichen planus the basal cell layer is ill-defined, and in pemphigoid it is intact. Epidermolysis bullosa and lichen planus can be differentiated by their skin manifestations. The lesions of erythema multiforme are characterized by a diffuse inflammatory infiltrate that may be perivascular in the deeper portions of the connective tissue. Edema of the epithelium is also noted. The characteristic skin lesions of erythema multiforme will also aid in the differential diagnosis. Although the clinical findings and the pattern of the inflammatory infiltrate in graft versus-host-disease and lichen planus are similar, the clinical history should serve to distinguish between them.

DEVELOPMENTAL MEMBRANE LESIONS

ADENOMATOID HYPERPLASIA

Clinical Features

This lesion is an asymptomatic, firm, sessile, local enlargement on the hard palate, soft palate, or rarely on the retromolar pad.[98] In the few reports in which the specific site on the palate has been documented, the lesion has occurred on only one side of the midline. Covering mucous membrane is normal. The lesion has not been reported in children or adolescents.

Histologic Features

On microscopic examination, the lesion is covered by a normal layer of stratified squamous epithelium (Fig. 57–20). Within the subjacent dense connective tissue are clusters of microscopically normal minor salivary gland acini, in numbers greater than normal for site. Mucus pooling and adipose tissue may also be noted. An inflammatory cell infiltrate is not a significant component of the lesion.

Differential Diagnosis

The clinical differential diagnosis includes a benign or malignant neoplasm of minor salivary glands, necrotizing sial-

ometaplasia that has not undergone ulceration, and a torus palatinus. The microscopic features differentiate adenomatoid hyperplasia from a salivary gland neoplasm and from necrotizing sialometaplasia. The torus palatinus is a bony enlargement that is found on the midline of the hard palate. On microscopic examination, this lesion is composed of dense, viable bone.

WHITE SPONGE NEVUS

Clinical Features

This autosomal dominant condition is characterized by asymptomatic, raised, white, shaggy patches on the oral mucous membranes.[99] While buccal mucosa is the most common site, the tongue, floor of mouth, and anterior faucial pillars may be affected. Nasal, esophageal, vaginal, anal, and penile mucosa have also been affected. The oral lesions may be present at birth or shortly thereafter.[100] Exacerbations and remissions have been reported.

Histologic Features

Microscopic examination shows an acanthotic stratified squamous epithelium which is markedly parakeratotic (Fig. 57–21). Individual, prematurely keratinizing cells are found in variable numbers scattered throughout the spinous cell layer. In addition, epithelial cells, each with a pyknotic nucleus and clear cytoplasm, are found in clusters throughout the epithelial layers. An inflammatory component is not a significant feature. Malignant change has not been reported.

Differential Diagnosis

Leukoplakia, candidiasis, chemical burn, and lichen planus should be considered in the differential diagnosis. The clini-

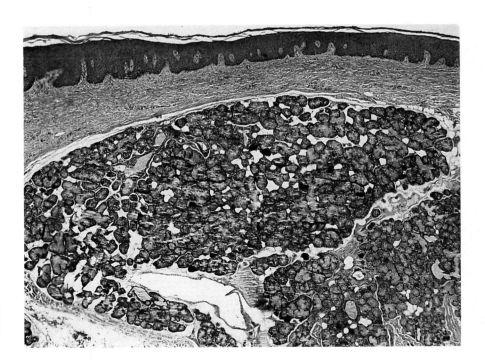

Figure 57–20. Adenomatoid hyperplasia. A large but otherwise normal minor salivary gland lobule is seen in the connective tissue beneath a hyperkeratotic layer of stratified squamous epithelium. (H&E, ×30.)

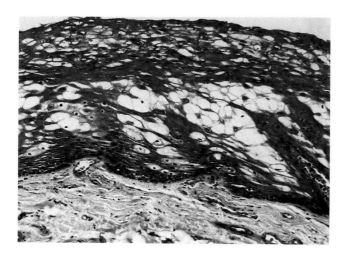

Figure 57–21. White sponge nevus. Clusters of large, vacuolated epithelial cells with pyknotic nuclei are seen. (H&E, ×180.)

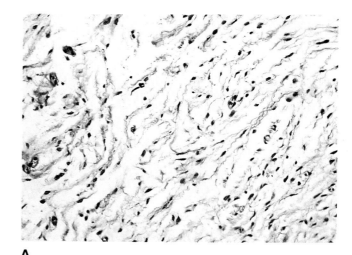

A

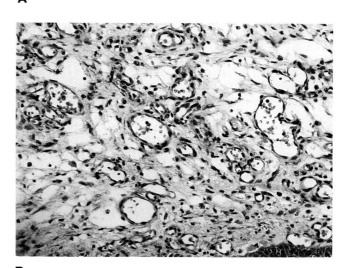

B

Figure 57–22. A. Lymphangiomas of the alveolar ridges in neonates. Loose connective tissue demonstrates vascular slits that do not contain blood cells. (H&E, ×400.) **B.** Lymphangiomas of the alveolar ridges in neonates. Photomicrograph demonstrates some well formed blood vessels containing red blood cells. (H&E, ×190.)

cal features of these conditions, as well as the histomorphology, should enable the appropriate diagnosis to be made. While the oral lesions of pachyonychia congenita, hereditary benign intraepithelial dyskeratosis, and dyskeratosis congenita may resemble those of white sponge nevus, the presence of extraoral anomalies, as well as the microscopic features, aid in the differential diagnosis.

LYMPHANGIOMAS OF THE ALVEOLAR RIDGES IN NEONATES

Clinical Features

These congenital soft tissue lesions are blue-domed and fluid-filled. They are found only on the mucous membranes of the mandibular and maxillary alveolar ridges in the posterior regions.[101] More than one has never been reported in each quadrant. They are present in 3.7% of all newborn black infants, but have not been described in other races. The condition resolves without treatment.

Histologic Features

The lesions are covered by a normal layer of stratified squamous epithelium. The subjacent tissue is composed of vascular slits, with little supporting fibrous connective tissue stroma (Fig. 57–22). Some slits contain red blood cells, but most are empty. No inflammatory infiltrate is seen.

Differential Diagnosis

Lymphangiomas of the alveolar ridges should not be confused with eruption cysts, mucoceles, or gingival cysts. Unlike eruption cysts, no teeth are found beneath lymphangiomas after they are removed or after spontaneous remission. Although mucoceles have a clinical appearance similar to lymphangiomas, mucoceles do not occur on the alveolar ridges. Gingival cysts are similar to lymphangiomas on clinical examination; however, they have never been reported in infants. The microscopic features of eruption cysts, muco-

celes, and gingival cysts should also differentiate them from lymphangiomas.

GINGIVAL CYST

Clinical Features

This odontogenic cyst is a well-circumscribed, elevated, round, fluid-filled enlargement on the attached gingiva in the canine and premolar region. The overlying mucous membrane may be normal or blue-grey in color. Although the overwhelming majority of these lesions occur on the buccal surface of the alveolar ridge,[102] they have also been reported on the lingual surface. Most do not exceed 0.6 cm in diameter.[103] The mandible is more frequently affected than the maxilla and the lesion is most common in the

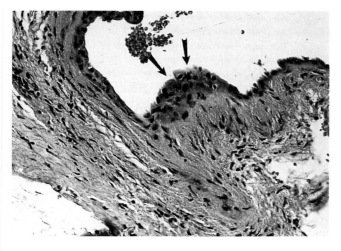

Figure 57–23. Gingival cyst. The lining is composed of a thin layer of epithelium with occasional plaque-like thickenings (arrows). (H&E, ×260.)

fifth and sixth decades of life. While in most cases these cysts are solitary, two adjacent to one another have been reported.[104] When removed, a depression in the underlying alveolar bone may be found.

Histologic Features
On microscopic examination, the gingival cyst is lined by a thin layer of flattened squamous or cuboidal epithelial cells, some of which have vacuolated cytoplasm[103] (Fig. 57–23). There is no evidence of keratinization or rete peg formation. Along the wall are intermittent, plaque-like epithelial thickenings, which sometimes display a swirling pattern.[103,105] The surrounding connective tissue wall is free of inflammatory cells.

Differential Diagnosis
The gingival cyst should be differentiated from the mucocele, lymphangiomas of the alveolar ridges in neonates, and the eruption cyst. The mucocele is similar in clinical appearance to the gingival cyst, but the mucocele has not been reported on the attached gingiva. Lymphangiomas of the alveolar ridges in neonates may also resemble the gingival cyst in clinical appearance; however, the lymphangioma is congenital. The eruption cyst occurs on the alveolar ridge over the crown of a deciduous or permanent tooth. The microscopic features of these lesions should serve to distinguish them from one another.

LEUKOEDEMA

Clinical Features
Leukoedema is an asymptomatic, diffuse-white or grey-white lesion of the oral mucosa.[106] The condition is most common bilaterally on the buccal mucosa, and the mucosal surface of the lips may also be affected. The hard palate and gingiva have not been reported affected. On stretching the mucosa, the white appearance may disappear, but returns after relaxation. In one report, 90% of all blacks examined had the condition, and only 43% of white individuals were affected.[106]

Histologic Features
On microscopic examination, the acanthotic surface epithelium is covered by a layer of parakeratin of varying thickness[106,107] (Fig. 57–24). Cells of the spinous cell layer are large and pale, and rete ridges are broad. No inflammatory infiltrate has been described.

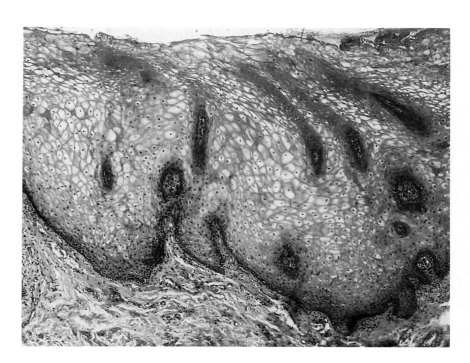

Figure 57–24. Leukoedema. The epithelium demonstrates many pale epithelial cells, each with a small, darkly stained nucleus. (H&E, ×65.) (Courtesy of Dr. Charles E. Tomich, Indianapolis, IN.)

Differential Diagnosis

Other conditions that solely manifest as white oral lesions include idiopathic leukoplakia, white sponge nevus, lichen planus, and candidiasis. Biopsy as well as clinical characteristics should serve to differentiate between these disorders. Hereditary benign intraepithelial dyskeratosis, dyskeratosis congenita, and pachyonychia congenita are also characterized by white lesions of the oral mucous membranes. However, each of these conditions manifests extraoral abnormalities as well: ophthalmologic abnormalities in hereditary benign intraepithelial dyskeratosis, and abnormalities of the skin and skin appendages in dyskeratosis congenita and pachyonychia congenita.

PRE-NEOPLASTIC MEMBRANE LESIONS

LEUKOPLAKIA (HOMOGENEOUS LEUKOPLAKIA)

Clinical Features

Leukoplakia is a clinical term that denotes a white patch or plaque that cannot be rubbed off, and clinically or microscopically cannot be diagnosed as a specific oral condition.[108] Proposed etiologic factors include smoking, alcohol, local trauma, and *Candida* infection. The most common intraoral site is the buccal mucosa, followed by the mandibular mucosa and sulcus, and palate.[108] Leukoplakia occurs with highest frequency in the fifth, sixth, and seventh decades of life.[108] Because leukoplakia is only a clinical description, biopsy is essential to determine the diagnosis.

Histologic Features

On microscopic examination from a variety of intraoral sites, Waldron and Shafer[108] showed that 80% were hyperorthokeratotic, hyperparakeratotic, and acanthotic without evidence of epithelial dysplasia[108] (Fig. 57–25). However, al-

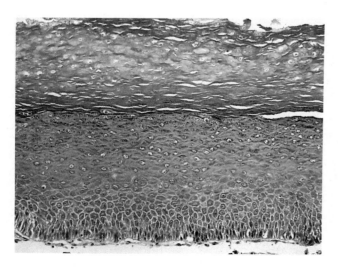

Figure 57–25. Leukoplakia (homogeneous leukoplakia). The epithelium is markedly hyperorthokeratotic and the epithelium is not dysplastic. (H&E, ×120.)

most 20% demonstrated findings ranging from mild epithelial dysplasia to squamous cell carcinoma. In 3.1%, infiltrating squamous cell carcinoma was found. Other investigators have shown a transformation rate of leukoplakia to squamous cell carcinoma of up to 6% over time.[109] If dysplasia was found on initial biopsy, carcinoma developed in approximately 15%.[109,110] The site at highest risk for dysplasia or squamous cell carcinoma was the floor of mouth, where almost 43% showed dysplasia or carcinoma.[108] In almost 25% of cases of leukoplakia on the tongue, dysplasia or carcinoma was also found. *Candida* has been found in 3% of leukoplakias.[111]

Differential Diagnosis

The differential diagnosis includes lichen planus, candidiasis, hairy leukoplakia, cheek or tongue chewing, white sponge nevus, pachyonychia congenita, dyskeratosis congenita, and hereditary benign intraepithelial dyskeratosis. Lichen planus, when white, can be distinguished on microscopic examination from leukoplakia by a normally maturing epithelium, individually dyskeratotic cells, loss of the basal cell layer and replacement by an eosinophilic band, and the dense, band-like infiltrate of lymphocytes immediately subjacent to the epithelium. Chronic hyperplastic candidiasis is characterized by a normally maturing epithelium that supports clusters of polymorphonuclear neutrophils. Characteristic hyphae are present in the epithelium. In addition, the lesions of chronic hyperplastic candidiasis can be removed with a tongue blade, leaving a bleeding surface. Hairy leukoplakia and tongue or cheek chewing are distinguished from leukoplakia by their hairlike projections of parakeratin and enlarged and vacuolated epithelial cells in the upper spinous cell layer. White sponge nevus, pachyonychia congenita, dyskeratosis congenita, and hereditary benign intraepithelial dyskeratosis are genetic disorders with microscopic findings different from leukoplakia. Leukoplakia is usually found in one intraoral site, although these disorders can be found in multiple sites. No evidence of dysplasia is noted on microscopic examination. White sponge nevus has no associated abnormalities, but the other three of these conditions can be diagnosed based on abnormalities in other body sites.

ERYTHROPLAKIA

Clinical Features

Erythroplakia is a red, velvety, flat or slightly elevated patch on oral mucous membranes that cannot be rubbed off and does not represent a specific or non-specific inflammatory disorder.[112] It is far less common in the oral cavity than its white counterpart, leukoplakia.[112] Erythroplakia represented less than 1% of all accessions of two oral pathology biopsy services.[112] In males, the most common location for erythroplakia is the floor of mouth,[112,113] and in females, the mandibular alveolar mucosa, gingiva, and mandibular sulcus are the most common sites.[112] The condition is most common in the sixth and seventh decades of life. Erythroplakic lesions may be very small or cover a large surface of oral mucous membrane. They may be well-delineated from the surrounding normal mucosa or margins may be

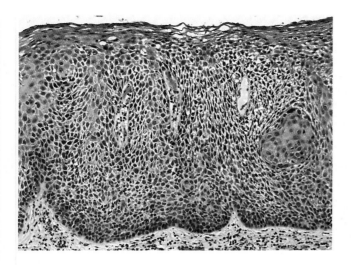

Figure 57–26. Erythroplakia. Carcinoma in situ is noted. (H&E, ×140.)

ill-defined. The area affected may be only mildly erythematous, with other regions bright red.

Histologic Features

There is little if any overlying keratin. Blood vessels are found close to the surface.[112] Fifty-one percent of erythroplakias biopsied are invasive carcinoma.[112] Forty percent demonstrate carcinoma in situ or severe epithelial dysplasia, and 9% show mild to moderate epithelial dysplasia (Fig. 57–26). Individual cell keratinization is rarely seen until invasion occurs.[112] Size of the lesion does not correlate with microscopic severity; small lesions are as likely to be invasive squamous cell carcinoma as large ones.[112,113]

Differential Diagnosis

Lesions of atrophic candiasis, trauma, and erosive lichen planus resemble erythroplakia. Biopsy and special stains for fungal forms will serve to distinguish atrophic candidiasis from erythroplakia. In addition, dysplastic epithelium is not found in candidiasis. Trauma from the edge of a denture or from a sharp tooth, for example, can be excluded from the differential diagnosis by elimination of the source of irritation. Erosive lichen planus can be distinguished from erythroplakia by its microscopic features.

SPECKLED LEUKOPLAKIA (NODULAR LEUKOPLAKIA)

Clinical Features

Speckled leukoplakia is a lesion of oral mucous membranes characterized by white patches interspersed with areas of erythema.[114,115] The lesions are frequently nodular. Because there are so few reports of this condition, its frequency is unknown; however, it is likely much less frequent than either leukoplakia or erythroplakia. Almost two-thirds are found on the buccal mucosa at the commissure.[114,116] The average age of occurrence is 54 years, and three fifths of reported lesions occur in males.[114]

Histologic Features

The mucous membrane in speckled leukoplakia is covered by a layer of hyperparakeratotic and/or hyperorthokeratotic stratified squamous epithelium[114,117] (Fig. 57–27). The ep-

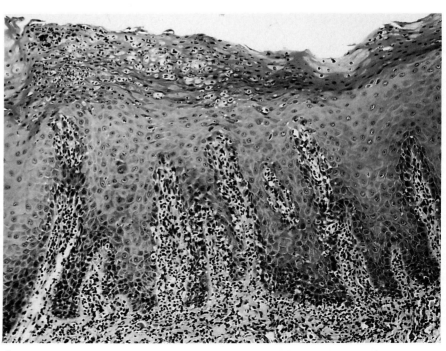

Figure 57–27. A. Speckled leukoplakia (nodular leukoplakia). The epithelium is normally maturing, there is a chronic inflammatory cell infiltrate in the connective tissue, and microabscesses in the superficial layers. (H&E, ×210.)

A

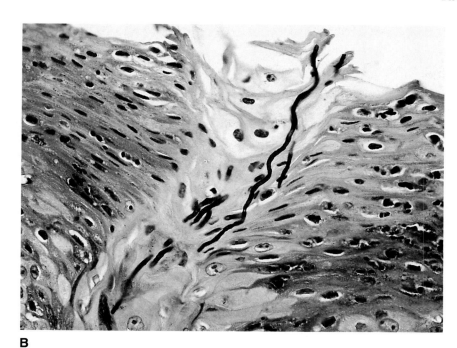

B

Figure 57–27. B. Speckled leukoplakia (nodular leukoplakia). *Candida* is seen in the epithelium. (PAS-D, ×400.)

ithelium exhibits regions of both epithelial hyperplasia and epithelial atrophy.[114] Dysplasia is found in 50 to 70% of all specimens.[114,117] Squamous cell carcinoma has been reported more frequently in speckled leukoplakia than in homogeneous leukoplakia.[118] Five of the 35 cases reported by Pindborg et al.[114] were diagnosed as carcinoma. Small abscesses may be present immediately beneath the surface of the lesion.[115] *Candida* has been found in the majority of speckled leukoplakias studied.[116,117] It is not known whether the presence of *Candida* is a cause of speckled leukoplakia or whether it is a secondary invader. An inflammatory infiltrate consisting of lymphocytes and plasma cells is found in the underlying connective tissue.[117]

Differential Diagnosis

The clinical and microscopic features of speckled leukoplakia resemble those of chronic hyperplastic candidiasis. Because the relationship between these two lesions is unknown, biopsy should be performed when treatment with antifungal therapy has been unsuccessful in order to determine whether epithelial dysplasia or carcinoma is present.

REFERENCES

1. Lynch DP, Crago CA, Martinez, MG. Necrotizing sialometaplasia. A review of the literature and report of two additional cases. *Oral Surg Oral Med Oral Pathol.* 1979; 47:63–69.
2. Chaudhry AP, Yamane GM, Salman L, et al. Necrotizing sialometaplasia of palatal minor salivary glands: A report on 2 cases. *J Oral Med.* 1985; 40:2–6.
3. Dunlap CL, Barker BF. Necrotizing sialometaplasia. Report of five additional cases. *Oral Surg Oral Med Oral Pathol.* 1974; 37:722–727.
4. Rossie KM, Allen CM, Burns RA. Necrotizing sialometaplasia:

A case with metachronous lesions. *J Oral Maxillofac Surg.* 1986; 44:1006–1008.
5. Brooks JK, Balciunas BA. Geographic stomatitis: Review of the literature and report of five cases. *J Am Dent Assoc.* 1987; 115:421–424.
6. Banoczy J, Szabo L, Csiba A. Migratory glossitis. A clinical–histologic review of seventy cases. *Oral Surg Oral Med Oral Pathol.* 1975; 39:113–121.
7. Littner MM, Gorsky M, Moskona B, Harel-Raviv M. Migratory stomatitis. *Oral Surg Oral Med Oral Pathol.* 1987; 63:555–559.
8. Eidelman E, Chosack A, Cohen T. Scrotal tongue and geographic tongue: Polygenic and associated traits. *Oral Surg Oral Med Oral Pathol.* 1976; 42:591–596.
9. Hall WH, Finegold S. A study of 23 cases of Reiter's syndrome. *Ann Interm Med.* 1953; 38:533–550.
10. Hancock JAH: Surface manifestations of Reiter's disease in the male. *Br J Vener Dis.* 1960; 36:36–39.
11. McCord WC, Nies KM, Louie JS. Acute venereal arthritis. Comparative study of acute Reiter syndrome and acute gonococcal arthritis. *Arch Intern Med.* 1977; 137:858–862.
12. Weathers DR, Baker G, Archard HO, Burkes EJ Jr. Psoriasiform lesions of the oral mucosa (with emphasis on "ectopic geographic tongue"). *Oral Surg Oral Med Oral Pathol.* 1974; 37:872–888.
13. van der Wal N, van der Kwast WAM, van Dijk E, van der Wall I. Geographic stomatitis and psoriasis. *Int J Oral Maxillofac Surg* 1988; 17:106–109.
14. Hietanen J, Salo OP, Kanerva L, Juvakoski T. Study of the oral mucosa in 200 consecutive patients with psoriasis. *Scand J Dent Res.* 1984; 92:50–54.
15. Buchner A, Begleiter A. Oral lesions in psoriatic patients. *Oral Surg Oral Med Oral Pathol.* 1976; 41:327–332.
16. Schmitz JF. A clinical study of inflammatory papillary hyperplasia. *Oral Surg Oral Med Oral Pathol.* 1964; 14:1034–1039.
17. Bhaskar SN, Beasley JD, Cutright DE. Inflammatory papillary hyperplasia of the oral mucosa: report of 341 cases. *J Am Dent Assoc.* 1970; 81:949–952.
18. Guernsey LH. Reactive inflammatory papillary hyperplasia

of the palate. *Oral Surg Oral Med Oral Pathol.* 1965; 20:814–827.

19. Ralph JP, Stenhouse D. Denture-induced hyperplasia of the oral soft tissues. Vestibular lesions, their characteristics and treatment. *Br Dent J.* 1972; 132:68–70.

20. Nordenram A, Landt H. Hyperplasia of the oral tissues in denture cases. *Acta Odontol Scand.* 1969; 27:481–491.

21. Cutright DE. The histopathologic findings in 583 cases of epulis fissuratum. *Oral Surg Oral Med Oral Pathol.* 1974; 37:401–411.

22. Archard HO, Glass NM. Degenerative changes in the superficial epithelium of chronic hyperplastic oral mucosa: Clinicopathological and histochemical study. *J Dent Res.* 1970; 49:1118–1124.

23. Chen S-Y. Ultrastructure of eosinophilic bodies in the degenerative surface epithelium of chronic hyperplastic lesions. *Oral Surg Oral Med Oral Pathol.* 1977; 43:256–266.

24. Phillips RL, Shafer WG. An evaluation of the peripheral giant cell tumor. *J Periodontol.* 1955; 26:216–222.

25. Giansanti JS, Waldron CA. Peripheral giant cell granuloma: Review of 720 cases. *J Oral Surg.* 1969; 27:787–791.

26. Katsikeris N, Kazarantza-Angelopoulou E, Angelopoulos AP. Peripheral giant cell granuloma. Clinicopathologic study of 224 new cases and review of 956 reported cases. *Int J Oral Maxillofac Surg.* 1988; 17:94–99.

27. Bhaskar SN, Cutright DE, Beasley JD III, Perez B. Giant cell reparative granuloma (peripheral): report of 50 cases. *J Oral Surg.* 1971; 29:110–115.

28. Eversole LR, Rovin S. Reactive lesions of the gingiva. *J Oral Path.* 1972; 1:30–38.

29. Buchner A, Hansen LS. The histomorphologic spectrum of peripheral ossifying fibroma. *Oral Surg Oral Med Oral Pathol.* 1987; 63:452–461.

30. Andersen L, Fejerskov O, Philipsen HP. Calcifying fibroblastic granuloma. *J Oral Surg.* 1973; 31:196–200.

31. Lehner T. Pathology of recurrent oral ulceration and oral ulceration in Behçet's syndrome: light, electron and fluorescence microscopy. *J Pathol.* 1969; 97:481–494.

32. Brody HA, Silverman S Jr. Studies on recurrent oral aphthae, I. Clinical and laboratory comparisons. *Oral Surg Oral Med Oral Pathol.* 1969; 27:27–34.

33. Cohen L. Ethiology, pathogenesis and classification of aphthous stomatitis and Behçet's syndrome. *J Oral Pathol.* 1978; 7:374–352.

34. Ship II, Morris AL, Durocher RT, Burket LW. Recurrent aphthous ulcerations and recurrent herpes labialis in a professional school student population. *Oral Surg Oral Med Oral Pathol.* 1960; 13:1191–1202.

35. Ship II, Merritt AD, Stanley HR. Recurrent aphthous ulcers. *Am J Med.* 1962; 32:32–43.

36. Graykowski EA, Barile MF, Lee WB, Stanley HR. Recurrent aphthous stomatitis. Clinical, therapeutic, histopathologic and hypersensitivity aspects. *JAMA.* 1966; 196:637–644.

37. Miller MF, Garfunkel AA, Ram C, Ship II. Inheritance patterns in recurrent aphthous stomatitis: Twin and pedigree data. *Oral Surg Oral Med Oral Pathol.* 1977; 43:886–889.

38. Nowparast B, Howell FV, Rick GM. Verruciform xanthoma. A clinicopathologic review and report of fifty-four cases. *Oral Surg Oral Med Oral Pathol.* 1981; 51:619–625.

39. Neville SW, Weathers DR. Verruciform xanthoma. *Oral Surg Oral Med Oral Pathol.* 1980; 49:429–434.

40. Graff SG, Burk JL Jr, McKean TW. Verruciform xanthoma. First case reported in a black person. *Oral Surg Oral Med Oral Pathol.* 1978; 45:762–767.

41. Shafer WG. Verruciform xanthoma. *Oral Surg Oral Med Oral Pathol.* 1971; 31:784–789.

42. Zegarelli DJ, Zegarelli-Schmidt EC, Zegarelli EV. Verruciform xanthoma. A clinical, light microscopic, and electron microscopic study of two cases. *Oral Surg Oral Med Oral Pathol.* 1974; 35:725–734.

43. Knapp MJ. Oral tonsils: Location, distribution, and histology. *Oral Surg Oral Med Oral Pathol.* 1970; 29:155–161.

44. Knapp MJ. Pathology of oral tonsils. *Oral Surg Oral Med Oral Pathol.* 1970; 29:295–304.

45. Buchner A, Hansen LS. Lymphoepithelial cysts of the oral cavity. A clinicopathologic study of thirty-eight cases. *Oral Surg Oral Med Oral Pathol.* 1980; 50:441–449.

46. Guinta J, Cataldo E. Lymphoepithelial cysts of the oral mucosa. *Oral Surg Oral Med Oral Pathol.* 1973; 35:77–79.

47. Buchner A, Hansen LS. Amalgam pigmentation (amalgam tattoo) of the oral mucosa. A clinicopathologic study of 268 cases. *Oral Surg Oral Med Oral Pathol.* 1980; 49:139–147.

48. Peters E, Gardner DG. A method of distinguishing between amalgam and graphite in tissue. *Oral Surg Oral Med Oral Pathol.* 1986; 62:73–76.

49. McGinnis JP Jr, Greer JL, Daniels DS. Amalgam tattoo: Report of an unusual clinical presentation and the use of energy dispersive X-ray analysis as an aid to diagnosis. *J Am Dent Assoc.* 1985; 110:52–54.

50. Cataldo E, Mosadomi A. Mucoceles of the oral mucous membrane. *Arch Otolaryngol.* 1970; 91:360–365.

51. Harrison JD. Salivary mucoceles. *Oral Surg Oral Med Oral Pathol.* 1975; 39:268–278.

52. Standish SM, Shafer WG. The mucous retention phenomenon. *J Oral Surg Anesth Hosp Dent Pract.* 1959; 17:15–22.

53. Eversole LR. Oral sialocysts. *Arch Otolaryngol Head Neck Surg.* 1987; 113:51–56.

54. Jenson JL, Howell FV, Rick GM, Correll RW. Minor salivary gland calculi. A clinicopathologic study of forty-seven new cases. *Oral Surg Oral Med Oral Pathol.* 1979; 47:44–50.

55. Allan JH, Chippendale I. Sialolithiasis of the minor salivary glands. *Oral Surg Oral Med Oral Pathol.* 1969; 27:780–785.

56. Schidt M, Greenspan D, Daniels TE, Greenspan J. Clinical and histologic spectrum of oral hairy leukoplakia. *Oral Surg Oral Med Oral Pathol.* 1987; 64:716–720.

57. Greenspan D, Greenspan JS, Conant M, et al. Oral "hairy" leucoplakia in male homosexuals: Evidence of association with both papillomavirus and a herpes-group virus. *Lancet.* 1984; 2:831–834.

58. Ficarra G, Barone R, Gaglioti D, et al. Oral hairy leukoplakia among HIV-positive intravenous drug abusers: A clinicopathologic and ultrastructural study. *Oral Surg Oral Med Oral Pathol.* 1988; 65:421–466.

59. Rindum JL, Schidt M, Pindborg JJ, Scheibel E. Oral hairy leukoplakia in three hemophiliacs with human immunodeficiency virus infection. *Oral Surg Oral Med Oral Pathol.* 1987; 63:437–440.

60. Greenspan D. Oral hairy leucoplakia in two women, a haemophiliac, and a transfusion recipient. *Lancet.* 1986; 2:978–979. (letter).

61. Eversole LR, Jacobsen P, Stone CE, Freckleton V. Oral condyloma planus (hairy leukoplakia) among homosexual men: A clinicopathologic study of thirty-six cases. *Oral Surg Oral Med Oral Pathol.* 1986; 61:249–255.

62. Silverman S Jr, Migliorati CA, Lozada-Nur F, et al. Oral findings in people with or at high risk for AIDS: A study of 375 homosexual males. *J Am Dent Assoc.* 1986; 112:187–192.

63. Greenspan D, Greenspan JS, Hearst NG, et al. Relation of oral hairy leukoplakia in infection with the human immunodeficiency virus and the risk of developing AIDS. *J Infect Dis.* 1987; 155:475–481.

64. Belton CM, Eversole LR. Oral hairy leukoplakia: Ultrastructural features. *J Oral Pathol.* 1986; 15:493–499.

65. Kanas RJ, Abrams AM, Recher L, et al. Oral hairy leukoplakia:

A light microscopic and immunohistochemical study. *Oral Surg Oral Med Oral Pathol.* 1988; 66:334–340.

66. Greenspan JS, Greenspan D, Lennette ET, et al. Replication of Epstein-Barr virus within the epithelial cells of oral "hairy" leukoplakia, an AIDS-associated lesion. *N Engl J Med.* 1985; 313:1564–1570.

67. Kanas RJ, Abrams AM, Jensen JL, et al. Oral hairy leukoplakia: Ultrastructural observations. *Oral Surg Oral Med Oral Pathol.* 1988; 65:333–338.

68. Hjørting-Hansen E, Holst E. Morsicatio mucosae oris and suctio mucosae oris. An analysis of oral mucosal changes due to biting and sucking habits. *Scand J Dent Res.* 1970; 78:492–499.

69. Sewerin I. A clinical and epidemiologic study of morsicatio buccarum/labiorum. *Scand J Dent Res.* 1971; 79:73–80.

70. van Wyk CW, Staz J, Farman AG. The chewing lesions of the cheeks and lips: Its features and prevalence among a selected group of adolescents. *J Dent.* 1977; 5:193–199.

71. Barker DS, Lucas RB. Localised fibrous overgrowths of the oral mucosa. *Br J Oral Surg.* 1967; 5:86–92.

72. Weathers DR, Callihan MD. Giant-cell fibroma. *Oral Surg Oral Med Oral Pathol.* 1974; 37:374–384.

73. Shafer WG, Hine MK, Levy BM. *A Textbook of Oral Pathology.* 4th ed. Philadelphia: WB Saunders Co; 1983:139–140.

74. Weathers DR, Callihan MD. Giant-cell fibroma. *Oral Surg Oral Med Oral Pathol.* 1974; 37:374–384.

75. Houston GD. The giant cell fibroma. A review of 464 cases. *Oral Surg Oral Med Oral Pathol.* 1982; 53:582–587.

76. Abbey LM, Page DG, Sawyer DR. The clinical and histopathologic features of a series of 464 oral squamous cell papillomas. *Oral Surg Oral Med Oral Pathol.* 1980; 49:419–428.

77. Greer RO, Goldman HM. Oral papillomas. Clinicopathologic evaluation and retrospective examination for dyskeratosis in 110 lesions. *Oral Surg Oral Med Oral Pathol.* 1974; 38:435–440.

78. Syrjanen SM, Syrjanen KJ, Lamberg MA. Detection of human papillomavirus DNA in oral mucosal lesions using in situ DNA-hybridization applied on paraffin sections. *Oral Surg Oral Med Oral Pathol.* 1986; 62:660–667.

79. Green TL, Eversole LR, Leider AS. Oral and labial verruca vulgaris: Clinical, histologic and immunohistochemical evaluation. *Oral Surg Oral Med Oral Pathol.* 1986; 62:410–416.

80. Eversole LR, Laipis PJ, Merrell P, Choi E. Demonstration of human papillomavirus DNA in oral condyloma acuminatum. *J Oral Pathol.* 1987; 16:266–272.

81. Eversole LR, Laipis PJ, Green TL. Human papillomavirus Type 2 DNA in oral and labial verruca vulgaris. *J Cutan Pathol.* 1987; 14:319–325.

82. Eversole LR, Laipis PJ. Oral squamous papillomas: Detection of HPV DNA by in situ hybridization. *Oral Surg Oral Med Oral Pathol.* 1988; 65:545–550.

83. Cummer CL. Leukoplakia (leukokeratosis) of the palate, papular form. *JAMA* 1946; 132:493–498.

84. Thoma KH. Stomatitis nicotina and its effect on the palate. *Amer J Orthodont Oral Surg.* 1941; 27:38–47.

85. Schwartz DL. Stomatitis nicotina of the palate. Report of two cases. *Oral Surg Oral Med Oral Pathol.* 1965; 20:306–315.

86. Reddy CRRM, Raju MVS, Ramulu, Reddy PG. Changes in the ducts of the glands of the hard palate in reverse smokers. *Cancer.* 1972; 30:231–238.

87. Farman AG, van Wyk CW, Staz J, et al. Central papillary atrophy of the tongue. *Oral Surg Oral Med Oral Pathol.* 1977; 43:48–58.

88. van der Waal I, Beemster G, van der Kwast WAM. Median rhomboid glossitis caused by *Candida? Oral Surg Oral Med Oral Pathol.* 1979; 47:31–35.

89. Martin HE, Howe ME. Glossitis rhombica mediana. *Ann Surg.* 1938; 107:39–49.

90. Wright BA. Median rhomboid glossitis: Not a misnomer. Review of the literature and histologic study of twenty-eight cases. *Oral Surg Oral Med Oral Pathol.* 1978; 46:806–814.

91. Baughman RA. Median rhomboid glossitis: A developmental anomaly? *Oral Surg Oral Med Oral Pathol.* 31:56–65.

92. Redman RS. Prevalence of geographic tongue, fissured tongue, median rhomboid glossitis, and hairy tongue among 3,611 Minnesota schoolchildren. *Oral Surg Oral Med Oral Pathol.* 1970; 30:390–395.

93. Shklar G, McCarthy PL. The oral lesions of lichen planus. *Oral Surg Oral Med Oral Pathol.* 1961; 14:164–181.

94. Andreasen JO. Oral lichen planus. I. A clinical evaluation of 115 cases. *Oral Surg Oral Med Oral Pathol.* 1968; 25:31–42.

95. Krutchkoff DJ, Eisenberg E. Lichenoid dysplasia: A distinct histopathologic entity. *Oral Surg Oral Med Oral Pathol.* 1985; 30:308.

96. Silverman S Jr, Gorsky M, Lozada-Nur F. A prospective follow-up study of 570 patients with oral lichen planus: Persistence, remission, and malignant associaton. *Oral Surg Oral Med Oral Pathol.* 1985; 60:30–34.

97. Andreasen JO. Oral lichen planus. II. A histologic evaluation of ninety-seven cases. *Oral Surg Oral Med Oral Pathol.* 1968; 25:158–166.

98. Arafat A, Brannon RB, Ellis GL. Adenomatoid hyperplasia of mucous salivary glands. *Oral Surg Oral Med Oral Pathol.* 1981; 52:51–55.

99. Jorgenson RJ, Levin LS. White sponge nevus. *Arch Dermatol.* 1981; 117:73–76.

100. Stiff RH, Ferraro E. Hereditary keratosis. *Oral Surg Oral Med Oral Pathol.* 1969; 28:697–701.

101. Levin LS, Jorgenson RJ, Jarvey BA. Lymphangiomas of the alveolar ridges in neonates. *Pediatrics.* 1976; 58:881–884.

102. Wysocki GP, Brannon RB, Gardner DG, Sapp P. Histogenesis of the lateral periodontal cyst and the gingival cyst of the adult. *Oral Surg Oral Med Oral Pathol.* 1980; 50:327–334.

103. Buchner A, Hansen LS. The histomorphologic spectrum of the gingival cyst in the adult. *Oral Surg Oral Med Oral Pathol.* 1979; 48:532–539.

104. Wescott WB, Correll RW, Craig RM. Two fluid-filled gingival lesions in the mandibular canine-first premolar area. *J Am Dent Assoc.* 1984; 108:653–654.

105. Bhaskar SN. Gingival cyst and the keratinizing ameloblastoma. *Oral Surg Oral Med Oral Pathol.* 1965; 19:796–807.

106. Sanstead HR, Lowe JW. Leukoedema and keratosis in relation to leukoplakia of the buccal mucosa in man. *J Nat Cancer Inst.* 1953; 14:423–433.

107. Archard HO, Carlson KP, Stanley HR. Leukoedema of the human oral mucosa. *Oral Surg Oral Med Oral Pathol.* 1968; 23:717–728.

108. Waldron CA, Shafer WG. Leukoplakia revisited. A clinicopathologic study 3256 oral leukoplakias. *Cancer.* 1975; 36:1386–1392.

109. Silverman S Jr, Gorsky M, Lozada F. Oral leukoplakia and malignant transformation. A follow-up study of 257 patients. *Cancer.* 1984; 53:563–568.

110. Bánóczy J. Follow-up studies in oral leukoplakia. *J Max-Fac Surg.* 1977; 5:69–75.

111. Renstrup G. Occurrence of *Candida* in oral leukoplakias. *Acta Path Microbiol Scand B.* 1970; 78:421–424.

112. Shafer WG, Waldron CA. Erythroplakia of the oral cavity. *Cancer.* 1975; 36:1021–1028.

113. Mashberg A, Meyers H. Anatomical site and size of 222 early asymptomatic oral squamous cell carcinomas. A continuing prospective study of oral cancer. II. *Cancer.* 1976; 37:2149–2137.

114. Pindborg JJ, Renstrup G, Poulsen HE, Silverman S Jr. Studies

in oral leukoplakias. V. Clinical and histologic signs of malignancy. *Acta Odont Scand*. 1963; 21:404–414.

115. Pindborg JJ. *Oral Cancer and Precancer*. Bristol: John Wright and Sons, Ltd; 1980:42–43.

116. Jepsen A, Winther JE. Mycotic infection in oral leukoplakia. *Acta Odontol Scand*. 1965; 23:239–256.

117. Renstrup G. Occurrence of *Candida* in oral leukoplakias. *Acta Path Microbiol Scand B*. 1970; 78:421–424.

118. Pindborg JJ, Renstrup G, Jølst O, Roed-Petersen B. Studies in oral leukoplakia: A preliminary report on the period pervalence (*sic*) of malignant transformation in leukoplakia based on a follow-up study of 248 patients. *J Am Dent Assoc*. 1968; 76:767–771.

SECTION X
Disorders of the Appendages

CHAPTER 58
Inflammatory Reactions of the Pilosebaceous Unit

Wilma F. Bergfeld

The inflammatory disorders of the pilosebaceous unit, for this chapter, are divided into folliculitis, acute and chronic types, and the inflammatory alopecias, nonscarring and scarring.

In general, this chapter deals with inflammatory folliculitis as an acute, chronic, and granulomatous inflammation, which partially or totally destroys the hair follicle, resulting frequently in reparative fibrosis. Specific entities discussed are staphylococcal folliculitis, such as impetigo of Bockhart, disseminated and recurrent infundibulofolliculitis, folliculitis barbae, furuncles and carbuncles, and folliculitis decalvans. In addition, fungal folliculitis, *Demodex* folliculitis, acne vulgaris and rosacea, and foreign body folliculitis are discussed briefly. The disorders of keratinization are dealt with only in their relationship to folliculitis (Table 58–1).

Other inflammatory alopecias include nonscarring types, such as alopecia areata, follicular mucinosis, follicular eczema, and the inflammatory scarring alopecias, such as lupus erythematosus, lichen planopilaris, and pseudopelade.

FOLLICULITIS

Folliculitis clinically appears as inflammatory papule, pustule, or boggy indurated plaques with draining sinuses and localized cellulitis. These inflammatory lesions can be seen anywhere there are pilosebaceous units and may be localized or diffuse.

Histologically, folliculitis can be broadly divided into superficial and deep folliculitis, with acute, chronic, granulomatous, or mixed inflammatory infiltrate resulting in reparative fibrosis (Table 58–2).

The etiology of folliculitis varies from infectious agents to foreign body inflammatory responses to hair fibers, sebum, follicular contents, parasites, mites, and disorders of keratinization (Table 58–3). Frequently, the etiologic cause of the folliculitis can be demonstrated with special stains, cultures, electron microscopy, and immunohistochemistry (Table 58–4).

Acute Folliculitis

Acute folliculitis is predominantly a neutrophilic folliculitis, with partial or complete destruction of the follicle and adjoining sebaceous lobule. The follicular epithelium demonstrates spongiosis, necrosis, and exocytosis of acute inflammatory cells with intra- and perifollicular abscess formation. The acute superficial folliculitis involves the infundibular area of the follicle and is classically represented as impetigo of Bockhart, whereas the deeper, acute folliculitis involves primarily the deeper portions of the hair follicle and frequently demonstrates partial total disruption of the hair follicle and abscess formation. Follicular epithelial remnants are commonly observed in areas of acute inflammation. Special stains can demonstrate the causative organism (Table 58–4). Adjacent to the folliculitis, a localized cellulitis can be observed. The adjacent small vessels have varied perivascular inflammatory infiltrate, which include lymphocytes, neutrophils, rarely plasma cells, and associated leukocytoclastic vasculitis. The classic deep folliculitis appears as a furuncle or carbuncle (Fig. 58–1).

Chronic Folliculitis

Chronic folliculitis can also be superficial or deep. The inflammation is primarily a lymphocytic, inflammatory infiltrate with occasional plasma cells or mixed granulomatous inflammation. Again, the follicle can show a variety of changes from partial, complete disruption of the follicle and surrounding reticular dermis with obvious follicular and connective tissue necrosis to granulomatous inflammation with epithelioid cells and foreign body giant cells. Small pockets of neutrophilic abscesses occasionally are observed. In more chronic, long-standing, deep folliculitis, a spectrum of granulation tissue and reparative fibrosis is present. This form of folliculitis can be seen in cystic acne vulgaris, fungal folliculitis, *Demodex* folliculitis, and follicular occlusive disorders, such as hidradenitis suppurativa. Hair foreign body reactions with chronic folliculitis are seen in pseudofolliculi-

TABLE 58–1. FOLLICULITIS

Superficial	Deep
Acute inflammation	Acute and mixed inflammation
Staphylococcal folliculitis	Staphylococcal folliculitis
Impetigo Bockhart	Furuncle, carbuncle
Folliculitis barbae	Folliculitis decalvans
Disseminant and recurrent	Folliculitis barbae
infundibulofolliculitis	Perifolliculitis capitis
Fungal folliculitis	abscedens et suffodens
Seborrheic folliculitis	Dissecting cellulitis of scalp
Parasitic folliculitis	Erosive pustular folliculitis
Eosinophilic folliculitis	Hidradenitis suppurativa
Demodex folliculitis	Keratinizing defect
Acne vulgaris	Acne vulgaris
Acne rosacea	Foreign body reaction
Psoriasis vulgaris	Folliculitis keloidalis nuchae
	Pseudofolliculitis

TABLE 58–2. HISTOLOGIC FEATURES OF FOLLICULITIS

Hair follicle—sebaceous gland
  Partial or total disruption of hair follicle
  Spongiosis, necrosis, inflammation
Inflammation
  Intra-, inter-, and perifollicular cell types
    Acute: neutrophils, eosinophils
    Chronic: lymphocyte
    Granulomatous
    Mixed: acute, chronic, granulomatous

TABLE 58–3. FOLLICULITIS: COMMON ETIOLOGIES

Bacterial
Fungal
Mixed infections
Viral
Demodex
Foreign material
Sterile

tis and pseudofolliculitis and folliculitis keloidalis nuchae (Fig. 58–2).

Deep Folliculitis

Deep folliculitis, which involves an inflammatory process of the hair follicle below the infundibular, occurs clinically as papules, pustules, crusts, plaques, and associated deep abscesses with sinus tracts. Those entities producing a deep folliculitis are differentiated one from the other by their site of predilection. For example, folliculitis barbae occurs most frequently on the face, folliculitis decalvans on the scalp, folliculitis keloidalis nuchae on the neck, acne vulgaris

and cystic acne vulgaris on the face and trunk, and hidradenitis in the intertriginous areas.

Histologically, the early lesion, a papule or pustule, occurs with a chronic predominantly lymphocytic perifollicular infiltrate with occasional histiocytes, plasmacytes, and neutrophils. When a pustule develops, there is obvious follicular spongiotic necrosis and exocystosis of neutrophils into the follicular epithelium, with interfollicular abscess formation (Fig. 58–3).

Older lesions, indolent, erythematous plaques with draining sinuses, show destruction of the follicle with follicular epithelial remnants, keratin, and hairs surrounded

TABLE 58–4. FOLLICULITIS SECONDARY TO INFECTIOUS ORGANISMS

Agent	Special Stains	Organism	Other
Bacterial	Gram-Weigert	Gram-positive: Blue	Culture
	Brown-Brenn	Gram-negative: Red	
Fungal	Gomori methenamine silver (GMS)	Fungus: Black	Culture
	Periodic acid-Schiff (PAS)	Fungus: Red	
	Gram-Weigert	*Actinomyces:* Blue	
	Brown-Brenn	*Nocardia:* Blue	
	Alcian blue	Capsule: Blue	
		Fungus: Blue	
	Mucicarmine	Capsule: Red	
	PAS	Fungus: Red	
	Giemsa	Histoplasma: Red-Blue	
Demodex	H & E	*Demodex:* Pink-Red	
	PAS		
Viral	H & E		Culture
			Electron microscopy
			Immunohisto-chemistry

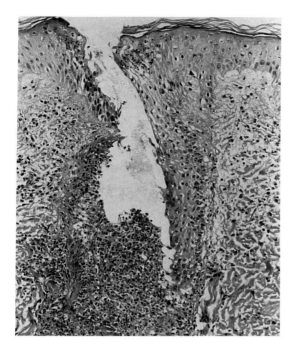

Figure 58–1. Acute suppurative folliculitis. (H&E, ×20.)

by a chronic granulomatous inflammation, with giant cells containing keratin and fragmented hair. Neutrophilic abscesses may be numerous throughout the granulomatous inflammation. Stroma surrounding the follicular inflammation demonstrates granulation tissue and reparative fibrosis. Chronic perivascular inflammation also is noted, and leukocytoclastic vasculitis is observed rarely. The causative agent frequently can be demonstrated with special stains for infectious agents or polarization for foreign material.

SPECIFIC FOLLICULITIS

Staphylococcal Folliculitis

Impetigo of Bockhart is caused by staphylococci and clinically occurs with small pustules, many of which are pierced by a small hair. Histologically, a subcorneal and follicular infundibular abscess is noted and is accompanied by localized upper dermal cellulitis. Gram stains and cultures confirm the diagnoses (Fig. 58–4).

Disseminant and Recurrent Infundibular Folliculitis

Disseminant and recurrent infundibular folliculitis primarily involves the trunk and extremities and appears as pruritic, minute papules that resemble chronic gooselike accentuations of hair follicles. Histologically, the infundibular portion of the hair follicle is spongiotic and surrounded by lymphocytic inflammatory infiltrate. The etiology is unknown, but staphylococci frequently are demonstrated.

Furunculosis

Furunculosis is a deep folliculitis that may begin as a superficial, acute folliculitis. Clinically, the furuncle appears as an erythemated papulonodule lesion that may be isolated or disseminated. Histologically, the deep folliculitis involves the hair follicle beneath the infundibulum. An acute, chronic, granulomatous, or mixed inflammatory infiltrate is present. Clinically, when there are multiple communicating furuncles or local involvement of multiple follicles, a carbuncle is diagnosed. Similar histologic changes can be seen in sycosis barbae and folliculitis decalvans and represents a deep staphylococcal infection demonstrated by gram stain. Gram-negative deep folliculitis is rare. In chronic

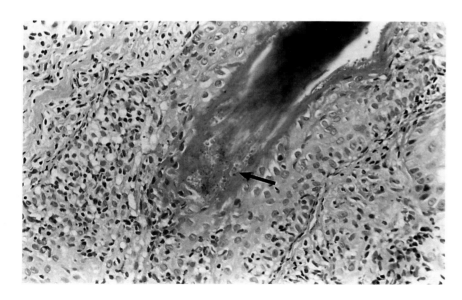

Figure 58–2. Chronic fungal folliculitis (Arrow: fungal spores). (H&E, ×40.)

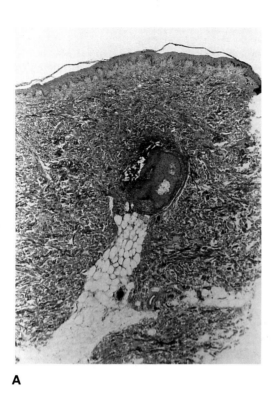

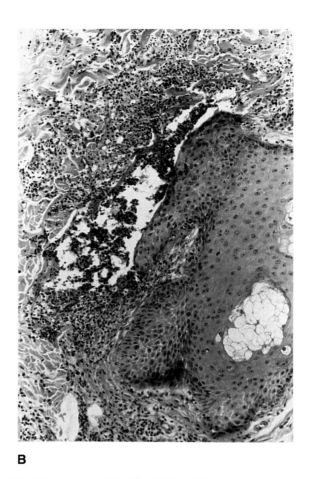

A

B

Figure 58–3. A. Chronic deep folliculitis. (H&E, ×4.) **B.** Chronic deep folliculitis. (H&E, ×40.)

granulomatous folliculitis, organisms are rare and frequently are not demonstrated with special stains or with cultures.

Fungal Folliculitis

Clinically, fungal folliculitis also involves hairbearing skin and occurs as a superficial or deep folliculitis with acute,

chronic, granulomatous, or mixed inflammatory infiltrates. In fungal folliculitis, hyphae and spores are found in the keratin layers of the hair follicle or the hair. In a deep, acute, and chronic folliculitis, such as Majocchi's granuloma (fungal folliculitis of women's legs) or kerion (deep folliculitis of the scalp, especially seen in children), fungal organisms are readily identified by special stains and may be seen, not only in the keratogenous areas of the follicle but also on or lining the hair fibers. As in all deep folliculitis,

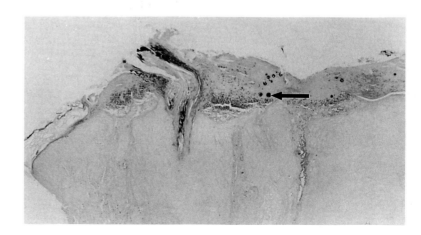

Figure 58–4. Staphylococcal folliculitis (Arrow: bacterial granules). (Gram stain, H&E, ×10.)

on resolution, scarring is frequently a sequela. Frequent fungal organisms that induce deep folliculitis include *Trichophyton, Microsporum, Candida,* and *Pityrosporum.* Cultures frequently are useful for verification of the specific organism. *Pityrosporum* are difficult or impossible to culture and are better diagnosed on PAS stain, where they appear as blastospores within the keratin of the follicle or within the follicular abscess.

Parasitic Folliculitis

Demodex Folliculitis

Demodex folliculitis occurs usually as a superficial, chronic, parasitic folliculitis or, rarely, an acute suppurative folliculitis. Within the hair follicle, a vermiform mite is identified. *Demodex folliculorum,* with its elongated body, is at present the most common in the infundibular area, and *Demodex brevis,* with a short body, is localized in the sebaceous canal (Fig. 58–5). These mites are saprophytic organisms and may induce an inflammatory response. Some researchers believe that *Demodex* is the primary elicitor of acne rosacea.

Acne Vulgaris and Acne Rosacea

The acneiform eruptions of acne vulgaris and acne rosacea occur as inflammatory papules, pustules, and nodulocystic lesions. Specifically, acne is observed in sites where pilosebaceous units are found.

Histologically, inflammatory acne resembles acute superficial and deep folliculitis. Special stains reveal mixed organisms within the follicular abscesses and include *P. acnes,* staphylococci, and *Pityrosporum.* It is theorized, however, that acne is primarily a disorder of follicular keratinization and not a primary infection (Fig. 58–6).

The chronic forms of papular acne are all basically a lymphocytic folliculitis and perifolliculitis and rarely a granulomatous folliculitis. Granulomatous folliculitis is the most common presentation of papular acne rosacea.

Acne rosacea differs from acne vulgaris in that it primarily involves the central face and is not associated with comedones but causes telangiectasias. Acne vulgaris has a spectrum of lesions including comedones, and it is most commonly present on the face, shoulders, upper chest, and back in young adults. A variant of acne rosacea includes perioral dermatitis of debatable etiology.

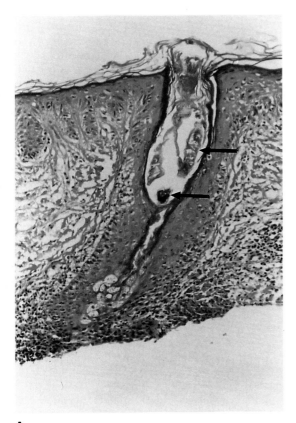

A

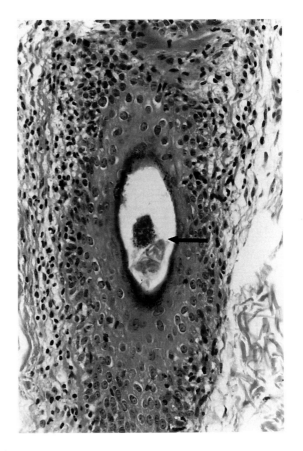

B

Figure 58–5. A. Demodex folliculitis. (H&E, ×20.) **B.** Demodex folliculitis (Arrow: cross section demodex mite). (H&E, ×40.)

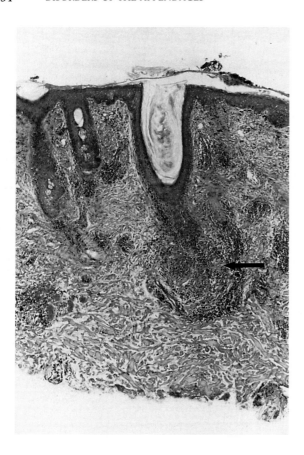

Figure 58–6. Acne vulgaris, chronic granulomatous folliculitis (Arrow: granulomatous inflammation). (H&E, ×10.)

Eosinophilic Pustular Folliculitis

Eosinophilic pustular folliculitis is a rare disorder first reported from Japan as an unusual papular eruption involving primarily the face, trunk, and extremities. Histologically, eosinophilic pustular folliculitis demonstrated edema, spongiosis, and destruction of the follicle by a moderate to intense infiltrate of eosinophils, with prominent interfollicular and subcorneal eosinophilic abscesses. It occurs clinically as superficial pustules. This disorder was noted to be associated with blood eosinophilia. The etiology of this disorder is unclear but it is thought to be associated with a hypersensitivity response and possibly eosinophilic cellulitis, or Well's syndrome.

Disorders of Keratinization with Secondary Folliculitis

Folliculitis has been observed in follicular keratinizing disorders, such as monilethrix and as ichthyosis. Folliculitis appears to be secondary to localized follicular plugging and an inflammatory response to infectious organisms, keratin, hair, and other fibers.

Folliculitis and Transepidermal Elimination Disorder

The transepidermal elimination disorders, such as perforating folliculitis, elastosis perforans serpiginosum, and reactive perforating collagenosis, clinically and histologically appear as an acute or chronic granulomatous folliculitis. Histologically, the dilated, hyperplastic follicular structure is filled with keratogenous debris, parakeratotic cells, curled hair, eosinophilic elastoid fibers, or degenerate collagen. Focal disruption of the lower half of the follicle results in acute and chronic granulomatous inflammation.

Erosive Pustular Folliculitis

Erosive pustular dermatosis–folliculitis, also known as folliculitis decalvans or pyoderma of the scalp, represents a suppurative folliculitis with destruction of the follicles and adnexal structures and end-stage scarring. Immunologic studies provide evidence of defective lymphocytes, increased immunoglobulins, abnormal neutrophilic chemotaxis, and hypocomplementemia. Several reports implicate staphylococci as initiators of this suppurative, destructive folliculitis.

ALOPECIA

The alopecic disorders can be broadly classified histologically as inflammatory or noninflammatory in type (see Table 58–5). Common features are (1) diminished follicles, (2) follicular cysts, and (3) chronic superficial changes of actinic damage. More specific features include alterations of tissue

Chemical and mechanical acne generally are seen on the extremities and trunk and occasionally on the face and are indistinguishable from acne vulgaris.

Steroid acne, another acneiform eruption, usually is generalized, occurs as papules and pustules with rare comedones, and histologically resembles acne vulgaris.

Foreign Body Folliculitis

Folliculitis secondary to spiral hair fibers can be seen in folliculitis barbae, pseudofolliculitis, and folliculitis keloidalis nuchae. Clinically, acneiform papules, pustules, and papulonodular lesions with or without fistulous tracts occur, predominantly on the face and neck. Superficial and deep acute and chronic folliculitis is present. However, also noted are hair fiber granulomas, which are fragmented hair fibers outside the follicle, and occasionally secondary infectious folliculitis, both superficial and deep in type. In chronic foreign body folliculitis, there is evidence of granulomatous inflammation, granulation tissue, and fibrosis. The fibrotic areas may contain keloidal collagen.

TABLE 58–5. ALOPECIA: CLASSIFICATION

Inflammatory		Noninflammatory
Alteration of hair follicle cycle	Destruction (damage) of hair follicle	Involution Scarring Nonscarring
Involution Nonscarring	Involution *Scarring*	

TABLE 58–6. INFLAMMATORY NONSCARRING ALOPECIA

Altered or Damaged Follicles
Alopecia areata
Follicular mucinosis
Follicular eczema
Keratinizing disorders

androgen/telogen ratios, miniaturization of follicles, presence or absence of inflammation, and end-stage scarring. In reviewing the biopsies, it is important to identify concomitant disease, such as *Demodex* folliculitis, seborrheic folliculitis, and even psoriasis vulgaris. Alopecia results from alteration of the follicle growth cycle, with acute or gradual involution of the follicle with or without inflammation, follicular destruction, or alterations and scarring. The inflammatory, nonscarring alopecias considered in this chapter are alopecia areata, follicular mucinosis, follicular eczema, and briefly the keratinizing disorders, such as psoriasis and pityriasis rubra pilaris (Table 58–6).

Alopecia Areata

Alopecia areata is hypothesized to be the result of an autosomal dominant, autoimmune disease and is commonly associated with other autoimmune diseases. Clinically, it is a heterogeneous disorder and has been described in the literature as alopecia areata, alopecia totalis, and alopecia universalis. The acute histologic findings of alopecia areata include sparse to moderate lymphocytic peribulbar inflammation surrounding catagen and anagen follicles, increased catagen follicles, and a focal lymphohistocytic vasculitis in the subcutaneous fat. Adjacent to the peribulbar inflammation, mast cells, plasma cells, and occasionally eosinophils can be observed (Fig. 58–7).

In chronic alopecia areata, there may be changes similar to those seen in the acute form. In addition, miniaturization of the follicle and associated decreased density of follicles are observed. Reversal of the tissue antagen/telogen ratio and an increased number of miniaturized telogen follicles is common. Other more subtle changes include melanophages within the fibrous tracts of the subcutaneous tissue and focal hyalinization of the catagen adventitial sheath and vitreous membrane (Table 58–7).

Follicular Mucinosis/ Alopecia Mucinosis

Clinically, the lesions of follicular mucinosis and alopecia mucinosis are similar and occur as group follicular erythematous papules or plaques. These lesions are devoid of hair and frequently are located on the head and neck and rarely on the extremities and trunk. The lesions may be isolated or disseminated. When follicular mucinosis is associated with a T cell lymphoma or mycosis fungoides, it is considered alopecia mucinosis. In this instance, a benign, chronic, perifollicular, inflammatory infiltrate contains atypical lymphoid cells similar to those seen in T cell lymphoma.

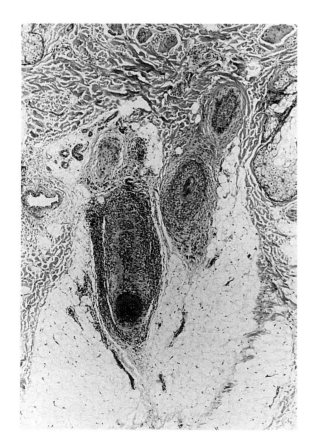

Figure 58–7. Alopecia areata, lymphocytic peribulbar inflammation. (H&E, ×20.)

TABLE 58–7. ALOPECIA AREATA: HISTOLOGIC FEATURES

Acute
Lymphocytic, peribulbar inflammation surrounding catagen and anagen follicles
Increased catagen follicles
Lymphocytic vasculitis focally

Chronic
Miniaturization follicles
Decreased hair follicles
Increased telogen and catagen follicles
Hyalinization of fibrous tracts and catagen follicles
Melanin incontinence within anagen fibrous tracts
Occasional mast cells and eosinophils
Occasional acute findings

Histologically, follicular alopecia mucinosis demonstrates similar changes of mucin, hyaluronic acid, collected in intra- and intercellular areas of trichilemmal sheaths, sebaceous glands, and follicle. When in abundance, the mucin pools in the follicular infundibulum resemble cystic degeneration of the follicle. Frequently, the mucin is accompanied by a chronic lymphocytic perifollicular infiltrate and folliculitis with plasma cells. Differential diagnosis includes follicular eczema.

Follicular eczema has many similarities to follicular mucinosis, with its clinical presentation of flesh-colored to erythematous papules, most commonly on the trunk and extremities of the young, and it is frequently associated with atopic dermatitis. Histologically, it differs from follicular mucinosis by the absence of follicular mucin, hyaluronic acid.

Inflammatory Scarring Alopecia

Inflammatory scarring alopecia primarily represents an acute or chronic, superficial and deep folliculitis. The inflammation is intense, and there are disruption, destruction of the follicle, and moderate to marked connective tissue destruction with resultant scarring alopecia. Briefly, inflammatory scarring alopecia can be divided into three major groups, acne vulgaris (papulonodular type), folliculitis, and immune modulated disorders (Table 58–8).

Lupus Erythematosus

Lupus erythematosus clinically and histologically is characterized as acute, subacute, and chronic. The classic presentation of chronic lupus erythematosus is that of a discoid psoriasiform alopecic patch plaque with prominent follicular plugging, and a relatively uncommon presentation is clinically a noninflammatory, smooth, hairless alopecic patch of varied size similar to that seen in end-stage lichen planopilaris, pseudopelade, or alopecia areata. The acute and subacute lupus forms of erythematosus cause a classic clinical erythema and scaling, with histologic changes of a superficial lichenoid dermatitis with vacuolopathy.

Histologically, the classic, chronic, discoid lupus erythematosus lesion of the scalp reveals basilar vacuolopathy and an interfacing lichenoid lymphocytic infiltration with

TABLE 58–8. INFLAMMATORY SCARRING ALOPECIA: ETIOLOGIES

Damaged Follicle (Inflammation)	Involution
Acne vulgaris	Autoimmune phenomena
Folliculitis	Pseudopelade
Infections	? Bullous pemphigoid
Parasitic	? Epidermolysis bullosa
Autoimmune phenomena	
Lupus erythematosus	
Lichen planopilaris	
Mixed inflammatory	
destructive alopecia	
Pseudopelade	

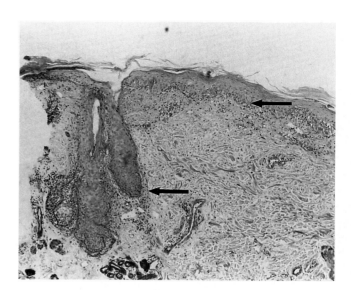

Figure 58–8. Lupus erythematosus, chronic (Arrow: interface lichenoid infiltrate and chronic folliculitis). (H&E, ×4.)

epidermal apoptosis and fibrin deposition at the dermal–epidermal junction (Fig. 58–8). These changes involve both the superficial and follicular epithelium. Direct immunofluorescence of the superficial and follicular epithelium reveals immunoreactants in the linear, finely granular pattern containing IgG, C3, and occasionally IgM. The associated inflammation is primarily lymphocytic and appears as a lymphocytic folliculitis of telogen follicles. Rarely an associated leukocytoclastic vasculitis is observed (Table 58–8). In the thicker plaques, lymphocytic, lobular panniculitis and lymphocytic vasculitis can be observed. Lupus profundus is diagnosed when the histologic features include the superficial features of lupus erythematosus and a lymphocytic panniculitis.

The noninflammatory alopecic lesions of chronic lupus erythematosus demonstrate none of the superficial findings of lupus erythematosus, only chronic lymphocytic inflammatory infiltrates within the adventitial dermis of the fibrous tracts, the vertical streaks or streamers. Occasionally, a remnant of a telogen follicle is present that may demonstrate linear immunoreactants similar to the pattern identified in lupus erythematosus. Focal hair granulomas can be observed within the fibrous tracts, usually at the dermal–subcutaneous junction as an end result of an inflammatory destructive alopecia. Debates might arise about whether this noninflammatory form of lupus erythematosus is actually an inflammatory pseudopelade.

In the more chronic forms of lupus erythematosus, clinically and histologically, the hair follicles are destroyed, and there is resultant reparative fibrosis and scarring. Scarring is interpreted as scar when elastic fibers are absent from the dermis that is fibrosed or hyalinized.

Lichen Planopilaris

Lichen planopilaris is a chronic, inflammatory, destructive alopecia that occurs on the scalp and other hairy areas of

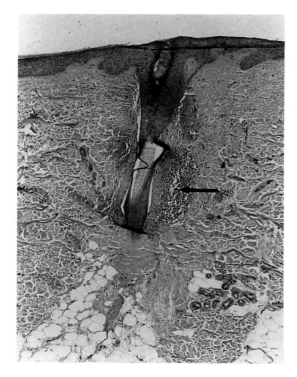

Figure 58–9. Lichen planopilaris, chronic folliculitis. (H&E, ×10.)

the adventitial dermis adjacent to the follicular basement membrane.

In the chronic form of lichen planopilaris, the inflammatory infiltrate appears to destroy the telogen follicles, which results in fibrosis and scar, similar to the end-stage of chronic lupus erythematosus (Table 58–9).

Mixed Inflammatory Scarring Alopecia

Mixed inflammatory scarring alopecia (MISA) is a term I have coined and represents an alopecic condition in which lupus erythematosus, lichen planopilaris, and inflammatory pseudopelade overlap, clinically and histologically. Clinically, MISA appears as small alopecic patches void of follicular plugging, which coalesce and form large alopecic areas. Clinically, this lesion has many similarities to alopecia areata and pseudopelade. This condition is unusual and is seen primarily in middle-aged females.

Histologically, there is a chronic inflammatory obstructive folliculitis, demonstrating changes similar to those of chronic lupus erythematosus and lichen planopilaris. A marked to dense perifollicular, lichenoid lymphocytic infiltrate, with focal destruction of the follicles, destructive folliculitis, prominent vacuolopathy, and lymphocytic exocytosis, is present. Within the reticular dermis, focal lymphocytic perivascular inflammation and vasculitis can be noted. Other findings include chronic inflammation within the midreticular fibrous tracts of the hair follicles and, rarely, hair foreign body granulomas. Direct immunofluorescence of involved skin demonstrates a mixed deposition of immunoreactants, globular and linear, a mixed pattern of lupus erythematosus, and lichen planopilaris (Table 58–10).

the body. Clinically and histologically, lichen planopilaris can resemble lupus erythematosus, and it appears as hyperkeratotic follicular plugs surrounded by mild erythema and, infrequently, as a psoriasiform plaque. This disorder is seen in older individuals, males more than females. A histologically moderate lymphocytic interfacing inflammatory infiltrate surrounding the superficial and follicular epithelium, or chronic folliculitis, is observed. Basilar vacuolopathy and exocytosis of lymphocytes are prominent. Civatte bodies are observed within the lichenoid infiltrate within the papillary dermis. Nonspecific changes of follicular plugging, mild lymphocytic perivascular infiltrates, and chronic dermal inflammation also are noted (Fig. 58–9). Direct immunofluorescence of the involved skin demonstrates globular deposition of IgG, IgM, and IgA and fibrinogen within

Pseudopelade of Brocq

Pseudopelade of Brocq shares many similarities with the noninflammatory lupus erythematosus, end-stage lichen planus, and mixed inflammatory destructive alopecia. Differentiating pseudopelade from these entities can be done if a hair follicle is present for direct immunofluorescence. On direct immunofluorescence immunoreactants, IgG, IgM,

TABLE 58–9. DISCOID LUPUS ERYTHEMATOSUS: HISTOLOGIC FEATURES

Acute	Chronic
Epidermal changes of lupus erythematosus	Scar
Intense perifollicular lymphocytic (lichenoid) infiltrate surrounding telogen follicles	Reactive fibrosis
	Loss of elastic fibers
Follicular plugging telogen follicle	Absence or diminished hair follicles
Lymphocytic vasculitis	
Lymphocytic mixed panniculitis may or may not be present	
Direct Immunofluoresence of follicle shows linear, fine granular IgG, C3, BMZ	
Elastic fibers intact	

TABLE 58–10. LICHEN PLANOPILARIS: HISTOLOGIC FEATURES

Acute	Chronic
Lacks epidermal changes of DLE	Scar
Intense perifollicular lymphocytic (lichenoid) infiltrate around telogen follicles(s)	Diminished or absent hair follicles
Follicular plugging of telogen follicle(s)	
Direct immunoflorescence (follicle) shows globular deposition of IgG, IgM, IgA, and fibrinogen within the papillary dermis	

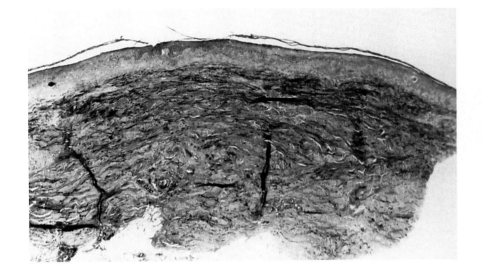

Figure 58–10. Pseudopelade, end stage (Arrow: elastic fibers). (Elastic stain, ×10.)

TABLE 58–11. MIXED INFLAMMATORY ALOPECIA: HISTOLOGIC FEATURES

Acute	Chronic
Intense perifollicular lymphocytic (lichenoid) infiltrate round telogen follicles	Scar
Focal lymphocytic vasculitis	Absent or diminished hair follicles
Lymphocytic infiltrate within expanded fibrous tracts	Hair fiber granuloma
Direct immunofluoresence shows mixed pattern of DLE, LLP, and pseudopelade	

TABLE 58–12. PSEUDOPELADE: HISTOLOGIC FEATURES

Inflammatory	Noninflammatory
Absence or rare hair follicle	Absence of hair follicle (total involution)
Patchy lymphocytic infiltrate within expanded fibrous tracts	
Occasional chronic, lymphocytic perivascular dermal infiltrate	Scarring may or may not be present
Scarring may or may not be present	
DIF: Follicular membranes linear IgM, C3	

TABLE 58–13. FOLLICULITIS: DISTINGUISHING HISTOLOGIC FEATURES AND DIFFERENTIAL DIAGNOSIS

	Hair Follicle		Inflammation					
	Anagen	Telogen	Lym	Plasma	Mast	Eos	Neut	Giant Cells
Infectious folliculitis	±	+	+	+	±	+	+	+
Alopecia areata	+	−	+	−	+	+	−	−
DLE	−	+	+	±	±	−	−	−
LPP	−	+	+	±	−	−	−	−
Pseudopelade	−	±	+	−	−	−	−	−

Lym, Lymphocyte.
Eos, Eosinophil.
Neut, neutrophil.

and C3 are observed in a linear distribution along the basement membrane zone of the hair follicle. Histologically, pseudopelade can occur as an inflammatory or noninflammatory alopecia. When it is inflammatory, hair follicles are absent. If a rare hair follicle is present, there is a patchy, lichenoid perifollicular inflammatory infiltrate with prominent vacuolopathy of the basilar area. Without the presence of hair follicles, the most common finding is a patchy, lymphocytic infiltrate within the midreticular expanded fibrous tracts (Fig. 58–11). Scarring is variable.

Noninflammatory pseudopelade demonstrates a total absence of hair follicles, total involution, and an absence of inflammatory infiltrate. On light microscopy, scarring often is seen (Table 58–12).

BIBLIOGRAPHY

Folliculitis

Cove JH, Cunliffe WJ, Holland KT. Acne vulgaris. Is the bacterial population size significant? *Br J Dermatol.* 1980;102:277–288.

Ecker RI, Winkelmann RK. *Demodex* granuloma. *Arch Dermatol.* 1979;115:343–344.

Golitz L. Follicular and perforating disorders. *J Cutan Pathol.* 1985;12:282.

Graham JH, Barroso-Tobila C. Dermal pathology of superficial fungus infections. In: Baker RD, ed. *The Pathologic Anatomy of Mycoses. Handbuch der speziellen pathologischen Anatomie and Histologie.* New York; Springer-Verlag; 1971;3.

Gross KG. Pseudofolliculitis barbae; shaving bumps of blacks. *J Assoc Milit Dermatol.* 1982;8:4.

Lavker RM, Leyden JJ, McGingley KT: The relationship between bacteria and the abnormal follicular keratinization in acne vulgaris. *J Invest Dermatol.* 1981;77:325–330.

Marks R. Histogenesis of the inflammatory component in rosacea. *Proc R Soc Med.* 1973;66:742.

Mehregan AH. Inflammation involving the pilosebaceous complex. In: *Pinkus Guide to Dermatohistopathology.* 4th ed. Norwalk, CT: Appleton-Century-Crofts; 1986;227–240.

Mehregan AH, Coskey RJ. Perforating folliculitis. *Arch Dermatol.* 1968;97:394.

Montagna W, Bell M, Strauss JS, eds. Sebaceous glands and acne vulgaris. *J Invest Dermatol* 62:117, 1974.

Montgomery H. Acne necrotica miliaris of the scalp. *Arch Dermatol Syph.* 1937;36:40–44.

Moyer DG, Williams RM. Perifolliculitis capitis abscedens et suffodiens. *Arch Dermatol.* 1962;85:378–384.

Mullanax MG, Kierland RR. Granulomatous rosacea. *Arch Dermatol.* 1970;101:206.

Noble WC, Presbury D, Connor BL. Prevalence of streptococci and staphylococci in lesions of impetigo. *Br J Dermatol.* 1974; 91:115–116.

Norm MS. *Demodex folliculorus:* incidence, regional distribution, pathogenicity. *Dan Med Bull.* 1971;18:14.

Nutting WB. Hair follicle mites (*Acari demodicidae*) of man. *Int J Dermatol.* 1976;15:79.

Ofuji S, Uehara M. Follicular eruptions of atopic dermatitis. *Arch Dermatol.* 1973;107:54.

Owen WR, Wood C. Disseminated and recurrent infundibulofolliculitis. *Arch Dermatol.* 1979;115:174.

Pinkus H. Furuncle. *J Cutan Pathol.* 1979; 6:517–518.

Pye RJ, Peachey RD, Burton JL. Erosive pustular dermatosis of the scalp. *Br J Dermatol.* 1979;100:559–566.

Rufli T, Murncunagli Y. The hair follicle mites *Demodex folliculorum* and *Demodex brevisi* biology and medical importance. *Dermatologica.* 1981;162:1.

Suter L. Folliculitis decalvans. *Hautarzt.* 1981;32:429–431.

Takematsu H, Nakamura K, Igarashi M, et al. Eosinophilic pustular folliculitis. Report of two cases with a review of the Japanese literature. *Arch Dermatol.* 1985;121:917.

Wheeland RG, Thurmond RD, Gilmore WA, Blackstock R. Chronic blepharitis and pyoderma of the scalp: an immune deficiency state in a father and son with hypercupremia and decreased intracellular killing. *Pediatr Dermatol.* 1983;1:134–142.

Inflammatory Alopecia

Bergfeld WF. Alopecia; histologic changes. *Adv Dermatol.* 1989; 4:301–322.

Bergfeld WF, Valenzuela R, Beutner EH, Lichen planus. In: Beutner EH, Chrozelski TP, Kumar V, eds. *Immunopathology of the Skin.* 3rd ed. New York: Wiley; 1987;647–658.

Binnick AN, Wax FD, Clendenning WE. Alopecia mucinosa of the face associated with mycosis fungoides. *Arch Dermatol.* 1978;114:791.

Braun-Falco O, Imai S, Schmoeckel C, Steger O, Bergner T. Pseudopelade of Brocq. *Dermatologica 86.* 1987;172:16–23.

Copeman PWM, Schroeter A, Kierland RR. An unusual variant of lupus erythematosis or lichen planus. *Br J Dermatol.* 1980; 83:269–270.

Gay Prieto J. Pseudopelade of Brocq: its relationship to some forms of cicatricial alopecias and to lichen planus. *J Invest Dermatol.* 1955;24:323–335.

Headington JT, Mitchell A, Swanson N. New histopathological findings in alopecia areata studied in transverse sections. *J Invest Dermatol.* 1981;76:325.

Ioannides G. Alopecia: a pathologist's view. *Int J Dermatol.* 1982; 21:23.

Lever WF, Schaumburg-Lever G. *Inflammatory diseases of the epidermal appendages and of cartilage.* 6th ed. In: *Histopathology of the Skin.* Philadelphia: Lippincott; 1983:198–210.

Marks R, Griffiths A. the epidermis in pityriasis rubra pilaris. *Br J Dermatol.* 1973;89 (suppl 9):19.

Messenger AG, Slater DN, Buenden SS. Alopecia areata: alterations in the growth cycle and correlation with follicular pathology. *Br J Dermatol.* 1986;114:337–347.

Perret C, Wiesner-Menzel L, Happle R. Immunohistochemical analysis of T-cell subsets in the peribulbar and intrabulbar infiltrates of alopecia areata. *Acta Derm Venereol (Stockh).* 1984;64:26.

Pinkus H. Alopecia: clinicopathologic correlations. *Int J Dermatol.* 1980;19:245.

Pinkus H. Alopecia mucinosa. Inflammatory plaques with alopecia characterized by root-sheath mucinosis. *Arch Dermatol.* 1957; 76:419.

Pinkus H. Alopecia mucinosa. Additional data in 1983. *Arch Dermatol.* 1983;119–698. Commentary.

Pinkus H. Differential pattern of elastic fibers in scarring and nonscarring alopecias. *J Cutan Pathol.* 1978;5:93.

Traupe H, Happle R. Alopecia ichthyotica. A characteristic feature of congenital ichthyosis. *Dermatologica.* 1983;167:225–230.

Van Scott EJ. Morphologic changes in pilosebaceous units and anagen hairs in alopecia areata. *J Invest Dermatol.* 1958;31:35–43.

CHAPTER 59

Noninflammatory Reactions of the Pilosebaceous Unit and Disorders of the Hair Shaft

Wilma F. Bergfeld

This chapter reviews selected noninflammatory alopecic conditions, trichodystrophies, and follicular hamartomas.

ALOPECIA BIOPSY (SCALP)

An excisional scalp biopsy to assess an alopecic condition should be at least a 4 mm full-thickness biopsy, and a full-thickness excisional biopsy is preferred. If a punch biopsy is done, a diagonal biopsy is desired in straight-haired individuals and a perpendicular biopsy in curly-haired individuals. The biopsy specimens can be sectioned vertically or horizontally and are stained with hematoxylin and eosin, periodic acid-Schiff (PAS), and elastic fiber stains for the best interpretation. The PAS stain allows for easy identification of catagen follicles because of their apoptotic changes and staining of vitreous membrane. The elastic fiber stain identifies the presence or absence of scarring and fibrous tracts with ARO-bodies of Pinkus.

ANDROGENETIC ALOPECIA

Androgenetic alopecia (Fig. 59–1, Table 59–1), known also as common baldness, hereditary baldness, and pattern baldness, is an autosomal dominant disorder that has been noted in males and females. The age of onset is usually puberty but can be seen as late as in the 60s. The female pattern alopecia differs from the male clinically in that it is a more diffuse, central hair loss with retention of the frontal hairline, whereas the male pattern demontrates multiple, patchy areas of hair loss over the central scalp.

The acute histologic findings include a decrease in anagen hair follicles, with relative increase in telogen follicles with diminished or hypertrophic sebaceous lobules. In males, vellus hair follicles are commonly observed. The hair follicles vary in their follicular diameters and prominent follicle miniaturization. In chronic androgenetic alopecia, there is a distinctive reduction of follicles, increased telogen

follicles, miniaturizatized follicles, and involution of follicles.

A reversal of the anagen/telogen follicle ratio is common. Hypertrophied collagen with or without associated elastic fibers can be observed in late, chronic stages. Histologically, the varied picture of androgenetic alopecia correlates with the varied clinical presentations.

TRICHOTILLOMANIA

Trichotillomania (Fig. 59–2, Table 59–2) is a psychologic disorder in which the involved individual extracts hair traumatically from the hairy areas in a bizarre pattern. This disorder is seen most commonly in young and old women and represents a serious psychologic problem.

Histologic changes in acute trichotillomania demonstrate perifollicular hemorrhage surrounding telogen follicles, follicular ectasia, and evidence of fractured fibers and trichomalacia. In the later stages, there is evidence of a reversal of the androgen/telogen ratio and perifollicular fibrosis, primarily around telogen follicles. The end result of chronic trichotillomania is a scarring alopecia. Frequently, the chronic stages of trichotillomania appear to mimic androgenetic alopecia.

TRACTION ALOPECIA

Traction alopecia is clinically and histologically similar to trichotillomania. It is the end result of repetitive chemical or physical damage to the follicle, with resultant perifollicular inflammation and scarring.

NONINFLAMMATORY PSEUDOPELADE

Noninflammatory pseudopelade (Fig. 59–3, Table 59–3) clinically occurs with small, 2 to 4 mm, to large alopecic areas, especially prominent on the parietal and vertex area of the

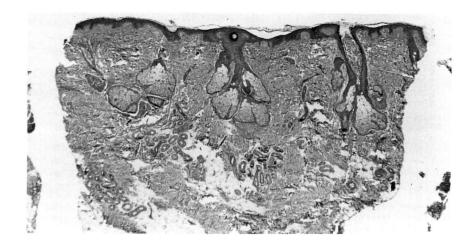

Figure 59–1. Androgenic alopecia. (H&E, 4.)

TABLE 59–1. ANDROGENETIC ALOPECIA

Acute	Chronic
Decreased hair follicles	Marked decreased hair follicles
Relative increased telogen follicles	Occasional increased sebaceous lobules
Increased vellus follicles	Numerous fibrous tracts—involution
Varied follicular size, miniaturization	Occasional scarring
Increased fibrous tracts (telogen effluvium)	
Minimal inflammation	
Nonscarring	

scalp. This is a rare, self-limiting disorder that affects females more than males. Histologically, there is a decrease or absence of hair follicles and adnexae, which is rarely associated with chronic inflammation within the residual fibrous tracts. If present, the fibrous tracts are hyalinized. Elastic fiber stains demonstrate variable presence of elastic fibers. When elastic fibers are absent, a scarring, permanent alopecia is suspected. However, even when elastic fibers are present, permanent alopecia may result. An autoimmune etiology is suspected and partially supported by immunohistologic tests.

EFFLUVIUM

Alopecia can result from increased shedding, or effluvium, of hair, which results in diminished density, or alopecia. An effluvium represents a disruption in the hair follicle growth cycle, usually of the anagen cycle, with a premature shunting of anagen to telogen follicle.

Anagen Effluvium

An anagen effluvium (Fig. 59–4) is acute alteration of growth of the majority of all active, anagen follicles, which results

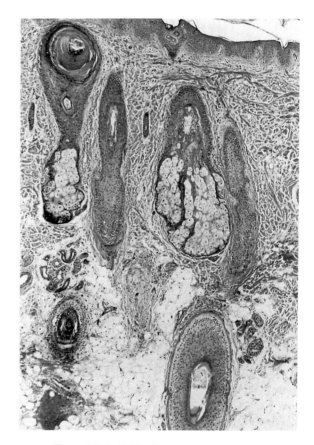

Figure 59–2. Trichotillomania. (H&E, ×10.)

TABLE 59–2. TRICHOTILLOMANIA/TRACTION ALOPECIA

Acute	Chronic
Increased catagen follicles	Increased telogen follicles
Follicular ectasia with pigment casts	Decreased total number hair follicles
Trichomalacia—fragmented hair fibers	Scar, frequently perifollicular
Perifollicular hemorrhage	

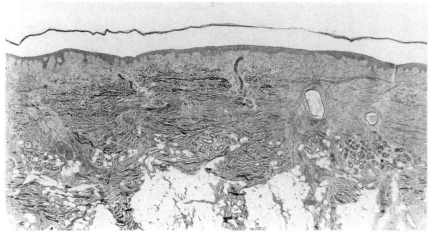

A

PSEUDOPELADE

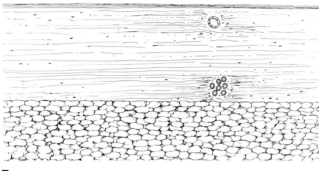

B

Figure 59–3. Pseudopelade, noninflammatory type.

TABLE 59–3. PSEUDOPELADE, NONINFLAMMATORY

Absent or rare follicles

Minimal chronic lymphocyte infiltrates within fibrous tracts

Eosinophilic, compacted collagen with diminished or ectatic sweat ducts and gland

Occasional loss of elastic fibers (scarring)

Epidermal changes: actinic damage

in an acute loss (80 to 90%) of hair. Hair pulls demonstrate tapering of proximal hair (Fig. 59–5), called "exclamatory hair." Histologically, the anagen/telogen ratio is normal. Rarely, a tapered hair will be observed within a hair follicle.

Telogen Effluvium

The telogen effluvium (Fig. 59–6) is a result of premature conversion of 20 to 35% anagen to telogen follicles, which results in shedding and hair loss of a similar percentage, that is, 20 to 35%. Histologically, the anagen/telogen ratio is reversed, with a relative increase in telogen follicles. In the chronic state, empty fibrous tracts, streamers, or in-

creased catagen follicles can be observed. If the fibrous tract is sclerotic or expanded, a permanent alopecia is suspected.

AUTOIMMUNE ALOPECIA

Many alopecic conditions are hypothesized as being secondary to immunlogic events within or around the hair follicle. Such alopecias include alopecia areata, discoid lupus erythematosus, lichen planopilaris, pseudopelade, scleroderma, bullous pemphigoid, and epidermolysis bullosa.

Scleroderma (Localized)

Localized scleroderma is a self-limiting, scarring alopecia that involves the scalp and face, the coup de sabre. It is frequently associated with morphea scleroderma and localized lipodystrophy. Histologically, the dermal connective tissue is hypertrophied and shows increased eosinophilic staining. Adnexal structures are diminished, atrophic, or absent. A lymphoplasmocytic vasculitis may be present in the early stages. Dermal elastic fibers are intact but separated by the hyperplastic collagen.

EFFLUVIUM ANAGEN   CATAGEN   TELOGEN   ANAGEN

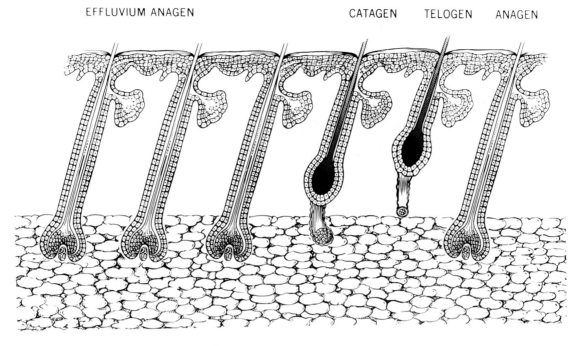

Figure 59–4. Anagen effluvium.

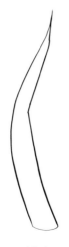

Figure 59–5. Tapered hair, or exclamatory hair.

Bullous pemphigoid and dermolytic epidermolysis bullosa, subepidermal bullous disorders, may occur in hairy areas with a clinical presentation of alopecia erosions and secondary cutaneous infection. Both disorders can produce an end-stage scarring alopecia. The diagnosis is made on light microscopy and confirmed on direct immunofluorescence. Further discussions of these disorders appear in Chapter 10.

TRICHODYSTROPHIES AND HAIR DYSPLASIAS

Trichodystrophies represent structural abnormalities of the hair shaft, which result in fragile hair (Tables 59–4, 59–5, 59–6, 59–7). Broadly classified, the trichodystrophies are divided into congenital and acquired types. The clinical presentation of both types is short, dry, lusterless, and sparse hair with associated partial or complete alopecia.

The acquired trichodystrophies are alterations of the hair shaft induced by a variety of chemical and physical factors, such as permanent waving, bleaching, extensive sunlight exposure, combing, brushing, and drying, and are are rarely associated with systemic diseases. Congenital trichodystrophies, on the other hand, are rare disorders of follicular keratinization and frequently are associated with metabolic disorders, developmental abnormalities, and mental retardation.

Monilethrix

Monilethrix is a congenital, autosomal dominant disorder with an occasional rare recessive form that is usually a generalized hair disorder. This disorder is rarely associated with mental retardation or metabolic developmental abnormalities. The fragile hair shaft has multiple nodular swellings (beaded hair) similar to a pearl necklace. The nodes represent normal hair (Fig. 59–7), whereas the internodal areas are constricted abnormal hair usually without medulla, similar to Pohl-Pinkus marks or exclamatory pointed

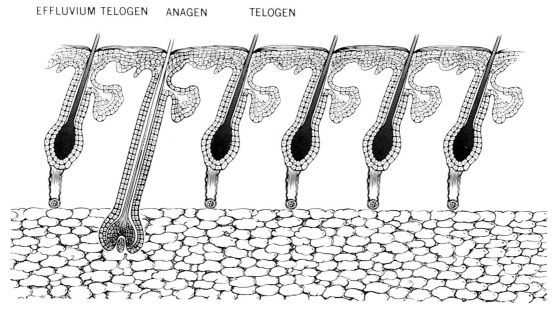

EFFLUVIUM TELOGEN   ANAGEN   TELOGEN

Figure 59–6. Telogen effluvium.

TABLE 59–4. CONGENITAL TRICHODYSTROPHIES

Fragile Hair	Fragility Absent
Monilethrix	Pili annulati
Pseudomonilethrix	Woolly hair
Trichorrhexis nodosa	Pili canaliculi
Trichorrhexis invaginata	
Pili torti	
Trichothiodystrophy	
Pili bifurcati	

hair. Fractures are noted within the internodal area. This is the reverse of pseudomonilethrix in which the nodal swellings represent the abnormal areas.

Monilethrix clinically appears as alopecia or hypotrichosis, with prominent follicular hyperkeratosis (Fig. 59–8). Histologically, abnormal hair can be noted within the dilated follicle and frequently is surrounded by chronic inflammatory infiltrate.

TABLE 59–6. TRICHODYSTROPHIES

Nodal swellings (beaded)	Decreased diameter hair
Monilethrix	Pohl-Pinkus
Pseudomonilethrix	Exclamation mark hair
Trichorrhexis nodosa	Androgenic alopecia
Trichorrhexis invaginata	Hypoplasia
Bayonet trichorrhexis nodosa	**Other**
Pohl-Pinkus marks	Pili annulati
Infestations	Pili bifurcati
Piedra	Pili canaliculi
Nits	Trichomalacia
Trichomycosis axillaris	Trichothiodystrophy
Twisted Hair	Multiple hairs
Pili torti	Pili multigemini
Corkscrew hair	Trichostosis spinulasia
Woolly hair	
Fractures	
Trichoclasis	
Trichoschisis	
Trichoptilosis	
Trichorrhexis nodosa	

TABLE 59–5. ACQUIRED TRICHODYSTROPHIES

Fragile Hair	Fractures
Trichorrhexis nodosa	Trichoptilosis
Trichomalacia	Trichoschisis
Spiral hair	Trichoclasis
Bayonet hairs	Pili bifurcati
Pohl-Pinkus mark	

Pseudomonilethrix

Pseudomonilethrix is a nodal trichodystrophy similar to monilethrix and has been shown to be an autosomal dominant disorder with late onset. It may be localized or generalized. The hair demonstrates nodal swellings, the abnormal

TABLE 59-7. SYSTEMIC DISEASES, MALFORMATION, AND TRICHODYSTROPHIES

Disease	Hair Dystrophy	Other Defects, Comments
Monilethrix	Beaded hair	Autosomal dominant, recessive forms ectodermal defects, follicular hyper-keratosis
Bjornstad's syndrome	Pili torti	Neurosensory hearing loss, mental retardation
Menkes	Pili torti	Defect in copper metabolism
Arginosuccinic aciduria	Trichorrhexis nodosa	Mental retardation
Biotin deficiency	Trichorrhexis nodosa	Biotin-responsive mental states and hair regrowth
Netherton's syndrome	Trichorrhexis invaginata	Ichthyosis, atopias
Trichothiodystrophy	Trichoschisis, banded appearance; polarized light	Sulfur-deficient hair, mental retardation, Pollitts syndrome, BIDS syndrome: ichthyosis IBIDS syndrome: short stature ichthyosis PIBIDS syndrome: photosensitivity

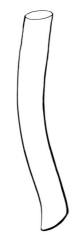

Figure 59-7. Normal hair.

areas, with normal internodal zones. Transverse fractures occur within the abnormal nodal swelling. This is the reverse finding of monilethrix.

Trichorrhexis Nodosa

Trichorrhexis nodosa (Fig. 59–9) is the most common tricho-dystrophy and can be congenital or acquired. The hair shaft has multiple nodal swellings that develop transverse fractures, leaving brushlike ends.

Congenital trichorrhexis nodosa is a generalized tricho-dystrophy and is rarely localized. Nodal swellings can be seen anywhere in the hair at which sites fractures occur. This results in hypotrichosis or alopecia.

Acquired trichorrhexis nodosa can be divided into two

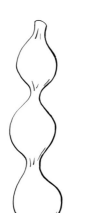

Figure 59-8. Monilethrix.

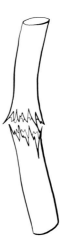

Figure 59-9. Trichorrhexis nodosa.

categories: trichorrhexis nodosa associated with other trichodystrophies and metabolic disorders, and trichorrhexis nodosa resulting from chemical and physical damage to the hair. Three types of traumatic TN are described: proximal nodal swellings found in the black race, distal nodes found in the white race, and localized nodes on nonscalp hairy areas probably secondary to physical trauma. Differential diagnosis includes the other nodal trichodystrophies and pediculosis, dandruff, and hair casts.

Trichorrhexis Invaginatum (Bamboo Hair)

Trichorrhexis invaginatum (Fig. 59–10) is a rare trichodystrophy that was first described by Netherton as an autosomal recessive disease most frequently found in females and associated with ichthyosis and atopy. This hair disorder occurs as a nodal swelling in which there is invagination of the distal hair into the proximal end, a ball and glove configuration. Transverse fractures occur within the node, resulting in short hair. This is usually a generalized hair disorder that may resolve at puberty.

Trichonodosis

Trichonodosis (Fig. 59–11) is seen in people with long, curly hair in which distal portions of the hair shaft develop knots that appear as nodal swellings. These knots fracture with normal hair care.

Pohl-Pinkus Marks

Pohl-Pinkus marks (Fig. 59–12) represent an acquired trichodystrophy and occur as hair shaft constrictions or narrowing. These changes are described as secondary to systemic disease, to antimitotic drugs, and to emotional stress. These constrictions are similar to that seen in the nail, Beaus'

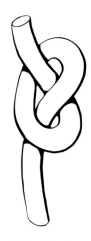

Figure 59–11. Trichonodosis.

lines, and are similar to the constricted, tapered end seen in the exclamatory pointed hair of alopecia areata.

Bayonet Hair

Bayonet hair is an acquired, pigmented nodal swelling of the hair shaft that may demonstrate some fragility and fracture with trauma. The significance of this defect is unknown.

Exclamatory Point Hair

The exclamatory point hair shaft is observed in acute alopecia areata and is the result of a tapered or abrupt narrowing or constriction of the hair, probably secondary to an insult on the dermal papillae. This tapered area is easily fractured or separated. If the entire hair is intact, a normal diameter of the hair is noted a short distance from the taper on both the proximal and distal ends.

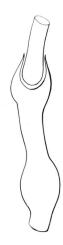

Figure 59–10. Trichorrhexis invaginata.

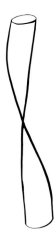

Figure 59–12. Pohl-Pinkus marks, or tapered hair.

Pili Torti

Pili torti (Fig. 59–13) is the second most common trichodystrophy and may occur as a congenital, familial, or sporadic and possibly acquired disorder. The characteristic of this trichodystrophy is a twisted (tort) hair that may be 90°, 180°, or even 360° and can be seen with regular versus irregular frequency. Fractures occur at the site of the tort. This disorder is common in light-haired females. Acquired pili torti has been reported as a result of inflammation and retinoid therapy. In addition, pili torti has been associated with other trichodystrophies, such as trichorrhexis nodosa, pili canaliculi, hypohidrotic ectodermal dysplasia, monilethrix, and Menkes' syndrome.

Menkes' Syndrome (Kinky Hair)

Menkes' syndrome is a recessive, sex-linked defect of copper metabolism that results in kinky hair and progressive neurologic degeneration, bony and vascular abnormalities, and early death. The kinky hair is light in color, with multiple trichodystrophies described as trichorrhexis nodosa and pseudopili torti.

Woolly Hair

Woolly hair (Fig. 59–14) is a light-colored, thin, tangled, and curly hair shaft that is the result of its oval diameter. It is the common hair of the black race and can be observed as a hereditary or a familial disorder. It has been described as an autosomal recessive disorder. This unusual curled, oval hair shaft is seen associated with trichorrhexis nodosa and pili torti.

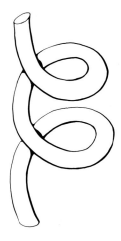

Figure 59–14. Woolly Hair, Menkes' syndrome.

Fractures

Trichoptilosis
Trichoptilosis (Fig. 59–15) is a distal longitudinal fracture of the hair, known as split ends, and is seen in long-haired people.

Trichoschisis
Trichoschisis (Fig. 59–16) represents a transverse fracture of hair and is seen frequently with monilethrix and trichothiodystrophy.

Trichoclasis

Trichoclasis is an oblique or transverse fracture with irregular borders and can be seen in a variety of trichodystrophies.

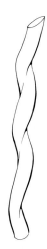

Figure 59–13. Pili torti.

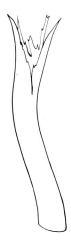

Figure 59–15. Trichoptilosis.

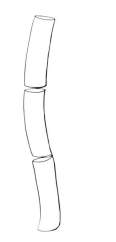

Figure 59–16. Trichoschisis.

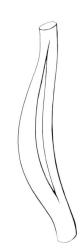

Figure 59–18. Pili bifurcate.

Pili Annulati

Pili annulati (Fig. 59–17) is a trichodystrophy that does not induce increased fragility of the hair shaft. It is an autosomal dominant with variable penetrance and is seen only sporadically. Examination of the hair shaft demonstrates light hair with normal diameter. On polarized light, it demonstrates light and dark bands, that is, ringed hair. The dark bands are the result of air bubbles in the cuticle and cortex. The reflected light gives these bands unusual highlights. Fragility is not evident, however. Trichorrhexis nodosa and fractures of the dark bands have been noted.

Pseudopili annulati has been reported as a result of sun damage in light-haired individuals and represents pseudopili torti, or twisted hair, which results in alternating highlights.

Pili Bifurcati

Pili bifurcati (Fig. 59–18) is a trichodystrophy and represents a longitudinal bifurcation of the hair at regular intervals, with each bifurcation being fully encased in its own cuticle. This appears to be primarily an isolated congenital defect, but acquired forms are suspected. The structural defect of the bifurcation produces increased fragility of the hair. This hair disorder may be localized and is associated with trichotillomania, pseudopelade, and pili torti.

Pili Canaliculi

Pili canaliculi, or triangle hair (Fig. 59–19), is a grooved hair that on transverse section demonstrates a triangular

Figure 59–17. Pili annulati.

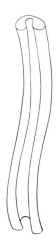

Figure 59–19. Pili canaliculi, or grooved hair.

shape. It has been called spun-glass hair or uncombable hair because of its clinical presentation. Unusual highlights and the inability of the hair to align itself gives an uncombed appearance. The triangular hair shaft can be seen in tissue if the hair shafts are inadvertently sectioned transversely. Pili canaliculi has been associated with many of the other trichodystrophies.

Trichothiodystrophy

Another congenital, generalized trichodystrophy that results in fragile hair with multiple fractures is trichothiodystrophy. The hair shaft diameter varies, and there is obvious longitudinal grooving, scarce cuticle coverage, and small nodal swellings that may undergo transverse fractures. Polarized light reveals clear and dark zones and a braided appearance and is the result of diminished sulfur and sulfuric amino acids, that is, cysteine, within the hair. Trichothiodystrophy is associated with other congenital abnormalities, such as ichthyosis, nail dystrophies, mental retardation, ocular and dental abnormalities, and reduced fertility.

Trichomalacia

Trichomalacia is an acquired softening of the hair shaft within the follicle and is observed as fragmented shaft or a pigmented amorphous material within the ectatic follicle. This softening of the hair is primarily seen in trichotillomania and alopecia areata.

PILOSEBACEOUS HAMARTOMAS

Trichostasis Spinulosis

Trichostasis spinulosis is an acquired follicular keratinizing defect that appears as a comedone containing multiple vellus hair. This disorder occurs as a dilated pore, with tufted, white hair usually present in the elderly on the forehead, nose, and cheek. Trichostasis spinulosis also has been observed within seborrheic keratosis, keratosis pilaris, and eruptive hair cysts.

Pili Multigemini

Pili multigemini is a rare follicular hamartoma in which one follicular dermal papilla separates into several buds, which produce multiple (6 to 8) hairs. On cross section, multiple hairs are bound by the external root sheath and display unusual shapes; triangular, stellate, oval, and grooved. This disorder is frequently seen on the face and would appear similar to trichostasis spinulosis.

BIBLIOGRAPHY

Alopecias

Abell E. Pathology male-pattern alopecia. *Arch Dermatol.* 1984;120:1607–1608.

Abell E. Immunofluorescent staining techniques in the diagnosis of alopecia. *South Med J.* 1977;90:1407–1410.

Bergfeld WF. Alopecia: histologic changes. *Adv Dermatol.* 1989;4:301–321.

Bergfeld WF. Hair disorders. In: Rakel RE, ed, *Conn's Current Therapy.* Philadelphia: WB Saunders Co; 1987:625–628.

Ioannides G. Alopecia: a pathologist's view. *Int J Dermatol.* 1982;21:23.

Kligman AM. Pathologic dynamics of human hair loss. I: telogen effluvium. *Arch Dermatol.* 1961;83:175.

LaChapelle JM, Pierard SE. Traumatic alopecia in trichotillomania: a pathogenic interpretation of histologic lesions in the pilosebaceous unit. *J Cutan Pathol.* 1977;4:51.

Lattanand A, Johnson WC. Male pattern alopecia. A histopathologic and histochemical study. *J Cutan Pathol.* 1975;2:58.

Lever WF, Schaumburg-Lever G. *Connective Tissue Disease, Histopathology of the Skin.* 6th ed. Philadelphia: JB Lippincott Co; 1983:445–471.

Maguire HC, Kligman AM. Common baldness in women. *Geriatrics.* 1963;8:329.

Mehregan AH. Histopathology of alopecias. *Cutis.* 1978;21:249–253.

Mehregan AH. Trichotillomania: a clinicopathologic study. *Arch Dermatol.* 1970;102:129.

Messenger AG, Slater DN, Bueden SS. Alopecia areata: alterations in the growth cycle and correlation with follicular pathology. *Br J Dermatol.* 1986;114:337–347.

Muller SA, Winklemann RK. Trichotillomania: a clinicopathologic study of 24 cases. *Arch Dermatol.* 1972;105:535.

Orfanos CE, ed. *Haar und Haar Krankheiten.* Stuttgart, New York: Gustav Fischer; 1979.

Pinkus H. Differential patterns of elastic fibers in scarring and nonscarring alopecia. *J Cutan Pathol.* 1978;5:93.

Trichodystrophies

Camacho-Martinez F, Ferrando J. Hair shaft dysplasias. *Int J Dermatol.* 1988;27:71–80.

Dupre A, Bonafe JL. *Les Dysplasies Pilaires.* Paris: Laboratoires Lutsia; 1979.

Ferrando J, Fontarnau R, Gratacos MR, et al. Pli canaliculi ("cheveux incoiffables" ou "cheveux en fibre de verre"). Dix-nouveaux cas avec etude au microscope electronique a balayage. *Ann Dermatol Venereol (Paris).* 1980;107:243–248.

Greene SL, Muller SA. Netherton's syndrome: report of a case and review of the literature. *J Am Acad Dermatol.* 1985;13:329–337.

Hays SB, Camisa C. Acquired pili torti in two patients treated with synthetic retinoids. *Cutis.* 1985;35:466–468.

Hutchison PE, Cairns RJ, Wells RS. Woolly hair: clinical and general aspects. *Trans St John's Hosp Dermatol Soc.* 1974;60:160–177.

Jordan RE. Subtle clues to diagnosis by immunopathology—scarring alopecia. *Am J Dermatopathol.* 1980;2:157–159.

Leonard JM, Gummer CL, Dawber RPR. Generalized trichorrhexis nodosa. *Br J Dermatol.* 1980;103:85–90.

Mehregan AH, Thompson WS. Pili multigemini: report of a case in association with cleidocranial dysostosis. *Br J Dermatol.* 1979;100:315–322.

Mortimer PS. Unruly hair. *Br J Dermatol.* 1985;113:467–473.

Mortimer PS, Gummer CL, English J, et al. Acquired progressive kinking of hair: report of six cases and review of literature. *Arch Dermatol.* 1985;121:1031–1033.

Price VH, Odom RB, Ward WH, et al. Trichothiodystrophy: sulfur-deficient brittle hair as a marker for a neuroectodermal symptom complex. *Arch Dermatol.* 1980;116:1375–1384.

Ricci MA, Tunnessen WW, Pergolizzi JM, et al. Menkes' kinky hair syndrome. *Cutis.* 1982;30:55–70.

Rodrigues-Pichardo A, Moreno JC, Ferrando J, et al. Woolly hair. A proposito de cinco observaciones. *Med Cutan Ibero Lat Am.* 1983;11:393–398.

Rook A, Dawber R. Defects of the hair shaft. In: Rook A, Dawber R, eds. *Diseases of the Hair and Scalp.* Oxford: Blackwell Scientific; 1982:179.

Schoenfeld RJ, Lupulescu AP. Crimped "spun glass" hair in siblings with twelve year follow-up of an earlier case. In: Orfanos CE, Montagna W, Stuttgen G, eds. *Hair Research: Status and Future Aspects.* Berlin: Springer-Verlag; 1981:424–429.

Stroud JD. Hair shaft anomalies. Hair disorders. *Dermatol Clin.* 1987;5:581–594.

Weary PE, Hendricks AA, Warner F, et al. Pili bifurcati: new anomaly of hair growth. *Arch Dermatol.* 1973;108:403–407.

Young MD, Jorizzo JL, Sanchez RC, et al. Trichostasis spinulosa. *Int J Dermatol.* 1988;24:575–580.

CHAPTER 60
Inflammatory Reactions of the Nail

Ruth Hanno

Inflammatory reactions of the nail unit are not, in many instances, precisely defined histologically. This may be due in part to a lack of experience in reading these biopsies, resulting from clinicians' reluctance to approach the nail unit surgically, patients' reluctance to have their nails biopsied, and technical problems with properly embedding and cutting the fibrous nail tissue. In addition, the difficulty in histologic diagnosis of nail biopsies may result because the nail unit may frequently respond to a specific insult with a nonspecific eczematous response. In a study of 20 patients with acquired inflammatory nail dystrophies, excluding fungal infection, we were able to make a specific diagnosis in only 8 specimens, the remainder showing eczematous changes that could not be further subclassified.

Despite these problems, the histopathology of inflammatory nail disorders has in certain entities been quite thoroughly documented, in large part owing to the original work of Zaias in the 1960s,[2,3] continued by others more recently.[4,5]

TYPE OF BIOPSY

The type of nail biopsy required depends on the clinical situation.[6] In general, an inflammatory process of unknown etiology is best sampled with a longitudinal nail biopsy, a technique first described by Zaias in 1967.[7] In this procedure (Fig. 60–1), an incision is made from the proximal nail fold to the hyponychium to the depth of the underlying bone. A parallel incision is made 2 to 3 mm from the initial incision, and the longitudinal sample of tissue outlined by this is disected off. The incisions can be made either along the lateral edge of the nail plate, which minimizes subsequent cosmetic defect, or in a central area, which may be necessary to encompass the pathologic portion of the nail. The nail plate can be removed before the biopsy, which makes processing of the specimen simpler. However, disruption of the underlying tissue may result from traumatic nail avulsion. No sutures may be used,[7] or the proximal portion of the incision may be sutured and the rest left to heal

secondarily.[1] If the specimen is properly embedded on edge, this technique allows for pathologic examination of the entire nail unit (Fig. 60–2).

In specific situations, a more limited biopsy may be adequate. In examination of a nail unit for candidal paronychia or other paronychial process, a simple shave biopsy of proximal or lateral nail fold may suffice. Shave biopsy of proximal nail fold has been advocated also in evaluation of collagen vascular disease.[8,9] To diagnose a dermatophyte infection, a shave or punch biopsy of nailbed or deep nail plate may be useful. Punch biopsy of matrix has been advocated as an alternative to longitudinal nail biopsy in nonspecific inflammatory nail disease.[10]

If the nail plate is left on during the biopsy process, it must be softened before cutting by fixation in 5% trichloracetic acid and 10% formalin or by placement in distilled water before formalin fixation.[11]

HISTOLOGIC FEATURES OF THE NORMAL NAIL UNIT

The nail unit is made up of the proximal nail fold, matrix, bed, and hyponychium.[12] Each area has a characteristic morphology, which is altered in inflammatory disease.

The normal proximal nail fold is considered an extension of the skin from the dorsal surface of the fingers and toes. It keratinizes with a granular layer, as does the skin with which it is contiguous, but Zaias points out that it differs from dorsal skin in that it is thinner and devoid of hair follicles.[12] The cuticle is the horny layer of the proximal nail fold, which adheres to the surface of the nail plate, protecting the delicate matrix area from contamination by external irritants.

The nail matrix is contiguous with the ventral proximal nail fold and differs from it morphologically. The matrix is made up of basaloid cells with their orientation directed diagonally and distally.[12] These cells mature with flattening of their nuclei and increasing eosinophilia. As they mature

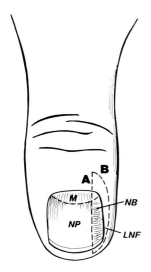

Figure 60–1. Technique of the longitudinal nail biopsy. Dotted lines A and B represent the first and second longitudinal incisions, respectively. NP = nail plate; LNF = lateral nail fold; M = matrix; NB = nailbed.

into the nail plate, nuclear fragments normally are lost. Thus, nail matrix matures without keratohyaline granules. The proximal portion of the matrix forms the superficial portion of the nail plate, and the distal matrix forms the deep nail plate.[12]

Distally, the matrix is contiguous with the proximal portion of the nailbed. The nailbed is characterized by deep epidermal rete ridges, which are aligned longitudinally and parallel. The nailbed epithelium is firmly attached to the overlying nail plate. Nailbed epithelium normally has a scanty horny layer and matures without a granular layer on light microscopy. The thin parakeratotic keratin produced by the nailbed is dragged forward by the overlying nail plate. In pathologic states, such as inflammatory dystrophies and after nail plate avulsion, the nailbed keratinizes with a granular layer, and its horny layer can become quite thick.

The hyponychium is a small piece of skin underlying the free portion of the nail plate. It extends from the distal nailbed to the distal groove of the fingertip, which marks the area where the normal plantar and volar epidermis with its prominent skin markings resumes. The hyponychium is usually only visible grossly in nail biters and those with closely clipped nails. It keratinizes like the contiguous skin with a distinct granular layer. It is important

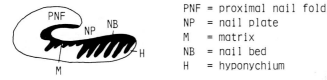

PNF = proximal nail fold
NP = nail plate
M   = matrix
NB = nail bed
H   = hyponychium

Figure 60–2. Diagram of the nail unit as seen on properly embedded longitudinal biopsy specimen.

pathologically because of its early involvement in dermatophyte infections of the nail unit.

PSORIASIS

Zaias has carefully documented the histologic correlates of the various clinical manifestations of psoriasis of the nail unit[3,12] (Table 60–1). Pitting, the most common manifestation of psoriasis on the nails, apparently results from psoriatic foci in the nail matrix. Specifically, psoriatic foci in the proximal matrix produce abnormal parakeratotic keratin in the superficial plate, which sloughs as the nail plate moves forward, resulting in pits. Psoriatic foci in more distal matrix, which forms the deep nail plate, result in deep defects, which clinically appear as white spots or leukonychia. Psoriatic involvement of the entire matrix produces the crumbling of the nail plate seen in severe psoriatic disease. Onycholysis, so-called oil spots under the nail plate, and subungual hyperkeratosis are due to psoriatic foci in the nailbed and hyponychium.

In a nail biopsy of a patient being evaluated for psoriasis, it is useful to be able to visualize both matrix and bed.[13] Histologic parameters to be documented to confirm a diagnosis of nail unit psoriasis include a focal parakeratosis of the keratin layer of the matrix and nailbed accompanied by neutrophilic fragments, equivalent to Munro microabsesses of the skin (Fig. 60–3). Accumulation of PAS-positive glycoprotein in the horny layer is also a helpful feature and is more common in nail psoriasis than in that of the glaborous skin[11] (Figs. 60–4, 60–5). The other features of psoriasis, such as hyperplasia of the epithelium and proliferation of upper dermal vessels, also are seen but are accompanied by more spongiotic changes than are seen in classic skin psoriasis.[11] Extreme care must be taken to rule out fungal infections in patients with nail changes suggestive of psoriasis, since clinically and histologically, in the absence of special stains, the changes can be identical.[4]

LICHEN PLANUS

Lichen planus can be a devastating nail disease, since permanent anonychia can result.[14,15] Since nail disease may occur in the absence of skin disease and since early aggressive therapy with corticosteroids can be beneficial, it is a disease in which nail biopsy can be extremely worthwhile.

TABLE 60–1. HISTOLOGIC CORRELATES OF PSORIATIC NAILS

Clinical Finding	Histologic Features
Pits	Psoriasis of proximal matrix
"Oil spots"	Psoriasis of distal matrix
Crumbling	Psoriasis of entire matrix
Onycholysis	Nailbed/hyponychial psoriasis
Subungual hyperkeratosis	Nailbed psoriasis

From refs. 3, 12.

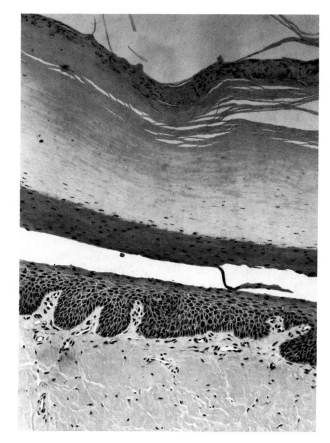

Figure 60–3. Psoriatic focus in the nail matrix showing deep and superficial areas of parakeratosis of adherent nail plate fragments with intervening orthokeratosis. Note neutrophilic debris in superficial parakeratotic nail fragments. (H&E, ×100.)

As with psoriasis, Zaias was the first to correlate the histopathologic changes in lichen planus with the clinical findings[14] (Table 60–2). Thinning and longitudinal ridges of the nail plate result from lichen planus lesions of the matrix. Severe matrix involvement results in complete disappearance of the nail plate, with subsequent adhesion of the proximal nail fold to the exposed nailbed, so-called pterygium formation. Nailbed lichen planus results in subungual keratoses and onycholysis.

On biopsy, lichen planus of the nails is similar histologically to that seen on glaborous skin. A dense lichenoid lymphocytic infiltrate can be seen directly abutting all areas of the nail unit apparatus (Fig. 60–6). Other histologic features, as in skin lichen planus, consist of thick orthokeratotic keratin, hypergranulosis of the matrix and bed epithelium, increased eosinophilia of keratinocytes, and sawtooth acanthosis of nailbed epithelium (Figs. 60–7, 60–8).

Twenty nail dystrophy of childhood has had conflicting pictures on biopsy. Some investigators have documented changes of lichen planus histologically,[16] suggesting that this is a severe form of lichen planus confined to the nail unit. Others have documented nonspecific eczematous changes histologically.[17]

DARIER'S DISEASE

In 1973, Zaias and Ackerman[18] carefully documented the nail unit changes in Darier's disease. Since then, little work has been done on the histopathology of the distinctive nail changes in this disease, perhaps because skin changes usually are concomitant, and nail biopsy is not needed diagnostically. Specific histopathology of Darier's disease of the glabrous skin (suprabasilar acantholysis) was seen by Zaias

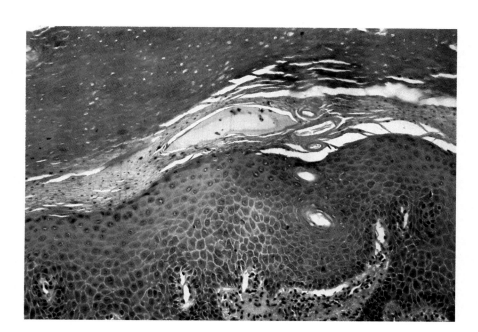

Figure 60–4. Psoriasis of the nailbed showing dilated subepithelial blood vessels, parakeratosis, and serumlike proteinaceous-exudate within the horny layers, with neutrophilic fragments. (H&E, ×250.)

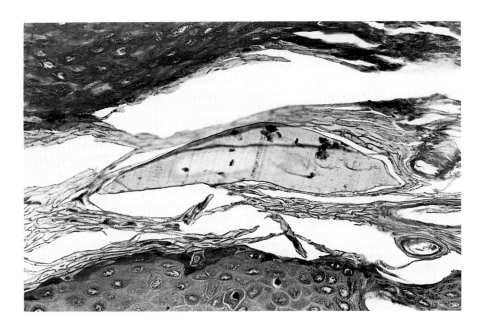

Figure 60–5. High power of neutrophilic debris trapped in serumlike exudate of Figure 60–4. (H&E, ×400.)

TABLE 60–2. HISTOLOGIC CORRELATES OF CLINICAL FINDINGS IN LICHEN PLANUS

Clinical Finding	Histologic Feature
Thinning of plate	Matrix lichen planus, partial
Longitudinal ridging	Matrix lichen planus, partial
Anonychia with pterygium	Severe matrical involvement
Onycholysis	Nailbed/hyponychial lichen planus
Subungual papules	Nailbed lichen planus

From ref. 14.

and Ackerman only in the proximal nail fold. They found that the longitudinal red keratoses of Darier nails were due to epithelial hyperplasia in the nailbed and that the white longitudinal streaks, which they considered later lesions, were due to epithelial hyperplasia accompanied by multinucleate giant cells and nuclear atypia of nailbed epithelium. In a single case of Darier's nail, Hanno et al. failed to observe the multinucleate giant cells reported by Zaias and Ackerman but did confirm the finding of epithelial hyperplasia of the nailbed, with hyperchromatism and mild atypia of occasional nailbed keratinocytes[1] (Fig. 60–9).

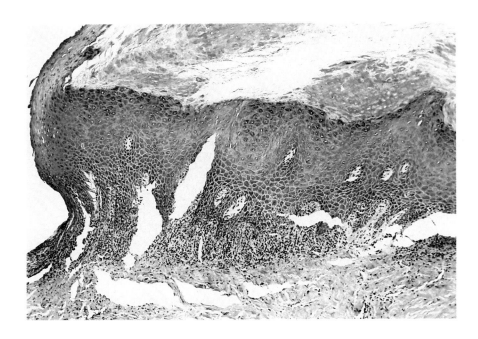

Figure 60–6. Lichen planus of the nail showing orthokeratotic hyperkeratosis, hypergranulosis, and lichenoid infiltrate abutting the nailbed epithelium. (H&E, ×65.)

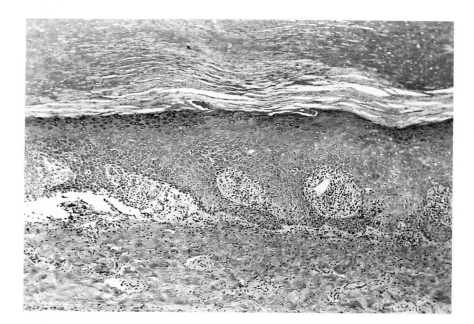

Figure 60–7. Lichen planus of the nail showing sawtooth pattern of nailbed epithelium and subepidermal lichenoid infiltrate. (H&E, ×65.)

FUNGAL INFECTIONS

Nail biopsy, either longitudinal or punch or shave biopsy of nailbed, hyponychium, or deep nail plate, is extremely important in the diagnosis of distal subungual onychomycosis, the most common type of dermatophyte infection of the nail unit.[12] Scher and Ackerman demonstrated fungal elements in nailbed biopsy of patients with repeatedly negative KOH and cultures.[4] Fungal hyphae usually are found in the cornified cells of the thickened nailbed and in the lower portion of the nail plate (Fig. 60–10). Simple scrapings for KOH and culture may sample a too superficial portion of the nail plate for consistently accurate diagnosis. The less common proximal subungual onychomycosis and su-

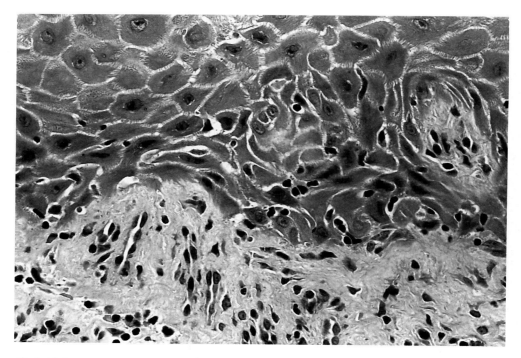

Figure 60–8. High power of basal layer of nailbed in lichen planus, showing degeneration of basal cells and infiltration by lymphocytes (H&E, ×400.)

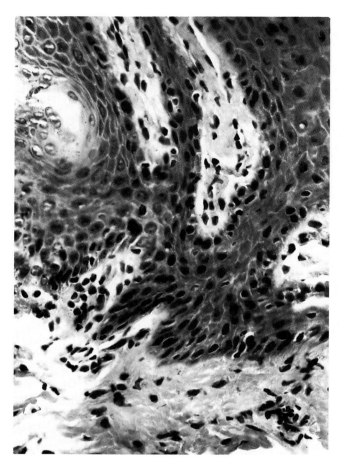

Figure 60–9. Nailbed in Darier's disease showing hyperplasia, hyperchromatism, and mild atypia of keratinocytes. (H&E, ×250.)

perficial white onychomycosis can be diagnosed by examination of the nail plate as it emerges from the proximal nail fold and from the superficial nail plate scrapings, respectively. Candidal infection most commonly involves the paronychial area, and a shave specimen from the nail fold may be diagnostic. True candidal invasion of the nail plate, as seen in mucocutaneous candidiasis, is diagnosed easily by biopsy of almost any portion of the nail unit, which usually manifests massive mycologic involvement, accompanied by a florid inflammatory, pustular reaction.

Biopsy diagnosis of bacterial nail infections is usually not performed, since culture is so much more effective. Scabies[19] and herpetic infections occasionally can be diagnosed by biopsy examination of the paronychial or subungual skin.

MISCELLANEOUS ACQUIRED INFLAMMATORY DYSTROPHIES

Not infrequently, patients have acquired nail dystrophies of unknown origin unaccompanied by skin changes. In our series, 12 of 20 cases of acquired inflammatory nail disease that underwent longitudinal biopsy showed only nonspecific eczematous changes, including hyperkeratosis with parakeratosis of nailbed epithelium, acanthosis and spongiosis, dermal fibrosis, and a nonspecific inflammatory dermal lymphoid infiltrate of the nailbed with exocytosis into the epidermis[1] (Fig. 60–11). It is unclear what these cases represent. They may demonstrate an end-stage of a specific disease that could have been detected earlier in the course, a posttraumatic dystrophy, eczema in the absence of the usual clinical picture, or a fungal infection despite negative culture and stains. It is realistic to recognize

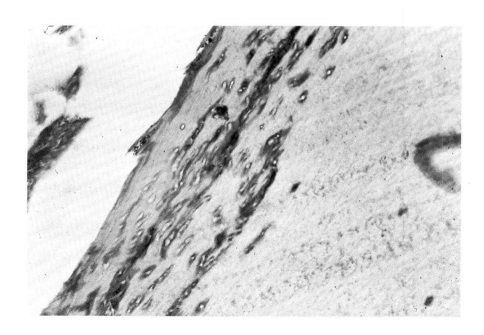

Figure 60–10. Fungal hyphae in deep portion of nail plate. (PAS, ×400.)

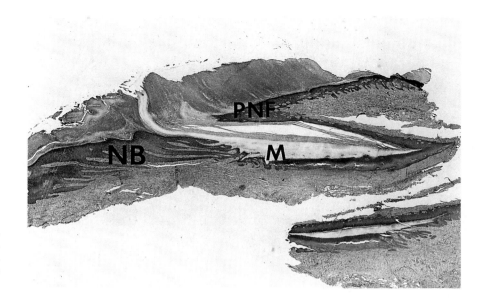

Figure 60–11. Nail unit biopsy showing non-specific eczematous changes. Note prominent subepithelial fibrosis and hyperkeratosis. NB = nailbed; M = matrix; PNF = proximal nail fold. (H&E, ×15.)

that not all inflammatory nail disorders will fit into a previously documented diagnostic pattern, such as psoriasis, lichen planus, or infection, and that a specific histologic diagnosis of inflammatory disease is even less likely when a single nail only is clinically involved.[1] However, it is important to biopsy a single nail dystrophy unresponsive to therapy, since Bowen's disease or malignant melanoma may masquerade as chronic nail inflammation until biopsy is undertaken.[20,21]

REFERENCES

1. Hanno R, Mathes BM, Krull EA. Longitudinal nail biopsy in the evaluation of acquired nail dystrophies. *J Am Acad Dermatol.* 1986;14:803–809.
2. Zaias N, Alvarez J. The formation of the primate nail plate. An autoradiographic study in squirrel monkeys. *J Invest Dermatol.* 1968; 51:120–136.
3. Zaias N. Psoriasis of the nail. *Arch Dermatol.* 1969;99:567–579.
4. Scher RK, Ackerman AB. The value of nail biopsy for demonstrating fungi not demonstrable by microbiologic techniques. *Am J Dermatopathol.* 1980;2:55–56.
5. Kouskoukis CE, Scher RK, Ackerman AB. The problem of features of lichen simplex chronicus complicating the histology of diseases of the nail. *Am J Dermatopathol.* 1984;6:45–49.
6. Baran R, Sayag J. Nail biopsy—why, when, where, how? *J Dermatol Surg.* 1976;2:322–326.
7. Zaias N. The longitudinal nail biopsy. *J Invest Dermatol.* 1967;49:406–408.
8. Schnitzler L, Baran R, Civatte J, et al. Biopsy of the proximal nail fold in collagen disease. *J Dermatol Surg.* 1976;2:313–315.
9. Thompson RP, Harper FE, Maize JC, et al. Nailfold biopsy in scleroderma and related disorders. *Arthritis Rheum* 1984;27:97–103.
10. Scher R. Biopsy of the matrix of a nail. *J Dermatol Surg Oncol.* 1980;6:19–21.
11. Omura EF. Histopathology of the nail. *Dermatol Clin.* 1985;3:531–541.
12. Zaias N. *The Nail in Health and Disease.* New York: Spectrum; 1980.
13. Lewin K, Dewit S, Ferrington RA. Pathology of the fingernail in psoriasis. *Br J Dermatol.* 1972;86:555–563.
14. Zaias N. The nail in lichen planus. *Arch Dermatol.* 1970;101:264–271.
15. Scott MJ Jr, Scott MJ Sr. Ungual lichen planus. *Arch Dermatol.* 1979;115:1197–1198.
16. Scher RK, Fischbein R, Ackerman AB. Twenty nail dystrophy: a variant of lichen planus. *Arch Dermatol.* 1978;114:612–613.
17. Wilkinson JD, Dawber RPR, Bowers RP, et al. Twenty nail dystrophy of childhood. *Br J Dermatol.* 1979;100:217–221.
18. Zaias N, Ackerman AB. The nail in Darier-White disease. *Arch Dermatol.* 1973;107:193–199.
19. Scher RK. Subungual scabies. *Am J Dermatopathol.* 1983;5:187–189.
20. Patterson RH, Helwig EB. Subungual malignant melanoma. *Cancer.* 1980;46:2074–2087.
21. Mikhail GR. Bowen's disease and squamous cell carcinoma of the nail bed. *Arch Dermatol.* 1974;110:267–270.

CHAPTER 61
Inflammatory Reactions of the Sweat Unit

James E. Fitzpatrick

The apocrine and eccrine sweat gland units are infrequently the primary targets of inflammation. The apocrine gland is actually a part of the pilosebaceous apparatus, since it typically empties into the infundibular portion of the hair follicle above the entrance of the sebaceous duct. Thus, inflammatory changes of the apocrine duct and glands are inevitably associated with concomitant pathologic alterations of the hair follicle because of this close anatomic relationship. Fox-Fordyce disease and hidradenitis suppurativa, which are presented as examples of inflammatory reactions of the apocrine sweat unit, both demonstrate changes of the pilosebaceous apparatus. In contrast, eccrine glands are atrichial, and histologic changes may occur in the absence of follicular disease. Disorders of the eccrine sweat gland unit to be discussed include miliaria, drug-induced changes, pressure-induced changes, and infectious diseases.

FOX-FORDYCE DISEASE (APOCRINE MILIARIA)

In 1902, Fox and Fordyce described this pruritic papular eruption of the axillae that now bears their names.[1] This chronic disorder typically develops in postpubertal women, although prepubescent girls and males also have been reported with the disease.[2] This disease characteristically involves the axillae but may also involve other apocrine-bearing areas, such as the pubic area, areolae, and umbilicus. Studies by Shelley and Levy have demonstrated localized apocrine anhidrosis secondary to occlusion of the apocrine duct.[3] The pathogenesis of this obstruction is not understood, but therapeutic responses to both estrogen and testosterone have incriminated hormonal factors.

Histologic Features
Histologic examination of a typical lesion reveals follicular hyperkeratosis of the infundibulum, with keratinous obstruction of the terminal intraepidermal apocrine duct. Epithelium proximal to the obstruction demonstrates lympho-

cytic spongiosis with occasional microvesicle formation.[3] Rare sections may demonstrate actual rupture of the duct contiguous with the areas of spongiosis.[4] The dermal apocrine duct and glands usually are not involved, although occasional mild inflammation and cystic dilatation may be noted. Dermal changes are not specific and consist of mild chronic inflammation and occasional fibrosis. In the typical case, not all of these changes are seen in a single section, and multiple levels are needed. The histologic differential diagnosis includes other causes of spongiotic folliculitis, including disseminate and recurrent infundibulofolliculitis, follicular atopic dermatitis, and keratosis pilaris. However, the presence of follicular hyperkeratosis associated with lymphocytic spongiosis of the apocrine duct is characteristic, and a definitive diagnosis can be made.

HIDRADENITIS SUPPURATIVA

Hidradenitis suppurativa is a chronic, suppurative, inflammatory disorder first described by Verneuil in 1854, but it was not reported in the English literature until 1933.[5] Brunsting emphasized the association of this condition with acne conglobata and dissecting cellulitis of the scalp and noted that there were many similarities.[6] The lesions typically appear after puberty in the axillae, inguinal regions, and perianal area, although other sites with apocrine glands may be involved. Early lesions are tender, deep-seated erythematous nodules, with late lesions consisting of abscesses, fistulas, sinus tracts, and scars. The pathogenesis is unknown, but experimental studies suggest that hormonally induced follicular occlusion of the pilosebaceous apparatus results in secondary bacterial infection of the apocrine gland.[7]

Histologic Features
Histologic examination of early, experimentally produced lesions reveals plugging of the follicular infundibulum associated with keratin plugs of the intraepidermal apocrine duct. The proximal duct and gland are dilated and filled

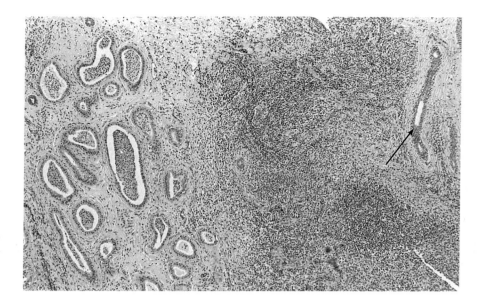

Figure 61–1. Hidradenitis suppurativa. Diagnostic features shown are a dermal abscess associated with intraglandular abscess of apocrine glands. Note the involved apocrine duct on the far right (arrow). (H&E, ×40.) (*Courtesy of L. Golitz.*)

with neutrophils.[7] Secondary changes that are present in developed lesions include both acute and chronic folliculitis and apocrine adenitis associated with dermal abscesses, foreign body reaction, granulation tissue, and fibrosis. Destruction of hair follicles and apocrine gland necrosis frequently are observed (Figs. 61–1, 61–2). Sinus formation and transepidermal elimination of elastic fibers also may be seen, but these are believed to be nonspecific secondary changes.[8] The differential diagnosis includes acne conglobata, dissecting cellulitis of the scalp, furuncles, and carbuncles. In earlier lesions, the presence of follicular hyperkeratosis associated with neutrophilic abscesses in the dermis and apocrine glands is sufficient to make a diagnosis. Late lesions reveal less specific changes, such as destruction of adnexal structures, foreign body reaction, granulation tissue, fibrosis, and sinus formation.

MILIARIA

Eccrine miliaria (prickly heat) is seen in four different clinical forms depending on the location of the ductal blockage and the type of infiltrate. An intracorneal poral blockage produces miliaria crystallina, an intraepidermal ductal blockage produces miliaria rubra, and an intradermal blockage produces miliaria profunda. If the infiltrate is predominantly neutrophils, the clinical result is miliaria pustulosa.[9] Experimental studies have attributed the blockage to an overgrowth of resident micrococci that presumptively produce a toxin capable of damaging the luminal lining cells.[10] However, other studies have shown that a variety of techniques designed to produce superficial injuries also may produce similar lesions.[11–13]

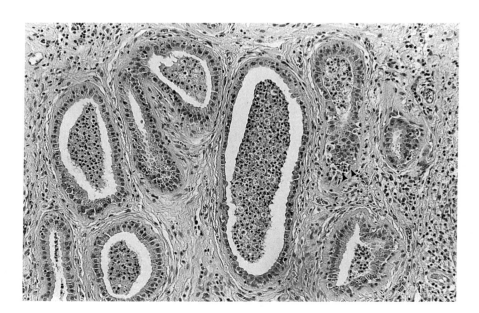

Figure 61–2. In this higher magnification, there is mild dilatation of the apocrine glands associated with neutrophils within the lumen. Note the neutrophils within the wall of the gland associated with early necrosis (arrowheads). (H&E, ×100.) (*Courtesy of L. Golitz.*)

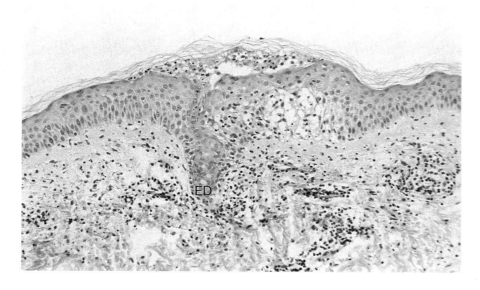

Figure 61–3. Miliaria rubra. Typical lymphocytic spongiosis associated with the acrosyringium. In this biopsy specimen, there is also a subcorneal vesicle with an infiltrate of neutrophils and lymphocytes that is contiguous with the ductal lumen (ED). (H&E, ×100.) (*Courtesy of J. Aeling.*)

Histologic Features

Miliaria crystallina is characterized by a subcorneal blister associated with an underlying eccrine duct. Multiple sections may reveal an apparent blockage of the ductal lumen by PAS-positive, diastase-resistant material. Inflammatory cells are typically absent, but older lesions may demonstrate mild lymphocytic spongiosis.[14] The earliest lesions of miliaria rubra demonstrate an apparent blockage of the intraepidermal duct by a PAS-positive, diastase-resistant plug associated with paraductal lymphocytic spongiosis with occasional neutrophils (Fig. 61–3). Older lesions demonstrate an overlying cap of parakeratosis and inflammatory cells.[15] Occasionally, colonies of cocci may be identified within this cap.[13] Miliaria profunda is identical except the inflammatory changes involve the lower portion of the epidermis and upper dermis. Miliaria pustulosa reveals a heavy accumulation of acute inflammatory cells in either a subcorneal or intraepidermal location (Fig. 61–4). The histologic findings in miliaria are sufficiently diagnostic that a definitive diagnosis can be made, although multiple sections usually are needed because the changes are so focal.

DRUG-INDUCED CHANGES OF THE ECCRINE SWEAT GLAND

The eccrine sweat gland and duct appear to be particularly susceptible to the effects of cytotoxic drugs, probably secondary to increased concentrations in sweat. Harrist et al.[16] were the first to describe neutrophilic eccrine hidradenitis secondary to induction chemotherapy. Although initially believed to be associated only with acute myelogenous leukemia and cytarabine therapy, more recent reports suggest that this disorder may be associated with other forms of

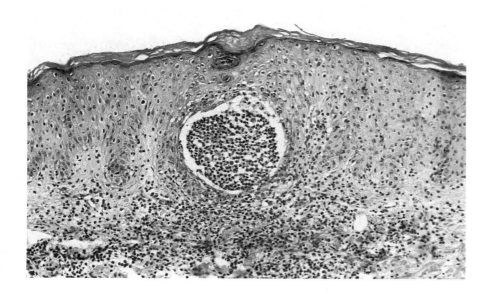

Figure 61–4. Miliaria pustulosa. Ductal lumen occluded by eosinophilic material and a few neutrophils above an intraepidermal abscess. (H&E, ×100.)

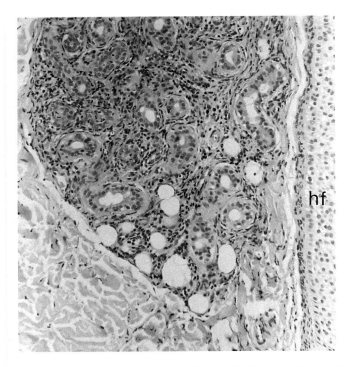

Figure 61–5. Neutrophilic eccrine hidradenitis. Heavy infiltrate of predominantly neutrophils surrounding the eccrine glands and coiled dermal duct. There is vacuolar alteration of the epithelial lining. Note that the adjacent hair follicle (hf) is not affected. (H&E, ×100.)

cancer and cytotoxic drugs.[17,18] The lesions are clinically erythematous papules and plaques that resolve spontaneously.

Histologic Features

Biopsies are characterized by the infiltration of the eccrine coil by a mild to heavy infiltrate of neutrophils with some mononuclear cells. There is associated vacuolar alteration and variable necrosis of the secretory epithelium (Fig. 61–5). Focal mucinous changes of the surrounding adipose

cuff also may be present. The eccrine duct may be normal or demonstrate nuclear pyknosis and cytoplasmic eosinophilia of the epithelial cells lining the duct. Nonspecific changes that may also be present include vacuolar alteration of the epidermis with necrotic keratinocytes and dermal hemorrhage.[18] The histologic differential diagnosis includes sweat gland necrosis secondary to coma and infectious eccrine hidradenitis. The heavier infiltrate of neutrophils and absence of associated necrosis of the epidermis, pilosebaceous apparatus, and vascular endothelium are helpful in excluding the former. Infectious eccrine hidradenitis is histologically very similar, although there is quantitatively less necrosis of the eccrine glands.

Necrosis of the eccrine duct in the absence of changes of the eccrine coil is also seen as a nonspecific finding from a variety of different cytotoxic drugs. The changes are typically most prominent in the acrosyringium and consist of dyskeratosis of the ductal lining producing the appearance of squamous metaplasia (Fig. 61–6). Typically, the epidermis and hair follicle also demonstrate vacuolar alteration of the basal keratinocytes, suggesting a generalized cytotoxic effect.[19]

PRESSURE-INDUCED BULLAE AND SWEAT GLAND NECROSIS

Blisters secondary to coma are frequently but not exclusively associated with drug-induced comas. The lesions are not thought to be related to toxic effects of the medication alone but rather the result of pressure-induced ischemia.[20] However, the possibility that certain drugs may act synergistically to produce these effects has not been excluded.

Histologic Features

Biopsies of developed lesions typically demonstrate variable changes of the epidermis, adnexal structures, and dermis. The epidermis demonstrates eosinophilic keratinocytes with variable karyolysis or pyknosis of the nuclei with the formation of intraepidermal or subepidermal bullae. The pilosebaceous units often demonstrate necrosis of the sebaceous

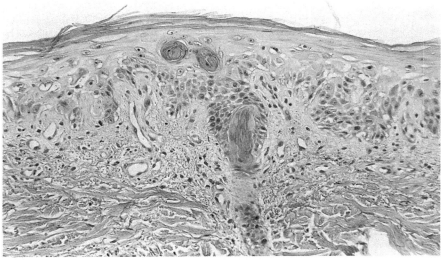

Figure 61–6. Methotrexate-induced dyskeratosis of the acrosyringium. The vacuolar alteration of the basal keratinocytes with necrotic keratinocytes and dilated vascular spaces in the absence of a significant infiltrate are helpful additional histologic features suggestive of cytotoxic drug-induced changes. (H&E, ×100.)

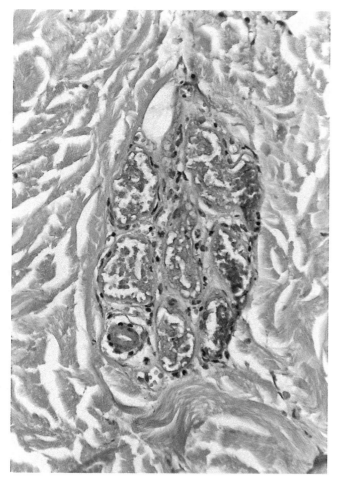

Figure 61–7. Sweat gland necrosis secondary to coma. The eccrine gland and coiled dermal duct demonstrate extensive necrosis with an infiltrate of only several neutrophils. In this specimen, the pilosebaceous unit demonstrated less extensive changes, and the epidermis demonstrated focal full thickness necrosis. (H&E, ×100.) (*Courtesy of L. Golitz.*)

glands and hair follicles. The most characteristic changes are the dramatic necrosis of the sweat ducts and glands. Characteristically, there is increased eosinophilia of the cytoplasm associated with either pyknosis of karyolysis of the nuclei. The cell membranes and basement membranes are often indistinct and smudged. The associated infiltrate may be virtually absent or be composed of neutrophils and lymphocytes[21] (Fig. 61–7). The dermis may demonstrate pyknotic changes of the fibroblasts and vascular endothelium. Hemorrhage frequently is present around involved vessels.[20]

INFECTIONS OF THE SWEAT GLANDS

Primary infection of sweat glands is a rare event not usually seen in healthy individuals. Multiple sweat gland abscesses secondary to *Staphylococcus* species is typically seen in undernourished infants, although apparently healthy infants

also may get this disorder. The primary lesion is a skin-colored or erythematous, dome-shaped nodule that is characteristically multiple. Biopsies demonstrate abscesses centered around eccrine glands, which may demonstrate variable degrees of necrosis. The infiltrate is composed primarily of neutrophils, although lymphocytes and macrophages may be present. Cocci may be demonstrable within the abscess.[22] The presence of eccrine involvement and absence of follicular involvement are histologic findings that exclude furunculosis.

Infectious eccrine hidradenitis secondary to *Serratia* infection has been reported in a hemodialysis patient.[23] The lesions were mildly pruritic erythematous papules. Multiple biopsies demonstrate a mixed infiltrate of neutrophils, lymphocytes, and occasional eosinophils arranged around the eccrine ducts and eccrine glands, with focal intraglandular abscesses.

REFERENCES

1. Fox GH, Fordyce JA. Two cases of a rare papular disease affecting the axillary region. *J Cutan Dis.* 1902;20:1–5.
2. Mevorah B, Duboff GS, Wass RW. Fox-Fordyce disease in prepubescent girls. *Dermatologica.* 1968;136:43–56.
3. Shelley WB, Levy EJ. Apocrine sweat retention in man. II: Fox-Fordyce disease (apocrine miliaria). *Arch Dermatol.* 1956;73:38–49.
4. Macmillan DC. Fox-Fordyce disease. *Br J Dermatol.* 1971;84:181.
5. Lane JE. Hidrosadenitis axillaris of Verneuil. *Arch Dermatol Syphilol.* 1933;28:609–614.
6. Brunsting HA. Hidradenitis and other variants of acne. *Arch Dermatol Syphilol.* 1952;65:303–315.
7. Shelley WB, Cahn MM. The pathogenesis of hidradenitis suppurativa in man. *Arch Dermatol.* 1955;72:562–565.
8. Hyland CH, Kheir SM. Follicular occlusion disease with elimination of abnormal elastic tissue. *Arch Dermatol.* 1980;116:925–928.
9. Shelley WB. Miliaria. *JAMA.* 1953;152:670–673.
10. Holzle E, Kligman AM. The pathogenesis of miliaria rubra: role of the resident microflora. *Br J Dermatol.* 1978;99:117–137.
11. Shelley WB, Horvath PN, Weidman FD, Pillsbury DM. Experimental miliaria in man. I: production of sweat retention anidrosis and vesicles by means of iontophoresis. *J Invest Dermatol.* 1948;11:275–291.
12. Shelley WB, Horvath PN. Experimental miliaria in man. II: production of sweat retention anidrosis and miliaria crystallina by various kinds of injury. *J Invest Dermatol.* 1950;14:9–20.
13. O'Brien JP. The etiology of poral closure. An experimental study of miliaria rubra, bullous impetigo and related diseases of the skin. *J Invest Dermatol.* 1950;15:95–152.
14. Dobson RL, Lobitz WC. Some histochemical observations on the human eccrine sweat glands. II: the pathogenesis of miliaria. *Arch Dermatol.* 1957;75:653–666.
15. Sulzberger MB, Zimmerman HM. Studies on prickly heat. II: experimental and histologic findings. *J Invest Dermatol.* 1946;7:61–68.
16. Harrist TJ, Fine JD, Berman RS, et al. Neutrophilic eccrine hidradenitis. *Arch Dermatol.* 1982;118:263–266.
17. Beutner KR, Packman CH, Markowitch W. Neutrophilic eccrine hidradenitis associated with Hodgkin's disease and chemotherapy. *Arch Dermatol.* 1986;122:809–811.
18. Fitzpatrick JE, Bennion SD, Reed OM, et al. Neutrophilic eccrine hidradenitis associated with induction chemotherapy. *J Cutan Pathol.* 1987:272–278.

19. Fitzpatrick JE, Hood AF. Histopathologic reactions to chemotherapeutic reagents. *Adv Dermatol.* 1988;3:161–184.

20. Arndt KA, Mihm MC, Parrish JA. Bullae: a cutaneous sign of a variety of neurologic diseases. *J Invest Dermatol.* 1973; 60:312–320.

21. Mandy S, Ackerman AB. Characteristic traumatic skin lesions in drug-induced coma. *JAMA.* 1970;213:253–256.

22. Mopper C, Pinkus H, Iacobelli P. Multiple sweat gland abscesses of infants. *Arch Dermatol.* 1955;71:177–183.

23. Moreno A, Barnadas MA, Ravella A, de Moragas JM. Infectious eccrine hidradenitis in a patient undergoing hemodialysis. *Arch Dermatol.* 1985;121:1106–1107.

Index

Page numbers in **bold** indicate major discussions.